UICC International Union Against Cancer

UICC MANUAL OF CLINICAL ONCOLOGY

EIGHTH EDITION

Editor
Raphael E. Pollock

Associate Editors
James H. Doroshow
David Khayat
Akimasa Nakao
Brian O'Sullivan

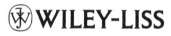**WILEY-LISS**

A JOHN WILEY & SONS, INC., PUBLICATION

Copyright © 2004 by John Wiley & Sons, Inc. All rights reserved.

Published by John Wiley & Sons, Inc., Hoboken, New Jersey.
Published simultaneously in Canada.

For general information on our other products and services please contact our Customer Care Department within the U.S. at 877-762-2974, outside the U.S. at 317-572-3993 or fax 317-572-4002.

Wiley also publishes its books in a variety of electronic formats. Some content that appears in print, however, may not be available in electronic format.

Library of Congress Cataloging-in-Publication Data:

UICC manual of clinical oncology.–8th ed. / editor, Raphel E. Pollock; associate
    editors, James H. Doroshow ... [et al.].
        p. : cm.
    At head of title: UICC International Union Against Cancer.
    Rev. ed. of: Manual of clinical oncology. 7th ed 1999.
    Includes bibliographical references and index.
    ISBN 0-471-22289-5 (cloth: alk. paper)
    1. Cancer–Handbooks, manuals, etc. I. Pollock, Raphael E. II. International Union
against Cancer. III. Manual of clinical oncology.
    [DNLM: 1 Neoplasms–Handbooks. QZ 39 U33 2003]
    RC262.5.M36 2004
    616.99'4–dc21   2004043069

Printed in the United States of America

10 9 8 7 6 5 4 3 2

CONTENTS

◼◼◼◼ PREFACE

The eighth edition of the *UICC Manual of Clinical Oncology* represents a thoroughly revised version of this standard text, which now has been translated into twelve languages. Many of the chapters have been rewritten and all have been carefully updated. New chapters have been added to the manual as the basic science underlying the contemporary practice of oncology continues to evolve rapidly.

Since publication of the previous edition of this manual, the need to approach oncology patients and their diseases using multimodality strategies has become more and more apparent. Indeed, it is the rare malignant problem that is treated utilizing only one form of therapy. This perspective is embodied in the new edition, which stresses the careful prospective integration of treatments as being in the best interest of the oncology patient. Predictably, integration of molecular approaches in both diagnosis and therapy in oncology will continue to progress as we move into the future.

The target readership for this manual consists of physicians-in-training in oncology and in the many subspecialty disciplines involved with multimodality cancer treatment programs, as well as practicing physicians and others throughout the world who care for cancer patients, often under less than optimal conditions. Each of the disease-site chapters in this edition of the manual has been updated to incorporate cancer staging as presented in the *UICC's TNM Classification of Malignant Tumours*, Sixth Edition (2002).

I would like to take this opportunity to thank the authors, my co-editors, and the staff at UICC and at John Wiley & Sons for their superlative efforts in behalf of this project. A special thanks is extended also to the Swiss Cancer League for their ongoing support of the *UICC Manual of Clinical Oncology*. Finally, and most importantly, I would like to thank our readers, whose efforts on behalf of oncology patients worldwide offer the very best hope for a future free of malignant disease.

Head, Division of Surgery   RAPHAEL E. POLLOCK
Professor and Chair, Department of Surgical Oncology
University of Texas
M. D. Anderson Cancer Center
Houston, Texas

Frederick R. Appelbaum, Fred Hutchinson Cancer Research Center, University of Washington School of Medicine, Seattle, Washington

Ijaz I. Arshad, Albany Medical College, Division of Medical Oncology, Albany, New York

G. Auclerc, Medical Oncology Department, Salpétrière Hospital, SOMPS, Paris, France

Riccardo A. Audisio, Whiston Hospital, Prescot, Merseyside, United Kingdom

Andrew Bayley, University of Toronto, Princess Margaret Hospital, Department of Radiation Oncology, Toronto, Ontario, Canada

J. L. Benedet, British Columbia Cancer Agency, Division of Gynecologic Oncology, Vancouver, British Columbia, Canada

J. Bloch, Medical Oncology Department, Salpétrière Hospital, SOMPS, Paris, France

P. Bloch, Medical Oncology Department, Salpétrière Hospital, SOMPS, Paris, France

Lisa M. Bodnar, Albany Medical College, Division of Medical Oncology, Albany, New York

Diane C. Bodurka, University of Texas, M. D. Anderson Cancer Center, Houston, Texas

Melissa L. Bondy, University of Texas, M. D. Anderson Cancer Center, Department of Epidemiology, Division of Cancer Prevention, Houston, Texas

Ron Burkes, University of Toronto, Princess Margaret Hospital, Department of Medical Oncology, Toronto, Ontario, Canada

B. H. Burmeister, Princess Alexandra Hospital, Department of Radiation Oncology, South Brisbane, Australia

Didier Buthiau, Medical Oncology Department, Salpétrière Hospital, SOMPS, Paris, France

Shine Chang, Office of Preventive Oncology, Division of Cancer Prevention, National Cancer Institute, National Institutes of Health, Bethesda, Maryland

Christopher H. Crane, University of Texas, M. D. Anderson Cancer Center, Houston, Texas

Steven A. Curley, University of Texas, M. D. Anderson Cancer Center, Department of Surgical Oncology, Houston, Texas

Nicole M. Daignault, Emory University, Medical School—South Clinic, Atlanta, Georgia

Rory R. Dalton, Department of Pathology, Medical College of Georgia, Augusta, Georgia

Louis J. Denis, Oncology Center Antwerp, Antwerp, Belgium

John DiGiovanni, University of Texas, M. D. Anderson Cancer Center, Department of Carcinogenesis, Smithville, Texas

James H. Doroshow, City of Hope National Medical Center, Department of Medical Oncology and Therapeutics Research, Duarte, California

Michael J. Edwards, University of Arkansas for Medical Sciences, Arkansas Cancer Research Center, Little Rock, Arkansas

Joshua D. I. Ellenhorn, City of Hope National Medical Center, Department of General and Oncology Surgery, Duarte, California

Douglas B. Evans, University of Texas, M. D. Anderson Cancer Center, Houston, Texas

Betty R. Ferrell, City of Hope National Medical Center, Department of Nursing Research and Education, Duarte, California

Michele Follen, University of Texas, M. D. Anderson Cancer Center, Department of Gynecological Oncology, Houston, Texas

M. A. Gil-Delgado, Medical Oncology Department, Salpétrière Hospital, SOMPS, Paris, France

Theresa A. Gillis, Oncology Rehabilitation Services, Helen F. Graham Cancer Center, Christiana Care Health System, Newark, Delaware

Robert J. Ginsberg, University of Toronto, Princess Margaret Hospital, Department of Surgical Oncology, Toronto, Ontario, Canada

Aron Goldhirsch, European Institute of Oncology, Center for Cancer Control and Palliative Care, Milan, Italy

Mary K. Gospodarowicz, University of Toronto, Princess Margaret Hospital, Department of Radiation Oncology, Toronto, Ontario, Canada

Keith Griffiths, University College of Medicine, Cardiff, Wales, United Kingdom

P. A. Groome, Kingston Regional Cancer Centre, Kingston General Hospital, Radiation Oncology Unit, Kingston, Ontario, Canada

James G. Gurney, University of Minnesota, Department of Pediatrics, Division of Pediatric Epidemiology, Minneapolis, Minnesota

Lee J. Helman, National Cancer Institute, National Institutes of Health, Pediatric Oncology Branch, Bethesda, Maryland

Wuan Ki Hong, University of Texas, M. D. Anderson Cancer Center, Department of Thoracic/Head and Neck Oncology, Houston, Texas

Jonathan Irish, University of Toronto, Princess Margaret Hospital, Department of Surgical Oncology, Toronto, Ontario, Canada

S. A. N. Johnson, Taunton and Somerset Hospital, Department of Hematology, Taunton, Somerset, England

Javed Khan, National Cancer Institute, National Institutes of Health, Advanced Technology Center, Pediatric Oncology, Gaithersburg, Maryland

David Khayat, Medical Oncology Department, Salpétrière Hospital, SOMPS, Paris, France

Fadlo R. Khuri, Winship Cancer Institute, Emory University, School of Medicine, Atlanta, Georgia

Yasuhiro Kodera, Department of Surgery, Nagoya University, Graduate School of Medicine, Nagoya, Japan

Brian I. Labow, Massachusetts General Hospital, Division of Surgical Oncology, Boston, Massachusetts

Anne Lee, Pamela Youde Nethersole Eastern Hospital, Clinical Oncology Department, Hong Kong

Lawrence Leichman, Albany Medical College, Division of Medical Oncology, Albany, New York

Scott M. Lippman, University of Texas, M. D. Anderson Cancer Center, Department of Clinical Cancer Prevention, Houston, Texas

Glenn Liu, University of Wisconsin, Comprehensive Cancer Center, Madison, Wisconsin

Caroline Lohrisch, British Columbia Cancer Agency, Vancouver, British Columbia, Canada

W. J. Mackillop, Kingston Regional Cancer Centre, Kingston General Hospital, Radiation Oncology Unit, Kingston, Ontario, Canada

Anne T. Mancino, University of Arkansas for Medical Sciences, Arkansas Cancer Research Center, Little Rock, Arkansas

Kim Margolin, City of Hope National Medical Center, Departments of Medical Oncology and Therapeutics Research and Hematology and Bone Marrow Transplant, Duarte, California

Alvin A. Martin, University of Louisville, James Graham Brown Cancer Center, Louisville, Kentucky

Keiichi Maruyama, Department of Surgical Oncology, National Cancer Center Hospital, Tokyo, Japan

Gordon B. Mills, University of Texas, M. D. Anderson Cancer Center, Houston, Texas

Akimasa Nakao, Department of Surgery, Nagoya University, Graduate School of Medicine, Nagoya, Japan

D. Nizri, Medical Oncology Department, Salpétrière Hospital, SOMPS, Paris, France

Brian O'Sullivan, University of Toronto, Princess Margaret Hospital, Department of Radiation Oncology, Toronto, Ontario, Canada

Xavier Paoletti, European Organization for Research and Treatment of Cancer (EORTC), Data Center, Central Office, Brussels, Belgium

David Payne, University of Toronto, Princess Margaret Hospital, Department of Radiation Oncology, Toronto, Ontario, Canada

Stephen Peiper, Department of Pathology, Medical College of Georgia, Augusta, Georgia

Martine Piccart, Institute Jules Bordet, Brussels, Belgium

Peter W. T. Pisters, University of Texas, M. D. Anderson Cancer Center, Department of Surgical Oncology, Houston, Texas

Raphael Pollock, University of Texas, M. D. Anderson Cancer Center, Houston, Texas

M. G. Poulsen, Princess Alexandra Hospital, Department of Radiation Oncology, South Brisbane, Australia

Paula Trahan Rieger, University of Texas, M. D. Anderson Cancer Center, Houston, Texas

O. Rixie, Medical Oncology Department, Salpétrière Hospital, SOMPS, Paris, France

Lazzaro Repetto, Oncology Unit, Istituto Nazionale di Riposo e Cura per Anziani, Rome, Italy

H. Ian Robins, University of Wisconsin Medical Center, Comprehensive Cancer Center, Madison, Wisconsin

M. A. Rocher, Medical Oncology Department, Salpétrière Hospital, SOMPS, Paris, France

Sanziana Roman, Yale School of Medicine, Department of Surgery, New Haven, Connecticut

Anita L. Sabichi, University of Texas, M. D. Anderson Cancer Center, Department of Clinical Cancer Prevention, Houston, Texas

Alberto Sbanotto, European Institute of Oncology, Center for Cancer Control and Palliative Care, Milan, Italy

David T. Scadden, Massachusetts General Hospital, Dana-Farber/Harvard Cancer Center, Harvard Medical School, Boston, Massachusetts

Elena Scaffidi, European Institute of Oncology, Center for Cancer Control and Palliative Care, Milan, Italy

Lillian Siu, University of Toronto, Princess Margaret Hospital, Department of Medical Oncology, Toronto, Ontario, Canada

David A. Sloan, University of Kentucky, Lexington, Kentucky

B. M. Smithers, Princess Alexandra Hospital, Department of Radiation Oncology, South Brisbane, Australia

Sarah Elizabeth Snell, University of Louisville, James Graham Brown Cancer Center, Louisville, Kentucky

George Somlo, City of Hope Comprehensive Cancer Center, Department of Medical Oncology, Duarte, California

C. Soubrane, Medical Oncology Department, Salpétrière Hospital, SOMPS, Paris, France

J.-P. Spano, Medical Oncology Department, Salpétrière Hospital, SOMPS, Paris, France

Wiley W. Souba, University of Texas, M. D. Anderson Cancer Center, Houston, Texas

Charles A. Staley, Emory University, Medical School—South Clinic, Atlanta, Georgia

Richard Sylvester, European Organization for Research and Treatment of Cancer (EORTC), Data Center, Central Office, Brussels, Belgium

J. Taieb, Department of Gastroenterology, Salpétrière Hospital, SOMPS, Paris, France

Zhao-You Tang, Liver Cancer Institute, Fudan University, Shanghai, China

Patrick Therasse, European Organization for Research and Treatment of Cancer (EORTC), Data Center, Central Office, Brussels, Belgium

Guillermo Tortolero-Luna, University of Texas, M. D. Anderson Cancer Center, Houston, Texas

Robert Udelsman, Yale School of Medicine, Department of Surgery, New Haven, Connecticut

Martine Van Glabbeke, European Organization for Research and Treatment of Cancer (EORTC), Data Center, Central Office, Brussels, Belgium

Charles J. Vecht, Department of Neurology, Medical Center, The Hague, The Netherlands

Vittorio Ventafridda, European Institute of Oncology, Center for Cancer Control and Palliative Care, Milan, Italy

Anne-Thérèse Vlastos, University of Texas, M. D. Anderson Cancer Center, Houston, Texas

Suryanarayana V. Vulimiri, University of Texas, M. D. Anderson Cancer Center, Department of Carcinogenesis, Smithville, Texas

John N. Waldron, University of Toronto, Princess Margaret Hospital, Department of Radiation Oncology, Toronto, Ontario, Canada

Alan S. Wayne, National Cancer Institute, National Institutes of Health, Pediatric Oncology Branch, Bethesda, Maryland

Jun S. Wei, National Cancer Institute, National Institutes of Health, Advanced Technology Center, Pediatric Oncology, Gaithersburg, Maryland

Craig C. Whiteford, National Cancer Institute, National Institutes of Health, Advanced Technology Center, Pediatric Oncology, Gaithersburg, Maryland

Robert A. Wolff, University of Texas, M. D. Anderson Cancer Center, Houston, Texas

Vittorina Zagonel, Department of Oncology and Oncology Unit, Fatebenefratelli Hospital, Rome, Italy

CHAPTER 1

The Natural History and Biology of Cancer

GLENN LIU and H. IAN ROBINS

University of Wisconsin, Comprehensive Cancer Center, Madison, Wisconsin

INTRODUCTION

Cancer is one of the most feared diseases throughout the entire world. Much of this fear is caused by the lack of effective treatment for most nonoperable metastatic tumors. Fortunately, some progress has occurred with regard to therapy over the past four decades. Improvements in surgical techniques, radiotherapy, and chemotherapy have increased survival since the mid-twentieth century. However, it now appears that a plateau has been reached with the use of these modalities. Hence, new strategies (e.g., biological modulators and immunotherapy) for combating neoplastic diseases in the new millennium will most certainly be grounded in an increased understanding of the biology and natural history of cancer.

Health care workers are often faced with difficult decisions regarding cancer detection, prognosis, and use of appropriate and effective treatment. For example, we may elect to follow a 0.8 cm (T1N0M0) breast cancer after surgery, while giving adjuvant chemotherapy in a patient with a 6 cm mass (T3N0M0) breast primary. We base this decision on our understanding of the biology of cancer, which takes into account many important factors (size, grade, histology, stromal invasion, etc.). Knowing and predicting the biological behavior of a cancer is what allows us to decide on the best appropriate management. Unfortunately, at times a T1N0M0 tumor will do much more poorly than a T3N0M0 cancer, illustrating the complexities involved in predictive factorial analysis and the need for an increased understanding of tumor biology.

Surgeons, radiation oncologists, and medical oncologists need to understand the natural history of cancers to provide appropriate therapies. Additionally, oncologic social workers, psychiatrists, and nurses also need to understand the natural history

UICC Manual of Clinical Oncology, Eighth Edition. Edited by Raphael E. Pollock
ISBN 0-471-22289-5 Copyright © 2004 John Wiley & Sons, Inc.

of cancer to appropriately deal with the complexities of disease management. Finally, researchers must understand the biology of cancer to develop novel therapeutic tools and conduct relevant laboratory studies. In this chapter, many of the major principles of the natural history and biology of cancer will be outlined in order to provide a knowledge base for the chapters to follow.

NATURAL HISTORY OF CANCER

An understanding of the natural history of cancer provides insights into the biology of cancer, which in turn is a requisite to approaching prevention and therapy. Clearly, neoplasia is a disease most often seen in the very young or the old, but, in general, cancer incidence increases with age. It is estimated that by age 85 years, the incidence approaches 2,500 per 100,000 persons. Beyond this, the incidence of certain cancers is increased with exposure to carcinogens such as cigarette smoke, chemicals, and radiation. Other environmental factors must also play an important role, as the prevalence of certain cancers varies by country (e.g., colon cancer in western countries, gastric cancer in Japan, nasopharyngeal cancer in Southern China, and oral cancer in India), and studies on migrants from those countries develop adjusted incidences of cancer comparable with the indigenous rates. Lastly, we understand that genes are important, as certain mutations are correlated with a high risk for specific cancers.

Given that age, environmental exposure, and genetics are relevant, two concepts regarding cancer development must be true: (1) cancer must have a long latent period, and (2) there must be a multistage process in carcinogenesis. With this being said, it can implied that it takes a long time to develop a cancer, with an average time period in an adult being approximately 20 years (from normal cell to visualization of neoplastic disease). This development has been well characterized in certain cancers (i.e., colon, breast, and cervical cancer), with precancerous lesions showing hyperplasia, then metaplasia or dysplasia. These lesions then can become carcinoma *in situ*, early invasive, and, finally, metastatic. This evolution has implications with regard to cancer detection and, hence, forms the basis of our current screening recommendations. The multistage process in cancer development implies that specific sequential changes must occur during the evolution of cancer. Whereas genetics may start this process from a later sequence, it is the environmental factors that complete the carcinogenesis. Because environmental factors are potentially controllable events, this has been a primary focus in cancer prevention. Taken collectively, it is clear that an understanding of tumor biology has importance both in clinical practice and in cancer epidemiology.

CANCER AS A CELLULAR DISEASE

In the nineteenth century, the pathologist Virchow stated, while examining tumors microscopically, that "every cell comes from another cell." This established early on that cancer was a cellular disease. Although much information has been learned since then, the underlying concept remains true.

We know that the fundamental unit of organization of all biologic material is the cell. In multicellular organisms, cells are organized into tissues and organs. Growth of cells may occur by an increase in the number of cells, an increase in the size of cells, or both. In higher animals, growth in cell number usually exceeds growth in size. Growth in cell number is the most significant component of human development. The average human adult is composed of about one quadrillion (10^{15}) cells derived from a single fertilized ovum. After humans reach maturity, the number of cells present remains essentially constant. Maintenance of cellular constancy, however, is a very dynamic process. Cell division occurs at a brisk rate, and approximately one trillion (10^{12}) human cells die each day, and must be replaced. The most active sites of cellular replication occur in the gastrointestinal tract, bone marrow, and skin. Thus, in the adult animal or human, the number of new cells produced is equal to the number of cells that die (Fig. 1.1). This basic equation is fundamental to our understanding of normal and abnormal cellular growth.

Three subgroups of cells comprise every cell population (Fig. 1.2). Cycling cells occupy the first group, continuously proliferating, moving from one mitosis to the next. Terminally differentiated cells, which irreversibly leave the growth cycle are destined to die without dividing again, comprise the second group. The third

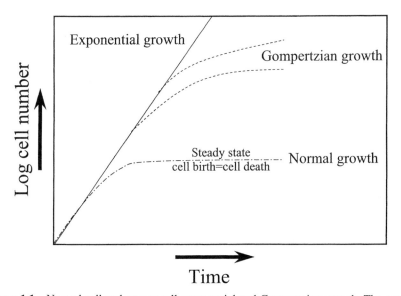

Figure 1.1 Normal cell and cancer cell exponential and Gompertzian growth. The growth kinetics as exhibited by increasing number of cancer cells with time is depicted. Note that the vertical axis represents the log of the cell number. Initial cancer cell growth *in vitro* is exponential, and is believed to be similar *in vivo*. As the developing cancer increases in mass, the growth kinetics are reduced from exponential rates. This latter growth curve can be described by an equation relating increasing cancer cell mass and time, that is, a Gompertzian curve.

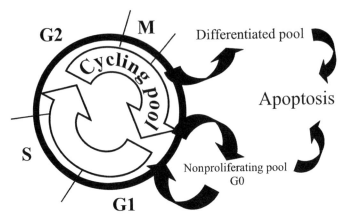

Figure 1.2   A depiction of the cell cycle. Cells continuously divide from one mitosis (M) to the next, passing through G_1, S (DNA synthesis), and G_2 phase. Some cells leave the cell cycle temporarily, entering a G_0 state (nonproliferative pool) from which they can be rescued by appropriate mitogenic stimuli. Other cells leave the cell cycle permanently, and become part of the terminally differentiated pool. Cells enter programmed cell death (apoptosis) from either the differentiated or nonproliferative pools (G_0).

subpopulation of nonproliferating cells is not cycling, do not die, but can reenter the cell cycle if an appropriate stimulus is applied (G_0 cells). During the normal cycling processes, proliferating cells progress through four different phases that are defined as G_1, S phase, G_2, and mitosis.

Nonproliferating (G_0 cells) are normally present in most tissues of living animals. For example, in the liver, most cells are in the G_0 phase. If, however, approximately two-thirds of the liver is removed surgically, the remaining nonproliferating (G_0) cells will reenter the cell cycle, proliferate, and restore the liver to its approximate original size. A similar phenomenon occurs in bone marrow. Knowledge of this is important to radiation and medical oncologists, who often introduce therapeutic procedures for the treatments of cancers that deplete maturing bone marrow cells, and stimulate protected (G_0) stem cells to reenter the cell cycle and eventually repopulate the bone marrow.

Growth in number of any population of cells can occur by any one of three mechanisms. In the first, shortening of the length of the cell cycle results in more cells being produced per unit time. In the second, decreasing the rate of cell death will also result in more cells being retained in the organism. In the third, moving G_0 cells into the cell cycle will result in more cells produced per unit time. Each of these mechanisms appears important in normal and cancer cell growth. In general, a complex web of proteins like cyclins, kinases, and other peptides controls the cell cycle. Abnormal ratios of stimulatory and inhibitory signals cause the cell's internal "switch" to turn on (relative increase in stimulatory to inhibitory signals) and to advance through the cell cycle without end. The end result is excessive proliferation of the cell and a closer step toward the development of cancer.

All cells, normal as well as cancer cells, may have their cell cycle characterized by the time required to double the cell population (cell doubling time). In normal cells, this doubling time is well regulated and controlled. However, in cancers, the cell and volume (or mass) doubling times of the primary tumor and its distant progeny, or metastases, may vary widely and relatively autonomously. One of the fastest growing neoplastic diseases (i.e., Burkitt's lymphoma), a mean volume doubling time of less than three days is present. Intermediate is a volume doubling time of 17 days for Ewing's sarcoma, and 155 days for a breast carcinoma. At a slow extreme is a volume doubling time of more than 600 days for certain adenocarcinomas of the colon and rectum. The cell and volume doubling times of cancers are real measures of the aggressiveness of a cancer, because they are dynamic measurements. Other measurements such as the mitotic index or the degree of anaplasia may be visualized by a pathologist at the level of the light microscope, but provide less sensitive measures of cancer aggressiveness.

In general, 1 gm of tumor cells (1 cm^3) contains approximately 10^9 cells and would have required 30 doublings to obtain that volume if had arisen from a single cell. Theoretically, another 10 doublings will result in a tumor weighing about 1 kg if left untreated and exponential growth continued. However, although a given tumor may have arisen from a single cell, not all the cells will behave in the exactly the same manner. We know that tumors do contain quiescent cells (do not divide) as well as other cells that may have differentiated further and spontaneously perform apoptosis. Also, parts of a tumor may undergo necrosis secondary to lack of nutrients or adequate blood supply. All this changes the growth toward a Gompertzian curve (Fig. 1.1) and can have importance in predicting tumor biology.

CANCER AS A TEMPORAL DISEASE

Each cancer, and each patient bearing a cancer, exhibits a chronological record of significant events. These events are set in motion by a process called initiation, which results in significant, irreversible changes in a host cell (usually a stem cell), leading to the development of cancer. If attempts to alter these processes are not made, or if attempts to alter them are made but fail, eventually clinical cancers will result that will lead to the death of the host. The summation of these temporal processes is designated as the natural history or biological progression of a cancer. This process is illustrated in Figure 1.3.

The phases of the temporal growth of a cancer may be categorized into the pre*clinical* and clinical phases. The preclinical phase is the latent period, which encompassed the tumor induction time. During this period, a number of now-recognizable molecular and cellular events occur in a chronological order. These changes result in the production of a cancer that can produce symptoms and be clinically detectable. The duration of this preclinical phase may be as short as a few months after initiation (e.g., Burkitt's lymphoma) or as long as many years (e.g., colon, lung, breast, or urinary bladder cancers). It has been estimated that the mean preclinical phase for most human cancers may be 8–20 years, but may be as long as

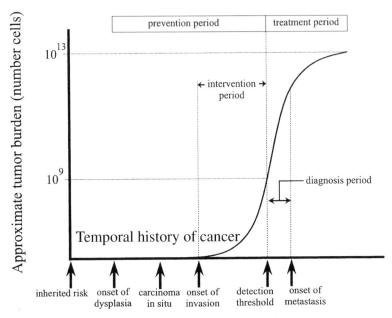

Figure 1.3   Cancer as a temporal disease. This figure summarizes the time course necessary to develop a cancer, including onset of dysplasia, carcinoma *in situ*, and finally acquisition of an invasive phenotype through further genetic mutations. Each stage in the development of a neoplasm has implications in prevention, detection, and treatment of neoplastic diseases. (Modified from Kohn and Liotta, 1995.)

30–40 years. During the preclinical phase, it is not possible to recognize any molecular or cellular abnormalities suggestive of cancer in a patient. The patient will have no signs or symptoms of the latent disease process. Estimates exist that the preclinical phase may occupy as much as 75% of the time of the natural history of a developing cancer. The insidious nature of this preclinical phase permits a cancer to grow without the development of signs or symptoms leading toward an early diagnosis. Again, about 30 volume doublings from the initial cancer cell are necessary to produce a cancer mass containing 1 billion (10^9) cancer cells. As a crude estimation, it is recognized that the accumulation of 10^{13} cells in a given patient usually correlates with a lethal event. During the latter portion of the preclinical phase, small cancers may develop micrometastases, worsening the prognosis upon diagnosis.

In this regard, Figure 1.4 relates tumor doubling to size. If a cancer has metastasized prior to the time it has reached a detectable size (prior to 20–25 doublings), surgical cure is not likely. This raises the specter of the need for effective adjuvant therapies, to be discussed later. Obviously, the tumor doubling time also has significant implications for cancer screening, which may change as the technology for detecting smaller tumors improves.

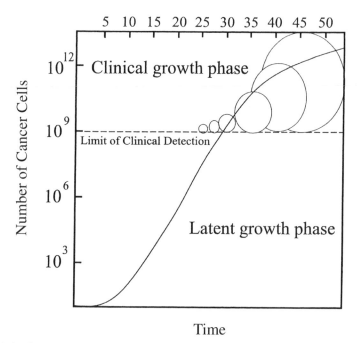

Figure 1.4 Growth curve of a hypothetical cancer. This diagram emphasizes that the preclinical phase (latent period) of growth occupies the majority of time (75%) of development of a cancer, and that by the time a cancer is diagnostically detectable it is very late in its natural history. Approximately 30 volume doublings have occurred prior to development of symptoms or signs leading to diagnosis. During the clinical phase of growth, with only a few additional volume doublings, the cancer burden to the host can become overwhelming. The larger number of cell doublings prior to diagnosis permits time for development of micro-metastases, as well as resistant clones of malignant cells. (Adapted from Hill and Tannock, 1998).

The clinical phase of the natural history of a cancer begins at the point when the cancer is definitively diagnosed. It is at this point when symptoms may appear in a patient, and where therapy is required in an attempt to cure or palliate the patient with cancer. Knowledge concerning the clinical phases of cancers is much more comprehensive. This later phase generally occupies only the last portion (~25%) of the natural history of an individual cancer. If the cancer is not successfully eradicated during this phase, a patient will die.

CANCER AS A MULTIPLE-STAGE DISEASE

The term *carcinogenesis* is used to describe the cascade of events that converts a normal cell into a cancer. It is visualized currently as a multiple-stage process

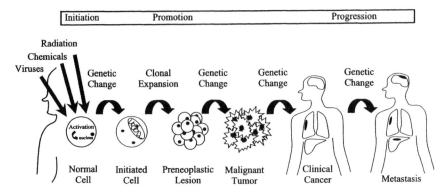

Figure 1.5   Multistage, temporal model of cancer development. This diagram presents the three stages of cancer development and depicts their time of occurrence in relationship to progression from a normal cell to a malignant clinical cancer. (Modified from Weisburger and Horn, 1991).

propelled by genetic damage and epigenetic changes (Fig. 1.5). Three main stages can be described depicting the sequential chronological events in carcinogenesis. The three stages are as follows: initiation and promotion (which occur in the latent phase), and progression (which begins the clinical phase of cancer). These terms describe conceptual changes within the cell, and by no means are reflective of the whole process of carcinogenesis. However, they do aid us in understanding neoplasia and how carcinogens play a role in tumor development.

Initiation

The stage of cancer initiation begins in cells, usually stem cells, through mutations from exposures to incomplete carcinogens (e.g., chemical, ultraviolet or x-radiations, or viruses). Initiating agents are only capable of beginning this first stage. Initiating agents are believed to change irreversibly the base composition or structure of component nuclear DNA and through this process begin the cancer development. Mutated cells can exhibit an altered responsiveness to their microenvironment and a selective growth advantage in contrast to surrounding normal cells, but in general are phenotypically identical to their noninitiated cell counterparts. It is also recognized that many potential initiation events are reversed by cellular DNA repair mechanisms. A number of characteristics describe the initiation stage of cancer. This process appears to be rapid and accomplished within fractions of seconds. Only single steps are required to confer initiation, and the process appears to be irreversible. At present, no threshold has been identified for the stage of initiation. In the present environment in which humans reside, exposure to potential initiating agents is inevitable, and their effects may be additive. It has been speculated that during the course of an individual's lifetime, many of the cells in their bodies may undergo the process of initiation, but those initiated cells either do not progress further, die, or become neutralized by immunologic mechanisms.

Promotion

The stage of cancer promotion involves alteration of gene expression, selective clonal expansion, and proliferation of initiated cells. This stage is characterized by reversibility, unlike initiation and progression. For example, focal lesions can regress upon discontinuation of the promoting agent; however, these lesions can reappear upon reinstitution of the promoting agent, confirming that initiation is irreversible. Promotion is dependent on many factors that continually change. For example, the exposure to environmental factors (including amount, frequency, and type), the age of the host, and dietary composition all plays a role. Given the reversibility and the fact that many promoters exert their influences on cellular receptors, a threshold limit must be present that encourages initiated cells to clonally expand. Although initiation is a major step in the multistage carcinogenesis theory, it is important to note that continual promotion of uninitiated cells can also be a risk factor in cancer development. By stimulating proliferation, the possibility of acquiring a genetic error is increased and can result in tumorigenesis.

Thus, the promotion stage exhibits characteristics of reversibility, it is prolonged in duration, it may require multiple steps, a dosage threshold may be present, it appears to be nonadditive, and it results in the expansion of a clone of initiated cells. The extent of human exposures to promoting agents may be variable. It appears clear that the several features of initiation and promotion that have been identified emphasize that they are distinct and different stages. Many of the characteristics of initiation and promotion have been known for more than 50 years, and have been referred to as two-stage carcinogenesis in which tumor initiation (mutation) is followed by tumor promotion (epigenetic changes). Recent concepts have been modified, as it is viewed that two-stage carcinogenesis, while conceptually important, is too simplistic. Other data suggest that there may be six or more independent mutational events preceding the formation of cancer.

Progression

The last stage is called progression. This stage is characterized by further molecular changes, additional enlargement of the primary cancer mass, the breaking off of cells from this mass and movement into adjacent tissues and organs, and the penetration of individual cancer cells or small clumps of cells into the circulatory system, with transport of these and entrapment in distant tissues and organs. These entrapped cancer cell clumps often establish residence in the new tissue sites and continue to grow, a process known as metastasis. A most characteristic feature of progression is the development of measurable changes in nuclear karyotype. Accompanying the change in karyotype is increase in growth weight of the cancer mass, increasing cellular autonomy, invasiveness, and metastatic capacity. The stage of progression concludes the pre-clinical phase of cancer evolution, and provides a transition into the clinical phase of cancer formation. If cancers can be diagnosed prior to the time of formation of generally undetectable micrometastases, then cures by the methods of surgery (or, where appropriate, radiation therapy) can occur with a high degree of likelihood. However, if micrometastases occur prior to the diagnosis of cancer, then cures (although possible in certain malignancies like testicular cancer) occur much less frequently. Attempts to control metastatic cancers must then rely upon systemic forms of therapy, including enhancement of host immunologic defense mechanisms, external biologic and immunologic therapies, or the introduction of chemotherapeutic or hormonal modes of therapies.

CANCER AS A MOLECULAR DISEASE

Overwhelming data now exist demonstrating that cancer is the result of genomic changes and that multiple mutations need to occur in order for malignant transformation to take place. For instance, Ames first observed that known carcinogens are also mutagens. Consistent with this idea is the fact that patients with defective DNA repair mechanisms are at increased risk for developing multiple types of cancers. Finally, the familial pattern of certain malignancies (implying that cancers can be inherited like other genetic traits) and the fact that tumors are clonal suggest that the underlying defect lies within DNA. That being said, for a cell to undergo malignant transformation, many distinct genetic events must occur. Although some of these changes can be inherited (germline mutations), the majority must be acquired throughout the lifetime of the organism.

Any type of mutation (i.e., point mutations, insertions or deletions, translocations, or amplifications) can lead to the development of cancer. Genes that are involved in the transcription or cell-signal transmission of growth-promoting stimuli are called *oncogenes* (e.g., *myc*, *ras*, *fos*, *src*), and abnormal expression of these genes can lead to excessive cellular proliferation and malignant transformation. This can occur via amplification of the gene or translocation of the gene to a different regulatory element, leading to increased translation of stimulatory proteins. On the other hand, genes that suppress malignant transformation, known as *tumor suppressor genes* (e.g., *Rb* [retinoblastoma gene], *p53*, *DCC* [deleted in colon cancer gene]) need to be either lost or inactivated by mutation to allow malignant transformation to occur. In brief, it is the imbalance between the stimulatory and the inhibitory signals that results in the cell's continuous movement around the cell cycle. Any additional genetic events can then potentially complete the malignant transformation.

Another important aspect in tumorigenesis that has received focused attention in recent years is apoptosis. Apoptosis (programmed cell death) is a cellular process important in normal cellular physiology and is used during embryogenesis, the development of immune tolerance, down-regulation of the immune system after infections and sepsis, and elimination of damaged cells (e.g., cells with mutated or aberrant DNA). An "abnormal" apoptosis tendency may in fact be a requisite step in cancer formation. In general, the number of cellular mitoses that a cell can accomplish is a well-controlled event dictated by several factors, such as telomere length, activity of suppressor genes, and the variable expression of apoptosis-triggering receptors (i.e., Fas and Fas ligand). For example, as a cell divides, it loses small portions at the end of each chromosome during each DNA synthesis phase. Fortunately, these ends are usually comprised of variable segments of base pair repeats called telomeres, which do not encode any relevant genes. As more divisions occur, however, eventually the telomeres will be lost and further mitosis takes place, resulting in the elimination of vital genes and cell death. Thus, the longer the telomere, the more replication a cell undergoes before dying. Likewise, cells that are able to "lengthen" the telomeres by the expression of the enzyme telomerase can achieve immortality (i.e., stem cells and tumors). Other agents, like the tumor suppressor gene *p53*, also act to trigger apoptosis in cells with damage to their DNA. Not surprisingly, people with a homozygous loss of the *p53* tumor suppressor are predisposed to developing multiple cancers by the accumulation of damaged DNA. Other genes inhibit apoptosis and, when overexpressed, can result in a failure of programmed cell death. This type of genetic pathology (e.g., *bcl*-2) is associated with certain hematological malignancies like follicular B-cell lymphoma and chronic lymphocytic leukemia. It may also be related to the presence of a more chemo-/hormonal-resistant phenotype, as it has been found to be a poor prognostic indicator in colon cancer, prostate carcinoma, and neuroblastoma.

It is now thought that apoptosis may also be responsible for tumor invasion, tumor-induced immunosuppression, and possibly cancer cachexia. For example, Fas ligand (FasL) has been found to be expressed on tumor cells and to trigger activated lymphocytes (which express the Fas receptor) to undergo apoptosis. This can lead to deletion of tumor-specific cytotoxic T cells, helping to give insights on why immune-based therapies have not yielded the results we initially expected, or why cancers can escape immune surveillance. Also, as most normal body cells express the Fas receptor, potentially the development of functional FasL on tumors can aid in local invasion and establishment of metastasis. Finally, soluble FasL has been found in the serum of patients in sepsis as well as certain malignancies such as leukemia. The sepsis syndrome and tumor cachexia can perhaps be explained by the presence of functional, circulating FasL.

In summary, we know that many steps (some prerequisite events) contribute to cancer development and progression. The discussion above is an oversimplification, as we are only beginning to understand the complexities involved in cancer formation. With time, we predict that advances in the knowledge of tumor biology will be followed by a new era in cancer therapeutics.

THE MALIGNANT NATURE OF CANCER: INVASION AND METASTASIS

We have already discussed the many steps required to allow a normal cell to transform into a tumor cell (initiation, promotion, and progression) and the implication this process has on screening recommendations and in risk reduction strategies. While important, the hallmark of cancer is its ability to invade and metastasize. Every so often, one sees a patient with a large tumor (sometimes as large as a basketball). These "benign" tumors obviously have the ability to overproliferate but, unlike other cancer cells, do not invade or metastasize. It would appear that these tumors have not yet acquired the ability to invade thereby implying that additional events need to be present to develop into a cancer. This observation is also seen with *in situ* breast cancers. In general, we view *in situ* breast cancer as a clonal disease with no metastatic potential. Patients can also be observed with large *in situ* neoplasms containing a small focus of invasive cancer implying that it has become "more malignant" in character. In theory, additional genetic events must have occurred to allow the *in situ* cancer to obtain invasive capabilities. This conjecture has been confirmed in some molecular studies. Again, the time it takes to progress from a preinvasive to an invasive cancer has direct implications for screening and therapy.

Simplistically, to metastasize, a cancer cells must first detach itself from the primary tumor, then invade a blood or lymphatic vessel. It can then travel to new site to set up a new colony. Although this may appear relatively easy, there exist many barriers that fortunately impede the metastatic process at each step. These

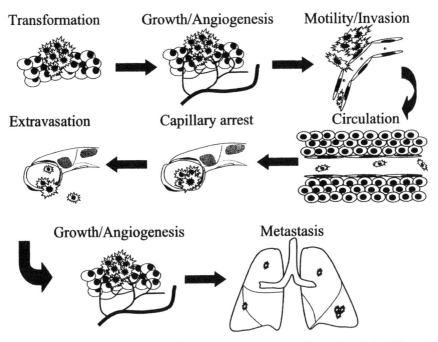

Figure 1.6 Invasion and metastasis. To metastasize, a tumor cell must detach itself from the primary tumor. It must then evade through the basement membranes to enter the circulation system. At this point, the tumor cell needs to avoid immune detection, lodge itself in a distal capillary, and transgress the endothelial boundaries to regain access to the extracellular stroma. Within the new microenvironment, appropriate stimulation must be present to encourage angiogenesis and proliferation. If successful, a new metastasis will be developed. (Modified from Fidler, 1997.)

barriers are relevant in that they have since become targets for novel therapeutic interventions.

Figure 1.6 illustrates invasion and metastasis. For an epithelial carcinoma to metastasize to the lungs, it must (1) gain mobility (secretion of motility factors) and (2) detach from its primary site by loosening the adhesion (loss of E-cadherin) that it has for neighboring cells. It then needs to (3) breach its basement membrane (using degradative enzymes) only to encounter (4) another basement membrane at the endothelial cell before it can successfully enter the blood stream. The cancer cell must then (5) avoid immune detection as it navigates the circulatory system before finally lodging in a capillary bed. The cell must then successfully (6) retract the endothelial cells and (7) repenetrate the endothelial basement membrane, before establishing a new colony. For this colony to survive, adequate nutritional support with growth factors and oxygen must be provided by (8) formation of a new blood supply (angiogenesis). Not surprisingly, probably fewer than 1 in 10,000 cancer cells that reach circulation actually survive to form a distant metastasis.

Entrance of cancer cells into the lymphatics is the second major route of distant cancer cell metastasis formation. This mode of spread of cancer cells into local lymphatic channels may sometimes block these channels and lymph nodes. This blockage of regional lymph nodes forms the basis for *en bloc* cancer surgery. At one time it was believed that lymph nodes served as filters for cancer cells. However, experimental investigations have demonstrated that cancer cells can pass through lymph nodes. In certain types of cancers, the number of lymph nodes involved in metastases is a critical measure of prognosis and likelihood for the development of other metastases found to be involved.

Body tissues or organs (e.g., bone, cartilage, or serosa) can impede the local extension of tumor growth. Cancers spreading by local extension often follow paths of least resistance (e.g., blood vessels, nerves, tissue planes). Where cancer cells have free access to serosal cavities, such as in ovarian cancer, cells may be disseminated in the free fluid and subsequently implant distant from the ovary of origin onto the abdominal serosa or mesentery. It has been demonstrated that implantation of cancer cells may occur during the process of surgery if a scalpel, other instrument, or surgical gloves become covered with cancer cells. These cells may be transferred to another part of the body or the wound. This mode of spread has led to the development of meticulous cancer surgical techniques such as the "no touch" techniques used to minimize this transfer problem. Occasionally, metastases may become evident later in a surgical scar formed following a cancer operation. Such metastases, in addition to direct introduction by the surgical process, may also occur because cancer cells circulating in the blood stream or lymph channels became lodged in damaged capillary structures of the wound and continued to proliferate.

Knowledge of routes of spread of particular cancer types provides the basis for staging or measuring the extent of disease in individual patients during the clinical phase of cancer growth and development. This knowledge is also applied to the design of appropriate therapies for patients classified as having identical stages of cancer.

Patterns of sites of metastases differ considerably for different primary cancers, and for different parts of a particular organ in which a cancer arises. Certain organs appear prone to metastasis formation depending upon the site of the primary cancer, while very few metastases occur in some organs (e.g., muscle, skin, thymus, and spleen). From many organs bearing a cancer, the lung capillaries are the first to receive venous blood, as well as lymphatic fluid through the thoracic duct, and thus the lungs are common sites for metastases. It has been demonstrated experimentally in mice that it is possible to select cancer cells that have specific predilections for growth as metastases in particular organs, so-called organo-tropism.

Detailed knowledge concerning the most significant mechanisms responsible for the occurrence of metastases is incomplete, but has been advancing rapidly. By the time the cancers develop to the stage of progression, cellular karyotypic instability has advanced, and individual cancer cells within a cancer mass have become heterogeneous with respect to each other. Other significant changes in the properties of cancer cells (e.g., cell-to-cell adhesion) must also have occurred, favoring successful metastatic development. For a given tumor to grow and metastasize within an organism, it must then avoid the host's immune system. Thus, for metastatic tumors, it can be inferred that the host's immune system must have failed to recognize the neoplasm as abnormal or foreign. Whether this failure is from lack of antigenic stimulation by the tumor (and thus no immune recognition is formed) or by clonal deletion of tumor-specific T cells by the tumor is a subject of much debate. Interest in this field has led many laboratories to study cancer vaccines and immunotherapies.

In addition to alterations in immunologic mechanisms, clotting mechanisms may be significantly perturbed, leading to a predisposition for intravascular clot formation. This may be the result of secretion of procoagulant mediators by tumors, increased platelet counts, and abnormalities in the production of clotting factors by the liver. Experimental studies have been directed toward development of interventions designed to enhance immunologic mechanisms, restore coagulation functions, and inhibit unrestricted growth of cancer cells.

Many clinical investigations have been conducted to explore the use of effective cancer drug therapies as an adjuvant to surgery and/or radiation therapy. These so-called adjuvant therapies have been directed at patients with known cancers with no clinical evidence of metastasis formation. Use of these therapies has been partially successful in patients with breast and colon cancers, but not yet been established in many other malignant diseases. Such adjuvant therapies may be limited by a variety of factors including: (1) cancer cell heterogeneity, that is, populations of cells within a given cancer resistant to the antineoplastic therapy; (2) an adequate biological milieu to deliver therapy (e.g., lack of a microvasculature to deliver chemotherapy, or tissue hypoxia creating relative resistance to ionizing irradiation); and (3) the efficacy of the therapy itself. Additionally, cancer regrowth after effective therapy in both the adjuvant and metastatic setting often heralds the emergence of a neoplasm resistant to therapy. This concept is illustrated in Figure 1.7.

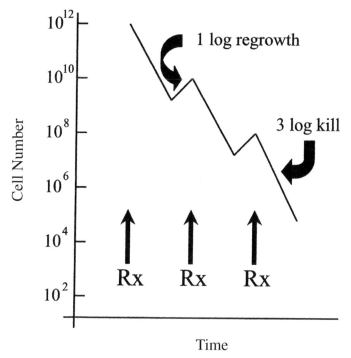

Figure 1.7 The relationship of therapy (Rx) and regrowth to cell numbers. If one assumes that a population of cancer cells does not evolve resistance to a given Rx, then a constant proportion of cell will be destroyed with each cycle of treatment. To produce a cure, cell killing must exceed regrowth. Once resistance develops, the amount of regrowth may then exceed the proportion killed.

IMPORTANCE OF TUMOR BIOLOGY

Much has been learned over the past decade about the environmental signals that need to be present to allow a cancer cell to divide, grow, differentiate, invade, and metastasize. These signals, in the form of cytokines, hormones, and peptides, bind to cellular receptors and activate a second messenger system that results in a modification of transcriptional factors dictating cell behavior. Known as signal transduction, abnormal expression of these signal transduction molecules is what causes tumor cells to behave the way that they do. Targeting of these molecules to restore normal cellular physiology has therefore been an area of focus in cancer therapy this past decade. A better understanding of tumor biology has also led researchers to target the individual steps required in invasion and metastasis. For example, special metalloproteinase inhibitors to prevent cancer cells from penetrating through the basement membranes are being studied. Also, antiangio-genesis inhibitors (e.g., vascular-endothelial growth factor [VEGF] inhibitors, thalidomide, endostatin) are actively being studied to prevent metastatic tumors from developing a blood supply as well as established tumors from growing larger. As emphasized in the introduction, although current therapies may have reached a plateau, advances in tumor biology have opened many therapeutic possibilities, placing us closer to developing effective cancer treatments.

CLINICAL SEQUELA OF MALIGNANCY

As cancers increase in size, they can destroy and invade surrounding normal tissues, resulting in compromised function and pain. Most advanced cancers cause morbidity because of local progression or the development of new lesions. Metastases in vital organs (i.e., liver, lung, bone marrow, or brain) can severely compromise organ function and lead to organ-specific symptoms. In addition to direct effects of cancers in sites of primary origin, or in sites of metastasis formation, cancers may have additional indirect effects of clinical significance. These include impairment of nutritional balance, significant metabolic disturbances, continued immunologic compromise, progressive weakness of the host, and enhanced susceptibility to life-threatening infections. Exact mechanisms producing such effects are not clearly understood, but may be related to the production of toxins by the continually expanding and heterogenous cancer burden, or may involve the trapping of certain essential nutritional elements (e.g., essential amino acids, vitamins) by the expanding cancer at the expense of the host. For example, certain cancers elaborate specific hormones, which mimic the action of normal body hormones. Lung cancers can often produce antidiuretic hormone (ADH) and adrenal corticotropic hormone (ACTH); the elaboration of these hormones may result in significant metabolic derangements. A frequent accompaniment of advancing cancer is suppression of appetite and distaste for food. A hormone-like substance elaborated by the growing cancer can mediate these effects. The secretions of such known and unknown hormones and the resultant clinical effects are called paraneoplastic syndromes. These often may be the most dominant and visible effects of advanced cancers in humans.

CONCLUSION

Over the past two decades, rapidly advancing knowledge of the natural histories of cancers and the specific characteristics of their stages have developed from biologic, cellular, and molecular levels of investigations, and the interdigitation of these three levels of comprehension. These new understandings have provided more specific methods designed in the preclinical phase to prevent cancer formation, and into the clinical phase to enhance management of these diseases in patients. The concept of the irreversibility of initiating agents has led to major efforts toward limiting human exposures to these agents (e.g., limiting radiation exposure from diagnostic radiology procedures, ultraviolet radiation from sunlight, and exposure to known human chemical carcinogens in the work place, in pharmaceutical products, and in dietary sources). Additional efforts at removing exposures to promotion agents has led to educational efforts to limit exposures to cigarette smoke, alcohol, dietary fat, and certain drugs or chemicals. A search for agents designed to modify the stage of promotion has led to the new science of cancer chemoprevention exemplified by the use of vitamin A analogs (e.g., 13-*cis*-retinoic acid and inhibition of continued development of upper airway cancers) and vitamin D analogs (in preventing prostate cancer). Understanding of the karyotypic instability present in the stage of progression and its relationship in some circumstances to actions by oncogenic viruses has led to development of immunization methods (e.g., hepatitis B vaccination and attempts to prevent hepatic cancers). Attempts have been made to inhibit the formation and growth of metastases by interfering with altered blood coagulation processes as well as by development of antiangiogenic therapies. Finally, adjuvant treatments have been actively designed in attempts to target each individual step necessary in the formation of metastases in patients with early clinical cancers. As new knowledge concerning the natural history of cancer and tumor biology is gained and applied, it should serve us well in designing novel approaches for neoplastic diseases.

FURTHER READING

Compagni A, Christofori G (2000) Recent advances in research on multistage tumorigenesis. *Br J Cancer* 83:1–5.

Desai PB (1994) Understanding the biology of cancer: has this any impact on treatment? *J Cancer Res Clin Oncol* 120:193–199.

Fidler IJ (1997) Molecular biology of cancer: invasion and metastasis. In *Cancer: Principles and Practice of Oncology*, 5th edition. Devita VT, et al (eds.) Lippincott-Raven Publishers, Philadelphia.

Heimbrook DC, Oliff A, Gibbs JB (1997) Essentials of signal transduction. In *Cancer: Principles and Practice of Oncology*, 5th edition. Devita VT, et al (eds.) Lippincott-Raven Publishers, Philadelphia.

Hill RP, Tannock IF (1998) Introduction to cancer biology. In *The Basic Science of Oncology*, 3rd edition. Tannock IF, Hill RP (eds.) McGraw-Hill, New York.

Holmes FF, Wilson J, Blesch KS, Kaesberg PR, Miller R, Sprott R (1991) Biology of cancer and aging. *Cancer* 68(11 Suppl):2525–2526.

Kastan MB (1997) Molecular biology of cancer: the cell cycle. In *Cancer: Principles and Practice of Oncology*, 5th edition. Devita VT, et al (eds.) Lippincott-Raven Publishers, Philadelphia.

Kerbel RS (2000) Tumor angiogenesis: past, present and the near future. *Carcinogenesis* 21:505–515.

Kohn EC, Liotta LA (1995) Molecular insights into cancer invasion: strategies for prevention and intervention. *Cancer Res* 55:1856–1862.

Loeb KR, Loeb LA (2000) Significance of multiple mutations in cancer. *Carcinogenesis* 21:379–385.

Pitot HC, Dragan YP (1991) Facts and theories concerning the mechanisms of carcinogenesis. *FASEB J* 5:2280–2286.

Ruoslahti E (1996) How cancer spreads. *Sci Am* 275:72–77.

Sagano H (1999) The cancer problem: carcinogenesis and prevention from the viewpoint of the natural history of cancer. *Anticancer Res* 19:3787–3790.

Slingerland JM, Tannock IF (1998) Cell proliferation and cell death. In *The Basic Science of Oncology*, 3rd edition. Tannock IF, Hill RP (eds.) McGraw-Hill, New York.

Weinberg RA (1996) How cancer arises. *Sci Am* 275:62–70.

Weisburger JH, Horn CL (1991) The causes of cancer. In *American Society Textbook of Clinical Oncology*. Americal Cancer Society, Atlanta, GA.

Zanke BW (1998) Growth factors and intracellular signaling. In *The Basic Science of Oncology*, Tannock IF, Hill RP (eds.) 3rd edition. McGraw-Hill, New York.

CHAPTER 2

Carcinogenesis

SURYANARAYANA V. VULIMIRI and JOHN DiGIOVANNI

The University of Texas, M. D. Anderson Cancer Center, Department
of Carcinogenesis, Science Park Research Division, Smithville, Texas

BACKGROUND AND HISTORICAL PERSPECTIVE

Human exposure to certain chemicals or substances was first related to an increased incidence of cancer independently by two English physicians. In 1761, Dr. John Hill observed an increased incidence of nasal cancer among snuff users. Fourteen years later, Dr. Percival Pott observed that chimney sweeps had an increased incidence of scrotal cancer and attributed this to occupational exposure to soot and coal tar. It was not until a century and a half later, in 1918, that two Japanese scientists, Yamagiwa and Ichikawa, confirmed these earlier observations by demonstrating that multiple topical applications of coal tar to rabbit ears produced skin carcinomas. The importance of this experiment was two-fold: (1) it was the first demonstration that a chemical or substance could produce cancer in animals, and (2) it confirmed Percival Pott's initial observation and established a relationship between human epidemiology studies and animal carcinogenicity. In the 1930s, Kennaway and co-workers isolated a single active carcinogenic chemical from coal tar and identified it as benzo[a]pyrene (B[a]P), a polycyclic aromatic hydrocarbon (PAH) resulting from the incomplete combustion of organic molecules.

The concept that cancer involves an alteration in the genetic material of a somatic cell (somatic mutation theory) and that cancer was related to chromosomal abnormalities was first introduced by Theodor Boveri in 1914. By 1934, Furth and Kahn had isolated single cell clones from a tumor and found that injection of these cells into a healthy host could reproduce the original disease, thus demonstrating that cancer is a stable heritable cellular alteration. In the 1950s and 1960s, James and Elizabeth Miller observed that a wide variety of structurally diverse chemicals could produce cancer in animals and suggested that these chemicals required metabolic activation to reactive electrophilic intermediates that bind covalently to

UICC Manual of Clinical Oncology, Eighth Edition. Edited by Raphael E. Pollock
ISBN 0-471-22289-5 Copyright © 2004 John Wiley & Sons, Inc.

nucleophilic centers on proteins, RNA, or DNA. The Millers termed this the electrophile theory of chemical carcinogenesis. In 1964, Brookes and Lawley demonstrated that covalent binding of carcinogenic PAH to DNA correlated best with carcinogenic potency. Subsequently, many chemical carcinogens were shown to bind covalently to DNA in various animal model systems and to produce mutations in both prokaryotic and eukaryotic cells. Chemicals that exert their action by binding to DNA are called *genotoxic carcinogens*. In contrast, chemicals that induce carcinogenesis by epigenetic mechanisms are termed *nongenotoxic carcinogens* (e.g., 2,3,7,8-tetrachlorodibenzo-*p*-dioxin [TCDD]).

FACTORS CONTRIBUTING TO THE INCIDENCE OF HUMAN CANCER

Epidemiological studies indicate that a majority of human cancers occur as a result of exposure to environmental agents or factors, as shown in Figure 2.1. Environmental factors include smoking, diet, cultural and sexual behavior, occupation, exposure to radiation (natural or medical), and exposure to agents or substances in air, water, and soil. Elucidation of the relationship between exposure to a particular environmental factor and incidence of a specific cancer in a given community has been aided through studies of specific populations that have been stratified according to a number of variables including occupation, race, and lifestyle. Although cancer incidence is associated to a major extent with cigarette smoking and exposure to dietary substances, human carcinogenesis in many cases may involve interactions between several etiologic factors.

For the purposes of this chapter, the term *carcinogenesis* is defined as a process wherein the normal physiologic function of living cells is altered, resulting in abnormal and uncontrolled growth of a particular organ or tissue. The newly formed mass of tissue, which is morphologically and genetically different from normal tissue and has autonomous growth, is called a *neoplasm*. An agent that either induces or causes a series of genetic or epigenetic events in normal cells,

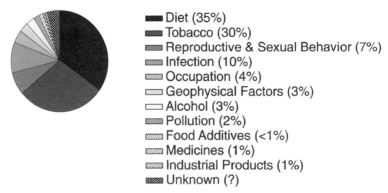

- Diet (35%)
- Tobacco (30%)
- Reproductive & Sexual Behavior (7%)
- Infection (10%)
- Occupation (4%)
- Geophysical Factors (3%)
- Alcohol (3%)
- Pollution (2%)
- Food Additives (<1%)
- Medicines (1%)
- Industrial Products (1%)
- Unknown (?)

Figure 2.1 Factors contributing to the incidence of human cancer. (Adapted from Doll and Peto, 1981.)

resulting in a significant increase in the incidence of a neoplasm of a given or multiple histologic type compared with normal untreated individuals, irrespective of whether the control individual has a high or low incidence of neoplasms of that kind, is termed a *carcinogen*.

Carcinogens can be broadly categorized as (1) biological carcinogens (e.g., viruses, such as human immunodeficiency virus [HIV] or hepatitis B virus [HBV]), (2) physical carcinogens (e.g., ultraviolet [UV] rays and ionizing radiation); and (3) chemical carcinogens (e.g., B[a]P and aflatoxin B_1 [AFB_1]). Because the majority of human carcinogens are chemical in nature, the remainder of this chapter is devoted to chemical carcinogenesis.

DIVERSITY OF CHEMICAL CARCINOGENS

Chemical carcinogens may be divided into three major classes: (1) organic chemicals, (2) inorganic chemicals, and (3) hormones. Organic carcinogens belonging to several classes, such as PAHs (e.g., B[a]P), *N*-nitrosamines (e.g., 4-(methylnitrosamine)-1-(3-pyridyl)-1-butanone [NNK]), aromatic amines (e.g., 4-aminobiphenyl [4-ABP] and 2-naphthylamine), heterocyclic aromatic amines (e.g., 2-amino-1-methyl-6-phenyl-imidazo-[4,5-b]pyridine [PhIP]), alkyl halides (e.g., vinyl chloride, cyclophosphamide), nitro aromatics and heterocyclics (e.g., 2-nitroflourene and nitrofurans), azo dyes and diazo compounds (e.g., 3-methyl-4-amino azobenzene), alkylating agents (e.g., bis(chloromethyl)ether) and mycotoxins (e.g., AFB_1) are known to be carcinogenic from epidemiologic and experimental studies. For example, B[a]P and similar PAHs, which are found in tobacco smoke, combustion emissions, and coal tar, are associated with both lung cancer and skin cancer. Another tobacco-specific carcinogen, NNK, has been shown to be a lung carcinogen. Aromatic amines (e.g., 2-naphthylamine and 4-ABP) used in the chemical and dye industries, induced bladder cancer in essentially 100% of workers involved in dye purification. Exposure to vinyl chloride is associated with an increased risk of hemangiosarcoma of the liver whereas benzene is known to induce acute myelogenous leukemia after prolonged exposure.

Inorganic chemicals that are carcinogenic in humans include arsenic (found in the copper mining and smelting industry), which is associated with skin, lung, and liver cancer. Chromium and chromates, used in the tanning and pigmenting industry, and nickel are also associated with cancers of the nasal sinus and lung.

Hormones, which are also organic carcinogens, are discussed as a separate class in this chapter since their mechanism(s) may be more like those of nongenotoxic carcinogens. In addition, other polypeptide growth factors (e.g., insulin-like growth factor-1 [IGF-1], growth hormone, transforming growth factor-α [TGF-α]) that are carcinogenic in experimental animals belong to this category. A dramatic example of hormonal carcinogenesis in humans involves the use of the synthetic estrogenic compound diethylstilbestrol (DES) in pregnant women to avert a threatened spontaneous abortion. A small percentage of the female offspring of mothers treated with DES during pregnancy developed clear cell carcinomas of the vagina, usually within a few years after puberty. Prolonged use of oral contraceptives containing synthetic steroidal estrogens is associated with the development of liver cell adenomas and has been linked to increased incidence of premenopausal breast cancer in some but not all epidemiologic studies. Similarly, administration of estrogens and androgenic steroids are associated with increased risk of developing endometrial and hepatocellular carcinomas, respectively. Finally, recent evidence has suggested that endometrial cancer may be induced by long-term treatment with the antiestrogen tamoxifen.

IDENTIFICATION AND CLASSIFICATION OF HUMAN CHEMICAL CARCINOGENS

The primary factors involved in the determination of carcinogenic potential are hazard identification and risk estimation, which form the basis of cancer risk assessment. Traditionally, carcinogen identification involved epidemiologic detection of human cancer risks. At present, the primary factor used in risk assessment for human cancer is tumor incidence in two-year bioassays in rodents. Each bioassay involves the chronic administration of a compound for a majority of the rodent's life span and the assessment of the incidence of tumors at all sites. Each study includes two doses of the compound, the maximum tolerated dose (MTD) and one-half the MTD, a solvent-treated control group and an untreated control group. The compound is administered by the route through which human exposure is most likely to occur. The animals should be susceptible but not hypersensitive to the tested effect. The two strains typically used in these studies are the B6C3F1 mouse and the F344 rat, which have high spontaneous rates of certain tumor types, limiting their predictive value and utility in risk estimation for these sites. Approximately 50 animals per dose per sex per species are used to approach statistical relevance for the dose-response data needed for use in risk assessment.

Based on weight of evidence for carcinogenicity from epidemiologic studies in humans and from the results obtained in animal studies, human carcinogens are classified into five major groups by the Environmental Protection Agency (EPA) and the International Agency for Research on Cancer (IARC). These groups are as follows:

- Group 1: Human carcinogens—sufficient epidemiologic evidence in humans to indicate that a particular agent is carcinogenic (e.g., aflatoxin, benzene, estrogens)
- Group 2A: Probable human carcinogens—limited human data and sufficient animal evidence (e.g., benz[a]anthracene, diethylnitrosamine, polychlorinated biphenyls)
- Group 2B: Possible human carcinogens—inadequate or no human data, but sufficient animal data (e.g., styrene, TCDD, urethane)
- Group 3: Not classifiable as to human carcinogenicity—lack of or an inadequate amount of human as well as animal data (e.g., 5-azacytidine, diazepam)

- Group 4: Noncarcinogenic to humans—lack of evidence in humans and no evidence for carcinogenicity of the putative agent in at least two adequate animal tests in two different species (e.g., caprolactam).

METABOLIC ACTIVATION OF CHEMICAL CARCINOGENS

According to the Millers' electrophilic theory of carcinogenesis, all chemical carcinogens that are not themselves chemically reactive must be converted metabolically to a chemically reactive form. The active metabolite is an electrophilic reagent, which reacts with nucleophilic groups in cellular macromolecules such as DNA to initiate carcinogenesis. Such carcinogens are called *indirect carcinogens* (e.g., B[a]P, NNK, and 4-ABP). In contrast, chemicals that are highly reactive and can bind to DNA directly without metabolic activation are called *direct carcinogens* (e.g., β-propiolactone, cyclophosphamide, and bis(chloromethyl) ether). These carcinogens spontaneously decompose to produce a highly reactive electrophilic intermediate that can alkylate DNA and produce base modifications such as O^6-alkylguanine, N^7-alkylguanine. Both direct and indirect carcinogens covalently modify DNA, producing adducts with various DNA bases.

The metabolic activation of chemical carcinogens is carried out primarily by the cytochrome(s) P450 enzymes (CYP), a class of enzymes that display a characteristic absorbance maximum at 450 nm when reduced with carbon monoxide, present in the endoplasmic reticulum of most cells. In humans, the CYP superfamily consists of approximately 60 genes, which are grouped based on sequence identity into families (1, 2, 3, . . .), subfamilies (A, B, C, . . .), and individual P450s (1, 2, 3, . . .) (e.g., 1A1, 1A2, 1B1, etc.). The CYP enzymes, also called phase I enzymes, play a central role in catalyzing a variety of reactions such as oxidation, reduction, oxygenation, dealkylation, desulfuration, dehalogenation, and hydroxylation, whereby nonpolar or hydrophobic compounds (e.g., drugs, chemical toxicants, and carcinogens) are converted to potentially reactive products through the formation of more reactive intermediates or converted to less toxic compounds. For example, the parent or primary carcinogen B[a]P, which is inactive per se, is metabolically activated by the enzymes CYP1A1 and epoxide hydrolase (EH), in a two-step reaction, to an intermediate metabolite or proximate carcinogen B[a]P-7,8-diol. This reactive intermediate is further metabolized to several B[a]P 7,8-diol 9,10-epoxide (BPDE) isomers, of which the (+) *anti*-BPDE is the ultimate carcinogen or metabolite. However, B[a]P is also metabolized by CYP enzymes into an array of metabolites including phenols, quinones, epoxides, and dihydrodiols. Aromatic amines such as benzidine, which contain a primary or secondary amine group, are metabolically activated through *N*-hydroxylation by CYP1A2 followed by esterification resulting in a reactive ultimate carcinogenic metabolite that can covalently modify DNA. Nitrosamines, such as the tobacco-specific nitrosamine NNK, are activated by P4502E1 in a one-step reaction to an unstable, hydroxylated intermediate that spontaneously decomposes to a carbonium ion capable of alkylating DNA.

As noted previously, the oxidation of indirect carcinogens, known generally as phase I metabolism, in most cases renders them more hydrophilic and prepares them as substrates for the conjugating enzymes, known as phase II metabolizing enzymes. These enzymes conjugate the metabolites produced during phase I metabolism with a variety of small ligands and include methyl transferases, sulfotransferases, glucuronyltransferases, and glutathione-S-transferases (GSTs). Of particular importance is conjugation with glutathione (GSH) catalyzed by GSTs. In general, conjugation reactions lead to less toxic/carcinogenic and more readily excretable metabolites; however, this is not always the case, as seen with aromatic amines such as benzidine. Both acetylation and sulfation of the N-hydroxyl substituent introduced during phase I metabolism by CYP1A2 lead to more chemically reactive and ultimate carcinogenic metabolites.

It should also be stressed that pathways other than those involving CYP enzymes may be involved in the metabolic activation of certain chemical carcinogens. In this regard, cyclooxygenase-dependent co-oxidation of carcinogens may be important for the metabolic activation of certain aromatic carcinogens in some extrahepatic tissues, especially the urinary bladder.

CARCINOGEN-DNA ADDUCTS, MUTATIONS, AND CARCINOGENESIS

As noted previously, DNA adducts are usually formed between reactive carcinogen metabolites and the bases of DNA, which can be quite specific for a given carcinogen. For example, the reactive metabolites of PAHs (e.g., B[a]P) predominantly bind to the N^2-position of guanine (G) or the N^6-position of adenine (A); aromatic amines (e.g., 4-ABP) bind to C^8 of A or G; mycotoxins (e.g., AFB_1) bind to N^7 of A or G forming bulky DNA adducts. In contrast, alkylating agents (e.g., MNU) are less specific and react at different sites and with all DNA bases. In addition, reactive oxygen species (ROS), produced as a result of carcinogen exposure, can lead to oxidative DNA damage, forming simple base modifications (e.g., 8-oxodeoxyguanosine and thymine glycol). Endogenous DNA damage as a result of oxidation of DNA bases, depurination, deamination, depyrimidination, single-strand breaks, or alkylation may also occur during normal cellular metabolism.

It is generally accepted that DNA adduct formation is the first step in tumor initiation during carcinogenesis. The biological potential of a given DNA adduct depends on its mutagenic potential, ability to be repaired, location within a target gene, and the nature of the target gene. For example, formation of BPDE-dGuo adducts in mutational hot spots of the $p53$ tumor suppressor gene in lung cancer patients substantiates the association between tobacco carcinogen-induced DNA damage and lung cancer. The presence of DNA adducts in target tissues often correlates with cancer status. Also, in experimental animal systems, extensive research has shown that the presence of a given carcinogen-DNA adduct in a particular target tissue correlates with the biologic effect of that carcinogen. Total

DNA adduct levels, and in some cases specific DNA adducts, have been correlated with *in vitro* mutations, chromosomal aberrations, and generally with carcinogenicity. Thus, quantitation of DNA adducts in human cells may provide a useful parameter of risk assessment in monitoring human carcinogen exposure. DNA adducts can be easily measured in target tissues or surrogate tissues (e.g., lymphocytes, uroepithelial cells and buccal mucosal cells) by several analytical methods such as ^{32}P-postlabeling, high-performance liquid chromatography (HPLC), immunological methods (e.g., enzyme-linked immunosorbent assay and slot-blot analysis) and gas chromatography/mass spectrophotometry. The presence and extent to which DNA adducts form often correlates with genetic risk factors such as DNA repair capacity and polymorphisms in drug metabolizing enzymes.

Cell replication in the presence of carcinogen DNA damage is generally considered to be the period when such damage produces critical effects such as cytotoxicity and mutagenesis. Extensive studies of different carcinogenic compounds have revealed a strong correlation between mutagenicity and carcinogenicity. Thus, carcinogens, by virtue of their ability to form specific DNA adducts, are able to induce a spectrum of mutations. The spectrum of mutations induced by chemical carcinogens include point mutations, frameshift mutations as a result of base deletions and/or insertions, chromosomal aberrations, aneuploidy, and polyploidy with varying degrees of specificity that are usually dose-dependent. The efficiency and the spectrum of mutational activity of chemical carcinogens are assayed *in vitro* using both bacterial and mammalian cell systems and cell-free systems. The mutagenicity of DNA adducts depends on the type of adduct formed, the extent to which it is repaired, the DNA sequence context and the DNA polymerases involved. For example, mutagenesis of the $(+)$-*anti*-BPDE metabolite was very recently examined in bacteria with site-directed vectors containing a single $(+)$ *anti*-BPDE-trans-N^2-dGuo adduct. Depending on the sequence context around the DNA adduct, both transversion and transition point mutations ($G \rightarrow T$, $G \rightarrow A$, and $G \rightarrow C$) were observed. Alterations in DNA sequences caused by carcinogen-induced mutations may have far-reaching consequences and may be life threatening if the mutations occur in proto-oncogenes and tumor suppressor genes.

ONCOGENES AND TUMOR SUPPRESSOR GENES INVOLVED IN HUMAN CANCER

Oncogenes

Certain normal cellular genes, termed proto-oncogenes, appear to be target genes for chemical carcinogens and their alteration is strongly associated with tumor formation and carcinogenesis. Proto-oncogenes function in a tightly regulated manner to control normal cellular proliferation and differentiation. However, when these genes are altered by a mutation, sequence deletion, virus integration, chromosomal translocation, gene amplification, or promoter insertion, they have the ability to transform cells *in vitro*. The altered forms of these genes are called *oncogenes*. Both proto-oncogenes and oncogenes are dominant in nature with broad tissue specificity and are rarely involved in germline inheritance for cancer development. Somatic mutations in both proto-oncogenes and oncogenes can be activated during all stages of carcinogenesis.

Proto-oncogenes can be activated to oncogenes either qualitatively or quantitatively. Qualitative changes include alterations in the coding region of the gene such as occurs with point mutations. For example, in hallmark studies by Barbacid and co-workers, it was observed that rat mammary carcinomas induced by methylnitrosourea contained an activated c-Ha-*ras* gene with a point mutation in codon 12 ($G^{35} \rightarrow A$ transition mutation), whereas those mammary carcinomas induced by 7,12-dimethylbenz[a]anthracene (DMBA) contained $A^{182} \rightarrow T$ transversion mutations in codon 61, providing evidence that the point mutations in *ras* genes are related to the type of carcinogenic agent used. Quantitative changes in proto-oncogenes include gene amplification, an increase in the number of copies of a given gene, which leads to overexpression of the gene or chromosomal translocation which may lead to aberrant expression of the proto-oncogene. Amplification of the proto-oncogene c-*myc*, a late progression-related event, has been detected in human or murine carcinomas, leukemias, and sarcomas. Translocation of c-*myc* from chromosome 8 to an immunoglobulin region in either chromosome 2, 14, or 22 is a consistent feature found in a majority of Burkitt's lymphoma tumor biopsies or cell lines derived from these tumors. According to one model, such a juxtaposition allows for the deregulation of c-*myc* expression, as it is no longer under proper cellular regulation but rather under the control of the immunoglobulin promoter and is therefore constitutively expressed. However, the actual mode(s) of such deregulation is not fully understood.

About a hundred potential cellular and viral oncogenes have now been identified. Most oncogene protein products appear to function in one way or another in cellular signal transduction pathways in which cells receive and process information and ultimately effect a biologic response. These signal transduction pathways often consist of external signals, receptors, transducer proteins, second messengers, amplifier proteins, and internal effectors, all of which are involved in the regulation of cellular function and/or gene expression.

Oncogenes fall into six main categories, all of which are molecules involved in signal transduction, including: (1) growth factors (e.g., *wnt-1*, *-2*, and *-3*, *hst*, *fgf-5*, *TGF*-α and *sis*; (2) growth factor receptors (e.g., *erb*B, *fms*, *kit*, *met*, *neu* [*erb*B-2], *ret*, *ros*, and *trk*; (3) cytoplasmic tyrosine kinases (e.g., *bcr-abl*, *fes*, and *jak*) and src family kinases (e.g., *src*, *frg*, *fyn*, *hck*, *lck*, *lyn*, *yes*, and *yrk*); (4) serine-threonine kinases (e.g., *mos*, *PKC*-β1, -γ, -ε and -ζ, and *raf*-1); (5) G proteins/GTPases (e.g., Ha-*ras*, Ki-*ras*, and N-*ras*); and (6) nuclear proteins, which include thyroid hormone receptors (e.g., *erb* A) and transcription factors (e.g., *ets*, *fos*, *jun*, L-*myc*, *myc*, N-*myc*, *rel*, and *tal*-1).

Tumor Suppressor Genes

Tumor suppressor genes and the proteins they encode function as negative regulators of cell growth. Their function is in direct contrast to the dominant transforming oncogenes, which act as positive regulators of cell growth. Tumor suppressor genes also have considerable tissue specificity, however, unlike onco-genes, they are frequently involved in germline inheritance and these mutations may not come into play until the stage of progression. Accordingly, tumor suppressor genes have been termed antioncogenes, recessive oncogenes, and growth suppressor genes. When tumor suppressor genes are lost by deletion or inactivated by point mutation, they are no longer capable of negatively regulating cellular growth. Generally, if one copy of the tumor suppressor gene is inactivated, the cell is normal, but if both copies are inactivated, loss of growth control can occur and cancer can develop. The concept that loss of genetic material is involved in carcinogenesis was derived from somatic cell fusion experiments. Many of the hybrid cells resulting from the fusion of a tumor cell to a normal cell are nontumorigenic. These experiments suggested that the normal cell is contributing genes to the tumor cell that impose normal growth restraints on the latter and that cancer is a recessive trait. Subsequently, it was determined that these tumor cells contained specific chromosomal deletions and such deletions were "corrected" in the normal-tumor cell hybrids because the previously deleted chromosome is now contributed by the normal cell. Further, by using microcell fusion experiments that allow for the selective introduction of specific chromosomes or a portion of a chromosome into these tumor cells, it was possible to determine which chromo-some or portion of a chromosome suppressed the tumorigenic phenotype and restored normal growth control. Additional evidence has come from the work of Knudson, who postulated that two mutational events are necessary for the devel-opment of retinoblastoma. This work led to the eventual identification of the retinoblastoma gene and the discovery that both copies of the gene (two mutational events) are inactivated and/or deleted in retinoblastoma tumors. This deletion involves a specific locus termed *Rb*.

Several tumor suppressor genes (indicated in the parentheses) have been identified through the analysis of families with inherited conditions such as Li-Fraumeni syndrome (*p53*), melanomas (*INK4a/ARF*), retinoblastoma (*Rb*), stomach cancers (*E-cadherin*), von Hippel-Lindau syndrome (*VHL* or *3p25*), hereditary nephroblastomas or Wilms's tumor (*WT1*), Cowden's disease (*PTEN/MMAC1*), familial breast and ovarian carcinomas (*BRCA1* and *2*), familial adenomatous polyposis (*APC, MCC*), and nonpolyposis cancer of the large intestine (*MSH2, MLH1, PMS1,* and *PMS2*).

The *p53* tumor suppressor gene is quite unique in that it regulates cell cycle, apoptosis, senescence, DNA repair, cell differentiation, and angiogenesis. In addition to being associated with Li-Fraumeni syndrome, this tumor suppressor gene is either mutated or deleted in many different types of human cancers and it has been shown to be a target of several types of carcinogens. In particular, a strong relationship between UV exposure and *p53* mutations exists with regard to human skin cancer. Epidemiologic and clinical studies have implicated UV radiation in sunlight as the agent responsible for the induction of most human skin cancers. Analysis of a large number of skin tumors (including both basal cell carcinoma and squamous cell carcinoma) has revealed the presence of UV signature mutations (i.e., C→T and CC→TT) in various exons of this gene at a relatively high percentage (60–100% of tumors). In addition, *p53* mutations have been detected in sun-damaged skin prior to the development of any tumors, suggesting that loss of *p53* may be an early event in human skin cancer.

Tumor suppressor genes are inactivated by either point mutations or by DNA methylation. Recent studies have shown that mutational hotspots in the *p53* gene found in lung cancers are hotspots for the formation of deoxyguanosine adducts by the reactive diol epoxide metabolite of B[a]P (BPDE-dGuo). These data support the hypothesis that the *p53* gene may be an important target for human chemical carcinogens. The extent to which other tumor suppressor genes may be targets for chemical carcinogens remains to be determined. The CpG sites in the *p53* tumor suppressor gene are known to be targets for methylation. Several tumor suppressor genes such as *VHL*, *Rb*, and *p16^{INK4a}* are known to be silenced by methylation in human tumors.

THE CELL CYCLE

The cell cycle is a tightly regulated process during which the cell replicates its DNA in the S, or synthetic phase, and divides during the M, or mitotic phase. As shown in Figure 2.2A, both S and M phases are separated by two G, or growth phases, a G1 phase preceding S phase and a G2 phase preceding M phase. During cell cycle

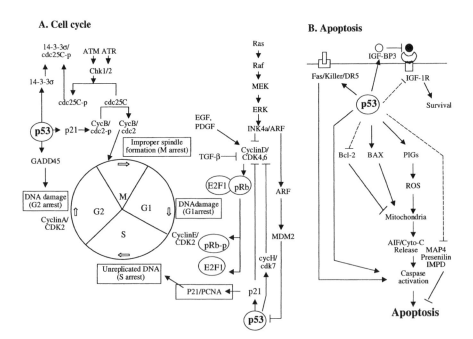

Figure 2.2   Cell cycle (A) and apoptosis (B).

progression these are feedback controls, cellular mechanisms that can arrest the cell cycle at specific checkpoints (e.g., G1/S and G2/M) until some processes are complete. Protein kinase complexes involving regulatory and catalytic subunits termed cyclins and cyclin-dependent kinases (CDKs), respectively, govern cell cycle progression. The rapid synthesis and degradation of cyclins and other cell cycle–dependent proteins allows the cell cycle to progress normally. Levels of different cyclins such as D, E, A, and B peak respectively, during the G1, G1/S, S/G2, and G2/M phases of the cell cycle and bind to different sets of CDKs. In the G1 phase, D-type cyclins are synthesized during sustained mitogenic stimulation leading to phosphorylation of the retinoblastoma protein (pRb), which is bound to the transcription factor E2F. Phosphorylated pRb (pRb-p) releases E2F, and the free E2F initiates transcription of genes involved in DNA replication. Growth factors such as epidermal growth factor (EGF) and platelet-derived growth factor (PDGF) are also positive regulators of cyclins.

CDKs are negatively regulated by functionally related proteins called CDK inhibitors (CKI) belonging to two families, that is, INK4 (e.g., p16, p15, p18, and p19) and CIP/KIP (e.g., p21, p27, and p57) families. If DNA damage is detected before the start of S phase, the G1 checkpoint will be activated. Upon exposure to genotoxic agents, the wild-type (wt) p53 of the cell is activated, which in turn up-regulates the CKI p21$^{WAF/Cip1}$. In the p21-dependent mechanism, p21 binds and inactivates cyclin-CDK complexes involved in G1 progression, leading to hypophosphorylation of pRb, E2F sequestration, and cell cycle arrest at the G1/S phase transition. p21 also binds to the proliferating cell nuclear antigen (PCNA) and prevents PCNA from mediating recognition of the DNA primer-template complex by inhibiting DNA polymerase δ, thus blocking elongation and leading to DNA replication arrest (S arrest). In the p21-independent pathway, p53 can bind to cyclin H and p36 Mat 1 protein and cause G1 arrest.

p16^{INK4a}, which belongs to the other family of CKI proteins coded by the *INK4a/ARF* locus, is transcriptionally activated by oncogenic processes leading to cell cycle arrest and apoptosis. The p16^{INK4a} protein inhibits CDK4-6/cycD kinases, thereby maintaining Rb and its homologues in the unphosphorylated state, thus preventing cell cycle progression. The p16^{INK4a}/Rb/cyclin D1 pathway has been shown to be altered in many human tumors. The other protein, p19^{ARF}, coded by the INK4a/ARF locus, associates with MDM2 and the sequestration and nucleolar localization of MDM2 by p19^{ARF} stabilizes p53 protein. The p19^{ARF}/p53 pathway is presumably deregulated in a large majority of human tumors either by (1) homozygous deletion of the entire *p53* locus (14% of tumors); (2) by intragenic mutation in the second exon (infrequent); or (3) by promoter methylation. p19^{ARF} is activated through the Ras-raf-MEK-ERK pathway also. Transforming growth factor-β (TGF-β) is another negative regulator of cyclin/CDK complexes. The delay in the entry into S-phase due to the G1/S arrest allows the cell to undergo DNA repair and progress through the cell cycle normally. If the DNA damage is excessive, the cells undergo programmed cell death or apoptosis. However, if the *p53* gene is mutated or absent, cell cycle continues even in the presence of DNA damage.

p53 mediates G2 arrest at least by inducing two genes, that is, the *14-3-3σ* gene and the *GADD45* gene. The product of the *14-3-3σ* gene sequesters the phosphorylated form of cdc25C, a phosphatase of the cyclin B/cdc2 complex necessary for the G2/M transition. p53 can also induce the *GADD45* gene, whose product can disrupt the cyclin B/cdc2 complex via a direct interaction with cdc2. In another mechanism following DNA damage, members of the PI-3K family of proteins including ATM and ATR are activated, which in turn activate chk1/2, leading to the phosphorylation of cdc25C generating a binding site for the 14-3-3σ proteins, thereby causing G2 arrest. p53-induced p21 can also inhibit cyclin B1/Cdc2, thereby causing G2 arrest. p53 is also involved in a mitotic spindle checkpoint, thereby preventing cell cycle progression.

In cancer cells, there is frequent overexpression of positive regulators (e.g., cyclins D1 and E, CDKs 4 and 6, and c-myc) or reduced or lack of expression of negative regulators (e.g., p16, p27, and pRb). The choice between growth arrest and apoptosis depends on the cell type, the oncogenic composition of the cell, the extracellular stimuli and the intensity of the stress conditions, the level of *p53* expression, and its interaction with specific proteins.

APOPTOSIS

Apoptosis is a process of cell death resulting from cell injury and is characterized by cell shrinkage, membrane blebbing, chromatin condensation, and nuclear fragmentation. It differs from necrosis in that the latter is caused by severe damage to the environment of the cell as a result of ischemia or physical trauma. In the event of unrepairable and irreversible DNA damage induced by chemical carcinogens, cells undergo apoptosis to avoid replicating a damaged DNA template, which may lead to mutations. p53 protein plays a central role in apoptosis. As shown in Figure 2.2B, apoptosis is triggered by p53 protein involving both sequence-specific transactivation (SST)-dependent and -independent mechanisms. In the SST-dependent pathway, p53 activates apoptotic target gene products in the plasma membrane that belong to signal transduction pathways (e.g., insulin-like growth factor 1–binding protein-3 [IGF-BP3] and Fas/Apo-1, KILLER/DR5), which signal to the mitochondria. There are other proteins, known as apoptotic effector proteins or internal sensors, present in the cell (e.g., proteins coded by Bax and p53-induced gene-3 [PIG3]), which signal the mitochondria, causing a release in apoptosis-inducing factors (AIF) or cytochrome *c*. Notably, PIG3 mediates its action through elevation of ROS. Cytochrome *c* in turn stimulates a family of intracellular cysteine aspartyl proteases (caspases), which rapidly degrade cellular organelles, characterized by morphological changes, nuclear condensation, plasma membrane blebbing, and DNA fragmentation. In the SST-independent pathway, apoptosis is induced by repression of both survival promoting genes such as IGF-1 receptor (IGF-1R) and presenilin or the inhibitors of apoptosis (e.g., bcl-2) as well as by direct activation of caspases by p53.

Apoptosis plays a pivotal role during cellular development and homeostasis and in many diseases, including acquired immunodeficiency syndrome (AIDS) and neurodegenerative disorders. Also, apoptosis is a major protective mechanism against cancer. Cancer is characterized by an uncontrolled proliferation of malignant cells, whereas apoptosis is a counterweight to proliferation. Thus, disruption of apoptosis is a key event in several kinds of cancers (e.g., follicular lymphomas, carcinomas with p53 mutations, and hormone-dependent cancers). In follicular lymphoma, a chromosomal translocation of the immunoglobulin heavy chain locus to *bcl-2* gene on chromosome 18 causes overexpression of bcl-2 in the cells of B-cell lineage, thereby preventing apoptosis. Also, increased bcl-2 expression in certain acute lymphoblastic and myelogenous leukemias is associated with increased resistance to chemotherapy. Thus, knowledge of the mechanisms involved in the apoptotic process in cancer patients or cell lines may be valuable in understanding the resistance of cancer cells to chemotherapy. It is also important in designing rational new therapies, which can induce apoptosis in cancer cells.

MULTISTAGE CARCINOGENESIS

The multistage nature of the carcinogenic process was first established using the mouse skin model of chemical carcinogenesis. In this model, epidermal neoplasia can be induced by two different protocols, that is, complete carcinogenesis and two-stage carcinogenesis protocols. In the first protocol, a single large dose or more commonly, multiple low-dose application of a genotoxic carcinogen (e.g., B[a]P), is used to induce tumors on the backs of susceptible strains of mice. In two-stage carcinogenesis protocols, subcarcinogenic doses of a carcinogen (e.g., B[a]P or DMBA) are followed by multiple applications of a noncarcinogenic agent that possesses the ability to induce epidermal hyperplasia (e.g., 12-*O*-tetradecanoyl-phorbol-13-acetate [TPA] or benzoyl peroxide [BzPo]). In the two-stage model of mouse skin carcinogenesis, three mechanistic stages can be defined: initiation, promotion, and progression. The characteristics of each of these stages are described in the following sections. Figure 2.3 shows the mouse skin model of multistage carcinogenesis and summarizes the major events that occur during the three mechanistically distinct stages described previously.

Initiation

The initiation stage of multistage carcinogenesis in mouse skin is effected by a single, subcarcinogenic dose of either a direct acting [e.g., *N*-methyl-*N'*-nitro-*N*-nitrosoguanidine (MNNG)] or indirect acting (e.g., B[a]P or DMBA) carcinogen. During initiation, chemical carcinogens such as MNNG or B[a]P either spontaneously decompose or are metabolically activated, respectively, to a reactive intermediate as described previously. The reactive carcinogenic intermediates then react with the DNA of epidermal cells of the skin to form DNA adducts. It

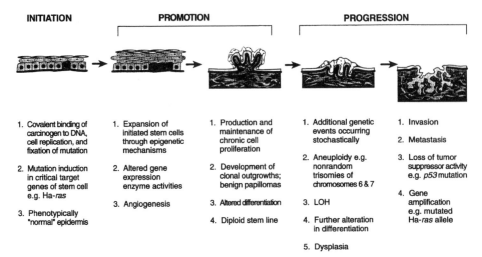

INITIATION **PROMOTION** **PROGRESSION**

1. Covalent binding of carcinogen to DNA, cell replication, and fixation of mutation

2. Mutation induction in critical target genes of stem cell e.g. Ha-*ras*

3. Phenotypically "normal" epidermis

---

1. Expansion of initiated stem cells through epigenetic mechanisms

2. Altered gene expression enzyme activities

3. Angiogenesis

---

1. Production and maintenance of chronic cell proliferation

2. Development of clonal outgrowths; benign papillomas

3. Altered differentiation

4. Diploid stem line

---

1. Additional genetic events occurring stochastically

2. Aneuploidy e.g. nonrandom trisomies of chromosomes 6 & 7

3. LOH

4. Further alteration in differentiation

5. Dysplasia

---

1. Invasion

2. Metastasis

3. Loss of tumor suppressor activity e.g. *p53* mutation

4. Gene amplification e.g. mutated Ha-*ras* allele

Figure 2.3   Multistage carcinogenesis in mouse skin.

is generally believed that the target cells for tumor initiation in this model system are epidermal stem cells and that DNA adducts produce mutations in a critical gene involved in controlling epidermal proliferation and/or differentiation. In the mouse skin model, the Ha-*ras* gene appears to be a critical target gene for some skin tumor initiators such as the PAHs. Mutations in certain codons of this gene (e.g., G^{38} of codon 13 for B[a]P; A^{182} of codon 61 for DMBA) lead to its activation. The hallmarks of skin tumor initiation in this model system are twofold: (1) the initiation stage is phenotypically silent, that is, the initiated skin behaves as normal skin unless it is challenged with chemical tumor promoters or other types of promoting stimuli such as wounding; and (2) the initiation stage is cumulative and irreversible, that is, one can fractionate the initiating dose without loss of tumor initiation and one can delay the start of tumor promotion without loss of tumor initiation. These latter points helped contribute to our initial understanding that the early stages of carcinogenesis in this model system were irreversible and involved a stable alteration in genetic material.

Promotion

The promotion stage of mouse skin carcinogenesis occurs as a result of exposure of the initiated skin to repetitive promoting stimuli. The endpoint of the promotion stage in the mouse skin model is the formation of squamous papillomas, which are exophytic, noninvasive lesions consisting of hyperplastic epidermis folded over a core of stroma. Tumor-promoting stimuli are very diverse in this model system and include various chemicals such as the phorbol esters (e.g., TPA), organic peroxides (e.g., BzPo), and okadaic acid. In addition, UV light, repeated abrasion, full-thickness skin wounding, and certain silica fibers when rubbed on the skin all function as skin tumor promoters. The tumor promotion phase of multistage carcinogenesis involves the clonal expansion of initiated cells. By definition and observation, tumor-promoting agents are not mutagenic like carcinogens but rather act through epigenetic mechanisms causing an alteration of the expression of genes whose products are associated with hyperproliferation, tissue remodeling, and inflammation. At some point, the developing papilloma constitutively expresses some or all of these genes and thus becomes tumor promoter-independent. The identification of the mechanisms by which tumor promoters elicit altered gene expression has been intensively pursued over the last decade, particularly because the identification of these critical events offers a target for chemoprevention strategies (see "Inhibition of Chemical Carcinogenesis" below).

A hallmark of the tumor promotion stage of mouse skin carcinogenesis is that it is reversible in the early stages until tumors become promoter-independent. However, once the papillomas that develop acquire additional genetic changes that allow them to grow autonomously, tumor promotion is no longer reversible. Changes in gene expression can occur directly as a result of tumor promoter action on skin epidermal cells as well as indirectly as a result of the paracrine action of a factor secreted from a nonepithelial skin cell resulting in the activation, or sometimes inactivation of specific signal transduction pathways. These paracrine factors may be produced as a function of direct tumor promoter action on the secreting cell or as a result of activation of the secreting cell by a keratinocyte factor elicited in response to tumor promoters.

The nature of the initial interaction of tumor promoters with the cell depends on the type of promoter. For example, TPA acts through one or more of the isoforms of protein kinase C, whereas okadaic acid acts by inhibiting phosphatases, causing a net increase in the level of phosphorylated proteins, an effect similar to the activation of kinases. However, for compounds such as BzPo, free radicals, including ROS, play a role in their tumor-promoting action. Regardless of the disparity in initial signalling events, the key biologic and molecular changes elicited by tumor promoters (including increased DNA synthesis, induction of ornithine decarboxylase [ODC], induction of growth factors and cytokines, and increased production of eicosanoids) are all similar, and lead to activation of additional signalling pathways via receptors specific for these molecules. This overall alteration of signal transduction and gene expression creates an environment conducive for the selection and growth of the initiated cell population. Some of the growth factors and cytokines whose expression is altered by tumor-promoting stimuli include: (1) transforming growth factor-α (TGF-α); (2) TGF-β; (3) interleukins 1 and 6; (4) tumor necrosis factor-α; (5) granulocyte macrophage colony stimulating factor; (6) vascular endothelial growth factor; and others.

Progression

Tumor progression or malignant conversion, as it is sometimes referred to in this model system, occurs when papillomas convert into SCCs. Most, if not all, SCCs that appear during a two-stage carcinogenesis protocol in mouse skin arise from pre-existing papillomas. The hallmark of tumor progression in the mouse skin model is the accumulation of additional genetic changes in cells that comprise premalignant papillomas. Because all SCCs arise from pre-existing papillomas in the two-stage carcinogenesis model, these lesions can be considered true premalignant lesions. Several genetic alterations have been linked to tumor progression in the mouse skin model system. For example, nonrandom trisomies of chromosomes 6 and 7 have been associated with the progression of papillomas to SCCs. γ-Glutamyltranspeptidase expression is elevated in SCCs, as is expression of α6β4 integrin and keratin 13. Elevated expression of certain proteases (e.g., stromelysin), TGF-β, and inactivation of the *p53* tumor suppressor gene occurs in some SCCs. Loss of the normal Ha-*ras* allele also occurs in later stages of progression. In addition, many of the changes in gene expression detected in papillomas persist in SCCs and may also contribute, in a permissive way, to the malignant phenotype of these tumors.

In concluding this section on multistage carcinogenesis, it should be emphasized that studies using the mouse skin model have shown that the carcinogenic process results from a series of stepwise changes that involve both genetic and epigenetic processes.

MULTISTAGE CARCINOGENESIS AND HUMAN CANCER

The concept of multistage carcinogenesis is particularly important in terms of human cancer for several reasons. First, outside of occupational settings, human exposure to chemical carcinogens usually occurs at very low dose levels that, alone, are insufficient to produce cancer. Second, there is considerable evidence from both human epidemiologic and experimental animal studies that certain human carcinogens exhibit a strong tumor-promoting activity. Tobacco smoke is an example of a human carcinogen with a strong tumor-promoting activity component. Thus, lung cancer is a good example of multistage carcinogenesis in humans. Genomic alterations such as loss of heterozygosity and microsatellite alterations, autocrine-paracrine loops, alterations in oncogenes and tumor suppressor genes, tumor angiogenesis, aberrant promoter methylation, and inherited predisposition to lung cancer are sequential events in the development of lung cancer. Lung cancer can be broadly categorized as small cell lung cancer (SCLC), which accounts for 20–25% of bronchogenic carcinomas, whereas the remainder consists of non–small cell lung cancer (NSCLC). Again, the NSCLCs may be subdivided into adenocarcinoma, squamous cell carcinoma, and large cell carcinoma.

With constant exposure to cigarette smoke carcinogens, the respiratory epithelial cells accumulate persistent DNA damage and eventually become neoplastic and invasive. DNA adducts formed by the activated metabolites of cigarette smoke carcinogens contribute to the first step toward cancer induction. Formation of specific DNA adducts in proto-oncogenes, such as *ras* (K-*ras*, N-*ras*, and Ha-*ras*), which code for guanosine triphosphate (GTP) binding proteins, confers oncogenicity. For example, K-*ras* is activated in 15–20% of NSCLC (90% in adenocarcinomas), but rarely in SCLC. About 70% of these mutations are G → T transversions induced by bulky DNA adducts formed by PAH carcinogen metabolites such as BPDE. *Myc* is another oncogene overexpressed in both NSCLC and SCLC, either by amplification or loss of transcriptional control. The tumor suppressor gene *Bcl-2*, which protects cells from apoptosis, is overexpressed in both SCLCs (75–95%) and NSCLCs (10–35%). The other tumor suppressor gene, p53, which is inactivated in several cancers, is mutated in 75–100% of SCLCs and ~50% of NSCLCs. Thus, the multistep nature of human lung tumorigenesis may involve the activation of proto-oncogenes as well as the inactivation of one or more tumor suppressor genes.

Loss of heterozygosity (LOH) is yet another molecular event involved in the induction and progression of lung cancer. Sequential LOH occurs in the order of 3p → 9p → 8p → 5q → 17q. Among the autocrine systems in lung cancer, expression of gastrin-releasing bombesin-like peptides (GRP/BN) in human respiratory tissues is associated with a proliferative response of bronchial epithelial cells to GRP/BN and with prolonged cigarette smoking, may be a risk factor for developing lung cancer. As indicated previously, mouse skin carcinogenesis also involves a number of sequential cellular, biochemical, and genetic events. Although the exact sequence of events may differ between tissues and species, the overall concept appears to be directly applicable to human cancer.

MODIFYING FACTORS IN CARCINOGENESIS

Several factors, such as exposure to other chemical agents, capacity to metabolize carcinogens, DNA repair capacity, age, gender, hormonal factors, immunological status, trauma, radiation, viruses, diet, nutrition and lifestyle, and genetic constitution of the individual are known to modulate the carcinogenesis process not only in experimental animals but in humans as well. A few of these factors are discussed in this section.

The ability of an individual to metabolize chemical carcinogens can be influenced by simultaneous exposure to other chemicals, by genetic constitution, or both. Many dietary and environmental chemicals that humans are exposed to can increase or decrease the activities or amounts of the enzymes that activate (phase I) or detoxify (conjugative or phase II enzymes) chemical carcinogens. For example, certain chemicals found in vegetables (e.g., isothiocyanates) can enhance the detoxification and excretion of certain chemical carcinogens. In addition, certain chemicals called polyphenols, which are found in green tea, can block carcinogen activation through inhibition of metabolizing enzymes and thereby block carcinogenesis. Some of these types of chemicals are being studied as potential chemopreventive agents as discussed in the next section.

Population studies have identified variants in genes encoding phase I and phase II metabolizing enzymes that can significantly influence individual cancer risk. Because these variants have a much higher frequency than the more rare allelic losses or variants associated with cancer syndromes, they may account for a significant component of the attributable risk of cancer in human populations. For example, certain variants in CYPs, GSTs, and acetyltransferases have been shown in some epidemiologic studies to be associated with increased risk for specific cancers. As a specific example, a significant number of studies have shown an increased risk of lung cancer in smokers who lack the GSTM1 allele. Because GSTM1 is important for detoxifying certain types of reactive carcinogenic intermediates, the lack of this enzyme may be detrimental in an exposed population.

Another important determinant of whether or not a cell becomes initiated by a chemical carcinogen is DNA repair. Inhibition of the excision repair system allows a greater chance that the carcinogenic damage will not be repaired, thus a greater likelihood of mutation induction and cancer initiation. A number of genetic diseases, including xeroderma pigmentosum (XP), Fanconi's anemia, Bloom's syndrome, ataxia-telangiectasia, and porokeratosis Mibelli, are associated with DNA repair defects. Individuals afflicted with any of these heritable syndromes have a higher if not invariable incidence of cancer, and this increase in susceptibility to certain types of cancer is attributed to a compromise in their ability to repair DNA damage. For example, in XP patients, the oversensitivity of the skin to UV light leads to skin cancer, a consequence of a defect in the ability of cells in these individuals to excise UV-induced DNA damage. In addition, other studies have provided evidence that variation in DNA repair capacity within the general population can also influence the risk of skin and other types of cancer.

Diet, nutrition, and lifestyle are important modifying factors of carcinogenesis in humans. Dietary intake (fat, protein, and calories) has been associated with cancers of the breast, colon, endometrium, and gallbladder. Considerable experimental evidence has demonstrated that carbohydrates and lipids are effective promoting agents in the development of neoplasms in several tissue types and in different species. Elevated risks of several neoplasms in humans result from excessive intake of alcoholic beverages. Ethanol is metabolized directly to acetaldehyde, which has been shown to be mutagenic. However, no evidence exists that ethanol or alcoholic beverages are complete carcinogens in any system. In contrast, chronic ethanol administration after initiation may act to enhance hepatic carcinogenesis in rats. Ethanol, when given simultaneously with a carcinogenic agent, acts as a cocarcinogen in several other organs in experimental animals. In support of the promoting action of ethanol in humans, risk of cancer of the oral cavity and pharynx increases markedly when an individual smokes tobacco and abuses alcoholic beverages. Further, individuals who have been infected with the hepatitis B virus and drink alcoholic beverages excessively may be more susceptible to the development of hepatic neoplasms. In general, it appears that many diet- and/or lifestyle-associated cancers result not from direct carcinogenicity of the dietary or lifestyle factor, but rather that these factors act as cocarcinogens and/or tumor promoters and thus either modify the action of other carcinogens or promote the development of spontaneously initiated cells.

INHIBITION OF CHEMICAL CARCINOGENESIS

Chemoprevention (administration of one or several naturally occurring or synthetic anticarcinogenic compounds) or dietary intervention are ways to approach cancer control when the disease results from exposure to environmental carcinogenic agents. Micronutrients present in food are the most desirable class of cancer chemopreventive agents because epidemiologic studies suggest that consumption of fresh fruits and yellow-green vegetables reduces the human cancer incidence and mortality due to stomach, colon, breast, prostate, and even lung and bladder cancers. A wide range of such micronutrients present in food has been shown to possess potent cancer chemopreventive effects in experimental animal models of carcinogenesis. Fruits, vegetables, common beverages, and several herbs and plants have been shown to be rich sources of cancer chemopreventive agents. At present, about 30 classes of chemicals with cancer chemopreventive effects have been described that may have practical implications in reducing cancer incidence. Moreover, the existence of a wide chemical diversity of chemopreventive agents enhances the likelihood that a variety of approaches can be made to cancer chemoprevention using these compounds.

In addition to identifying potentially useful inhibitors of cancer development, cancer chemoprevention studies have also been important in increasing the understanding of the mechanisms of carcinogenesis. For example, agents such as antioxidants, protease inhibitors, mixed function oxidase inhibitors, prostaglandin synthesis inhibitors, and anti-inflammatory agents, among others, have been shown to inhibit carcinogenesis, suggesting the involvement of these events or pathways in the carcinogenesis process.

Given the multistage nature of carcinogenesis and our advancing knowledge of the critical processes involved at each stage, strategies for the inhibition of chemical carcinogenesis have focused on stopping the carcinogenic process at the earliest possible point in the pathway through mechanism-based approaches. As shown in Figure 2.4, potential targets for inhibition of the initiation stage include (1)

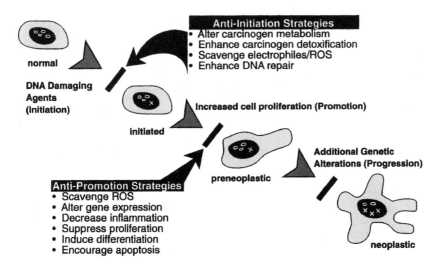

Figure 2.4 Anti-initiation and antipromotion strategies for the inhibition of carcinogenesis.

modifying carcinogen activation by inhibiting the enzymes responsible for that process (e.g., epigallocatechin gallate [EGCG], selenium, phenethylisothiocyanate [PITC], and indole-3-carbinol [I3C] and coumarins such as bergamottin, imperatorin, and isopimpinellin); (2) enhancing carcinogen detoxification by altering the activity of detoxifying enzymes (e.g., oltipraz, dallylsulfide [DAS], s-allyl-cysteine, N-acetyl cysteine, EGCG, resveratrol, and glucarolactone); (3) directly scavenging DNA-reactive electrophiles (e.g., riboflavin, EGCG, and ellagic acid); and (4) enhancing DNA repair processes (e.g., caloric restriction [CR], EGCG, and selenium).

Targets for blocking the processes involved in the promotion stage of carcinogenesis include (1) scavenging ROS (e.g., antioxidant vitamins C and E), selenium, green tea polyphenols, and CR; (2) altering the expression of genes involved in cell signalling, proliferation, apoptosis, and differentiation (e.g., retinoids such as 4-hydroxyphenyl retinamide [4-HPR] and CR); (3) decreasing inflammation (e.g., glucocorticoids, indomethacin, flubriprofen, sulindac, vitamins C and E, piroxicam, glycyrrhetinic acid, and ibuprofen); (4) suppress proliferation (e.g., difluoromethylornithine [DFMO], dehydroepiandrosterone [DHEA], selenium and tamoxifen); (5) induce differentiation (e.g., 4-HPR, 13-cis-retinoic acid, and calcium); and (6) encourage apoptosis (e.g., DHEA).

Of the several chemopreventive agents mentioned above, oltipraz, vitamins C and E, 4-HPR, DFMO, DHEA, and selenium are currently in human clinical trials. It should be noted that most of the chemopreventive agents that are currently undergoing clinical trials target primarily the tumor promotion stage of the overall carcinogenesis process. In this regard, two fundamental concepts of carcinogenesis in humans, "multistage carcinogenesis" and "field cancerization," have influenced clinical researchers in applying cancer chemoprevention to patients. In studying the process of multistage carcinogenesis in humans and two-stage carcinogenesis in rodents, it is accepted that exactly when initiation takes place in human cells is unknown. However, once a cell is initiated, it is an irreversible process. In contrast, tumor promotion requires repeated exposure and is a reversible process (at least in its early stages). In addition, preventive agents can arrest growth of benign tumors. Finally, tumor progression is characterized by an irreversible change of tumors from benign to malignant, and then further malignant changes such as metastasis that are often observed in the process of human carcinogenesis may occur. Thus, inhibition of tumor promotion, rather than of initiation or tumor progression, has been considered the more practical way to apply chemoprevention strategies.

The term "field cancerization" signifies multiple carcinogenesis in an area of epithelium preconditioned by an as yet unknown carcinogenic agent. The high recurrence rate in oral cancer supports this concept. For example, cancers of the aerodigestive tract and the lung are typical examples of field cancerization. The cases of "field cancerization" are 5% of the annual incidence of second primary cancers in patients with squamous carcinomas of the head and neck. Thus, many clinical trials involving potential chemopreventive agents are aimed at preventing the occurrence of second primary cancers.

Although targeting the tumor promotion stage of the carcinogenic process appears to be a highly effective strategy aimed at the chemoprevention of human cancer, agents that target the initiation stage should not be abandoned. For example, oltipraz has been used in a randomized, placebo-controlled phase IIa clinical trial in China as a chemopreventive agent for AFB_1-induced hepatocellular carcinoma. It has been shown that intermittent, high-dose oltipraz blocks the phase 1 activation of AFB_1, whereas sustained low-dose oltipraz increased phase 2 conjugation of aflatoxin, causing increased excretion of AFB_1-mercapturic acid metabolite in the urine.

Although it is likely that tumor promotion plays an important role in human carcinogenesis, there are clear examples of complete carcinogenesis through repetitive exposures to carcinogenic agents (e.g., tobacco smoke, UV light). In addition, humans are constantly exposed to low levels of carcinogens through air, water, and food. Except for very unusual situations, humans are likely not exposed to sufficient quantities of carcinogens in single doses to lead to carcinogenesis or even initiation. Any modifying factor that reduces the effective dose of a carcinogen (i.e., DNA adducts) in a specific target tissue may have a dramatic effect on overall cancer incidence, especially if the initiation process requires cumulative exposure to reach a threshold. Therefore, understanding specific dietary constituents that may reduce or block metabolic activation or DNA adduct formation of carcinogens is an important goal. Such information could lead to the development of specific chemopreventive agents, to specific dietary recommendations regarding food containing substantial quantities of certain types of chemicals, or to approaches using mixtures of agents (e.g., a broad-spectrum P450 inhibitor plus an antioxidant and/or an electrophile trapping agent) that block more than one stage of the carcinogenic process.

Recently, the availability of genetically altered mice, either through the over-expressing of an oncogene or inactivation of a tumor suppressor gene, has provided investigators with new models to study the carcinogenesis process and for testing chemopreventive strategies. For example, the heterozygous *Min* (multiple intestinal neoplasia) mouse (*Min* $+/-$), developed as a model for human colon cancer, carries a mutation in the tumor suppressor gene, adenomatous polyposis coli (*Apc*). This mouse has been shown to develop multiple, grossly detectable adenomas through-out the small intestine (rarely in colon) in 1–3 months. Although human familial adenomatous polyposis differs from that of *Min* mice in having more adenomas in the colon and duodenum, the *Min* mouse model should offer the advantage of studying both carcinogenesis and anticarcinogenesis processes involving *Apc* in colon cancer. Also, in mice developed by crossing $Apc^{\Delta 716}$ mice (has a mutation at codon 716 of mouse *Apc* gene) with cyclooxygenase-2 (COX-2) knockout mice, the number and size of intestinal polyps were reduced dramatically, suggesting that COX-2 plays a pivotal role in Apc-related carcinogenesis and that COX-2 inhibitors may have great promise as chemopreventive agents in colon carcinogenesis.

Knockout mice for the tumor suppressor gene *p53* also have shown promise as a model for chemopreventive studies. It is important to note that caloric restriction caused a 75% delay in spontaneous lymphoma development in $p53_{-/-}$ mice compared with *ad libitum*–fed p53 null mice. In addition, the DHEA analogue

16-α-fluoro-5-androsten-17-one also suppressed spontaneous lymphoma development and lengthened survival time in p53$_{-/-}$ mice, suggesting that the loss of p53 function, which increases susceptibility to cancer, may be offset, at least in part, by preventive regimens. Also, heterozygous p53-knockout (p53$_{+/-}$) mice, which have one of the alleles inactivated, may be analogous to hereditary human syndromes such as Li-Fraumeni syndrome. These p53$_{+/-}$ mice have also been shown to be more susceptible than p53$_{+/+}$ mice to low-dose, chronic carcinogenic regimens (physical and chemical) that more closely mimic human exposures. Thus, genetically altered animal models involving carcinogen-induced cancer are essential to further our understanding of the influence of diet on chemical carcinogenesis, and future progress may be facilitated by the integration of these animals into cancer prevention studies.

CONCLUSION

A majority of human cancers are attributed to lifestyle and involve exposure to chemical carcinogens through diet, smoking, and occupation. Chemical carcinogenesis in rodents is a multistep process, divided broadly into three stages referred to as initiation, promotion, and progression. A majority of the chemical carcinogens form DNA adducts and induce mutations in critical genes, thereby either activating oncogenes (e.g., *ras*) or inactivating tumor suppressor genes (e.g., *p53*). In addition, many tumors display alterations in cell cycle regulation and/or apoptotic mechanisms. Human cancer also occurs via a multistep process involving the progressive accumulation of genetic alterations. Lung carcinogenesis induced by tobacco is an excellent example of multistage chemical carcinogenesis in humans. There are many factors that may impact the process of chemical carcinogenesis, including age, gender, genetic composition, and cumulative exposure to environmental and dietary agents. Chemoprevention strategies aimed at blocking the carcinogenic process during the promotion stage appear to be very promising.

FURTHER READING

Barbacid M (1986) Oncogenes, mutagens and cancer. *Proc. Am. Ass. Cancer Res.* 27:435.

Bowden GT (1997) Proto-oncogenes as potential targets for the action of carcinogens. In *Comprehensive Toxicology*, Vol. 12. Sipes IG, McQueen CA, Gandolfi AJ (eds.) Elsevier Science, New York, pp. 55–81.

Dandekar S, Sukumar S, Zarbl H, Young LJT, Cardiff RD (1986) Specific activation of the cellular Harvey-*ras* oncogene in dimethylbenzanthracene-induced mouse mammary tumors. *Mol Cell Biol* 6:4104–4108.

DiGiovanni J (1992) Multistage carcinogenesis in mouse skin. *Pharmacol Ther* 54:63–128.

DiGiovanni J (1997) Genetic determinants of cancer susceptibility. In *Comprehensive Toxicology*, Vol. 12. Sipes IG, McQueen CA, Gandolfi AJ (eds.) Elsevier Science, New York, pp. 425–451.

Doll R, Peto R (1981) *The Causes of Cancer.* Oxford University Press, Oxford, England.

Escobar MR (1989) Oncogenic viruses. In *The Pathobiology of Neoplasia*. Sirica AE (ed.) Plenum Press, New York, pp. 81–109.

Fujiki H, Komori A, Suganuma M (1997) Chemoprevention of cancer. In *Comprehensive Toxicology* Vol. 12, Sipes IG, McQueen CA, Gandolfi AJ (eds.) Elsevier Science, New York, pp. 453–471.

Hursting SD, Fischer SM, Wargovich MJ, DiGiovanni J (1999) Nutritional modulation of the carcinogenesis process. In *Nutritional Oncology*. Academic Press, pp. 91–104.

Mulcaby T (1989) Radiation carcinogenesis. In *The Pathobiology of Neoplasia*. Sirica AE (ed.) Plenum Press, New York, pp. 111–129.

Pitot HC, Dragan YP (1996) Chemical carcinogenesis. In *Casarett and Doull's Toxicology: The Basic Science of Poisons*, 5th ed. Klaassen CD (ed.) McGraw-Hill, New York, pp. 201–267.

Smart RC (1994) Carcinogenesis. In *Introduction to Biochemical Toxicology*, 2nd ed. Hodgson E, Levi PE (eds.) Appleton & Lange, Norwalk, CT, pp. 381–414.

Sukamar S, Notario V, Martin-Zanca D, Barbacid M (1983) Induction of mammary carcinomas in rats by nitroso-methyl-urea involves the malignant activation of the H-*ras*-1 locus by single point mutations. *Nature* 306:658–661.

Sukumar S (1990) An experimental analysis of cancer: role of ras oncogenes in multistep carcinogenesis. *Cancer Cells* 2:199–204.

Zarbl H, Skumar S, Arthur AV, Martin-Zanca D, Barbacid M (1985) Direct mutagenesis of Ha-*ras*-1 oncogene by *N*-nitroso-*N*-methylurea during initiation of mammary carcinogenesis in rats. *Nature* 315:382–385.

CHAPTER 3

Genomics, Microarrays, and Proteomics

CRAIG C. WHITEFORD, JUN S. WEI, and JAVED KHAN

Advanced Technology Center, Pediatric Oncology Branch, Center for Cancer Research, National Cancer Institute, National Institutes of Health, Gaithersburg, Maryland

GENOMICS

The Human Genome Project (HGP) was launched in 1990, and has completed the sequencing of the human genome (http://www.genome.gov/). In addition, it has aimed to generate complete sets of full-length cDNA clones for all of the estimated 30,000–40,000 genes (http://mgc.nci.nih.gov/). Many of the resources, generated by both the public and the private sectors (http://www.celera.com/), are available to investigators (http://genome.cse.ucsc.edu/, http://www.ncbi.nlm.nih.gov/, http://www.ensembl.org/), and have stimulated the explosion of techniques on the use of "genomics" in cancer research.

The term *genomics* was initially applied in the 1930s, to describe the scientific discipline of mapping, sequencing, and analyzing genomes. Genomics can be divided into "structural genomics" and "functional genomics." Structural genomics includes high-resolution genetic, physical, and transcript mapping of an organism and ultimately the complete DNA sequence. Functional genomics refers to the development and application of global (genome-wide or system-wide) experimental approaches to assess gene function by using the information and reagents provided by structural genomics (1).

Because cancer is a genetic disease occurring as a result of progressive accumulation of genomic aberrations, genomics afford a powerful approach that promises to unlock many of the mechanisms involved in oncogenesis. Neoplastic cells have accumulated numerous genetic abnormalities, including aneuploidy, chromosomal rearrangements, amplifications, deletions, gene rearrangements, and loss or gain of function mutations. Traditional techniques such as cytogenetics and,

UICC Manual of Clinical Oncology, Eighth Edition. Edited by Raphael E. Pollock
ISBN 0-471-22289-5 Copyright © 2004 John Wiley & Sons, Inc.

Southern, Northern, and Western analysis, have been successfully used to identify translocations, losses or gains of large chromosomal regions, and increasing numbers of genes involved in cancer. However, these methods provide either very low-resolution information, as in the case of cytogenetics, or target only one specific gene or chromosome region at a time, and do not provide insight into global nonrandom genomic changes that occur in cancers.

Several techniques have emerged for genome-wide screening of alterations of copy number and structure of chromosomal regions including fluorescent *in situ* hybridization (FISH) (2), spectral karyotyping (SKY) (3), and comparative genomic hybridization (CGH) (4) (termed *molecular cytogenetics*). Although these techniques allow a genome-wide detection of chromosomal structure alterations, newer and more powerful techniques have been developed to detect aberrations in genes at the sequence, expression, and protein levels. A detailed discussion of molecular cytogentics analysis is outside the scope of this chapter and is reviewed in the literature (5).

The structure and biological behavior of a cell is determined by the pattern of gene expression within that cell. In any given cell, it has been suggested that only a fraction, perhaps 10,000, of the genes are being actively transcribed (6,7). Genomic approaches to cancer investigations encompass sequencing-based technologies and genome-wide differential expression analysis (Fig. 3.1). The former includes sequencing of entire genomes, high-throughput mutation detection, sequencing cDNA libraries, identification of single-nucleotide polymorphisms (SNPs) and the serial analysis of gene expression (SAGE). Because all disease-related genomic changes will eventually be manifested by alterations in gene expression reflected in the mRNAs (transcriptome) and proteins (proteomics; *prote*ins expressed by a given gen*ome*), monitoring of gene expression is a logical approach to decipher the biological processes involved in oncogenesis.

In this chapter, we will primarily focus on the current techniques used in high-throughput molecular profiling and their applications to cancer research.

Sequence-Based Technologies

Genomic Sequencing Sequencing provides the highest resolution physical map of the whole genome. The HGP has stimulated rapid advancements of sequencing technology such that it may soon be possible to sequence the entire 3 billion base pairs of each individual cancer in a high-throughput manner. In 1999, an initiative aimed at identifying the genes that cause cancer was established in the United Kingdom, named the Cancer Genome Project (CGP, http://www.sanger.ac.uk/CGP/). The CGP aims to use the human genome sequence, generated by the HGP, with high-throughput mutation detection techniques to identify somatically acquired sequence variants/mutations, and hence identify genes critical in the development of human cancers. Because small intragenic mutations are commonly found in both recessive oncogenes (tumor suppressor genes) and dominantly acting oncogenes, the detection of this type of mutation will lead to the identification of both classes of oncogenes. The project aims to

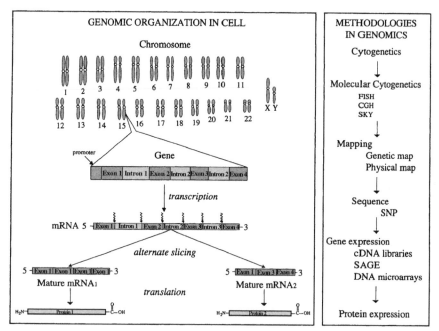

Figure 3.1 Genomic investigation of cancer. The human genome is contained within 23 chromosomal pairs comprising 3.2 billion pairs of the four nucleotides (adenosine [A], cytidine [C], guanosine [G], and thymidine [T]). Genomic sequence contains a promoter region, exons, containing the coding regions, and introns. The introns are spliced out following transcription and alternate splicing can generate several different mRNAs and protein products. Shown are the genome-wide approaches of investigating cancer, going from low-resolution chromosomal structure analysis including cytogenetics to molecular cytogenetics, mapping to the sequencing of the genome. In parallel to the sequencing of the human genome, many SNPs are being detected and catalogued and may contribute to the phenotypic differences found in many patients and their cancers. Finally, several methods are available as discussed in the text for detecting which genes are actively being transcribed and translated into proteins. [Modified from Null et al. (60)]

polymerase chain reaction (PCR) amplify promoter regions, exons, and flanking splice junctions of all human genes of the tumor and normal DNA from individual patients, then use conventional high-throughput methods to detect differences in the PCR fragments and sequence those that are different between tumor and normal. This method may identify both activating (dominant) and inactivating (recessive) mutations in cancer.

cDNA Libraries   cDNA libraries, representing expressed genes, can be generated from normal tissues, tumor, or microdissected individual cells and can be "normalized" to remove common housekeeping genes (8). Sequencing of these cDNA libraries generates "expressed-sequence tags" (ESTs) from which expression profiles of individual cancers can be determined. The National Cancer Institute (NCI) of the National Institutes of Health (NIH) has recently embarked on the Cancer Genome Anatomy Project (CGAP), which catalogues the gene expression profiles based on sequencing of cDNA libraries derived from normal, precancer, and cancer cells (http://cgap.nci.nih.gov/). Their website includes tools to compare expression profiles between different cDNA libraries. Disadvantages of sequencing cDNA libraries include the cost of sequencing, both in terms of money and labor, the presence of redundancy of highly expressed genes, and the lack of sensitivity in detecting genes that are expressed at low level. A recent NIH initiative known as the Mammalian Gene Collection (MGC) that supports and co-ordinates the production and sequencing of full-length (open reading frame) cDNA libraries (http://mgc.nci.nih.gov/). In addition to the sequence information, these clones are also commercially available to investigators and provide a useful resource for functional studies of differentially expressed genes.

Sequencing DNA Chips   Aside from standard dideoxy nucleotide sequencing techniques (9), newer hybridization-based high throughput DNA sequencing methods have been developed. For example, high-density DNA sequencing chips have been developed by Affymetrix (Santa Clara, CA), in which short oligonucleotide ($\sim$25 nucleotides) are manufactured onto chips using a modification of semiconductor photolithographic process. Currently, it is possible to produce arrays containing 100,000–400,000 oligonucleotides within a 1.28 cm^2 area. Four oligonucleotides are designed to interrogate a single base position. One sequence is complimentary to the reference or known sequence, the other three sequences are identical except in this single position (usually in the center of the oligonucleotide), which is substituted with each of the three other possible bases (Fig. 3.2). Therefore, in order to sequence 1,000 base pairs, a chip containing 4,000 DNA sequences ($4 \times 1,000$; one sequence for each base pair) is required (10). The target DNA to be sequenced is PCR amplified and labeled with a fluorescent tag, and hybridized onto the DNA sequencing chip. The probe containing the correct sequence will produce the brightest intensity (Fig. 3.2). Using this strategy, it is possible to sequence a DNA sample as well as detect mutations and polymorphisms (see below). These methods have numerous applications, for example, investigators have designed chips for successfully detecting mutations in all exons of the BRCA1 mutation (11), mutations in the HIV-1 (12), and in Mycobacterium sequences that contribute to drug resistance (13).

Single Nucleotide Polymorphisms   SNPs are the most common genetic variations in the genome and occur once every 100–300 bases in human. A SNP is defined as a stable substitution of a single base with a frequency of more than 1% in at least one population. It is postulated that the presence of SNPs may explain many phenotypic differences among individuals, including incidence, severity, and response to treatment of a variety of, if not all, human diseases. It is expected that association of specific SNPs to diseases will accelerate the identification of disease genes for a given population. SNPs are detected by PCR amplification of the region

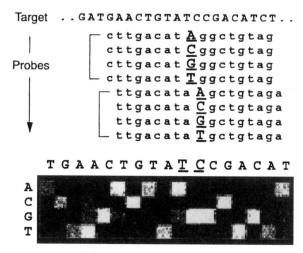

Figure 3.2 Sequencing CHIPS. Shown is a general tiling strategy using a 17mer sequencing chip. On the top is shown the target sequence and below the sequence of the probes on the sequencing chip. Each central base pair sequence of the probe is represented by all four possible base pairs, shown bold and underlined. Following this set, the probe the next nucleotide is interrogated with the next set of sequences. Below this is shown the raw image where the brightest signal corresponds to probe that forms the most stable duplex, and hence the correct sequence can be read. This method can be used for sequencing, genotype analysis, and the detection of SNPs. [Modified from Lipshutz et al. (10)].

of interest followed by sequencing. Non–gel-based high-throughput methodologies such as DNA chips, as outlined above, can be used for screening populations.

An example is the presence of SNPs in the promoter and coding regions of the β2 adrenergic receptor, which determine responses to inhaled beta-agonist drugs in patients with asthma (14,15). Currently, high throughput screening and cataloging of SNPs of candidate genes in coding, noncoding (5′ and 3′ UTR), and promoter regions are underway (16). In addition, a "dbSNP" database has been established that serves as a central repository for both single-base nucleotide substitutions and short deletion and insertion polymorphisms (http://www.ncbi.nlm.nih.gov/SNP/). This has been implemented as a collaborative effort between the National Human Genome Research Institute (NHGRI), and the National Center for Biotechnology Information (NCBI). The dbSNP uses a looser definition for SNPs, such that there is no requirement or assumption about minimum allele frequency of 1%.

Serial Analysis of Gene Expression SAGE is a technique that utilizes high-throughput sequencing technologies to obtain a quantitative profile of cellular gene expression. The technique does not directly measure the expression level of a gene, but the frequency of a "tag," which represents the transcription product of a gene. In this method, mRNA from a sample is reverse transcribed, converted to double-stranded cDNA, and digested with restriction enzymes such as NIaIII. The most 3'-end of the cDNA (up to the most 3' NIaIII site) is then extracted and ligated to a linker, which has a recognition site for a type IIS restriction enzyme (e.g., Bsmfl) that cuts a certain number of bases away from the recognition sequence. These tags are blunt-ended, ligated to each other to form ditags, and PCR amplified. Cleavage of this PCR product with NIaIII then releases the ditags, which are isolated, concatenated, subcloned into an appropriate vector, and sequenced (Fig. 3.3). Each mRNA species is thus represented by a 9–11 base nucleotide sequence (depending on the type IIS restriction enzyme used) (17,18), and sequencing, from both directions within a vector, can provide information on as

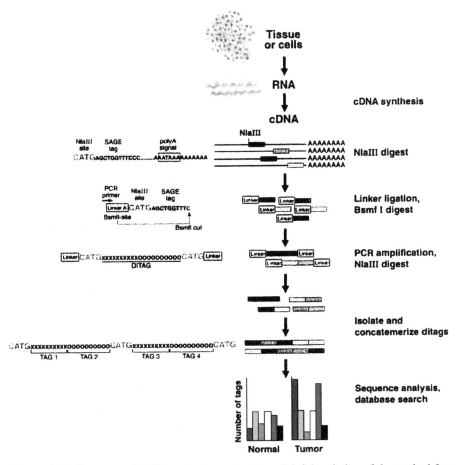

Figure 3.3 Summary of SAGE technology, showing a brief description of the method for generating a SAGE sequence database. mRNA purified from cells are reverse transcribed to cDNA, using a series of reactions SAGE ditags are made concatemerized, cloned, and sequenced. Finally, the sequence data is entered into a database from which differential "tag" counts, hence relative gene expression, can be calculated. [Used with permission from Polyac et al. (61)].

many as 60–70 different genes. The data generated by SAGE analysis is a list of tags, with their corresponding frequencies, and thus is a digital representation of cellular gene expression.

In the first application of SAGE, the authors sequenced 1,000 tags generated from the pancreas, which revealed a gene expression pattern characteristic for this tissue, and identified new pancreatic transcripts (17). This technique has also been used to identify genes induced by the p53 tumor suppressor gene (19). Further applications of SAGE include the identification of differentially expressed genes in cancers and the generation a catalogue of expression profile for each cancer. As a part of CGAP's goal to create a Tumor Gene Index, SAGE was added as a strategic analytic technique. This database archives SAGE tag counts, and contains online query tools to generate virtual Northerns (http://www.ncbi.nlm.nih.gov/SAGE/). It is now the largest source of public SAGE data to which investigators can submit their data. To date, more than 4 million tags from 95 different libraries have been deposited on the National Center for Biotechnology Education/CGAP SAGEmap website.

Although SAGE has the potential to generate genome scale expression profiles, DNA microarrays have a particular advantage for their ability to analyze multiple samples, thereby generating a large amount of gene expression data for statistical analysis.

DNA MICROARRAY TECHNOLOGIES

Overview

DNA microarray is a recently developed high-throughput technology for monitoring gene expression at the transcription level. It is akin to performing tens of thousands of northern blots simultaneously, and has the potential to interrogate the expression level of an entire genome in parallel. The first reported DNA microarray was fabricated on nylon membranes using complementary DNA (cDNA) clones (20). Since then, many large-scale DNA microarray platforms have been developed.

The DNA probes on the microarrays can be double-stranded cDNA, short (25 mers) or long (50–70 mers) oligonucleotides of known sequences, that are immobilized on a solid support, such as a glass microscope slide. An ideal DNA microarray should be able to query all of the genes expressed in an organism. For cDNA arrays, the probes are PCR amplified from plasmid cDNA clones, purified, and robotically printed onto coated glass slides (21). Oligonucleotide arrays have the advantage over cDNA microarrays due to the lack of requirement for physical clones. Oligonucleotides can be either previously synthesized and printed on glass slides, or can be synthesized directly on the surface of silicon or glass slides. Several print-ready oligonucleotide (60–70 mers) sets are commercially available for human, mouse, and other organisms (http://www.cgen.com, http://www.operon.com).

Affymetrix Inc. has developed gene expression arrays, GeneChips[TM], by chemically synthesizing short oligoneucleotides (25 mers) on silicon surface using photolithography technology, a technique routinely used in making silicon

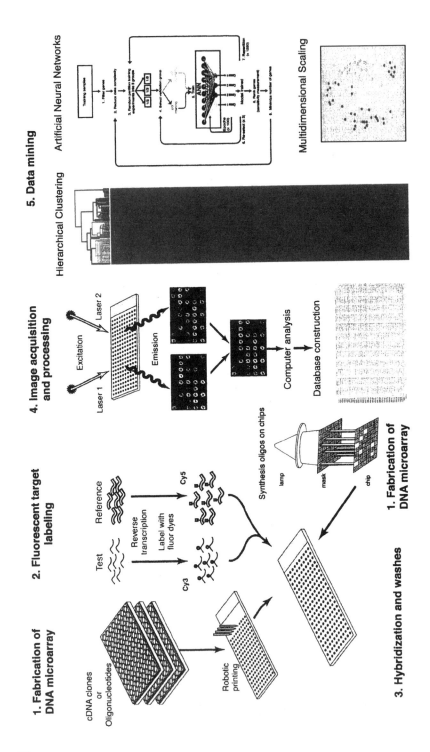

50

computer chips (10). Originally, they were designed to detect single-nucleotide mutations, but now also have applications for gene expression profiling studies (22–24). As an alternative, a single nucleic acids can be delivered by ink-jet onto glass surfaces, and longer oligonucleotide (∼60 mers) synthesis occurs directly on the slides, which can be utilized for expression analysis (25).

The targets used in DNA microarray experiments are prepared from total RNA or purified mRNA extracted from cell or tissue samples. During the reverse transcription (RT) reactions, targets of experimental and reference RNA populations are labeled with dUTP-conjugated fluorescent dyes, either Cy3 or Cy5. Then they are combined and applied on microarray slides for hybridization. After hybridization, the slides are scanned and a digital image is acquired for both dyes (Fig. 3.4).

DNA Microarray Data Analysis

A detailed description of the data analysis tools currently being developed is beyond the scope of this chapter. We will briefly describe in this section a broad overview of the analytical tools available for image analysis, data mining, clustering, classification, and visualization of microarray data.

Image analysis software, such as DeArray developed by Chen et al. (26), is used to calculate gene expression ratios for all the printed spots. Although ratio-based analysis is an easy and effective way to compare many samples in a large study, single-color-intensity-based analysis is an alternative way to determine expression levels for individual genes. This type of analysis uses intensities from only one channel, instead of ratio, to measure the gene expression levels in a sample without the requirement for a reference sample. The advantage of intensity-based analysis is

----

Figure 3.4 Summary of the DNA microarray technology. (1) Fabrication of DNA microarray: Purified cDNA products or oligonucleotides are printed onto glass slides using robots. Alternatively, prefabricated oligonucleotide DNA arrays (e.g., GeneChips™ can be used. (2) Fluorescent labeling of targets; Total RNA extracted from reference and test samples is fluorescently labeled by reverse transcription utilizing nucleotides tagged with either Cy3 or Cy5 respectively. (3) Hybridization: The probe mixture is hybridized to the microarray on the DNA microarrays. (4) Image acquisition and processing: Fluorescence intensities at target spots are measured using laser confocal microscopes with the appropriate excitation lasers and emission filters. Each of the images is arbitrarily assigned a pseudo-color (i.e., Cy5 = red and Cy3 = green). A normalization process is performed to compensate for differential efficiencies of labeling and detection of Cy3 and Cy5. The two fluorescent images thus constitute the raw data from which differential gene expression ratio values are calculated. All the measurements are stored in a database for further processing. (5) Data mining: Biological information is extracted in this step using a variety of data mining tools. The relationships between genes and experiments can be visualized by hierarchical clustering, while multidimensional scaling allows visualization of the similarity of expression profiles between experiments. Algorithms such as artificial neural networks can classify cancers. [Modified from Khan et al. (28) and Duggan et al. (62)].

that it avoids the overestimation of the expression of a gene if the signal in the reference channel is weak due to failure of hybridization or low expression of the gene in the reference sample. Affymetrix has used single-color hybridization in their GeneChips (27), and we have reported its successful implimentation for cDNA microarrays (28).

The expression ratios, mean intensities for each spot, and other information used as quality controls, such as normalization constant and spot size, can be imported into a database for further analysis. Each microarray experiment generates thousands of data points and the first step of data analysis is to reduce the complexity of the data, visualize relationships between samples or genes, and to develop data mining tools to extract biologically relevant information.

A simple visualization tool is the pseudo-color-coding of the gene expression ratios (29). As a convention in the DNA microarray field, red represents overexpression whereas green represents underexpression. Because human perception is much more sensitive to the color patterns than numbers, the patterns of gene expression level can be easily recognized, with different shades representing the gene expression levels.

Starting from the raw data, filtering steps are taken to eliminate the inherent "noise" in the system. Next, analytical tools, including hierarchical clustering dendrograms and multidimensional scaling (MDS) can be utilized to "plot" or visualize the relationships among the tumors or genes in the form of a map according to distance matrices calculated from correlation coefficient or Euclidean distances (29).

Sample classification methods, from gene expression data, can be generally grouped into two broad categories, supervised or unsupervised. Supervised classification utilizes existing knowledge such as cancer diagnosis or prognosis to rank genes according to their significance to the classifications using various scoring methods (i.e., Golub score, gene weight, etc.) (28,30–32). This reduces the list of genes to a smaller subset with which one can more accurately classify these cancers and which can be used to develop small easily affordable diagnostic or prognostic arrays (28,33). In addition, it is a powerful way to discover the genes that distinguish one group of cancer from another or from normal tissues. In this way, one may identify the most relevant genes within a cancer and potential new targets for therapy. Unsupervised classification, such as hierarchical clustering and self-organizing maps (SOMs), classifies cancers without prior knowledge of cancers (34,35) This approach is useful for discovering new subclasses within a cancer (class discovery).

Applications of DNA Microarrays

Tumor Diagnosis Currently, tumors are diagnosed on the basis of clinical presentation, routine histology, immunohistochemistry, and electron microscopy. However, the histological appearance may not reveal the genetic aberrations or underlying biologic processes that contribute to the malignancy. Monitoring global gene expression levels by DNA microarrays provides an additional tool for elucidating tumor biology as well as the potential for molecular diagnostic classification of cancer (28). Several studies have demonstrated that gene expression profiling using DNA microarrays is able to classify tumors with high accuracy and to discover new cancer classes (28,29,31,32,36). Therefore, DNA microarray holds the promise to facilitate clinical diagnostics and therapies, and to predict of cancer prognosis in the future.

Elucidation of Downstream Targets Monitoring the temporal and global changes in gene expression using DNA microarray profiling methods has also been effective in identifying targets of transcription factors (TFs). An example is the investigation of the molecular effects of tumor-specific chromosome translocations that encode chimeric TFs. These chimeric TFs are thought to exert their oncogenic effects through the dysregulation of gene expression, and DNA microarrays provide an opportunity to observe the broad effects of oncogenic transcription factors on gene expression and potentially elucidate their role in oncogenesis. An example is the PAX3-FKHR chimeric oncogene that is found in the skeletal muscle cancer, alveolar rhabdomyosarcoma (ARMS), and results from a t(2;13). This translocation is found in the majority of ARMS, and leads to the fusion of the DNA binding domain of PAX3, a gene involved in muscle differentiation, with the trans-activation domain of FKHR. The PAX3-FKHR gene retains the DNA binding specificity of PAX3 and potentially acts by increasing expression of genes containing PAX3 binding sites. Investigators, using murine cDNA microarrays, have found that the PAX3-FKHR gene triggers cells into a myogenic differentiation pathway producing a population of rhabdomyoblasts that may eventually lead to the development of fully malignant muscle cancer upon accumulation of other genetic aberrations (37). Since this report, DNA microarrays have been used to profile the downstream effect of a growing number of oncogenes and tumor suppressor genes (38,39).

Other applications of DNA microarrays have been used to determine the molecular effects of environmental factors (i.e., nutrition, carcinogens, toxins, and drugs) not only by *in vitro* tissue culture, but also *in vivo* where investigators can monitor gene expression in specific organs such as liver (40–44). The advantage of using DNA microarrays for these kinds of studies is not only in identifying pathways that lead to cellular damage, but also the possible detection of changes in gene expression that may proceed any phenotypic alterations, such as low-level exposure to a drug or an environmental hazard.

Comparative Genomic Hybridization Arrays DNA microarray platforms have also been used to identify genomic regions that are amplified or deleted in cancers at a higher resolution than that possible by standard CGH of 5–10 megabases (MB). In this application, genomic fragments such as BAC clones (bacterial artificial chromosomes) from specified chromosome regions are printed on glass slides. Differentially labeled cancer and normal genomic DNA is hybridized onto these DNA chips, allowing the detection of gains and losses in these regions at a resolution of less than 1 MB (45,46). cDNA microarrays have also been utilized for CGH-array analysis in which the differentially labeled genomic DNA is hybridized onto cDNA expression arrays, allowing direct identification of genes that are amplified or deleted (47–49).

DNA microarrays are therefore a powerful technology that enables researchers to study biological systems as a whole, in extremely high-throughput fashion and generating detailed molecular profiles of each cancer. The next challenge is the development of web-based bioinformatic, statistical, and pattern recognition tools that will enable a more detailed processing of the vast amounts of information that is currently being generated. Many cancers still remain incurable, and the knowledge we are learning from DNA microarray experiments will revolutionize our understandings of the mechanisms of oncogenesis and, it is hoped, will ultimately impact on the morbidity and mortality of this common disease.

Tissue Arrays

After identification of potential tumor markers using either cDNA microarrays or proteomic analysis (see below) from tumor tissue or cell lines, one can validate the putative markers in larger sets of tumor samples. Before the advent of tissue arrays, it was possible to perform histological analysis of one cancer at a time on one slide. Tissue arrays are generated by taking several cylindrical 600-micron tumor biopsies, from multiple tumor donor paraffin blocks, and placing them into a recipient block. In this way, several hundred tumors can be arrayed onto one block. Sections (6–8 μm) can be cut from this recipent block to prepare regular histological slides. One can thus perform routine hematoxylin and eosin staining, immunohistochemistry, FISH, and in situ hybridization on several hundred samples in one experiment. Tissue arrays are therefore ideal for examining putative diagnostic or prognostic tumor markers over a large panel of tumors (50).

PROTEOMICS

In parallel with advances in genomic analysis and DNA microarrays, the global analysis of cellular proteins, termed *proteomics*, has become a key area of research in the "postgenomic" era. Genomic alterations result in changes in the transcriptome, which are ultimately transmitted to changes within the proteome. Because proteins are the functional effectors of the expressed genes, proteomic analysis is required for a complete understanding of the biological processes in human diseases. Other changes detected by proteomic approaches include the detection of post-translational modifications of the proteins, such as phosphorylation and glycosylation, which are not readily apparent from the DNA sequence, or gene expression changes, and can only be determined only by proteomic methodologies.

Traditionally, the term *proteomics* has been applied to the large-scale biochemical analysis of proteins, usually by two-dimensional gel electrophoresis. In this chapter, we will also review the newer techniques of mass spectrometry, protein chips, and protein sequencing (Fig. 3.5).

Tumor Sampling

Solid tumors are often heterogeneous, consisting of a mixture of cellular lineages, including nonmalignant stromal, precancerous, and malignant cells. Due to this "contamination" with nonmalignant cells, it is not ideal to perform proteomic analysis on whole tumor biopsies. To obtain pure populations of malignant or pre-malignant cells, researchers have applied mechanical forces or calcium starvation to disrupt intracellular adhesion and isolate cells by immunoaffinity methods, such as, immunomagnetic beads and fluorescence-activated cell sorting.

Although these methods are able to isolate pure populations of cells, they are time intensive and delays in protein extraction can lead to artifactual changes, due to protein degradation or other changes resulting from disruptions of cell-cell interactions and to the vascular circulation prior to protein extraction. Therefore, a rapid method that allows for the direct procurement of the desired cells from a tissue or tumor without the need for cellular disruption are advantageous. One of the most widely used of these techniques is laser capture microscopy (LCM), in which individual cells are captured and isolated from a stained tissue section. An infrared laser melts a thermosensitive film onto the surface of the preselected cells, and the captured cells are removed for further analysis. The extricated cells maintain their morphology, and the DNA, RNA, and protein integrity remains intact (51).

Two-Dimensional Electrophoresis

The most common proteomic analysis is performed on the soluble hydrophilic cytoplasmic proteins obtained by standard cell lyses methods. With the advent of newer solubility reagents and detergents, it is now also possible to solubilize hydrophobic membrane-associated proteins. In addition, proteins can be extracted from specific compartments such as the nucleus and mitochondria. Once solubilized, the most commonly used method for the separation of proteins from a complex mixture is high-resolution two-dimensional electrophoresis (2DE), first described by O'Farrell (52). In the first dimension of 2DE, the proteins are separated according to their charge by an isoelectric focusing (IEF) strip, and in the second dimension proteins are separated according to their molecular weights using a polyacrylamide gel. Upon separation on a 2D gel, the proteins are visualized by direct staining methods such as Coomassie, silver staining or the Sypro series of fluorescent protein dyes (53). The gels are then scanned by a high-resolution CCD camera and a computer-based imaging software such as Melanie (http://us.expasy. org/melanie/) or PDQuest (Bio-Rad Laboratories, Hercules, CA) then analyzes the images generated to identify differentially expressed proteins.

Image analysis software uses the digital image 2D gels to quantify the spot intensities and normalizes images to a reference sample image. Upon normalization, the software can calculate intensity ratios tumor/reference of each spot and identify the differentially expressed ones (54).

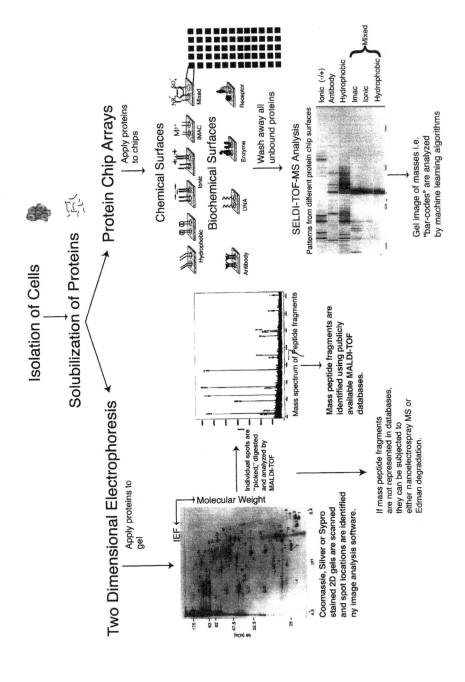

Isolation of Cells

Solubilization of Proteins

Protein Chip Arrays

Apply proteins to chips

Chemical Surfaces

Hydrophobic Ionic IMAC Mixed

Biochemical Surfaces

Antibody DNA Enzyme Receptor

Wash away all unbound proteins

SELDI-TOF-MS Analysis

Patterns from different protein chip surfaces

Ionic (-/+)
Antibody
Hydrophobic
Imac
Ionic
Hydrophobic
Mixed

Gel image of masses i.e. "bar-codes" are analyzed by machine learning algorithms

Two Dimensional Electrophoresis

Apply proteins to gel

Molecular Weight

IEF

pH

Mr [kDa]
175
83
62
47.5
32.5
25

Coomassie, Silver or Sypro stained 2D gels are scanned and spot locations are identified ny image analysis software.

Individual spots are "picked," digested and analyzed by MALDI-TOF

Mass spectrum of peptide fragments

Mass peptide fragments are identified using publicly available MALDI-TOF databases.

If mass peptide fragments are not represented in databases, they can be subjected to either nanoelectrospray MS or Edman degradation.

Protein Identification

One of the most significant improvements in proteomic analysis is the mass spectrometric identification of 2DE gel isolated proteins. These methods will largely replace classical protein sequencing (Edman degradation), because they are high throughput, and require less protein and can handle complex protein mixtures. Differentially expressed spots are located and cut out by an integrated robotic spot picker and placed into an individual well of a 96-well plate. The individual protein spots are then digested into peptide fragments with a site-specific proteolytic enzyme, such as trypsin. The masses of each peptide fragment are then determined by matrix associated laser desorption/ionization-time of flight (MALDI-TOF) mass spectrometer. The peptide mass fingerprints obtained from the mass spectrometer are then compared with "virtual" fingerprints of theoretical tryptic cleavages of protein sequences found in MALDI-TOF databases such as Mascot (http://www.matrixscience.com/), MassSearch (http://cbrg.inf.ethz.ch/Server/Server Booklet/MassSearchEx.html), or MS-Fit (http://falcon.Ludwig.ucl.ac.uk/). Each protein has an unique tryptic peptide fragmentation pattern and therefore can only be correctly identified if this information is available within the database. To aid identification of proteins not represented in the databases, it is possible to separate the generated peptide mixtures with reverse phase high-pressure liquid chromatography (RP-HPLC), and fractionated peptides are partially sequence by MALDI-PSD (post-source decay). The data generated by MALDI-PSD is used to search publicly available PSD databases such as MS-Tag and Ms-Seq from ProteinProspector (http://prospector.ucsf.edu/) or PepFrag (http://prowl.rockefeller. edu/PROWL/pepfragch.html). If the PSD spectrum does not lead to an identification, then *de novo* sequencing of single peptides is possible using either nano-electrospray tandem mass spectrometry or standard Edman degradation sequencing (55).

Figure 3.5   Schematic representation of proteomic analysis. Protein is extracted from cell lines, or microdisected from the tumor or tissue of interest followed by solubilization. The proteins can be analyzed by either two-dimensional electrophoresis (2DE) or protein chip arrays. Proteins applied to 2DE gels are first separated according to their charge on an isoelectric focusing (IEF) strip and then separated according to their molecular weight on an SDS-PAGE gel. The gels are stained and spots are located by image analysis software and picked. Picked spots are subjected to trypsin digestion and peptide fragments are analyzed on a MALDI-TOF mass spectrometer. Mass peptide fingerprints can be matched and identified in the publicly available MALDI-TOF databases. Individual spots can also be partially sequenced by nanoelectrospray MS. Proteins applied to protein chip arrays are incubated on various surfaces, consisting of many different binding surfaces, and then unbound proteins removed. The chips are then read in a SELDI-TOF mass spectrometer and gel images of the protein masses then can by analyzed by machine learning algorithms. [Modified from Chambers et al. (53) and Merchant et al. (63)].

Antibody Arrays In these arrays, the antibodies are robotically printed onto a coated substrate and act as the probes, and the proteins act as the targets. Like DNA microarrays, these arrays have the potential of analyzing hundreds or thousands of proteins at one time. Antibody arrays are similar to a large-scale version of an enzyme-linked imunosorbent assays that are widely used in clinical diagnostics. Proteins from two different cell lysates, for example, normal and diseased state, can be differentially labeled with fluorochromes such as Cy3 and Cy5, and compared on the same array to determine the relative abundance of specific proteins or its phosphorylated counterpart depending on the specificity of the antibody (56). However, this system is dependent upon well-characterized antibodies as far as antigen specificity and is still under development.

Surface Enhanced Laser/Desorption Ionization Time of Flight Mass Spectrometry (SELDI-TOF-MS) Other commercially available protein arrays have been developed, for example, ProteinChip array from Ciphergen Biosystems (Palo Alto, CA) (Fig. 3.5). These arrays contain bait spots (1 mm diameter) that have either a chemical (anionic, cationic, hydrophobic, or hydrophilic) surface or a biochemical (antibody, nucleic acid, or receptor) surface, which is designed to capture specific proteins of interest. The whole protein lysate from a sample is loaded directly to the array, followed by a wash to remove unbound proteins. The array is then placed into a ProteinChip reader, a SELDI-TOF-MS, which allows the instantaneous and precise measurement of the molecular weights of all the proteins bound to individual bait surfaces on the chips. Tumor protein expression profiles can be represented in a form of a "bar code," which is a graphical representation of the proteins from a spot according to their molecular weight and quantity. This bar code upon profiling of multiple samples can be regarded as a "protein fingerprint" of the tumor. Using sophisticated pattern recognition software, such as machine learning algorithms, protein fingerprints are being identified as potential diagnostic markers for bladder, prostate, and ovarian cancers and other diseases (57). Although these protein arrays hold great promise for diagnostic purposes, this method does not directly reveal the identity of the proteins within a fingerprint that determine the diagnosis.

Application of Proteomics to Cancer Research

Early detection of cancer leads to a better prognosis for the patient. Therefore, the ability to detect early serological or secreted markers for cancer prior to the development of symptoms may improve the outcome for these patients. Recently, proteomic analysis has been utilized to investigate differentially expressed proteins in human luminal and myoepithelium of breast cells. Page et al. (58) identified known differentially expressed proteins such as cytokeratin, muscle-specific enzymes, and contractile intermediate filaments, but also found several that could not identified, using existing databases, and may represent novel putative tumor markers (58).

Other studies have used proteomics approaches to identify secreted proteins within urine such as psoriasin, a calcium binding protein, which may be used as potential diagnostic markers for bladder squamous cell carcinoma (SCC) (60). Ostergaard et al. have constructed a web-based proteomic database to provide a resource for the research community to aid in the discovery of tumor markers in bladder cancer (http://proteomics.cancer.dk). Proteomic analysis has also been applied to various different tumor types, including lung, kidney, colon, prostrate, and hepatic cancers (52). Proteomics continues to be a rapidly evolving field providing increasingly useful tools for deciphering the mechanisms involved in the malignant process.

CONCLUSIONS

The HGP, together with the rapid increase in computer processing power, has fueled an extraordinary advancement in high-throughput investigations of cancer at the DNA, RNA, and protein level. Future benefits of these methods include improved cancer diagnosis according to new molecular markers, increased understanding of biological behavior, the accurate prediction of prognosis, and the identification of new markers or targets for cancer.

REFERENCES

1. Hieter P, Boguski M (1997) Functional genomics: it's all how you read it. *Science* **278**: 601–602.
2. Pinkel D, Straume T, Gray JW (1986) Cytogenetic analysis using quantitative, high-sensitivity, fluorescence hybridization. *Proc Natl Acad Sci USA* **83**: 2934–2938.
3. Schrock E et al. (1996) Multicolor spectral karyotyping of human chromosomes. *Science* **273**: 494–497.
4. Kallioniemi A et al.(1992) Comparative genomic hybridization for molecular cytogenetic analysis of solid tumors. *Science* **258**: 818–821.
5. Forozan F, Karhu R, Kononen J, Kallioniemi A Kallioniemi OP (1997) Genome screening by comparative genomic hybridization. *Trends Genet* **13**: 405–409.
6. Lander ES et al. (2001) Initial sequencing and analysis of the human genome. *Nature* **409**: 860–921.
7. Venter JC et al. (2001) The sequence of the human genome. *Science* **291**: 1304–1351.
8. Soares MB et al. (1994) Construction and characterization of a normalized cDNA library. *Proc Natl Acad Sci USA* **91**: 9228–9232.
9. Sanger F, Nicklen S, Coulson AR (1997) DNA sequencing with chain-terminating inhibitors. *Proc Natl Acad Sci USA* **74**: 5463–5467.
10. Lipshutz RJ, Fodor SP, Gingeras TR, Lockhart DJ (1999) High density synthetic oligonucleotide arrays. *Nat Genet* **21**: 20–24.

11. Hacia JG, Brody LC, Chee MS, Fodor SP, Collins FS (1996) Detection of heterozygous mutations in BRCA1 using high density oligonucleotide arrays and two-colour fluorescence analysis. *Nat Genet* **14**: 441–447.

12. Kozal MJ et al. (1996) Extensive polymorphisms observed in HIV-1 clade B protease gene using high-density oligonucleotide arrays. *Nat Med* **2**: 753–759.

13. Gingeras TR et al. (1998) Simultaneous genotyping and species identification using hybridization pattern recognition analysis of generic Mycobacterium DNA arrays. *Genome Res* **8**: 435–448.

14. Israel E et al. (2000) The effect of polymorphisms of the beta(2)-adrenergic receptor on the response to regular use of albuterol in asthma. *Am J Respir Crit Care Med* **162**: 75–80.

15. Drysdale CM et al. (2000) Complex promoter and coding region beta 2-adrenergic receptor haplotypes alter receptor expression and predict in vivo responsiveness. *Proc Natl Acad Sci USA* **97**: 10483–10488.

16. Cargill M et al. (1999) Characterization of single-nucleotide polymorphisms in coding regions of human genes. *Nat Genet* **22**: 231–238.

17. Velculescu VE, Zhang L, Vogelstein B, Kinzler KW (1995) Serial analysis of gene expression. *Science* **270**: 484–487.

18. Zhang L et al. (1997) Gene expression profiles in normal and cancer cells. *Science* **276**: 1268–1272.

19. Polyak K, Xia Y, Zweier JL, Kinzler KW, Vogelstein B (1997) A model for p53-induced apoptosis. *Nature* **389**: 300–305.

20. Drmanac S, Drmanac R (1994) Processing of cDNA and genomic kilobase-size clones for massive screening, mapping and sequencing by hybridization. *Biotechniques* **17**: 328–329, 332–326.

21. Schena M, Shalon D, Davis RW, Brown PO (1995) Quantitative monitoring of gene expression patterns with a complementary DNA microarray. *Science* **270**: 467–470.

22. Li H et al. (1999) Novel strategy yields candidate Gsh-1 homeobox gene targets using hypothalamus progenitor cell lines. *Dev Biol* **211**: 64–76.

23. Nau ME et al. (2000) Technical assessment of the affymetrix yeast expression GeneChip YE6100 platform in a heterologous model of genes that confer resistance to antimalarial drugs in yeast. *J Clin Microbiol* **38**: 1901–1908.

24. Yoshioka K et al. (2000) Determination of genes involved in the process of implantation: application of GeneChip to scan 6500 genes. *Biochem Biophys Res Commun* **272**: 531–538.

25. Blanchard A, Kaiser R, Hood L (1996) High-density oligonucleotide arrays. *Biosens Bioelectron* **6**: 687–690.

26. Chen Y, Dougherty ER, Bittner ML (1997) Ratio-based decisions and the quantitative analysis of cDNA microarray images. *Biomedical Optics* **2**: 364–374.

27. Lockhart DJ et al. (1996) Expression monitoring by hybridization to high-density oligonucleotide arrays. *Nat Biotechnol* **14**: 1675–1680.

28. Khan J et al. (2001) Classification and diagnostic prediction of cancers using gene expression profiling and artificial neural networks. *Nat Med* **7**: 673–679.

29. Khan J et al. (1998) Gene expression profiling of alveolar rhabdomyosarcoma with cDNA microarrays. *Cancer Res* **58**: 5009–5013.

30. Brown MP et al. (2000) Knowledge-based analysis of microarray gene expression data by using support vector machines. *Proc Natl Acad Sci USA* **97**: 262–267.

31. Golub TR et al. (1999) Molecular classification of cancer: class discovery and class prediction by gene expression monitoring. *Science* **286**: 531–537.

32. Bittner M et al. (2000) Molecular classification of cutaneous malignant melanoma by gene expression profiling. *Nature* **406**: 536–540.

33. Alizadeh AA et al. (2000) Distinct types of diffuse large B-cell lymphoma identified by gene expression profiling. *Nature* **403**: 503–511.

34. Eisen MB, Spellman PT, Brown PO, Botstein D (1998) Cluster analysis and display of genome-wide expression patterns. *Proc Natl Acad Sci USA* **95**: 14863–14868.

35. Toronen P, Kolehmainen M, Wong G, Castren E (1999) Analysis of gene expression data using self-organizing maps. *FEBS Lett* **451**: 142–146.

36. Hedenfalk I et al. (2001) Gene-expression profiles in hereditary breast cancer. *N Engl J Med* **344**: 539–548.

37. Khan J et al. (1999) cDNA microarrays detect activation of a myogenic transcription program by the PAX3-FKHR fusion oncogene. *Proc Natl Acad Sci USA* **96**: 13264–13269.

38. O'Hagan RC et al. (2000) Gene-target recognition among members of the myc superfamily and implications for oncogenesis. *Nat Genet* **24**: 113–119.

39. Arvand A, Welford SM, Teitell MA, Denny CT (2001) The COOH-terminal domain of FLI-1 is necessary for full tumorigenesis and transcriptional modulation by EWS/FLI-1. *Cancer Res* **61**: 5311–5317.

40. DeRisi JL, Iyer VR, Brown PO (1997) Exploring the metabolic and genetic control of gene expression on a genomic scale. *Science* **278**: 680–686.

41. Nuwaysir EF, Bittner M, Trent J, Barrett JC, Afshari CA (1999) Microarrays and toxicology: the advent of toxicogenomics. *Mol Carcinog* **24**: 153–159.

42. Sato H, Sagai M, Suzuki KT, Aoki Y (1999) Identification, by cDNA microarray, of A-raf and proliferating cell nuclear antigen as genes induced in rat lung by exposure to diesel exhaust. *Res Commun Mol Pathol Pharmacol* **105**: 77–86.

43. Feng X, Jiang Y, Meltzer P, Yen PM (2001) Transgenic targeting of a dominant negative corepressor to liver blocks basal repression by thyroid hormone receptor and increases cell proliferation. *J Biol Chem* **276**: 15066–15072.

44. Feng X, Jiang Y, Meltzer P, Yen PM (2000) Thyroid hormone regulation of hepatic genes in vivo detected by complementary DNA microarray. *Mol Endocrinol* **14**: 947–955.

45. Pinkel D et al. (1998) High resolution analysis of DNA copy number variation using comparative genomic hybridization to microarrays. *Nat Genet* **20**: 207–211.

46. Bruder CE et al. (2001) High resolution deletion analysis of constitutional DNA from neurofibromatosis type 2 (NF2) patients using microarray-CGH. *Hum Mol Genet* **10**: 271–282.

47. Pollack JR et al. (1999) Genome-wide analysis of DNA copy-number changes using cDNA microarrays. *Nat Genet* **23**: 41–46.

48. Heiskanen MA et al. (2000) Detection of gene amplification by genomic hybridization to cDNA microarrays. *Cancer Res* **60**: 799–802.

49. Hui AB, Lo KW, Yin XL, Poon WS, Ng HK (2001) Detection of multiple gene amplifications in glioblastoma multiforme using array-based comparative genomic hybridization. *Lab Invest* **81**: 717–723.

50. Kononen J et al. (1998) Tissue microarrays for high-throughput molecular profiling of tumor specimens. *Nat Med* **4**: 844–847.

51. Emmert-Buck MR et al. (1996) Laser capture microdissection. *Science* **274**: 998–1001.

52. O'Farrell PH (1975) High resolution two-dimensional electrophoresis of proteins. *J Biol Chem* **250**: 4007–4021.

53. Chambers G, Lawrie L, Cash P, Murray GI (2000) Proteomics: a new approach to the study of disease. *J Pathol* **192**: 280–288.

54. Lopez MF (2000) Better approaches to finding the needle in a haystack: optimizing proteome analysis through automation. *Electrophoresis* **21**: 1082–1093.

55. Gevaert K, Vandekerckhove J (2000) Protein identification methods in proteomics. *Electrophoresis* **21**: 1145–1154.

56. Haab BB, Dunham MJ, Brown PO (2001) Protein microarrays for highly parallel detection and quantitation of specific proteins and antibodies in complex solutions. *Genome Biol* **2**, RESEARCH0004.

57. Liotta L, Petricoin E (2000) Molecular profiling of human cancer. *Nat Rev Genet* **1**: 48–56.

58. Page MJ et al. (1999) Proteomic definition of normal human luminal and myoepithelial breast cells purified from reduction mammoplasties. *Proc Natl Acad Sci USA* **96**: 12589–12594.

59. Ostergaard M, Wolf H, Orntoft TF, Celis JE (1999) Psoriasin (S100A7): a putative urinary marker for the follow-up of patients with bladder squamous cell carcinomas. *Electrophoresis* **20**: 349–354.

60. Null AP, Muddiman DC (2001) Perspectives on the use of electrospray ionization Fourier transform ion cyclotron resonance mass spectrometry for short tandem repeat genotyping in the post-genome era. *J Mass Spectrom* **36**: 589–606.

61. Polyak K, Riggins GJ (2001) Gene discovery using the serial analysis of gene expression technique: implications for cancer research. *J Clin Oncol* **19**: 2948–2958.

62. Duggan DJ, Bittner M, Chen Y, Meltzer P, Trent JM (1999) Expression profiling using cDNA microarrays. *Nat Genet* **21**: 10–14.

63. Merchant M, Weinberger SR (2000) Recent advancements in surface-enhanced laser desorption/ionization-time of flight-mass spectrometry. *Electrophoresis* **21**: 1164–1177.

CHAPTER 4

Genetic Predisposition to Cancer

GORDON B. MILLS and PAULA TRAHAN RIEGER

University of Texas, M. D. Anderson Cancer Center, Houston, Texas

Five to ten percent of all cancers occur in individuals who have inherited mutations in cancer predisposition genes. Cancer predisposition genes have been identified that account for the majority of hereditary breast, ovary, and bowel cancer, as well as for a spectrum of less common tumors. Family history provides the cornerstone for identifying high-risk individuals. Genetic testing can then be used to determine whether a high-risk individual carries a gene mutation. Identification of appropriate management approaches, including chemoprevention, early detection, and prophylactic surgery, is needed to decrease the physical and psychological distress of individuals with a genetic predisposition to cancer.

CANCER: A GENETIC DISEASE

Cancer is caused by changes in the function or expression of critical genes as a consequence of mutation, translocation, amplification, deletion, or heritable epigenetic processes. In general, the accumulation of five to nine genetic changes must occur within a given cell to allow the cell to acquire the characteristics needed to escape normal growth control mechanisms and to develop into a malignant tumor. These genetic changes preferentially occur in a subset of human genes related to cellular development, cell differentiation, cell proliferation, cell survival, cellular senescence, and genetic repair. The majority of genetic changes leading to tumorigenesis are acquired by mutation of genes in somatic cells, giving rise to what are commonly known as sporadic tumors. These changes can be the consequence of a number of insults, including environmental toxins such as those in cigarette smoke, DNA damage due to ultraviolet radiation, or the low, but significant, spontaneous mutation rate associated with DNA replication and repair.

UICC Manual of Clinical Oncology, Eighth Edition. Edited by Raphael E. Pollock
ISBN 0-471-22289-5 Copyright © 2004 John Wiley & Sons, Inc.

TABLE 4.1. Examples of Familial Cancer Syndromes with Identified Genetic Mediators

Syndrome	Responsible Gene/Class	Chromosome Location	Potential Function	Common Tumors	Rare Tumors	Nonmalignant Manifestations
Li Fraumeni	P53 Class A	17p13	Cell cycle progression Apoptosis	Leukemia	Sarcomas	
Breast/ovary	BRCA1 Class C	17q21	DNA repair (?)	Breast (early onset) Ovary	Prostate Bowel (?)	
Breast/ovary	BRCA2 Class C	13q12	DNA repair (?)	Breast (early onset) Ovary	Male breast cancer Pancreas Ocular melanoma	
FAP/Gardner's	APC Class A	5q22	Cell adhesion	Colon	Desmoid Small intestine Thyroid Liver	Colon Polyps Osteomas
HNPCC	MLH1 MSH2 PMS1 PMS2 GTBP Class C	3q21 2p16 2q 7p 2p16	Mismatch repair Mismatch repair Mismatch repair Mismatch repair Mismatch repair	Colon Endometrium	Ovary Breast Renal Small bowel	
Gorlin's	Patched/PTC Class A	9q22	Receptor	Basall cell	Medulloblastoma Primitive neuroectoderm	Ovarian fibroma Developmental defects Hamartoma
MEN1	MENIN Class A	11q13	Unknown	Parathyroid Pituitary Enteropancreatic Adrenal	Pancreatic	
MEN2	RET Class B	10q11	Tyrosine kinase receptor	Medullary thyroid Pheochromacytoma	Parathyroid	Parathyroid Mucosal Neuromas Skeletal abnormalities Hirschsprung

Syndrome	Gene / Class	Locus	Function	Tumors		Features
Cowden's	MMAC1/PTEN Class A	10q23	Phosphatase	Breast Basal cell Thyroid	Endometrium (?) Ovarian (?) Renal cell (?) Brain	Facial papule Keratoses Benign breast lumps Trichilemmoma Thyroid hypertrophy
RB	RB Class A	13q14	Cell cycle progression	Retinoblastoma Sarcoma	Melanoma	
Denys-Drash/ WAGR	WT1 Class A	11q13	Transcription factor	Wilms		Gonadal abnormalities Aniridia Retardation
VHL	VHL Class A	3p25	Unknown RNA elongation (?)	Kidney Adrenal Neural		Retinal angiomas Cysts
Hereditary papillary	MET Class B	7q32	Tyrosine kinase receptor	Kidney		
Ataxia telangiectasia	ATM Class C	11q23	DNA repair P13 kinase family	Leukemia	Breast	Ataxia Telangiectasia
Peutz-Jeghers	STK11/LKB1 Class A	19q13.3	Serine kinase	Colon	Sex chord Stroma	Hamartomas Hyperpigmentation
Dysplastic nevi Syndrome	P16/15 Class A CDK4 Class A	9p21 12q14	Kinase inhibitor Cyclin-dependent kinase	Melanoma		Dysplastic Nevi
NF1 Neurofibro- matosis	NF1 Class A	17q11	Guanine exchange factor	Schwann cell Glia	Adrenal	Café au lait Neurofibroma
NF2 Neurofibro- matosis	NF2 Class A	22q12	Cytoskeleton	Schwann cell		Café au lait

Class A, loss of function mutations in growth regulators; Class B, gain of function mutations in growth regulators; Class C, regulators or mediators of genomic stability.

Inherited germline genetic changes predispose a number of individuals to the development of cancer. Mutations in the currently identified inherited cancer predisposition genes (Table 4.1) are all relatively rare. These inherited germline genetic changes probably play a major role in the development of about 5–10% of all solid tumors and a smaller proportion of cases of leukemia and lymphoma. In addition to the rare, high-penetrance cancer predisposition genes currently identified (Table 4.1), it is also likely that an additional set of relatively common, low-penetrance cancer predisposition genes remain to be identified that may contribute to a much higher proportion of cancers than do the high-penetrance cancer predisposition genes currently identified.

The known cancer predisposition genes can be subcategorized into three classes, depending on functional role and the type of mutation (Table 4.1). A small group of cancer predisposition genes would normally be classified as oncogenes. These cancer predisposition genes exhibit mutations resulting in a "gain of function" that increases the activity of the gene product or releases the gene product from normal regulatory control. The majority of cancer predisposition genes undergo loss of function mutations (Table 4.1). In order for the effects of these genes to be expressed, the normal copy of the gene must also be lost or inactivated. This class of cancer predisposition genes can be further subdivided into those genes that regulate cell cycle progression, apoptosis, and cellular senescence and those genes that detect or repair DNA damage. As indicated in Table 4.1, abnormalities in cancer predisposition genes result in a very discrete pattern of susceptibility to cancer, however, the reasons underlying the sensitivity in specific cell lineages and resistance in other cell lineages remain unknown.

THE COMMON HEREDITARY CANCER SYNDROMES

In the United States and Western countries, there is a high prevalence of breast, colorectal, and prostate cancers. For this reason, hereditary cancer syndromes that encompass these diseases are seen more frequently in clinical practice and will be briefly reviewed here. As shown in Table 4.1, cancer predisposition genes have been discovered for hereditary breast and ovarian cancer, and hereditary colorectal cancers. The search continues for genes associated with hereditary prostate cancers.

Hereditary Breast and Ovarian Cancer

Syndromes of breast cancer susceptibility have been linked to mutations in several genes. The breast cancer 1 (*BRCA1*) and breast cancer 2 (*BRCA2*) genes currently account for the majority of hereditary breast and ovarian cancers. Rare genetic conditions such as the Li-Fraumeni syndrome, Cowden disease, Muir-Torre syndrome, Peutz-Jeghers, and ataxia telangiectasia can also lead to increased risk of breast cancer. The precise functions of the *BRCA1* and *BRCA2* genes remain unknown, however, both function as tumor suppressor genes and have similar protein partners, suggesting related functions. Their most likely function is in transcriptional regulation and in transcription-coupled DNA repair.

BRCA1 is located on chromosome 17q (long arm) and is thought to account for 30–45% of breast cancer cases in families with a high incidence of early-onset breast and ovarian cancer. To date, more than 600 mutations and sequence variations have been detected according to the Breast Cancer Information Core. Details are available on the Internet at http://www.nhgri.nih.gov/Intramural_research/Lab/transfer/Bic/.

BRCA2 is located on chromosome 13q and appears to account for about 35% of families with early-onset breast cancer. To date, more than 150 different mutations and sequence variants have been identified. Thus, although *BRCA1* and *BRCA2* mutations account for a significant percentage of hereditary breast cancer, it is believed that other, as yet undiscovered genes such as breast cancer 3 (*BRCA3*) may also increase susceptibility to breast and other cancers. Alternatively, groups of high-frequency, low-penetrance cancer predisposition genes may explain the remaining families. In contrast, it is believed that *BRCA1* and *BRCA2* mutations account for the majority of familial ovarian cancers.

The lifetime risk for developing breast cancer in *BRCA1*-linked families is relatively high. In the general population, the cumulative incidence for breast cancer by age 50 is 2%, whereas in women with an alteration in *BRCA1*, the risk may be as high as 50%. Some mutations may carry a lower penetrance than others may; thus, lifetime risk for breast cancer may range from 60% to as high as 85% in some families. The penetrance may also be influenced by the co-inheritance of modifier genes. In the general population, the lifetime risk for ovarian cancer is in the range of 1–2%. In women with an alteration in *BRCA1*, the lifetime risk may range from 15% to 45%. There may also be a small but significant increased risk for prostate cancer in men and colon cancer in men and women with *BRCA1* mutations. Recent studies have also indicated that primary peritoneal carcinomatosis and fallopian tube carcinoma should be considered a clinical component of the hereditary breast-ovarian cancer syndrome, and may be associated with both *BRCA1* and *BRCA2* tumors. This becomes an important consideration when prophylactic oophorectomy is performed in high-risk women, suggesting that prophylactic oophorectomy may not provide complete protection and also that the tubes should be removed as part of any prophylactic procedure.

A lifetime risk of breast cancer similar to that in families with *BRCA1* mutations is seen in families with *BRCA2* alterations, although some data indicate that the onset of breast cancer may be at an older age. Ovarian cancer is also seen in women carrying mutations in *BRCA2*, although to a lesser extent than with *BRCA1*. Estimates for the lifetime risk of ovarian cancer range from 10% to 20% in women with *BRCA2* mutations. Other cancers that may be associated with *BRCA2* mutations include pancreatic, fallopian tube, laryngeal, uterine, and male breast cancers as well as leukemia. The estimated lifetime risk of breast cancer for male carriers of *BRCA2* mutations is roughly 6%.

BRCA1 and *BRCA2*-associated breast cancer may have different clinical, histological, immunophenotypic, and prognostic implications than sporadic breast cancer. Thus far, several studies have confirmed that *BRCA1*-associated tumors exhibit a phenotype characterized by high tumor grade and estrogen receptor negativity. They often carry a somatic p53 mutation, and may also be of the typical or atypical medullary type. The latter two characteristics have not been seen in all studies. Some studies have shown that there is a lower frequency of *erbB-2* overexpression, evaluated by immunohistochemistry, in *BRCA1*-associated tumors. Even though the histopathologic features of *BRCA1*-associated tumors would seem to confer an adverse prognosis, studies to date have not consistently shown an adverse effect of *BRCA1* mutations on outcome. At this point in time, the evidence is not yet strong enough to recommend any modification of standard therapy. A specific phenotype has not yet been consistently described for *BRCA2*-associated breast cancers, nor have studies conclusively shown a different prognosis when compared with age-matched sporadic breast cancer patients, however, only few breast cancers have been analyzed to date.

Several groups have studied ovaries prophylactically removed from members of hereditary breast ovarian cancer syndrome families who had undergone prophylactic oophorectomies and whose *BRCA1* and *2* status was known. Some studies have found differences in micropapillae, invaginations, stromal activity, and behavior in tissue culture, however, whether the effects of *BRCA1* or *BRCA2* mutations are manifest in normal ovarian epithelium remains controversial. There is the potential that the effects of *BRCA1* or *BRCA2* may also be evident in the heterozygous state due to haploinsufficiency. Whether haploinsufficiency occurs and whether this contributes to the propensity for cancer development due to DNA instability is unclear at this time.

For a carrier of an alteration in either *BRCA1* or *BRCA2* who is as yet unaffected with cancer, the most optimal strategy for management is not yet known. Options include heightened surveillance, chemoprevention, and prophylactic surgery (Table 4.2). It is not known whether increased surveillance will reduce breast cancer-related mortality in women at high risk, but data from younger women in the general population suggest that early detection and treatment are as likely to be effective in *BRCA* carriers as in noncarriers. *BRCA* tumors have the same radiological appearance as cancers from noncarriers. Alternative screening strategies such as the use of magnetic resonance imaging (MRI) or ultrasound for screening are under study, particularly as *BRCA1*-related tumors tend to occur more frequently in premenopausal women where the performance of mammography is suboptimal.

Oral contraceptives have been proven to protect against the development of ovarian cancer in the general population. Indeed, oral contraceptives provide definitive proof of the concept that a major life-threatening cancer can be prevented by a simple, relatively nontoxic approach. Several studies have evaluated the relationship of oral contraceptive use with the development of ovarian cancer in women with proven abnormalities in *BRCA1* and *BRCA2*. Although one recent study has failed to identify a protective effect, the preponderance of the epidemiological evidence is that oral contraceptives do decrease the incidence of ovarian cancer in these women. Although follow-up prospective trials are needed, oral contraceptives represent a reasonable temporizing step in women who have completed their families. There may be a slight increase in the incidence of breast cancer in women with abnormalities in *BRCA1* and *BRCA2* who receive exogenous estrogens, however, ovarian cancer is much more difficult to detect and treat than breast cancer and is thus much more lethal, making this a reasonable approach.

Retinoids are under investigation in prevention studies for a multitude of cancers, including breast and ovarian cancer, because they have been shown to inhibit cellular proliferation and to induce cellular differentiation. The retinoid 4HPR (fenretinide, a synthetic retinoic acid derivative) was selected for use in breast cancer prevention studies because of its low toxicity profile and prevention efficacy in preclinical studies. A randomized trial of fenretinide in Milan demonstrated a potential decrease in the occurrence of a second breast malignancy in premenopausal women, and in preliminary results, a potential decrease or delay in the development of ovarian cancer. There was no major activity in other population groups. It is now being assessed in combination with tamoxifen in a phase II breast cancer prevention trial. Prospective chemoprevention trials with oral contraceptive pills and retinoids will be important to determine whether these drugs are effective in selected populations, such as women who are carriers of a genetic change that predisposes for the development of breast or ovarian cancer.

Tamoxifen has now received regulatory approval to decrease the incidence of breast cancer in women at increased risk for breast cancer as determined by the Gail model. Initial results of a study to determine the effect of tamoxifen on women with a mutation of *BRCA1* or *BRCA2* were presented in May 2001. The study was based on sequencing of *BRCA1* and *BRCA2* in 288 cases of participants of the Breast Cancer Prevention Trial (BCPT). Nineteen cases of mutations in either *BRCA1* or *BRCA2* were identified. Of the eight women with an inherited mutation in BRCA1 who developed breast cancer, five had received tamoxifen and three had not. The risk ratio suggests no reduction in breast cancer incidence in women with mutations in *BRCA1* based on small numbers of events. In the BCPT, tamoxifen had no effect on the incidence of estrogen receptor–negative breast cancer. Women who are *BRCA1* positive tend to develop estrogen receptor–negative tumors. In women who are *BRCA2* carriers, the genetic data suggest that the reduction in breast cancer incidence due to tamoxifen was similar to the reduction in incidence due to tamoxifen of estrogen receptor–positive tumors, however, there were insufficient events to demonstrate statistical significance. Although the numbers are small, this is the first prospective study evaluating the efficacy of chemoprevention of breast cancer in a *BRCA1/2*-positive population.

Data are beginning to emerge that support the use of prophylactic surgery to manage risk in women who are carriers of a mutation in either *BRCA1* or 2. The precise degree of risk reduction associated with prophylactic mastectomy or oophorectomy has not yet been determined for individuals who carry a mutation that predisposes for breast or ovarian cancer. Nevertheless, it is clear that some risk remains after prophylactic surgery. Hartmann and colleagues, in a retrospective study of 639 women with a family history of breast cancer who underwent bilateral prophylactic mastectomy at the Mayo Clinic between 1960 and 1993, showed that prophylactic mastectomy was associated with a reduction in the incidence of breast

TABLE 4.2. Management of Selected Cancer Predisposition Syndromes

Syndrome/Gene	Penetrance	Testing	Prevention	Screening	Prophylactic Surgery
Breast/Ovarian BRCA1 BRCA2	Breast 40%–60% Ovary 20%–40% Breast 30%–50% Ovary 10%–30%	Management options may not be altered by test results Test results have high false-negative rate Full-length sequencing method of choice	No known chemoprevention methods Birth control pill decreases risk of ovarian cancer by approximately 50%, conflicting studies. Tamoxifen may prevent development of breast cancer in BRCA2 carriers. Further research needed.	*Breast cancer:* Breast self exam, begin age 20 Clinical breast exam, annual age 25 Mammography, annual age 30 *Ovarian cancer:* Transvaginal ultrasound, annual age 30–35 years CA125, annual age 30–35 years *Prostate cancer:* Digital rectal exam, annual age 50	Prophylactic mastectomy may decrease risk by 20-fold Prophylactic oophorectomy may decrease risk 2 to 20-fold Further research needed
Cowden's PTEN/MMAC1	Breast 15% DCIS and ductal carcinoma Basal cell Thyroid Ovary (rare) Renal cell (rare) Brain (rare)	Genetic testing now available	None known	*Breast cancer:* Breast self exam, begin age 20 Clinical breast exam, annual age 25 Mammography, annual age 30 *Basal cell carcinoma:* Dermatological exams *Thyroid:* Physical exam	Prophylactic mastectomy has been standard. May not be needed due to low frequency and good outcome. However, may improve quality of life as patients have multiple lumps and biopsies.

Syndrome/Gene	Lifetime risk of cancer	Genetic testing	Chemoprevention	Surveillance	Surgery
Familial adenomatous polyposis (FAP) APC	Nearly 100%	Genetic testing part of the standard management of affected families	Ongoing clinical trials to evaluate the use of chemoprevention agents (e.g., NSAIDs) in this disease. Celecoxib approved as add-on therapy.	Flexible sigmoidoscopy, begin annually at 10–11 years. Surveillance for extracolonic neoplasms, e.g., upper gastrointestinal tract adenomatous polyps	Prophylactic colectomy performed after appearance of adenomatous polyps
Hereditary nonpolyposis colorectal cancer (HNPCC) MLH1, MSH2, PMS1, PMS2, GTBP	Colorectal cancer— 60–75% Metachronous colorectal cancer— 30–50% Endometrial cancer— 30–50% Ovarian cancer— 3.5-fold increase (<10%)	Management options may not be altered by test results. Test results have high false-negative rate. Optimal testing method not yet defined	Ongoing clinical trials to evaluate the use of chemoprevention agents (e.g., NSAIDs) in this disease	*Colon cancer:* Colonoscopy every 1–3 years, beginning at 30–35 years *Endometrial cancer:* Transvaginal ultrasound, annually, at 30–35 years OR Endometrial biopsy, annually, at 30–35 years	Subtotal colectomy with ileorectal anastomosis should be considered in HNPCC-associated mutation carriers who have colon cancer and as prophylaxis in selected HNPCC-associated mutation carriers with adenomas at the time of surveillance.
MEN II RET	Lifetime risk of 90% for medullary thyroid cancer; parathyroid, 10–20%; pheochromocytoma 40–60%	Genetic testing part of the standard management of affected families	None currently available	Pentagastrin testing, historical	Thyroidectomy, generally done during childhood

cancer of at least 90%. In a small subset of 16 women with proven inherited mutations in either *BRCA1* or *BRCA2*, none have developed breast cancer, with an average 16.1 years follow up. The data indicate that bilateral prophylactic mastectomy yields a significant reduction in breast cancer risk in *BRCA1/2* mutation carriers, ranging from 69% to 79%. In July 2001, Meijers-Heijboer and colleagues published results from a prospective study of 139 women with BRCA1 or BRCA2 mutations who were enrolled in a breast cancer surveillance program at the Rotterdam Family Cancer Clinic. Seventy-six of the women underwent prophylactic mastectomy, and the other 63 remained under surveillance. There were no cases of breast cancer observed after prophylactic mastectomy, with a mean follow-up of 2.9 years. There were eight breast cancers in women who had not undergone prophylactic surgery after a mean follow-up of 3 years. Although the numbers are small and the follow-up early, prophylactic bilateral total mastectomy appears to markedly reduce the incidence of breast cancer at 3 years of follow-up.

The risk of ovarian cancer in *BRCA* carriers is estimated to be 10–45%, which is more than 10-fold that of the 1–2% risk in the general population. The effectiveness of ovarian cancer screening using CA-125 blood levels and transvaginal ultrasound in this high-risk population is not known and is the topic of several prospective studies. Two large prospective studies are underway to determine the efficacy of these modalities in low-risk women. Results are expected in 2008. Prophylactic oophorectomy, thus, remains a reasonable option for carriers to consider, however, it is clear that primary peritoneal carcinoma occurs at a higher frequency in *BRCA1* and *BRCA2* mutation carriers and that prophylactic oophorectomy does not prevent primary peritoneal carcinomatosis. Several studies complicated by a lack of genetic testing or small sample size have suggested that prophylactic oophorectomy decreases the incidence of ovarian cancer (including primary peritoneal carcino-matosis) by between 2- and 10-fold. Strikingly, prophylactic oophorectomy not only decreases the incidence of ovarian cancer but also decreases the incidence of breast cancer by up to 70%. This effect appears independent of whether women receive hormonal supplementation. Modeling studies have attempted to determine the cost benefit of interventions for *BRCA1* and *BRCA2* patients.

With concerns about the quality of the data supporting the assumptions used to build the models, it appears that prophylactic oophorectomy and mastectomy will improve survival and that maximal cost benefit occurs if these procedures are performed sometime in the range of 40–45 years of age. Further studies will be needed to justify these conclusions and to integrate the efficacy of screening into the algorithms.

Other Hereditary Syndromes that Predispose to Breast Cancer

Cowden's syndrome is one of a large number of genetic syndromes associated with dermatoses. It is characterized by mucocutaneous lesions, trichilemmomas, acral keratoses, papillomatous papules, mucosal lesions, macroencephaly, and Lhermitte-Duclos disease. Some individuals may exhibit fibroids, lipomas, fibromas, hamar-tomas, or thyroid adenomas. Individuals with Cowden's syndrome exhibit an increased frequency of breast cancer, gastrointestinal cancers, and thyroid disease. Breast cancers, which occur in 25–50% of mutation carriers, tend to occur at an earlier age and also have a greater propensity to be bilateral. Cowden's is a rare syndrome and accounts for only a very few cases of hereditary breast cancers. Cowden's syndrome is caused by inherited mutations in the PTEN tumor suppressor gene located at 10q23. PTEN functions to dephosphorylate membrane phosphatidylinositols as well as intracellular proteins. PTEN, which inhibits signaling through the phosphatidylinositol 3 kinase pathway, is a critical regulator of cell proliferation and cell survival.

The Li Fraumeni syndrome, caused by mutations in the p53 tumor suppressor gene on chromosome 17p, is also rare. The most common components of the syndrome are childhood leukemias and lymphomas, brain tumors, and sarcomas. Premenopausal breast cancers are a relatively uncommon component of this syndrome, which accounts for about 1% of all familial breast cancers. The age of the breast cancers can be very young, warranting screening initiation at age 20–25. Indeed, this syndrome, in contrast to *BRCA1* or *BRCA2*, contributes to breast cancers under the age of 25. p53 plays a critical role in regulating cell cycle transit and apoptosis, particularly in response to DNA damage. As noted above, p53 interacts with *BRCA1*, suggesting that they may both function in a complex, which surveys genomic stability. Mutations in p53 are the most common genetic abnormality in sporadic tumors, further indicating the importance of this tumor suppressor gene.

Hereditary Colon Cancers

About 1 in 18 individuals will be diagnosed with colorectal cancer in their lifetime. Highly penetrant cancer susceptibility syndromes account for about 5% of colorectal cancers. The most common syndrome is hereditary nonpolyposis colon cancer (HNPCC), with familial adenomatous polyposis (FAP) being much less frequent.

HNPCC   HNPCC is evidenced by early-onset colorectal cancer (diagnosis before the age of 50 years), and extracolonic tumors such as uterine, ovarian, stomach, and small intestine tumors and transitional cell tumors of the renal pelvis and ureter. Individuals with HNPCC do not have evident polyps, however, they do develop adenomas that tend to develop at an early age, have villous components, and are more dysplastic than adenomas detected in the general population. Individuals who have HNPCC have inherited a germline mutation in one of the several genes responsible for repairing DNA mismatches. Mismatch repair genes allow for accurate transmission of genetic information from a cell to its progeny by recognizing abnormal base pairs and correcting the sequence on one strand to restore normal base pairing. These errors are most frequently found in "microsatellites." Mutations in the following genes have been found to cause HNPCC: *hMSH2* (found on chromosome 2p (short arm)), *hMLH1* (found on chromosome 3p), *hPMS1* (found on chromosome 2p), *hPMS2* (found on chromosome 7p), and *hMSH6* (found on chromosome 2p). Microsatellites are stable stretches of DNA throughout the genome that are repetitive, and usually do not encode for proteins. Most cancers in patients with HNPCC show a high degree of microsatellite instability (MSI). MSI provided clues for the discovery of genes associated with this syndrome in the early 1990s.

Testing tumor for microsatellite instability is often used as a prescreen to determine whether full sequencing for genes associated with HNPCC should be performed. Because evidence exists that a low percentage (15%) of tumors associated with *MLH1* or *MSH2* mutations are MSI-low or MSI-stable, other methodologies have been investigated to determine whether a family might test positive for an HNPCC-associated gene. As most mutations in mismatch repair genes render the mRNA unstable and thus result in a loss of protein expression, immunohistochemistry is being used as a rapid and inexpensive screen. Studies have show that loss of protein expression detected by this technique correlates well with an *MSH2* and *MSH6* gene defect, however *MLH1* mutation detection is not as efficient. Therefore, the best approach at this time appears to be a combination of MSI analysis and immunohistochemistry in families suspected of HNPCC.

There is a 70–75% risk of developing colorectal cancer by age 65 years in carriers of mutations in the HNPCC-related genes. In some families, the penetrance may be as high as 90%. The median age at diagnosis is less than 50 years. In many families, synchronous cancers of the colon (several tumors presenting at the same time) and metachronous tumors (several tumors presenting at different times) have been documented. The risk for endometrial cancer ranges from 20% to 50% by age 70 years, as compared with a population risk of 3%. Some studies have shown a better prognosis of patients, with HNPCC-related colorectal and endometrial cancers compared with sporadic cancers.

The International Collaborative Group on HNPCC defined criteria for identifying the syndrome; these are currently known as the "Amsterdam criteria." The criteria for the syndrome are histologically verified colorectal cancer in three or more relatives, one of whom is a first-degree relative of the other two; colorectal cancer involving at least two generations; and one or more colorectal cancer cases diagnosed before 50 years of age. A limitation of these criteria has been the omission of endometrial and other extracolonic tumors. The Bethesda criteria for HNPCC includes the Amsterdam criteria as well as colon cancer cases before 40 years, and the noncolonic tumors associated with HNPCC.

Because individuals who harbor a genetic mutation associated with HNPCC have a greatly increased lifetime risk for colorectal cancer, they must be managed differently than the population in general. Cancer risk associated with HNPCC may actually be reduced by colonoscopy with polypectomy on a regular basis. Vasen et al. have estimated a 7 year increase in life expectancy for HNPCC mutation carriers who undergo colonoscopy every 2–3 years. Screening recommendations thus include full colonoscopy every 1–3 years starting between 20- and 25-years of age and annual screening of the endometrium beginning between 25- and 35-years of age (Table 4.2). The optimal method for screening the endometrium is undetermined, but current methods include endometrial aspiration, biopsy, or ultrasonography. Because of insufficient data on the effectiveness of screening for other cancers associated with the syndrome, such as ovarian cancer, no consensus recommendations on screening for these cancers are available. However, some experts do recommend screening for ovarian or urinary tract cancers in families with HNPCC.

The consensus panel also recommended consideration of subtotal colectomy with ileorectal anastomosis when colon cancer is diagnosed and as a prophylactic measure for some mutation carriers, that is, those not willing or able to undergo annual colonoscopy. Rectal cancer warrants consideration of proctocolectomy because of the remaining high risk of another cancer in the colon, particularly the right colon. Women with an HNPCC mutation should consider the option of prophylactic hysterectomy and oophorectomy between the ages of 35 and 40 years or at completion of child-bearing.

Current cancer chemoprevention trials are evaluating the use of agents such as retinoids or nonsteroidal antiinflammatory agents (NSAIDs) and are being extended to persons at risk for developing colorectal cancer and to those known to have mutations in a cancer predisposition gene. NSAIDs provide the greatest promise of effect at this time for chemoprevention of cancers in HNPCC families. Elevated prostaglandin levels are found in colon cancers and their precursor lesions, adenomatous polyps. Agents such as aspirin and other NSAIDs, which inhibit the generation of these arachidonic acid metabolites, are associated with a decreased risk of developing or dying from colon cancer. Early studies indicate that aspirin suppresses the accumulation of mutations due to mismatch repair deficiency, thus reducing the incidence of colorectal cancer in persons with HNPCC mutations.

FAP FAP is a rare syndrome characterized by hundreds to thousands of polyps carpeting the colon that inevitably progress to colon cancer. Polyps usually begin to appear in an affected person's late teens and twenties, and if untreated (generally by prophylactic colectomy), death from colon cancer will occur in virtually all cases by age 50 years. Congenital hypertrophy of the retinal pigment epithelium is a useful diagnostic marker for the syndrome and consists of pigmented lesions in the retina that can be detected by fundoscopic examination. Individuals with a variant form of FAP known as Gardner's syndrome also exhibit sebaceous cysts, lipomas, desmoid tumors, fibromas, facial bone osteomas, and impacted or supernumerary teeth.

Mutation of the *APC* gene is the cause of FAP. As are most genes associated with hereditary cancer syndromes, the *APC* gene is large, and a wide spectrum of mutations has been observed. However, genotype-phenotype correlations have begun to be identified. The majority of mutations in *APC* have been observed in the 5′ half of the gene, with a large number in a defined region within exon 15.

Internationally accepted screening guidelines for individuals at risk for FAP include flexible sigmoidoscopy every 2 years from age 10 to 14 years until 40 years of age and then every 3–5 years until age 60. Polyps may become symptomatic earlier in childhood, in which case screening should be initiated at an earlier age. Once the individual is found to have polyposis, colonoscopy and polypectomy are performed every 6–12 months. Prophylactic colectomy is generally recommended for individuals with classical FAP when the polyps can no longer be monitored and managed adequately with colonoscopy. Every effort is made to put this surgery off until a child has gone through puberty. The most frequent surgery is colectomy with ileorectal anastomosis. After subtotal colectomy for the treatment of cancer or prophylaxis, mutation carriers still have a risk for rectal cancer that should be monitored with endoscopic examination every 6–12 months.

Approximately 50–90% of FAP patients who undergo a colectomy will also develop duodenal adenomas. However, only about 5% of this group will develop a duodenal cancer. Thus, optimal upper gastrointestinal tract management for FAP patients is not entirely clear inasmuchas removal of duodenal adenomas is not practical and early detection and treatment are of unproven benefit. There is also a predisposition for hepatoblastomas, brain tumors, and thyroid cancer associated with FAP, but only a small number of individuals develop these extracolonic tumors.

Chemoprevention in FAP is being actively studied. The NSAID sulindac has demonstrated a significant impact on the reversal of rectal adenomas, but no benefit in the reversal of upper gastrointestinal adenomas. Some pediatric gastroenterology specialists are using NSAIDs to control colorectal adenomas in children affected by FAP in order to forestall the inevitable surgery until the child is older. In 2000, Celebrex^{TM} (celecoxib) became the only drug federally approved for reducing the number of polyps in patients with FAP. Although this is an important advance in FAP treatment, some key points must be kept in mind. First, Celebrex is approved only as add-on therapy and does not replace standard care. Second, although polyps are generally a precursor to colon cancer, it is not known whether reducing the number of polyps will actually reduce the likelihood of developing colon cancer, obviate the need for prophylactic surgery, and improve quality of life and outcome.

Attenuated Familial Adenomatous Polyposis AFAP is also due to mutations in the *APC* gene. In AFAP, however, the age at onset of cancer is generally much older (over 40 years of age) than in classical FAP and the number of polyps is far fewer. The colon polyps occur predominantly on the right side of the colon and tend to range in number from 0 to approximately 100. Surveillance consists of colonoscopy every other year from about age 25 to 30 years, and then annually thereafter. Chemoprevention trials are exploring the effectiveness of sulindac and other NSAIDs in persons affected by AFAP.

APC Variants The I1307K variant of the *APC* gene, which confers an increased risk of colorectal tumors, including multiple adenomas and carcinomas, was recently discovered. This variant has been found to be present in 6% of persons of Ashkenazi Jewish heritage. Thus far, the I1307K variant has not been reported in other populations. The variant is believed to double the population risk of colorectal cancer among carriers as compared with the general population, but the risk of colorectal cancer associated with the I1307K variant is much lower than the high risk seen in *APC* mutations associated with classical FAP. This and possibly other variants in the *APC* gene may improve our understanding and eventually our ability to treat or prevent at least a subset of sporadic cancers.

IDENTIFICATION OF INDIVIDUALS AT RISK FOR CARRYING INHERITED CANCER PREDISPOSITION GENES— THE IMPORTANCE OF PEDIGREE

Family history remains the best screening approach for identifying individuals at high risk for developing cancer due to the inheritance of a mutated cancer predisposition gene and is the cornerstone of clinical cancer genetics. Characteristics suggestive of the presence of a cancer predisposition gene in a family pedigree include an increased number of cancers and unexpectedly early age of onset of tumors. In addition, multiple tumors in a single individual, rare tumors (such as sarcomas or childhood cancers), identifiable patterns of cancers predictive of a cancer syndrome, nonmalignant manifestations of a cancer gene syndrome, and ethnic background that may correlate with a potential "founder" effect may also be seen. Validation of a patient's family history remains paramount and problematic. A patient may not be aware of all of the cases of cancer in a family. Especially in more distant and older generations, the presence of cancer in a family member was often not discussed among the family. Age of onset, which is critically important, may not be readily available. Further, in many instances, family members have wrongly attributed death to a metastatic cancer site rather than to the original primary cancer. It is advisable to ask the patient to validate the family history or pedigree through discussions with a number of relatives. Historical reporting of some types of cancer such as breast cancer appears to be relatively reliable, whereas distinguishing between the many causes of abdominal cancer including bowel, ovary, uterus, cervix, or kidney is comparatively unreliable. Thus, an attempt should be made to obtain pathology reports on all reported cases of cancer in the family. Because of medical privacy laws, this will generally require the written permission of the person affected with cancer or the living next of kin to obtain copies of records. Practice guidelines, to assist oncologists in identifying high-risk families, were initially published by the National Comprehensive Cancer Network (NCCN) in 1999. Although it is critical to obtain an accurate history of cancer in family members, it is also important to ascertain whether individuals in the family demonstrate other constitutional changes. As indicated in Table 4.1, individuals carrying germline mutations in the known cancer predisposition genes may also demonstrate noncancer-related phenotypic changes that are likely to indicate the presence of a cancer predisposition syndrome. For example, multiple bowel polyps would be suggestive of the multiple hamartoma syndromes associated with familial adenomatosis polypi/Gardner's syndrome or Cowden's disease with associated mutations in *APC* or MMAC1/PTEN, respectively. Hyperpigmentation might be a clue to the presence of a Peutz Jegher's syndrome with associated mutations in *STK11/LKB1* (Table 4.1).

When evaluating a family history, a number of characteristics suggest that a family is more likely to harbor a mutated cancer predisposition gene. The first and foremost characteristic of a pedigree predictive of the presence of an inherited cancer predisposition syndrome is a higher than expected incidence of specific types of cancer in the family. Initially, the analysis should consist of looking for multiple cases of the same type of tumor such as breast cancer. However, as demonstrated in Table 4.1, the majority of cancer predisposition genes predispose individuals to the development of cancers in several different cell lineages. For example, an excess of breast and ovarian cancer would suggest that the family might carry an abnormality in *BRCA1* or *BRCA2* (Table 4.1). A high frequency of bowel and endometrial cancer would suggest that a family might have a mutation in the genes that make up the HNPCC syndrome (Table 4.1). It is important, however, to remember that familial clustering of cancers in common cancers such as bowel, lung, prostate, and breast can occur by chance or due to environmental influences so that a strong family history does not necessarily indicate the presence of a mutated cancer predisposition gene.

As noted above, development of a sporadic tumor usually requires mutations in a number of different genes. This need for accumulation of multiple mutations in a single cell results in most sporadic cancers occurring at a relatively late age. Tumors due to the inheritance of a cancer predisposition gene tend, however, to occur at an earlier age. This characteristic remains the hallmark suggestive of the presence of a mutated cancer predisposition gene in the family and its presence should always alert the clinician to scrutinize the family history more closely.

Given that the chance of a single individual developing multiple primary tumors is relatively low, a history of multiple primaries in a single individual is sufficiently predictive of a mutated cancer predisposition gene to require a more thorough evaluation of the patient's pedigree. Patients may have tumors in paired organs such as the breast, which would be suggestive of one of the hereditary breast/ovary syndromes or in the kidney, which could be suggestive of Wilms, papillary renal carcinoma, or Von Hippel Lindau syndromes. Further, primaries in multiple organs, especially if they cannot be explained by another mechanism, such as radiation- or chemotherapy-induced tumors, may be suggestive of the presence of a mutated cancer predisposition gene. For example, a single patient with endometrial and colon cancer raises concern about the HNPCC group of familial predisposition genes. Similarly, a patient with both breast and ovarian cancer is strongly supportive of the inheritance of an abnormality in one of the genes that predispose to the breast/ovarian hereditary cancer syndromes (Table 4.1).

A number of cancer predisposition syndromes exhibit "founder" affects and are more common in certain ethnic groups. Abnormalities in *BRCA1* and *BRCA2* are present in about 1 in 1,000 individuals when assessed in a mixed population. Individuals of Dutch, Icelandic, French Canadian, or Ashkenazic Jewish origin may have, because of founder effects, as much as a 20-fold increase in the incidence of mutations in *BRCA1* or *BRCA2*. A similar increased incidence of a potential deleterious change in the *APC* gene (termed I1307K) has been identified in individuals of Ashkenazic Jewish origin. Mutations within a specific ethnic background likely occurred by chance in a germ cell many generations ago and, due to the limited effect of adult cancers on reproductive fitness, were "fixed" and spread in that ethnic population. Knowledge of the patient's ethnic origin may provide an additional clue suggesting the presence of a mutated cancer predisposition gene, thus modifying the interpretation of the family pedigree. Further, as the genetic changes found in a given ethnic background are often limited to specific sites in the cancer predisposition gene, the patient's ethnic background could guide the genetic testing approach to be used.

GENETIC COUNSELING IN A HIGH-RISK CLINIC

The field of human clinical cancer genetics is changing rapidly with the discovery of new cancer predisposition genes and new options for care and management of high-risk patients. Because highly specialized skills are necessary to obtain and validate pedigrees, and to educate and counsel patients, it is preferable to evaluate patients in a high-risk clinic that uses a multidisciplinary approach combining ancillary and medical staff with expertise in cancer genetics and in cancer care. Members of the multidisciplinary team include genetic counselors with additional training in cancer management, nurse practitioners with additional training in genetics, clinical geneticists, medical oncologists, and surgical oncologists. In addition, access to psychologists and psychiatrists, diagnostic imaging expertise, molecular diagnostics, and an ethicist is important. Due to the potential negative psychological sequelae of learning that one is either positive or negative for a mutation, inclusion of both psychologists and psychiatrists in the team for consultation is an important step. Support from individuals skilled in cancer screening, particularly diagnostic imaging and molecular diagnostics, is critical to the long-term success of the program. Finally, given the lack of consensus about appropriate approaches to the management of patients, concerns about genetic confidentiality, and the lack of precedents for many of the issues that arise, an ethicist should be available to provide support to the rest of the team.

Comprehensive services should include determinations of the individual's reasons for seeking cancer risk counseling; data collection that provides an in-depth review of the family history (a minimum of three complete generations with pathology reports) and patterns of transmission of cancers within the family; risk assessment as outlined above; determination of the client's level of knowledge regarding hereditary cancer syndromes and cancer genetics, self-perception of risk for developing cancer, and the motivation for seeking predisposition genetic testing; recommendations for management of risk (i.e., surveillance, chemoprevention, prophylactic surgery); evaluation of the appropriateness of testing; education regarding the testing process and the benefits, risks, limitations, costs, and potential outcomes that may result from testing; and disclosure of test results and their implications. All counseling should include an evaluation of the patient's psychosocial status, support systems, ability to receive and cope with test results, and referrals as appropriate for medical or surgical means of early detection or prevention of cancer. It is considered standard practice in many centers that provide cancer genetic counseling, that individuals receive a follow-up letter or other contact after counseling that documents clearly the information provided regarding family history, risk assessment, implications of testing and/or known results, and recommendations for management of risks. It is also critically important to attempt to obtain documentation of the cancers in the family through securing pathology records or death certificates as reviewed previously. Table 4.3 provides an over view of important issues that are addressed in cancer genetic counseling and services provided.

Many individuals are "information seekers" and want as much information as possible to guide future decisions. Information about a person's chance of developing cancer may provide important directions for patient care. Furthermore, high-risk patients have questions related to the best options for management (Table 4.2). Even when the best medical management option is not known, identifying one's risk and the potential options may provide empowerment allowing the individual to make decisions based on the best information available. For many patients, awaiting the results of ongoing trials to define the best mode of care is not an

TABLE 4.3. The Cancer Genetic Counseling Process

Process	Information to be Reviewed
Assessment and information gathering	
Reason for referral	Patient concerns and questions about family history
	Empowerment/ability to make informed decisions
	Information on risk for self and children
	Risk management options
	Physician recommendation
Family history	Collect information on three generations when possible
	Minimum: parents, siblings, aunts, uncles, grandparents
	Cancers in the family: age at diagnosis, bilaterality in paired organs, more than one primary tumor
	Relevant genetic testing results
	Verification by pathology report or death certificates of cancers in the family
Personal history	Past medical history and screening practices
	History relevant to cancer risk assessment (e.g., gynecologic history for breast/ovarian cancer)
	Lifestyle factors (e.g., smoking, alcohol, carcinogen exposure)
Patient perception of risk for cancer	Beliefs about cancer and its causation
	Patient perception of lifetime risk for developing cancer and probability of altered gene in the family that is responsible for cancer

TABLE 4.3   (*Continued*)

Process	Information to Be Reviewed
Patient concerns about risk counseling	Fears of discrimination
	Impact on family dynamics
	Lack of definitive methods to decrease risk
Social, emotional, and cultural concerns	Cultural beliefs
	Support systems
	Economic Factors
Evaluation and analysis of data	
Family history	Assess family for characteristics seen with hereditary cancer syndromes
	Estimate of probability that family would test positive for alteration in cancer predisposition gene
Focused physical examination	Dependent on syndrome present in the family e.g., eye exam for FAP
Laboratory testing	Dependent on syndrome present in the family
Communication of genetic and risk information	
Natural history of condition	Discussion of types of cancer seen in the family
	Explanation of hereditary cancer syndrome present
Inheritance patterns	Review of autosomal dominant transmission of cancer predisposition genes
Discussion of risk for developing cancer	Populational risk and estimated risk for patient
	Review in terms of several types of risk (e.g., in terms of relative risk, lifetime risk)
Ramifications and appropriateness of cancer predisposition genetic testing	Benefits, risk, limitations, costs of testing
	Potential answers that may be obtained
	Who in the family is best to test
Strategies for managing risk	Lifestyle changes
	Options for screening and detection
	Signs and symptoms of cancer
	Chemoprevention
	Prophylactic surgery
Supportive counseling	
Discussion of patient and family questions and concerns	Common concerns include potential risk for children, potential for discrimination due to cancer predisposition genetic testing
Providing emotional and social support	Determination of existing coping patterns and support systems
	Teaching new coping strategies as required
	Assisting patient in discussing genetic testing results with family
	Allow patient and family to voice fears and concerns
Referral for additional counseling and support as needed	Available support systems for patients with extreme anxiety and distress

option as they feel that they must take action in the immediate future. Wanting to do all that is possible to remain cancer free for themselves or for their children can drive utilization of approaches that have not been medically proven to be beneficial. Concerns about risks for children and relatives are paramount for many individuals who have already developed cancer. In general, genetic testing has a significant potential to contribute to patient management when the family has a 10% probability of carrying a mutation in a gene. However, genetic testing may be appropriate for lower-risk individuals who have a cancer and are deciding between management options, are contemplating prophylactic surgery, individuals from specific ethnic groups and for patients who "just need to know."

GENETIC TESTING—TECHNOLOGY

Genetic testing for many of the cancer predisposition syndromes remains controversial (Table 4.2). At a minimum, the patient must be counseled as to the ramifications of testing and the potential interpretation of test results. Patients must be able to understand what testing can and cannot tell them, hence the patient must be informed of the potential of obtaining a false negative, a false positive, or uninformative results. The person counseling the patient should understand the limitations of the particular technology utilized (Table 4.3). The American Society of Clinical Oncologists does not recommend testing unless the results have the potential to alter the patient's medical management. However, knowing one's mutation status, whether or not there are specific proven medical management options, may provide the patient with information that will improve their quality of life.

In most cases, genetic testing should be considered experimental and be performed under an informed consent approved by an institutional review board. However, as genetic testing approaches are validated, appropriate management techniques developed and safeguards against genetic discrimination put in place, genetic testing will likely become a component of general medical practice. An individual's risk of developing cancer will be one piece of the process in designing individualized screening and prevention programs.

In the broadest sense, genetic tests are defined as the analysis of human DNA, RNA, chromosomes, proteins, and other gene products to detect disease-related genotypes, mutations, phenotypes, or karyotypes. The tests may be helpful in identifying those at risk of getting the disease in question, identifying carriers of mutated genes, and establishing diagnoses or prognoses. A number of different techniques are utilized for genetic testing.

Interpretation of testing results can be complex. Mutations that have been identified to track with disease in several families are the easiest to interpret. Clearly, they predispose an individual to the development of cancer. Nevertheless, the degree of penetrance and age of onset of cancer induced by a particular mutation may vary between families and between individuals in a family. Mutations that result in a truncated protein generally can be expected to result in a predisposition to cancer. However, a significant portion of the carboxyterminus of *BRCA2* can be deleted with no apparent ill effect. Mutations that result in a change in the identity of a single amino acid (missense mutations) in the resultant protein product are most difficult to interpret. Such changes may represent polymorphisms of no or limited consequences. When the same missense mutation is found in a number of different cancer prone families and is found to track with the disease, it likely predisposes to tumor development. When a missense mutation has not been seen before or has not been demonstrated to track with disease, the mutation must be categorized as being of "unknown significance." Further analysis of these missense mutations are required to determined if the mutation segregates with cancer or if it is found in a significant number of nonaffected individuals in the general population, making it a likely polymorphism. Mutations that result in a change in the nucleotide sequence without a change in protein sequence due to "third codon wobble" can generally be assumed to be without consequence. However, recent data indicates that these may alter mRNA splicing and may thus contribute to disease development. Mutations found in introns, particularly those in splice acceptor and donator sites, must be assessed further to determine whether they track with disease in several families. Similar examination is necessary for mutations in promoter regions.

Emerging technologies such as gene sequencing CHIPs (arrays of short nucleotide sequences on a solid matrix which can detect all potential sequences in a gene), tandem mass spectrometry (linking HPLC and mass spectrometry to give extremely accurate size measurement), and functional assays (assessing function of a patients gene in model systems such as yeast) may prove to be more accurate and less expensive than current approaches. More important, functional assays, such as studying function of the gene product in yeast, have the potential to distinguish significant mutations from polymorphisms. These new technologies will need to mature prior to being instituted as "first line" approaches, replacing current sequencing technology. It is important to note, however, that *p53* sequencing CHIPs are commercially available and that CHIPs have been developed that can detect the majority of point mutations and small inserts even in large genes such as *BRCA1*.

GENETIC TESTING—GOOD NEWS, BAD NEWS, AND NO NEWS

The interpretation and presentation of positive test results to the patient is relatively straightforward. Patients should be told that they are at an increased risk for the development of cancer and offered a menu of management options. The risk level should be presented so as to reflect the range of penetrance for abnormalities in the cancer predisposition gene and, where possible, the penetrance for the specific mutation. Where clinical studies have identified appropriate management options (Table 4.2), they can be offered to the patient. However, where the appropriate medical approach has not been defined, the alternative options should be described to the patient in a nondirective manner, allowing the patient to make his or her own informed decision. It is important to note that the patient's decision will likely be tempered by his or her own exposure to family members who have developed cancer and, despite extensive education during the counseling process, to previous convictions and education. Although a positive test result would normally be considered bad news, many people find an explanation for the number of cancers in their family as a positive and empowering event, thus resulting in this being "good" news. Further, as indicated above, a number of interventions are now available for individuals with an inherited predisposition to cancer, empowering the client.

The interpretation and presentation of test results that do not indicate the presence of a mutation is more complex, particularly if the individual tested does not have cancer. Indeed, it is preferable, but not always possible, to test a family member who is afflicted with cancer. However, even in families at high risk for cancer, sporadic cases of cancer, particularly common cancers such as breast cancer, can occur and confuse the issue (see individual 103 in Figure 4.1). A failure to detect a mutation could be indicative that mutations in the tested genes are not present in the family. Alternatively, it may suggest that a genetic change is present in the family and was not inherited by the tested individual. A failure to detect a mutation in the cancer predisposition gene may indicate that the mutation is outside of the region tested, not detected by the technique used, or that a mutation is present in an, as yet unidentified, cancer predisposition gene that induces a similar syndrome. *BRCA1* and *BRCA2* (and potential *BRCA3, 4, 5,* or *6*) provide excellent examples. Full-length sequencing for *BRCA1* may miss up to 30% of the mutations in *BRCA1*. This could be due to deletions of large regions of the gene, the complete gene, changes in introns, silent changes in exons that alter mRNA splicing and mutations in distant enhancers. Furthermore, sequencing of *BRCA1* alone will clearly miss all mutations in *BRCA2* and any other related phenocopy syndromes. Thus, there is a high potential for false negative results in testing. There is controversy as to whether a negative test result decreases the chance that a mutation is present in the family. However, conditional probability suggests that the predicted likelihood of a mutation in a cancer predisposition gene in a family based on family history is not markedly altered by a negative test result. Rather, a negative test result suggests that the mutation in the family is not detectable by the technology utilized. Thus, in most cases, patients can only be given "bad news" (they have a genetic abnormality) or "no news" (we don't know if there is a genetic abnormality in the family). In either case, medical management and advice may not change markedly as a consequence of genetic testing. The patient, regardless of test results, may continue to be considered to be at high risk and would continue to be offered intensive screening or prophylactic surgery. Indeed, this lack of new options decreases the attractiveness of genetic testing for many patients (Table 4.3).

There are exceptions to the "no news" category. When the identity of the mutation present in a family is known, it is possible, with a high degree of accuracy, to determine whether any person in the family has or has not inherited the specific mutation. Thus, the patient could potentially receive "good news." Furthermore, in cases where the likely location of a specific mutation can be predicted due to the

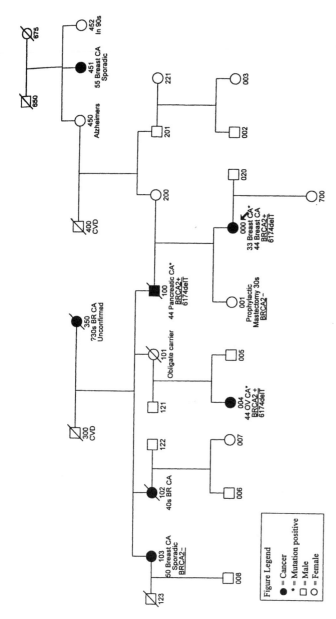

Figure 4.1 This is a typical *BRCA2* family pedigree. There are a number of salient points demonstrated in this pedigree. The proband, 000, originally sought counseling because she was concerned about the potential risk her daughter, 700, might have for developing breast cancer. Individual 001 had a prophylactic mastectomy prior to testing negative based on her concern about her risk for developing cancer. Studies have shown that more than 95% of women who have had a prophylactic mastectomy have been very pleased with the outcome and "would do it again" or would "recommend the procedure to family members" under similar circumstances. Individual 101 died without developing a cancer. As both her daughter, 004, and her brother, 100, have tested positive for a mutation in *BRCA2*, she would be an obligate carrier (must have the mutation in *BRCA2*). This demonstrates that penetrance is <100% and that the phenotype can skip a generation. Individual 100 has tested positive for a mutation in the *BRCA2* gene and passed it on to his daughter, 000. It is always important to assess the paternal side of the family as mutations in *BRCA1* or *BRCA2* have an equal likelihood of being passed by either the mother or the father. Individual 103 has a sporadic breast cancer in a family with a known mutation. The age at onset is later than for other individuals in the family. If this person had been tested first, it could have resulted in a false-negative result for the family.

phenotype, hot spots accounting for the majority of inherited cases, or mutations prevalent in specific ethnic backgrounds, it may be possible to indicate that negative results essentially rule out the likelihood of a mutation being present in the tested gene in that patient. This may have important consequences for the patient, allowing decreased surveillance or potentially abrogating the need for prophylactic surgery (Table 4.3). It may have a major effect on the patient's concerns about reproduction and about the concern of having passed on a high risk to one's children.

VARIATION IN PENETRANCE

The degree of penetrance and the severity of the syndromes associated with cancer predisposition genes can vary widely between families and between individuals in the same family. This makes it necessary in many cases to communicate the likelihood of developing cancer to a high risk individual with a very wide confidence interval. In our breast/ovarian cancer clinic, patients routinely over-estimate their risk and are relieved to discover that developing and dying of cancer in not inevitable. The bad news that they carry an abnormality in a cancer pre-disposition gene such *BRCA1* or *BRCA2* can be tempered by the knowledge that developing and dying from cancer is not inevitable.

Although it is possible to indicate to a patient what the expected frequency of cancer is for individuals with a given cancer predisposition syndrome, it is usually not possible to determine which individuals and, importantly, when a specific individual will develop cancer (Tables 4.1 and 4.2). Patients find it particularly difficult to relate statistical risks of developing cancer to their own likelihood of developing cancer in the near future or even in their lifetime. The patient's response to counseling is frequently driven by the patient's past experience as well as by their prior knowledge. These preconceptions have proven particularly recalcitrant to patient education. Approaches ranging from intensive counseling to the develop-ment of interactive computer driven education programs are under investigation to provide more efficient and convincing patient education.

PSYCHOSOCIAL CONSEQUENCES

There are many psychosocial implications associated with cancer predisposition testing. Several factors such as beliefs about cancer and its prognosis, life history, and the level of fear and anxiety present, are known to influence how patients perceive personal risk and their comprehension of risk information. In the United States, uncertainties regarding the potential for genetic discrimination by insurance companies or by employers remain, despite the passage of legislation. Diligent measures within the clinical setting to safeguard patient information specific to genetic testing must be maintained and patient's wishes respected. The full spectrum of psychological reactions to the results of genetic testing has not yet been fully elucidated, and thus remains an area of active research. Family dynamics are important and should be discussed prior to initiation of testing, as results obtained for one family member may have potential impact upon others within the family. Some family members may wish to know their status, whereas others most definitely will not want to know. This can obviously lead to conflict within the family. Potential negative sequellae that may result from testing include heightened fear and anxiety, depression, changes in family relationship, guilt over transmission of a mutated gene, guilt over not receiving a mutated gene (survivor guilt), changes in functional status, and changes in body image and self perception. Within the context of the patient's beliefs about health care and their cultural orientation, the multidisciplinary team must strive to support patients following provision of test results by reinforcing existing coping mechanisms, teaching new ones, providing the necessary information to empower patient decision making, and referral to mental health professionals when warranted. There are also potential benefits that may be obtained from testing. These include relief from the uncertainty of not knowing one's risk status, targeting of aggressive screening measures and prevention strategies to those at the highest risk, and providing information on the potential for children to have inherited a predisposition to develop cancer. It is important to reinforce that the presence of a mutated cancer predisposition gene within the family does not mean that every family member will inherit this mutation, or that they will develop cancer.

THE FUTURE

The completion of the human genome project and the maturation of multicenter groups such as the Cancer Genetics Network are rapidly increasing our ability to determine the identity of genes that predispose to tumor development. Further, the completion of epidemiological and intervention trials are beginning to provide options for management of patients, which will prevent the development of tumors or allow detection at an early curable stage. As indicated above, a new generation of testing approaches may improve the accuracy and decrease the cost of genetic testing. In the United States, many of the questions around genetic confidentiality are being answered by the passage of state and federal laws as well as the by passage of time. Overall, it is clear that the identification and management of individuals with abnormalities in cancer predisposition genes will improve rapidly.

FURTHER READING

American Society of Clinical Oncology (1996) Statement of the American Society of Clinical Oncology: genetic testing for cancer susceptibility. *J Clin Oncol* 14:1730–1736.

Aziz S, Kuperstein G, Rosen B, Cole D, Nedelcu R, McLaughlin J, Narod, SA (2001) A genetic epidemiological study of carcinoma of the fallopian tube. *Gynecol Oncol* 80:341–345.

Bertwistle D, Ashworth A (1998) Functions of the BRCA1 and BRCA2 genes. *Curr Opin Genet Dev* 8:14–20.

Boland CR, Thibodeau SN, Hamilton SR, Sidransky D, Eshleman JR, Burt RW, Meltzer SJ, Rodriguez-Bigas MA, Fodde R, Ranzani GN, Srivastava S (1998) A National Cancer Institute Workshop on Microsatellite Instability for cancer detection and familial predisposition: development of international criteria for the determination of microsatellite instability in colorectal cancer. *Cancer Res* 58:5248–5257.

Burke W, Petersen G, Lynch P, Botkin J, Daly M, Garber J, Kahn MJ, McTiernan A, Offit K, Thomson E, Varricchio C (1997) Recommendations for follow-up care of individuals with an inherited predisposition to cancer. I. Hereditary nonpolyposis colon cancer. Cancer Genetics Studies Consortium. *JAMA* 277:915–919.

Burke W, Daly M, Garber J, Botkin J, Kahn MJ, Lynch P, McTiernan A, Offit K, Perlman J, Petersen G, Thomson E, Varricchio C (1997) Recommendations for follow-up care of individuals with an inherited predisposition to cancer. II. BRCA1 and BRCA2. Cancer Genetics Studies Consortium. *JAMA* 277:997–1003.

Collins FS (2001) Contemplating the end of the beginning. *Genome Res* 11:641–643.

Cummings S (2000) The genetic testing process: how much counseling is needed? *J Clin Oncol* 18(21 Suppl):60S–4S.

de la Chapelle A, Peltomaki P (1998) The genetics of hereditary common cancers. *Curr Opin Genet Dev* 8:298–303.

Geller G, Botkin JR, Green MJ, Press N, Biesecker BB, Wilfond B, Grana G, Daly MB, Schneider K, Kahn MJ (1997) Genetic testing for susceptibility to adult-onset cancer: the process and content of informed consent. *JAMA* 277:1467–1474.

Giardiello FM, Brensinger JD, Petersen GM, Luce MC, Hylind LM, Bacon JA, Booker SV, Parker RD, Hamilton SR (1997) The use and interpretation of commercial APC gene testing for familial adenomatosis polyposis. *N Engl J Med* 336:823–827.

Hartmann LC, Schaid DJ, Woods JE, Crotty TP, Myers JL, Arnold PG, Petty PM, Sellers TA, Johnson JL, McDonnell SK, Frost MH, Jenkins RB (1999) Efficacy of bilateral prophylactic mastectomy in women with a family history of breast cancer. *N Engl J Med* 340:77–84.

King MC, Hale K, Dalakishvili K, Walsh T, Owens K, Lee M, Tait J, Wieand S, Costantino J, Wickerham, DL, Wolmark N, Fisher B, Ford L (2000) Tamoxifen and breast cancer incidence among women with BRCA1 or BRCA2 mutations: a genomics resequencing project embedded in the breast cancer prevention trial. Presented May 13, 2001, at American Society of Clinical Oncology Annual Meeting.

Meijers-Heijboer H, Bert van Geel B, van Putten LF, Henzen-Logmans SC, Seynaeve C, Menke-Pluymers MBE, van den Ouweland AMW, Niermeijer MF, Brekelmans TM, Klijn JG (2001) Breast cancer after prophylactic bilateral mastectomy in women with a BRCA1 or BRCA2 mutation. *N Engl J Med* 345:159–164.

Modan B, Hartge P, Hirsh-Yechezkel G, Chetrit A, Lubin F, Beller U, Ben-Baruch G, Fishman A, Menczer J, Ebbers SM, Tucker MA, Wacholder S, Struewing JP, Friedman E, Piura B; National Israel Ovarian Cancer Study Group (2001) Parity, oral contraceptives, and the risk of ovarian cancer among carriers and noncarriers of a BRCA1 or BRCA2 mutation. *N Engl J Med* 345:235–240.

Nathanson KL, Weber BL (2001) "Other" breast cancer susceptibility genes: searching for more holy grail. *Hum Mol Genet* 10:715–720.

National Society of Genetic Counselors (1997) Predisposition genetic testing for late-onset disorders in adults *JAMA* 278:1217–1220.

Offit, K (Ed) (1998) *Clinical Cancer Genetics: Risk Counseling and Management.* Wiley-Liss, New York, p. 30.

Olopade OI, Fackenthal JD (2000) Breast cancer genetics: Implications for clinical practice. *Hematol Oncol Clin North Am* 14:705–725.

Phillips KA (2000) Immunophenotypic and pathologic differences between BRCA1 and BRCA2 hereditary breast cancers. *J Clin Oncol* 18(21s):107s–112s.

Ponder BA (2001) Cancer Genetics. *Nature* 411:336–341.

Robson M (2000) Are BRCA1- and BRCCA2-associated breast cancers different? Prognosis of BRCA1-associated breast cancer. *J Clin Oncol* 18(21s):113s–118s.

Rodriguez-Bigas MA, Boland CR, Hamilton SR, Henson DE, Jass JR, Khan PM, Lynch H, Perucho M, Smyrk T, Sobin L, Srivastava S (1997) A National Cancer Institute Workshop on Hereditary Nonpolyposis Colorectal Cancer Syndrome: meeting highlights and Bethesda guidelines. *J Natl Cancer Inst* 89:1758–1762.

Schrag D, Kuntz KM, Garber JE, Weeks JC (1997) Decision analysis—effects of prophylactic mastectomy and oophorectomy on life expectancy among women with BRCA1 or BRCA2 mutations. *N Engl J Med* 336:1465–1471.

Struewing JP, Hartge P, Wacholder S, Baker SM, Berlin M, McAdams M, Timmerman MM, Brody LC, Tucker MA (1997) The risk of cancer associated with specific mutations of BRCA1 and BRCA2 among Ashkenazi Jews. *N Engl J Med* 336:1401–1408.

Vasen HFA (2000) Clinical diagnosis and management of hereditary colorectal cancer syndromes. *J Clin Oncol* 18(21s):81s–92s.

CHAPTER 5

Cancer Epidemiology

SHINE CHANG

Office of Preventive Oncology, Division of Cancer Prevention, National Cancer Institute, National Institutes of Health, Bethesda, Maryland

MELISSA L. BONDY

University of Texas, M. D. Anderson Cancer Center, Department of Epidemiology, Division of Cancer Prevention, Houston, Texas

JAMES G. GURNEY

University of Minnesota, Department of Pediatrics, Division of Pediatric Epidemiology, Minnneapolis, Minnesota

CANCER EPIDEMIOLOGY

This chapter provides an overview of epidemiologic methods, including study designs, potential biases, and statistical measures of effect, with examples from the literature to illustrate the concepts. Information in this chapter should help clinicians and other health professionals better understand the approaches used in epidemiologic research on the causes and consequences of cancer and to interpret and communicate research findings to their patients.

CENTRAL CONCEPTS OF EPIDEMIOLOGY

Epidemiology is a scientific methodology for conducting health-related research and can be defined as the comparative study of the distribution and determinants of disease and other health-related conditions within defined human populations. Distribution of disease refers to the identification, description, and interpretations of the patterns of cancer occurrence, and determinants refers to the factors that may cause or contribute to the occurrence, prevention, control, and outcome of cancer (1,2). Historically, the field of epidemiology focused on identifying and controlling

UICC Manual of Clinical Oncology, Eighth Edition. Edited by Raphael E. Pollock
ISBN 0-471-22289-5 Copyright © 2004 John Wiley & Sons, Inc.

sources of infectious diseases and outbreaks, but now, especially in industrialized countries, the focus includes chronic diseases such as cancer. Epidemiologic studies on smoking and lung cancer in the 1950s were instrumental in developing the study designs and statistical methodologies used today in cancer research. Over the last decade, the field has evolved with contributions from the Human Genome Project, where molecular genetic markers have been incorporated into epidemiologic studies. This new area is called *molecular epidemiology.* Epidemiology incorporates aspects of research from biological, clinical, social, and statistical sciences. Two central concepts of epidemiology are:

1. *Disease is not randomly distributed.* Measurable factors influence the patterns and causes of disease within a defined population.
2. *Disease causation is multifactorial.* Few individual agents are necessary or sufficient to cause disease. Disease results from a multitude of endogenous and exogenous factors. Identifying and measuring the relative contribution and interaction of these factors is the principal role of analytic epidemiology.

SURVEILLANCE AND DESCRIPTIVE STUDIES

Public health surveillance involves the systematic collection, analysis, and interpretation of outcome-specific health data, and timely dissemination to prevent and control disease or injury. Cancer surveillance systems are essential to plan, implement, and evaluate public health practices (3); they provide data on disease incidence and mortality on a population basis for policy makers and researchers. The U.S. National Cancer Institute established the Surveillance, Epidemiology, and End Results (SEER) in 1973, and now includes five state and six large metropolitan cancer registries (http://seer.cancer.gov) (4).

The SEER registry collects cancer incidence information on about 14% of the U.S. population. These data serve as the primary source of our understanding of the distribution of and trends in cancer in the United States. Because SEER ascertains and describes virtually every new case of cancer in its reporting area, these population-based data offer information on the entire spectrum of malignant disease, and is more representative of cancer trends in the United States than data from individual hospitals, which are limited by referral patterns, specialized patient populations, and small case sizes. For epidemiologists, an additional benefit of population-based registries is that, unlike clinical data, researchers can clearly delineate the populations that gave rise to the cases and use them for calculating reliable incidence rates.

Annually, in January, the American Cancer Society publishes its *Cancer Statistics*, available on its website (http://www.cancer.org/). *Cancer Statistics* estimates cancer occurrence in the United States, including the numbers of deaths, new cases, and survival, as well as behaviors that affect risk of developing cancer and use of screening tests. A resource available for international cancer incidence, prevalence, mortality, and survival data is the International Agency for Research on

Cancer (IARC; http://www-dep.iarc.fr/). Several IARC-designed software packages permit online calculation of cancer trends by geographic region, age, and gender. In addition, IARC has available on its website the Automated Childhood Cancer Information Systems, a database of childhood cancer in Europe.

ANALYTIC STUDY DESIGNS

Some epidemiologic studies, such as randomized intervention trials and randomized controlled clinical trials, follow the principles of scientific experimentation in which a treatment or intervention of interest and the control condition are randomly assigned (5). Despite some beliefs to the contrary, well-designed and well-conducted nonexperimental (i.e., observational) studies also can provide accurate estimates of treatment effects (5–7).

Nonexperimental analytic studies assess the causal influence of potential risk factors unable to be evaluated experimentally because the experiment would be unethical or impractical. Thus, epidemiologists must employ several observational study designs to identify causal risk factors and quantify the contribution that the risk factors have on disease incidence on populations with "naturally" occurring exposures. A subtle point is that the exposure must vary enough between study groups to be useful in comparisons. Cohort and case-control studies are two analytic observational approaches commonly employed by epidemiologists.

Cohort Studies

Cohort studies evaluate participants who are initially free of a specific disease of interest and whose exposure status can be classified. Subjects are followed for a defined time period to ascertain endpoints, such as new cases of or death from disease. The disease rate in the exposed group is then compared statistically with the rate in the unexposed group to generate a rate comparison, relative rate ratio (i.e., relative risk), which indicates the increase or reduction in risk associated with the exposure of interest. A prospective cohort study resembles a clinical trial, but subjects are not randomly allocated to an exposure arm. Rather, as mentioned above, exposure (or lack of exposure) occurs "naturally" and the investigator uses variations in natural exposure levels to evaluate differences in the risk of subsequent disease occurrence during some follow-up period.

An example of a notable cohort is the Nurses' Health Study that began in 1976 with over 120,000 U.S. registered nurses. The initial goal of the cohort was to evaluate the effect of oral contraceptives and risk of breast cancer (8). However, since its inception, prospective data from the Nurses' Health Study have provided insights into many health outcomes like heart disease and other types of cancer, in addition to revealing important clues about the role of estrogens and the etiology of breast cancer. The importance of cohort studies is that the participants can be followed over time, which permits efficient study of relatively common diseases with a reasonably short latency period from exposure to disease onset. Cohort studies are usually impractical for rare cancers, as statistically meaningful results could be achieved only by assembling and following a large number of at-risk individuals for a very long time. Cohort studies may be *prospective*, involving active follow-up of subjects in real time or *retrospective*. Retrospective cohort studies use historical records to identify the study population and to reconstruct their exposure and subsequent disease experience.

Case-Control Studies

For relatively rare diseases such as cancers, case-control studies provide a more efficient strategy than cohort studies to evaluate potential causal associations. A cancer case-control study identifies and recruits individuals diagnosed with cancer from a defined population and time period. A similar group of individuals without the disease, but from the same population defined by time period, geographic location, and eligibility criteria that gave rise to the cases, are recruited to serve as the comparison population. The investigators, as completely and accurately as possible, use self-report, health records, and biological specimens to reconstruct the cases' prediagnosis exposure experience. Similarly, a "reference" date, substituting for a diagnosis date, is assigned to each control, whose exposure experience prior to that date is reconstructed. The exposure frequency among the case group is then compared statistically to the exposure frequency among the control group. The resultant statistic, known as an odds ratio (OR), is analogous to a relative risk and is a measure of the strength of the association between the exposure and the disease.

Cluster Investigations

It is not uncommon for clinicians to encounter concerns from patients about multiple cancer occurrences in their community (i.e., a cancer cluster). The implication, of course, is that a shared environmental exposure is responsible for the cluster of cancer cases. Cluster investigations use standard epidemiologic study designs, primarily case-control studies, to ascertain whether or not an unusual number of cancer cases have occurred in a specific area (i.e., spatial cluster) or time period (i.e., temporal cluster) or both (i.e., space-time cluster) (9,10). The latter, for instance, would be an excess of childhood leukemia in a neighborhood or school over a specific time period. Public health agencies have the responsibility to investigate cancer clusters and communicate findings to the public (9). In the United States, clinicians are well advised to refer cluster inquiries to local health departments or the U.S. Centers for Disease Control and Prevention (http://www.cdc.gov or http://www.atsdr.cdc.gov). Such investigations, however, rarely produce evidence that a true cancer cluster exists (11).

MOLECULAR EPIDEMIOLOGY

Classical or traditional epidemiology, as discussed above, permits epidemiologists to evaluate risks and causal roles of environmental factors in cancer. Molecular epidemiology, a hybrid of epidemiology and molecular genetics, enables researchers to assess biological characteristics that may influence cancer susceptibility. The concept that risk of cancer from a given exposure differs between subgroups of a population is known in the epidemiologic vernacular as *effect modification*; biostatisticians often refer to this heterogeneity of effect as *interaction*. With the advent of polymerase chain reactions and other advanced laboratory methods, epidemiologists can incorporate molecular markers into their studies to identify specific suspect endogenous or exogenous host factors at the biochemical or molecular level (12). Such studies aim to determine the roles, including interactions, of environmental and genetic factors in the initiation and progression of the carcinogenic process. The approach of incorporating genetic markers in epidemiologic studies of cancer etiology shows promise for reducing cancer risk and providing strategies for prevention. Molecular epidemiology is certainly accompanied by challenges, however, such as ensuring the appropriate interpretation of molecular testing and resolving associated ethical, legal, and social concerns.

From molecular epidemiology has come the identification of biomarkers that may provide information on the extent of exposure to carcinogens. Perera and Weinstein (13) delineated four categories of biomarkers that help predict risk: internal dose, biologically effective dose, response, and susceptibility. Biomarkers represent a valuable research tool for detecting early changes caused by exposures, and they identify individuals with particularly high risk of cancer development. Describing and determining the occurrence of suitably selected biomarkers has led to tremendous progress in research on the mechanisms of cancer initiation and promotion, and has begun to make possible the assessment of cancer risk in healthy individuals. The knowledge that gene defects (e.g., gene mutations and changes in their expression) underlie carcinogenesis has resulted in focused efforts to detect such aberrant genes and their associated proteins.

The addition of molecular parameters to population-based studies should help identify genes and pathways involved in cancer development due to environmental exposures and to identify susceptible or resistant subpopulations. In turn, information about molecular mechanisms of carcinogenesis should improve risk assessment. The exponential growth of scientific technology and information promises rapid future expansion of knowledge about identity of potential genes and cancer pathways.

Current studies of molecular epidemiology are based upon an understanding of the complex, multistage process of carcinogenesis and heterogeneous responses to carcinogenic exposures. Quantitative methods to measure human exposures to carcinogens improve continuously and have been successfully applied in a number of epidemiological studies. Genetic predispositions to cancer, both inherited and acquired, have been, and continue to be, identified. The combined approach of correlating inherited genetic polymorphisms with other cancer risk factors is showing considerable promise. For instance, this type of study illustrates the hope that, in the future, molecular epidemiologists will be able to develop an individual's risk profile for specific diseases, including assessment of multiple biomarkers. The field has the near-term potential to have a significant impact on regulatory quantitative risk assessments, which may aid in the determination of allowable exposures. Molecular epidemiological data may also aid in the identification of individuals who will benefit most by cancer prevention strategies.

Investigators who conduct molecular epidemiology studies employ traditional designs, including case-control and cohort studies, with inclusion of one or more biological markers to determine exposure associations with disease outcome. Scientists agree that chronic diseases, including cancer, likely result from gene-environment interactions. In fact, some researchers have said that "genetics is the loaded gun, and the environment pulls the trigger." Many are concerned about the question of nature versus nurture, and how to evaluate the contribution of each component. A recent large study of twins, although statistically limited, concluded that environment plays a substantial role in causing sporadic cancers, but still requires genetic potential for cancer to occur (14).

Methodological challenges of epidemiological studies, as described below, such as accurate measurement of disease and exposure, appropriate selection and recruitment of study samples, reducing the influence of potential competing risk factors (i.e., confounders), and optimizing precision of effect measures, also apply to studies in the rapidly growing and promising field of molecular epidemiology. A serious concern lies with assuring an adequate sample size for study. Often, the prevalence of a genetic polymorphism or other biomarker is either quite low or quite high. Hence, the number of cases required to detect an association tends to be very large. Because cancers are relatively rare, it is often necessary to combine data from several studies to obtain adequate statistical power to draw meaningful conclusions. All of these issues speak to the need for investigators to exercise caution when interpreting their study data and discussing the implications of their results (15).

BIAS AND ITS CONTROL IN EPIDEMIOLOGICAL STUDIES

To varying degrees, all human studies are susceptible to bias, that is, producing inaccurate measures of the effect of a treatment or exposure on disease. An important goal of any study is to make every effort feasible to minimize the effect of bias.

Three general types of bias can occur: (1) confounding bias, when an extraneous factor distorts (increases or decreases) the true magnitude of the exposure-disease association; (2) information (misclassification) bias, when information collected on exposure, treatment, disease, or other study factors is inaccurate or incomplete; and (3) selection bias, when subjects who are sampled, recruited, enrolled, and complete the study are unrepresentative of the population at risk, in that they inaccurately reflect the exposure-disease relation in the population of interest (i.e., target population).

Confounding Bias

In clinical trials, investigators use randomization to reduce the probability that an extraneous factor will cause bias in the results because such "nuisance" factors should be randomly and evenly distributed among treatment groups. Absent randomization, however, confounding is a potential threat to the validity of results derived from observational studies. For a factor to exert a confounding influence it must be associated with, or a marker for, the disease of interest and it must occur at a differing frequency between the exposure (or treatment) groups. When these two conditions hold, the extraneous factor may bias the exposure-disease association.

Statistical methods to correct (i.e., control, adjust for) confounding, such as pooled stratified analysis or multivariate regression analysis, are at hand, but effective only if data on the potentially confounding variables are collected and accurate. Thus, for statistical analysis, observational studies often collect data on many factors that are not directly related to the cause-effect relation being investigated. Design strategies can also minimize or eliminate confounding. For example, a study of asbestos exposure and lung cancer could avoid confounding from smoking status by recruiting only nonsmokers.

Information Bias

The most important threat to the validity of epidemiologic research of cancer is inaccurate or incomplete information on study participants' exposure relevant to etiology. It is usually impossible, especially in retrospective studies, to directly measure exposure dose and duration during a time that is thought to be biologically relevant to cancer initiation. As such, indirect or surrogate measures of exposure are used in lieu of direct measures. For instance, a proxy for blood levels of cotinine, a biomarker of tobacco use, could be self-reported recall of smoking behavior. Such proxy measures may usefully approximate real exposure, but can provide only imprecise information on dose, duration, and exposure time period. When exposure measures are equally inaccurate between study groups (i.e., nondifferential error), the cause-effect relation may be attenuated or completely obscured. Nondifferential misclassification of exposure has no doubt been one reason why few environmental agents have been firmly established as known risk factors for cancer.

Differential information bias occurs when the accuracy and completeness of exposure information differs between comparison groups. Recall bias in case-control studies, for example, can occur when cases remember exposures differently than controls. For example, cases may be more likely to accurately report relatives having a disease of interest compared with controls, leading to an underestimation of positive family history in the control families and thus a biased estimate of the effect of family history. From a practical standpoint, however, some investigators suggest that recall bias may be more theoretical than factual (16).

Selection Bias

Because all human studies include some element of sampling from larger populations of interest (i.e., target populations), selection bias is a potential source of error. Selection bias occurs when exposure or disease frequency among study participants is unrepresentative of the target population. Case-control studies are susceptible to this bias because it is difficult to identify and recruit controls who provide an accurate accounting of baseline exposure frequency in the population that gave rise to the cases. Cohort studies and randomized trials, on the other hand, are susceptible to selection bias from attrition. If participants who are lost during the follow-up period represent a different outcome experience than those who remain in the study to completion, the final results may be biased. For this reason, great effort must be expended in prospective studies to assure the most complete follow-up possible of study participants.

Epidemiologic studies strive to provide the most accurate and precise risk estimate of an exposure-disease association. Criteria commonly used to evaluate study results and to help guide judgments on the likelihood that an association is indeed causal and not merely a random or chance finding (i.e., statistical), include:

1. *Strength of the exposure-disease association.* Large relative risks are less likely than small relative risks to result from chance or uncontrolled confounding (although this does not preclude other sources of error).
2. *Temporal relation between exposure and disease onset.* Studies are stronger when they can establish that the exposure appropriately preceded the biological onset of disease.
3. *Biological coherence.* When a plausible biological mechanism and/or when experimental evidence from animal studies supports the hypothesized relation, there is greater confidence in the observed relation.
4. *Dose response gradient.* If exposure intensity or duration is associated with increased disease frequency when it is hypothesized that such a dose gradient should exist, the results appear more coherent and believable.
5. *Consistency of results within and across studies.* If multiple reports evaluating the same type of exposure show similar effects, and/or if multiple studies using different target populations and study designs report consistent results, there is greater evidence to favor a true relation.

These concepts, which are widely applied, were originally derived from two papers by Sir Austin Bradford Hill, recently reprinted in a monograph on philosophy and epidemiologic reasoning in causal inference (17).

STATISTICAL MEASURES IN EPIDEMIOLOGY

Epidemiologic analyses generally focus on estimating effect measures, the strength or magnitude of an exposure-disease association, rather than statistical hypothesis testing using a *P* value (2). *P* values provide a measure of probability for observing the study results, or results more extreme than those observed, if indeed no true association exists. *P* values provide no direct information, however, on the strength, direction, or precision of an effect measure. Nor do *P* values supply information on the extent to which an association (or lack of an association) can be explained by confounding or other bias.

Effect measures for dichotomous outcomes, such as disease occurrence versus no disease, are often estimated using one of several ratio measures of the *relative risk* (2,16). In a cohort study, where disease rates can be directly calculated, the ratio of the incidence rate of a cancer among those exposed to an agent can be compared with the rate of the specific cancer type among those not so exposed. The ratio is 1 : 1 if the rates are the same in the two comparison groups, a relative risk of 1.0, suggesting no association between exposure and disease. If the exposed group has a higher incidence rate than the unexposed group, the ratio will be larger than 1, suggesting an excess risk due to exposure. If the rate is lower in the exposed compared with the unexposed groups, the ratio will be less than 1, suggesting a protective effect from exposure. The further the effect measure is away from the "null" value of 1.0 in either direction, the stronger the association. Notice that a relative risk of 2.0 (2-fold increased risk compared with the reference group) is equivalent in strength to a relative risk of 0.5 (half the risk of the reference group). In case-control studies, incidence rates of disease cannot be calculated directly. Thus, exposure frequencies are compared between diseased groups and comparable nondiseased groups. The resultant *odds ratio* is an effect measure on a ratio scale and, as mentioned previously, is functionally equivalent to a relative risk. Other types of ratio-based relative risks are rate ratios, hazard ratios, standardized mortality ratios (SMR), standardized incidence ratios (SIR), and proportional mortality ratios.

Confidence intervals are used to measure the precision of an effect measure, like relative risks and odds ratios. Like *P* values, confidence intervals are functions of the variability of the data and the size of the sample. Roughly speaking, a confidence interval provides a likely range in which the true effect measure lies within some level of confidence (often calculated as a 95% confidence interval).

Relative risks are important to help judge whether an association is causal, and to estimate the degree to which risk of disease is increased (or decreased) by exposure. Relative risks, however, do not measure the "absolute" risk from exposure. In other words, a relative risk does not measure the number of excess cancers that are likely to be caused by an exposure.

Attributable risk measures provide estimates of the actual rate (or number, or percentage) of cases "due to" exposure, assuming there is a causal relation (17). Thus, attributable risks indicate the proportion of the disease preventable, if the exposure were removed from the population at risk. Estimating attributable risk for specific exposures is used to understand the importance of that exposure in a larger public health context.

THE GLOBAL CANCER BURDEN

Estimates of the global cancer burden have been made for 1975, 1980, 1985, and 2000 (18). These estimates are for all forms of cancer but specifically exclude nonmelanoma skin cancer, which is poorly registered on incidence statistics and only infrequently fatal. In men, there were an estimated 5.3 million new cases diagnosed in 2000, an increase of 1.5 million incident cases diagnosed in 1985. As for mortality worldwide, there were 4.7 million cancer deaths among men. Lung cancer is the most common form of cancer in men, with an estimated 902,000 new cases in 2000 (18). The estimated number of cases of lung cancer increased 35% over the 5-year period from 1995 to 2000. Other forms of cancer that have increased notably are colorectal cancer, prostate cancer, bladder cancer, melanoma, and lymphoma, particularly non-Hodgkin's lymphoma. Although some of these increases could be due to better surveillance or poor precision in the estimation of rates, there may well be a real etiologic component to the trends.

In women, it was estimated that there were 4.7 million new cases of cancer in 2000, an increase of almost a million new cases over the estimate for 1995. Breast cancer is the most common form of cancer in women, with an estimated 1 million new cases in 2000, an increase of 94% over the last 25 years. A similar increase has taken place in oral cavity cancers, colorectal cancers, and lymphomas. However, the largest relative increase of cancer in women has been in lung cancer, which increased from 126,700 new cases in 1975 to 337,000 in 2000, an increase of 266% (not accounting for population changes). This can almost entirely be explained by changes in smoking patterns in women in many parts of the world (18).

The estimated number of new cases of cancer worldwide increased from 5.9 million in 1975, to 6.4 million in 1980, to 7.6 million in 1985 (18). Assuming that the age-specific rates remain constant at the 1985 levels, it was estimated that there were 8.4 million new cases in 1990 and would be 10.3 million new cases in the year 2000. It could be deduced that the number of new cases of cancer worldwide would have doubled between 1970 and 2000. Beyond 2000, the absolute numbers of cases of cancer will likely increase as the post-World War II "baby boom" generation reaches ages at which the age-specific rates of cancer start to increase. In many countries, this generation is the first whose numbers were not reduced by a great war and the first to have benefited from the advances in medical care and treatment witnessed in the second half of this century. Most members of this generation are still alive at age 50 compared with the same situation in many countries for the preceding generations.

GEOGRAPHIC AND TEMPORAL VARIATION IN CANCER RISK

The importance of acknowledging the large international variation in cancer occurrence throughout the world has led to the designation of initial observations on cancer epidemiology as geographical pathology. There are still many interesting aspects to the geographic epidemiology of different forms of cancer worldwide. Descriptive studies are important in epidemiology to determine the rate of disease in different groups. We have learned a great deal from migrant studies, as well as ecologic studies where exposure and disease can be evaluated on a population level rather than an individual level. For example, when the exposure is fairly common (e.g., smoking, sunlight exposure, dietary fat intake), one can look at these exposures nationally and plot them against the incidence of the disease in that nation. If one plots dietary fat consumption by country with the incidence of breast cancer, one might find evidence for an increased rate of breast cancer in countries with high dietary fat intake. This association might not be causal, but provides hypothesis-generating data for further investigations (8).

Another type of comparison that can be used for hypothesis-generating studies are from data generated through cancer mapping. Geographic variation can be seen from cancer mortality or incidence maps using computer generated mapping programs, a strategy where small areas (e.g., county level) might show spatial clusters of common tumor types. The NCI has published an atlas of cancer mortality maps at the county and state level for two time periods. These data and maps can be found on the NCI website (http://seer.cancer.gov). These cancer maps uncovered high oral cancer rates among women in the United States in the rural South and prompted investigators to conduct cases-control studies. North Carolina researchers identified an excess of cases associated with the long-standing practice of snuff-dipping, which led to a smokeless tobacco prevention program.

CANCER RISK FACTORS

Epidemiology provides compelling evidence that a large proportion of human cancer may be avoidable. Different populations throughout the world experience different levels of different forms of cancer and these levels change with time. Groups of immigrants acquire the cancer pattern of their new home, sometimes within decades (as demonstrated by immigrants to Australia) or sometimes requiring generations, as in the case of breast cancer in Japanese immigrants to the United States. Further, groups of individuals in a community with some characteristic that differentiates them from other members of the same community (such as Seventh Day Adventists, Mormons, African Americans in parts of the United States, etc.) have markedly different cancer patterns. Partly from evidence such as this, the environmental theory of carcinogenesis has developed, and it is held by many that upwards of 80–90% of cancer may be attributable to environmental factors (19). "Environment" is broadly defined to include a wide range of lifestyle factors including dietary, social, and cultural practices.

Therefore, in theory, the majority of cancers diagnosed each year may be avoidable, but specific avoidable causes of many common cancers have not yet been clearly identified, nor how risk factors may work in combination. A prerequisite of cancer prevention lies in identifying the determinants of cancer risk. Cancer control embraces a number of important elements with the aim of reducing the incidence of cancer and, failing primary prevention, reducing morbidity and mortality either by finding disease at an earlier and more curable stage, or by improving survival through improvements in therapy. A number of disciplines are involved in this pursuit, including epidemiology, clinical science, behavioral science, and health education and communication.

TOBACCO

Tobacco smoking remains the largest single avoidable cause of premature death world wide and is the single most important human carcinogen (20). It is estimated that at least 16% of all cancers in developed countries are related to tobacco use, with a higher proportion of tobacco-related cancers among men (25%) than women (4%). Cancers that have been linked to tobacco use include those of the oral cavity, pharynx, larynx, lung, bladder, pancreas, kidney, renal pelvis, and endometrium. However, for endometrial cancer, reduced risk, rather than increased risk, is thought to result from antiestrogenic effects of tobacco use rather than exposure to the more than 55 carcinogenic compounds identified by the International Agency for Research on Cancer (21). For more than 40 years, it has been clear that prevention of smoking would lead to substantial reductions in death associated with lung and other cancers, but also with heart disease, bronchitis, emphysema, and a number of other conditions. Despite this knowledge, the problem of tobacco-related disease has increased in many parts of the world. It is estimated that 1.1 billion people smoke daily, the majority of whom (80%) live in developing countries where tobacco use started within the past 30 years, more recently than in industrialized countries.

The mechanisms that influence addiction to tobacco are complex. Since the 1950s, manufacturers have sought to reduce cigarette levels of tar and nicotine, the component that drives addiction and smoking behaviors. As suggested by reports of associations between smoking quit-rates and specific polymorphisms in the dopamine receptor gene (DRD2) (22), a key receptor in the mesolimbic dopaminergic reward system, the genetic susceptibility of individuals to tobacco addiction varies considerably. Just as multiple factors affect behavior, susceptibility to tobacco-related cancers is also likely to vary under the influence of multiple factors, which helps explain why not all tobacco users get cancer.

Gender and ethnicity are important risk factors, as women relative to men and African Americans compared with white Americans appear to have higher risk of bladder cancer associated with tobacco use. Age is also an important factor, as the majority of smokers initiate during their teenage and early adult years. Smokers who start earlier tend not to quit and to smoke more heavily, putting themselves at higher risk. Synergistic effects with tobacco use have been observed with asbestos and crystalline silica in occupational settings, and with alcohol, as alcohol acting as a solvent may facilitate absorption of tobacco products. Much evidence suggests that diets, particularly those high in the intake of fruits and vegetables, may impede the formation of smoking-related DNA adducts, reduce the DNA damage from tobacco carcinogens, and promote other anticarcinogenic mechanisms that prevent cellular damage and reduce risk.

In the past decade, tobacco research has come to include the evaluation of exposure to environmental (passive) tobacco smoke and a diversity of adverse health events, including lung cancer. On the basis of 30 epidemiologic studies, the United States Environmental Protection Agency (EPA) concluded that environmental tobacco smoke was a human lung carcinogen and the body of evidence is increasing for greater risk of lung cancer in nonsmokers who are exposed to environmental tobacco smoke (23). Environmental tobacco smoke tends to have more carcinogens than smoke inhaled through filters but is diluted with ambient air. However, the focus on passive smoke inhalation in epidemiologic research and health policy in Western countries cannot be allowed to divert attention from the major public health issue of active cigarette smoking: smokers are at much higher risk of cancer than those who involuntarily inhale some of their cigarette smoke. In any program of cancer control, top priority should be given to control of tobacco; this is likely to have the greatest impact on reducing cancer incidence, and cancer mortality, than any other strategy currently known.

VIRUSES AND INFECTION

The contribution of viruses to the public health burden of cancer incidence is greatest in young to middle age individuals, with the age-incidence curve peaks before middle age (24). It has been estimated that the attributable risk associated with viruses and cancer is about 15%, second only to tobacco use (25). There is now strong evidence that human papilloma virus (HPV) is causally related to an increased risk of cervix cancer in women, that Epstein-Barr virus (EBV) is causally related to an increased risk of nasopharyngeal cancer and Burkitt's lymphoma, that human T-lymphotropic virus type 1 (HTLV-1) is causally related to adult T-cell leukemia and some types of non-Hodgkin's lymphoma, that hepatitis B is causally related to an increased risk of primary liver cancer, and that human immunodeficiency virus (HIV) infection is causally related to Kaposi's sarcoma and some forms of non-Hodgkin's lymphoma (25).

Long latency periods between infection and cancer diagnosis and the fact that only a portion of the infected develop cancer suggest that viral agents may increase the risk of individuals for developing cancer but are not the sole determinant for developing the disease. Great geographic variation in both infection rates and the rates of viral-related cancer worldwide suggest that much infection-related cancer could be prevented by control of viral infection. This is no trivial matter, as infection rates are high in many parts of the world and the types of cancers associated with viral infection often have poor prognosis and few successful treatment options. Obviously, effective vaccination programs against these viral infections, such as that now available for hepatitis B, would have a considerable impact on reducing the global burden of these forms of cancer.

In addition to infection from viral agents, bacterial infection has also been linked to cancer risk in the example of *Helicobacter pylori* (*H. pylori*) infection and increased risk of gastric cancer, one of the most common cancers worldwide (26). Incidence rates of gastric cancer vary geographically, particularly for the intestinal type, which is typically accompanied by chronic atrophic gastritis and intestinal metaplasia. Both chronic atrophic gastritis and intestinal metaplasia, possible precursors to gastric cancer, are thought to result from *H. pylori* infection, suggesting an important role for *H. pylori* infection in gastric carcinogenesis.

Other evidence comes from epidemiologic investigations, linking areas with high rates of *H. pylori* infection to regions with high rates of gastric cancer. Risk factors for *H. pylori* infection are associated more with socioeconomic factors like overcrowding, family size, and bed sharing, than with ethnicity, and no consistent associations have been demonstrated for lifestyle behaviors, like smoking, tobacco use, or diet. Although the association between *H. pylori* infection and gastric cancer is complex, evidence continues to build, necessitating greater efforts to control and reduce *H. pylori* infection as a means to reduce cancer risk, particularly among children, for whom infection rates are high and nearly 100% by adulthood in areas of high infection rates. Thus, control of *H. pylori* infection, as well as other infectious agents associated with cancer risk, is well warranted.

SUNLIGHT EXPOSURE

Exposure to sunlight has been well established as the major agent in the development of skin cancer, particularly solar ultraviolet (UV) A and B wavelengths. Exposure to UVA can result in DNA base damage, strand breaks, and DNA-protein cross-links, whereas exposure of DNA to UVB mainly results in dimerizations between adjacent pyrimidines, which may predispose for *p53* mutation hotspots (27). Such knowledge of the underlying molecular mechanisms for sunlight's role in skin carcinogenesis contributes to efforts in prevention and control in human populations, but other information is necessary for successful public health interventions.

In the past decade, a rapid rise in the worldwide incidence of skin cancer is hypothesized to result in part from the migration of Caucasian populations to areas for which their skin is not adapted. This hypothesis is supported by several reports linking skin cancer incidence with solar radiation at different geographical latitudes (28), where locales with greater annual sun exposure tend to have higher incidence of skin cancer. In general, human skin can be categorized by two characteristics, its susceptibility to sunburns and its ability to tan without burning, that together correlate with susceptibility to skin cancer (29). However, many other factors also contribute to skin cancer risk, such as age at exposure, ethnicity, skin color, lifestyle, occupation, and individual genetic susceptibility.

Although sunlight is a major risk factor in general, important differences between the subtypes of skin cancer suggest differences in carcinogenic pathways. There are three main types of skin cancer: squamous cell cancer (SCC), which develops from stem cells in the follicular and interfollicular region of the dermis; basal cell carcinoma (BCC), which arises from basal cells in the skin and follicular infundibulum; and melanoma, which develops mainly from melanocytic nevi. For BCC, the most common form of human skin cancer worldwide, most lesions develop on the face. However, nearly a third of BCC lesions occur on skin that is typically protected from the sun, and it rarely appears on sun-exposed sites like the forearms and the backs of hands, as SCC does. Some research suggests that exposure during childhood and adolescence, both intermittent sun exposure and severe sun burns, predisposes for adult BCC (30) and melanoma (31), whereas adult sunlight exposure tends to be associated with SCC risk.

Melanoma incidence has increased worldwide over the past 30 years, particularly for lesions appearing on women's legs and men's torsos, where sunlight exposure tends to be more intermittent. By far, melanoma is the rarest type of skin cancer, but its mortality rates can be high without early detection and treatment. Such efforts can be directed towards groups at high risk, such as those with pale skin, red or blond hair, who freckle easily, particularly those with higher numbers of nevi from sun exposure during childhood.

Two major hypotheses have emerged to explain variation in skin cancer incidence related to sun exposure: first, that the pattern of exposure (i.e., intermittent or steady) and total accumulated exposure contribute to risk independently; and second, that exposure before age 10 years strongly determines lifetime risk, although sun exposure in adulthood may influence the manifestation of outright cancer. The strongest support for the importance of childhood sun exposure comes from studies of risk of skin cancer associated with age of immigration to Australia, where early age at immigration predicts increased risk (32). Also, intermittent sun exposure with sunburn in childhood has been associated with increased BCC risk later in life. Complementary to those findings, other research suggests that adult exposures may help promote skin carcinogenesis through response to short term exposure to sunlight.

The main factor responsible for the dramatic increases in skin cancer rates is generally held to be the increased levels of recreational sun exposure (as during sunbathing sessions or outdoor recreational activities) that has taken place as a result of the economic improvement of many white communities. Since 1980, the suntanning fashion has fostered the large-scale marketing of sunbeds (33). In 1995, nearly half of Swedish women 15–35 years old reported regular exposure to sunbeds (34). Repeated exposure to sunbeds is suspected to increase the risk of both melanoma and nonmelanoma skin cancers, but further studies are needed to correctly assess the magnitude of risk associated with the so-called "UVA suntanning" (35). The important message is to avoid overexposure to sunlight and, in particular, to avoid sunburns at all times and to be particularly careful to protect children (36). There have been several very effective campaigns, especially in Australia and New Zealand, where sun exposure can be intense and of high annual duration, suggesting the possibility of achieving population-wide success in skin cancer prevention and control.

DIET

Diet and nutritional factors became the focus of serious attention in the etiology of cancer from the 1940s onward (37). Initially dealing with the effect of feeding specific diets to animals receiving chemical carcinogens, research turned to the potential of associations with human cancer risk. This was conducted through international comparisons of estimated national per capita food intake data with cancer mortality rates. Strong correlations were consistently reported from these data, particularly between higher dietary fat intake and increased rates of breast cancer (38). As dietary assessment methods improved, and certain methodologic difficulties were identified and overcome, the science of nutritional epidemiology emerged (39).

Initially, the focus of attention in human studies has largely been centered on associations with fat intake and the intake of vitamins in the diet. As the complexity of the association with cancer for fats and fatty acids has unfolded, research interest has broadened to include other foods and food components. In general, high consumption of fruits and vegetables is associated with a reduced risk of a number of forms of cancer, including leukemia, lung, oral, pancreatic, laryngeal, esophageal, bladder, and gastric cancer. The major exceptions have been the lack of strong association with hormonally related forms of cancer such as those of the prostate, breast, ovary, and endometrium (40). Reduced risk associated with consumption of dark green, leafy vegetables and red and yellow fruits and vegetables that have high levels of micronutrients thought to have antioxidant and other anticarcinogenic properties has identified several food components that are of interest. Compounds like phytoestrogens found in soybean products and lycopene and other carotenoids found in high concentrations in tomatoes and other fruits and vegetables have been featured in a number of recent studies and more interest has developed toward testing these food compounds as chemopreventive agents in prevention trials (41,42). However, not only are the micronutrient compounds in foods piquing interest, but how foods may be metabolized (e.g., glycemic index) and how food is prepared (e.g., grilled meats) have become suspect as well. Thus, the interest surrounding the potential for diet and nutrition to play a key role in determining cancer risk has grown tremendously since the last century and is flourishing at a rapid pace.

ALCOHOL CONSUMPTION

The strongest evidence of a direct causal role for alcohol consumption in carcinogenesis comes chiefly from investigations of cancers of the oral cavity, pharynx, larynx, and esophagus (43). To assess alcohol's effect independently from the strong confounding effect of tobacco use, the most important risk factor for these cancers, studies have evaluated risk associated with alcohol consumption among groups of nonsmokers, although carefully conducted studies among smokers suggest a synergistic effect for alcohol consumption linked to tobacco use (44). Another confounding factor commonly associated with alcohol consumption is poor diet, particularly diets low in fruit and vegetable consumption. Such modification of alcohol's effect on cancer risk suggests the importance of antioxidant or other anticancer properties contained in fruits and vegetables, such as vitamin A, which is depleted from liver stores by alcohol.

For risk of liver cancer, evidence exists for a modest effect of alcohol in general. However, risk appears to be synergistically enhanced by viral hepatitis infection. As for whether alcohol-induced liver cirrhosis also increases risk of liver cancer, the literature is not clear because not all alcoholics with liver cancer have cirrhosis. Problems of epidemiologic studies that rely on data from heavy consumers of alcohol include underreporting of intake by alcoholics and the differences between alcoholics and the majority of people consuming alcohol, but it is plausible that heavy drinkers, but not moderate consumers, may consume the quantities of alcohol necessary to demonstrate an association with liver cancer.

A number of investigations suggest a role for alcohol in the development of pancreatic and colon cancers, as well as hormonally responsive cancers of the breast and prostate. However, in contrast to cancers of the oral cavity, pharynx, larynx, and esophagus, the mechanistic pathways for alcohol may be different for breast and prostate cancer (45). Both acute and chronic intake have been shown to increase circulating estrogens and to decrease circulating androgens in both men and women, which is consistent with the increased breast cancer risk observed for higher consumption of alcohol (46). However, only heavy alcohol intake, not moderate consumption, has been associated with increased prostate cancer risk, suggesting an alternative pathway than the putative increased androgen exposure mechanism. In general, the influence of the type of alcohol consumed remains unclear. Mouthwash with more than 25% alcohol has been associated with higher risk of mouth cancer and studies for some cancers suggest that distilled liquors may have more potent effects than other types of alcohol. Other studies suggest that other compounds in alcoholic beverages may modify alcohol's carcinogenic effects. Ethyl carbamate and acetaldehyde, a by-product of alcohol metabolism, are both carcinogens in animals. Conversely, a compound in wine and beer that has received much recent attention for several of its anticarcinogenic properties is resveratrol (47), found in high concentrations in grape skins. Although high consumption of alcohol is clearly not recommended in regards to cancer risk, it remains unresolved whether more moderate consumption increases risk sufficiently to cause concern.

OBESITY

Several large-scale prospective studies assessing the long-term effects of obesity have shown that obesity increases the risk of developing some forms of cancer. An American Cancer Society study described the pattern of mortality related to relative weight for 900,000 subjects followed for 21 years (48). Larger body size was associated with higher mortality from cancer of the liver, gallbladder, pancreas, kidney, esophagus, colon and rectum, non-Hodgkin's lymphoma, and multiple myeloma. Obese women also had an increased risk of cancer of the cervix, ovary, uterus, and breast, whereas obese men had an increased risk of stomach and prostate cancer. The Danish Record-Linkage Study compared a cohort of nearly 44,000 obese persons with the Danish population as a whole and found that the cohort had an increased incidence of cancers of the esophagus, liver, pancreas, colon, prostate, and kidney (49). More recent studies indicate a clear association among women between obesity and the increased risk of endometrial, renal cell, gallbladder, and colorectal cancer. Among men, obesity may be associated with greater risk of colon cancer, renal cell cancer, gallbladder cancer, and esophageal and gastric cardia adenocarcinoma. Lung cancer is the one neoplasm that the obese may be less prone to develop than leaner individuals, possibly because of smoking-related effects on resting energy expenditure, although some have argued that residual confounding by smoking or weight loss due to presymptomatic disease may bias reported findings. The relationship between breast cancer and obesity is less clear. Among postmenopausal women, the obese have a greater risk of breast cancer than their leaner counterparts, whereas among premenopausal women, the obese appear to experience modest protection from breast cancer compared to leaner women (50). For postmenopausal women, the effect of obesity and breast cancer risk appears to be greater among those who have never used hormone replacement therapy, supporting the hypothesis that in the absence of ovarian sources of estrogens, increased risk is derived from excess estrogen converted from adrenal hormones in the fat tissue of heavier women.

For prostate cancer, although some have reported increased risk associated with tallness, no strong relationship for either risk or mortality has been consistently demonstrated with adult obesity, usually measured as body mass index (BMI) ≥ 30 kg/m^2. Typically, the components of BMI, height and weight, are easy to recall accurately, easy and inexpensive to measure, and are generally recorded in a variety of documents, all considerations for conducting research in large populations. For these reasons, BMI is the most widely used measure of body composition in epidemiological studies and serves as the basis for the National Heart, Lung, and Blood Institute/National Institutes of Health and World Health Organization clinical definitions for underweight, normal, overweight, and obesity (51,52). However, using BMI to quantify obesity and body composition is inherently limited. People with vastly different height and weight can have the same BMI. BMI is correlated with both lean mass and fat mass. BMI also provides no information about the ratio of lean to fat mass or about body fat distribution, which has metabolic implications for steroid hormone balance. Thus, it is possible that characterizing body composition using only BMI may mask associations between carcinogenesis and specific components of obesity.

Other measures of body composition, particularly the ratio of waist and hip circumferences and skin-fold thickness, have also been used in epidemiologic research. Ratio measures must be interpreted carefully within the context of underlying body size distributions of the study sample, whereas assessing body composition using skin-fold thicknesses requires special training for accurate measurement. Recent work identifying hormones, growth factors, and cytokines that are associated with specific components of body composition present new opportunities for better mechanistic investigations. Overall, although the mechanisms underlying the obesity-carcinogenesis relationship are not fully understood, they are likely to be highly complex, as both obesity and cancer are multifactorial diseases involving many genetic pathways.

PHYSICAL ACTIVITY

The most consistent evidence supporting a role for physical activity in the prevention of cancer comes from studies of colon cancer. As reviewed by Colditz et al. (53), nine of nine case-control studies and six of seven cohort studies consistently reported significantly reduced risk of colon cancer due to physical activity independent of BMI effects and across different populations. In general, a dose-response pattern exists for levels of physical activity increasing by either intensity, frequency, or duration resulting in greater risk reduction for colon cancer risk. Hypothesized mechanisms include reduced exposure time to carcinogens passing through the gut in people who exercise, as exercise increases gut motility and reduces bowel transit time. For breast cancer, rapidly emerging support comes from epidemiologic studies in the United States, Asia, and Europe as reviewed by McTiernan et al. (54) for a protective effect of physical activity among both premenopausal and postmenopausal women measured at different times during the lifecycle and at different levels of intensity. Likewise, but among far fewer studies than for either colon or breast cancer, a pattern is surfacing for reduced risk of endometrial cancer associated with physical activity among both premenopausal and postmenopausal women. Other investigations report protective effects associated with physical activity for both prostate cancer and testicular cancer, albeit less consistently than that of colon and breast cancer.

For colon, breast, and endometrial cancers, the impact on cancer risk of physical activity may be influenced directly from biochemical factors important in the carcinogenic pathway (e.g., growth factors, hormones, immune function) and indirectly through obesity prevention and control. Physical activity lowers levels of insulin, glucose, and triglycerides, and raises HDL cholesterol, which may protect against proliferation of colon and breast cancer lesions. Exercise appears to increase the number and/or the activity of macrophages, natural killer cells, and their regulating cytokines, although epidemiological data on immune function are limited. Physical activity may also prevent cancer indirectly by producing physiological changes in hormone profiles that are thought to influence tumorigenesis. High levels of exercise delay menarche and reduce the number of ovulatory cycles, thereby reducing lifetime exposure to endogenous estrogen and consequently reduce the risk for estrogen-dependent cancers (55). Exercise may also reduce the risk of hormone-dependent cancers by increasing the production of sex hormone binding globulin (SHBG) in men and women, lowering levels of circulating bioavailable testosterone and estradiol.

Epidemiological research on physical activity has been limited in past by poor quantification, although more recent studies have improved efforts to capture at a minimum the intensity level of physical activities, as well as the frequency and duration of time spent doing physical activities. Data on the types of activities can also be used to calculate metabolic values associated with specific activities based on standardized expenditure values. Other approaches have attempted to use more direct measurement devices or even biological markers, like doubly labeled water, to quantify physical activity. Ultimately, because it is a modifiable lifestyle factor, physical activity holds great promise for a large positive impact on public health overall, in addition to reducing cancer incidence.

OCCUPATIONAL EXPOSURES

Occupational exposures have been estimated to account for approximately 4% of all cancers (56). To date, many occupational risk factors for cancer have been identified through epidemiological research, particularly the identification of chemicals commonly used in industrial settings that have been shown to be carcinogenic to humans. The most comprehensive source of occupational exposures associated with cancer is maintained in a series of monographs published by the International Agency for Research on Cancer. Another useful resource is the annual report on carcinogens published by the U.S. National Toxicology Program. These compiled reports reflect a considerable body of work conducted by scientific researchers in a number of disciplines, including toxicology, cancer biology, and epidemiology.

Epidemiological studies, including retrospective cohort and nested case-control studies, have been used to identify increased cancer risk associated with single occupational exposures, particularly when the exposure-disease relationships are clear (57), as for benzene exposure in rubber hydrochloride workers. Development of rare histopathologic types of cancer in occupational settings has also revealed occupational carcinogens. One example is the development in studies of workers exposed to vinyl chloride of angiosarcoma of the liver (58), a rare (<1% of all hepatic cancers) subtype of hepatic cancers. More difficult to characterize are occupational carcinogens that are mixtures, because individual components of mixtures may be hard to identify. Exposure assessment methods may not be available, and exposure duration may be short, transient, or both. Measuring solvent exposure accurately in occupational settings may be a challenge, as concentrations of individual components may vary considerably between exposure episodes (59). These issues have impeded research on the relationships between cutting and lubricating oils and bladder cancer, the most common occupational cancer, and between diesel exhaust and lung cancer, the second most common occupationally related cancer. Other useful research has resulted from the evaluation of large occupational cohorts, like farmers, laundry and dry cleaning workers, and painters. However, cohort studies require long follow-up for development of disease and large sample sizes, such that sufficient numbers of cancers of the same organs can be analyzed (60). Moreover, because of the necessity for follow-up, results from cohort studies are vulnerable to the influence of secular trends and exposure may vary considerably for workers with the same job titles.

Today, with an improved safety profile in the workforce apparent in many industrialized countries, it is important to ensure that exposure to known carcinogenic hazards in the workplace is not transferred to the preindustrialized countries. Such countries should be encouraged to maintain the standards of protection in place in industrialized countries. Specifically, for identified carcinogens, legislation should clearly define exposure restrictions and dose limits. Ensuring that these regulations are followed would lead to reductions in occupational cancers.

RADIATION

To initiate carcinogenesis, ionizing radiation can damage DNA directly or indirectly by causing the formation of highly reactive free radicals that can damage DNA or induce chromosomal instability in nearby cells not directly damaged by radiation (i.e., the "bystander" effect). Unlike other types of exposures, radiation exposure tends to induce DNA strand breaks that lead to chromosomal rearrangements like translocations, inversions, additions, and deletions. Exposure to ionizing radiation in humans has been most consistently associated with leukemia and cancers of the breast, thyroid, and lung (61). Evidence has come from studies of radiotherapy-treated patients, residents exposed to environmental radon, workers with occupational exposure to radiation, and for the largest part, survivors of the Japanese atomic bomb (United Nations Scientific Committee on the Effects of Atomic Radiation) and the nuclear accident at Chernobyl in 1986 (62). Some studies have focused on children, as excess risk of cancer appears to be inversely related to age at exposure. From long-term studies of the Japanese atomic bomb survivors, a linear dose-response pattern has emerged for exposure to ionizing radiation and risk of solid cancers and a linear-quadratic dose-response relationship has appeared for leukemia except for the highest levels of exposure (63). However, these findings from the Japanese atomic bomb survivors are based on a single, acute radiation exposure and do not reflect the low-level, chronic, or fractionated exposures that occur more commonly in contemporary occupational and environmental settings. For low-level ionizing radiation exposures, less high-quality epidemiological data exist. This is due in part to lack of good dosimetry information, inadequate ascertainment of cancer outcomes, possible screening biases, short length of follow-up for cancer development, and small samples sizes (62).

HORMONES

A large number of studies have investigated the role of oral contraceptive usage in breast cancer risk. Initially, there appeared to be consistent evidence supporting an increased risk of breast cancer in young women associated with current prolonged use (over 5 years) of oral contraceptives, defining young as less than 35 years and perhaps less than 45. However, a recent study by Marchbanks et al. (64) of findings from the Women's Contraceptive and Reproductive Experiences (Women's CARE) study the investigators found no association between past or present use of oral contraceptives and breast cancer. This was a well-conducted, population-based study of 4,575 women with breast cancer and 4,682 controls. The importance of this finding for public health is enormous, because more than 75% of the women in the study had used oral contraceptives. Thus, even a small risk associated with such a common exposure could account for a substantial number of new cases of breast cancer. These findings are reassuring to women who used oral contraceptives, and there was no difference by dose of estrogen (low or high).

A 1996 meta-analysis of 54 epidemiologic studies of oral-contraceptive use and the risk of breast cancer showed that women had a slightly increased risk of breast cancer while taking oral contraceptives, as compared with the risk among nonusers (relative risk [RR] = 1.24; 95 percent confidence interval [CI] = 1.15–1.33) (64). The risk diminished steadily after cessation of use, with no increase after 10 years. This meta-analysis had the virtues of large size and inclusion of data from studies conducted around the world, both published and unpublished. The findings from this study provide strong support for two main conclusions. First, breast cancers diagnosed in women who had used combined oral contraceptives were less clinically advanced than those diagnosed in women who had never used these contraceptives: long-term users had lower relative risk for tumors that had spread beyond the breast versus localized tumors compared with women who never used contraceptives (RR = 0.88, 95% CI = 0.81–0.95). There was no obvious association in the results for recency of use between women with different background risks of breast cancer, including women from different countries and ethnic groups, women with different reproductive histories, and those with or without a family history of breast cancer. Other features of hormonal contraceptive use such as duration of use, age at first use, and the dose and type of the hormone within the contraceptives had little additional effect on breast cancer risk once recency of use had been taken into account. Further reassuring news is that the relative risks are small and the period-at-risk appears confined to times of life when the incidence of breast cancer, although not negligible, has not reached the highest levels attained in the latter part of the sixth and seventh decades of life.

The other important, and increasingly common in industrialized countries, source of exogenous hormones is hormonal replacement therapy (HRT), and several important recent studies have addressed breast cancer risk and HRT use. To quantify the relationship between the use of HRT in postmenopausal women and the risk of breast cancer, the follow-up in the Nurses' Health Study was extended to 1992. There were 1,935 cases of invasive breast cancer recorded during 725,550 woman-years of follow-up among postmenopausal women. The risk of breast cancer was slightly, but statistically significantly, increased among women who were currently using estrogen alone (RR = 1.32; 95% CI = 1.14–1.54) as compared with postmenopausal women who had never used hormones. The risk of breast cancer was also significantly increased, albeit only modestly, among women who were currently using estrogen plus progestin (RR = 1.41; 95% CI = 1.15–1.74). Among current HRT users, use of such therapy for 5–9 years was associated with higher risk (RR = 1.46, 95% CI = 1.22–1.74), with a similar risk for 10 years of use. This effect of duration of use for 5 or more years was greater among older women (RR for women aged 60 to 64 = 1.71; 95% CI = 1.34–2.18). The relative risk of death from breast cancer was also increased among women who had taken estrogen for 5 or more years (RR = 1.45; 95% CI = 1.01–2.09).

From the recent studies of HRT use and cancer, results are consistently suggesting a risk with increasing use of the drugs. Past studies suggested that postmenopausal hormone treatments might be effective in preventing or reducing some of the negative long-term effects of aging, such as heart disease and osteoporosis. However, the results from a large multicenter clinical trial (67), showed increases in breast cancer, coronary heart disease, stroke, and blood clots in the lungs and legs for women on estrogen-progestin therapy for an average of 5.2 years. The trial, part of the Women's Health Initiative (WHI), also found fewer cases of hip fractures and colon cancer among women taking the combined therapy. However, because overall the harm was greater than the benefit, the trial was stopped 3 years ahead of schedule. The WHI randomized trial for estrogen-alone drugs in women who have had their uterus removed is continuing.

Previous studies looking at the effect of postmenopausal hormones on ovarian cancer risk have been inconsistent. Some reported increased risk with estrogen use whereas others reported either no effect or a protective one. Most of these earlier studies were relatively small and limited by incomplete information about ovarian cancer risk factors. Two recent large studies found a link between hormone use and ovarian cancer. A large prospective study published in 2001 (68) showed that postmenopausal estrogen use for 10 or more years was associated with increased risk of ovarian cancer mortality, and a recent Swedish study (69) reported that estrogen use alone and estrogen-progestin used sequentially (i.e., progestin used on average 10 days per month) may be associated with an increased risk for ovarian cancer. In contrast, estrogen-progestin used continuously (i.e., progestin used on average 28 days per month) seemed to confer no increased ovarian cancer risk.

In a study of ovarian cancer risk of women who participated in the Breast Cancer Detection and Demonstration Project, and used estrogen-only replacement therapy, particularly for 10 or more years, were at significantly increased risk of ovarian cancer in this study (70). Women who used short-term, estrogen-progestin-only replacement therapy were not at increased risk, but risk associated with short-term and longer-term estrogen-progestin replacement therapy warrants further investigation.

RISK FACTORS FOR CHILDHOOD CANCER OCCURRENCE

Environmental risk factors for adult cancer generally involve long latency periods from exposure commencement to clinical onset of disease. Cigarette smoking illustrates this point: smoking usually starts during adolescence, but associated malignancies do not become apparent for many decades after smoking is initiated. However, the genetic processes that go awry and lead to childhood cancer are likely to be different from that of adult malignancies, as suggested by a shorter time for the carcinogenic process to occur in children. Infancy, when embryonal neoplasms such as neuroblastoma predominate, is the age when cancer incidence rates are highest during childhood (71). It is reasonable to surmise, therefore, that many childhood cancers result from aberrations in early developmental processes.

To our dismay from a prevention standpoint, the current evidence to support a major etiologic role for environmental or other exogenous factors in childhood cancer is minimal. A comprehensive review of epidemiologic studies of childhood cancer is available elsewhere (16). The major types of childhood cancer and the few risk factors that are reasonably well documented are shown in Table 5.1. Many other factors are suspected to increase or decrease risk, but are not well established. However, even the known risk factors explain only a small proportion of childhood cancer cases.

TABLE 5.1. Known Risk Factors for Selected Childhood Cancers[*]

Cancer Type	Risk Factor	Comments
Acute lymphoid leukemia	Ionizing radiation	Although primarily of historical significance, prenatal diagnostic x-ray exposure increases risk. Therapeutic irradiation for cancer treatment also increases risk.
	Race	White children have a 2-fold higher rate than black children in the U.S.
	Genetic conditions	Down syndrome is associated with an estimated 20-fold increased risk. Neurofibromatosis type 1, Bloom syndrome, ataxia telangiectasia, and Langerhans cell histiocytosis, among others, are associated with an elevated risk.
Acute myeloid leukemias	Chemotherapeutic agents	Alkylating agents and epipodophyllotoxins increase risk
	Genetic conditions	Down syndrome and neurofibromatosis 1 are strongly associated. Familial monosomy 7 and several other genetic syndromes are also associated with increased risk.
Brain cancers	Therapeutic ionizing radiation to the head	With the exception of cancer radiotherapy, higher risk from radiation treatment is essentially of historical importance.
	Genetic conditions	Neurofibromatosis 1 is strongly associated with optic gliomas, and, to a lesser extent, associated with other central nervous system tumors. Tuberous sclerosis and several other genetic syndromes are associated with increased risk.

TABLE 5.1 (*Continued*)

Cancer Type	Risk Factor	Comments
Hodgkin's disease	Family history	Monozygotic twins and siblings of cases are at increased risk.
	Infections	Epstein-Barr virus is associated with increased risk.
Non-Hodgkin's lymphoma	Immunodeficiency	Acquired and congenital immunodeficiency disorders, and immunosuppressive therapy, increase risk.
	Infections	Epstein-Barr virus is associated with Burkitt's lymphoma in African countries.
Osteosarcoma	Ionizing radiation	Cancer radiotherapy and high radium exposure increase risk.
	Chemotherapy	Alkylating agents increase risk.
	Genetic conditions	Increased risk is apparent with Li-Fraumeni syndrome and hereditary retinoblastoma.
Ewing's sarcoma	Race	White children have about a 9-fold higher incidence rate than black children in the U.S.
Neuroblastoma		No known risk factors
Retinoblastoma		No known nonhereditary risk factors
Wilms' tumor	Congenital anomalies	Aniridia and Beckwith-Wiedemann syndrome, as well as other congenital and genetic conditions, increase risk.
	Race	Asian children reportedly have about half the rates of white and black children.
Rhabdomyosarcoma	Congenital anomalies and genetic conditions	Li-Fraumeni syndrome and neurofibromatosis 1 are believed to be associated with increased risk. There is some concordance with major birth defects.
Hepatoblastoma	Genetic conditions	Beckwith-Wiedemann syndrome, hemihypertrophy, Gardner's syndrome, and family history of adenomatous polyposis increase risk.
Malignant germ cell tumors	Cryptochidism	Cryptochidism is a risk factor for testicular germ cell tumors.

*Derived from the National Cancer Institute's SEER Pediatric Cancer Monograph (71).

CONCLUSION

There is strong evidence that cancer is, and will be for the immediate future, a major public health problem; that the majority of human cancers may be avoidable; and that several of the avoidable causes have already been identified. In global terms, the greatest impacts would be from the control of tobacco smoking and the prevention of breast and prostate cancers. Whereas tobacco control could be achieved using a series of government and societal actions, prospects for the prevention of breast cancer are more remote. In this regard, ongoing intervention trials of selective estrogen receptor modulators (SERMs), such as tamoxifen and raloxifene, in healthy women have a unique role in being the only available intervention with a reasonable probability of success against this common condition. Other important reductions could be brought about by vaccination against hepatitis B and human papilloma virus and control of *H. pylori*. Failing primary prevention, screening for cancers of the breast, cervix, and colon could have a significant effect on reducing mortality from these common diseases. Screening for other forms of cancer will emerge as public health strategies once there has been proper evaluation. With the expansion in the absolute numbers of cases of cancer set to continue in the new millennium, the role of prevention in cancer control strategies will increase in importance. The time has come to focus on the implementation of current knowledge in populations where many thousands, if not millions, of frequently premature deaths could be avoided.

REFERENCES

1. Szklo M, Nieto FJ (2000) *Epidemiology: Beyond the Basics*. Gaithersburg, MD: Aspen Publishers.
2. Rothman KJ, Greenland S (1998) *Modern Epidemiology*, 2nd ed. Philadelphia: Lippincott-Raven Publishers.
3. Thacker SB (2002) Surveillance. In *Field Epidemiology*. Gregg MB (ed.) New York, NY: Oxford University Press.
4. Ries LAG, Kosary CL, Hankey BF, Miller BA, Harras A, Edwards BK (eds.) (1997) SEER Cancer Statistics Review, 1973–1994. National Cancer Institute. NIH Publication No. 97-2789, Bethesda, MD.
5. Weiss NS (1996) *Clinical Epidemiology: The Study of the Outcome of Illness*, 2nd ed. New York: Oxford University Press.
6. Benson K, Hartz AJ (2000) A comparison of observational studies and randomized, controlled trials. *N Engl J Med* 342:1878–1886.
7. Concato J, Shah N, Horwitz RI (2000) Randomized, controlled trials, observational studies, and the hierarchy of research designs. *N Engl J Med* 342:1887–1892.
8. Adami HO, Hunter D, Trichopoulos D (2002) *Textbook of Cancer Epidemiology*. New York, NY: Oxford University Press.
9. Brownson RC (1998) Outbreak and cluster investigations. In *Applied Epidemiology*. Brownson RC, Petitti DB (eds.) New York, NY: Oxford University Press, pp. 71–104.

10. Rothman KJ (1990) A sobering start for the cluster busters' conference. *Am J Epidemiol* 132(1 Suppl):S6–13.

11. Alexander FE (1999) Clusters and clustering of childhood cancer: A review. *Eur J Epidemiol* 15:847–852.

12. Perera FP (2000) Molecular epidemiology: on the path to prevention? *J Natl Cancer Inst* 92:602–612.

13. Perera FP, Weinstein IB (1982) Molecular epidemiology and carcinogen-DNA adduct detection: new approaches to studies of human cancer causation. *J Chronic Dis* 35: 581–600.

14. Lichtenstein P, Holm NV, Verkasalo PK, Iliadou A, Kaprio J, Koskenvuo M, Pukkala E, Skytthe A, Hemminki K (2000) Environmental and heritable factors in the causation of cancer—analyses of cohorts of twins from Sweden, Denmark, and Finland. *N Engl J Med* 343:78–85.

15. Vineis P, Malats N, Lang M, d' Errico A, Caporaso N, Cuzick J, Bofetta P (eds) (1999) *Metabolic Polymorphisms and Susceptibility to Cancer.* Lyon, France: IARC.

16. Little J (1999) *Epidemiology of Childhood Cancer.* Lyon, France: IARC.

17. Greenland S (ed.) (1987) *Evolution of Epidemiologic Ideas: Annotated Readings on Concepts and Methods.* Newton Lower Falls, MA: Epidemiologic Resources, Inc.

18. Parkin DM (2001) Global cancer statistics in the year 2000. *Lancet Oncol* 9:533–543.

19. Doll R, Peto R (1981) The causes of cancer: quantitative estimates of avoidable risks of cancer in the United States today. *J Natl Cancer Inst* 66:1191–1308.

20. Kuper H, Adami HO, Boffetta P (2002) Tobacco use, cancer causation and public health impact. *J Intern Med* 251:455–466.

21. International Agency for Research on Cancer (1986) *Tobacco: A Major International Health Hazard.* Lyon: IARC.

22. Wu X, Hudmon KS, Detry MA, Chamberlain RM, Spitz MR (2000) D2 dopamine receptor gene polymorphisms among African-Americans and Mexican-Americans: a lung cancer case-control study. *Cancer Epidemiol Biomarkers Prev* 9:1021–1026.

23. USDHHS (United States Department of Health and Human Services) (1989) *Reducing the Health Consequences of Smoking: 25 Years of Progress. A Report of the Surgeon General.* US Government Printing Office, Washington, DC.

24. Doll R (1978) Prevention: some future perspectives. *Prev Med* 7:486–497.

25. Lancaster WD, Piccardo JC (2002) Viral agents. In *Encyclopedia of Cancer*, 2nd ed. Bertino JR (ed) San Diego, CA: Academic Press.

26. Yamaguchi N, Kakizoe T (2001) Synergistic interaction between *Helicobactor pylori* gastritis and diet in gastric cancer. *Lancet Oncol*, 2:84–94.

27. Tommasi S, Denissenko MF, Pfeifer GP (1997) Sunlight induces pyrimidine dimers preferentially at 5-methylcytosine bases. *Cancer Res* 57:4727–4730.

28. Giles GG, Marks R, Foley P (1988) The incidence of nonmelanomic skin cancer in Australia. *Br Med J* 296:13–17.

29. Vitaliano PP, Urbach F (1980) The relative importance of risk factors in nonmelanoma carcinoma. *Arch Dermatol* 116:454–456.

30. Rosso S, Zanetti R, Martinez C, Tormo MJ, Schraub S, Sancho-Garnier H, Franceschi S, Gafa L, Perea E, Navarro C, Laurent R, Schrameck C, Talamini R, Tumio R, Wechscler J (1996) The multicentre south European study 'Helios' II: different sun exposure patterns

in the aetiology of basal cell and squamous cell carcinomas of the skin. *Br J Cancer* 73:1447–1454.

31. Kaskel P, Sander S, Kron M, Kind P, Peter RU, Krahn G (2001) Outdoor activites in childhood: a protective factor for cutaneous melanoma? Results from a case-control study in 271 matched pairs. *Br J Dermatol* 145:602–609.

32. Elwood M, Jopson J (1997) Melanoma and sun exposure: an overview of published studies. *Int J Cancer* 73:198–203.

33. Autier P, Dore JF, Lejeune F, Koelmel KF, Geffeler O, Hille P, Cesarini JP, Lienard D, Liabeuf A, Joarlette M, Chemaly P, Hakim K, Koeln A, Kleeberg U (1994) Cutaneous malignant melanoma and exposure to sunlamps or sunbeds: an EORTC multicenter case-control study in Belgium, France and Germany. *Int J Cancer* 58:809–813.

34. Boyle P, Veronesi U, Tubiana M, Alexander FE, Calais da Silva F, Denis LJ, Freire JM, Hakama M, Hirsch A, Kroes R, La Vecchia C, Maisonneuve P, Martin-Moreno JM, Newton-Bishop J, Pinborg JJ, Saracci R, Scully C, Standaert B, Storm H, Blanco S, Malbois R, Bleehen N, Dicato M, Plesnicar S (1995) European School of Oncology Advisory Report to the European Commission for the "Europe Against Cancer Programme": European Code Against Cancer. *Eur J Cancer* 9:1395–1405.

35. Tomatis L, Day NE, Heseltine F, et al. (1990) *Cancer: Causes, Occurrence and Control.* International Agency for Research on Cancer, Scientific Publication no. 100, Lyon, France.

36. Autier P, Dore JF, Lejeune D, Koelmel KF, Geffeler O, Hille P, Cesarini JP, Lienard D, Liabeuf A, Joarlette M, Chemaly P, Hakim K, Koeln A, Kleeberg U (1994) Recreational exposure to sunlight and lack of information as risk factors for cutaneous malignant melanoma. Results of a European Organisation for Research and Treatment of Cancer (EORTC) case-control study in Belgium, France and Germany. *Melanoma Res* 4:79–85.

37. Armstrong B, Doll R (1975) Environmental factors and cancer incidence and mortality in different countries, with special reference to dietary practices. *Int J Cancer* 15:617–631.

38. Willett WC (1990) *Nutritional Epidemiology.* Oxford University Press, Oxford.

39. Steinmetz KA, Potter JD (1991). Vegetable, fruit, and cancer I. Epidemiology. *Cancer Causes Control* 2:325–358.

40. Blot WJ, Li J-Y, Taylor P, Guo W, Dawsey S, Wang G-Q, Yang CS, Zheng S-F, Gail M, Li G-Y, Yu Y, Liu B, Tangrea J, Sun Y-h, Liu F, Fraumeni JF, Zhang Y-H, Li B (1993) Nutrition intervention trials in Linxian, China: supplementation with specific vitamin/mineral combinations, cancer incidence, and disease-specific mortality in the general populaton. *J Natl Cancer Inst* 85:1483–1492.

41. Alpha-Tocopherol, Beta-Carotene Cancer Prevention Study Group (1994) The effect of vitamin E and beta carotene on the incidence of lung cancer and other cancers in male smokers. *N Engl J Med* 330:1029–1035.

42. Hennekens CH, Buring JE, Manson JE, Stampfer MJ, Rosner B, Cook NR, Belanger C, LaMotte F, Gaziano JM, Ridker PM, Willett WC, Peto R (1996) Lack of effect of long-term supplementation with beta-carotene on the incidence of malignant neoplasms and cardiovascular disease. *N Engl J Med* 334:1145–1149.

43. International Agency for Research on Cancer (1988). Monographs on the Evaluation of Carcinogenic Risk of Chemicals to Humans, Vol. 44. *Alcohol Drinking.* IARC, Lyon, France.

44. Longnecker MP (1995) Alcohol consumption and risk of cancer in humans: an overview. *Alcohol* 12:87–96.

45. Dennis LK, Hayes RB (2001) Alcohol and prostate cancer. *Epidemiol Rev* 23:110–114.

46. Sarkar DK, Liehr JG, Singletary KW (1995) Role of estrogen in alcohol promotion of breast cancer and prolactinomas. *Alcoholism Clin Exp Res* 25:230S–236S.

47. Bhat KP, Pezzuto JM (2002) Cancer chemopreventive activity of resveratrol. *Ann N Y Acad Sci* 957:210–229.

48. Calle EE, Rodriguez C, Walker-Thurmond K, Thun MJ (2003) Overweight, obesity, and mortality from cancer in a prospectively studied cohort of U.S. adults. *N Engl J Med* 348:1625–1638.

49. Moller H, Mellemgaard A, Lindvig K, Olsen J (1994) Obesity and cancer risk: a Danish record-linkage study. *Eur J Cancer* 30:344–350.

50. Ballard-Barbash R (1994) Anthropometry and breast cancer: body size—a moving target. *Cancer* 74:1090–1100.

51. NCI/NHLBI Obesity Education Initiative Task Force Members (1998) *Clinical Guidelines on the Identification, Evaluation, and Treatment of Overweight and Obesity in Adults.* National Heart, Lung, and Blood Institute, Baltimore, MD, pp. 1–137.

52. WHO Consultation on Obesity (1998) Global prevalence and secular trends in obesity. In: *Obesity. Preventing and Managing the Global Epidemic.* Geneva: World Health Organization, pp. 17–40.

53. Colditz GA, Cannuscio CC, Frazier AL (1997) Physical activity and reduced risk of colon cancer: implications for prevention. *Cancer Causes Control* 8:649–667.

54. McTiernan A, Ulrich C, Slate S, Potter J (1998) Physical activity and cancer etiology: associations and mechanisms. *Cancer Causes Control* 9:487–509.

55. Bernstein L, Ross RK, Lobo RA, Hanisch R, Krailo MD, Henderson BE (1987) The effects of moderate physical activity on menstrual cycle patterns in adolescence: implications for breast cancer prevention. *Br J Cancer* 55:681–685.

56. Doll R, Peto R (1981) *The Causes of Cancer.* Oxford: Oxford University Press.

57. Ward E (1995) Overview of preventable industrial causes of occupational cancer. *Environ Health Perspect* 103(Suppl 8):197–203.

58. Doll R (1988) Effects of exposure to vinyl chloride. An assessment of the evidence. *Scand J Work Environ Health* 14:61–78.

59. Zaebst D, Clapp D, Blade LM, Marlow DA, Steenland K, Hornung RW, Scheutzle D, Butler J (1991) Quantitative determination of trucking industry workers' exposures to diesel exhaust particles. *Am Ind Hyg Assoc J* 52:529–541.

60. Carpenter L, Roman E (1999) Cancer and occupation in women: identifying associations using routinely collected national data. *Environ Health Perspect* 107(Suppl 2): 299–303.

61. Boice JD Jr, Land CE, Preston DL (1996) Ionizing radiation. In: Schottenfeld D, Fraumeni JF (eds) *Cancer Epidemiology and Prevention*, 2nd ed. New York: Oxford University Press, pp. 319–354.

62. Moysich KB, Menezes RJ, Michalek AM (2002). Chernobyl-related ionizing radiation exposure and cancer risk: an epidemiologic review. *Lancet Oncol* 3:269–279.

63. United Nations Scientific Committee on the Effects of Atomic Radiation (UNSCEAR) (2000) Report to the General Assembly. *Sources and Effects of Ionizing Radiation.* Vol 1: Sources. Vol 2. Effects. (United Nations Publication Sales No. E.00.IX.3).

64. Marchbanks PA, McDonald JA, Wilson HG, Folger SG, Mandel MG, Daling JR, Bernstein L, Malone KE, Ursin G, Strom BL, Norman SA, Weiss LK (2002) Oral contraceptives and the risk of breast cancer. *N Eng J Med* 346:2025–2032.

65. Collaborative Group on Hormonal Factors in Breast Cancer (1996) Breast cancer and hormonal contraceptives: collaborative reanalysis of individual data on 53,297 women with breast cancer and 100,239 women ithout breast cancer from 54 epidemiological studies. *Lancet* 347:1713–1727.

66. Hulka BS, Liu ET, Lininger RA (1994) Steroid hormones and risk of breast cancer. Cancer 74:1111–1124.

67. Writing Group for the Women's Health Initiative Investigators (2002) Risks and benefits of estrogen plus progestin in healthy postmenopausal women: principal results from the Women's Health Initiative randomized controlled trial. *JAMA* 288:321–333.

68. Rodriguez C, Patel AV, Calle EE, Jacob EJ, Thun MJ (2001) Estrogen replacement therapy and ovarian cancer mortality in a large prospective study of US women. *JAMA* 285:1460–1465.

69. Riman T, Dickman PW, Nilsson S, Correia N, Nordlinder H, Magnusson CM, Weiderpass E, Persson IR (2002) Hormone replacement therapy and the risk of invasive epithelial ovarian cancer in Swedish women. *J Natl Cancer Inst* 94:497–504.

70. Lacey JV Jr, Mink PJ, Lubin JH, Sherman ME, Troisi R, Hartge P, Schatzkin A, Schairer C (2002) Menopausal hormone replacement therapy and risk of ovarian cancer. *JAMA* 288:334–341.

71. Ries LAG, Smith MA, Gurney JG, Linet M, Tamra T, Young JL, Bunin GR (eds) (1999). Cancer Incidence and Survival Among Children and Adolescents: United States SEER Program 1975–1995. National Cancer Institute, SEER Program. NIH Pub. No. 99-4649. Bethesda, MD. The publication and additional data available on the SEER website at http://seer.cancer.gov/publications/.

■■■■■ CHAPTER 6

The Chemoprevention of Cancer

FADLO R. KHURI

Winship Cancer Institute, Emory University, School of Medicine, Atlanta, Georgia

WUAN KI HONG

University of Texas, M. D. Anderson Cancer Center, Department of Thoracic/Head and Neck Oncology, Houston, Texas

ANITA L. SABICHI and SCOTT M. LIPPMAN

University of Texas, M. D. Anderson Cancer Center, Department of Clinical Cancer Prevention, Houston, Texas

INTRODUCTION

Cancer chemoprevention is the arrest, reversal, or delay of carcinogenesis with pharmacologic agents. The U.S. Food and Drug Administration's (FDA's) recent, high-profile approvals of the two molecular-targeting drugs tamoxifen and cele-coxib have firmly established cancer chemoprevention in the arena of standard cancer control modalities. In 1998, tamoxifen, a selective estrogen-receptor modula-tor (SERM), became the first drug explicitly approved for cancer risk reduction, specifically for reducing breast cancer risk. In 1999, celecoxib, a selective cyclooxy-genase-2 (COX-2) inhibitor, was approved as an adjunct to standard surveillance and treatment in the setting of familial adenomatous polyposis (FAP).

This chapter will review the following critical areas of chemoprevention research: the biology of chemoprevention, including the seminal biological and molecular concepts of multistep and multifocal carcinogenesis; key design concepts of clinical and translational chemoprevention trials; major chemopreventive agents under development; and trials of various chemopreventive agents in the head and neck, lung, colorectal region, skin, cervix, breast, bladder, prostate, and other regions and sites of epithelial carcinogenesis.

UICC Manual of Clinical Oncology, Eighth Edition. Edited by Raphael E. Pollock
ISBN 0-471-22289-5 Copyright © 2004 John Wiley & Sons, Inc.

BIOLOGY OF CHEMOPREVENTION

Epithelial carcinogenesis is a complex multistep process occurring over decades and influenced by many exogenous and endogenous factors. Carcinogenesis involves the accumulation of specific molecular alterations, which can vary depending on carcinogen exposure and genetic susceptibility. Understanding this complex biology is crucial to the development and design of clinical chemoprevention trials.

Carcinogenesis also is multifocal, involving either multiple genetically distinct clones (field carcinogenesis) and/or the lateral spread of genetically related preinvasive clones. Examples of field carcinogenesis include skin exposure to UV irradiation, colon exposure to bile and fatty acids, or head-and-neck, lung or bladder exposure to tobacco carcinogens. Intervention within multistep carcinogenesis and throughout a wide tissue field is the essence of chemoprevention.

CHEMOPREVENTION TRIAL DESIGNS

Chemoprevention trials are characterized by their trial populations and endpoints. Chemoprevention trials based in the general population are called primary, conducted in healthy, generally high-risk subjects; secondary trials are conducted in patients with premalignant lesions; and tertiary trials are conducted in patients with a prior cancer. Depending on the endpoint (toxicity, surrogate [for cancer] activity, or cancer), there are three major phases of clinical prevention study—phase I (toxicity), phase II (surrogate endpoint), and phase III (cancer)—and each phase can involve any of the three types of study populations (Table 6.1).

Phase I

The first step in clinical chemopreventive drug development is a phase I trial, which can be of two types: phase Ia (single-dose application) and phase Ib (continuing dose application). Phase Ia trials are designed to assess the acute toxicity and pharmacokinetics (i.e., absorption, distribution, metabolism, and elimination) of single administrations of various, usually escalating, drug dose levels, beginning with a dose suggested by preclinical study. These trials generally involve 20–30

TABLE 6.1. Chemoprevention Trial Designs

Phase	Major Features
Ia	Single-dose trial to characterize acute toxicity, pharmacokinetics
Ib	Repeated daily-dose study to characterize chronic toxicity/pharmacokinetics/efficacy
IIa	Dose de-escalation and fixed-dose trials, activity, surrogate endpoints
IIb	Randomized, comparative, surrogate endpoint
III	Randomized, cancer-incidence endpoint

fasting and nonfasting subjects. The toxicity limit is that acceptable to generally healthy subjects (e.g., $\leq$ grade 2 of the NCI Common Toxicity Criteria).

Phase Ib trials are designed to assess the toxicity and pharmacokinetics of repeated administrations of various, usually escalating, dose levels of an agent. Phase Ib trials generally are short term (~3 months) and primarily are designed to assess drug toxicity and safety and to define the optimal dose and schedule. These trials include relatively nontoxic agents, oral administration, a daily schedule, and frequently pharmacokinetic studies. Whereas classic phase I therapy trials define the maximal tolerated dose (MTD), phase I prevention trials are designed to determine the maximum dose with only minimal toxicity in most subjects. Randomized phase I studies are desirable to control for the minor subjective effects often reported by subjects on placebo. Phase Ib trials can include evaluations of potential surrogate endpoint biomarkers (SEBs).

Phase II

Phase II trials, including phase IIa and IIb designs, are relatively short-term assessments of drug activity with respect to SEs, which can be either premalignant lesions or SEBs. Phase IIa trials are preliminary, generally nonrandomized single-arm assessments of drug activity and technical feasibility. Phase IIa prevention and typical phase II therapy designs have many similarities, such as the frequent incorporation of two-stage designs. De-escalation designs to find the lowest, least-toxic biologically active dose, however, are fairly common in phase IIa prevention trials and virtually nonexistent in phase II therapy trials.

Phase IIb trials are pivotal to the long-term success of chemopreventive drug development because they have the potential to at least partly replace phase III trials in the FDA process of evaluating and approving cancer prevention agents. Large-scale phase III trials (which are further discussed below) require several years, many thousands of subjects, and many millions of dollars to assess their cancer endpoints. Phase IIb trials require much shorter terms, smaller sample sizes, and less expense to assess their preinvasive endpoints, which are surrogates for the phase III cancer endpoint. Therefore, phase IIb trials potentially can allow more agents to be tested in a more cost-effective manner (versus phase III testing), possibly indispensable advantages in an era of uncertain budgets for cancer research.

Phase IIb prevention trials are randomized comparative assessments of drug effects on surrogate endpoints (SEs). The crux of phase IIb trial designs is to establish preinvasive SEs that are directly linked to clinical benefit. The phase III cancer endpoint is the standard primary endpoint for determining clinical benefit, as recognized by the FDA when it approved tamoxifen for breast cancer risk reduction in the primary, secondary, and tertiary prevention settings. Phase II premalignant lesion endpoints are precursors to cancer, and some, such as FAP, are considered to be diseases in themselves. Significantly arresting, reversing, or delaying an important disease lesion in a phase IIb trial can provide a clinical benefit, as documented by FDA approvals of several phase IIb agents for controlling FAP. No association has been established to date between controlling a precursor lesion and subsequently reduced cancer incidence. Such associations have been demonstrated in other settings, however, including that between controlling cholesterol and subsequently reduced cardiovascular disease.

Premalignant lesion SEs are associated with a wide spectrum of cancer risks, and those associated with a moderate-to-high risk have been referred to as intraepithelial neoplasias (IENs). Even within IENs, however, associated cancer risks can vary substantially. Therefore, actual cancer risks are being redefined by molecular markers, such as loss of heterozygosity. For example, these markers can indicate lower risks in severely dysplastic oral IENs, which generally are thought to be very high risk, or higher risks in hyperplastic oral IENs, which generally are thought to be low risk.

Phase II studies have focused mainly on tissue sites or lesions (e.g., oral leukoplakia) that can be directly visualized and easily sampled. Less accessible sites or lesions (e.g., prostatic intraepithelial neoplasia, or PIN) present great difficulties in mapping and imaging the at-risk epithelial field. The FDA has accepted certain IENs for drug approval, including actinic keratoses, superficial bladder tumors, and FAP.

There are a number of pros and cons associated with FDA approvals based on phase IIb testing. Chemoprevention in IENs could reduce cancer risk and the morbidity associated with screening and therapy. A major FDA concern, however, is that preventive agents approved and widely used on the basis of phase IIb IEN results may lead healthy high-risk people away from standard screening practices with proven cancer risk reduction benefits. Another concern is that the short terms and small scales of phase IIb trials render them incapable of detecting potential slow-developing or relatively rare but serious adverse drug effects. Also, phase IIb trials typically would not provide comprehensive risk-benefit profiles, such as the complex tamoxifen profile provided by the phase III Breast Cancer Prevention Trial (BCPT).

Phase III

Phase III trials are randomized, controlled, and considered to be definitive because they provide the highest level of evidence of a chemopreventive agent's effect on cancer risk. Definitive phase III trials are very large scale ($>1,000$ to $>10,000$ patients per two-arm trial) and long term, depending on the event rate in the control arm and estimated treatment effect in the experimental arm. The efficiency of these trials can be enhanced by variant designs, such as factorial designs, which allow more than one intervention/hypothesis to be tested within the same trial population. These trials use a placebo control or positive control, such as tamoxifen, which is the comparative standard treatment (established in the BCPT) for testing raloxifene in the Study of Tamoxifen and Raloxifene (STAR). Phase III trials should be double blind so as to control for investigator bias and other potential endpoint-ascertainment problems. In addition to definitively answering primary endpoint questions, phase III trials have the ability to address a host of important prespecified secondary endpoint questions. Secondary endpoint analyses of phase III trials have generated provocative hypotheses for definitive testing in new phase III trials. Phase III trials also have the potential to validate SEs (i.e., to link SE modulation to cancer outcome). SE validation can be disease and drug specific.

Chemoprevention, especially phase III chemoprevention, commonly faces greater difficulties in recruitment (especially minority and special population recruitment) and compliance than do cancer therapy trials. Whereas therapy trial participation is based on the exigencies of present disease, chemoprevention trial entry and compliance are motivated generally by the perception of risk (among relatively healthy people), which often differs from actual risk. The intent-to-treat policy requires that all randomized patients must be included in the primary analysis. Therefore, noncompliance is a major issue in large, long-term phase III prevention trials. This problem is exacerbated by the use of oral medications, self-reported compliance, and noncompliant "drop-ins" (placebo-arm members who take the intervention agent) in trials involving over-the-counter agents, such as nonsteroidal anti-inflammatory drugs (NSAIDs), vitamins or minerals. Frequently, a placebo run-in period is designed into phase III prevention trials to remove the expensive randomization of noncompliers. Approximately 10–15% of run-in subjects will be detected as noncompliers and removed prior to randomization.

After their promise is suggested by epidemiologic and/or *in vitro* and *in vivo* animal data, chemopreventive drugs ideally would be developed in a clinical sequence from phase I to IIa to IIb to III trials. No agent has been developed in this ideal clinical sequence, however, with several jumping the queue to phase III testing, such as occurred with β-carotene, which went directly from strong epidemiologic evidence into phase III testing for lung cancer prevention. The phase III β-carotene results dramatically refuted the epidemiologic β-carotene data. Although this β-carotene experience did not lead to the ideal sequence of clinical testing, it has led to requiring far more comprehensive rationales (than epidemiology alone) before starting new definitive, costly phase III trials. There are three major levels of evidence currently accepted for phase III rationales—molecular targeting and mechanism data, preclinical animal and *in vitro* data, and secondary-endpoint data generated in other phase III trials. The rationale for tamoxifen in the phase III BCPT included compelling supportive data from all three major levels of rationale.

CHEMOPREVENTIVE AGENTS

Epidemiologic, preclinical *in vivo* and *in vitro*, and clinical studies have identified several thousand potential cancer chemopreventive agents. Major classes of these agents include the retinoids, NSAIDs, SERMs, 5-α-reductase inhibitors, and pharmacological micronutrients. This section will highlight a few of the most active chemopreventive agents under intensive study at the present time.

Retinoids

Retinoids are a class of compounds that includes natural vitamin A and its synthetic and natural analogs. Retinoids are among the best-studied classes of chemopreventive agents. Retinoids operate through activation of signal transduction pathways to maintain orderly growth, differentiation, and apoptosis of epithelial cells. Data from clinical and laboratory studies suggest that vitamin A and other retinoids have cancer-preventive effects in a number of epithelial sites, including the skin, bladder, breast, and oral cavity.

The synthetic retinoid 13-*cis*-retinoic acid (13cRA) is active in reversing oral premalignant lesions. Although significant toxicity was incurred in initial studies using high-dose 13cRA, subsequent studies defined active drug regimens with acceptable toxicity profiles. Retinoids also have been studied in preventing second primary tumors in subjects after definitive treatment for primary cancer of the skin, lung or head and neck.

N-(4-hydroxyphenyl)retinamide (4-HPR) is an exciting synthetic retinoid with potent apoptosis-inducing effects in malignant and premalignant epithelial cells. 4-HPR induces apoptosis by a different mechanism from that of classic retinoic-acid signaling (involved in most natural-retinoid effects) and has shown laboratory activity in natural-retinoid-resistant cancer cells of the head and neck.

NSAIDs

A large body of epidemiologic and preclinical data suggest that the regular use of aspirin or other NSAIDs in humans reduces the risk of colon cancer and precursor adenomatous polyps. The epidemiologic data also indicate that this benefit may not be evident until after at least a decade of regular NSAID consumption. The U.S. Physicians' Study, employing a 2-by-2 factorial design to assess aspirin and β-carotene, did not show a reduction in colon polyps or cancer incidence in the aspirin-treated group. Major molecular targets of NSAIDs are the cyclooxygenases (COX) and lipoxygenases (LOX). NSAIDs can be nonselective COX inhibitors (e.g., aspirin), selective COX-2 inhibitors (e.g., celecoxib), and LOX modulators, such as 15-LOX-1 inducers (e.g., sulindac sulfone). COX- and-LOX-modulating NSAIDs have shown activity in colorectal carcinogenesis.

SERMs

Tamoxifen, raloxifene, and other SERMs are intensively studied agents for the prevention of breast cancer. Tamoxifen, a nonsteroidal triphenylene derivative, has established efficacy in primary, secondary, and tertiary breast cancer prevention. Tamoxifen has both pro- and antiestrogenic effects. In the breast, it acts as an antiestrogenic agent, and it has been shown to reduce the likelihood that post-menopausal women who have had breast cancer will develop a recurrence or a second primary cancer. In the uterus, however, tamoxifen acts as a proestrogenic agent, and it has been shown to slightly increase the risk of developing uterine cancer. Because of this increased risk, the newer agent raloxifene, a compound similar to tamoxifen in its antiestrogenic activity in breast tissue but without any evidence of proestrogenic activity in uterine or other tissue, is being evaluated in the large-scale phase III Study of Raloxifene and Tamoxifen (STAR).

5-α Reductase Inhibitors

5-α reductase inhibitors can inhibit the conversion of testosterone to the active metabolite dihydrotestosterone, which is felt to play a crucial role in prostate cancer development. The 5-α reductase inhibitor finasteride currently is being tested clinically in the large-scale phase III Prostate Cancer Prevention Trial (PCPT), which is discussed further in the "Major Chemoprevention Clinical Trials" section below.

Pharmacological Micronutrients

Selenium A number of epidemiological studies have suggested an inverse correlation between estimated intake or blood and serum levels of selenium and the incidence of cancers including breast, colon, prostate, lung, and bladder. Selenium is an essential nonmetallic trace element, which has potent antioxidant and antiproliferative properties. It can also induce apoptosis and promote differentiation. Studies in animal models have shown that carcinogen-induced tumor formation can be inhibited by dietary supplementation with selenium. A trial by Clark et al. suggested the chemopreventive potential of selenium in humans. After 4.5 years of treatment and 6.4 years follow-up, selenium at 200 mcg/day (in high-selenium brewers yeast tablets) significantly reduced overall cancer incidence and mortality and the incidences of lung, prostate, and colorectal cancers.

The primary endpoint of the Clark study was skin cancer. The results of the primary endpoint analysis were negative, without even a trend toward reduction in the rate of skin cancer. Lung, colorectal, and prostate cancer development were secondary endpoints. Therefore, the statistical significance of the reductions in these cancers must be viewed with caution in as much as these are secondary-analysis results, which are prone to an increased type I (false-positive) statistical error rate.

Vitamin E (alpha-tocopherol) A study conducted in Basel, Switzerland, followed 2,974 men prospectively and found that simultaneously low levels of lipid-adjusted vitamin E and plasma vitamin C were associated with a significantly increased risk for lung cancer. Low vitamin E levels in smokers were related to an increased risk for prostate cancer. The authors concluded that low plasma levels of vitamin E and other micronutrients (vitamin C, retinol, and β-carotene) are related to increased risk of overall and lung cancer mortality, and that low levels of vitamin E in smokers are related to an increased risk of prostate cancer mortality.

The ATBC Prevention Study assessed the effects of vitamin E, or alpha-tocopherol (AT), (50 mg, alone or combined with β-carotene) on lung cancer incidence. The primary ATBC analysis showed that AT was negative, neither increasing or reducing the incidence of lung cancer in the ATBC population of high-risk male smokers. A secondary ATBC analysis showed a significant reduction in the risk of prostate cancer in patients receiving AT. Based largely on the secondary ATBC results, AT (400 mg) currently is being evaluated in the very large-scale definitive phase III Selenium and Vitamin E Cancer Prevention Trial (SELECT) in the prostate (discussed below in the "Major Chemoprevention Clinical Trials" section).

Lycopene Although disappointing results occurred with β-carotene in lung-cancer prevention (discussed above), studies of other carotenoids, such as alpha-carotene and lycopene, are generating encouraging results. The Health Professionals follow-up study assessed dietary intake for 1 year in a study cohort, finding that tomato-based foods (tomatoes, tomato sauce, and pizza) and strawberries were primary sources of lycopene (a nonprovitamin-A carotenoid with potent antioxidant activity) and were associated with lower prostate cancer risk. The combined weekly intake of greater than 10 servings versus less than 1.5 servings of tomato (the fruit, tomato sauce and juice, pizza) was inversely associated with the risk of prostate cancer. This study also found that the intake of greater than 10 servings per week of lycopene-rich foods was inversely associated with advanced (stage C and D) prostate cancer. The authors concluded that the intake of lycopene or other compounds found in tomatoes may reduce prostate cancer risk. A follow-up study demonstrated that lycopene could be measured in the prostate at concentrations that were biologically active in laboratory studies. These findings support the hypothesis that lycopene may contribute to reduced prostate-cancer risk by direct effects within the prostate.

Calcium Studies in both rats and humans suggest that calcium and several other micronutrients in the diet may have preventive effects on colon carcinogenesis. Dietary calcium precipitates some of the cytotoxic agents that may promote colon cancer, such as fatty acids and secondary bile acids. Short-term (4 months) administration of 2,000–3,000 mg of calcium has favorably altered the bile acid profile in individuals with a history of resected adenocarcinoma of the colon.

Colon cancers arise in mucosa with abnormalities of increased proliferative rates and/or decreased rates of cell death (apoptosis) that lead eventually to the formation of adenomas. Proliferation of the epithelial lining of the colon is altered in patients at risk for colon cancer and has been studied as a marker of drug effects in many human calcium trials in the colon. Five small, uncontrolled clinical trials have found that calcium has decreased proliferation within the colonic epithelial layer. The results of three large, randomized, placebo-controlled trials differed one from the other with respect to calcium effects on proliferation: decreased, increased, and no effect on the proportion of proliferating cells in the colonic mucosa crypts. A recent large randomized calcium trial (the Polyp Prevention Study) reported a statistically significant 19% reduction in adenomas.

Multiple Vitamin-Mineral Supplements People in the Huixian and Linxian regions of China have low intake and blood levels of various micronutrients. Several large studies have shown that a strikingly high incidences of esophageal and gastric cancers occur in these regions. These observations led to several prevention trials. Subjects from Huixian received supplements of retinol, riboflavin, and zinc for 13.5 months. There was no overall difference in the occurrence of premalignant lesions or prevalence or severity of dysplasia in the gastrointestinal tract between those who received the intervention and those who did not.

In Linxian, the efficacies of four different nutrient combinations were tested in reducing the incidences of esophageal and gastric cancers. The four nutrient combinations were retinol plus zinc, riboflavin plus niacin, ascorbic acid plus molybdenum, and β-carotene plus selenium plus alpha-tocopherol. There was a 13% reduction in total cancer deaths, a 4% reduction in esophageal cancer deaths, and a 21% reduction in gastric cancer deaths in the group that received β-carotene plus alpha-tocopherol plus selenium. Gastric cancer mortality is a major health problem in many parts of the world, and its reduction in this Linxian trial has important global public-health implications. None of the other nutrient combinations significantly reduced gastric or esophageal cancer deaths. It is not known which nutrient(s) (β-carotene, alpha-tocopherol, or selenium) was responsible for the observed protection, and the applicability of these results to populations with adequate nutritional status or to other tumor sites may be limited.

A second Linxian trial was designed to determine whether a multivitamin/multimineral preparation plus β-carotene could reduce esophageal and gastric cardia cancers in over 3,000 residents with esophageal dysplasia. After 6 years of intervention, cumulative esophageal/gastric cardia cancer death rates were 8% lower, esophageal cancer mortality was 16% lower, and total cancer mortality was 4% lower in the supplemented group. Surprisingly, stomach cancer mortality was 18% higher in the supplemented group. None of these results were statistically significant.

MAJOR CHEMOPREVENTION CLINICAL TRIALS

Over 80 randomized chemoprevention trials have been reported to date, including phase II trials for the reversal of premalignancy in the head and neck, lung, colon, skin, esophagus, bladder, and cervix and phase III trials to prevent cancers of the head and neck, lung, colon, skin, breast, esophagus, and stomach.

Head and Neck Cancer Prevention

Premalignancy   Oral leukoplakia is a premalignant condition that manifests as white patches in the mouth or throat. These lesions are directly related to tobacco exposure (often chewed), and, depending upon their severity, have a 10–40% chance of transforming into cancer. Surgery and radiotherapy are not recommended for oral leukoplakia, in as much as these lesions usually return after local treatment. Oral leukoplakia is responsive to chemopreventive treatment with various retinoids, including 13-*cis*-retinoic acid (13cRA) at high (induction) and low (maintenance) doses. The lesions relapse at a high rate, however, after 13cRA treatment stops. Prolonged 13cRA treatment delayed progression, although lesions became resistant over time, and lesion progression, or drug resistance, was associated with persistent genotypic alterations and cancer development. In addition to trials of low-dose 13cRA for maintenance, newer trials of 13cRA plus interferon-α and 4-HPR in oral and laryngeal leukoplakia also have been conducted and achieved positive results.

Head and Neck Cancer–Related SPTs Three phase III trials have been completed in the chemoprevention of second primary tumors (SPTs) associated with head and neck cancer. The first of these studies tested high-dose 13cRA and achieved a marked decrease in the incidence of SPTs in patients after treatment for advanced primary head and neck cancer. Common treatment side effects included conjunctivitis, cheilitis, hypertriglyceridemia, and severe drying and cracking of the skin. Approximately 80% of the patients needed to have their dosage lowered in order to complete the treatment. The two other phase III retinoid trials in this SPT setting involved different retinoids (etretinate or retinyl palmitate) and did not achieve a lower incidence of SPTs in the retinoid group. Ongoing studies are experimenting with newer retinoids and lower doses of previously tested retinoids, such as 13cRA, in an effort to find the safest and most effective drug and drug dosage for head and neck SPT chemoprevention. The Head and Neck Cancer Second Primary Tumor Prevention Trial (HNSCC-SPT) randomized 1191 patients to 13cRA at 30 mg per day for 3 years versus placebo. No effect was seen for the low dose of 13cRA in terms of second primary prevention.

Lung Cancer Prevention

Lung Premalignancy In contrast with positive studies in premalignancy and SPTs of the head and neck, lung cancer chemoprevention studies have been discouraging. Several such studies have been completed to date, producing no clinical/histologic activity of various retinoids, vitamin B-12, or β-carotene in this model.

Lung Cancer–Related SPTs Two large phase III trials in preventing SPTs associated with lung cancer have been completed. The EUROSCAN trial evaluated retinyl palmitate and/or N-acetylcysteine (NAC) (in a 2-by-2 factorial design) and found no significant drug effects. The Lung Intergroup Trial (LIT) of 13cRA found no overall effect in the 1,166 evaluable patients, but there was a significant RA-smoking interaction causing harm in the subgroup of current smokers and benefit in the subgroup of nonsmokers in a post hoc secondary (subgroup) analysis. The LIT investigators are planning continued follow-up of their patients to assess the potential long-term beneficial effect of 13cRA in nonsmokers (former and never), as well as the biological mechanisms of the potential harm in current smokers and the natural history of SPT development in patients with resected early stage non-small cell lung cancer.

Primary Lung Cancer As mentioned in the "Chemoprevention Trial Designs" section above, two phase III studies, the ATBC and CARET, found that β-carotene not only did not decrease lung cancer incidence but actually increased it in smokers.

These trials were based on strong prior epidemiologic data indicating that β-carotene could protect against lung cancer development. The phase III primary negative/harmful β-carotene findings emphasize the need for rigorous confirmation of epidemiological data. This is an important issue for current community medical practice with respect to chemoprevention, which now involves prescriptions and advice to take agents, such as vitamin E, selenium, and raloxifene, for preventing certain cancers without definitive proof that these agents can prevent cancer. The three agent examples just given are currently in definitive phase III testing to determine their effectiveness in the settings of prostate (vitamin E and selenium) or breast cancer (raloxifene) prevention.

The issue of smoking cessation remains paramount to prevention of lung and other tobacco-related cancers. Data indicate that smoking cessation, however, is not always sufficient to remove increased cancer risk. Many smokers remain at increased risk for 5 or 10 years after stopping the habit. Therefore, chemoprevention offers a potential approach for further reducing former smokers' level of cancer risk.

Colorectal Cancer Prevention

Several colon and rectal cancer chemoprevention trials of various agents, including NSAIDs, calcium salts, and vitamin/micronutrient combinations, have been completed (see "Chemopreventive Agent" section). Extensive studies of calcium have been conducted in this setting, with encouraging results. The most promising agents in this setting are NSAIDs, which were suggested for colorectal chemoprevention by results of population-based analyses showing that long-term NSAID supplementation lowered risk of colon cancer. Sulindac and celecoxib are the NSAIDs with established activity in randomized (phase IIb) clinical trials in colorectal carcinogenesis (FAP). Celecoxib (a selective COX-2 inhibitor) has been FDA approved for reducing the IEN burden of adenomatous polyps in FAP patients, a disease characterized by germline mutations in the APC gene and virtually a 100% risk of colorectal cancer by age 50. The celecoxib reduction in polyp burden was significant but rather modest. Combinations of several drugs (including celecoxib) may be more effective than is celecoxib alone in FAP.

Skin Cancer Prevention

Retinoids have significantly reduced the incidence of skin cancers in patients at extremely high risk, such as xeroderma pigmentosum patients and renal transplant recipients. Recently, molecularly targeted treatment of a DNA-repair defect reduced the skin cancer rate in xeroderma pigmentosum patients.

Several phase III chemoprevention studies also have been conducted in other skin cancer risk settings. A placebo-controlled randomized trial of topical all-*trans*-retinoic acid (ATRA) successfully reversed actinic keratoses, which have a low rate of malignant transformation. Systemic etretinate therapy was studied in two randomized trials involving actinic keratosis patients. Both studies showed significant regression of actinic keratosis lesions in treated patients compared with those receiving placebo. Retinoids have not been as effective in other populations at high risk for developing skin cancers. One large phase III randomized study showed that oral retinol was effective in preventing squamous cell cancers but not basal cell cancers in patients with prior actinic keratoses. Three other agents—13cRA, carotene, and selenium—were tested in three separate phase III trials, none of which achieved protective effects against skin cancer development.

Breast Cancer Prevention

The program of clinical tamoxifen testing in breast cancer incidence and risk reduction is a paradigm of beneficial clinical cancer chemoprevention. Tested in over 50,000 women, tamoxifen has produced remarkably consistent prevention/risk reduction results in the narrow range of from 43% to 49% and is approved by the U.S. FDA in the three distinct settings of healthy high-risk women (primary prevention), ductal carcinoma *in situ* (secondary), and early stage breast cancer (tertiary). The major completed phase III tamoxifen prevention trials in the breast are the BCPT in 13,388 high-risk, healthy women; adjuvant trials conducted by the Early Breast Cancer Trialists' Cooperative Group and involving over 36,000 breast cancer patients; and the National Surgical Adjuvant Breast and Bowel Project B-24 trial involving 1,804 ductal carcinoma *in situ* patients. Estimates based on the BCPT suggest that tamoxifen could prevent up to 500,000 primary breast cancers in the United States over 5 years. The Study of Tamoxifen and Raloxifene (STAR) is an ongoing intergroup assessment of the standard control arm of tamoxifen versus the experimental arm of raloxifene in 22,000 postmenopausal high-risk women. STAR excludes premenopausal high-risk women because no safety data on raloxifene in these women were available either when or soon after STAR was activated.

The retinoid 4-HPR, which has fewer side effects than many other studied retinoids, also has undergone phase III chemoprevention study in breast cancer. Although a recently completed chemoprevention trial of 4-HPR failed to show an overall benefit in the prevention of breast SPTs, a post hoc subset analysis indicated that premenopausal women on 4-HPR did have fewer SPTs.

Prostate Cancer Prevention

The Southwest Oncology Group (SWOG), a cooperative group consisting of cancer treatment and research institutions from across the United States and other parts of the world, completed accrual of over 24,000 men into its phase III Prostate Cancer Prevention Trial (PCPT) of finasteride, or Proscar. Finasteride currently is accepted treatment for benign prostatic hypertrophy. The PCPT met its accrual goal (over 18,000 evaluable men) on time in 1997, 3 years after study activation, establishing that large-scale chemoprevention trials can be conducted in the multiple-institution setting of a cooperative group. The primary endpoint question of the finasteride effect on prostate cancer incidence is expected to be analyzed in 2004, when all the male subjects will have completed their prescribed period of treatment and follow up.

Secondary analyses from the phase III trials of selenium in skin-cancer prevention (discussed above) and vitamin E (alpha-tocopherol) in the phase III ATBC Prevention Study (discussed above) have made selenium and vitamin E highly attractive agents for chemopreventive testing in the prostate. These two prespecified secondary analyses from large phase III trials led to the recently activated SWOG-coordinated Intergroup Selenium and Vitamin E Cancer Prevention Trial (SELECT), which will involve 32,400 men at high risk of prostate cancer due primarily to age (50 years or older for African Americans [who are at higher risk than men of other ethnic backgrounds]; 55 years or older for all other men). The SELECT anticipates accrual to be completed in 5 years from activation in July 2001. The trial employs a 2-by-2 factorial design (four arms—selenium, vitamin E, selenium plus vitamin E, placebo) to administer study agents to men for 7 (minimum) to 12 (maximum) years.

Bladder Cancer Prevention

Clinical interest in retinoids for preventing bladder cancer was raised by positive retinoid studies in animals and population-based studies showing that vitamin A protects against bladder cancer. To date, a few small trials have been completed in this setting, showing some potential benefit of low-dose, long-term retinoids in preventing recurrence of superficial bladder tumors. In one informative study, very high doses of vitamins A, C, and E, zinc, and paradoxene supplements were more effective than the recommended dietary allowance of multivitamins in reducing the rate of superficial bladder tumor recurrence. Currently ongoing clinical and translational studies of 4-HPR, DFMO, and celecoxib will establish the effects of these promising agents on bladder carcinogenesis.

Esophageal and Stomach Cancer Prevention

Five large placebo-controlled chemoprevention trials in esophageal and gastric carcinogenesis have been conducted in regions of China with unusually high rates of esophageal/gastric cancers. In four of these five trials, multiple natural compounds, including retinol, β-carotene, vitamin E, and selenium, were tested (see "Chemopreventive Agents" section). In one of the trials, a small reduction in gastric cancer rates was achieved, but all five trials suffered from problems of high drop-out rates and poor study compliance. Therefore, the jury is still out on whether high multivitamin supplementation can effectively reduce the risk of gastric or esophageal cancer in high-risk populations.

Cervical Cancer Prevention

Cervical carcinogenesis is a well-defined process: the premalignant lesion dysplasia develops and proceeds through mild, moderate, and severe stages before developing into invasive cancer. Seven of eight chemoprevention trials that have been conducted in cervical dysplasia produced negative results with several agents, including folic acid, β-carotene, and interferon. One of the eight trials was a positive phase IIb trial of the retinoid tretinoin in 301 women. Tretinoin was significantly active in moderate dysplasia but not in severe dysplasia. Other ongoing retinoid trials are designed to confirm the early, promising results with tretinoin in this setting.

FUTURE DIRECTIONS

After three decades of extraordinary effort, cancer chemoprevention came of age near the very end of the 20th century with the FDA approvals of tamoxifen for breast cancer risk reduction (1998) and celecoxib for the control of FAP (1999). The continued and future progress of cancer chemoprevention in the 21st century will rely heavily on the following major areas of study: phase III trials (for definitive primary endpoint analyses; new study leads from promising secondary analyses; and complex risk-benefit assessment technologies integrating multiple, differing clinical outcomes); clinical-laboratory (translational) premalignant model systems; infectious diseases that cause cancer; pharmacologic smoking cessation (especially in people with genetic predispositions for smoking addiction); and molecular studies of carcinogenesis and drug mechanisms to develop novel chemopreventive targets and drugs (Table 6.2).

New molecular technologies will be extremely useful for developing and studying new targets of drug activity, existing candidate surrogate endpoint biomarkers, novel imaging techniques to monitor agent activity, and preclinical drug-testing models, such as gene targeting/knockout models, and molecular genetic risk models for identifying high-risk prevention trial cohorts. The activities of celecoxib in FAP and tamoxifen in women with *BRCA*2 mutations illustrate the potential of chemoprevention to benefit individuals with extremely high molecular genetic risk.

TABLE 6.2. Molecular-Targeting Agents

Receptor-selective retinoids
Selective estrogen-receptor modulators (SERMs)
Cyclooxygenase-2 (COX-2) inhibitors
Lipoxygenase (LOX) modulators
Epidermal growth factor receptor (EGFR) inhibitors
Farnesyl transferase inhibitors (FTI)
Difluoromethylornithine (DFMO)
P53 gene delivery/targeting
Protein kinase C inhibitors
Histone deacetylase inhibitors
Vitamin D analogs
5-α-reductase inhibitors
Matrix metalloproteinase inhibitors

The future of cancer chemoprevention is bright. In the United States, for example, from the National Cancer Institute to individual institutions across the country, preventing major epithelial cancers is an important focus of oncology research and funding support. Steadily, chemoprevention is rising to its rightful place beside screening and early detection, surgery, and chemo- and radiotherapy as a widely accepted standard approach for controlling the devastating consequences of major cancers.

FURTHER READING

Albanes D, Heinonen OP, Taylor PR et al. (1996) Alpha-tocopherol and beta-carotene supplements and lung cancer incidence in the alpha-tocopherol, beta-carotene cancer prevention study: effects of base-line characteristics and study compliance. *J Natl Cancer Inst* 88:1560–1570.

Auerbach H, Hammond EC, Garfinkel L (1979) Changes in bronchial epithelium in relation to cigarette smoking, 1955–1960 vs. 1970–1977. *N Engl J Med* 300:381–386.

Baron JA, Beach M, Mandel JS et al. (1999) Calcium supplements for the prevention of colorectal adenomas. *N Engl J Med* 340:101–107.

Blot WJ, Li J-Y, Taylor PR et al. (1993) Nutrition intervention trials in Linxian, China: supplementation with specific vitamin/mineral combinations, cancer incidence, and disease-specific mortality in the general population. *J Natl Cancer Inst* 85:1483–1492.

Bostick RM (1997) Human studies of calcium supplementation and colorectal epithelial cell proliferation. *Cancer Epidemiol Biomarkers Prev* 6:971–980.

Clark LC, Combs Jr GF, Turnbull BW et al. (1996) Effects of selenium supplementation for cancer prevention in patients with carcinoma of the skin. A randomized controlled trial. *JAMA* 276:1957–1963.

Clinton SK, Emenhiser C, Schwartz SJ et al. (1996) Cis-trans lycopene isomers, carotenoids and retinol in the human prostate. *Cancer Epidemiol Biomarkers Prev* 5:823–833.

Fisher B, Costantino JP, Wickerham DL et al. (1998) Tamoxifen for prevention of breast cancer: report of the National Surgical Adjuvant Breast and Bowel Project P-1 study. *J Natl Cancer Inst* 90:1371–1388.

Fisher B, Dignam J, Wolmark N et al. (1999) Tamoxifen in treatment of intraductal breast cancer: national surgical adjuvant breast and bowel project B-24 randomised controlled trial. *Lancet* 353:1993–2000.

Giardiello FM, Hamilton SR, Krush AJ et al. (1993) Treatment of colonic and rectal adenomas with sulindac in familial adenomatous polyposis. *N Engl J Med* 328:1313–1316.

Giovannucci E, Egan KM, Hunter DJ et al. (1995) Aspirin and the risk of colorectal cancer in women. *New Engl J Med* 333:609–614.

Greenberg ER, Baron JA, Stukel TA et al. and the Skin Cancer Prevention Study Group (1990) A clinical trial of β carotene to prevent basal-cell and squamous-cell cancers of the skin. *N Engl J Med* 323:789–795.

Greenberg ER, Baron JA, Tosteson TD et al. and the Polyp Prevention Study Group (1994) A clinical trial of antioxidant vitamins to prevent colorectal adenoma. *N Engl J Med* 331:141–147.

Gupta RA, DuBois RN (2000) Combinations for cancer prevention. *Nat Med* 6:974–975.

Hennekens CH, Burning JE, Manson JE et al. (1996) Lack of effect of long-term supplementation with beta carotene on the incidence of malignant neoplasms and cardiovascular disease. *N Engl J Med* 334:1145–1149.

Hong WK, Sporn MB (1997) Recent advances in chemoprevention of cancer. *Science* 278:1073–1077.

Hong WK, Endicott J, Itri LM et al. (1986) 13 *cis* retinoic acid in the treatment of oral leukoplakia. *N Engl J Med* 315:1501–1505.

Hong WK, Lippman SM, Itri LM et al. (1990) Prevention of second primary tumors with isotretinoin in squamous-cell carcinoma of the head and neck. *N Engl J Med* 323:795–801.

Hong WK, Spitz MR, Lippman SM (2000) Cancer chemoprevention in the 21st century: genetics, risk modeling, and molecular targets. *J Clin Oncol* 18:9s–18s.

Hoque A, Albanes D, Lippman SM et al. (2001) Molecular epidemiologic studies within the selenium and vitamin E cancer prevention trial (SELECT). *Cancer Causes Control* 12:627–633.

Kelloff GJ, Johnson JR, Crowell JA et al. (1995) Approaches to the development and marketing approval of drugs that prevent cancer. *Cancer Epidemiol Biomarkers Prev* 4:1–10.

Khuri FR, Kim ES, Lee JJ et al. (2001) The impact of smoking status, disease stage, and index tumor site on second primary tumor incidence and tumor recurrence in the head and neck retinoid chemoprevention trial. *Cancer Epidemiol Biomarkers Prev* 10:823–829.

Khuri FR (2003) Secondary primary cancers of the head and neck. In *Clinical Hematology and Oncology*. Philadelphia: Churchill Livingstone, pp. 1012–1016.

Kraemer KH, Digiovanna JJ, Moshell AN et al. (1988) Prevention of skin cancer in xeroderma pigmentosum with the use of oral isotretinoin. *N Engl J Med* 318:1633–1637.

Kucuk O, Sarkar FH, Sakr W et al. (2001) Phase II randomized clinical trial of lycopene supplementation before radical prostatectomy. *Cancer Epidemiol Biomarkers Prev* 10:861–868.

Kurie JM, Lee JS, Khuri FR et al. (2000) N-(4-hydroxyphenyl) retinamide in the chemoprevention of squamous metaplasia and dysplasia of the bronchial epithelium. *Clin Cancer Res* 6:2973–2979.

Lee JJ, Hong WK, Hittelman WN et al. (2000) Predicting cancer development in oral leukoplakia: ten years of translational research. *Clin Cancer Res* 6:1702–1710.

Lee JJ, Liu D, Lee JS et al. (2001) Long-term impact of smoking on lung epithelial proliferation in current and former smokers. *J Natl Cancer Inst* 93:1081–1088.

Li J-Y, Taylor P, Li B et al. (1993) Nutrition intervention trials in Linxian, China: multiple vitamin/mineral supplementation, cancer incidence, and disease-specific mortality among adults with esophageal dysplasia. *J Natl Cancer Inst* 85:1492–1498.

Li M, Lotan R, Levin B et al. (2000) Aspirin induction of apoptosis in esophageal cancer: a potential for chemoprevention. *Cancer Epidemiol Biomarkers Prev* 9:545–549.

Lippman SM, Brown PH (1999) Tamoxifen prevention of breast cancer: an instance of the fingerpost. *J Natl Cancer Inst* 91:1809–1819.

Lippman SM, Hong WK (2001) Molecular markers of the risk of oral cancer (editorial). *N Engl J Med* 344:1323–1326.

Lippman SM, Lee JS, Lotan R et al. (1990) Biomarkers as intermediate endpoints in chemoprevention trials. *J Natl Cancer Inst* 82:555–560.

Lippman SM, Batsakis JG, Toth BB et al. (1993) Comparison of low-dose isotretinoin with beta carotene to prevent oral carcinogenesis. *N Engl J Med* 328:15–20.

Lippman SM, Benner SE, Hong WK (1994) Cancer chemoprevention. *J Clin Oncol* 12:851–873.

Lippman SM, Lee JJ, Sabichi AL (1998) Cancer chemoprevention: progress and promise. *J Natl Cancer Inst* 90:1514–1528.

Lippman SM, Lee JJ, Karp DD et al. (2001) Randomized phase III intergroup trial of isotretinoin to prevent second primary tumors in stage I non-small-cell lung cancer. *J Natl Cancer Inst* 93:605–618.

Lotan R, Xu XC, Lippman SM et al. (1995) Suppression of retinoic acid receptor-beta in premalignant oral lesions and its up-regulation by isotretinoin. *N Engl J Med* 332:1405–1410.

Mao L, El-Naggar AK, Papadimitrakopoulou V et al. (1998) Phenotype and genotype in advanced premalignant head and neck lesions after chemopreventive therapy. *J Natl Cancer Inst* 90:1545–1551.

Mao L, Lee JS, Kurie JM et al. (1997) Clonal genetic alterations in the lungs of current and former smokers. *J Natl Cancer Inst* 89:857–862.

Mayne ST, Lippman SM (2001) Retinoids, carotenoids, and micronutrients. In *Cancer: Principles and Practice of Oncology*, 6th ed. DeVita VT, Hellman S, Rosenberg SA (eds), Baltimore, MD: Lippincott Williams & Wilkins, pp 575–590.

Meyskens F, Surwit E, Moon TE et al. (1994) Enhancement of regression of cervical intra-epithelia neoplasia II (moderate dysplasia) with topically applied all-trans retinoic acid: a randomized trial. *J Natl Cancer Inst* 86:539–543.

Moon TE, Levine N, Cartmel B et al. (1997) Effect of retinol in preventing squamous cell skin cancer in moderate-risk subjects: a randomized, double-blind, controlled trial. *Cancer Epidemiol Biomarkers Prev* 6:949–956.

Muto Y, Moriwaki H, Ninomiya M et al. (1996) Prevention of second primary tumors by an acyclic retinoid, polyprenoic acid, in patients with hepatocellular carcinoma. Hepatoma Prevention Study Group. *N Engl J Med* 334:1561–1567.

Omenn GS, Goodman GE, Thornquist MD et al. (1996) Effects of a combination of beta carotene and vitamin A on lung cancer and cardiovascular disease. *N Engl J Med* 334:1150–1155.

Pastorino U, Infante M, Maioli M et al. (1993) Adjuvant treatment of stage I lung cancer with high dose vitamin A. *J Clin Oncol* 11:1216–1222.

Ruffin IV MT, Koyamangalath K, Rock CL et al. (1997) Suppression of human colorectal prostaglandins: determining the lowest effective aspirin dose. *J Natl Cancer Inst* 89:1152–1160.

Shin DM, Mao L, Papadimitrakopoulou VM et al. (2000) Alteration of p53 gene and protein expression and biochemo-preventive therapy in patients with advanced premalignant lesions of the head and neck. *J Natl Cancer Inst* 92:69–73.

Shin DM, Khuri FR, Murphy B et al. (2001) Combined interferon-, 13-cis-retinoic acid and tocopherol in locally advanced head and neck squamous cell carcinoma: novel bioadjuvant phase II trial. *J Clin Oncol* 19:3010–3017.

Shureiqi I, Lippman SM (2001) Lipoxygenase modulation to reverse carcinogenesis. *Cancer Res* 61:6307–6312.

Shureiqi I, Chen D, Lee JJ et al. (2000) 15-LOX-1: a novel molecular target of nonsteroidal anti-inflammatory drug-induced apoptosis in colorectal cancer cells. *J Natl Cancer Inst* 92:1136–1142.

Shureiqi I, Cooksley CD, Morris J et al. (2001) Effect of age on risk of second primary colorectal cancer. *J Natl Cancer Inst* 93:1264–1266.

Shureiqi I, Xu X, Chen D et al. (2001) Nonsteroidal anti-inflammatory drugs induce apoptosis in esophageal cancer cells by restoring 15-lipoxygenase-1 expression. *Cancer Res* 61: 4879–4884.

Slaughter DP, Southwick HW, Smejkal W (1953) 'Field cancerization' in oral stratified squamous epithelium: clinical implications of multicentric origin. *Cancer* 6:963–968.

Soria J-C, Moon C, Wang L et al. (2001) Effect of *N*-(4-Hydroxyphenyl)retinamide on hTERT expression in the bronchial epithelium of cigarette smokers. *J Natl Cancer Inst* 93: 1257–1263.

Steinbach G, Lynch PM, Phillips RK et al. (2000) The effect of celecoxib, a cyclooxygenase-2 inhibitor, in familial adenomatous polyposis. *N Engl J Med* 342:1946–1952.

The Alpha-Tocopherol, Beta Carotene Cancer Prevention Study Group (1994) The effect of vitamin E and beta carotene on the incidence of lung cancer and other cancers in male smokers. *N Engl J Med* 330:1029–1035.

The Alpha-Tocopherol, Beta Carotene Cancer Prevention Study Group (1994) The effect of vitamin E and beta carotene on the incidence of lung cancer and other cancers in male smokers. *N Engl J Med* 330:1029–1035.

van Zandwijk N, Dalesio O, Pastorino U et al. (2000) Euroscan, a randomized trial of vitamin A and *N*-acetylcysteine in patients with head and neck cancer or lung cancer. *J Natl Cancer Inst* 92:977–986.

Veronesi U, De Palo G, Marubini E et al. (1999) Randomized trial of fenretinide to prevent second breast malignancy in women with early breast cancer. *J Natl Cancer Inst* 91: 1847–1856.

Vokes EE, Weichselbaum RR, Lippman SM, Hong WK (1993) Head and neck cancer. *N Engl J Med* 328:184–194.

Xu X-C, Sneige N, Liu X et al. (1997) Progressive decrease in nuclear retinoic acid receptor-β messenger RNA level during breast carcinogenesis. *Cancer Res* 57:4992–4996.

Yarosh D, Klein J, O'Connor A et al. (2001) Effect of topically applied T4 endonuclease V in liposomes on skin cancer in xeroderma pigmentosum: a randomised study. *Lancet* 357:926–929.

CHAPTER 7

Screening and Early Detection

DAVID A. SLOAN

University of Kentucky, Lexington, Kentucky

The early detection of cancer is a critical strategy in reducing cancer-specific mortality. Whether screening is appropriate for a given cancer is dependent upon a number of factors. An understanding of the principles of cancer screening and an appreciation for the specific biology and epidemiology of a particular type of cancer is essential in determining the benefit of screening large populations of individuals for a specific cancer. In this chapter, the essential principles of cancer screening are discussed first in a general sense and then are examined in the setting of four common cancer models.

Cancer screening refers to the process by which a large number of people within a population undergo one or more tests that are designed to find occult cancer. The principal reason for detecting preclinical disease is to initiate treatment at an earlier time point in the natural history of the cancer. Only if earlier treatment results in improved outcomes will the screening have been worthwhile. Different outcomes can be measured, although the most important is often the most difficult to achieve: namely, a reduction in cancer-specific mortality. Deciding whether to screen for a particular cancer involves consideration of the biology and natural history of the cancer, the prevalence of the cancer, and the degree of morbidity and mortality the cancer causes in a population. The decision to initiate screening is also dependent on the quality of the screening test or tests available. Finally, there are financial, ethical, and societal issues that must be resolved.

Screening programs by definition are large-scale events that for the most part involve considerable expenditure. In view of the increasing competition for health care resources within society, compromises are invariably necessary. What is best for the individual in terms of screening for cancer is not always best for society as whole when the cost-effectiveness of the screening is rigorously examined.

UICC Manual of Clinical Oncology, Eighth Edition. Edited by Raphael E. Pollock
ISBN 0-471-22289-5 Copyright © 2004 John Wiley & Sons, Inc.

Cancer screening is an important tool that can alleviate the pain and suffering caused by cancer within society. Screening programs for a few cancers such as those for breast and cervix have been shown to be effective, but controversies continue to surround screening issues for most if not all cancers. Even with regard to breast and cervical cancer, unresolved and controversial issues persist.

The general principles of cancer screening are discussed in the first half of this chapter. These include the biologic basis for cancer screening, the determinants of a good cancer screening test, screening biases, the measurement of outcomes related to screening, and, finally, societal and financial issues associated with screening. In the latter half of the chapter, four models for cancer screening are examined in detail. For cervical, breast, colorectal, and prostate cancer, the history and current status of screening are examined in light of the general principles of cancer screening. The status of screening for these four cancers in terms of efficacy is very different, but the discussion of each of these models should serve to reinforce the fundamental principles of cancer screening.

GENERAL PRINCIPLES OF CANCER SCREENING

Biologic Basis of Screening

Screening may not be appropriate for a cancer even if a good screening test is available. For screening to be appropriate, the biology of the cancer must be such that there is a protracted preclinical stage during which distant metastasis is uncommon. Because the presence of distant metastasis is generally synonymous with incurability for almost all cancer types, it is important that cancers be detected early in their natural history, *before* the cancer has spread beyond the site of the primary tumor. Therefore, tumors that tend not to metastasize until they have reached a certain size (e.g., breast cancer) are best suited for screening.

The longer the asymptomatic preclinical phase, the more opportunity there will be to detect asymptomatic cancer through a screening program. If a cancer is very slow growing, even if an initial screen test fails to detect it, a subsequent screen may find it and still permit a cure. Colon cancer, for example, is associated with a long preclinical phase, a prolonged process that progresses from hyperplasia through adenomatous neoplasia, dysplasia, carcinoma *in situ*, and ultimately to invasive cancer. This multistep progression probably takes as long as 10 to 15 years. The preclinical stage is further lengthened, then, if the cancer in question is associated with a recognizable precancerous condition (e.g., cervical cancer preceded by cervical dysplasial). If a diagnosis of cancer or even precancer can be made early, the biology of the cancer should be such that early treatment will decrease mortality. Treatment of early disease must therefore be effective if screening is to be worth the effort expended.

Another consideration is the prevalence of the cancer. If the cancer is rare, then it is unlikely that mass screening programs will be of value. It is not surprising, then, that the most widely studied cancers in terms of screening are among the most common (e.g., breast, colon, prostate, and cervical cancer). It is estimated that one

Is the cancer appropriate for screening?

- ☐ common cancer

- ☐ a high prevalence in preclinical state

- ☐ associated with substantial morbidity and mortality

- ☐ long disease-detectable, nonmetastatic preclinical phase

- ☐ preclinical detection of cancer permits improved treatment outcomes

- ☐ effective screening test(s) available

Figure 7.1   Checklist of the important characteristics of a cancer that would make the cancer suitable for screening.

woman in eight will develop breast cancer in her lifetime and that one man in ten will develop prostate cancer. In the case of prostate cancer, autopsy studies have shown that as many as 30% of men 50 years of age or older have demonstrable evidence of prostate cancer, although most prostate cancers are probably of little biologic significance. This point underscores the fact that the mere prevalence of cancer may not reflect its true aggressiveness. Similarly, papillary carcinoma of the thyroid, which, although a very common finding at autopsy, is, in fact, a rare cause of death from cancer. Figure 7.1 summarizes the conditions that should be met in deciding whether to screen a population for a specific type of cancer.

Screening Test Determinants

The screening test is the most critical component of a screening program. It may be a single test (e.g., the Pap smear for cervical cancer) or it may be a combination of tests (e.g., clinical breast examination and mammography for breast cancer). In contrast to diagnostic tests, which are generally employed when patients develop symptoms, screening tests are generally deployed before any symptomatology is manifested. Screening tests focus on the preclinical phase of cancer in a population. Different types of tests may focus on different time points in the natural history of the cancer. For example, screening clinical breast examination (CBE) is used to detect palpable tumors, whereas mammography usually identifies nonpalpable tumors. A molecular test (e.g., *BRCA-1* or *BRCA-2* gene determination for breast cancer or the *c-K-ras* test for colon cancer) will be positive at a much earlier time point. Figure 7.2 lists the criteria by which the quality of the screening test should be measured. A good screening test should first and foremost be associated with high sensitivity and high specificity. Sensitivity refers to the probability of obtaining positive results if cancer is truly present. Specificity is the probability of obtaining negative results if there is in fact no cancer present. The predictive value of a screening test is another important parameter. The positive predictive value (PPV) is a measure of the accuracy of a test in gauging the likelihood that

Is the screening test a good one?

- ☐ high sensitivity
- ☐ high specificity
- ☐ inexpensive
- ☐ risk-free
- ☐ simple
- ☐ easy to administer
- ☐ lends itself to mass implementation
- ☐ leads to early treatment and reduced cancer-specific mortality
- ☐ low psychological and financial costs attached to workup of false positives

Figure 7.2   Checklist of the important characteristics of a screening test that would make the test suitable for use in a cancer screening program.

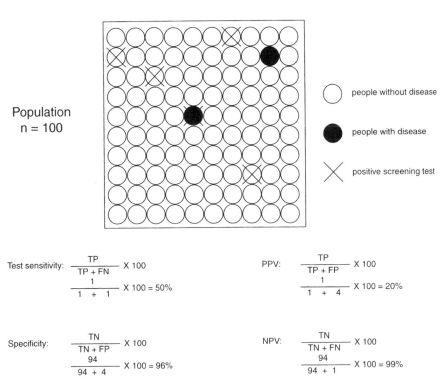

Population
n = 100

◯ people without disease

● people with disease

✕ positive screening test

Test sensitivity: $\dfrac{TP}{TP + FN}$ X 100

$\dfrac{1}{1 + 1}$ X 100 = 50%

PPV: $\dfrac{TP}{TP + FP}$ X 100

$\dfrac{1}{1 + 4}$ X 100 = 20%

Specificity: $\dfrac{TN}{TN + FP}$ X 100

$\dfrac{94}{94 + 4}$ X 100 = 96%

NPV: $\dfrac{TN}{TN + FN}$ X 100

$\dfrac{94}{94 + 1}$ X 100 = 99%

Figure 7.3   Hypothetical population of 100 people, two of whom have preclinical cancer. A hypothetical screening test is positive for five individuals, only one of whom actually has cancer. The formulas for determining test sensitivity, specificity, positive predictive value (PPV), and negative predictive value (NPV) are provided along with the numbers applicable to the hypothetical example illustrated.

disease or cancer is actually present when the test is positive. For example, a PPV of 10% means that there is a 1 in 10 chance that disease is present. On the other hand, negative predictive value (NPV) is the accuracy of a test in determining the absence of disease. Figure 7.3 presents a hypothetical population of 100 people, two of whom have subclinical cancer. The results of the available hypothetical screening test are positive for five people, only one of whom actually has cancer. When these numbers are used, hypothetical values for sensitivity, specificity, PPV, and NPV can be generated.

Screening tests vary in nature (Fig. 7.4). Some, such as the CBE for breast cancer detection, the digital rectal examination (DRE) for prostate cancer, the pelvic exam and visualization of the cervix for cervix cancer and the complete skin examination for skin cancer, are simply focused physical examinations. Such tests, although simple and "low-tech," are subjective but nonetheless have great merit; however, the quality of physical examination can be quite variable. More objective are screening tests that consist of imaging studies such as chest radiograph, mammogram, or transrectal ultrasound (TRUS). Imaging tests such as these or screening cytologic tests such as the Pap smear are still subject to interpretation by specialists. The literature clearly shows that specialists never come close to 100% agreement when viewing images, be they mammograms, ultrasounds, or cytologic slides. Most objective are laboratory tests such as the prostate-specific antigen (PSA) or Hemoccult test. However, even though such laboratory tests are more objective, they are still fraught with problems of interpretation. For example, a "cutoff" point needs to be agreed upon at which "positives" are distinguished from "negatives." If Hemoccult specimens are rehydrated before the chemical testing is done, the likelihood of positive results will quadruple. The serum level for the "cutoff" point for the PSA test will affect the sensitivity and specificity of the test. For the four models of cancer screening that are discussed, the established screening tools are shown in Figure 7.5.

How easy is the screening test to administer? How readily do healthy people submit to the screening test? There is a not surprising reluctance on the part of

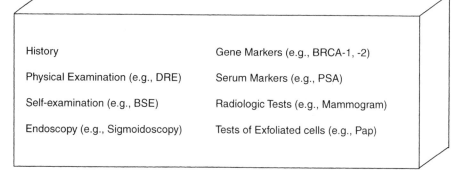

Figure 7.4 Various screening tools that are available for use by clinicians in screening people for occult cancer.

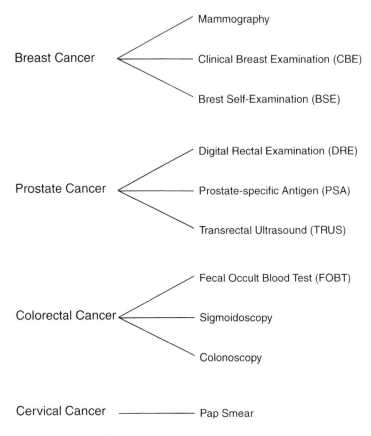

Figure 7.5 Commonly employed screening tests for breast, cervical, colorectal, and prostate cancer.

many people to provide stool samples for fecal occult blood testing (FOBT). Mammograms are associated with some discomfort and apprehension on the part of women. Some screening tests are associated with risks. Although the risk of radiation associated with screening mammography is minuscule, the risks associated with screening colonoscopy are significant (e.g., 0.1% incidence of bowel perforation). How difficult is it to ensure that a screening test is done well? Although it may be fairly easy to ensure the quality of a serum test, ensuring that a standard high level of quality accompanies every mammogram and Pap smear is much more difficult. The quality of mammography performed as part of the widely quoted Canadian breast screening studies has, for example, been harshly criticized.

A screening test needs to be incorporated into a sound administrative structure that ensures that the screening is carried out in a safe and orderly manner. Rigorous attention needs to be paid to the quality control of the particular test, the accurate recording of test results, and the notification of patients and physicians to make certain that all patients with positive test results are appropriately investigated.

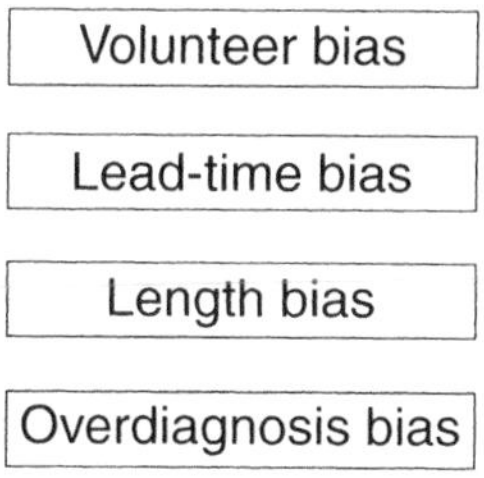

| Volunteer bias |

| Lead-time bias |

| Length bias |

| Overdiagnosis bias |

Figure 7.6   Typical biases encountetred in the course of evaluating scientific studies for the purpose of determining the efficicacy of cancer screening programs.

Screening Biases

As screening programs are implemented and subsequently evaluated, a degree of caution needs to be exercised. Unfortunately, screening programs may appear more effective than they truly are because of one or more potential biases (Fig. 7.6). The first is a volunteer bias inserted into a screening program because of the characteristics of people volunteering for a screening study. Women volunteering for a mammography screening program, for example, are more likely than matched controls to perform breast self-examination, which in turn "contaminates" or overestimates the impact of mammography. One recent study found that women who exercise regularly and eat a healthier diet were more likely to use screening services. Patients undergoing screening sigmoidoscopy in one case-control study had a 30% reduction in the risk of cancer of the rectum. The author observed a strong correlation between the number of sigmoidoscopies performed and the number of periodic health examinations undergone; people willing to be screened for rectal cancer appeared more likely to seek medical attention.

Lead-time bias refers to the "advantage" that a screened population has in having cancer detected at an earlier time point in the natural history of the cancer. If the cancer of patient A is diagnosed earlier than that of patient B because of screening but both die of cancer at the same time, patient A will appear to have had a longer survival time, but in fact the mortality data will be unchanged. Lead-time bias can be illustrated in a simple scenario in which two people get on the same bus, one passenger boarding the bus 20 minutes outside of the city center terminal and the other passenger 10 minutes from city center. Both travelers disembark at the same time but their respective traveling times are quite different.

Length bias is not to be confused with lead-time bias. Length bias refers to the phenomenon that screening programs will tend to detect slower-growing cancers and miss rapidly growing, more aggressive cancers. Many screening studies show that a screened population has a higher percentage of early tumors than a non-screened population. An excellent example of this phenomenon is colon cancer FOBT screening: many studies show significantly more early tumors and significantly fewer advanced tumors in FOBT-screened patients. Indolent cancers such as colon cancer with a long preclinical phase are therefore ideal for screening detection from this standpoint. It follows that the survival rates of patients whose cancers are detected by screening may well be better than those of patients whose cancers are not detected by screening, thus artificially enhancing the benefit of screening to the observer.

Over-diagnosis bias refers to the danger of diagnosing cancer in a large percentage of the population when in fact the cancer is a significant cause of morbidity and mortality for only a small proportion of the population. The examples of prostate cancer and papillary thyroid cancer have already been provided. Another example may be ductal carcinoma *in situ* (DCIS), a cancer that exhibits a wide spectrum of biologic the explosion in diagnosis precipitated by widespread mammography screening of aggressiveness.

Efficacy of Screening: Outcome Measurements

Screening programs are costly ventures that consume resources and require years of effort. It is crucial that the benefits of screening outweigh any "risks" or "negatives" associated with the screening program (Fig. 7.7). What sorts of risks might accompany a screening test? Imaging studies such as chest radiographs or mammograms expose people to very small amounts of ionizing radiation. Much more important as a source of screening-related morbidity are the possible adverse effects related to the diagnostic workup of patients whose tests are positive. For example, although prostate screening tests such as DRE and PSA are associated with minimal morbidity, the potential morbidity of the many prostate biopsies

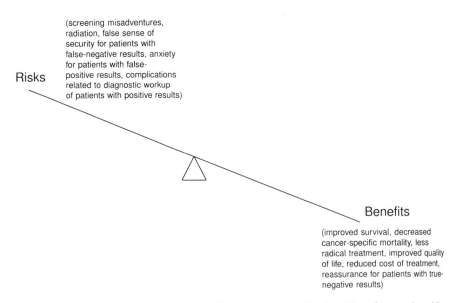

Figure 7.7 The benefits of cancer screening should outweigh the risks of screening if a cancer screening program is worthwhile.

necessitated by screening is much greater. Similarly, the colonoscopies performed as a result of positive FOBTs (up to 10% of screened people are FOBT positive) are associated with real risks (perforation, hemorrhage, risks related to sedation). If such complications occur among patients with false-positive results, the efficacy equation of the screening test is negatively affected. Most breast biopsies performed because of screening mammograms yield positive results, but show the presence of benign disease, not cancer. Again, although biopsy-related complications are few, they do occur. Further, more than workup complications must be considered. Even if the procedures are complication free, they consume medical resources, occupy physician time, cause pain for patients, and keep patients away from work. It is also important not to overlook the psychological trauma inflicted on people who are told they have test results that are indicative of cancer. Depending on the PPV of the screening test, varying numbers of people will ultimately be proved to be cancer free yet left with the emotional scars of the diagnostic testing procedures. A recent study concluded that as many as 50% of women suffered short-term anxiety and depression (as measured with the Hospital Anxiety and Depression Scale) when recalled to mammography centers because of abnormal screening mammograms. With the previously mentioned problem of over-diagnosis bias, many patients suffer the trauma of being told that they have cancer even though the cancer may have little biologic significance. Nevertheless, the patients are forced to live with the diagnosis of cancer. Another "hidden" risk of screening is the false sense of security that some patients might receive as a result of negative test results. Colorectal screening studies have shown that only a minority of colon cancers actually result in detectable fecal blood at any given point in time. A person testing negative might not return for follow-up testing, a problem that plagues all screening programs.

What are the potential benefits of a screening test that would justify the previously discussed risks? One hopes to see patients with earlier diagnosed cancers treated with greater effect in terms of cancer cure. Improved survival is obviously sought, but one also hopes to see patients treated with less debilitating and less mutilating treatments. Small breast cancers that are diagnosed earlier, for example, are more likely to be amenable to breast-conserving treatments. Making an earlier diagnosis of breast cancer may also mean that adjuvant chemotherapy may be rendered unnecessary and that the patient may be spared the morbidity and inconvenience associated with such treatment. Improved quality of life for screened patients then might be enough to justify a screening program even if reduced mortality is not demonstrated.

It is apparent at this point in the discussion that the effectiveness of any screening program needs to be rigorously measured. What yardsticks are available? Most screening programs result in the diagnosis of an increased number of cancers among screened populations. However, simply diagnosing more cancers is not a satisfactory measure unless treatment leads to reduced mortality and, particularly, reduced cancer-specific mortality. Reduced cancer-specific mortality is clearly the bottom line for any screening program. Screening programs can also be evaluated in terms of quality-of-life measures, as has already been alluded to in the discussion of breast cancer treatment. Finally, the costs associated with a screening test are easily measured.

As one reviews the cancer screening literature, three primary types of outcome studies are seen: historical studies, case-control studies, and prospective randomized trials (PRTs). A case-control study is a retrospective analysis comparing the outcomes of patients who have been screened with those of unscreened controls. Although the literature is replete with case-control studies, a much more satisfactory measure of screening effectiveness is the PRT. A PRT should negate the effects of volunteer, lead-time, and length bias as people are randomly assigned to screening and nonscreening groups. Both groups can then be evaluated in terms of the outcome measures already discussed: numbers of cancers diagnosed, survival, cancer-specific mortality, years of life saved, quality-of-life measures, and financial costs. PRTs, unfortunately, are hampered by various problems including compliance issues and the contamination of the control group by outside factors such as the availability of screening tests themselves. Although one might hope that a PRT would settle any debate about screening efficacy, this is often not the case, as the situation with breast cancer screening for younger women illustrates (Fig. 7.8).

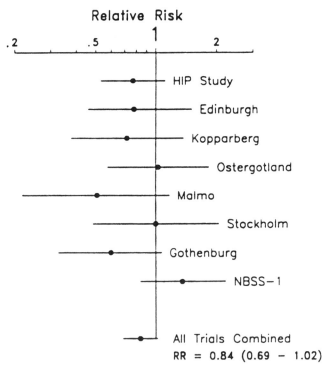

Figure 7.8   Relative risks and 95% confidence intervals from all breast cancer screening randomized clinical trials that have included women ages 40 to 49 years at entry. The last line shows meta-analysis results. (From Smart et al. *Cancer* 75:1619–1626, 1995.)

Cost and Societal Issues

The morbidity and mortality caused by cancer show little signs of diminishing in spite of substantial improvements in treatment regimens. For a society, the cost of cancer treatment is enormous in terms of health care resources, workplace losses, and individual suffering. Because the societal and financial costs of cancer treatment are greatest when disease is most advanced, there is a compelling reason to invest resources at the "front end" of cancer management. The essential purpose of screening programs is to make an early diagnosis of cancer in a large number of people, the goal being to reduce both cancer morbidity and cancer mortality. Unfortunately, there are many barriers to achieving this goal for the common cancers that plague society. These barriers are financial, educational, societal, racial, and ethical.

There are formidable financial barriers to screening. Screening tests vary widely in cost. Although the test materials themselves may be inexpensive, the "downstream costs," as one author has termed them, may be very high. While a Hemoccult test may cost only a few dollars, by the time one adds the associated costs bundled into a colorectal cancer screening program (administrative costs, diagnostic workup costs) the expenses are considerable. For people over the age of 50, current recommendations include flexible sigmoidoscopy every 5 to 10 years, with some experts advocating a screening colonoscopy for all individuals aged 60 or greater. If the current sigmoidoscopy guidelines alone were adhered to in the United States, the estimated cost would be well over $1 billion U.S. per year. If the prostate cancer screening guidelines that some groups have recommended were implemented on a large scale, the cost would be staggering and health care facilities would be overwhelmed by patients. Such a scenario underscores the point that health care institutions need to have adequate infrastructures to support screening programs. Health care workers are needed to administer screening tests, interpret the tests, conduct the workups of those with positive results, and treat all patients who have newly diagnosed cancer. In the current climate of aggressive cost controls and judicious resource allocation, politicians, government departments, health care institutions, employers, physician organizations, and interested parties in society need to work together to prioritize screening-related issues. Cost-effectiveness analyses and cost-benefit analyses need to be looked at carefully. For example, by calculating the cost of a given screening program per year of life saved, public health authorities can compare the cost-effectiveness of various screening programs. One government agency has set as an arbitrary benchmark $40,000 per year of life saved by screening, and it is only if the cost of a screening program is below this figure that the screening program is believed to be justified. Ideally, carefully designed multicenter PRTs measuring a number of endpoints should be carried out to determine the efficacy of a given screening program.

Education is a multilevel barrier to effective screening. Volunteers for screening programs tend to consist of people who are on the whole better educated and from higher socioeconomic groups. The poorly educated population may not recognize the importance of screening or of following physicians' recommendations if their test results are positive. The education pendulum can also swing the other way, however. One study showed that women under the age of 50 greatly overestimated both their risk of developing breast cancer and the effectiveness of breast cancer screening. If the education of the general population is a barrier, the education of health care professionals is an even greater one. A substantial majority of physicians do not adhere to recommended screening guidelines in their individual practices. Data show that physicians are inadequately trained in the area of cancer screening; they do not know when to order a mammogram or how to do a proper CBE. A number of authors have made pleas for the improved cancer education of physicians and other health care professionals.

Racial barriers to screening clearly exist as well. African American men, for example, are less likely to take advantage of screening for prostate cancer, an unfortunate problem given the higher prostate cancer mortality rates in African Americans. One recent nursing study found that for African American men, specific obstacles included "would be embarrassed," "no way to get there," and "refuse to go." Studies have shown that there are barriers to breast cancer screening for African American women that include misconceptions about the etiology of breast cancer and fatalistic perspectives related to breast cancer outcomes. Screening programs clearly need to be sensitive to and need to address in creative ways these important barriers.

SPECIFIC MODELS FOR CANCER SCREENING

Cervical Cancer

Cervical cancer is the second most common cancer among women worldwide. Four of every five new cases are diagnosed in the developing parts of the world. Cervical cancer is ideal for screening because it has a very long preclinical phase during which precancerous and early cancerous changes can be easily diagnosed with a simple test, the Papanicolaou (Pap) smear. The Pap test has been used in screening programs for half a century. Although the test is inexpensive, a number of problems are associated with it, including quality issues related to cervical sampling, slide preparation, and cytologic interpretation. In one study in which two institutions traded 20,000 slides, the rate of under-calling *in situ* or invasive cancer was 34–57%. False-negative rates for the Pap test are usually 5–10%, although they can exceed 50%. Problems with the conventional Pap test have led recently to interest in a number of other possible screening tests that include human papilloma virus (HPV) DNA testing, liquid-based thin layer methods for cytologic evaluations, and cervicography. Screening intervals from 1 to 10 years with the Pap test have been used and there is good evidence that relatively long intervals of 3–5 years are associated with important reductions in cancer-specific mortality.

The evidence for the efficacy of Pap cytologic screening is based not on PRTs but on historic and case-control studies. Numerous studies have shown that the mortality rates associated with cervical cancer are up to 90% less for screened patients than for nonscreened patients. The primary problem with cervical cancer screening has been to achieve high rates of screening in the population of women most at risk for the disease. Recent efforts to study the use of lay health advisors have been shown to significantly reduce barriers to understanding among women in low literacy level and poor populations. Investigators have recently looked at the screening potential of self-collected vaginal swabs for HPV DNA testing. Such strategies may greatly increase cancer screening among high-risk populations. Cervical cancer screening is a unique model for cancer screening that is built on a simple, low-tech test; it has been shown to be efficacious for all ages of women in both developed and undeveloped countries. Cervical cancer screening is without question not only the oldest cancer screening program but also the most solidly entrenched.

Breast Cancer

Breast cancer is common and the prevalence of premalignant breast disease and *in situ* cancer is high. Small preclinical tumors tend not to have metastasized; thus, patients can benefit from screening. Screening tests for breast cancer include breast self-examination (BSE), clinical breast examination (CBE), and mammography. Mammography as a screening tool has continued to evolve in terms of technical sophistication, but the most notable study demonstrating its efficacy is more than three decades old. The Greater New York Health Insurance Plan (HIP) study randomized 62,000 women between the ages of 40 and 64 to control or to yearly CBE and mammography for 4 years. Over a 10-year period, 30% fewer deaths occurred among the screened women. Almost 300,000 women were enrolled in the Breast Cancer Detection Demonstration Project. This nonrandomized but prospective study found that the incidence of breast cancer in the screened group was higher (1.34 times the expected incidence) and that the mortality rate was only 80% of that expected. Evidence has continued to accumulate for the efficacy of breast cancer screening. In contrast to prostate and cervical cancer screening, breast cancer screening has been demonstrated by a number of recent PRTs to be effective, particularly for women between the ages of 50 and 69. Screening generally means mammography (at 1- to 3-year intervals, depending on the study), sometimes with CBE. For women between 50 and 69 years of age, the PRTs indicate a reduction of mortality from 15% to 30% as a result of screening programs. Even the casual reader is aware of the controversy that has raged over the efficacy of screening for women between the ages of 40 and 49. Figure 7.8 summarizes the PRTs for this age group. Meta-analysis of the available studies has shown a 16% reduction (not significant) in breast cancer mortality. If the first Canadian National Breast Screening Study (CNBSS) trial is excluded from the meta-analysis, the mortality reduction improves to 24%. Figure 7.8 shows that two of the PRTs showed no change in mortality at all, whereas the much-criticized Canadian study showed an increased risk of breast cancer in screened women. Screening mammography, although not particularly expensive, is associated with substantial downstream costs, including the cost of the large number of surgical consultations and biopsies that ensue (most of which are negative for cancer) and the anxiety caused for the numerous women with "false-positive" results from mammograms.

Although mammography is the dominant screening tool, the importance of CBE and BSE should not be overlooked. It has been estimated that most of the decrease in mortality in the screened population of the HIP study was because of CBE rather than mammography; in that study, 58% of the breast tumors were found with CBE alone. More recently, the second CNBSS trial randomized women between the ages of 50 and 59 to CBE and BSE or to mammography and BSE. The mammography group had significantly more node-negative small tumors, but there was no difference in the death rate from breast cancer at up to 7 years of follow-up. With regard to BSE and CBE, there is much room for improvement in terms of both patient and physician education. Greater efforts need to be devoted to improving physicians' understanding of the role of BSE, CBE, and mammography in breast cancer screening and in communicating positive clinical or mammographic findings to patients.

Colorectal Cancer

Colorectal cancer is an important cause of cancer deaths worldwide. Unfortunately, in spite of advances in adjuvant treatment, half of the patients with colorectal cancer die of the disease. Screening for colon cancer can be subdivided into screening for high-risk groups and screening for the general population. At-risk groups include patients with ulcerative colitis, patients with a history of polyps (including familial polyposis), and, to a lesser degree, patients with a history of colon cancer among first-degree family members. Because colorectal cancer largely affects older patients, screening programs have targeted those aged 50 and over. Current recommendations for screening the general population (aged 50 and over) are best summarized with the following: yearly DRE and FOBT in association with flexible sigmoidoscopy every 5 to 10 years.

Colon cancer appears ideal for screening in that the disease is common and is associated with a long preclinical phase. The polyp-to-cancer sequence is an established tenet of oncology, because most cancers appear to arise from preexisting polyps. Patients with multiple polyps are at increased risk for colon cancer, and aggressive prospective extirpation of polyps results in a reduction of colon cancer.

Aside from the DRE, which should always be part of a general physical examination for adult patients, two other screening tests are available. The simplest test is the FOBT, which tests tiny amounts of stool for traces of blood. Popularized by Greegor, the FOBT is a simple screening test that is nonetheless beset with some important drawbacks. The first problem with the FOBT is patient compliance. One author commented that a great effort was expended to achieve a rather poor compliance rate of 68%. The second problem is that, because most colon tumors are not detectably bleeding at any given point in time, they will not be detected with a single screening FOBT. The third problem relates to the cutoff point of the test. Rehydration of the specimens results in a much higher positivity rate. Rehydration detects more cancers but on the other hand also results in a great many more false-positive results. There is evidence, however, for the efficacy of FOBT. In the Minnesota Colon Cancer Control Study, *46,551* people between the ages of 50 and 80 were randomized to one of three groups: annual FOBT screening, biennial screening, and control. With a study follow-up of 13 years, a significant reduction of 33% in colon cancer mortality was found in the group undergoing annual screening (Fig. 7.9). The mortality rates of the biennial group were almost identical, however, to those of the control group. The incidence of metastatic disease was twice as high for the control group than for the annual screening group. It should be noted, however, that most FOBT studies have not demonstrated an unequivocal benefit for FOBT screening.

Screening sigmoidoscopy (flexible being preferable to rigid) has been advocated by many experts for people over the age of 50. Reductions of up to 30% in cancer-specific mortality have been suggested to result from periodic screening sigmoido-scopy, with intervals of up to 10 years. More complete colonic screening with colonoscopy is increasingly popular. Some authorities recommend a single colono-scopic screening at age 60, with others even suggesting age 50. A recent University of Michigan study estimated that the number of screening colonoscopies needed to save 1 year of expected life was from 2.9 to 6.0 depending on the screening regimen adopted. Endoscopic screening, although extremely sensitive and specific, is costly in terms of money and time and is associated with rare but significant complica-tions. Showing promise as potential screening tools are new strategies such as assays for altered DNA exfoliated into stool, the immunological fecal hemoglobin and albumin test, and the exciting virtual colonoscopy or three-dimensional computed tomography colography.

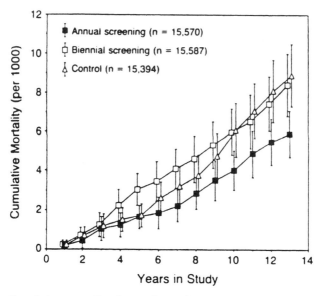

Figure 7.9 Cumulative mortality from colorectal cancer, according to FOBT screening group. (From Mandel et al. *N Engl J Med* 328:1366–1371, 1993.)

Prostate Cancer

Prostate cancer is a leading cause of cancer death for men and its incidence continues to rise. The prostate cancer screening model is unique in that, although three effective and quite different screening tools are in use, the efficacy of screening for this cancer is far from established. As Figure 7.10 shows, there is a spectrum for prostate cancer in terms of biologic aggressiveness. Prostate cancer is very commonly found at autopsy in men over the age of 50, but the mortality rates from prostate cancer are much lower than one would expect given the high prevalence of the disease. Most men with prostate cancer will not die of prostate cancer. On the other hand, though, for most men dying of prostate cancer the diagnosis was not made in time, when the disease was organ-confined and curable. This dichotomy has led to the dilemma of prostate cancer treatment: how to make an early diagnosis for patients with potentially lethal prostate cancer, but how *not* to over-diagnose and over-treat cancer that is biologically indolent and nonlethal. This dilemma has resulted in much confusion about how to screen effectively for prostate cancer.

The long preclinical phase and high prevalence of prostate cancer among men over the age of 50 would appear to make prostate cancer an ideal tumor for screening. Three screening tests have been implemented in prostate cancer screening programs: physical examination (i.e., DRE); PSA, a serologic test; and transrectal ultrasound (TRUS), an imaging study. The DRE is a focused physical examination that, like the CBE, while simple, is subjective and clearly operator dependent. The PPV of DRE is 24–35%. Data from the American Cancer Society Prostate Cancer Detection Project showed a sensitivity of 50% and a specificity of

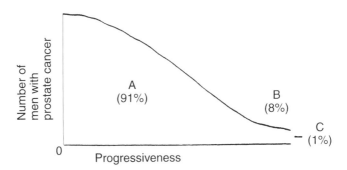

Figure 7.10 Latent, progressive, and rapidly progressive prostate cancers. (**A**) Non-progressive (latent): no need to screen-detect, as tumor will not progress. (**B**) Progressive: wothwhile to screen-detect as will eventually become symptomatic (and possibly fatal) and because screen-detection and early treatment can improve prognosis. (**C**) rapidly progressive: no need to try to screen-detect as tumor progresses so quickly that preclinical phase is very brief and death is likely outcome whether diagnosis is early or late. Percentages refer to relative weights of prostate cancer prevalence (27%), risk of diagnosis (2.31%), and risk of death (0.36) for 65- to 69-year old while men. (From Waterbor et al. *Cancer Causes and Control* 6:267–274, 1995.)

94% for DRE. The detection rate for DRE in prostate screening programs is less than 2%. Annual DREs are recommended for men more than 50 years of age (or younger if patients are high risk, e.g., positive family history, African American ethnicity), but, not surprisingly, compliance is a problem, and, furthermore, there are real questions about how effective DRE alone is in detecting cancer early.

In contrast to tumor markers such as carcinoembryonic antigen (CEA), PSA is produced by only one organ, the prostate. PSA is not specific, however, for cancer, and elevated PSA levels are seen in a number of benign prostatic conditions such as prostatitis and benign prostatic hypertrophy. The higher the PSA, however, the more specific for prostate cancer it becomes. PSA determination illustrates the cutoff point principle: deciding at which level the test is positive affects both the sensitivity and the specificity of the test. For PSA levels greater than 10 ng/mL, the specificity exceeds 90%. The value of the PSA as a test can be increased further by looking at PSA density, age-specific reference ranges, the free-to-total PSA ratio, and the rate of change of the PSA level over time. The sensitivity and specificity of PSA are similar to that of the DRE, although the specificity of PSA tends to be lower. The two tests often do not detect the same cancers; thus, the combination of the two tests is superior to either test alone (Fig. 7.11). For this reason, some groups, such as the American Urological Association and the American Cancer Society, have recommended that prostate cancer screening for men over the age of 50 (over the age of 40 if high risk) consist of a yearly DRE and PSA level determination.

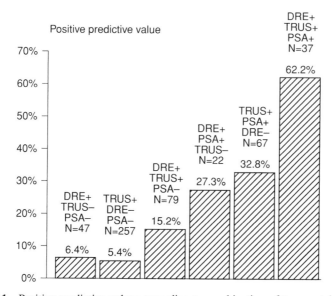

Figure 7.11 Positive predictive values according to combination of transrectal ultrasound (TRUS), digital rectal examination (DRE), and prostate-specific antigen (PSA) result. Positive PSA is defined as >4.0 ng/ml. (From Babaian et al. *Cancer* 69:1196–1200, 1992.)

The third screening test, TRUS, has been used for about 25 years. TRUS is an invasive test: an ultrasound probe placed into the rectum allows the user to detect areas of hypoechoicity within the prostate. In expert hands, TRUS can detect tumors much smaller than 1 cm. Because TRUS is invasive, expensive, and not reliable as a single-modality screening test, it is best reserved for prostate biopsy guidance for patients with abnormal PSA levels or DRE findings.

Prostate cancer screening detects many asymptomatic cancers, but does prostate cancer screening result in lowered mortality rates from prostate cancer? The answer to this bottom-line question is not available at this time. Multiple ongoing long-itudinal PRTs are currently underway. However, it will be several years before the results of these studies are known. This having been said, the initial analysis of the 1988 Quebec PRT for prostate cancer screening has recently been reported. In this study, 46,193 men aged 45 to 80 years were randomized to either screening or no screening, screening consisting of DRE and PSA with TRUS being done if abnormal DREs or PSAs. The prostate cancer death rate was significantly lower in the screened population. In the absence, however, of more definitive outcome data, most cancer organizations have not supported large-scale prostate cancer screening, although men are increasingly asked to be screened. An important concern associated with prostate cancer screening is financial: the cost of the screening tests themselves, the cost of numerous prostate biopsies generated by the screening process, and the staggering cost of treating all of the cancers diagnosed. Because widespread screening with the tools currently available would result in the detection of huge numbers of new prostate cancers and could overwhelm health care facilities, it seems prudent to channel patients into available multi-institutional PRTs.

CONCLUSION

The four models of cancer screening presented illustrate not only the general principles of screening but also the many problems that plague screening programs. Screening whole populations for a specific type of cancer, even if a simple screening test such as the FOBT exists, involves considerable expenditure. Thus, it behooves public health authorities to be certain of the efficacy of the particular screening program. That efficacy is best demonstrated by PRTs, although, as has been seen with breast cancer, PRTs do not necessarily quiet controversial issues in screening. As societies come to terms with controlling health care expenditures, cost-benefit analyses become an increasingly important part of decision making. As public health authorities increasingly take a bottom-line approach, controversial screening issues may ultimately be decided on the basis of cost-benefit analyses. For example, it can easily be demonstrated that with mammography a far greater amount of money must be spent to save 1 year of life for a woman between the ages of 40 and 49 than for a woman between the ages of 50 and 69. Other age-related issues arise. Patients at risk for cervical cancer and melanoma are younger than patients at risk for colon and prostate cancer. Should more of a society's resources be put into screening for cancers that afflict younger people? Do older patients who are near the ends of their lives and out of the work force have less of a right to cancer screening than younger patients? Other ethical issues also exist. For example, how much autonomy should individual practitioners have with regard to screening practices? A health maintenance organization in the United States recently undertook a large-scale educational effort to dissuade their physicians from screening patients for prostate cancer.

The many issues operative in cancer screening do not lend themselves to easy solutions. Consensus conferences at which experts present data and then develop a strategic plan for screening can serve to inflame rather than quiet controversy, as illustrated by recent discussions in the United States about breast cancer screening for younger women. To best serve their patients, individual practitioners should be aware of the general principles of screening, the risks and benefits associated with the different types of screening tests, the evidence for the efficacy of common screening tests, and the screening recommendations of national cancer organizations. Practitioners have a responsibility to their patients to select those individuals who are at risk; to be skilled in performing screening examinations such as CBE, DRE, pelvic examination with inspection of the cervix, and the Pap smear; and, to be at least aware of newer screening strategies such as molecular testing. Above all, physicians need to help patients understand the importance of complying with screening recommendations, and they need to be able to communicate screening test results to patients in an understandable and compassionate manner.

FURTHER READING

Benoit RM, Naslund MJ (1997) The socioeconomic implications of prostate-specific antigen screening. *Urol Clin North Am* 24:451–458.

Catalona WJ, Smith DS, Ratliff TL et al. (1991) Measurement of prostate-specific antigen in serum as a screening test for prostate cancer. *N Engl J Med* 324:1156–1161.

Ciatto S, Zappa M, Bonardi R, Gervasi G. (2000) Prostate cancer screening: the problem of overdiagnosis and lessons to be learned from breast cancer screening. *Eur J Cancer* 36:1347–1350.

Cupp MR, Oesterling JE (1993) Prostate-specific antigen, digital rectal examination, and Transrectal ultrasonography: their roles in diagnosing early prostate cancer. *Mayo Clin Proc* 68:297–306.

Cuzick J (1999) Screening for cancer: future potential. *Eur J Cancer* 35:1925–1932.

DeMay RM (1997) Common problems in Papanicolaou interpretation. *Arch Pathol Lab Med* 121:229–238.

Eckhardt S, Badellino F, Murphy GP (1994) UICC meeting on breast-cancer screening in pre-menopausal women in developed countries. *Int J Cancer* 56:2–5.

Eddy DM (1990) Screening for cervical cancer. *Ann Intern Med* 113:214–226.

Gohagan JK, Prorok PC, Kramer BS et al. (1994) Prostate cancer screening in the prostate, lung, colorectal and ovarian cancer screening trial of the National Cancer Institute. *J Urol* 152:1905–1909.

Harris R, Leininger L (1995) Clinical strategies for breast cancer screening: weighing and using the evidence. *Ann Intern Med* 122:539–547.

Inadomi JM, Sonnenberg A (2000) The impact of colorectal cancer screening on life expectancy. *Gastrointest Endosc* 51:517–523.

Jessup JM, Menck HR, Fremgen A, Winchester DP (1997) Diagnosing colorectal carcinoma: clinical and molecular approaches. *CA Cancer Clin* 47:70–92.

Labrie F, Candas B, Dupont A et al. (1999) Screening decreases prostate cancer death: first analysis of the 1988 Quebec prospective randomized controlled trial. *Prostate* 38:83–91.

Leitch AM (1999) Breast cancer screening: success amid conflict. *Surg Oncol Clin North Am* 8:657–672.

Mandel JS, Bond JH, Church TR et al. (1993) Reducing mortality from colorectal cancer by screening for fecal occult blood. *N Engl J Med* 328:1365–1371.

Miller AB, Chamberlain J, Day NE et al. (1990) Report on a workshop of the UICC project on evaluation of screening for cancer. *Int J Cancer* 46:761–769.

Miller AB, Baines CJ, To T et al. (1992) Canadian National Breast Screening Study: 1. Breast cancer detection and death rates among women aged 40 to 49 years. *Can Med Assoc J* 147:1459–1476.

Miller AB, Baines CJ, To T et al. (1992) Canadian National Breast Screening Study: 2. Breast cancer detection and death rates among women aged 50 to 59 years. *Can Med Assoc J* 147:1477–1488.

Nelson RL (1997) Screening for colorectal cancer. *J Surg Oncol* 63:249–258.

Rimer BK, Schildkraut J (1997) Cancer screening. In *Cancer: Principles and Practice of Oncology*, 5th edition. DeVita VT, Hellmann S, Rosenberg SA (eds.) Lippincott-Raven, Philadelphia.

Smith RA (2000) Breast cancer screening among women younger than age 50: a current assessment of the issues. *CA Cancer J Clin* 50:312–336.

Toribara NW, Sleisenger MH (1995) Screening for colorectal cancer. *N Engl J Med* 332:861–867.

Winawer SI, Flehinger BJ, Schottenfeld D et al. (1993) Screening for colorectal cancer with fecal occult blood testing and sigmoidoscopy. *J Natl Cancer Inst* 85:1311–1318.

Vogel VG (2000) Breast cancer prevention: a review of current evidence. *CA Cancer J Clin* 50:156–170.

Cancer Diagnosis: New Imaging

O. RIXE, J.-P. SPANO, D. NIZRI, M. A. GIL-DELGADO, J. BLOCH, P. BLOCH,
M. A. ROCHER, C. SOUBRANE, G. AUCLERC, D. BUTHIAU, and D. KHAYAT

Medical Oncology Department, Salpêtrière Hospital, SOMPS, Paris, France

When it comes to imaging, improvements in computer capabilities have extended the boundaries of what is possible. Techniques that have evolved as a result, such as helical computed tomography (CT), intraoperative magnetic resonance imaging (MRI), clinical positron emission tomography (PET), and fusion imaging, provide oncological physicians with more flexibility and accuracy in the diagnosis and assessment of tumors.

HELICAL COMPUTED TOMOGRAPHY

The word *tomography* is derived from the Greek words *tomos*, meaning to slice, and *graphein*, meaning to write. Tomography was computerized during the 1970s. A narrow beam of X rays sweeps across an area of the body and is recorded not on film but with a radiation detector as a pattern of electrical impulses. Data from many sweeps are integrated by a computer, which uses the radiation absorption figures to assess the density of tissues at thousands of points. Helical scanning is a breakthrough technology that has changed the medical communitys approach to CT procedures (1–53). Helical CT can improve lesion detection and cancer staging because it improves image quality. With helical CT, the pitch is defined as the ratio between table speed and collimator width (pitch = table speed [mm/sec]/collimator width [mm]). Increasing the pitch allows a greater volume of tissue to be scanned per unit time. Additionally, a pitch greater than one enables narrower collimation, which ultimately results in improved resolution. Another benefit of helical CT is the

UICC Manual of Clinical Oncology, Eighth Edition. Edited by Raphael E. Pollock
ISBN 0-471-22289-5 Copyright © 2004 John Wiley & Sons, Inc.

ability to obtain more consistent opacification of vessels with smaller volumes of contrast, primarily because of the shorter imaging times. Three new techniques, virtual endoscopy and three-dimensional (1) constructions, clinical measurement of volumes, and perfusion imaging, put this new level of precision to good use in the clinical setting.

Helical CT is particularly suitable for the study of anatomical cavities. New methods of image processing can produce virtual endoscopic images without the use of an endoscope (2). By combining contiguous table movement at a constant velocity during data collection with concomitant rotation of the tube and detectors at a constant speed and direction, helical CT enables the performance of single volumetric breath-hold acquisition of images of the thorax. Further calculation or interpolation reduces artifacts caused by patient movement. Similarly, respiratory motion artifacts can be eliminated. A high-quality three-dimensional image can be reconstructed from the contiguous slices. These reconstructions can be made volumetric by using a slice thickness formed by the summation of several adjacent sections, a technique known as multiprojection volume reconstruction (MPVR) (Fig. 8a.1). It is also possible to select minimum intensity or maximum intensity algorithms to obtain image projections of the cavities from their outside surface. So-called surface reconstructions appear in relief (Figs. 8a.2 and 8a.3).

The helical CT technique can be applied to resolve a number of clinical difficulties (Figs. 8a.4–8a.9). In the case of tracheobronchial endoscopy, it can be employed to visualize semi-distal lesions that can be seen only with a thinner endoscope (3–41). It can also be applied as an aid in brachytherapy. Virtual tracheobronchial endoscopy permits follow-up of endoprostheses (sensitivity 95%; specificity 79%) without additional risk to the patient, and it permits the surgeon to check on suture stability.

Virtual colonoscopy (42–49) means more comfort for patients as its application can decrease the need to perform barium enemas (see Fig. 8a.5). It permits easy follow-up after polypectomy and a more thorough way of diagnosing patients with nonspecific abdominal symptoms.

Virtual cystoscopy can aid in pretherapeutic planning, follow-up after treatment, or documenting the origin of a hematuria of dilation of the urinary tract (see Fig. 8a.4) (50–52).

The limits of helical CT include the visualization of artifacts and artificial stenoses, small lesions or mucosal changes that are sometimes not visible. It also only gives an outline image and endoscopic knowledge and experience are needed. The benefit is it is noninvasive. It eliminates the need to use an endoscopic probe.

According to the World Health Organization (WHO) criteria for therapeutic evaluation of the response to treatment, chemotherapy, radiotherapy, or immunotherapy should be assessed using clinical findings and one- or two-dimensional (surface) measurements. These measurements are subject to interpretation biases and other factors that influence accuracy. Helical CT adds a third dimension to cases to which the traditional bidimensional modalities are applied. The primary application of this more precise and direct measurement of volumes is the anatomical sizing of the volume of an organ (whole or part) or other specific

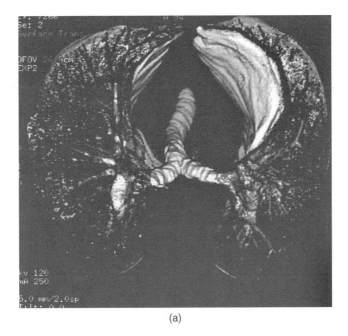

(a)

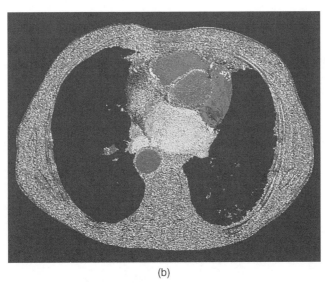

(b)

Figure 8a.1 (a) MIP reconstruction, with a slice thickness of more than 3 cm of tracheobronchial tract and pulmonary parenchyma, with helical CT; (b) volume rendering of mediastinal lymph nodes by helical CT.

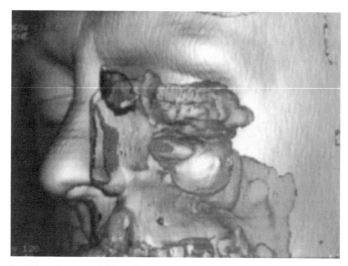

Figure 8a.2   3D surface modeling of the walls of the sinus cavities with thresholding at air density, based on CT sections.

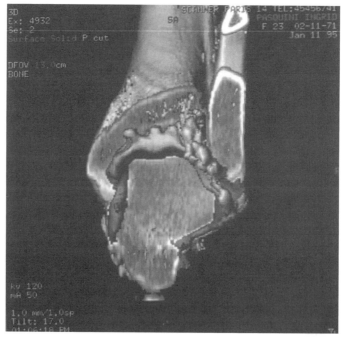

Figure 8a.3   3D reconstruction of bone by helical CT.

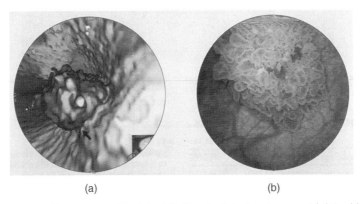

(a)   (b)

Figure 8a.4 Papillary tumor with virtual (left) and clinical cystoscopy (right) with a "sea-anemone like aspect." (Courtesy of Dr. Palau, *Virtual Endoscopy*, D. Buthiau, D. Khayat (eds.), © 2003, Springer).

structures. The chief clinical application relative to oncology is the evaluation of a tumor mass. The benefits of volumetric measurements are optimal before treatment, when knowledge regarding the tumor's size and position will influence prognosis (Fig. 8a.10). In fact, more accurate assessment of the tumor volume will be useful when predicting the tumor's reponse to treatment. The measurement of volume may

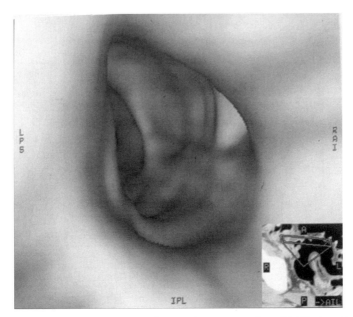

Figure 8a.5 Polypoid tumor corresponding to a degenerate polyp with 2D view (down right) by virtual colonoscopy.

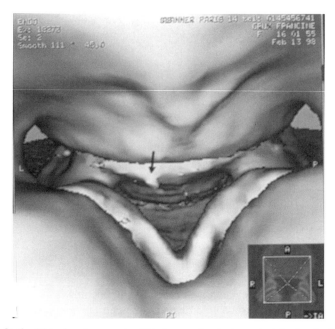

Figure 8a.6   Virtual endoscopy by CT of normal spinal canal at the level of L4–L5.

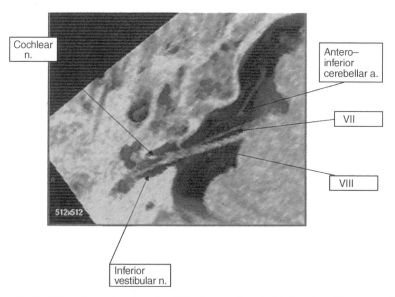

Figure 8a.7   3D endoscopic view by CD of acoustico-facial bundle. (Courtesy of Dr. Bensiman, *Virtual Endoscopy*, D. Buthiau, D. Khayat (eds.), © 2003, Springer).

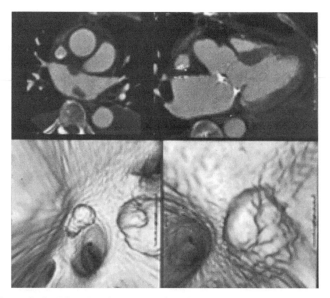

Figure 8a.8   Virtual endoscopy by CT of a pulmonary artery thrombosis.

also permit improved assessment of operability or determination of lesion volume before radiotherapy (54).

The advent of helical scanners now makes it possible to track a bolus of iodinated contrast medium through tissue. In reference to drug development, the study of blood flow in the tumor could be useful in measuring the impact of antiangiogenesis inhibitors. Ongoing research at the Centre of Imagery RMX and

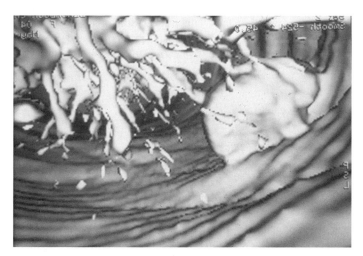

Figure 8a.9   CT intrathoracic virtual endoscopy, showing the pleural and wall direct extension of a lung carcinoma.

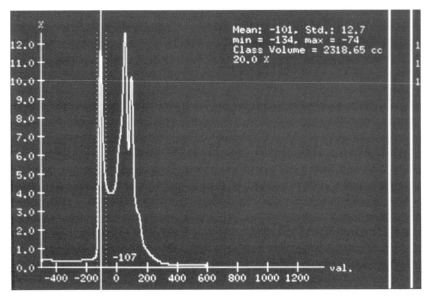

Figure 8a.10 Volume measurement and density histogram of hepatic metastasis by CT.

SOMPS (Paris, France) has made more practical use of this new capability with the development of quantitative imaging of blood flow and volume in tumors. We have optimized the method for application in cancer patients so that it can easily be incorporated into routine CT imaging protocols. The perfusion study protocol requires intravenous injection of 300 mg/mL non-ionic contrast agent at the dosage of 0.5 mL/kg body weight and 45 seconds of continuous CT scanning. Within minutes of the completion of the perfusion study, a map of tumor blood flow can be generated from the acquired images. This information on the development of blood flow in tumors can be applied to diagnosis, prognosis, and the evaluation of treatment response, especially the evaluation of post-therapeutic decrease of antiangiogenesis (55).

MAGNETIC RESONANCE IMAGING

Nuclear magnetic resonance (NMR) (56–59) imaging is more commonly referred to as magnetic resonance imaging (MRI). MRI developed into an important clinical modality between 1978 and 1985. The modality capitalizes on the fact that magnetic nuclei in a static magnetic field exhibit a characteristic resonance frequency that is proportional to the field strength and unique to nuclei of the same type and same environment. The net magnetization of the sample when irradiated by a radio wave at the resonance frequency could thus be manipulated to produce an induced NMR signal. Primarily, clinical MRI systems produce images of the distribution of hydrogen nuclei (mainly water) within the body. Other biologically important nuclei (carbon, nitrogen, and phosporus), as well as the imaging of hyperpolarized inert gases (helium and xenon), are under investigation. Recent developments in MRI have included chemical shift imaging (hydrogen-containing metabolites), blood flow imaging (MR angiography), ultra-high-speed imaging (echo planar), and imaging of brain function based upon magnetic susceptibility differences resulting from blood oxygenation changes during brain activity.

For a long time, oncologists have valued MRI's unique ability to image soft tissue and to differentiate benign and malignant tissue. As a result, it has become a major component of oncological diagnosis and therapy staging.

Dynamic imaging of extracellular fluid space contrast media after bolus injection may currently be the single most important component of an MR examination for the liver. This is true in a number of circumstances, particularly, the detection and characterization of tumors. Pratical imaging strategies can be applied in three different clinical situations: the characterization of incidental liver lesions, detection and characterization of hepatocellular carcinoma in cirrhosis, and detection of liver metastasis before surgical resection.

While MRI has been highly utilized for staging and prognosis, before now, it has not been suitable for intraoperative guidance. This can be attributed to many factors, including patient access. Advances in magnetics, like the development of the Signa SP (a vertical gap magnet) and the increasing speed at which modern systems can obtain images, have made it possible to use MRI intraoperatively. Surgeons can view MRI images in real-time while operating. Such technology stands to improve a surgeon's ability to better distinguish between malignant and benign tissue and to remove tissue accordingly.

As mentioned earlier, MRI provides excellent soft-tissue resolution (Fig. 8a.11) but poor source definition and CT provides excellent source localization but poor

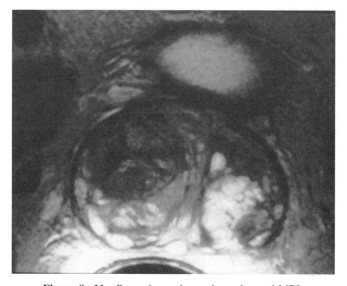

Figure 8a.11   Prostatic carcinoma by endorectal MRI.

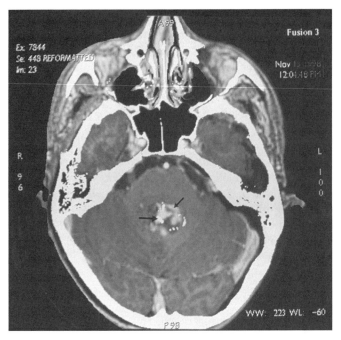

Figure 8a.12 Fusion image of CT and MRI of a fourth ventricle tumor (arrows).

soft-tissue visualization. The two fused together can generate a useful datatset that provides both source tissue resolution and source definition.

CT combined with MRI can provide anatomical answers by better defining tumor volume and its evolution under treatment (Fig. 8a.12). It might also increase the accuracy of radiotherapy by helping physicians to distinguish between the residual tumor and inflammatory or scar tissue. Because it requires good visualization of patient anatomy and localization of sources for dose calculations, CT-MRI fusion images can help to assure the quality of permanent brachytherapy implants.

Real endoscopy by imaging calls upon magnetic resonance imaging using an intraluminal receiver (see Figs. 8a.13–8a.15). This receiver acts as a miniature surface microreceiver connected to the entry of the MRI like a classical surface receiver.

The resolution is equal to or slightly better than optical endoscopy, but this technique adds the possibility of viewing tissues, not only their intraluminal contours but also their parietal thickness. Finally, real endoscopy by imaging assists in the performance of a "virtual" biopsy by spectroscopy, determining the zone to biopsy with forceps.

The patient is positioned within the MRI device. The entire zone to be analyzed is first visualized with a classical surface receiver (e.g., abdominal). Using endoscopy, the zone is then observed, in real time, by classical investigation. Once the endoscope is well positioned, one switches the machine over to the

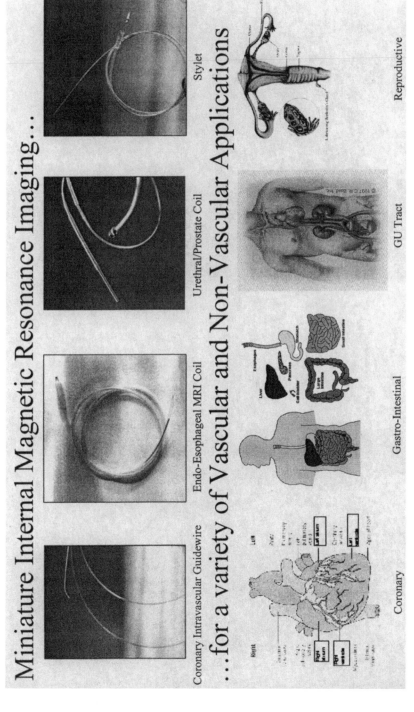

Figure 8a.13 Principle of direct endoscopy by MRI using different miniature surface coils.

169

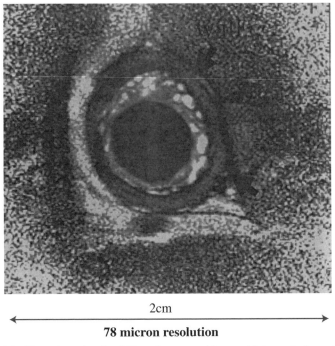

2cm

78 micron resolution

Figure 8a.14 Normal urethra by MR endoscopy with very high resolution, showing the different layers of the wall.

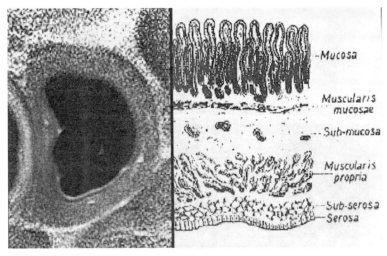

Figure 8a.15 MR endoscopy of normal esophagus showing all the layers of the wall and structures around the wall. (Courtesy of D. Buthiau, General Electric Medical Systems).

intraluminal receiver, which supplies almost real-time images. Our investigations are carried out on a General Electric Medical Systems MRI, with an intraluminal receiver from Surgi-Vision. The aims of real-time virtual endoscopy are:

- To obtain an increasingly fine spatial resolution (in the order of 50 to 70 μm).
- To investigate not only the intraluminal contents, but also their parietal thickness and the neighboring tissues.
- To serve as a pretherapeutic assessment, notably as a means of positioning and control.
- To allow complementary imaging to anatomical study, that is to say above all metabolic and functional.

The purpose of this technique is thus early diagnosis, allowing several means of assessment in the course of the same investigation, with the possibility of directed biopsy.

The potential applications of this method are yet to be studied. They are multiple, covering therapeutic as well as diagnostic fields. In this way, potentially, in nonvascular pathology, real endoscopy by imaging could extend to the diagnostic imaging of the esophagus and esophageal cancer, ureteric and gynecological imaging, and spinal investigations, as well as breast, rectal, prostate, and hepatic cancers. From a therapeutic point of view, it could contribute to the treatment of esophageal cancer, the treatment of incontinence, noninvasive spinal surgery, the thermal ablation of rectal and prostate cancers, and the assessment of radiotherapeutic positioning for prostate cancer and the thermal ablation of hepatic cancers (Table 8a.1).

Potential applications may also be envisaged in the vascular plane (Table 8a.2). From a diagnostic viewpoint, it could contribute toward the imaging of aortic plaques by a transesophageal approach, the study of plaques and coronary and peripheral vascular walls, and the assessment of vascular stenosis and obstruction.

TABLE 8a.1. Real Endoscopy by Imaging: Potential Clinical Applications (Nonvascular)

Diagnostic	Therapeutic
Imaging of the esophagus and esophageal cancer	Treatment of esophageal cancer
	Treatment of incontinence
Imaging of the ureter	Noninvasive spinal surgery
Spinal investigation	Thermal ablation of rectal and prostate cancers
Breast cancer	
Rectal cancer	Assessment of radio-therapeutic positioning for prostate cancer
Prostate cancer	
Hepatic cancer	Thermal ablation of hepatic cancer
Gynecological imaging	

TABLE 8a.2. Real Endoscopy by Imaging: Potential Clinical Applications (Vascular)

Diagnostic	Therapeutic
Imaging of aortic plaques by transesophageal approach	Angioplasty
Study of plaques, and coronary and peripheral vascular walls	Assistance in the placement of stents
Assessment of vascular stenosis and obstruction	Gene therapy

Its therapeutic contribution could include angioplasty, assistance in the placement of stents, and gene therapy.

Currently, the experimental scientists envisage a systematic clinical evaluation of this technique in all its fields of application. The limitations could include the cost, at the current stage of development of this modality.

POSITRON EMISSION TOMOGRAPHY

Positron emission tomography (PET) (60) is an unique diagnostic imaging modality that displays the metabolic function of the human body. PET scans produce images of the body that represent the functional rather than anatomical characteristics of disease, resulting in the early detection of abnormalities that are undetectable by other modalities. PET imaging with F-18 fluorodeoxyglucose (FDG), a metabolic tag, has proven to be a valuable imaging modality over the last few years. Its major indications are grading and staging of tumors, identification of epilectic foci, and the evaluation of three-vessel coronary disease.

PET imaging can be used to stage many common tumors such as bronchial carcinoma and lymphoma, but for these indications, whole-body PET capabilities are necessary. Whole-body imaging requires a higher level of efficiency, and the detection systems that have been developed over the past few decades can provide it. The newer systems are capable of producing tomographic whole-body PET scans in less than an hour.

Our investigation with a relatively large series of patients showed PET could be superior to the morphological picture modalities for tumor staging. These results concurred with studies conducted by other groups. There are two reasons for PET's superiority: (1) by detecting pathological FDG uptake, PET imaging can detect lesions smaller than 1 cm, which morphology cannot clearly classify as benign or malignant; and (2) the high external S/N ratio illuminated lesions, making reading the scans easier, which reduces the chances of making an error.

The realization of PET imaging has created a multitude of clinical indications, and the high cost of PET imaging machinery and installation has created a new consideration for health policy makers. Careful planning of the installation site and the logistics of radiopharmaceutical delivery is critical. For any public institution

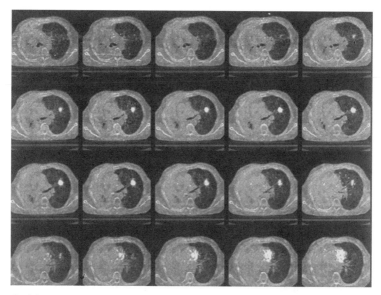

Figure 8a.16   PET-CT of lung cancer, showing the uptake of 18 FDG at the level of the left pulmonary lesion demonstrated by the CT-scan.

that wishes to introduce the technology cost efficiently, the optimization of funding ressources and national consensus of where to strategically place the equipment will need to be considered. The actual evolution of PET is the combination with CT, with anatomical and functional information, the "18 FDG" acting as "a new contrast agent" for the CT scanner (Fig. 8a.16).

OTHER TECHNOLOGIES

The oncologist's imaging tool kit has become a lot fuller and its depth and width continues to expand. Teleradiology is another new medical application derived from coupling physical sciences with computer applications. Teleradiology involves transmitting high-resolution medical images from one remote site to another and displaying the images effectively so that radiologists can perform the proper diagnosis.

The ability to electronically transmit radiologic images from one location to another provides convenience. Thus, teleradiology can be of benefit in many situations, not the least of which is the increased availability of radiologic expertise in remote areas.

The process of remotely displaying radiologic (x-ray) and other imaging studies for interpretation, consultation, or both requires use of a local area networks (LANs), wide area networks (WANs), picture archival and communication systems

(PACS), and compression DICOM (digital imaging and communication in medicine).

DICOM has allowed teleradiology to expand from a point-to-point technology to an Internet-like network. Recent developments in computer technologies have made it possible to store images digitally, therefore they can be transmitted digitally over phone lines.

PACS is the central component of any digitial imaging distribution system. It forms the basis for distributing information throughout an enterprise, regardless of its size; it can range from an enterprise-wide, high-perfomance network to a single workstation connected to the acquisition device by phone. The heart of a PACS-teleradiology system is its archive, the place where all the images can be stored and retrieved.

Another innovation in the optical sciences that may eventually find an application in the clinic is the construction of a table-top laser capable of generating a coherent beam of X rays. It has long been possible to generate X rays with lasers, but in the past, long physical distances were necessary to manipulate the light source in an appropriate manner.

As the intense light passes through a hollow glass tube filled with gas, electrons pull away from their atoms then snap back when their field is reversed. These electrons emit energy in the form of X-ray photons, a particle form of X-ray light. The work currently enables any researcher with a short-pulse laser to use the techniques to improve their view of biological processes. Attempts to alter and improve upon the way x-rays are obtained in the clinic are probably not far behind.

Technology is changing the ways of diagnosis. The physician may discover that she or he can have a more detailed picture of the disease process or may find the newer systems more convenient. However, it is the patient who is spared an invasive diagnostic procedure or whose prognosis was improved due to earlier diagnosis, and who will be most grateful for the innovations and changes in this realm.

BIBLIOGRAPHY

1. Henschke CI (2002) *New Imaging in Oncology*. Early Lung Cancer Action Project Symposium 12th International Congress on Anti-Cancer Treatment, Paris, February 6th.

2. Buthiau D, Khayat D (2003) *Virtual Endoscopy*. New York: Springer.

3. Ferretti G, Knoplioch J, Coulomb M, Brambilla C, Cinquin P (1995) Reconstruction 3D endoluminal de l'arbre trachéobronchique (bronchoscopie virtuelle). *J Radiol* 76:531–774.

4. Amiel M, Magnin IE, Friboulet D, Moll T, Revel D (1995) L'imagerie médicale en 3D: concepts, bases techniques, applications. *Rev Im Med* 7:107–116.

5. Johnson CD, Ahlquist DA (1999) Computed tomography colonography (virtual colonoscopy) a new method for colorectal screening. *Gut* 44:301–305.

6. Summers RM (1997) Navigation aids for real-time virtual bronchoscopy. *AJR* 168:1165–1170.

7. Summers RM, Feng DH, Holland SM et al. (1996) Virtual bronchoscopy: Segmentation method for real-time display. *Radiology* 200:857–862.

8. Summers RM, Shaw DJ, Shelhamer JH (1998) CT virtual bronchoscopy of simulated endobronchial lesions: Effect of scanning, reconstruction and display settings and potential pitfalls. *AJR* 170:947–950.

9. Ferreti GR, Khayat D, Buthiau D et al. (2003) Virtual bronchoscopy in oncology. In *Virtual Endoscopy*. Buthiau D, Khayat D (eds.). Springer, pp. 109–141.

10. Geiger B, Kikinis R (1994) Simulation of endoscopy. In *Medical Image Processing*, AAAI Spring Symposium Series, Stanford University.

11. Haponik EF, Aquino SL, Vining DJ (1999) Virtual bronchoscopy. *Clin Chest Med* 20:201–217.

12. Naidich DP, Harkin TJ (1995) Airways and lung: Correlation of CT with fiberoptic bronchoscopy. *Radiology* 197:1–12.

13. Pue CA, Patch ER (1995) Complications of fiberoptic bronchoscopy at a university hospital. *Chest* 107:430–432.

14. Colice GL, Chappel GJ, Frenchman JM, Solomon DA (1985) Comparison of computed tomography with fiberoptic bronchoscopy in identifying endobronchial abnormalities in patients with known or suspected lung cancer. *Am Rev Respir Dis* 131:397–400.

15. Henschke CI, Davis SD, Auh Y, Romano P, Westcott J, Berkmen YM, Kazam E (1987) Detection of bronchial abnormalities: Comparison of CT and bronchoscopy. *J Comput Assist Tomogr* 11:432–435.

16. Rapp-Bernhardt U, Welte T, Budinger M, Bernhardt TM (1998) Comparision of three-dimensional virtual endoscopy with bronchoscopy in patients with oesophageal carcinoma infiltrating the tracheobronchial tree. *Br J Radiol* 71:1271–1278.

17. Summers RM, Selbie WS, Malley JD, Pusanik LM, Dwyer AJ, Courcoutsakis NA, Shaw DJ, Kleiner DE, Sneller MC, Langford CA, Holland SM, Shelhamer JH (1998) Polypoid lesions of airways: Early experience with computer-assisted detection by using virtual bronchoscopy and surface curvature. *Radiology* 208:331–337.

18. Summers RM, Shaw DJ, Shelhamer JH (1998) CT virtual bronchoscopy of simulated endobronchial lesions: Effect of scanning, reconstruction, and display setting and potential pitfalls. *AJR* 170:947–950.

19. Stitik FP (1994) The new staging of lung cancer. *Radiol Clin North Am* 32:635–648.

20. Lewis JW, Pearlberg JL, Beaute GH (1990) Can computed tomography of the chest stage lung cancer? Yes and no. *Ann Thorac Surg* 49:591–596.

21. McLoud TC, Bourgouin PM, Greenberg RW, Kosiuk JP, Templeton PA, Shepard JA, Moore EH, Wain JC, Mathisen DJ, Grillo HC (1992) Bronchogenic carcinoma: Analysis of staging in the mediastinum witch CT by correlative lymph node mapping and sampling. *Radiology* 182:319–323.

22. Webb WR, Gatsonis C, Zerhouni EA, Heelan RT, Glazer GM, Francis IR, McNeil BJ (1991) CT and MR imaging in staging non-small-cell bronchogenic carcinoma: Report of the Radiologic Diagnostic Oncology Group. *Radiology* 178:705–713.

23. Naidich DP (1996) Staging of lung cancer: Computed tomography versus bronchoscopic needle aspiration. *J Bronchol* 3:69–73.

24. Wang KP (1994) Staging of bronchogenic carcinoma by bronchoscopy. *Chest* 106:588–593.

25. Prakash UBS, Stubbs SE (1991) The bronchoscopy survey: Some reflections. *Chest* 100:1660–1667.

26. Castro de FR, Lopez DF, Serda GJ, Lopez AR, Gilart JF, Navarro PC (1997) Relevance of training in transbronchial fine-needle aspiration technique. *Chest* 111:103–105.

27. Vining DJ, Ferretti G, Stelts DR, Ahn D, Ge Y, Haponik EF (1997) Mediastinal lymph node mapping using spiral CT and three dimensional reconstructions in patients with lung cancer: Preliminary observations. *J Bronchol* 4:18–25.

28. McAdams HP, Goodman PC, Kussin P (1998) Virtual bronchoscopy for directing transbronchial needle aspiration of hilar and mediastinal lymph nodes: A pilot study. *AJR* 170:1361–1364.

29. Haponik EF, Aquino SL, Vining DJ (1999) Virtual bronchoscopy. *Clin Chest Med* 20:201–217.

30. Solomon SB, White P Jr, Acker DE, Strandberg J, Venbrux AC (1998) Real-time bronchoscope tip localization enables three-dimensional CT image guidance for transbronchial needle aspiration in swine. *Chest* 114:1405–1410.

31. Bricault I, Ferretti G, Cinquin P (1998) Registration of real and CT-derived virtual bronchoscopic images to assist transbronchial biopsy. *IEEE Trans Medical Imaging* 17:703–714.

32. Higgins WE, Ramaswamy K, Swift RD, McLennan G, Hoffman EA (1998) Virtual bronchoscopy for three-dimensional pulmonary image assessement: State of the art and future needs. *Radiographics* 18:761–778.

33. Buthiau D, Khayat D (1998) *CT and MRI in Oncology.* New-York: Springer.

34. Buthiau D, Antoine E, Piette JC, Nizri D, Baldeyrou P, Khayat D (1996) Virtual tracheo-bronchial endoscopy: Educational and diagnostic value. *Surg Radiol Anat* 18:125–131.

35. Buthiau D, Blum A, Régent D (1996) Scanner hélicoïdal: Principes et perspectives cliniques. *Rev Med Interne* 17:243–254.

36. Buthiau D, Chaumier P, Piette O et al (1994) Scanner hélicoïdal en pathologie thoracique. In *Progrès en Scanner et IRM*, D Buthiau (ed.) Vigot, Paris, pp. 49–57.

37. Heiken JP, Brink JA, Vannier MW (1993) Spiral (helical) CT. *Radiology* 189:647–656.

38. Naidich DP (1994) Helical computed tomography of the thorax. *Radiol Clin North Am* 32:759–774.

39. Rémy J, Rémy-Jardin M, Giraud F, Wannebroucq J (1994) Le balayage spiralé volumique et ses applications en pathologie thoracique. *Rev Mal Resp* 11:13–27.

40. Rémy J, Rémy-Jardin M, Petyt L, Wannebroucq J (1994) La trachéobronchoscannographie sans contraste par reconstruction multiplanaires et tridimentionnelles surfaciques (RMP-3D) et volumiques (MIP). *Rev Im Med* 6:S210.

41. Merran S (1997) L'imagerie virtuelle: Applications à l'endoscopie virtuelle, *J Radiologie* 78 [3 Suppl]:9–12.

42. Schmutz G, Khayat D, Buthiau D et al. (2003) Virtual colonoscopy in oncology. In *Virtual Endoscopy* Buthiau D, Khayat D (eds). Springer, pp. 143–165

43. Fenlon HM, Ferrucci T (1997) Virtual colonoscopy: What will the issues be? *AJR* 169:453–458.

44. Dachman AH, Lieberman J, Osnis RB, Chen SYJ, Hoffmann KR, Chen CT et al. (1997) Small simulated polyps in pig colon: sensitivity of CT virtual colonography. *Radiology* 203:427–430.

45. Fenlon HM, Numes DP, Schroy PC et al. (1999) A comparison of virtual and conventional colonoscopy for the detection of colorectal polyps. *N Engl J Med* 341:1496–1503.

46. Fenlon H, McAnemy DB, Numes DP et al. (1999) Occlusive colon carcinoma: virtual colonoscopy in the preoperative evaluation of the proximal colon. *Radiology* 210:423–428.

47. Sonnenberg A, Delco F, Bauerfeind P (1999) Is virtual colonoscopy a cost-effective option to screen for colorectal cancer? *Am J Gastroeterol* 94:2268–2274.

48. Weishaupt D, Patak AM, Froehlich J et al. (1999) Focal tagging to avoid colonic cleansing before MRI colonography. *Lancet* 354:835–836.

49. Royster AP, Fenlon HM, Clarke PD, Numes DP, Ferrucci JT (1997) CT colonoscopy of colorectal neoplasms: two-dimensional and three-dimensional virtual-reality techniques with colonoscopic correlation. *AJR* 169:1237–1242.

50. Khayat D, Rixe O, Palau R et al. (2003) Virtual cystoscopy of the urinary tract. In *Virtual Endoscopy.* Buthiau D, Khayat D (eds.). Springer, pp. 143–165.

51. Vining DJ, Zagoria RJ, Liu K, Stels D (1996) CT cystoscopy: An innovation in bladder imaging. *AJR* 166:409–410.

52. Olcott EW, Nino-Murcia M, Rhee JS (1998) Urinary bladder pseudolesions on contrast-enhanced helical CT: Frequency and clinical implications. *AJR* 171:1349–1354.

53. Waterkeyn J, Bensimon JL, Buthiau D (2003) Virtual endoscopy in otorhinolaryngology. In *Virtual Endoscopy.* Buthiau D, Khayat D (eds.). Springer, pp. 81–108.

54. Buthiau D, Antoine EC, Nizri D, Stefani E, Lucien P, Cohen-Aloro G, Gozy M, Guinet F, Chiche B, Weil M, Khayat D (1996) The clinical measurement of volumes using helical CT. *Surg Radiol Anat* 18:227–231.

55. Buthiau D, Rixe O, Spano J-P, Bloch J, Bloch P, Piette JC, Khayat D. Imagerie et Angiogénére tumorale. *Bulletin de l'Académie de Médecine.* Nov 2004. (In press)

56. Buthiau D, Khayat D (eds.) (1998) *Progress in CT and MRI in Oncology.* New-York, Springer, pp. 380–391.

57. Buthiau D, Godeau P, Khayat D (2003) Real endoscopy by imaging. In *Virtual Endoscopy* Buthiau D, Khayat D (eds). Springer, pp. 189–192.

58. Alkadhi H, Kollias SS (2002) Morphological and functional MR characterization of intracranial brain tumors for treatment planning. *Symposium New Imaging in Oncology.* 12th International Congress on Anti-Cancer Treatment, Paris, February 6th.

59. Mardor Y (2002) The use of MR diffusion weighed imaging. *Symposium New Imaging in Oncology.* 12th International Congress on Anti-Cancer Treatment, Paris, February 6th.

60. von Schulthess GK (2002) Pet-CT: One year of experience in oncology. *Symposium New Imaging in Oncology.* 12th International Congress on Anti-Cancer Treatment, Paris, February 6th.

Cancer Diagnosis: Pathology

ALVIN W. MARTIN

University of Louisville, James Graham Brown Cancer Center, Louisville, Kentucky

RORY R. DALTON and STEPHEN PEIPER

Department of Pathology, Medical College of Georgia, Augusta, Georgia

Pathologic examination represents a unique consultation that is vital to the oncologist for proper diagnosis and management of patients with malignancies. Pathologists represent a source of information that helps to establish a diagnosis through interpretation of specimens obtained through biopsy or resection, and they collaborate with the oncologist to formulate a treatment plan, before, during, and after definitive surgical procedures. Once an operative specimen has been excised, the pathologist provides critical feedback to confirm any initial diagnosis and, in the case of a malignancy, a profile of the tumor that includes histological differentiation and nuclear grade, the extent of involvement of the primary site, completeness of the resection, and the stage (i.e., whether there is local, regional, or distant spread). The surgeon has the immediate firsthand opportunity to evaluate the gross pathology *in situ* and thus a unique knowledge of the surgical specimen that can furnish critical information to direct the orientation, dissection, and selection of areas for histopathologic analysis. Therefore, the process of evaluating a surgical specimen is a partnership and the patient is best served when there is effective communication between the surgeon and the pathologist. Once the diagnosis and stage have been ascertained, the pathologist has an armamentarium of special immunohistochemical, molecular genetic, and cytogenetic studies that can enhance understanding of the biological behavior of the process.

GROSS EXAMINATION AND SPECIMEN SUBMISSION

The gross examination of biopsies and surgical specimens is the foundation of the pathological analysis. Although small biopsies, such as mucosal, kidney and liver,

UICC Manual of Clinical Oncology, Eighth Edition. Edited by Raphael E. Pollock
ISBN 0-471-22289-5 Copyright © 2004 John Wiley & Sons, Inc.

may be submitted in part or *in toto* in a fixative, orientation of mucosal surfaces is critical to proper embedding and sectioning to optimize interpretation. A variety of different agents have been advocated for the preservation of tissue morphology, however, buffered formalin has emerged as the overwhelming favorite and the only practical choice. Previously, mercury-based fixatives (i.e., B5, Bouin's, Zenker's, etc.) gained popularity because of enhancement of sectioning and histopathologic staining. They have fallen from popularity because of (1) toxicity of mercury and difficulty in handling of wastes, (2) the archival tissues frequently cannot be used for immunohistochemistry, and (3) the archival tissues cannot be used for genetic analyses. Although it is advantageous to immediately place mucosal, liver, and part of kidney biopsies in fixative, it is highly desirable that excisional biopsies be submitted to the pathology laboratory unfixed, ideally wrapped in gauze wetted with sterile saline, and unsectioned. This is particularly critical to the evaluation of malignant lymphomas, because many monoclonal antibodies used for flow cyto-metric or immunohistochemical analysis cannot be applied to the study of fixed cells or paraffin-embedded tissues. It is often helpful to consult the pathology department regarding policies and procedures for the handling of special specimens and notify them in advance when tissues requiring nonroutine processing will be obtained so that appropriate processing can be anticipated and scheduled.

All major specimens should be submitted for pathological examination in the fresh state and held at 4°C until the initial analysis and dissection are performed. It is optimal that the specimen not be opened in the operating room, as this may obscure some pathologic findings and complicate the identification of surgical margins, typically done by inking the boundaries of the specimen.

The gross examination relies on the orientation of the surgical specimen. Although the landmarks of the excised tissue may be self-evident, it is highly desirable for the surgeon to mark critical structures as reference points for the gross examination. For example, it is helpful to define superior and lateral aspects of excisions and apical regions of tissues containing lymph nodes. Typically, the surgical pathologist will dissect lymph nodes from fresh tissues and then fix the resected tissues in neutral buffered formalin (NBF). Optimal fixation of a specimen is obtained in NBF with a window of time ranging from 4 to 18 hours, with 12 hours being a happy medium. If tissue is to be kept longer in a fixative before tissue processing, then it should be transferred to 70% ethanol after washing as a holding media until tissue processing can ensue. The gross description will first contain a general characterization of the specimen, including dimensions, overall appearance, and, in some instances, weight. The margins are then marked with ink, typically after fixation, to provide a reference point for determining whether the surgical margins are free of tumor. If the specimen has been opened prior to fixation, the ink may have access to regions of the tissue that are inside the boundaries of resection and evaluation of the surgical margins may be compromised. Because the colloidal ink is visible in histologic sections, it is possible to establish the distance of tumor from the point of resection by microscopic examination with a high degree of accuracy. The specimen is then dissected and the pathologic features of the tumor and other relevant processes are described. The submitted tissue is examined for macroscopic evidence of the presence of tumor. The size of the tumor, the distance of the tumor from the surgical margins, and involvement and effacement of normal architecture should be clearly characterized in the gross description portion of the pathology report.

This description represents a formal documentation of the characteristics of the specimen and should provide sufficient detail to present a clear picture of the nature and extent of the resected tissues and the involvement by pathological processes. As such, it represents an extension of the operative note. Tissues representative of the tumor, other disease processes, normal landmarks, surgical margins, and lymph nodes should be sectioned for the preparation of histologic slides. The tissues submitted for histological analysis should be clearly detailed in the "block description" of this section of the report. This is critical for documentation of the pathologic process in the event of future review. There are few formal guidelines for the submission of tumor tissues for histologic examination, but a rule of thumb is that one block should be submitted for each centimeter of diameter of the primary tumor. It is also important to exercise common sense in this process. For example, if tumors contain multiple types of gross appearance (i.e., cystic, hemorrhagic, solid, sclerotic, etc.), as may occur in ovarian tumors and sarcomas, it is critical to section the various areas so that the biologic differentiation of the malignancy can be determined from the microscopic examination. Using standard techniques, the process of tissue processing and embedding formalin-fixed tissues in paraffin takes approximately 12–14 hours. Sectioning and staining takes an additional 2–3 hours. Thus, if the pathologic interpretation is straightforward and special studies are not required, it is possible to receive a finalized diagnosis and report on the day after surgery. The goal for routine specimens is thus to have a turn around time (TAT) ranging from 24 to 48 hours. If the specimen requires special studies, TAT may lengthen commensurate with the studies needed.

INTRAOPERATIVE CONSULTATION (FROZEN SECTION)

Intraoperative consultation with the pathologist is a valuable tool that can serve several purposes in cancer diagnosis and treatment. Excellent and direct communication between the operating surgeon and the pathologist is essential if intraoperative consultation is to yield the maximum benefit. When called to examine a fresh specimen, the pathologist will select from gross examination, touch imprint preparation for cytological examination, and histological sections prepared from frozen tissue to answer the specific question asked by the operating surgeon. In addition to providing an intraoperative diagnosis, intraoperative consultation may be indicated for joint examination of a gross specimen, to provide the pathologist with orientation of a complex specimen, to determine if adequate tissue has been procured for diagnostic evaluation, and to allocate tumor for specialized diagnostic testing. Frozen section examination may also be used for the evaluation of resection margins. In this setting, the surgeon may elect either to submit small separate specimens from areas of concern or to have the pathologist select margins from the gross specimen. If the latter method is selected, the surgeon will gain more useful information if specific areas of interest are identified for frozen section analysis because a complete evaluation of circumferential resection margins by frozen section analysis is usually not practically possible.

The surgeon and pathologist should have a clear understanding of the strengths and weaknesses of frozen section diagnosis. Freezing tissue induces histological artifacts that limit the ability of the pathologist to provide the same detailed results that are available after fixation and standard histological processing for permanent sections. The characteristics of the tissue submitted may also limit the usefulness of frozen sections: tissues containing relatively more fat (breast, some skin excisions) do not freeze well and are technically difficult to examine. The size of the specimen is also an important consideration: with large specimens, the limited number of sections that can be examined invariably carries the risk of undersampling whereas for small specimens, the pathologist must be careful to preserve fresh tissue for subsequent specialized testing. Lastly, some diagnoses should only be made after careful examination of an entire specimen (follicular carcinoma of the thyroid, ductal carcinoma in situ of the breast) or rely heavily on specialized testing (soft tissue tumors, lymphoma).

MICROSCOPIC EXAMINATION

The microscopic examination of a well-fixed, well-stained hematoxylin and eosin (H&E) section continues the characterization of a disease process that the gross examination began. Although numerous ancillary studies are now available to aid the pathologist in solving a difficult diagnostic dilemma, the H&E remains the cornerstone of disease classification.

When a pathologist examines a slide microscopically, he or she will begin formulating a differential diagnosis. This differential diagnosis will encompass several categories.

1. Is the specimen adequate or inadequate? Adequacy of a specimen clearly depends on what question is being asked of the pathologist as well as what is present under the microscope. An extremely small biopsy that contains a carcinoma in a patient with a history of breast cancer can be adequate, whereas a biopsy that is quite generous in size but does not represent the lesion is not.

2. Is the sample representative of what the surgeon or clinician has submitted as documented on the surgical pathology request slip.

3. Is there any normal tissue that the pathologist can recognize and, if so, does it match the specimen submitted.

4. Is the tissue normal or is there a disease process?

5. If a disease process is present, can it be broken into a category such as an inflammatory process, a scar/repair process or a malignancy?

6. If this is an inflammatory process, is it an infectious process or a possible autoimmune disorder? If it is an infectious process, what are the features present to distinguish bacteria from fungal from viral? Is it acute or chronic active?

7. If it is a malignancy, is it invasive or noninvasive? How a pathologist decides whether a malignancy is present is a process that requires attention to detail at both the histological and cytological level. Cytological features of malignancy include loss of polarity of nuclei, chromatin openness, presence or absence of nucleoli, and anaplasia of the nucleus. Histological features include loss of cellular organization, crowding, increased mitotic activity, penetration of the basement membrane (*in situ* vs. invasive), and possible invasion of surrounding tissue structures and or vasculature. Though cytological features are important in arriving at a diagnosis of malignancy, histological features offer a tremendous amount of information in this regard.

8. If invasive, what type of malignancy is it?

Once a malignancy has been demonstrated, not only must the lineage of the tumor be determined, but, in the case of many cancers, various staging and prognostic features must be recorded. Obviously, if the sample is a resection specimen, all appropriate margins need to be inked and designated because, if a tumor is close to a margin, re-excision may be necessary.

Histological and nuclear grading of tumors offers powerful prognostic information in many tumors. Though a number of grading schemes are available for various tumors, the pathologist should use a scheme that all treating parties can understand. In addition, the pathologist must make every effort to maintain reproducibility with the chosen scheme. Nuclear grading encompasses morphological features that, in a well-differentiated or low-grade lesion, have more uniform and regular nuclei with more uniform and smooth chromatin, and small and regular nucleoli. In a poorly differentiated or high-grade lesion, the nuclei are less uniform and have more anaplastic features consisting of open chromatin and variation in size and shape of nucleoli, as well as more prominence of the nucleoli. Mitotic figures tend to increase in number in higher nuclear grade tumors. This type of thinking process is fairly typical of a microscopic examination.

Once the disease category has been established, does the pathologist need to do any additional testing on this sample to differentiate the diagnosis further? If the specimen displays characteristics of an infectious process, then perhaps special stains to help enumerate what type of organism is present are called for. A PAS stain may be used for determination of fungal organisms and Gram stain may be used for bacterial organisms. Stains to highlight destruction of blood vessels, such as an elastic stain (in case of an autoimmune disorder), may be necessary.

In some ways, characterization of benign lesions can be more difficult than characterization of a malignancy. When one thinks of a physician as a pathologist, one invariably links their skills as a surgical pathologist to their ability to make an accurate and reliable diagnosis of malignancy. The diagnosis of a malignancy has changed dramatically in the ensuing years in surgical pathology. The pathologist has a number of studies available to assist in diagnosis and disease classification. Once the pathologist has examined the H&E specimen and has determined that a malignancy is present, the lineage of the tumor must then be elucidated. In most instances, the presence of gland formation evident from the H&E section with perhaps a mucin stain is all that is required to render an appropriate diagnosis of adenocarcinoma. The challenge of malignancy arises when a small sample is present or when there is a large amount of necrosis and not enough viable material is present to give sufficient histological pattern for the pathologist to classify the tumor. Because treatment and prognosis can vary widely depending upon the type of malignancy, it behooves the pathologist to make as definitive a diagnosis as possible. It should always be kept in mind that if this sample has been distorted by crushing artifact during specimen procurement and/or processing or if large amounts of necrosis are present, the surgeon may have to retrieve more samples from the patient for further pathological interpretation.

The process known as immunohistochemistry (IHC) has greatly aided pathologists in the classification of tumors. IHC has gained acceptance as a mainstay of surgical pathology and is now considered state of the art in diagnostic pathology. IHC allows the pathologist to determine protein antigens that are expressed on the cell membrane, on the cytoplasm, or in the nucleus of tumor cells. These protein antigens then allow the "phenotype" of the tumor to be known so that classification can be provided. There is a wide array of antibodies available for the characterization of tumor antigens. A common problem arising in surgical pathology is a small biopsy sample that contains an undifferentiated tumor. Undifferentiated, in this instance, implies that there is insufficient histological or cytological features to allow exact tumor classification to be ascertained from this material. In such a situation, IHC can be particularly valuable. A pathologist at this point could select a panel of three antibodies directed at general antigens to allow for classification purposes. This general classification may vary depending on the situation, however, an example to start with would be to separate the tumor into (1) carcinoma, (2) melanoma, or (3) lymphoma. To allow this, a surgical pathologist could select the following menu for lineage determination. To phenotype the tumor as epithelial, a broad-spectrum cytokeratin cocktail could be chosen such as AE1/3; for melanocytic origin, S100 would be used; and for lymphoreticular origin, CD45 would be used (Table 8b.1) It must be stressed that it is the H&E tissue sample that has guided the differential diagnosis. IHC merely allowed the demonstration of protein antigens present to confer phenotype on the tumor, thus further aiding

TABLE 8b.1. Undifferentiated Malignancy

	CD45	S100	AE1/3
Malignant lymphoma	+	−	−
Melanoma	−	+	−
Carcinoma	−	−	+

TABLE 8b.2. Spindle Cell Lesions of Skin

	AE1/3	S100	Tyrosinase	Desmin	CD68	CD31
Squamus cell carcinoma	+	−	−	−	−	−
Melanoma	−	+	+	−	−	−
Atypical Fibroxanthoma	−	−	−	−	+	−
Leiomyosarcoma	−	−	−	+	−	−
Angiosarcoma	−	−	−	−	−	+

classification. (See Table 8b.2 for further examples of classification of tumors by IHC.)

This same process can be extended further, by utilizing a "panel" of selected antibodies that allow exclusion of one immunophenotype from another. This is illustrated in Table 8b.2. Spindle cell lesions of the skin can be a very challenging diagnostic dilemma for pathologists. Many times there are only small pieces of tissue to examine or too few histological clues are present to allow reliable separation of various tumor types from one another. IHC has allowed the phenotype of these tumors to be reliably determined, thus enabling appropriate tumor classification and treatment to be made.

Further refinement of lineage is possible with IHC. Tumors arising from different epithelium express different cytokeratins. This can be taken advantage of via IHC to profile a tumor by its pattern of expression of different cytokeratins and allows a metastatic lesion to be classified by tissue of origin. One must be careful in using this approach, as some epithelium has virtually identical keratin expression as others, however, with 20 different subsets available for study, many options are possible. This use of IHC would be particularly useful in separating lesions in a patient that has more than one primary tumor. An example would be in a patient who has both an ovarian surface epithelial tumor and a colonic adenocarcinoma. An adequate panel could be chosen to allow determination of which tumor a metastasis or recurrence is from, thus allowing appropriate therapy to be given (Table 8b.3).

IHC can be applied to various scenarios to allow lineage determination of tumors that are difficult to classify via standard microscopical examination. This is further illustrated in Tables 8b.4–8b.9. One could configure a number of different panels to solve various differential diagnostic dilemmas; however, the panels described here are the ones we typically use in our everyday practice of surgical pathology.

IHC has developed to the point where various prognostic factors may also be determined. Examples of these include the detection of estrogen (ER) and progesterone (PR) receptor and *neu* oncoprotein in breast cancer. These factors had previously been determined using biochemical assays such as ligand binding and enzyme immunoassay, which required not only fresh tissue but consumed tissue that could be used for diagnostic purposes. Although this would not be a problem for large resection specimens, it could be problematic in small samples. In addition, one always knows tumor is being assayed via IHC as the pathologist views

TABLE 8b.3. Keratin Subset Expression as a Way to Classify Metastatic Adenocarcinoma

CK7+/CK20+
  Transitional cell carcinoma
  Pancreatic (ductal)
  Ovarian (mucinous)

CK7+/CK20−
  Lung adenocarcinoma
  Breast (ductal)*
  Ovarian (serous)*
  Endometrial*
  Mesothelioma
  *Further Breakdown of CK7+/CK20−

ER/PR+	GCDFP-15+	CA-125+	Calretinin+
Breast	Breast	Ovary	Mesothelioma
Ovary		Endometrial	
Endometrial			

CK7−/CK20+
  Colon

CK7−/CK20−
  Hepatocellular
  Renal cell carcinoma
  Prostate

TABLE 8b.4. Differential Diagnosis of Hepatic Tumors

	Mucin Stain	AE3 (34βE12)	AE1/3	CAM 5.2	CEA	AFP
Hepatocellular carcinoma	−	−	−/+	+	−	+
Cholangiocarcinoma	+/−	+	+	+	+/−	−
Metastatic carcinoma	+/−	+/−	+	+	+/−	−/+

AE3, high molecular weight keratin; CAM 5.2, anti-cytokeratin; CEA, carcinoembryonic antigen; AFP, alpha feto protein.

TABLE 8b.5. Differential Diagnosis of Bladder, Kidney, and Prostate Origin

	AE1/3	AE3 (34βE12)	CK7/CK20	PSA	CEA
Prostate	+	−	−/−	+	−
Bladder	+	+	+/+	−	−/+
Renal	+	−	+/−	−	−

PSA, prostate specific antigen; see Table 8b.4 for other abbreviations.

TABLE 8b.6. Renal vs. Adrenal

	AE1/3	CAM 5.2	EMA	S100	Chromagranin	MART1
Renal cell carcinoma	−/+	+	+	+/−	−	−
Adrenal	−/+	+/−	−	−/+	−	+
Pheochromocytoma	−	−	−	+/−	+	−

EMA, epithelial membrane antigen. See previous tables for other abbreviations.

TABLE 8b.7. Lesions of the Nipple

	AE1/3	CK7	S100	Tyrosinase	Neu
Paget's disease	+	+	−	−	+
Melanoma	−	−	+	+	−
Squamus cell carcinoma	+	−	−	−	−

CK7, cytokeratin 7. See previous tables for other abbreviations.

TABLE 8b.8. Mesothelioma vs. Adenocarcinoma

	AE1	CEA	B72.3	CD15	CK5/6	Calretinin	Thrombomodulin
Adenocarcinoma	2+/− 4+	+/−	+/−	−/+	−	−	−
Mesothelioma	4+[*]	−	−	−	+	+	+/−

[*]Uniform + intense. See previous tables for other abbreviations.

TABLE 8b.9. Small Blue Round Cell Tumors

	NSE	CD45	Desmin	AE1/3	NF	CK20	CD
Small cell carcinoma	+/−	−	−	−/+	−	−	−
Merkel cell carcinoma	−/+	−	−	+	+	+	−
Lymphoma	−	+	−	−	−	−	−
Ewing's sarcoma/PNET	−/+	−	−	−	−	−	+
Rhabdomyosarcoma	−	−	+	−	−	−	−
Neuroblastoma	−	−	−	−	+	−	−
Desmoplastic small cell Tumor	+	−	+	+	−	−	−

NSE, neuron specific enolase; NF, neurofilament; PNET, primitive neuroectodermal tumor. See previous tables for other abbreviations.

not only the IHC reactions but also views the tumor on which the reaction is generated. Newer prognostic assays being developed that will use IHC determination are epidermal growth factor receptor (EGFR) and CD117 (*c-kit*) (Table 8b.10). Anti-EGFR compounds will be used initially to treat breast cancers, but will more

TABLE 8b.10. Prognostic Assays

Antigen	Tumor
ER/PR	Breast cancer/ovarian/endometrial
Neu	Breast
EGFR	Colon
CK117 (*c-kit*)	GIST (gastrointestinal stromal tumor)
p53	Colon
Ki-67	S-phase/cell cycle of tumors

than likely be expanded to other tumors, including colon cancers. Anti-CD117 therapy is being directed against gastrointestinal stromal tumors (GIST) and any sarcoma that is positive for this antigen.

FISH (FLUORESCENCE *IN SITU* HYBRIDIZATION)

FISH is a technique that allows for specific translocations and chromosome numbers to be detected on single-cell suspensions as well as frozen tissue sections and even on formalin-fixed, paraffin-embedded tissue sections. Standard cytogenetic analysis of tumors is fraught with difficulty, as viable tumor is needed. The advantage of the FISH technique is that one may use interphase cells from tissue that is no longer viable (Table 8b.11).

FISH uses a specific probe that is tagged with a fluorescent conjugate. This probe is then placed on the slide containing the sample and, with appropriate denaturation and heating, will anneal to the target DNA.

FISH probes are typically designed so that, when looking for a translocation, two probes are used. One probe is labeled with a red fluorochrome and the second probe is labeled with a green fluorochrome. When there are only normal chromosomes, one would view two red dots and two green dots in a nucleus under a fluorescent microscope in a sample that has been successfully stained via FISH. The dots would, of course, correspond to the areas of successful hybridization. If a chromosome translocation is present in which the probes overlap, typically a yellow dot will form where the red and green fluorochrome overlap each other. In addition, a smaller red dot and a smaller green dot will also be present in the nucleus, which represents segments of DNA that were not part of the translocation process.

FISH can be used in the following applications:

- Detection of structural chromosome abnormalities
- Detection of rearranged chromosomes
- Detection of numerical chromosomes
- Utilization of fresh, frozen, and formalin-fixed tissue sections
- Examination of interphase cells

TABLE 8b.11. Cytogenetic Abnormalities in Solid Tumors

Tumor	Cytogenetic Abnormality	Frequency
Ewing's sarcoma and primitive neuroectodermal tumor	+ (11;22) (q22;a12)	> 90%
Synovial sarcoma	+ (x;18) (p11;q11)	90%
Alveolar rhabdomyosaroma	+ (2;13) (q35; q14)	80–90%
Wilm's tumor	del 11p13 on T12	50%
Desmoplastic small round cell tumor	+ (11;22) (p13;q12)	90%
Lipoma	Rearrangement 8q11-q13	70%

FISH has the following advantages:

- Rapid results (2 days)
- Sensitivity and specificity is very high
- Large numbers of cells can be analyzed in a short period of time
- Direct correlation of morphology and chromosome abnormality is possible in same study
- It can be performed on small amounts of tissue/cells.

But there are a few disadvantages:

- One must know which abnormality to look for
- If DNA degrades, the test cannot be performed
- A fluorescent microscope is required
- Only neutral buffered formalin may be used as a fixative
- Community pathology experience is limited with this technique

SUMMARY

- The gross pathologic examination is a critical foundation for the histopathologic diagnosis. It is an extension of the surgical procedure, and documentation of landmarks optimizes the pathologic analysis.
- It is important for the surgeon to supply appropriate clinical information.
- The intraoperative consultation obtained through the frozen section analysis provides valuable insights into the nature of epithelial tumors, but is limited in the assessment of lymphomas and sarcomas. Understanding of the operative findings, reason for the frozen section, and how the results will impact the surgical approach provided by the surgeon will guide the pathologist to reach an appropriate diagnosis.

- The microscopic examination extends the gross pathologic observations to characterize tumors for evidence of malignancy, including: (1) loss of architecture, invasion, and metastasis; (2) the derivation of tissue of origin; (3) the degree of differentiation and nuclear grade of the tumor, reflecting the relative gap in differentiations and primitive nature of the malignant tumor (i.e., grade, stage); and (4) documents the status of clinical landmarks, such as surgical margins.

- Specialized studies using immunologic and genetic technologies can be used to refine the diagnostic characterization by detecting the expression of markers that are associated with specific tissues and the presence of genetic abnormalities that are emblematic of specific malignancies.

RECOMMENDED READING

Fletcher CDM (ed.) (2000) *Diagnostic Histopathology of Tumors*, 2nd ed. London: Churchill Livingstone. An in-depth presentation of the surgical pathology of tumors that includes gross specimen photographs and radiographs in addition to discussions of immunohistochemistry and molecular diagnosis.

Leonard DGB (2003) *Diagnostic Molecular Pathology*. Philadelphia: Saunders. A concise overview of current molecular diagnostic procedures in pathology.

Mills SE, Carter D, Greenson JK, Oberman HA, Reuter V, Stoler MH (eds.) (2004) *Sternberg's Diagnostic Surgical Pathology*. Philadelphia: Lippincott, Williams, and Wilkins. A comprehensive reference for surgical pathologists.

Rosai J (2004) *Rosai and Ackerman's Surgical Pathology*. St. Louis: Mosby. The standard reference for diagnostic surgical pathology with an emphasis on gross pathology.

Weidner N, Cote RJ, Suster S, Weiss LM (eds.) (2003) *Modern Surgical Pathology*. Philadelphia: Saunders. An excellent review of surgical pathology emphasizing contemporary tools available to the surgical pathologist for diagnosis and classification of malignant disease. The introductory chapters contain concise overviews of specimen handling, intraoperative consultation, and immunohistochemistry.

CHAPTER 9

The Role of Cancer Staging in Evidence-Based Medicine

W. J. MACKILLOP and P. A. GROOME

Kingston Regional Cancer Centre, Kingston General Hospital, Radiation Oncology Unit, Kingston, Ontario, Canada

M. K. GOSPODAROWICZ and B. O'SULLIVAN

University of Toronto, Princess Margaret Hospital, Department of Radiation Oncology, Toronto, Ontario, Canada

The term *cancer staging* refers to the classification of patients with cancer based on the anatomic extent of the disease. In this chapter, we will show how staging contributes to the creation and dissemination of knowledge about cancer, and how staging can be used to guide the treatment of individual patients and the management of cancer control programs. We will begin by considering why staging is necessary and how a staging system is constructed.

THE CLASSIFICATION OF CANCER

The classification of patients with cancer is challenging because there are many diverse types of cancer, and because each individual case progresses over time.

The Problem of Diversity

Cancer is a diverse group of diseases characterized by uncontrolled cellular proliferation, genetic variability, invasion, and metastasis. The prognosis and the potential benefits of treatment vary widely from case to case. Some system of classification is required to identify groups of cases, which share similarities in their clinical behavior. The classification of diseases may seem rather remote from

UICC Manual of Clinical Oncology, Eighth Edition. Edited by Raphael E. Pollock
ISBN 0-471-22289-5 Copyright © 2004 John Wiley & Sons, Inc.

clinical practice, but it is, in fact, at the heart of scientific medicine. Only when a specific clinical problem has been recognized and defined can we start to accumulate the information about it that is needed to answer the fundamental questions that face doctors and patients in day-to-day practice: what will happen if the disease is left untreated, what treatments may help, and which is best (1)? In the physical sciences, new knowledge may be sometimes created by the process of deduction without reference to the external world, but biological systems are not well enough understood to permit the valid use of deduction. Medical knowledge can only be created empirically by the process of induction, which allows us to infer what will happen in a specific set of circumstances in the future, based on what has been observed to happen in similar circumstances in the past (2). The predictive value of inductive inference depends not only on how many observations have been made, but also on how uniform the outcome was in those cases, and that is determined by the effectiveness of the system of classification used to define the group (3).

The classification of cancers presents particular challenges because of the large number of anatomic sites and tissues that may be affected by neoplasia, and because of the genetic plasticity associated with neoplasia. Several complementary systems of classification are available. Cancers are usually classified by their site of origin (4), and by their microscopic appearance (5). However, two cases that look alike from these points of view may prove to be very different when the phenotypic or genotypic characteristics of their tumor cells are studied in greater detail, and new techniques in immunology, biochemistry, and molecular genetics are now beginning to improve the classification of some types of cancer (6,7). In defining similar groups of cases, it is important to consider the characteristics of the patient as well as the cancer, and classification based on the patient's functional status is, therefore, also important (3).

The Problem of Progression

It is a defining characteristic of malignancy that the volume of the cancer and its anatomic extent increase over time. In general, as the anatomic extent of a cancer increases, the prognosis gets worse, the range of treatment options becomes more restricted, and the benefits of treatment diminish. A system of classification based on the extent of the disease is, therefore, required to create groups of clinically similar cases. *Staging* is the term used to describe the classification of cancers based on their anatomic extent.

Staging complements, rather than competes with, classifications based on inherent cellular characteristics. We are sometimes asked why, in the era of sophisticated molecular markers, we still need to classify cancers based on anatomic extent of the disease. The inherent cellular characteristics of a cancer do in part determine how far it will progress before it is detected. Cancers with faster growth rates and higher metastatic potential are less likely to be diagnosed at an early stage because there is a shorter window of opportunity to detect them before they spread. However, random events are involved in clonal evolution and metastasis, and the point in time at which a cancer first spreads may depend on chance alone. Factors entirely unrelated to cancer biology may also determine when the cancer is detected in a specific case. Some tumors are detected by screening, or are found incidentally by diagnostic tests done for other purposes. Others progress until symptoms develop, and many different factors determine how long it is after those symptoms develop before the diagnosis is made. Thus, a system of classification based only on the cellular characteristics of the tumor cannot be expected to create groups of cases that are uniform in their anatomic extent at the time of diagnosis.

THE DESIGN OF A STAGING SYSTEM

A staging system may be considered as a system of measurement in which certain attributes of the tumor are coded to become ranked variables (8). Like any other measuring system, a good staging classification must be valid, reliable, and practical (9), and its value will be maximized if the same system is used universally.

A clinically valid staging system is one that creates groups of cases requiring similar management or groups of cases that experience similar outcomes. To achieve this, the system has to reflect the clinical findings that identify important subgroups of cases. This requires a site-specific system that is tailored to the relevant anatomy, to the characteristic behavior of the specific cancer, and to the available treatment options. A valid system will be exhaustive, that is, it should be capable of reflecting the full range of possible presentations of each type of cancer. To retain its validity over time, the system also needs to be flexible enough to permit it to adapt to important changes in medical practice or medical knowledge (9).

A reliable staging system will as far as possible, ensure that identical cases will always be assigned to the same category. To achieve this end, cancer stage should be assigned based on objective assessment of measurable quantities. The reliability of the system will also be enhanced by a clear set of rules about when and how it is to be applied. The classification system should be unambiguous and accompanied by explicit rules for its application. To permit comparisons over time, the system of clinical experience should not be subject to frequent changes. A practical staging system will be suitable for day-to-day use in a wide range of clinical settings. To meet this requirement, the whole system needs to be easy to comprehend. This means it must be simple in concept and based on common principles that are applicable to all sites. It should not rely on extraordinary expertise or on diagnostic procedures that are not generally available. The system and the rules for its use should be readily accessible; it should be available in all major languages both in print and in electronic form, and the necessary documentation should not be expensive to buy (9).

In practice, the attributes listed above may sometimes conflict with one another, and compromises may be required. Attempts to make the system unambiguous and exhaustive should not be taken so far that it loses its simplicity. The requirement for stability over time should not preclude making changes that are required to keep the system clinically relevant when medical practice changes. A staging system has to be site-specific in order to provide a clinically valid description of different primary cancers that differ in their natural history, but common principles are required to keep the system coherent and comprehensible to the user. A good system will be precise enough to allow specialists to record important differences among cases, but it should not be so complicated as to become impractical for day-to-day use. A good system should be sufficiently reliable that results can be compared among observers, but it has to do this without the help of sophisticated technology in order to remain applicable to routine practice in a wide variety of settings (9).

To maximize the value of staging in communication, the same system should be used universally. Widespread acceptance will be facilitated if the system is valid, reliable, and practical, but a solid administrative infrastructure is also required to keep the system under continuous review and to revise it as necessary (9).

THE TNM CLASSIFICATION

The History of the TNM System

The TNM classification of malignant tumors is a mature system of anatomic staging that meets most of the criteria outlined in the preceding section. The TNM system evolved from the work of Pierre Denoix in the early 1940s (10). The first TNM classification for cancers of the breast and larynx was published in 1958 (11), and the first comprehensive *livre de poche*, which included classifications for 23 sites, was published in 1968 (12). A great effort has been made over the years to reconcile differences between the TNM system and other systems. Today, the TNM classification is used both by the International Union Against Cancer (UICC), and by the American Joint Committee for Cancer Staging (AJCC), and their systems are now identical (13,14). The TNM classifications for the gynecological malignancies are essentially identical to those of the International Federation of Gynecology and Obstetrics (FIGO) (13,15). The TNM classification of colorectal cancer is compatible with the Dukes' system and its modifications (13,16,17), and the TNM classification for the lymphomas is identical to the Ann Arbor system (13,18). The TNM classification is published today in a dozen languages, and is kept under continuous review by an international expert committee.

The UICC and AJCC have recently developed an evidence-based approach to the continuous review of the TNM system. The approach includes ongoing review of the literature for articles that (1) assess the validity and reliability of TNM staging, (2) describe new prognostic schemes based on extent of disease, or (3) present a criticism of the current system. Also, new proposals for changes to TNM staging that meet minimum quality criteria undergo a peer-review process, with recommendations presented to the international committee for their consideration. This new initiative formalizes the existing process of continuous review. Whenever possible, changes to the TNM system are made by creating new subgroups within the existing framework, thus preserving the ability to compare outcomes over time.

The Elements of TNM

The TNM system is based on a set of general rules that have been modified for application to specific primary sites (12). The system requires that the primary site be defined and the diagnosis confirmed microscopically before stage is assigned. As well as providing a vocabulary for describing most of the common cancers, the TNM system provides the syntax required to ensure that the language of stage is used correctly (12).

The system is based on the assessment of three components:

T—the extent of the primary tumor

N—the absence or presence and extent of regional lymph node metastases

M—the absence or presence of distant metastases

As shown in Table 9.1, the addition of numbers to these three components indicates the extent of the cancer.

If there is doubt about which T, N, or M category to assign to a case, then the lower, or less advanced category, should be chosen. After assigning T, N, and M categories, cases may be collected into stage groups. The TNM system provides rules for doing this, but acknowledges that other groupings may be better for specific purposes, and that clinicians may sometimes wish to create their own groups based on the T, N, and M categories. Although the system is simple in principle, the details vary from site to site, and no clinician is likely to retain all of this information in memory. Even very experienced oncologists often carry the UICC's *livre de poche* and refer to it daily in their practice.

TABLE 9.1. The TNM Classification

T—Primary tumor	
TX	Primary tumor cannot be assessed
T0	No evidence of primary tumor
Tis	Carcinoma *in situ*
T1, T2, T3, T4	Increasing size and/or local extent of the primary tumor
N—Regional lymph nodes	
NX	Regional lymph nodes cannot be assessed
N0	No regional lymph node metastasis
N1, N2, N3	Increasing involvement of regional lymph nodes
M—Distant metastasis	
MX	Distant metastasis cannot be assessed
M0	No distant metastasis
M1	Distant metastasis

In some sites, further subdivisions of the main categories are available to permit a greater degree of precision (e.g., T1a, 1b, or N2a, 2b). The category M1 may be further subdivided to specify sites of distant metastases. For details of site specific classifications, see References 13 or 14.

The Clinical and Pathologic TNM Classifications

There are, in fact, two important TNM classifications described for each site (12). The first is a *clinical classification* that is based on evidence arising from physical examination, imaging, endoscopy, biopsy, surgical exploration, and whatever other pretreatment examinations are relevant to that specific site. This classification is used in making initial treatment decisions, and provides some information about the prognosis. This type of classification can be applied in every case and provides a level playing field for comparisons of outcome between treatment strategies that involve surgery and those that do not.

The second is a *pathologic classification*, designated pTMN. This is based on the evidence obtained before treatment, supplemented or modified by the additional evidence acquired from surgery and from pathologic examination. The pTNM classification does not replace the TNM classification in operated cases; the preoperative TNM stage remains unaltered, and the pTNM stage is recorded separately. pTNM is used to guide decisions relating to postoperative treatment and provides additional information about the prognosis. Pathologic staging contributes to our understanding of how well clinical stage reflects the true anatomic extent of the cancer, and may be useful in assessing the value of new diagnostic techniques.

The TNM system is primarily intended for use in classifying newly diagnosed cases, but the same nomenclature can be used in modified form in other circumstances. The TNM classification may be applied to recurrent tumours, but the TNM and pTNM categories are then to be identified by the prefix r and recorded separately from the record of stage at diagnosis, which should not be changed. The extent of disease may also be assessed after chemotherapy or radiotherapy, but the TNM or pTNM categories assigned in this context are to be identified by the prefix y.

The Roles of Staging in Cancer Control

Table 9.2 summarizes the several important roles that staging plays in cancer control. We will now discuss each of these in turn.

THE ROLE OF STAGING IN RESEARCH

Staging plays a key role in studies of the effectiveness of cancer treatment, and in studies of the effectiveness of cancer control programs. It may also be important in studies of the etiology and natural history of cancer.

Research on the Effectiveness of Cancer Treatment

Experimental Studies The prospective, randomized controlled trial (RCT) is accepted today as the standard method of comparing the effectiveness of different

TABLE 9.2. The Uses of Staging in Cancer Control

In creating knowledge
- Permits clinical research to produce new information through the systematic observation of groups of similar patients
- Permits integration of information about similar patients from diverse sources

In disseminating knowledge
- Provides a common language for sharing information internationally
- Facilitates the teaching of new health-care workers, and the continued learning of those already in practice

In applying knowledge to the care of individual patients
- Permits the use of knowledge derived from past experience to guide medical decisions in the individual case
- Fosters a disciplined, multidisciplinary approach to the evaluation of cancer patients
- Facilitates communication with patients, and promotes their involvement in decisions about their care

In managing programs of cancer control
- Permits projections of workload needed for strategic planning and resource allocation
- Permits evaluation and improvement of cancer control programs

treatment strategies (19). In RCTs in oncology, stage is almost always one of the entry criteria used to create uniform groups of cases for study. Stage may also serve as a basis for stratification to ensure an even balance of prognostic factors between the arms of a trial. Routine recording of stage at a cancer treatment center permits estimation of the number of cases eligible to participate in proposed trials, and also provides a way of monitoring accrual to trials in progress. Information about the stage mix in the community reveals how well the sample in a trial represents the overall population, and this is useful in estimating the generalizability of its results.

Observational Studies Much of our knowledge about the results of cancer treatment still comes from retrospective, observational studies of the experience of individual institutions. Reviews of institutional experience are inferior to RCTs as a means of comparing the effectiveness of different treatments, but they are a means of learning from clinical experience, and are often the source of hypotheses that can later be tested in formal clinical trials. In the rarer malignancies, retrospective reviews may be the only source of information about the effectiveness of treatment, and their importance in that context cannot be overstated (20). However, the problem with such observational studies is that comparisons of outcomes between treatment groups in the same institution are usually confounded by selection bias, and comparisons of outcome among institutions are often further confounded by the problem of referral bias. The ability to control for stage goes some way toward reducing these problems and permits a more valid comparison of the results of competing treatment strategies. Reporting results by stage also gives a clearer idea of the subgroups of patients most likely to benefit from specific treatments.

Integrating Information About the Effectiveness of Treatment   Review articles and book chapters are the traditional way of bringing together information from diverse sources. In compiling these reports, stage is used to identify comparable groups, and to describe and compare outcomes achieved by different treatment strategies. There is, however, growing dissatisfaction with unstructured literature reviews because of a) the potential for bias in the choice of information to be included, and b) the lack of a valid process for combining data from different sources. This has led to a more structured approach, known as the "systematic review," which is now promoted worldwide by the Cochrane collaboration (21). Here the reviewer is forced to be explicit about the search process used to identify relevant material, and about criteria used to select the information to be included in the analysis. The results of different RCTs are combined by the formal process of meta-analysis. The trials combined in the process of meta-analysis need to have involved similar groups of patients. Information about stage is, therefore, necessary to select trials for inclusion in a meta-analysis.

Research on the Effectiveness of Cancer Control Programs

Population-based cancer registries were originally established to study the epidemiology of cancer, but they can also be used to study the epidemiology of cancer treatment. Like cancer incidence and mortality, patterns of cancer treatment and survival can be compared among communities, across socioeconomic strata, and over time. Registry-based observational studies (RBOs) of the management and outcome of cancer deal with unselected cohorts of cases and are, therefore, free of the problems of referral bias and selection bias that confound institution-based observational studies. RBOs and RCTs are complementary, rather than competing, methodologies; RCTs tell us how patients should be managed, whereas RBOs tell us what really happens in practice. RBOs can be used to describe how RCT results and treatment guidelines affect the management and outcome of cancer in the population.

Research on Economic Aspects of Cancer Care

It is increasingly recognized that information about the effectiveness and the cost of different types of treatment is necessary for rational allocation of resources. Economic information is important in decisions at many levels. It may be used to decide how much public money to spend on health programs as opposed to other publicly funded programs, how much to spend on cancer care as opposed to other health programs, how much to spend on early detection as opposed to treatment, and how much to spend on palliative care as opposed to active treatment. Economic analyses are now being built into some RCTs, but RBOs may be the ultimate way of addressing economic questions. In health economics, it is just as important to define the patient group studied in terms of the site and stage of the cancer as it is in any other type of cancer research.

Research on the Epidemiology and Natural History of Cancer

Gathering information about stage mix at the population level extends the scope of conventional epidemiological research in oncology by permitting the investigation of factors that are associated with more or less advanced stage at presentation. Staging also contributes to studies of the natural history of cancer. In the evaluation of putative markers of metastatic potential and putative predictors of response to therapy, it is important to control for stage to ensure that the study indicator really does provide more prognostic information than was provided by conventional approaches.

THE ROLE OF STAGING IN DISSEMINATING KNOWLEDGE

Stage as a Language

Stage provides a common language of communication among doctors worldwide. In day-to-day practice, doctors use the language of stage to communicate with one another and with their patients. Stage provides a framework for teaching and learning in undergraduate, postgraduate, and continuing medical education. Journal articles, textbooks, and treatment guidelines all rely on the language of stage in summarizing their management recommendations.

Potential Barriers to Communication

Because stage is used in creating, integrating, and disseminating the knowledge that guides the practice of oncology, the fidelity of information transfer along this path is very important (9). This depends on how consistently the language of stage is used from one observer to the next, from one clinical trial to the next, from one country to the next, from one year to the next, from one clinic to the next, and from one case to the next. Even when reliability has been given a high priority in designing a staging system, some inconsistency in its use is inevitable. It has been shown experimentally that the same clinician cannot always be relied upon to assign the same stage to identical cases on two separate occasions (intraobserver variation), and that there is a greater degree of variation in stage recorded by different clinicians observing the same cases (interobserver variation) (22). Errors in staging may be random or systematic. Although both are equally important in the management of the individual case, systemic error is the more serious problem in the analysis and interpretation of collective experience.

Stage Migration

One particular type of systematic error deserves special mention. Figure 9.1 illustrates a curious phenomenon that arises when staging investigations change over time, or vary from one place to another. It was described more than half a century ago by Bradford Hill, who called it "the problem of attributes" (1), but it is

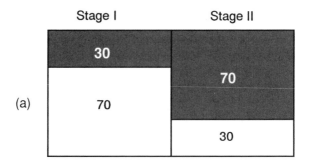

Stage I (n=100), 5 year survival=70/100=70%
Stage II (n=100), 5 year survival=30/100=30%
Overall Group (n=200), 5 year survival=100/200=50%

Stage I (n=80), 5 year survival=60/80=75%
Stage II (n=120), 5 year survival=40/120=33.3%
Overall Group (n=200), 5 year survival=100/200=50%

Figure 9.1 The problem of attributes: stage migration. The diagrams describe five-year survival in an imaginary cancer, which is classified using a simple two-stage system. Panels *a* and *b* show the results reported before and after the introduction of a new diagnostic test that "upstages" a subgroup of patients with an intermediate prognosis from stage I to stage II. The shaded areas indicate the patients who die of the disease. Survival "improves" in both subgroups, although overall survival is unchanged (1,25).

now more widely known as "stage migration" (23). Figure 9.1 shows how this problem might affect reports of the outcome of a cancer with an overall five-year survival of 50%, when it is classified using a very simple two-stage system. Based on the results of conventional staging investigations, half of the patients are assigned to a good prognosis group, stage I, which has a five-year survival of 70%, and the other half to a poor prognosis group, stage II, which has a five-year survival of 30% (Fig. 9.1a). Suppose that a new radiological technique is adopted that has a higher resolution than conventional techniques, and this reveals that 20% of the former stage I cases are more extensive than was thought, and actually belong to stage II. Let us assume, as seems reasonable, that this subgroup has a worse prognosis than the rest of the stage I patients, but a better prognosis than the stage II patients, say 50% survival at five years. When the information provided by the new radiological technique is used in assigning stage, this intermediate group is transferred from stage I to stage II. This leads to an "improvement" in survival in stage I, from 70% to 75%, and an "improvement" in survival in stage II from 30% to 33.3%, but the overall survival, of course, remains unchanged at 50% (Fig. 9.1b). There are many practical examples of this phenomenon, and in general changes in investigations that lead to systematic up-staging, improve results in each subgroup (20,24). The phenomenon of stage migration makes it hazardous to compare outcomes by stage in different series of cases that have not been investigated in the same way. The reader should always be suspicious of improvements in the outcome of subgroups that are not accompanied by any improvement in the outcome of the overall group.

There has so far been insufficient effort directed toward assuring the uniform use of the TNM system, and additional work is required in this area. It can be argued that the TNM system could be enhanced by gradually becoming more prescriptive with respect to the information that may, and may not, be used in assigning stage. One of the reasons why the FIGO system has been so widely accepted as a valid means of comparing the results of treatment of the gynecologic malignancies around the world is that it very clearly defines what information may *not* be used in assigning stage (15).

THE ROLE OF STAGING IN CLINICAL PRACTICE

What Is Involved in "Staging" the Patient?

In practice, "staging" involves three separate steps: assessment, classification, and recording. Assessment involves the gathering of information about the extent of disease from the clinical history, the physical examination, endoscopy and/or radiological investigation, and, in the case of pathologic classification, from surgical and histological evaluation. Classification involves the analysis of this information, and may require the reconciliation of apparently conflicting data. It culminates in a conscious judgment about the T, N, and M categories to be assigned to the case. This is followed by the act of recording the stage as a permanent part of the patient's record. This is usually the responsibility of the attending physician, although the stage assigned may reflect the combined views of several consultants.

It is sometimes thought that a commitment to staging implies that all cases of a particular cancer must be submitted to a given series of investigations whether or not they serve the needs of the individual patient. This is incorrect. Consider a patient who presents with cough, hemoptysis, and widespread bone pain, and who is found to have a large opacity at the right hilum on chest x-ray, malignant squamous cells in his sputum, and multiple hot spots on bone scan that are consistent with metastases. This patient would not benefit from the additional investigations that would be necessary to delineate the extent of the primary tumor, or to ascertain the status of the mediastinal lymph nodes. The TNM system does not mandate these investigations. Rather, the TNM system provides the X categories for use when the medically appropriate investigations do not yield sufficient information to permit classification. This case would be classified as TXNXM1. If a diagnosis of cancer is made in a patient who is not fit for any active treatment regardless of the stage of the disease, then it is perfectly correct to stage the patient, TXNXMX without any staging investigations at all (13).

The Role of Stage in Guiding Treatment Decisions

The way that knowledge is created dictates the way it must be applied. Almost all the knowledge about cancer treatment that has been created by clinical research trials is knowledge about specific stages of specific diseases. It can, therefore, only be used to guide the management of the individual patient once the site and stage of the cancer have been established. The staging of cancer is, therefore, necessary for the practice of evidence-based medicine (9).

Staging influences several aspects of the treatment decision. First, the stage of the cancer often determines whether the intent of treatment should be curative or palliative. Consider a patient who presents with dysphagia and weight loss and is found to have a squamous carcinoma of the esophagus and multiple metastases in the liver. Because metastatic squamous cancer of the esophagus is not curable by surgery, radiotherapy, or chemotherapy, the goals of therapy should be palliative. One of the great benefits of staging is that it avoids exposing patients to the morbidity of aggressive interventions that offer no chance of cure or long-term survival. Secondly, the clinical stage of the cancer often decides the choice of primary treatment in patients with potentially curable cancers. Many of the site-specific T and N classifications were designed to reflect the boundaries of resectability. The clinical stage of the cancer at presentation, therefore, often determines whether an attempt at radical surgery would be worthwhile. Similarly, in many operated cases, the pT and pN status of the cancer provides information about the potential value of adjuvant radiotherapy, or adjuvant systemic therapy, or both. Thirdly, the stage of the cancer may serve as a basis for planning the details of treatment once the modality has been chosen. The T and N categories may delineate the extent of the surgery required for complete resection, or may serve to define the anatomic volume that must be encompassed in a curative radiotherapy plan. pT and pN categories may help to define the volume to be treated with postoperative radiotherapy.

Of course, neither the clinical nor the pathologic stage can be equated with the true extent of the cancer. The subclinical extent of the disease often only becomes apparent when it is manifested later by the sites of progression or recurrence after treatment. However, stage provides a link with past experience that permits us to infer the true extent of the disease. This type of reasoning, in fact, led to the concept of adjuvant treatment that, in some situations, has proved to decrease failure rates and improve survival. It was the analysis of patterns of failure that showed that the pathologic involvement of the axillary lymph nodes in breast cancer (pN1) was strongly associated with a high risk of occult distant metastases in M0 cases. RCTs then showed that the risk of subsequent distant relapse was diminished when adjuvant systemic treatment was given to pN1 cases in the absence of any clinical evidence of distant metastasis.

The Role of Staging in Promoting Good Medical Practice

The process of staging itself fosters good medical decision making. It promotes a rational and disciplined approach to the evaluation of patients with cancer, and encourages the clinician to make a judgment about the extent of the disease before initiating treatment. It provides a means of summarizing the patient's status, which makes it easier to discuss the case with colleagues, either informally or in the setting of a multidisciplinary tumor conference. Routine staging readily identifies patients eligible for management according to clinical practice guidelines, or for participation in randomized trials. Staging also permits real-time audit of treatment decisions and retrospective audit of the process and outcome of treatment.

The Role of Staging in Promoting Autonomous Decision Making

In recent years, there has been a trend toward actively involving patients in decisions about their medical care. The ethical requirement for respect for the autonomy of the individual is now widely recognized, and is enshrined in the legal doctrine of informed consent. An autonomous decision is one that is made intentionally, without coercion, and with understanding. To help patients understand the decisions which they face, they not only need information, but also a conceptual framework in which to process it. The concept of stage is readily understood by the majority of patients, and provides a useful framework for discussion of the details of the individual case. Many patients ask doctors about the stage of their disease, and a clear answer can help them to understand the treatment options and to participate actively in discussions about their treatment. A knowledge of the stage of cancer also helps patients to distinguish information that is relevant to them from that which is not. This is important because patients recently diagnosed with cancer are often bombarded with the experiences of relatives and acquaintances, which are often entirely irrelevant to their own situation. Once patients know the stage of their disease, they are also empowered to seek additional information about it for themselves from other sources such as support groups, books, or the Internet (3).

Stage is an important determinant of the prognosis in almost every type of cancer. The prognosis may be important to patients not only in making treatment decisions, but also in making decisions about other aspects of their lives (25). Many patients ask about their chances of cure or survival, and they need an honest answer, whether the prognosis is good or bad. For many people, uncertainty is even more difficult to deal with than bad news, and the information about the prognosis provided by staging helps them to make the best possible plans for the future.

THE ROLE OF STAGING IN MANAGING CANCER CONTROL PROGRAMS

A knowledge of stage mix in a population can guide the management of cancer programs in the same way as a knowledge of stage in the individual case guides the individual treatment. In this final section, we will show how the routine use of staging is valuable both in the strategic planning of cancer programs and in their day-to-day management.

Cancer Staging and Strategic Planning

By studying trends in cancer incidence over many years, cancer registries have been able to predict the future incidence of cancer very accurately. This information is sometimes used as a basis for making long-term plans about the location and size of cancer treatment facilities, and for estimating future requirements for specialized equipment and personnel. However, a knowledge of incidence alone does not provide an optimal basis for this type of planning because the appropriate treatment of cancer is highly stage-dependent. Predictions should be based on projections of the incidence of cancer by stage, and, whenever possible, population-based cancer registries should, therefore, collect and compile information about stage. A knowledge of trends in caseload in terms of disease and stage mix can also help to anticipate the future workload of a specific treatment center. Projections of caseload can be integrated with projections of treatment patterns to estimate future requirements for equipment, manpower, and resources. However, this is only possible if the institutional cancer registry routinely collects and compiles information about stage.

Cancer Staging and Resource Allocation

A knowledge of case mix in terms of stage provides a basis for the rational allocation of resources at many levels. In publicly funded health-care systems, cancer control competes with other programs for limited health dollars. The more precisely societal needs for cancer treatment can be defined, the more likely it is that an appropriate slice of the available resources will be allocated to cancer treatment. Accurate descriptions of case mix in terms of site and stage may also serve as a rational basis for the allocation of resources within a cancer center or cancer program.

Cancer Staging and Quality Management

Managing any health-care program involves setting goals, developing processes, implementing them, evaluating what has been achieved, and modifying the program accordingly. Formerly, the planning and evaluation cycle was aimed at achieving static goals. It is now seen as more appropriate to strive for continuous quality improvement without setting fixed upper limits on achievement. The appropriate criteria for measuring the success of a cancer program depend on its purpose and on the target population, but no cancer program can be adequately evaluated without information about case mix including stage.

Programs of early detection, like mammographic screening for breast cancer, are intended to reduce cancer mortality, but the first indication of their success may be a decrease in the proportion of patients presenting with more advanced stages (26). Stage mix at presentation can be evaluated as an intermediate outcome of the program that may predict its long-term benefits. Because screening programs operate at the population level rather than at the level of individual institutions, evaluation of screening programs requires stage to be recorded in population-based registries.

Evaluation of cancer treatment programs requires consideration of access to the service, the quality of the service, and the outcomes achieved in specific groups of cases defined by stage. Stage is not an outcome measure here, but a means of defining the target population.

The overall effectiveness of any cancer treatment program is limited by the proportion of people who might benefit from it, that actually have access to it. Publicly funded health-care programs in many countries are designed to remove financial barriers to care. However, they do not guarantee access to care unless resources keep pace with demand for service, and if they do not, waiting lists may develop and operate as a form of implicit rationing. Monitoring of access is necessary to identify this type of problem (27). Access to care must also be examined carefully whenever centralized facilities are expected to provide services for dispersed populations, as is often the case with radiotherapy and other specialized forms of cancer treatment. Regional cancer services often create out-reach programs to overcome geographic access barriers, but these require ongoing evaluation to ensure their success (28). Measuring access to care at the population level requires a knowledge of the number of cases eligible for the service as well as the number who actually receive it. Eligibility is almost always stage-dependent, so monitoring access requires information about stage in the population. Monitoring access to service within cancer treatment centers is equally important. In any institution that manages cancer patients, it is appropriate to ask what proportion of its patients with stage II breast cancer get the opinion of a medical oncologist, what proportion of patients with stage I prostate cancer get the opinion of a radiation oncologist, and what proportion of patients with stage IV non–small-cell lung cancer are seen by a palliative care service. Such questions can only be addressed if stage is routinely recorded and compiled in the institutional registry.

It is known that there are large variations in the management of many different cancers, both within institutions, among institutions, and among societies. Wide variations in practice suggest that the management of cancer may often be suboptimal (29), but the extent to which these variations are appropriate or inappropriate can only be determined if information about stage has been collected. If stage is available, medical practice in a given region or in a given institution can be compared with practice elsewhere or with some standard deemed to be appropriate based on the scientific evidence available in the literature. However, when external standards are used to evaluate medical practice using only summary data about site, stage, and treatment, it should not be assumed that noncompliance in an individual case represents inappropriate management. Medical contraindications or patient preferences may sometimes make the standard approach inappropriate. It seems more reasonable to try to set targets based on experience of what is achievable in the field, for example, that more than 80% of patients with stage II breast cancer should receive systemic adjuvant treatment, or that less than 10% of patients with stage I breast cancer should have a bone scan (30).

There is currently great interest in the use of clinical practice guidelines to assist medical decision making and reduce practice variations (31). The extent to which this approach succeeds in changing the practice of oncology will only be evaluable if stage information is recorded in the appropriate registry (9). Evaluating treatment at the population level obviously requires capture of stage information in a population-based registry. Evaluating treatment within an institution can be achieved by recording stage routinely within an institution-based registry.

Individual consumers and particularly the sophisticated purchasers who operate on behalf of health insurance programs, now expect institutions to be able to describe not only how they manage their patients, but also what results they achieve. Monitoring cancer outcomes is the ultimate way of evaluating the success of any cancer control program, but a long time has to elapse before the outcome of the curative treatment of cancer can be evaluated in most diseases. For this reason, audit of outcome cannot be relied upon to optimize cancer treatment programs, and a lot of attention has to be directed toward audit of the treatment process along the lines described above. However, in the long term, survival achieved in a given region or institution can be compared with the outcome expected based on clinical trials and with outcomes achieved elsewhere, but fair comparisons require a knowledge of stage mix (9).

CONCLUSIONS

Cancer staging plays a central role in the scientific practice of oncology. The TNM system is a sophisticated tool for classifying cancer that provides a vital link between research and medical practice, and is appropriate for use in most cancers. Doctors who provide care for cancer patients should routinely record the stage of the disease in their patients' medical records using the TNM system. Institutions that provide care for cancer patients should ensure that stage is routinely and accurately recorded, and should regularly compile and report the management and outcome of cancer by stage. Agencies that certify doctors who treat cancer and accredit institutions that provide care for cancer patients should recognize the use of the TNM system as a standard of care.

REFERENCES

1. Hill BA (1937) *Principles of Medical Statistics*, 1st edition. The Lancet Limited, London, England.

2. Howson C, Urbach P (1989) *Scientific Reasoning*. Open Court Publishing Company, LaSalle, Illinois.

3. Mackillop WJ (2001) The importance of prognosis in cancer medicine in prognostic factors. In *Cancer*, 2nd edition. Gospodarowicz M, Henson DE, Hutter R, O'Sullivan B, Sobin L, Wittekind CH (eds.). Wiley-Liss, New York.

4. *Manual of the International Classification of Diseases, Injuries, and Causes of Death* (1975) World Health Organization, Geneva, Switzerland.

5. *International Classification of Diseases for Oncology* (ICDO), 2nd edition (1990) Percy C, Van Hollen V, Muir C (eds.). World Health Organization, Geneva, Switzerland.

6. Crump M, Gospodarowicz M (2001) Non-Hodgkin's malignant lymphoma. In *Prognostic Factors in Cancer*, 2nd edition. Gospodarowicz M, Henson DE, Hutter R, O'Sullivan B, Sobin L, Wittekind CH (eds.). Wiley-Liss, New York.

7. Brundage MD, Mackillop WJ (2001) Lung cancer. In *Prognostic Factors in Cancer*, 2nd edition. Gospodarowicz M, Henson DE, Hutter R, O'Sullivan B, Sobin L, Wittekind CH (eds.). Wiley-Liss, New York.

8. Sokal RR, Rohlf FJ (1969) Biometry. In *The Principles and Practice of Statistics in Biological Research*. Emerson R, Kennedy D, Park RB, Beadle GW, Whitaker DM (eds.). W.H. Freeman and Company, San Francisco, CA.

9. Mackillop WJ, O'Sullivan B, Gospodarowicz M (1998) The role of cancer staging in evidence-based medicine. *Cancer Prev Control* 2:269–277.

10. Denoix PF (1944) *Bull Inst Nat Hyg (Paris)*, 1:1–69.

11. International Union Against Cancer (UICC), Committee on Clinical Stage Classification and Applied Statistics (1958) *Clinical Stage Classification and Presentation of Results, Malignant Tumours of the Breast and Larynx*. UICC, Paris.

12. International Union Against Cancer (UICC) (1968) *TNM Classification of Malignant Tumours*. Geneva.

13. Sobin LH, Wittekind Ch (eds.). (2002) *UICC TNM Classification of Malignant Tumours*, 6th Edition, Wiley-Liss, New York.

14. Fleming ID, Cooper JS, Henson JS, Hutter RVP, Kennedy BJ, Murphy GP, O'Sullivan B, Yarbro JW (eds.) (1997) *AJCC Cancer Staging Manual*. Lippincott, Philadelphia.

15. International Federation of Gynecology and Obstetrics. (1991) Annual report on the results of treatment in gynecological cancer. *Int J Gynecol Obstet* 36:27.

16. Dukes CE (1940) Cancer of the rectum: an analysis of 1000 cases. *J Pathol Bacteriol* 50:527–539.

17. Nathanson SD, Schultz L, Tilley B, Kambouris A. (1986) Carcinoma of the colon and rectum. A comparison of staging classification. *Am Surg* 52:428–433.

18. Carbone PP, Kaplan HS, Musshoff K, Smithers DW, Tubania M (1971) Report of the Committee on Hodgkin's Disease Staging Classification. *Cancer Res* 31:1860–1861.

19. Sackett DL, Haynes RB, Guyatt GH, Tugwell P (1985) *Clinical Epidemiology: A Basic Science for Clinical Medicine*, 2nd edition, Little, Brown and Company, Boston, MA.

20. O'Sullivan B, Mackillop WJ (1986) An approach to the interpretation of the literature of head and neck cancer. *Clin Oncol* 5:411–433.

21. Bero L, Rennie D (1995) The Cochrane Collaboration. Preparing, maintaining, and disseminating systematic reviews of the effects of health care. *JAMA* 274:1935–1938.

22. Eapen L, Nair R, Lavigne B, Laewan A (1990) The TNM system for oral and oropharyngeal cancer—a study into the accuracy and reproducibility with which it is used. *Int J Radiat Oncol Biol Phys* 19:227.

23. Feinstein AR, Sosin DM, Wells CK (1985) The Will Rogers phenomenon: stage migration and new diagnostic techniques as a source of misleading statistics for survival in cancer. *N Engl J Med* 312:1604–1608.

24. Barbera L, Groome PA, Mackillop WJ, Schulze K, O'Sullivan B, Irish JC, Warde PR, Schneider KM, Mackenzie RG, Hodson DI, Hammond JA, Gulavita SPP, Eapen LJ, Dixon PF, Bissett RJ (2001) The role of computed tomography in the T classification of laryngeal carcinoma. *Cancer* 91:394–407.

25. Mackillop WJ, Quirt CF (1997) Measuring the accuracy of prognostic judgements in oncology. *J Clin Epidemiol* 50:21–29.

26. Winawer SJ, Fletcher RH, Miller L, Godlee F, Stolar MH, Multrow CD, Woolf SH, Glick SN, Ganaits TG et al. (1997) Colorectal cancer screening: clinical guidelines and rationale. *Gastroenterology* 112:594–642.

27. Mackillop WJ, Fu H, Quirt CF, Dixon P, Brundage M, Zhou Y (1994) Waiting for radiotherapy in Ontario. *Int J Radiat Oncol Biol Phys* 30:221–228.

28. Mackillop WJ, Groome PA, Zhou Y, Zhang-Salomons J, Holowaty EJ, Cummings B, Feldman-Stewart D, Paszat K, Dixon P (1997) Does a centralized radiotherapy system provide adequate access to care? *J Clin Oncol* 15:1261–1271.

29. Anderson TF, Mooney G (eds.). (1990) *The Challenges of Medical Practice Variations.* The MacMillan Press Ltd., London, England.

30. Hillner BE, McDonald K, Desch CE et al. (1997) Measuring standards of care for early breast cancer in an insured population. *J Clin Oncol* 15:1401–1408.

31. Browman GP, Levine MN, Mohide EA, Hayward RSA, Pritchard II, Gafni A et al. (1995) The practice guidelines development cycle: a conceptual tool for practice guidelines development and implementation. *J Clin Oncol* 13:502–512.

Principles of Surgical Oncology

SARAH ELIZABETH SNELL

University of Louisville, James Graham Brown Cancer Center, Louisville, Kentucky

ANNE T. MANCINO and MICHAEL J. EDWARDS

University of Arkansas for Medical Sciences, Arkansas Cancer Research Center, Little Rock, Arkansas

With the progressive evolution of new technologies and therapies, the importance of specialization and the personal commitment of an individual physician to a limited number of diseases is increasingly a practical concern for maintaining competence. This is especially true for the patient with cancer as it pertains to the intricacies of integrated multimodal cancer care. Surgery was the first effective treatment modality and remains a mainstay in the treatment of cancer; the surgical excision of solid tumors is still the most effective treatment for most tumors. However, optimal therapy today often involves surgery in association with chemotherapy and radiation therapy. Coordination of various oncologic disciplines involves significant surgical input and a refined knowledge of principles of surgical management. In addition, efficient diagnosis, staging, and follow-up all require specific knowledge to provide efficient, cost-effective, and compassionate care.

Within the world of medicine, the collective personal commitment of surgeons to their patients and personal mission are considered by some to be characteristic. This commitment and the associated character traits do not reflect personality so much as an attitude toward illness. That attitude is perhaps best characterized by actions that result from a prompt evaluation of treatment alternatives in the context of the biology of an individual patient's disease and overall general health. This assessment culminates in an acute therapeutic intervention with obvious, inherent treatment risks, most often outweighed by a profound therapeutic impact. To understand the state-of-the-art and the future of surgical oncology as a discipline, we begin with a historical perspective.

UICC Manual of Clinical Oncology, Eighth Edition. Edited by Raphael E. Pollock
ISBN 0-471-22289-5 Copyright © 2004 John Wiley & Sons, Inc.

HISTORICAL PERSPECTIVES

Although history documents the surgical treatment of tumors as early as ancient times, the modern era of elective surgery for visceral tumors began in Kentucky in 1809 when Ephraim McDowell removed a 22-pound ovarian mass from Mrs. Jane Todd Crawford. Skeptical citizens gathered around the house on that Christmas Day in Danville, Kentucky. They were convinced that Dr. McDowell had embarked on a course of intervention more akin to assault than what we now know as surgery. The citizens hung a rope from a tree threatening his hanging should his patient die (1). Ms. Crawford lived some 30 years following this first spectacularly successful elective abdominal operation. McDowell performed 13 other ovarian resections, documenting the feasibility of elective abdominal surgery. Realizing the full potential of the surgical intervention for the general populace, however, hinged on overcoming three hurdles: eliminating the pain associated with the operation, controlling infection, and developing quality surgical training programs.

Anesthesia

The inquisitive mind of Crawford Long at 27 years of age led to the first operation under inhalation sulfuric ether anesthesia in Jefferson, Georgia, on March 30, 1842. That day, a small tumor was removed from the posterior neck area of a 20-year-old man named James Venable. Mr. Venable later stated he "did not experience the slightest degree of pain." This, the primary event in the history of anesthesia, would not be recorded until 1848 (2). The first public demonstration of ether anesthesia by the dentist William Thomas Green Morton might have been viewed as a relatively insignificant sequel to Crawford Long's discovery had Long proceeded immediately with publication, and if it were not for Morton's surgical connections and relentless opportunism. Morton was schooled in dentistry in the early 1840s by Horace Wells. He subsequently learned that ether induced sufficient analgesia to make the practice of dentistry tolerable. Morton pursued animal experiments with ether anesthesia, and also experimented on himself. On September 30, 1846, a Boston merchant arrived at Morton's office with an infected tooth. Morton painlessly removed the tooth. That event was chronicled in the lay Boston press. Morton communicated his observations regarding his preclinical and clinical experiences to John Collins Warren, the Chief of the Surgical Service at the Massachusetts General Hospital at that time. An invitation for a demonstration of "anesthesia" was extended. Morton, who like Crawford Long was also 27 years young, administered ether at the Massachusetts General Hospital in 1846 while Warren ligated a congenital vascular malformation. Witnessing the efficacy of ether anesthesia and recognizing the seminal nature of the event, Warren exclaimed to his audience of colleagues, trainees, and students, "Gentlemen, this is no humbug." The limitation of pain as an obstacle to the evolution of surgery was about to be eliminated (3,4).

Infection

If Crawford Long and William Morton can be credited with making surgery tolerable, Joseph Lister should perhaps be credited with making surgery safe. Before the application of Lister's principles of antisepsis, operative mortality was almost prohibitive. Most patients died from complications of wound infections. After Lister developed and instituted his antiseptic methods of wound management, infection-related mortality reached acceptable levels.

Lister's achievement had its origin with the observations of Pasteur. Pasteur showed that fermentation did not occur in dust-free air. In developing his "germ theory," Pasteur showed that "organisms" were associated with alcoholic fermentation, but were distinct from other "organisms" associated with milk souring (5). After reading Pasteur's papers, Lister believed that the germ theory could be applied to the prevention of surgical wound infections and began his search for a chemical antiseptic. After experimenting with several substances, he discovered carbolic acid. He learned of the foul-smelling fluids use as a sewage disinfectant in the town of Carlisle in northern England. Lister finally prevented infection by treating wounds with carbolic acid in 1865. He eventually developed an antiseptic gauze dressing. Lister retreated the wound, his hands, and the instruments with carbolic acid throughout the course of an operation, and eventually designed a device to spray carbolic acid into the air surrounding the operative field (5,6).

German surgeons were the first to accept the antiseptic techniques of Lister. By 1880, the antiseptic technique was practiced throughout Great Britain as well. German researchers were also the first to show that surgeons could reduce wound infection rates by scrubbing their hands and instruments with soap and water prior to surgery, the first use of combined antiseptic and aseptic techniques. Although Lister's antiseptic methods were eventually supplanted by the aseptic technique, his principle of antisepsis was the fundamental basis of all modern efforts in preventing infection in surgical wounds.

SURGICAL TRAINING AND EDUCATION

The history of modern surgical training also originates in Germany. The German surgical education model was primarily based on the system founded by Bernhard Rudolf Konrad von Langenbeck (1810–1887). His perhaps greatest, and certainly most longstanding, contribution was his systematic method of training young surgeons. William S. Halsted recognized and concluded in his famous address delivered at Yale in 1904, entitled "The Training of the Surgeon," that German surgeons were the first to adopt antisepsis; he attributed this in large part to "the character of the scientific and practical training of surgeons in Germany" (7,8). The trainees, or "residents," in German programs in that time had access to quality research facilities, were exposed to a broad clinical experience, and served under the greatest surgical educators. The German surgical educators and their students were Halsted's models. Their mentorship was justifiably appropriate, for it was

Theodor Billroth, one of von Langenbeck's students, who between the years 1850 and 1880 successfully performed the first gastrectomy, the first laryngectomy, and the first esophagectomy (9,10).

Halsted sought to duplicate this German education model in the United States. He said, "We need a system, and we shall surely have it, which will produce not only surgeons, but surgeons of the highest type, men who will stimulate the first youths of our country to study surgery and to devote their energies and their lives to raising the standard of surgical science" (8). He committed to a system in which highly qualified trainees were selected for an extended course of study that included clinical, educational, and research experience. Trainees acquired graded levels of clinical responsibility as they advanced and were responsible for teaching the more junior house staff. Many of the surgeons trained by Halsted went on to leadership roles in surgery and disseminated his philosophy.

Halsted propagated Joseph Lister's principles of antiseptic surgery, promoted the careful handling of tissues and the minimization of blood loss, pioneered the use of surgical gloves, addressed fundamental problems of surgical science, and developed successful operations. In addition to the radical mastectomy for breast cancer, he made important contributions to thyroid and parathyroid surgery, hernia surgery, surgery of the gastrointestinal and biliary tracts, and vascular surgery. His meticulous technique made surgery safer and paved the way for increasingly complex procedures. But most importantly, Halsted created the educational platform for the dramatic progress of 20th-century American surgery. By the end of his career, Halsted had transformed surgery from a trade practiced by variably trained physicians to an academic specialty and profession characterized by prolonged and effective training and scholarship (11).

MILESTONES IN THE EVOLUTION OF SURGICAL ONCOLOGY

Although specific developments may be debated with regard to their relative significance and overall impact, certain "firsts" have signaled the beginning of new eras of improved therapeutic efficacy for particular malignancies. For example, the radical mastectomy became the treatment of choice for breast cancer just after 1900, when Halsted demonstrated the effective local control of chest wall disease for the first time. Other examples of initial resections for cancers of specific organs from the early 1900s include the radical prostatectomy by Hugh Young in 1904, the radical hysterectomy by Ernest Wertheim in 1906, and the abdominoperineal resection for rectal cancer by W. Ernest Miles in 1908 (4,12). During the period from 1910 to 1930, Harvey Cushing pioneered surgery for brain tumors. The first successful surgical resection for cancer of the esophagus was performed in 1913 by Franz Torek, even though a considerable operative mortality relative to the probability of cure by esophagectomy is still daunting today. The treatment of lung cancer began with Evarts Graham's first successful pneumonectomy in 1933. Successful surgical resections of lung tumors were made possible by developments that included intrathoracic anesthesia and effective methods of ligating the pulmonary artery and the bronchial stump. The modern treatment of pancreatic tumors began in 1935 when A.O. Whipple first performed a two-stage pancreaticoduodenectomy (12). Progress with the pancreaticoduodenectomy was, however, limited owing to an extraordinary complication rate that has been minimized only in the last 20 or 30 years as the procedure became increasingly refined and practiced by tertiary centers with a critical volume of experience. The last 25 years has witnessed the expansion of the field of reconstructive surgery as techniques of wound coverage and reconstruction evolved. Coupled with improvements in the ability to assess operative risk and manage postoperative complications, we now commonly schedule extirpative operative interventions not thought possible only a few years ago.

Although more complex procedures are now feasible, perhaps our most significant progress in recent years has been the development of approaches that minimize the magnitude of the associated surgical injury. The evolution of prospective randomized clinical trials to scientifically quantitate therapeutic impact has accelerated the refinement of operations and their integration with other treatment modalities. The progress and history of the National Surgical Adjuvant Breast and Bowel Project under the leadership of Bernard Fisher began in the 1960s and persists to the present (12). The precision of operations has also been more finely tuned by new technologies. Some recent advances include ultrasound and stereotactic guided surgery, precise staging through the use of lymphatic mapping, and limited access surgery by laproscopic, thorascopic, and increasingly complex endoscopic techniques. Such approaches pay the dividend of limited morbidity while preserving diagnostic and therapeutic efficacy. In perhaps no other surgical specialty or field of interest have these advances been as revolutionary as in the field of surgical oncology.

THE CURRENT STATUS AND FUTURE OF SURGICAL ONCOLOGY

The surgeon's current role in the field of oncology is multi-faceted. This includes the goals of cancer prevention, screening, diagnosis, staging, all aspects of treatment, monitoring for recurrence, and the development of new diseases. Also included is the pursuit and application of new knowledge from both basic scientific and clinical perspectives.

Cancer Prevention and Screening

In the mission to minimize the morbidity and mortality of cancer, prevention and early detection of malignancies are obvious top priorities. Certain tumors are more likely curable when detected and treated at an earlier, less advanced stage. Surgeons have historically initiated and supported educational programs for health professionals and public awareness programs to identify such patients. Surgeons must be knowledgeable of the natural history, etiology, and epidemiology of malignancies in order to reliably impact prevention and early detection.

"Screening" refers to the clinical application of simple tests to a selected population to segregate individuals who probably have the malignancy in question from those who most likely do not. It is important to recognize that screening programs are applied to an asymptomatic, apparently healthy population and must be evaluated to verify the magnitude of reduction of the morbidity and mortality of the targeted disease. Adherence to this principle often precipitates debate. For example, consider the proper age for screening women with mammography for breast cancer, a controversial screening issue in recent years. Although screening is effective and precisely defined for many diseases such as cervical cancer, not all cancers are suitable for screening. The prevalence and duration of the asymptomatic but clinically detectable disease state in the screened population may be insufficient to justify testing costs, especially in an increasingly hostile economic health-care environment with limited resources.

Unfortunately it is also clear, albeit less frequently recognized by the legal profession and lay public, that certain malignancies are governed by a biological nature characterized by incurability from the earliest possible date of clinical detection. Apparent increases in survival rates attributed to screening programs using fixed endpoint survival measures are often an illusion created by lead-time basis, with no real, long-term, overall survival impact. In the absence of effective therapy, it is hoped that this subset of cancers may eventually be prevented.

Two primary factors have limited the impact of preventive measures to date. First, our understanding of the process of malignant transformation for our most common cancers is currently, at best, a primitive science. The clinically relevant inciting event or factors for the origin of our most common tumors are simply not known. Secondly, adapting patterns of human behavior, especially in the context of substance addiction, has proven difficult, even when the malignancy-inducing behavior or habit has been precisely identified. The roles of tobacco and alcohol in lung and head and neck cancers, the duration of our knowledge of the deleterious effects of cigarette smoking, and the simultaneous dissemination of death and destruction over the globe by the tobacco industry, despite this understanding, must be considered. Nevertheless, some degree of cancer prevention has been achieved.

There is also significant and immediate potential for progress through our evolving understanding of the genetics of inheritable disease. Many cancers have a genetic basis, which has prompted screening examinations and diagnostic genetic evaluations. Multiple genes have been implicated in a variety of organ specific malignancies, for example, familial polyposis and other polyposis syndromes of the large bowel. Historically, serial colonoscopy in family members of affected kindred was used to screen and diagnose polyposis or adenocarcinoma. Genetic mutations of these diseases are now defined. As genetic testing becomes widely available, definitive one-time diagnostic genetic testing will progressively supplant serial screening colonoscopic examinations. The issue then becomes one of appropriate monitoring and the proper timing of the "preventative" surgical intervention.

Cancer Diagnosis

In most clinical situations, the diagnosis of cancer requires histopathological confirmation before initiating definitive treatment. Some malignancies are readily accessible for biopsy and may be diagnosed preoperatively. Others, such as small bowel and pancreatic lesions, are many times biopsied at the time of surgery with definitive resection after frozen section analysis. Multiple techniques of acquiring cells or tissue for diagnosis are available, and new methods of obtaining samples for analysis with less invasive approaches such as endoscopy and laproscopy have increased the role of biopsy procedures over recent years. Each approach has distinct advantages and disadvantages, but all originate in certain fundamental principles.

- Biopsied tissue should be representative of the lesion in question. Areas of hemorrhage, necrosis, and infection should be avoided when selecting the site for biopsy. Multiple specimens are most often helpful. Clamping, tearing, crushing and charring of tissue creates distortion of the pathological specimen and should be avoided.
- The choice of biopsy technique should satisfy the tissue sample needs of the pathologist. For some tumors, electron microscopy, flow cytometry, or other specialized techniques may be necessary. Sufficient tissue must be obtained and properly submitted. If biopsy specimens are immediately placed in formalin, the opportunity to perform diagnostic tests may be lost.
- Needle punctures and incisions should be carefully placed with consideration of the subsequent definitive surgical procedure. Incisions on the extremity generally should be placed in the direction of the underlying muscle, almost always longitudinally. Hematomas may increase the magnitude of subsequent surgery and enlarge required fields of radiation therapy; meticulous hemostasis is mandatory for optimum therapy. Drainage exit sites should also be carefully planned for similar reasons.
- Close cooperation should exist between the surgeon and pathologist. The surgeon should orient, label, and, when indicated, ink the specimen for the pathologist (4,13). The pathologist should always be provided with the relevant clinical information. With image-directed biopsy, the surgeon must ensure radiographic, clinical, and pathological correlation.

Certain specifics of each biopsy technique must be considered in choosing the optimum approach. Fine needle aspiration biopsy cytology involves the aspiration of cells through a small-caliber needle. The needle may be guided into the suspicious lesion by palpation or image-directed assistance. Cytologic analysis provides a tentative diagnosis of malignancy and allows the surgeon to proceed with the staging evaluation. However, in most cases, major surgical resections should not be undertaken solely on the basis of the conclusions of fine-needle aspiration biopsy cytology. A small risk of a false-positive diagnosis exists in the hands of even the most experienced cytopathologist. Fine-needle aspiration biopsy cytology diagnosis must nearly always be confirmed by definitive histological studies of tissue.

Core needle biopsy refers to obtaining a tiny piece of tissue in the hollow of a specially designed needle. This tissue may be histologically evaluated for architecture, and, if of adequate size and quality, usually provides definitive diagnosis. Some tumors, such as lymphomas, sarcomas, and other tumors of mesenchymal origin, are difficult to diagnose with small tissue cores. Incisional biopsy refers to the surgical removal of a larger portion of tissue that is often the preferred method of diagnosing tumors of mesenchymal origin.

Excisional surgical biopsy provides the pathologist with the entire lesion. As such, excisional biopsies are most useful if performed without compromising the outcome of the definitive operation. It is important to note that a diagnostic excisional biopsy makes no effort to achieve a gross or histological margin of normal tissue. Biopsy sites from procedures done with only "diagnostic intent" must be re-excised in as much as residual carcinoma may be found in a significant number of cases, even when the pathologist reported the diagnostic excision as having "negative margins"; definitive excisions must proceed with "therapeutic intent" on the part of the surgeon to be efficacious.

Preoperative Considerations and Staging

Cancer patients are often elderly and sometimes of poor nutritional status. The general condition of the patient must be thoroughly evaluated before treatment. Cardiac, pulmonary, renal, nutritional, and other assessments are necessary to prepare the patient for major surgery. Ensuring an adequate preoperative hydration is increasingly important in this era of outpatient mechanical cleansing of the bowel and the obligatory preoperative fasting for general anesthesia.

A preoperative mechanical cleansing bowel prep should be used for colon surgery, as well as for all patients undergoing extensive abdominal procedures. An unexpected *en bloc* partial colectomy or enterotomy may occasionally occur as part of the procedure. The recovery from ileus is also thought more tolerable by some if mechanical cleansing is accomplished preoperatively. Patients undergoing major liver resections also need preoperative cleansing to reduce the risk of postoperative encephalopathy.

Timing the surgical intervention in patients receiving chemotherapy or radiation is important to ensure that bone marrow suppression will not complicate the immediate postoperative period. Bleeding problems should be suspected by a history of suggestive symptoms or drug use including aspirin and preoperative chemotherapy. A screening complete blood cell count with differential is usually necessary. Baseline liver function tests and tumor markers, if applicable, should be obtained prior to surgery as trends in these levels may be monitored during follow-up. A chest X-ray film is usually indicated as a baseline and to identify potential other new primary cancers, metastases, or other pulmonary pathology.

Infection is a special consideration in immunocompromised patients with metastatic diseases and in patients receiving chemotherapy. The source of infection can vary, but must be identified and is usually best eliminated by "the four surgical Ds": drainage, debridement, diversion, and drugs (antibiotics). Patients recently treated with steroids, another special consideration, should receive steroid supplements to prevent an Addisonian crisis.

Cancer Therapy

For most of our solid tumors there is no more effective treatment modality than the proper operation for the particular stage of malignancy. The surgical treatment of cancer has the goals of cure, prolongation of life among uncured patients, the palliation of clearly defined symptoms, and the local control of disease as a measure to prevent subsequent complications. The operative summary should explicitly detail the intended goals. It is important to recognize that prophylactic surgery causes morbidity in an asymptomatic patient. To reliably help more patients than we harm, prophylactic interventions must proceed only after thoughtful consideration of the natural history of the disease and the individual patient's operative risk.

The extent of the appropriate local excision varies with the individual cancer type and the site of involvement. For many malignancies, definite surgical therapy requires only a wide local excision defined by a sufficient margin of normal tissue. The magnitude of surgical resection is modified when surgery is integrated with adjuvant treatment modalities. In some instances, effective adjuvant modalities have led to a decrease in the magnitude of surgery with preservation of function not possible without multimodal therapy. For example, our success in limb preservation function with sarcoma surgery entails integrated surgery and radiation therapy. Rationally integrating surgery with other treatments requires a careful consideration of all effective treatment options; this knowledge often distinguishes the differentiated surgical oncologist from more generally oriented surgeons (13).

In some diseases, such as ovarian cancer, extensive local metastases preclude the surgical excision of all gross disease. The debulking or cytoreduction of selected cancers may lead to enhanced local disease control. However, for most solid tumors, any significant patient benefit has been most often negated by associated surgical morbidity. Cytoreductive surgery is usually of significant benefit only for diseases that respond to other treatments to control small residual deposits of unresectable disease (4,13).

A significant percentage of patients with solid tumors have regional or distant metastases when they present with their first symptoms (4). Surgical resections designed to include regional lymphatic metastases can cure some patients. Lymph node metastases, depending on the specific organ site and disease, may or may not be an indication of systemic disease. The impact of surgery on long-term survival, and even cured fraction, in patients with regional nodal and metastatic disease is underestimated by most physicians. Patients with a limited number of pulmonary, hepatic, or cerebral metastases can also enjoy an extended life with surgical resection. For example, the resection of pulmonary metastases in sarcoma patients may benefit as many as 30% of carefully selected patients. Similarly, hepatic resection of colorectal metastases enhances long-term survival. Patients with solitary hepatic metastases from colorectal cancer have a long-term survival of about 30%, a magnitude of benefit dramatically exceeding the uniformly fatal result in untreated, age-matched cohorts.

Palliative surgery is defined as the surgical relief of intractable symptoms, it does not apply to the asymptomatic patient. The judicious use of surgery for the relief of pain can improve the quality of life for some patients. Palliative surgery also includes the removal of masses causing disfigurement, and operations for emergencies from complications related to hemorrhage, obstruction, or perforation. Perforations of an abdominal, pelvic, or thoracic viscus may result from direct tumor invasion or rarely from tumor lysis with systemic chemotherapy as tumors respond and disintegrate. Decompression of the central nervous system is another emergency situation that must be promptly addressed to preserve neurologic function.

Urinary obstruction is another relatively frequent complication. Urinary diversion must be carefully considered because it may sometimes only prolong patient suffering from an intractable, incurable malignancy. However, sometimes surgery may palliate symptoms due to urinary fistulas or injuries resulting from bladder irradiation. Fecal stream diversion should be similarly considered, but is more often beneficial from a palliative perspective. Locally advanced tumors of the aerodigestive tract may sometimes be managed by fulguration, laser surgery, or stents to establish patency without the disadvantage of a diverting cutaneous intestinal stoma. Feeding gastrostomies are sometimes required for feeding advanced head and neck cancer patients, or for palliative decompression with peritoneal carcinomatosis in the terminally ill.

Follow-Up Monitoring

One goal of follow-up monitoring is early detection of local, regional, or distant metastases to extend life after surgery or other therapy. Unfortunately, the impact of such screening programs has historically been poorly studied. Most screening programs are organized by intention, but without definitive scientific basis. Some patterns of follow-up practiced by some disciplines frankly defy logic. Consider the routine follow-up of pancreatic cancer patients with computerized tomograms of the abdomen and chest. The evidence to suggest that any treatment based on these findings offers significant therapeutic impact is lacking. Such patients are also frustrated by the anxiety associated with equivocal results and may suffer the unnecessary morbidity of invasive biopsies in an attempt to clarify diagnosis. Proper follow-up monitoring can only be prescribed in the context of a clear understanding of the natural history of the disease, and a realistic probability of therapeutic impact in the screened population.

During the last 25 years, long-term venous access for the administration of chemotherapy, nutritional support, and blood drawing has been progressively refined with numerous technological advances. The first silicone rubber catheter was introduced just over 25 years ago. Long-term vascular access devices take the form of external catheter devices and a variety of totally implantable venous access reservoirs or ports. Numerous studies have confirmed reliability and an acceptable complication rates for these devices. In recent years, there has been a virtually continuous series of modifications of existing vascular access devices, often with little, if any, significant improvement, but also in association with exaggerated claims and marketing fanfare on the part of the medical technology industry. An intensive educational program for patients, families, and caregivers of meticulous catheter maintenance is the key essential to achieve extended catheter function in the absence of complications (14). For further details of catheter selection, choice of site for venous access, and other aspects of management the reader is encouraged to review the details of the book by Alexander, a most comprehensive and excellent review of the state-of-the-art of long-term venous access (15).

Research

In 1971, the United States Congress approved legislation to address the issue of cancer diagnosis and therapy. The stated goal was to eliminate cancer as a disease in the immediate coming years. The outcome of this investment of funds, energy, and resources has been significant; however, the impact in terms of the goal of "curing" common solid tumors has been collectively disappointing. In spite of significant failure, a continued commitment to research has paid dividends in small steps, which collectively, over time, have enhanced cancer therapy with some degree of improvement of long-term survival, and certainly the minimization of associated treatment toxicities.

No previous time in the history of cancer treatment has witnessed as much breakthrough potential as today. Surgeons, although acknowledged for their clinical contributions in providing the most effective treatment modality for patients with solid tumors, have historically pursued, and greatly contributed to, the advancement of our understanding of the basic molecular and biologic nature of cancer. As in Halstead's day, surgeons are committed to a depth of knowledge and exploration vital to answering basic, translational, and clinical questions. Increasingly, answers to these questions support the concept of cancer as a disease caused by mutation in genes that regulate cell division. It has been just over 20 years since the cloning of the first tumor suppressor gene. Significant progress continues with the knowledge of the human genome. Novel technologies fuel the gradual elucidation of the genes and problems responsible for a given malignancy.

Efforts to realize the potential of gene therapy currently pursue a variety of approaches. Clinical trials of gene-based therapies now underway seek to augment immunotherapy and/or chemotherapy. These strategies include exploiting unique synergies between gene-based agents and other cancer therapeutics, drug sensitization with genes regulating drug delivery, and the use of drug resistance genes for organ protection from high doses of chemotherapy. *Ex vivo* and *in vivo* gene transfer, the regulation of gene expression, the inactivation of oncogene expression, and gene replacement of tumor suppressor genes are other strategies being studied to target underlying genetic lesions unique to the cancer cell. Significant effort has also been directed toward optimizing delivery systems and constructs for gene therapy. Early results with these strategies are encouraging with regard to the possibility of mediating tumor regression with acceptable toxicity (16).

Surgeons continue contributing to our understanding of tumor immunology. Hope grows that the cycle of scientific discovery, renewed enthusiasm, and heightened expectation, historically followed by disappointment, will finally be overcome by a critical mass of knowledge resulting in clinical relevance. Other efforts in the field of angiogenesis have also yielded some early encouraging results as a number of anti-angiogenic agents have been identified, and clinical trials targeting angiogenic factors have been initialed.

Novel Technologies

A detailed history and thorough physical examination are the keys to minimizing the unnecessary costs associated with extensive radiographic testing and staging evaluation. In recent years, clinicians, especially those from primary care and medical oncology specialities, have increasingly relied on various scans and other expensive imaging to evaluate potential sites of metastases. In many cases, these studies have not altered the treatment approach and often unnecessarily duplicate the operative findings for indicated operations. Surgeons must endeavor to educate other physicians as to the accuracy of operative staging, and uniformly document these findings as a regular part of the operative record. The surgeon must also be familiar with the likely patterns of metastasis to guide his or her operative exploration. Staging the disease is the most important factor in establishing the prognosis; it must be diligently and accurately pursued. All treating physicians should have a thorough knowledge of the natural history of the disease and appropriately investigate potential sites of metastases in order to practice safe and cost-efficient medicine.

Technological advances have had a dramatic, and sometimes unsettling, impact on clinical practice in recent years. For example, the recent development of image-guided core needle breast biopsy, by both stereotactic and ultrasound technologies, has provoked a major change in the diagnosis of mammographically detected abnormalities. Recent reports, including several by surgeons, document accuracy equivalent to needle-directed excisional breast biopsy and verify the validity of this approach, which is also more economically efficient. As a result, the next decade will likely witness the demise of the diagnostic surgical breast biopsy. Issues related to the credentialing and privileging processes, and the respective roles of surgeons and radiologists remain controversial (17). Incorporating the skills required of imaging, clinical management, and pathological interpretation are significant concerns for patient safety. Necessary modifications in resident training are being implemented in several surgical training programs. Practicing surgeons with limited imaging skills must endeavor to extend these skills in order to become significantly involved.

Lymphatic mapping and sentinel lymph node biopsy has supplanted elective lymph node dissection and become the standard approach for staging cutaneous melanoma. The validity of sentinel lymph node staging breast cancer has also been precisely defined (18,19). Axillary node status is the most important factor in the decision for adjuvant chemotherapy following surgical treatment; therefore, accurate determination of node status is vital. However, this can be determined more accurately with sentinel node biopsy with a decreased risk of both lymphedema and intercostal brachial nerve paresthesia if performed by an adequately trained and experienced surgeon. Data from 1999 and 2000 suggest that individual surgeon accuracy improves with greater than 20 sentinel lymph node biopsies performed; the false-negative rate for 1–20 cases in the largest reported study to date was 9.6%, versus 1.3% with greater than 20 cases (20). The American Society of Breast Surgeons has responded and issued a statement on credentialing and privileging providing specific criteria for local hospitals for safe implementation of this new and evolving technological approach (19,20); the immediate future will likely see an increasing role in this regard by other farsighted specialty societies.

DATA, INFORMATION, AND KNOWLEDGE MANAGEMENT

The information age is rapidly evolving. Universal access to accurate, understandable information, now available in a digital format, routinely empowers individuals with specific knowledge in a variety of industries in a matter of minutes. However, the conversion of "knowledge to power" resulting in cost-efficient medical practice is yet to become a practical reality. The health-care system today and in the recent past has been characterized by a host of efforts to "manage" health data to achieve efficiency. Organizations networking to share health information have, however, had limited impact in their quest to reduce costs. Although emphasizing their electronic capabilities, health-care data management networks are in the early stages of development.

Managed care and capitation systems are organized such that a primary care physician is to evaluate and direct the patient's care without the use of sophisticated, expensive resources and technologies unless they are warranted. This failed process has been referred to as having the physician act as the gatekeeper. In this role a generalist-trained physician manages health-care resource utilization. In order for this concept to function properly, the primary care physician must be knowledgeable of all the details and management specifics of a patient's particular illness. This concept works relatively well when applied to more common diseases that can be managed according to guidelines regarding standard medical practice. However, in cases where a generally trained physician is required to provide specialized care, this approach often results in delaying referral, and inefficient, costly, poor care. This is especially true for the more unusual disease diagnoses. The gatekeeper approach is a valid and functional hypothesis only if the primary physician is empowered with the specialized knowledge required to accomplish the goals of an efficient diagnosis, staging, therapy, and referral. From a cost standpoint, the physician certainly holds a tremendous sway in the financial future of any health-care entity—estimates are that physicians affect seven out of every eight dollars of health-care spending. This fact is the basis for the financial value to support the infrastructure of knowledge dissemination. By empowering the primary physician with specialized knowledge on a case-by-case basis, costs may be reduced.

To date, medical expertise has, been geographically organized, often with remarkable heterogeneity of medical practice even within tertiary centers. The opportunity to organize a multi-institutional consulting group of recognized medical specialists, and to provide timely consultations in the management of some of the more rare, and historically imprecisely and inefficiently managed diseases, is a concept yet to evolve in practical application. Information dissemination systems will allow such a group to provide specific recommendations for the treatment of a specific patient, who in years past would not have had efficient access to these physicians. In the next few years, within hours of a tissue biopsy and pathological diagnosis, a nationally recognized specialist will consult in the treatment of particular rare disease and provide a statement of clinical significance in the patient's medical record. This unsolicited consultation will empower the local primary physician with the knowledge of a highly experienced specialist and thereby prevent unnecessary diagnostic testing, facilitate therapeutic decision-making, and streamline referral from the primary physician, thus resulting in the most cost-effective, high-quality practice of medicine. This approach will provide unprecedented and unobtrusive opportunities for truly "managing care," while at the same time providing cost-effective quality care. These systems will dramatically change the clinical practice and referral in the near future.

The Future

What, then, is the future of the surgeon's role in the field of oncology? Some have suggested that the discipline has reached a peak and will be limited in future contributions. Such thinking has been consistently erroneous in the past, and remains so. As quickly as one surgical intervention becomes antiquated, technological and conceptual advances spur the application of new ideas and technologies in areas previously thought beyond surgical endeavor.

Surgeons have historically provided a leadership role in the care of patients with cancer. The scope of surgery's future leadership role, relative to the other oncologic disciplines, will be defined by the extent to which individual surgeons persist in acquiring a comprehensive and differentiated knowledge of specific malignancies. In this regard, individual surgeons are increasingly faced with two fundamental choices. Do we narrow our individual interests and scope of clinical expertise to more effectively contribute to promising research and the clinical implementation of technological advances? Or, do we maintain a broader surgical practice and delegate these responsibilities to other tangentially related specialties? Perhaps too often in the past strategies have been pursued that precipitated the involution of whole areas of clinical interest previously recognized within the purview of surgery. The resulting obligatory fragmentation of patient care has proven inconvenient for patients, and unnecessarily costly. In a world of tremendous economic pressures for the practice of medicine to conform to the efficiencies of business, strategies that eliminate redundancies have to be investigated. In some cases, the fragmentation of patient care in recent years occurred because surgeons failed to expand the scope of their discipline through their commitment to the implementation of novel technologies. Other decisions, such as the indication for adjuvant therapy, have sometimes been referred as a matter of convenience for the surgeon, resulting in inconvenience for the patient, and increased costs for the payor. Surgeons should be sophisticated concerning decisions regarding adjuvant therapy and the treatment of metastatic cancer. Such treatment may involve significant expense and morbidity for marginal benefit. One of the prime goals of the discipline of surgical oncology is the education of all physicians and surgeons in the comprehensive management of cancer. This is not to suggest that surgeons, or any other single discipline, should dominate the decision-making of oncologic management, but rather suggests that the surgical discipline must continue to occupy a central role in the treatment of solid tumors. Strong surgical representation is vital to ensure appropriate planned cancer care coordinated by multidisciplinary cancer teams. A successful cancer program is usually approved by the American College of Surgeons Commission on Cancer, certifying that such programs pass certain milestones in their care of their cancer patients.

The traditional role of surgery is being transformed. For many years, there has been an ongoing debate regarding the role of surgical oncologist relative to the general surgeon. The recent past has been characterized by a trend toward less "oncological surgery" and more "surgical oncology" (13). The surgical operation is only one intervention in an increasingly integrated therapeutic process requiring spcialized physicians. The role of the general surgeon is not necessarily diminished, but general surgeons must commit to an expanded and specialized knowledge in order to continue to participate and lead the integration of care.

REFERENCES

1. Flexner JT (1969) *Doctors on Horseback.* Dover Publications, New York, 10.
2. Long CW (1849) An account of the first use of sulphuric ether by inhalation as an anaesthetic in surgical operations. *South Med Surg J* 6:705–713.
3. Meade RH (1968) *An Introduction to the History of General Surgery.* WBC Saunders, Philadelphia.
4. Rosenberg SA (1997) Principles of cancer management: surgical oncology. In *Cancer: Principles & Practice of Oncology*, 5th edition. Lippencott-Raven, Philadelphia.
5. Fisher RB (1977) *Joseph Lister, 1827–1912.* Stein and Day, New York.
6. Guthrie D (1949) *Lord Lister, His Life and Doctrine.* E & S Livingstone, Edinburgh.
7. Billroth T (1924) *The Medical Sciences in the German Universities.* Macmillan, New York.
8. Halsted WS (1904) The training of the surgeon. *Bull Johns Hopkins Hosp* 15:267.
9. Heuer GW (1952) Dr. Halsted. *Bull Johns Hopkins Hosp* (Suppl), 90:1.
10. Nunn D (1989) William Stewart Halsted: A profile of courage, dedication, and scientific search for truth. *J Vasc Surg* 10:221–229.

11. Harvey AM (1981) The influence of William Stewart Halsted's concept of surgical training. *Johns Hopkins Med J* 148:215–236.

12. Olson JS (1984) *The History of Cancer.* (An annotated bibliography.) Greenwood Publishing Group, Westport, Connecticut.

13. Arnesjo B, Burn I, Denis L, Mazzeo F (1989) *Surgical Oncology (A European Handbook).* Springer-Verlag, Berlin.

14. Broadwater JR, Henderson MA, Bell JL, Edwards MJ, Smith GJ, McCready DR, Swanson RS, Hardy ME, Shenk RR, Lawson M, Ota DM, Balch CM (1991) Percutaneous subclavian catheterization for cancer outpatients. *Am J Surg* 60:676–680.

15. Alexander HR (ed.) (1994) *Vascular Access in the Cancer Patient: Devices, Insertion Techniques, Maintenance, and Prevention and Management of Complications.* JB Lippincott, Philadelphia.

16. Roth JA, Cristiano RJ (1997) Gene therapy for cancer: What have we done and where are we going? *J Natl Cancer Inst* 89:21–39.

17. Edwards MJ, Israel PA (1997) Beyond the credentialing and privileging controversy for image-guided breast biopsy. *Bull Am Coll Surg* 82:20–23.

18. Whitworth P, McMasters KM, Tafra L, Edwards MJ (2000) State-of-the-art lymph node staging for breast cancer in the year 2000. *Am J Surg* 180:262–267.

19. Edwards MJ, Whitworth P, Tafra L, McMasters KM (2000) The details of successful sentinel lymph node staging for breast cancer. *Am J Surg* 180:257–261.

20. Tafra L, McMasters KM, Whitworth P, Edwards MJ (2000) Credentialing issues with sentinel lymph node staging for breast cancer. *Am J Surg* 180:268–273.

Principles of Radiation Oncology

JOHN N. WALDRON and BRIAN O'SULLIVAN

University of Toronto, Princess Margaret Hospital, Department of Radiation Oncology, Toronto, Ontario, Canada

The discovery of X rays by Wilhelm Conrad Roentgen in 1895 was one of the most important events in the evolution of modern medicine. It was soon after this that X rays were first used for both diagnostic and therapeutic purposes. Radiation therapy is one of the major therapeutic modalities for the treatment of malignant disease. It is estimated that 50% of cancer patients will require radiation therapy at some point in their illness (1). This emphasizes the need for all physicians to be familiar with this form of treatment.

Radiation oncology represents the branch of medicine concerned with the application of radiation for the treatment of neoplastic disease. This application requires not only a sound knowledge of medicine and oncology but also expertise in the principles of radiation physics and radiation biology (2). In most countries, certification for the practice of radiation oncology requires 3–5 years of postgraduate training following medical school and internship. This training generally occurs in university-affiliated departments, with emphasis not only on the clinical aspects of radiation oncology but also on research and teaching.

Radiation oncology finds itself in an era of rapid change characterized by significant improvements in both the ability to detect and display the targets to be treated and the technical ability to precisely deliver radiation to these targets. This chapter is a summary of the general principles of the clinical practice of radiation oncology and the physical and biologic concepts on which these are based.

RADIATION PHYSICS—THE BASICS

Radiation is energy (3). The term *radiation* applies to the emission, propagation, and absorption of energy through space or a material medium in either wave or particle form. Radiation is propagated in two forms: photons or particles. Photons

UICC Manual of Clinical Oncology, Eighth Edition. Edited by Raphael E. Pollock
ISBN 0-471-22289-5 Copyright © 2004 John Wiley & Sons, Inc.

are "packages" of energy without mass or charge that behave as either particles or waves in terms of their interaction with each other or matter. Both X rays and gamma rays comprise photons differing only in their method of production. Particle radiation is propagated by units of mass. The most commonly used forms of particle radiation are electrons, protons, and neutrons. When radiation is absorbed, energy is transferred to matter. The final effect depends on the nature and energy of the radiation as well as the quality of the matter. If the energy of the incident radiation is sufficiently high, it causes ejection of orbital electrons from the atoms of the matter, resulting in a net deficit of charge termed *ionization*, hence the term *ionizing radiation*. It is this process of ionization of atoms and further effects produced by the ejected electrons that leads to the molecular damage ultimately manifested in the biological effects of radiation. Because radiation is essentially energy, the measure of the transfer of this energy to a given mass of material is the measure of radiation dose and is expressed as the SI unit the Gray (Gy). One Gray is equivalent to a 1 joule per kilogram energy deposition. The distribution of radiation dose within irradiated tissues is dependent on the energy and type of radiation (photon *vs.* electron *vs.* other particles), the volume and composition of tissue irradiated, and the distance from the source of radiation.

The distribution of radiation dose within tissue can be graphically illustrated using a depth dose curve, which plots the relative dose (percentage depth dose) as a function of depth from the irradiated surface. Figure 10b.1 illustrates such a plot for photon beams of increasing energies. As beam energy increases, so does the depth of maximum dose deposition while the rate of dose fall-off at depth decreases. The type and energy of radiation used can therefore influence the distribution of dose within tissue, as illustrated in Figure 10b.2. Whereas depth dose curves serve to illustrate the distribution of dose in one dimension (depth), a more clinically

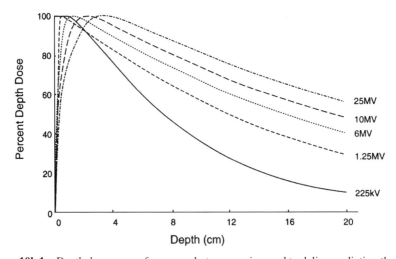

Figure 10b.1   Depth dose curves for some photon energies used to deliver radiation therapy.

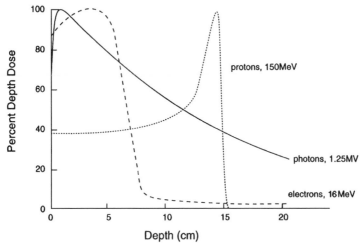

Figure 10b.2   Depth dose curves for electrons, photons, and protons.

practical method of depicting the distribution of dose within an irradiated volume of tissue is the isodose distribution. An isodose distribution represents a two-dimensional representation of dose within a plane through an irradiated volume by generating lines that connect points of equal dose (isodose curves). Three such distributions are illustrated in Figure 10b.3. By knowing the location of tumor and normal tissues within an isodose distribution, the radiation oncologist can then determine the dose of radiation these structures will receive.

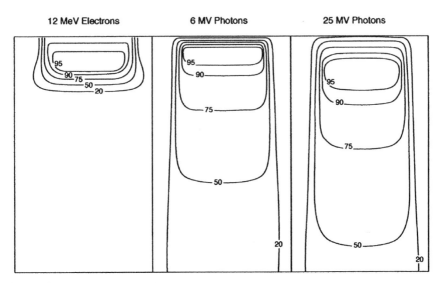

Figure 10b.3   Isodose curves for 10 × 10 cm beams of 12 MeV electrons, 6 and 25 MV photons.

RADIATION PHYSICS—CLINICAL APPLICATION

The clinical application of radiation for the treatment of malignant disease requires an appreciation of the methods of delivery of radiation and the process whereby they can be used to deliver radiation to a specifically defined volume of tissue.

Delivery of Radiation

There are three main methods by which radiation therapy is delivered clinically: teletherapy, brachytherapy and isotope therapy.

Teletherapy, more commonly known as external beam therapy, involves the delivery of radiation from a source located external to the body. This is the most common type of radiation therapy and utilizes delivery machines such as an X ray generator, cobalt-60 unit, and, most frequently, a linear accelerator.

Brachytherapy involves placement of the radiation source(s) in contact with the body whether the source(s) be physically implanted into the tissues (interstitial therapy), into existing cavities (intracavitary therapy), or approximated to the body surface (surface or contact therapy). Brachytherapy radiation sources consist of a variety radionuclides similar in principle to cobalt-60 that release radiation as they decay. The process of brachytherapy will be described in more detail later.

Isotope therapy consists of the administration, by either intravenous or oral routes, of radioactive isotopes that are selectively taken up by specific tumor-bearing tissue. The subsequent decay and release of radiation by these isotopes produces the desired clinical effect. The most common examples of isotope therapy include intravenous strontium-89 for the treatment of bone metastasis from carcinoma of the prostate and oral iodine-131 for the treatment of certain thyroid carcinomas. Isotope therapy research is presently examining the use of radioactive isotopes linked to antibodies for malignant cell antigens in the hope of specifically targeting malignant cells.

Treatment Planning for External Beam Therapy

The process of treatment planning is that which ensures a homogeneous dose of radiation is reproducibly delivered to a defined volume in order achieve tumor control with minimum effect on the surrounding normal tissues. This process requires the input and expertise of a large team of individuals, including the radiation oncologist, pathologist, radiologist, surgeon, dosimetrist, radiation thera-pist, and clinical physicist.

The first step in planning radiation therapy requires a decision as to the volume of tissue to be treated. The radiation oncologist makes this decision based on the known extent and biologic behavior of the tumor in question. The radiation oncologist then determines three separate and sequential volumes as defined by the International Commission on Radiation Units and Measurements (4) (Fig. 10b.4). First, the gross tumor volume (GTV), defined as the gross palpable or visible/demonstrable extent and location of malignant growth. The GTV is then expanded

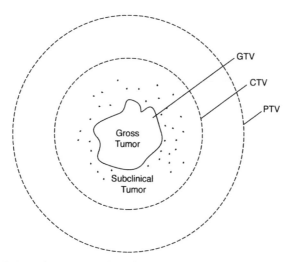

Figure 10b.4   Schematic representation of the ICRU volumes used for treatment planning. See text for details.

to define the clinical target volume (CTV), which contains the GTV plus areas at risk of harboring subclinical microscopic disease. Finally, the planning target volume (PTV), which contains the CTV and is a geometric concept used to select appropriate beam sizes and energies in order to deliver the prescribed dose to the entire CTV given variations in day-to-day delivery of radiation due to both organ and patient movement. Once the CTV has been defined, an arrangement of separate radiation beams can be designed to encompass it while minimizing the volume of uninvolved normal tissue irradiated. This may require the use of single or, more commonly, multiple beams. Beams may vary in size and shape, the energy of photons or electrons they deliver; and whether they move (dynamic) or not (static) during therapy. The orientation of beams is defined with the patient in a fixed treatment position, which may involve the use of certain supports or immobilization devices such as masks in order to ensure reproducibility.

Treatment Simulation

Radiation beams may be simulated using a fluoroscopic device called a simulator that reproduces the geometric relationship that will exist between the patient and the actual treatment machine. Using the simulator, the relationship between the various beams and the bone and tissue structure can be defined. The use of metal or wire markers placed on the patient can aid in defining the position of tumor and critical structures. Similarly, the use of barium or contrast at the time of simulation can define the position of visceral structures such as bowel or bladder. Although this process of fluoroscopic simulation has been a standard of treatment planning for decades and is still in widespread use, it is being replaced by computed tomography (CT)-based simulation and planning that should now be considered the standard of practice. CT simulation and planning is performed on dedicated, commercially available planning CT scanners. The patient is scanned in the treatment position and the CT data transferred to computer work stations at which the radiation oncologist can outline or contour the target and surrounding critical normal tissues or organs at risk (OAR) on the individual CT slices (Fig. 10b.5a).

Digitally reconstructed radiographs (DRRs) can be generated from the CT data, including a superimposed display of the contoured target(s) and, in a process similar to conventional simulation, virtual beams providing the radiation oncologist with a beam's eye view (BEV) of the target (Fig. 10b.5b). These beams can be manipulated in orientation and shape to achieve optimum target coverage and sparing of critical structures. This process can be assisted by using the CT data to reconstruct three-dimensional images of the target and OARs, which may then be viewed in any orientation (Fig. 10b.5c). Finally, the data can be transferred to a treatment planning program whereby dose distributions can be calculated in three dimensions, providing the oncologist with dose volume histograms (DVHs) specific to the target and any critical normal tissues. DVHs provide important information

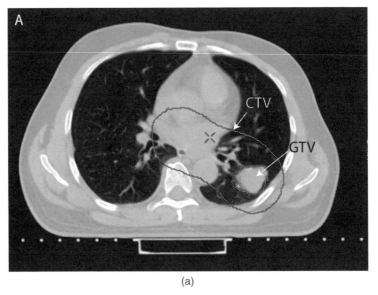

(a)

Figure 10b.5 Three-dimensional (3D) CT planning. (a) Target volumes are contoured on individual CT slices as shown for this patient with a lung tumour (GTV) including the mediastinum at risk of tumour spread (CTV). (b) Digitally reconstructed radiograph (DRR) from the contoured CT slices displays the GTV, CTV and radiation field as a beam's eye view. The dashed line indicates the level of the CT slice in panel A. (c) A 3D reconstruction of the GTV and normal tissues with the anterior radiation beam shown.

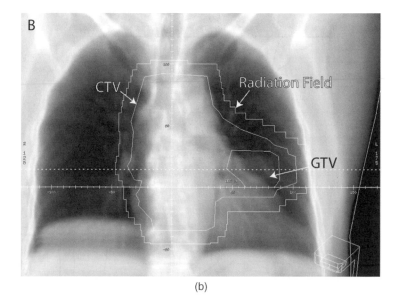

(b)

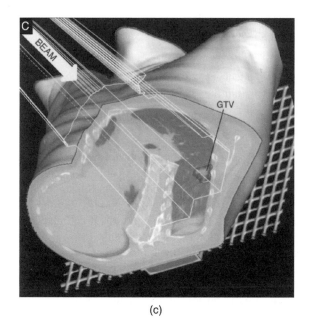

(c)

Figure 10b.5 (*Continued*)

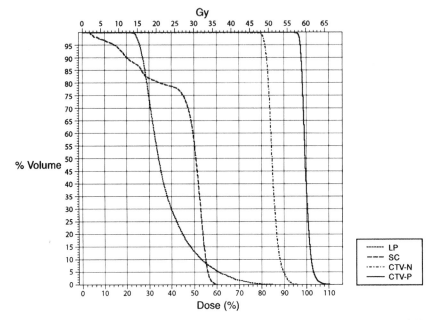

Figure 10b.6   Dose volume histograms for a head and neck cancer radiation plan to deliver 60 Gy to the primary tumour CTV (CTV-P), 50 Gy to the neck (CTV-N) and spare spinal cord (SC) and left parotid (LP). The vertical axis represents the percent volume of each of these structures receiving a given dose.

with respect to the adequacy of the coverage (or avoidance) of predefined (contoured) volumes within the irradiated tissues (Fig. 10b.6).

Treatment Delivery

The patient attends the radiation treatment unit for delivery of radiation. The planned treatment field(s) are reproduced on the treatment machine with reference to small tattoos or marks placed on the patient or immobilization device at the time of simulation. The field is often defined by collimation within the treatment machine and may be further modified with shielding, multileaf collimation, wedge filters, or missing tissue compensators placed in the path of the beam as needed to achieve the desired distribution of dose. The treatment machine is turned on for a length of time necessary to deliver the prescribed dose defined by the total dose, number of fractions, number and size of fields treated, and the known output of a given machine. Generally, this is no longer than a minute or two for each beam in a multibeam plan. The majority of patients are treated as outpatients and receive once-or twice-daily treatments Monday to Friday for a period of one to seven weeks. In order to assure accuracy in treatment delivery, X ray films are exposed with the beams from the treatment unit with the first treatment and as needed thereafter. These X rays are compared with the simulator films or DRRs taken during planning to ensure the CTV is being adequately treated and critical normal tissues are spared. Alternatively, this can be done with the use of a portal imager that electronically captures the treatment image of the relevant beams for review.

Advanced Treatment Planning

The introduction of advanced treatment planning and delivery systems has had a major impact on the delivery of radiation therapy. CT simulation and planning as described above has provided the ability to define complex targets in three dimensions. The visualization of targets has been improved by the ability to electronically fuse images obtained with other modalities such as magnetic resonance imaging (MRI) and positron emission tomography (PET) with the CT planning images. Linkage between dosimetry software and linear accelerator operating systems including multileaf collimators has allowed the development of a variety of treatment approaches. Among these is stereotactic radiation therapy, whereby small volumes (typically isolated brain lesions) can be treated within an accuracy of millimeters to very high doses with little dose to surrounding tissues. Powerful computer software now allows the variation of beam orientation and shape during treatment resulting in a modulation in radiation intensity across a beam (Fig. 10b.7a). By rapidly calculating the thousands of possible combinations

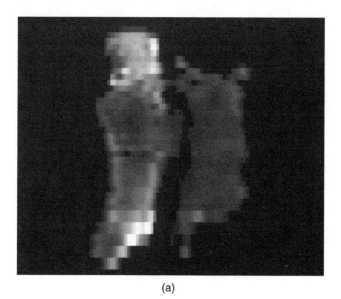

(a)

Figure 10b.7   Intensity modulated radiation therapy (IMRT). (a) An IMRT radiation field illustrating the variance of radiation intensity throughout the field. (b) 3D representation of targets and organs at risk for a head and neck cancer patient. CTV-P (primary tumor CTV), CTV-N (neck CTV), LP (left parotid gland), RP (right parotid gland), and spinal cord. (c) IMRT field and 3D structures superimposed illustrating distribution of radiation to targets. A typical IMRT plan would be composed of multiple fields from different angles.

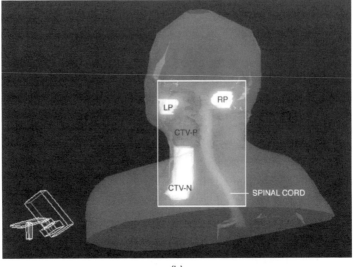

(b)

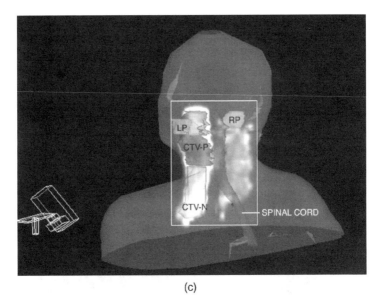

(c)

Figure 10b.7   (*Continued*)

of beam orientations and intensities, these programs can derive radiation treatment plans to optimally treat very complex volumes by a process known as intensity modulated radiation therapy (IMRT). This planning process, termed *inverse planning*, first requires the radiation oncologist to specify the clinical objectives by defining the target volumes and the organs at risk to be avoided (Fig. 10b.7b)

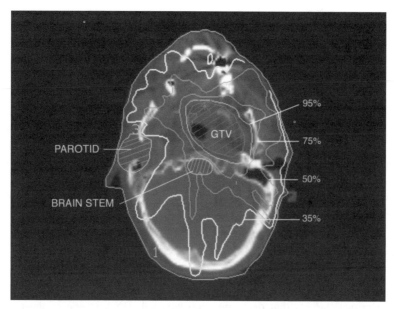

Figure 10b.8 Isodose curves displayed on CT slice of patient illustrated in Figure 10b.7. Note conformation of high dose to GTV and relative sparing of brain stem and right parotid gland achieved with IMRT.

along with specific instructions as to the doses of radiation to be delivered. The resultant sculpting of dose distribution within three dimensions permits an opportunity to spare critical normal tissues thereby allowing dose escalation to, and even within, the tumor (Fig 10b.8). It is important to recognize that since the process of IMRT planning is guided by the target volumes and predefined dose constraints provided by the radiation oncologist, its ultimate clinical benefit may be limited by the ability to clearly delineate tumor. In other words, the precise delivery of dose is of little benefit if it remains uncertain as to where to deliver dose. Imaging technologies such as MRI, PET, and magnetic resonance spectroscopy (MRS) may play a very important role in this regard and may allow the identification of not only the tumor itself but regions within the tumor that may be more resistant to radiation. Such areas, including hypoxic regions, areas of high cell density, or regions overexpressing genes associated with radiation resistance, could comprise a separate biologic target volume (BTV) that would be treated to higher dose (5). IMRT is now in clinical use in many centers and to date has most frequently been used for the treatment of prostate and head and neck malignancies (6).

RADIATION BIOLOGY

Our understanding of the biology of radiation has expanded rapidly over the last 50 years (7–9). Many insights have been gained by the careful isolation and study of a variety of radiation-sensitive cell lines from normal tissues and tumors of both humans and animals. Initial studies documented the effects of radiation at the cellular level and described the radiation survival curve on which many of the principles of contemporary clinical radiation fractionation regimes are based. In recent decades, with the emergence of molecular biology, attention has turned toward study of the effects of radiation at the molecular level. This has lead to the description of critical molecular targets damaged by radiation and the complex responses of the cell to this damage resulting in cell survival or death. Other clinical and laboratory research is describing the important influence of the cellular microenvironment on outcome following radiation. Altogether, progress in the field of radiation biology continues to lead to a variety of strategies for both the prediction and modification of outcome following cellular exposure to ionizing radiation.

Radiation Effects at the Molecular Level

Although any molecule within a cell can be damaged by radiation, it is likely that the vast majority of this damage has no consequence, and rather it is damage to certain critical targets that determine cell survival. DNA is one of these critical targets and evidence is now emerging that damage to other structures such as cellular microtubules or membrane systems may play a role. Ionizing radiation activates a wide variety of cellular biochemical pathways and it is likely that it is damage to these critical targets that serves as the triggering event. In general, these biochemical pathways involve the interaction of numerous cellular proteins in a complex and sequential fashion leading to a multitude of endpoints, including altered gene expression. Some of these genes are involved with DNA repair, which requires the interaction of a host of nuclear proteins that recognize, excise, align, and ligate the damaged strands. Other genes are involved with the progression of cells through their normal reproductive cycle (the cell cycle). Ionizing radiation induces cell cycle arrest at specific checkpoints with the hypothetical function to provide the cells both the time and environment in which to repair DNA damage before proceeding with replication. Irreparably damaged cells may be diverted into an autodestructive process known as apoptosis, which is an orderly and highly regulated process involving specific proteins that essentially results in the dismantling of the cell. As our understanding of the complex molecular biological effect of radiation expands, so will our ability to manipulate this process to therapeutic advantage with the identification of specific molecular targets.

Tumor Radiobiology

The response of a tumor to radiation is extremely complex. Tumor control requires the eradication of every malignant cell capable of reproduction. Some of the main factors that influence this outcome include: (1) the number of clonogenic cells that need to be eradicated (how big is the tumor?); (2) the rate at which these cells are reproducing during treatment (how fast is the tumor growing); and (3) how sensitive these cells are to ionizing radiation? For any given tumor, the outcome is very likely determined by a unique balance of these a factors. For example, a large tumor comprised of relatively radiation sensitive cells (e.g., a bulky mediastinal lymphoma) may be controlled with radiation, whereas a small carcinoma may not. Nevertheless some general conclusions can be made and, for a given histology, larger tumors are less likely to be controlled by radiation.

Tumors can respond to cell loss with accelerated cellular reproduction. Such a process is thought to occur during a prolonged course of radiation treatment and could unfavorably shift the balance of cell killing to reproduction such that the tumor is not controlled.

The radiation sensitivity of the cells comprising a tumor is influenced by a multitude of factors. Microenvironmental factors such as the oxygen level in which individual tumor cells exist can influence response to radiation in a profound manner. Because hypoxic cells are more resistant to radiation, the proportion of such cells within a tumor can influence outcome. Cells exposed to ionizing radiation can produce a variety of cytokines that could potentially influence tumor response to radiation. Cytokines are proteins secreted by cells that regulate cell behavior in an autocrine and/or paracrine manner by binding to cell surface receptors and initiating signal transduction pathways. The position of cells within the cell cycle is known to affect their radiation sensitivity, therefore, the proportion of cells actively cycling and the distribution of these cells within the cell cycle could affect outcome of a tumor.

The influence of microenvironment and cell cycle effects can be controlled for by studying cultures of cell lines establish from human tumors growing *in vitro* under controlled conditions. Radiation survival curves of such cultures demonstrate considerable variation in radiation sensitivity both between different tumor types and within a given type of tumor. This variation is thought to be due to differences in the intrinsic radiation sensitivity of the cells themselves. Factors that determine cellular intrinsic radiation sensitivity are likely genetic in origin and include those influencing signal transduction pathways resulting in cell cycle arrest, DNA repair and apoptotic cell death.

Normal Tissue Radiobiology-Acute and Late Effects

Normal tissue injury due to radiation is a consequence of cell loss and resultant structural and functional impairment. Therefore, for any given normal tissue, the rate and extent of cell killing dictates the pattern of radiation injury. The time course and severity of injury is dependent on total radiation dose, the daily fraction size, the overall time of radiation, and the volume and type of tissue irradiated. Tissues containing a large population of rapidly proliferating cells manifest injury within days or weeks of being irradiated. These tissues include mucosa, skin, and bone marrow in which injury is in part due to the loss of proliferating cells leading to the inability to replace the normal day to day cell loss. Such normal tissue injuries, occurring up to three months from completion of radiation, are termed *acute effects*. Some acute effects of radiation injury are noted in Table 10b.1. It

TABLE 10b.1. Acute Effects of Radiation Therapy

Normal Tissue Irradiated	Acute Effect (S)	Symptoms and Signs	Management
Skin	Erythema, dry and moist desquamation, epilation	Warmth, pruritis, pain	Drying agents, topical steroids, topical antibiotics for superinfection
Oropharyngeal mucosa	Mucositis	Dysphagia, odynophagia, thick secretions, halitosis with superinfection	Oral hygiene, viscous xylocaine, analgesics, antibiotics for superinfection
Esophagus	Esophagitis	Dysphagia, odynophagia	Viscous xylocaine, analgesics, antibiotics for superinfection
Lung	Pneumonitis	Cough, pleuritic chest pain, dyspnea	Observation if mild, systemic corticosteroids in severe cases, rule out pneumonia
Bowel	Gastroenteritis	Nausea, vomiting, cramping, diarrhea	Antiemetics if a significant volume of bowel included in the high dose volume, antidiarrheal agents, diet modification
Bladder	Cystitis	Frequency, dysuria, urgency	Urinary analgesic (pyridium), rule out infection
Rectum	Proctitis	Tenesmus	Stool softeners, analgesics
Bone marrow	Cytopenia	Fatigue, bleeding, febrile neutropenia	Transfusion, alteration in treatment time or volume if severe, role of cytokines

should be kept in mind, however, that not all acute effects of radiation therapy are due to cell loss. For example, patients will experience nausea and vomiting within hours of irradiation to a significant volume of the upper abdomen, somnolence can occur soon after cranial irradiation, acute edema and erythema can occur within an irradiated volume. The exact etiology of these acute radiation effects is poorly understood but may be related to radiation-induced cytokine release.

Normal tissue damage by radiation can manifest itself gradually over many months or years from the completion of treatment. The exact etiology of these late effects of radiation therapy is not known. They are likely the consequence of gradual loss of small vessel vasculature, parenchymal cell dysfunction, and fibrosis. The ability of a given normal tissue to withstand the effects of radiation is termed

TABLE 10b.2. The Late Effects of Radiation Therapy

Normal Tissue	Late Effect	Tolerance Dose (Gy)
Brain	Necrosis	50
Eye (lens)	Cataract	10
Eye (retina)	Retinopathy	50
Salivary gland	Xerostomia	32
Mandible	Osteoradionecrosis	60
Spinal cord (5 cm segment)	Paralysis	50
Lung	Pneumonitis/fibrosis	17
Heart	Pericarditis	45
Esophagus	Stricture	55
Liver	Hepatitis	30
Kidney	Nephritis	25
Small bowel	Stricture	45

Tolerance dose represents the dose (delivered in 2 Gy fractions once daily, Monday to Friday) known to produce a 5% incidence of the late effect within 5 years of completion of treatment. Unless otherwise stated, dose volumes are to whole organ.

its *tolerance* and is dependent on a number of factors including total dose, fraction size, and the volume of tissue irradiated. Radiation tolerance has been documented for a variety of normal tissues by careful clinical observation of large populations of individuals treated over many years (10). The tolerance limit of a tissue is defined as the radiation dose delivered in a standard fashion of 2 Gy once per day five days a week that produces a 5% chance of a severe late effect over the subsequent five years. Some tolerance doses for late effects are listed in Table 10b.2. The consequence of normal tissue radiation injury depends on the clinical importance of the tissues irradiated the extent of injury and the reserve capacity of the remaining unirradiated tissues. These factors in turn can be influenced by the age of the patient and comorbid disease.

CLINICAL USE OF RADIATION THERAPY

Indications

Radiation therapy can be given as a sole curative modality or in combination with surgery or chemotherapy for the treatment of malignant disease. The use of radiation therapy specific to any given cancer is discussed in the relevant chapters of this volume. Although certain generalizations can be made, there is considerable variability in the use of radiation therapy throughout the world. Alternate approaches exist for a variety to cancers such that the patient could be treated with radiation alone with surgery reserved for salvage, or the initial treatment could be surgery alone with radiation given either pre- or postoperatively in selected cases. The used of chemotherapy given concurrently with radiation therapy is becoming more commonplace for a wide variety of cancers. In many instances, the treatment approach chosen is often based on specific local patterns of practice and the availability of expertise rather than evidence based (11).

Principles of Dose and Fractionation

The goal of treatment is to achieve an optimum balance between the probability of tumor cure and normal tissue damage (the therapeutic ratio). The dose of radiation required to achieve an optimum therapeutic ratio depends on the tumor being treated and the nature of the normal tissues within the volume to be irradiated. Our appreciation of these optimal doses has evolved empirically by careful clinical observation. One such observation was that a higher total dose could be delivered with similar normal tissue effects if it was divided into smaller fractions separate in time and that, by delivering this higher dose, the likelihood of controlling the tumor increased. This phenomenon is thought to be due to a differential ability of tumor and normal tissue to repair the damage induced by the radiation between fractions given.

While there is considerable variation in dose and fractionation regimes in clinical use throughout the world, a useful historical standard for comparison would deliver a 2 Gy fraction once a day Monday to Friday. It is important to realize that once-daily, five-days-a-week treatment regimes were developed more for logistic than biologic reasons. Attempts to optimize the therapeutic ratio based on our understanding of radiobiology have lead to a variety of alternate fractionation strategies. One such strategy is hyperfractionation, which involves the delivery of two or more small daily fractions to a larger total dose over approximately the same time as a conventional regime. Hyperfractionation regimes often use small fraction size, usually <1.5 Gy, with an interfraction interval of at least six hours. This exploits the fact that most normal tissues are less sensitive to the late effects of a given total dose of radiation if it is delivered in small fractions with a sufficient interfraction interval for repair. In this way, the total dose delivered can be increased without increasing the risk of normal tissue damage. Clinical trials are underway comparing various hyperfractionation regimes to standard once-daily treatment for a variety of tumor sites. Preliminary results have been encouraging and many centers now consider hyperfractionation their standard treatment regime for some tumors. Another fractionation strategy is accelerated fractionation, in which the overall treatment time is reduced while the number of fractions, fraction size, or total dose remain similar. This is accomplished by treating more than once a day and/or treating on the weekends. This strategy attempts to counteract accelerated tumor repopulation during treatment.

Combining Radiation and Surgery

Radiation or surgery can be used alone for the treatment of selected cancers while the other reserved for the salvage of persistent or recurrent cancer. However, many tumors require a combination of radiation and surgery. Usually this involves the use of radiation following surgery in order to eradicate any residual disease. This approach has resulted in improved rates of organ preservation (e.g., breast cancer, rectal cancer, and sarcomas) by permitting less radical resections to be performed without compromising cure rates. Alternatively, preoperative radiation may sterilize the periphery of larger tumors, possibly allowing a more limited resection or even rendering an inoperable tumor operable. These two approaches have advantages and disadvantages and it often remains unclear which approach is superior for a given tumor.

Combining Radiation and Chemotherapy

Radiation and cytotoxic chemotherapy are often combined in the treatment of tumors. In most cases, chemotherapy is given with the intention of eradicating distant micrometastasis while the radiation treatment is addressing local control of the primary tumor. Such examples would be the treatment of node-positive breast cancer or rectal carcinoma with postoperative radiation to the primary site. Concurrent chemotherapy, delivered at the same time as the radiation, may provide an advantage in terms of local tumor control, however, it can also produce increased local toxicity (within the irradiated tissues) such that it is unclear whether the same result could not have been achieved without simply increasing the dose of radiation. Nevertheless, clinical evidence has emerged describing improved outcome for selected patients with malignancies of the cervix, lung, anal canal, head and neck, and esophagus treated with concurrent chemotherapy and radiation. Most of these approaches combine concurrent chemotherapy with once-daily radiation treatments. Combining aggressive accelerated or hyperfractionated radiation treatment schedules with cytotoxic chemotherapy may prove difficult due to unacceptable acute toxicity. Strategies to overcome this may include the use of highly conformal treatment approaches such as IMRT to spare normal tissues or, alternately, the selection of agents known not to enhance acute radiation toxicity. Trials in lung, cervix, and head and neck cancer patients have shown positive results using hyperbaric oxygen to sensitize hypoxic cells. However, given the logistical difficulties of treating patients in hyperbaric chambers, the unorthodox fractionation schemes required, and some increased normal tissue toxicity, these approaches have not been repeated and perhaps abandoned prematurely. Clinical studies using hypoxic cell radiosensitizers mimicking the radiosensitizing properties of oxygen (metronidazole, misonidazole, etanidazole, and nimorazole) have shown some improvement in outcome for selected subgroups of patients, however, toxicity has limited their use. In addition, compounds that are specifically toxic to hypoxic cells (tirapazamine and mitomycin-c) show promise. Finally, the use of biologic agents such as epithelial growth factor receptor (EGFR) inhibitors concurrently with radiation therapy represents an important emerging avenue of research.

The Palliative Role of Radiation Therapy

Approximately 50% of patients diagnosed with malignant disease will succumb to their illness. For these patients, attention should be given to palliation of the

TABLE 10b.3. Contrast Between Radiation Treatments of Palliative Versus Curative Intent

	Palliative Intent	Curative Intent
Goal of therapy	Reduction of some disease	Eradication of all disease
Clinical endpoint	Symptom control	Cure
Length of treatment	1 day to 2 weeks	4 to 7 weeks
Total dose	8 to 30 Gy	Greater than 50 Gy
Fraction size	Large (3–10 Gy) to reduce overall treatment time	Small (2.5 Gy or less) to reduce late effects
Volume treated	Gross symptomatic disease only	All tumor and potential areas of microscopic spread

symptoms of progressive disease. Every doctor should be familiar with the general principles of palliative medicine, including pain management. Differences exist between radiation treatment with palliative versus curative intent. Palliative treatments are of lower dose and shorter duration than curative treatments to minimize side effects and patient inconvenience (Table 10b.3.). In selected cases when the patient has minimal or slowly progressive disease a more prolonged course of treatment to a higher dose may be justified.

Radiation therapy can provide effective palliation of a variety of symptoms including pain, bleeding, and compression produced by expanding tumor. Palliative radiation therapy is most frequently employed for painful bone metastasis, and the cough or hemoptysis resulting from lung tumors. A short course of treatment (one to ten fractions) can produce clinical improvement in at least 70% of patients. Similarly, short courses of treatment can produce benefit for other palliative indications including compression of airways, viscera, or nervous system (nerves, brain, or spinal cord).

Clinical Brachytherapy

Brachytherapy involves placement of a radioactive source in physical contact with the patient. The major advantage of this approach is that the radiation dose delivered close to the source is very high and drops off as an inverse square of the distance from the source thus sparing tissues distant from the source. The most common use of brachytherapy involves the temporary placement of a source (usually cesium-137 or iridium-192) into an existing body cavity. This is termed *intracavitary therapy* and is most often used in the treatment of cervix cancer to provide a boost dose to the cervix following external beam treatment to the pelvis. Because of the rapid dose drop off with distance from the source, the cervix will receive a high dose while the bladder and rectum will be relatively spared. Intracavitary therapy can also be used in the treatment of esophageal, tracheobronchial and nasopharyngeal tumors.

Brachytherapy sources may be implanted into tissues (interstitial therapy) using catheters with remote afterloading to boost the operative bed in the treatment of breast and head and neck cancers as well as selected intra-abdomenal malignancies. Such techniques may also be used as part primary radiation treatment of oral or oropharyngeal malignancies. Permanent implants with gold seeds are used by many centers for the treatment of early carcinoma of the prostate as an alternative to surgery or a prolonged course of fractionated radiotherapy.

QUALITY ASSURANCE

An active continuous quality assurance program serves to ensure the provision and maintenance of high-quality care. This begins with a careful review of all clinical and laboratory findings. Ideally, the prescribed radiation therapy is validated by case presentation at a multidisciplinary tumor conference to ensure compliance with established treatment guidelines. Next, a review of the treatment plan and dosimetry by the radiation oncologist, therapist, and medical physicist is necessary prior to the initiation of treatment. Every patient must have verification films performed periodically during treatment. All elements of planning and delivery should be discussed at a regular quality review meeting to minimize errors in treatment, including verification of the irradiated volume. The radiation oncologist should personally assess every patient on a weekly basis for acute toxicity and tumor response if feasible. Equipment calibration and evaluation should take place on a regular basis. The introduction of new equipment or technologies such as CT simulation or IMRT requires strict attention to both the commissioning process and staff training prior to clinical use. Every department should regularly review its results and compare these to established benchmarks to ensure that any adverse systematic anomalies in clinical outcome are detected and appropriately investigated.

REFERENCES

1. Mackillop W, Groome P, Zhang-Solomons J et al. (1997) Does a centralized radiotherapy system provide adequate access to care? *J Clin Oncol* 15:1261–1271.
2. Perez C, Brady L (1998) *The Principles and Practice of Radiation Oncology*, 3rd ed. Philidelphia: Lippincott-Raven.
3. Johns H, Cunningham J (1983) *The Physics of Radiology*, 4th ed. Springfield: Thomas.
4. International Commission of Radiation Units and Measurements (ICRU) (1993) *Prescribing, Recording, and Reporting Photon Beam Therapy.* Bethesda, MD.
5. Ling CC, Humm J, Larson S et al. (2000) Towards multidimensional radiotherapy (MD-CRT): biological imaging and biological conformality. *Int J Radiat Oncol Biol Phys* 47:551–60.

6. Intensity Modulated Radiation Therapy Collaborative Working Group (2001) Intensity-modulated radiotherapy: current status and issues of interest. *Int J Radiat Oncol Biol Phys* 51:880–914.

7. Tannock I, Hill R (1998) *The Basic Science of Oncology*, 3rd ed. Toronto: McGraw Hill.

8. Hall E (1994) *Radiobiology for the Radiologist*, 4th ed. New York: Lippincott.

9. Coleman CN (2001) International Conference on Translational Research and Preclinical Strategies in Radio-Oncology (ICTR)—conference summary. *Int J Radiat Oncol Biol Phys* 49:301–309.

10. Emami B, Lyman J, Brown A et al. (1991) Tolerance of normal tissue to therapeutic irradiation. *Int J Radiat Oncol Biol Phys* 21:109–122.

11. O'Sullivan B, Mackillop W, Gilbert R et al. (1994) Contoversies in the management of laryngeal cancer: results of an international patterns of care survey. *Radiother Oncol* 31: 23–32.

Principles of Medical Oncology

JAMES H. DOROSHOW

City of Hope Comprehensive Cancer Center, Department of Medical Oncology and
Therapeutics Research, Duarte, California

The first successful systemic therapies for cancer were descriptions by Beatson of
the efficacy of oophorectomy for the treatment of breast cancer in 1895, and, much
later, the application of folate antagonist antimetabolites by Farber and alkylating
agents by Gilman, Goodman, and Karnofsky in the mid-1940s. Systemic cancer
therapy with cytotoxic drugs, hormonal agents, or biological response modifiers is
now capable of providing curative treatment for advanced Hodgkin's disease and
certain types of non-Hodgkin's lymphoma, acute myelogenous and lymphoblastic
leukemia, testicular cancer, gestational trophoblastic disease, and a variety of
childhood leukemias. Systemic therapies have also been clearly shown to improve
the survival of patients with breast, ovarian, and colorectal cancer as well as
osteosarcoma when utilized as postoperative adjunctive treatment. For patients with
all forms of lung cancer, and metastatic cancers of the breast, bladder, prostate,
head and neck, and gastrointestinal tract, systemic treatment with palliative intent
can frequently improve quality of life and reduce the symptoms of patients with
advanced disease.

Over the past half-century, several critical concepts in tumor biology and
pharmacology important in determining the effectiveness of systemic therapy for
cancer have been established. These include the role of tumor burden and cellular
heterogeneity; drug resistance; drug delivery and dose intensity; host factors; and
multimodality treatment in the success of chemo-, hormonal, or biological therapies
for cancer. These concepts provide the background for a more specific understanding of the mechanism(s) by which systemic agents alter the growth of tumor
cells.

UICC Manual of Clinical Oncology, Eighth Edition. Edited by Raphael E. Pollock
ISBN 0-471-22289-5 Copyright © 2004 John Wiley & Sons, Inc.

PRINCIPLES OF TUMOR BIOLOGY AND PHARMACOLOGY UNDERLYING SYSTEMIC CANCER TREATMENT

Tumor Burden and Tumor Cell Heterogeneity

Initial experimental therapeutic studies in murine leukemia models established the ability of many classes of antineoplastic agents to kill tumor cells according to first-order kinetics; that is, a given concentration of drug utilized for a particular time period will kill a fixed number of tumor cells. If each treatment course at a given dose is cytotoxic for a constant fraction of cells, the curability of the particular therapy depends on the number of courses delivered, the drug concentration applied, and the initial tumor burden. Although this concept has been unequivocally verified in many animal tumor models that undergo logarithmic tumor cell expansion, it is not clear how well it applies to much more slowly growing and genetically heterogeneous solid tumors in man. However, the model does, in part, form the basis for the rational use of postsurgical adjuvant chemotherapy, which is used to destroy microscopic residual disease after surgical excision or irradiation has removed or destroyed most or all macroscopically detectable tumor cells. It is assumed that the decreased tumor burden that follows surgery (which would assist fractional cell kill) as well as the potential for stimulation of cell cycle progression in the residual tumor cells will increase the cytotoxic potential of systemic treatments that frequently are more effective during active tumor cell proliferation.

A major factor that underlies the efficacy of all systemic cancer treatment is the genetic heterogeneity of all human tumors. Although most cancers may develop initially from a single malignant clone, all malignancies demonstrate genetic instability, which leads to a remarkable degree of biochemical heterogeneity that can be observed not only from metastatic site to metastatic site but from cell to cell in a single tumor mass. Thus, the enormous inherent variation in the expression of any one of the wide range of proteins that establish the innate sensitivity of malignant cells to systemic agents is probably responsible for both the unpredictability of the efficacy of treatment (from patient to patient but not in populations of patients) in the common solid tumors as well as the regrowth of clones of malignant cells after an initial response to treatment. Regrowth, thus, may represent the expansion of tumor cells that, prior to any systemic drug exposure, already expressed gene products capable of providing a growth advantage under the selective pressure of treatment with a cytotoxin.

The unequivocal demonstration of heterogenous populations of tumor cells in man has provided a critical rationale for the use of combinations of systemic agents with different sites of action that might circumvent at least some mechanisms of inherent drug insensitivity and for the use of surgical or radiotherapeutic tumor "debulking." In the latter instance, it has been predicted by Goldie and Coldman that the probability of a tumor possessing random mutations leading to insensitivity to systemic treatment is a function of the tumor cell burden. Thus, removal of tumor mass prior to systemic treatment may decrease not only the total body burden of cancer but also the percentage of tumor cells inherently resistant to treatment.

Tumor cell heterogeneity also plays a critical role in establishing the genetic makeup of the tumor cell with respect to growth regulation. Normal tissues undergo a regular process of growth and decay governed by the highly regulated expression of several critical cell cycle control genes, including *p53* and the cyclin genes, as well as the genes that regulate apoptosis (programmed cell death) such as the *bcl-2* and *bax* gene families. In many human tumors, alterations in the expression of these genes, which occurs as a regular feature of genetic instability, is intimately related to both their unregulated growth and their resistance to systemic treatment.

Drug Resistance

Antineoplastic chemotherapy is not uniformly successful because, as noted above, many types of cancer in man are either intrinsically resistant to treatment or acquire resistance during therapy, or because the chemotherapy cannot be successfully delivered in cytotoxic concentrations to the tumor. Mechanisms by which drug resistance can develop are, at least in part, specific to the mechanism of action of the class of agents being utilized. However, there are a wide variety of biochemical and physiological phenomena that have been observed either *in vitro* or *in vivo* that can modulate the effectiveness of several different antineoplastic drug classes. These include reduced drug uptake by the tumor cell; enhanced drug efflux; increased repair of drug-induced damage to DNA or other critical tumor cell targets; development of alternative routes for the synthesis of biologically important molecules when the primary synthetic pathway is blocked by a given drug; overexpression of the target gene product for a specific drug; production of an aberrant drug target that does not interact with a given agent, yet retains biochemical function sufficient to support tumor cell growth; enhanced intracellular metabolism or detoxification of the chemotherapeutic agent that limits tumor cell toxicity; overexpression or modification of cytoprotective gene products that alter tumor cell sensitivity to the anticancer agent; variations in the oxygenation state or blood supply of the tumor that can blunt the effectiveness of the drug directly or the delivery of the drug to the tumor itself; and factors in the normal tissues of the host that can significantly change the concentration of drug delivered to the tumor (such as alterations in renal or hepatic drug metabolism or variations in the tolerance of hematopoietic tissues to cytotoxic drug exposure).

Although the clinical relevance of each of these mechanisms is uncertain, samples of human tumors have been shown to express one or more of these phenotypic markers of drug resistance. As noted previously, the mutations that lead to expression of these characteristics occur prior to the recognition of a tumor and may become more prominent under the selective pressure of therapy. A tumor cell does not "begin" to express a resistance phenotype in the presence of a given drug; instead, cells with a particular phenotype emerge by a process of mutation/evolution and then are "selected" during therapy because cells lacking this phenotype are killed.

Drug Delivery and Dose Intensity

Certain characteristics of tumor masses can impede delivery of effective concentrations of drug to the entire tumor. A major impediment is size. Large tumor masses often contain areas of poorly vascularized tissue. Consequently, delivery of cytotoxic drugs to these areas of tumor via the blood will also be poor. The problem can be partially addressed by preferential administration of a drug to a region of the body involved by tumor. For example, infusion of agents metabolized by the liver directly into the hepatic artery permits the delivery of large concentrations of drug to the liver and tumors in the liver with limited exposure of the rest of the body to this same drug. Fluoropyrimidines (5-fluorouracil and 5-fluorodeoxyuridine) are the prototypical drugs that have a great pharmacologic advantage with hepatic artery infusion. Similarly, administration of drug directly into the peritoneum (cisplatin) or directly into the bladder (mitomycin C) allows for considerable local concentration of cytotoxic drug to tumors confined to those areas, with a much lower systemic exposure. Although the clinical utility of such regional approaches in curing cancer continues to be investigated, the pharmacologic advantage presented by this approach holds promise.

A corollary to the general problem of drug delivery is the issue of tumor sanctuaries. There are pharmacologically privileged sites in the body where tumor cells can lodge, but to which antineoplastic drugs cannot gain access. The blood–brain and the less-well-characterized blood–testis barriers are two clinically relevant examples. The blood–tissue barriers are constituted by components of vascular endothelium and basement membranes. The blood–brain barrier prevents large molecules and biologic agents from penetrating into the substance and supporting membranes of the brain. However, tumor can invade the blood–brain barrier and then spread within the substance of the brain or in the cerebrospinal fluid. This accounts for examples of central nervous system relapse of diseases such as acute lymphoid leukemia or small cell lung cancer despite complete suppression of systemic tumor growth by chemotherapy.

To the degree that first-order kinetics apply in man, or at least that a dose-response relationship exists for many of the systemic agents in common clinical practice, the efficacy of treatment is likely to be enhanced if a higher dose of drug is administered. Considerable preclinical data and clinical experience support the hypothesis that maximally effective therapy is achieved if maximally tolerated or even supralethal doses of chemotherapy are administered. The most striking example of this concept is the success of very high doses of chemotherapy for acute myeloid leukemia and lymphomas, with subsequent reinfusion of allogeneic or autologous bone marrow cells to avert or reduce infectious complications of prolonged marrow aplasia. The hematopoietic growth factors further enhance the ability to give high-dose chemotherapy with a reduction in the time required for recovery of bone marrow function. With improvements in supportive care techniques and the development of hematopoietic growth factors, it is now possible to administer doses of cytotoxic drugs heretofore considered lethal. With this approach, tumor regression and long-term tumor-free survival may be seen in refractory hematopoietic malignancies and even some epithelial tumors. Although the optimal dose intensity for each human tumor and each clinical situation is not defined, it is clear that administration of maximally tolerated dose intensity is an important concept in cancer chemotherapy.

Host Factors and Angiogenesis

The success of systemic therapies for cancers is clearly linked to a number of factors specific to the host organism bearing the tumor. Among these factors are nutritional status, functional capabilities, and integrity of major organ systems. The effects of some of these factors on the success of chemotherapy are easily understood. For example, the ability of an individual to withstand the toxic side effects of a drug is linked to the reserve in the organ systems that might be targets of the toxicity of that drug. Patients with dysfunction of an organ necessary for the metabolism or excretion of a cytotoxic are likely to suffer more toxicity from that drug. The folate antagonist methotrexate is dependent on the kidney for excretion. Individuals with abnormal renal function suffer considerably more toxicity with methotrexate than do individuals with normal renal function. This toxicity is directly related to enhanced systemic exposure to methotrexate because of diminished clearance. Algorithms for adjusting dose to achieve a "normal" exposure in patients with abnormal renal or hepatic function are not generally available; however, as described below, knowledge of the pharmacokinetics and routes of metabolism and excretion of every antineoplastic is required so that dosages can be appropriately adjusted for each agent in patients with abnormal organ function who require therapy.

Less clear, but nonetheless important, are generalized host factors. The functional capability or performance status of a patient has been repeatedly shown to be of great prognostic importance in determining the outcome of systemic cancer treatment. Performance status is presumably a reflection of overall organ function integrity. Patients with poor performance status suffer greater toxicity with almost all forms of cancer therapy; they have shorter survival even when reasonable doses of therapy are administered and optimal supportive care is provided.

In addition to the tolerance of normal tissues to the toxic side effects of chemotherapy, evidence has rapidly accumulated indicating that control of the host's vascular supply to tumors, mediated in part by angiogenic gene products produced by essentially all types of malignancies, is likely to become an increasingly important target for the development of novel therapeutic agents. A variety of endothelial growth factors (such as the vascular endothelial growth factor) and angiogenic peptides (including angiostatin and endostatin) have been shown to interact with receptors on the endothelial cell surface that play a critical role in transducing growth signals in blood vessels, leading to an enhanced blood supply for established tumors. The potential now exists, either with novel antiangiogenic molecules or antibodies, or as recently demonstrated with low doses of cytotoxic compounds, to interfere with this self-perpetuating cycle of tumor-induced angiogenesis. It is likely that in the very near future, a substantial addition to the systemic therapeutic approach to the control of human tumors will involve targeted interventions at the interface between the tumor cell and the blood supply necessary for its growth and dissemination.

Multimodality Therapy

Over the past decade, it has become increasingly clear for the common solid tumors in man that tumor destruction man be improved by the application of a number of modalities of therapy and that the judicious use of more than one modality is often important. The first clinical examples of this were obtained in pediatric oncology, where it was shown that the use of combination chemotherapy, surgical tumor removal, and local tumor site irradiation enhanced the cure of tumors such as Wilms' tumor, Ewing's sarcoma, and neuroblastoma. Application of these concepts in adult malignancies have been somewhat slower to develop but are now well established. The best example of the advantage of multimodality treatment in the treatment of adult malignancies is the clear demonstration of the importance of systemic therapy administered in concert with optimal local therapy for clinically localized breast cancer. For many years, women with breast tumors were known to be able to be cured with surgical removal of the breast. However, it was also known that many women died despite removal of all visible tumor, because of the presence of micrometastatic disease at the time of primary tumor treatment. The use of cytotoxic chemotherapy, hormonal therapy, or combinations of cytotoxic and hormonal therapy increases the cure rate in women with clinically localized breast cancer when such therapy is administered together with optimal local treatment of the primary tumor (irradiation or surgery). Such adjuvant chemotherapy has also now been demonstrated to increase cures in colorectal and ovarian cancers and lymphoma.

CHEMOTHERAPEUTIC AGENTS

Based on the fundamental principles of tumor cell biology and clinical pharmacology that form the underpinnings for the rationale use of systemic anticancer therapies, the choice of an appropriate chemotherapeutic agent is related to the inherent sensitivity of a specific disease to the various classes of drugs that are currently available and on the ability to administer these drugs either as single agents or in combination based on their combined toxicity for critical organ systems. The major classes of chemotherapeutic agents can be grouped by their underlying antineoplastic mechanism of action or source.

Alkylating Agents and Platinum Coordination Compounds

The first nonhormonal agents to be successfully utilized in the treatment of cancer were the alkylating agents, a large group of drugs with the ability to covalently bond DNA and other biologically significant molecules through an alkyl group consisting of one or more saturated carbon atoms. The common features of these compounds is that they are composed of mono- or bifunctional alkyl groups linked to a core structure that confers pharmacologic and toxicologic differences on the alkylating moieties. The simplest backbone for a bifunctional alkylating agent is that of nitrogen mustard (HN_2, mechlorethamine), which consists of a nitrogen atom (as NCH_3) linked to two chloroethyl groups. By contrast L-phenylalanine mustard (LPAM, melphalan) consists of the same bifunctional alkylating groups attached to the L-phenylalanine molecule; chlorambucil, cyclophosphamide, and ifosfamide are three other clinically useful alkylating agents that have substituted other side chains for the methyl group in HN_2. These four drugs have replaced nitrogen mustard in common clinical practice; cyclophosphamide and ifosfamide are distinct amongst this class of drugs because they require activation by hepatic microsomal enzyme systems to specific, short-lived metabolites that produce their cytotoxic action.

The common mechanistic feature of the alkylating agents is that, upon entering cells, the alkyl groups bind to electrophilic sites in DNA and other biologically active molecules; bifunctional alkylation of DNA can result in cross-links between strands of DNA, which impedes replication. Other biochemically important molecules are also alkylated by such agents, but the dominant effect seems to be DNA cross-linking. Both cyclophosphamide and chlorambucil are orally bioavailable and are used both intravenously and by mouth; melphalan and HN_2, because of either variable bioavailability or chemical reactivity, are best utilized by the intravenous route. Except for the requirement for hepatic metabolism of cyclophosphamide, which prolongs its primary elimination as well as the disappearance of its metabolites (8 hours), the elimination of the alkylating agents is rapid (<2 hours) in the blood due to chemical decomposition.

The toxicity of alkylating agents is primarily hematopoietic. Some alkylating agents have more prominent effects on granulocytes (HN_2); with other agents, platelet toxicity may be more pronounced (melphalan) although granulocytopenia occurs often; hematologic toxicity is most frequently observed 8–14 days after drug administration. In addition to hematologic toxicity, the cyclophosphamide metabolite acrolein can irritate the bladder mucosa, requiring strict attention to hydration and urine flow for its safe use; and ifosfamide metabolites, in addition to irritating the bladder, may produce renal tubular injury. All of the alkylating agents can produce alopecia, nausea, and vomiting, as well as gastrointestinal mucosal damage, gonadal dysfunction, and infertility. These agents are also those most closely associated with treatment-related second malignancies. Clear-cut evidence connects alkylating agents with the development of secondary leukemias, the frequency of which is related to the amount of alkylating agent received. The presumed mechanism of this effect is damage to normal bone marrow stem cells resulting in mutagenic changes.

Alkylating agents are among the most widely used antineoplastics and form an important part of curative therapy regimens for Hodgkin's disease and non-Hodgkin's lymphoma as well as important surgical adjuvant regimens for breast cancer. Alkylating agents are also the class of drugs whose doses can be most readily escalated; and the class with the steepest dose-response curves *in vitro*. Thus, these drugs are frequently employed as part of high-dose chemotherapy regimens administered with autologous or allogeneic bone marrow support.

There are several other families of alkylating drugs in which the classic nitrogen mustard backbone has been altered. The nitrosoureas are bifunctional alkylating agents linked to a nitrosourea moiety. Nitrosoureas are lipid soluble and appear to be among the most effective agents for the use in central nervous system (CNS) tumors. It is believed that their lipid solubility enhances penetration through the blood–brain barrier and hence delivery into the CNS. These agents have a unique pattern of toxicity for normal tissues, though their mechanism of tumor cell killing seems to be DNA cross-linking like the more classical alkylating agents. Nitrosoureas tend to exert their most pronounced toxic effects on the hematopoietic system at a later time than do classic alkylating agents. After nitrosourea therapy with carmustine (bischloroethylnitrosourea, BCNU) for example, the nadir of myelosuppression occurs at day 30–36, although drug disappearance from the circulation is rapid; furthermore, nitrosoureas appear to have the ability to damage bone marrow stem cells more effectively than other classic alkylating agents. Nitrosoureas are also associated with pulmonary interstitial fibrosis more commonly than other alkylating agents and can produce cumulative renal injury. Other alkylating species in clinical practice include busulfan, an alkane sulfonate widely used for the treatment of chronic myelogenous leukemia; temozolamide, which methylates DNA, and is orally active in the treatment of brain tumors; and dacarbazine (DTIC), which methylates as well as binds to DNA and is used to treat soft tissue sarcomas and malignant melanoma.

The serendipitous finding that platinum salts were toxic to bacteria led to the discovery that such salts are also quite effective antineoplastic agents. The prototype platinum coordination complex is the drug cisplatin (cis-diamminedichloroplatinum II). This rather simple molecule exerts effects similar to those of the alkylating agents. The chloride groups on cisplatin are labile and, in biologic systems, the sites on the platinum atom previously occupied by the chloride groups can be covalently linked to biologically important macromolecules. The primary target for cisplatin damage in proliferating cells is DNA. "Platinated" DNA contains intra- and interstrand cross-links that disrupt DNA function and replication. The clearance of cisplatin is primarily through endogenous inactivation via binding to biologic macromolecules, including protein sulfhydryls, and the half-life of the unchanged parent molecule in the plasma is short; hepatic metabolism and renal excretion play little role in the drug's elimination. The toxicity of cisplatin can be significant; severe nausea and vomiting, renal tubular impairment, damage to cochlear hair cells with high-frequency hearing loss, and peripheral nerve damage resulting in a sensorimotor neuropathy can accompany treatment. However, careful attention to enhanced intravenous hydration and urine output can largely ameliorate the nephrotoxicity of cisplatin; and the recent development of improved antiemetic regimens has dramatically reduced the emetogenic side effects of cisplatin administration. On the other hand, the myelotoxicity of cisplatin is modest. The introduction of cisplatin into oncologic therapeutics has led to a remarkable change in the therapy of disseminated testicular germ cell cancer (significantly increasing the curability of this disease), as well as the management of advanced ovarian, and small-cell and non-small-cell lung cancers, and squamous cancers of the head and neck.

Carboplatin (diammine 1,1-cyclobutanedicarboxylatoplatinum II) is an analogue of cisplatin in which the two chloride ligands are replaced by the carboxylate moiety. The DNA cross-linking species formed by carboplatin are identical to those formed with cisplatin, but the pharmacokinetics and spectrum of toxicity of this analogue are markedly different. The half-life of carboplatin is more prolonged (4–6 hours) than cisplatin, and the disposition of carboplatin is determined primarily by renal excretion. Carboplatin is substantially less toxic to the kidneys and has less propensity for causing nausea and vomiting. Similarly, no neurotoxicity is seen except at high doses of carboplatin. Unlike cisplatin, carboplatin is a potent bone marrow–suppressing agent. Platelets are more affected than are granulocytes. Generally speaking, carboplatin appears equivalent to cisplatin in terms of antitumor activity, except for the treatment of germ cell malignancies. The precise dose equivalents of these two drugs are uncertain, however. Furthermore, in combination chemotherapy, carboplatin presents the problem of myelosuppression, generally requiring dose reduction of both carboplatin and other myelosuppressive agents used at the same time.

Antimetabolites

A substantial group of highly effective chemotherapeutic drugs disrupt the intermediary metabolism of malignant cells. These compounds can inhibit important enzyme targets or serve as psuedo-substrates, resulting in the incorporation of a fraudulent component into biologically active molecules. Several antimetabolites are widely used as part of curative chemotherapeutic regimens for the treatment of childhood malignancies, the acute leukemias and lymphomas, and for the palliation of patients with common solid tumors.

Methotrexate Methotrexate is the most widely used folate antagonist and was the prototype of the antimetabolite class, first developed for the treatment of childhood leukemias in the late 1940s as structural analogues of folic acid. Methotrexate binds to and inhibits the enzyme dihydrofolate reductase (DHFR). DHFR is necessary for the genesis of reduced folates that serve as sources of methyl groups for the synthesis of thymidine and other biologically important molecules critical for DNA replication. Methotrexate is water soluble and is cleared by glomerular filtration with a terminal half-life of 8 hours. Impaired renal function can considerably alter the pharmacokinetics and toxicity of methotrexate. Because methotrexate impairs the genesis of reduced folates, methotrexate toxicity and efficacy can, in part, be inhibited by the concomitant administration of exogenous reduced folates, such as leucovorin (citrovorum factor). However, when the toxic effects of methotrexate such as renal dysfunction, myelosuppression, or mucositis have become clinically evident, reduced folates play little role in their resolution.

Methotrexate is a drug with broad activity in the treatment of acute lymphocytic leukemia (ALL), breast cancer, and head and neck cancer.

Fluoropyrimidines The fluoropyrimidines 5-fluorouracil (5-FU), 5-fluoro-deoxyuridine (FUdR), and capecitabine, after metabolic conversion and in the presence of reduced folates, bind to the DNA synthetic enzyme thymidylate synthase in the place of the normal substrate, uracil. Formation of a covalent complex between the fluoropyrimidine metabolite, fluorodeoxyuridylate, reduced folate, and thymidylate synthase inactivates the enzyme. Fluoropyrimidines can also be directly incorporated into RNA in place of uracil, leading to impaired RNA processing. 5-FU and FUdR are cleared rapidly by hepatic metabolism, principally by the enzyme dihydropyrimidine dehydrogenase (DPD), with a half-life in the plasma of 10–15 minutes; the large capacity of the liver to detoxify these drugs provides a pharmacologic advantage when they are infused directly into the liver (high local drug concentration with modest or no systemic drug exposure and toxicity). Hepatic artery infusion of fluoropyrimidines is modestly successful in the treatment of hepatic metastases from colorectal cancer. Recently, patients with partial or complete deficiencies of DPD have been described; these individuals are at markedly increased risk of developing severe side effects after treatment with a fluoropyrimidine. The toxicity of the fluoropyrimidines is manifested as reversible, usually mild myelosuppression, and potentially more severe diarrhea and stomatitis, with very occasional cerebellar dysfunction and minimal alopecia, principally occurring 8–14 days after completion of therapy. Fluoropyrimidines are important components of combination regimens utilized for breast cancer and are the most active compounds for the treatment of a wide variety of gastrointestinal malignancies. Because the binding of fluoropyrimidines to thymidylate synthase can be enhanced by increasing intracellular concentrations of reduced folates, the combination of 5-FU and leucovorin was evaluated and has been shown to be one of the most active regimens for the treatment of colorectal cancer in both the advanced disease and adjuvant settings. Treatment with this combination, however, is associated with an increased risk of severe mucositis or diarrhea. The orally active fluoropyrimidine, capecitabine, has recently become available based on its activity in advanced breast and gastrointestinal cancers. This drug is well absorbed from the gastrointestinal tract and is then converted enzymatically to 5-FU in a three-step process that relies on a final step catalzyzed by the enzyme thymidine phosphorylase, which is present to a greater degree in tumor rather than adjacent normal tissues. The multistep activation of capecitabine leads to a much more prolonged exposure to 5-FU in tumors than in plasma after capecitabine administration; however, the daily nature of the usual treatment schedules for this drug do lead to measurable 5-FU concentrations in plasma and, concomitantly, a spectrum of toxicity that is similar to that of a constant intravenous infusion of 5-FU. This includes the possibility of the development of palmar-plantar erythrodysesthesia (hand-foot syndrome) as well as typical mucosal and hematopoietic toxicities.

Cytosine Arabinoside Cytosine arabinoside (Ara-C) is a "fraudulent" nucleoside consisting of the purine cytosine linked to the sugar arabinose;

arabinose does not occur normally in man. Cytosine arabinoside is metabolized by enzymes necessary for the synthesis of cytosine triphosphate (CTP), which is incorporated into DNA. Incorporation of the fraudulent base Ara-CTP inhibits DNA replication and repair, and leads to impaired cellular proliferation, in part through the induction of apoptosis. The efficacy of Ara-C is directly related to a rate of formation of Ara-CTP, a process that can be enhanced by administering the drug in high doses. Ara-C is rapidly catabolized in the liver, peripheral tissues, and serum by the enzyme cytidine deaminase with a terminal half-life of 2 hours. The major toxicities of Ara-C are bone marrow suppression, stomatitis, and intrahepatic cholestasis. At high doses of Ara-C, CNS toxicity consisting of disorientation, cerebellar dysfunction, and coma may result. The primary use of Ara-C is in the treatment of acute myelogenous leukemia (AML).

Gemcitabine   Gemcitabine (2′-2′-difluorodeoxycytidine; dFdC) is a new cytidine analogue which, like Ara-C, is activated by deoxycytidine kinase and detoxified by cytidine deaminase. The mechanism of action of gemcitabine also depends on incorporation of its major intracellular metabolite into DNA. However, gemcitabine is a more potent inhibitor of ribonucleotide reductase, which leads to a decrease in all intracellular deoxynucleotide triphosphates, and, unlike Ara-C, an inhibitor of deoxyctidine deaminase that decreases the breakdown of its intracellular metabolites. Despite these known differences, a clear explanation for the different antineoplastic spectrum of action of gemcitabine, compared with Ara-C, remains to be determined. The dose-limiting toxicity of gemcitabine is myelosuppression, with neutropenia occurring more frequently than thrombocytopenia. Fever, skin rash, and flu-like symptoms may occur. Gemcitabine has been shown to improve the quality of life of patients with advanced pancreatic cancer and has palliative benefit in the treatment of non-small-cell lung cancer, ovarian cancer, and breast cancer.

Antitumor Antibiotics

Actinomycin D   Actinomycin D is a by-product of a species of *Streptomyces*; it is actively used for the treatment of childhood malignancies, particularly soft tissue sarcomas and neuroblastoma. The mechanism of action of actinomycin D is inhibition of RNA and protein synthesis that occurs after DNA intercalation, RNA chain elongation being principally affected. The drug is excreted in part by the kidney and into the bile as the unchanged parent molecule with a long terminal half-life of over 30 hours. The major toxicities of actinomycin D are myelosuppression, which may be severe, alopecia, nausea and vomiting, diarrhea and mucositis, and the potential for extravasation injury if the drug leaks from a vein into the surrounding soft tissues.

Mitomycin C   Mitomycin C was also isolated from a species of *Streptomyces* yeast. It is a unique molecule that combines quinone and aziridine moieties that both play important roles in its reductive intracellular activation to a potent alkylating species, as well as in the generation of reactive oxygen molecules. Under hypoxic conditions, reductive alkylation appears to be responsible for tumor cell killing. Mitomycin C is metabolized by the liver, and excreted in part by the kidney with a terminal half-life of 30–60 minutes. Its major toxicities include myelosuppression (which may be delayed up to 4–5 weeks after treatment), alopecia and stomatitis, hemolytic-uremic syndrome, extravasation injury, and the exacerbation of anthracycline cardiac toxicity. The major therapeutic role of mitomycin C is in the treatment of superficial bladder cancer, where it is used by direct instillation, and for the palliative therapy of gastrointestinal, breast, and non-small-cell lung cancers.

Bleomycin   Bleomycin is a complex mixture of peptides isolated from the *Streptomyces verticillus* fungus that plays an important role in the treatment of testicular germ cell neoplasms and non-Hodgkin's lymphoma. Bleomycin has a unique mechanism of tumor cell killing that involves the formation of a metal-bleomycin complex, which rapidly binds oxygen; the activated metal (usually ferrous iron)-oxygen-bleomycin complex is stabilized by and actively cleaves DNA producing both single- and double-strand breaks. The drug is metabolized by a hydrolase that is found in both normal and malignant cells but in low concentration in skin and in the lung, two organs that are particularly sensitive to bleomycin. Bleomycin is excreted in the urine with an elimination half-life in plasma of approximately 3 hours; the pharmacokinetics of the drug are markedly altered in patients with abnormal renal function. Bleomycin produces little myelosuppression, but its administration is frequently associated with fever and occasionally with an acute allergic reaction. The major side effect of bleomycin is a cumulative pulmonary toxicity, the etiology of which remains unclear; however, the clinical picture of bleomycin-induced lung damage is well known and is characterized by nonproductive cough and shortness of breath, with minimal findings on physical examination, and occasionally a patchy interstitial infiltrate on chest X ray. Pulmonary function studies demonstrate a reduced diffusion capacity especially in patients with a total dose of more than 240 mg. Discontinuation of the drug may lead to complete resolution of signs and symptoms of respiratory compromise over a period of months to years; however, all patients previously exposed to bleomycin are at risk of developing acute respiratory failure postoperatively if exposed to high oxygen tensions during the induction of anesthesia.

Topoisomerase Inhibitors and Agents with Pleiotropic Mechanisms of Action

Anthracyclines   The anthracyclines, doxorubicin and daunorubicin, were also isolated from *Streptomyces* species, and thus, are antitumor antibiotics. However, these drugs interact significantly with a wide range of biochemical systems in tumor cells; many of these interactions contribute to their broad antineoplastic activity. Anthracyclines appear to exert their antiproliferative activity, at least in part, by the following mechanisms: binding to the nuclear enzyme topoisomerase II to form a "cleavable complex" that interferes with the ability of the enzyme to reduce torsional strain in DNA; the generation of reactive oxygen species that interfere with mitochondrial function and that of other critical macromolecules; and activation of signal transduction pathways ultimately leading to the stimulation of apoptosis. The pharmacokinetics of doxorubicin and daunorubicin, as well as epirubicin, the anthracycline analogue most frequently used in Europe, demonstrate tri-exponential decay with a long terminal half-life in plasma of approximately 10 hours. All of the anthracyclines are metabolized primarily by the liver and excreted, in part, into the bile; individuals with liver dysfunction may exhibit considerably enhanced anthracycline toxicity because of delayed drug clearance. The toxicity profile of anthracyclines includes myelosuppression and damage to oral and gastrointestinal mucosa, resulting in stomatitis and diarrhea. Alopecia is a universal accompaniment of anthracycline administration. The anthracycline antibiotics are also potent vesicants; extravasation of these agents into soft tissues results in extensive necrosis and soft tissue damage. Consequently, great care must be exercised when anthracyclines are administered intravenously. Continuous infusion must be done through indwelling central venous catheters. A unique toxicity of the anthracyclines is cumulative, dose-dependent myocardial damage. Recent studies that have used either gated cardiac blood pool scanning or endomyocardial biopsy as endpoints for functional or histological confirmation of doxorubicin cardiac toxicity have demonstrated that the incidence of measurable heart damage begins to climb precipitously above a cumulative dose of 350 to 400 mg/m^2 if the drug has been administered by short intravenous infusion. Thus, in patients who begin therapy with normal cardiac function, several months of anthracycline can be administered with low risk of myocardial dysfunction. However, in individuals who have a history of hypertensive heart disease or prior left chest wall irradiation, the maximum safe dose of doxorubicin may be substantially lower. Data indicate that infusional therapy with anthracyclines (e.g., 96 hours continuous infusion) allows a higher cumulative dose to be administered with diminished risk of cardiac toxicity. A novel agent that appears to significantly ameliorate doxorubicin cardiac toxicity, dexrazoxane, has recently come into clinical practice. Anthracyclines have a broad range of neoplastic activity and form an important component of combination therapies for non-Hodgkin's lymphoma and Hodgkin's disease, breast cancer, osteogenic sarcoma, and a variety of pediatric solid tumors. Daunorubicin and doxorubicin are also among the most active drugs for the treatment of lymphoid and myeloid leukemias.

Podophyllotoxins Podophyllotoxin derivatives have been known for many years to possess antiproliferative effects. Etoposide (VP16) and teniposide (VM26) are the two podophyllotoxin derivatives now commonly used in clinical oncologic practice. These agents exert their anticancer activity through interaction with the enzyme topoisomerase II (topo II), which facilitates the uncoiling of DNA prior to DNA replication. VP16 and VM26 are metabolized by the liver; about 40% of a dose of etoposide is excreted by the kidney. The terminal half-lives of both drugs are from 8 to 10 hours in plasma after intravenous administration. VP16 is the most frequently used podophyllotoxin and can be administered either intravenously or orally. Recent data suggest that continuous low dose oral VP16 might be active when intermittent schedules have failed. The toxicity of these agents is primarily leukopenia and thrombocytopenia, as well as mild to moderate alopecia; at high doses stomatitis occurs. Because the primary toxicity of VP16 is hematopoietic, it has frequently been used in high-dose regimens requiring bone marrow reconstitution. A recently recognized late effect of VP16 is the development of secondary leukemia. VP16 is active in germ cell tumors, small-cell and non–small-cell carcinoma of the lung, Hodgkin's and non-Hodgkin's lymphoma, and myeloid and lymphoid leukemia.

Camptothecins Camptothecin and its derivatives are active cytotoxics that kill tumor cells through inhibition of the nuclear enzyme topoisomerase I, a distinct 100-kDa protein that, like topoisomerase II, plays a critical role in relieving torsional strain in DNA during replication; however, unlike topoisomerase II, the nuclear content of topoisomerase I does not vary significantly with the cell cycle. It has been postulated that this difference is important for explaining the activity of the topoisomerase I inhibitors in tumors with low growth fractions. The camptothecin derivatives topotecan and irinotecan (CPT-11) have now been introduced into clinical practice for the treatment of advanced ovarian and colorectal cancer, respectively. Topotecan is metabolized by a nonenzymatic process that produces a carboxylated derivative that is less active; about one-third of the drug is excreted into the urine. The major toxicity of topotecan is myelosuppression, especially neutropenia, that occurs approximately 10 days after administration. Topotecan has demonstrated moderate activity in patients with platinum-refractory ovarian cancer. Irinotecan is a prodrug that requires side chain cleavage by an esterase to produce its active metabolite SN-38; like topotecan, both irinotecan and SN-38 undergo hydrolysis of the lactone to produce a carboxylate metabolite. Whereas the excretion of the irinotecan parent drug is into the urine and bile, SN-38 is excreted by several mechanisms into the bile. In addition to neutropenia, treatment with irinotecan can produce two forms of diarrhea that may be dose-limiting. The early type of diarrhea, which occurs within hours of drug administration, is probably cholinergic and is associated with cramping and diaphoresis; it can be prevented by pretreatment with atropine. A more difficult to control, late-onset diarrhea is frequently seen after the second or third weekly dose of irinotecan; it can produce dehydration if not aggressively managed with loperamide and fluid replacement. Irinotecan clearly can produce objective remissions in patients with fluoropyrimidine-refractory colorectal cancer.

Antimicrotubule Agents

Vinca Alkaloids Derivatives of the periwinkle plant (*Vinca rosea*) were among the earliest antineoplastics discovered. The three most commonly utilized vinca alkaloids are vincristine, vinblastine, and vinorelbine. These drugs are complex molecules whose mechanism of action is based on disruption of microtubular function through microtubular aggregation. This results in disruption of the formation of the mitotic spindle and inhibition of cells progressing through the cell cycle at the stage of mitosis. Vinca alkaloids are metabolized primarily by the liver and their toxicity is considerably enhanced in individuals with severe hepatic dysfunction. The primary toxicity of vincristine is neurologic. Vincristine administration results in peripheral neuropathy and ileus. Ileus is thought to be due to damage to autonomic nerves supplying the gastrointestinal tract; peripheral neuropathies are related to nerve damage associated with microtubular disruption. Vinorelbine also produces constipation and peripheral neuropathy, but to a lesser extent than vincristine. Its dose-limiting toxicity is neutropenia. Vinca alkaloids are components of effective combination therapies for a wide variety of tumors. They are proven most active in hematologic malignancies and germ cell tumors. Vinorelbine, in particular, is active in breast cancer and non-small-cell lung cancer where it is frequently used. The primary toxicity of vinblastine is myelosuppression affecting both granulocytes and platelets. Neuropathy is an uncommon side effect of vinblastine administration.

Taxanes Paclitaxel is the lead compound in the taxane class of antimicrotubule agents; it was originally isolated from the bark of the Pacific yew, *Taxus brevifolia,* but is now available from semisynthetic approaches. This agent has a wide spectrum of antineoplastic activity and a unique mechanism of cytotoxicity. Paclitaxel interacts with microtubules, but rather than inhibiting their formation as the vinca alkaloids do, paclitaxel stabilizes microtubules and inhibits their dissolution, upsetting the dynamic balance between microtubular formation and dissolution upon which many intracellular processes are dependent. The most obviously affected process is mitosis. Although both paclitaxel and vinca alkaloids inhibit microtubular function, cells resistant to one class of drugs are not always resistant to the other. Paclitaxel is cleared primarily by the liver; dose adjustment is required for patients with moderate elevations of hepatic enzymes. The primary toxicities of paclitaxel are myelosuppression and peripheral neuropathy. Toxicities of paclitaxel that complicated its development are hypotension and anaphylactoid reactions, which appear to be related to the vehicle (Cremophor-EL) in which paclitaxel is prepared; the hypersensitivity reactions have been averted by pretreatment with antihistamines and corticosteroids. Paclitaxel is active in refractory ovarian cancer and in small-cell and non–small-cell lung cancer and breast cancer.

The taxane analogue docetaxel is a product of semisynthetic approaches to synthesis. Docetaxel shares the hepatic metabolism of paclitaxel but interacts differently with cells based on their level of *bcl-2* phosphorylation; this may explain the partial lack of cross-reactivity of docetaxel and paclitaxel. Docetaxel is very active in the treatment of breast, lung, and ovarian cancer. Because of its enhanced solubility, it is not prepared in the same vehicle as paclitaxel and thus does not produce the same incidence of immediate hypersensitivity reactions although they do occur; however, unlike paclitaxel, docetaxel can produce a capillary leak syndrome characterized by peripheral edema, ascites or pleural effusion, and weight gain observed in patients treated with cumulative doses >400 mg/m^2. Premedication with dexamethasone can decrease the severity and delay the onset of this syndrome.

Hormonal Agents

Beatson demonstrated in 1895 that oophorectomy would slow the progression of breast cancer. Since that observation, a variety of hormonal agents have been proven to be useful in the therapy of human cancers. The mechanisms by which hormonal therapy can favorably affect the growth of cancers may depend upon withdrawal or inhibition of secretion of endogenous hormones necessary for the sustenance of the growth of the cancer (e.g., estrogens, androgens), or by direct interference with the biochemical effects of endogenous hormones.

Estrogens, progestins, and androgens derived from the ovaries have been shown to be important in the progression of breast cancer and endometrial cancer. Removal of the ovaries or suppression of their function through the administration of gonadotropin-releasing hormone (GNRH) agonists plays a role in the suppression of those cancers. Prostate cancer and breast cancer in the male are dependent upon the secretion of androgens from the testes. Orchiectomy or inhibition of testicular antigen synthesis through the use of luteinizing hormone-releasing hormone (LH-RH) analogues plays an important role in the control of those cancers.

Adrenal-derived androgens and estrogens appear to be important in supporting the growth of prostate cancer and breast cancer. A number of agents such as aminoglutethimide (AG) and ketoconazole have been shown to inhibit enzymes necessary for the synthesis of adrenal androgens and estrogens. In addition, AG and other newer aromatase inhibitors such as anastrazole alter the peripheral conversion of androgens to estrogens (aromatization); because of the enhanced tolerance of the newer aromatase inhibitors, they have become important additions to the hormonal management of advanced breast cancer.

Another class of hormonal agents were originally classified as "antihormones." Tamoxifen, which is a nonsteroidal antiestrogen, and flutamide, a nonsteroidal antiandrogen, are the prototypes of this class of compounds. They exert their antiproliferative effects by a variety of mechanisms including, in the case of tamoxifen, alterations in the activation of the estrogen receptor gene, blockade of estrogen-stimulated progesterone receptor synthesis, and stimulation of other growth-regulating gene products such as transforming growth factor beta. Tamoxifen has been proven to be safe and beneficial in both the surgical adjuvant therapy of breast cancer and in the treatment of advanced disease. It is currently being evaluated as a chemopreventive agent for women at high risk for developing breast cancer. Tamoxifen, however, possesses both agonist and antagonist effects; while blocking the effects of estrogen on the breast, it is an estrogen mimic with respect to the uterus. This can lead to hyperplasia and an increased risk of endometrial cancer after long-term tamoxifen exposure. Other side effects include weight gain, hot flashes, and an increased risk of deep venous thrombosis.

Flutamide competes with natural androgen for binding to the androgen receptor. Flutamide is a modestly active agent in advanced prostate cancer; it is sometimes used in combination with either orchiectomy or LH-RH analogues in a so-called total androgen deprivation approach to the treatment of prostate cancer. The superiority of this approach over orchiectomy alone for advanced prostate cancer remains unclear.

Progestational agents are also effective in some forms of cancer. Endometrial cancer is suppressed in 40%–50% of cases by exogenous administration of progesterone or progesterone analogues. Progestational agents are also effective in advanced breast cancer, particularly in women whose tumors have previously responded to hormonal manipulation; these agents also have some activity in advanced prostate cancer. Although the cytotoxic mechanism of action of progestins is unclear, these drugs produce a characteristic spectrum of toxicity including weight gain, fluid retention, hot flashes, cholestasis, and an increased risk of thromboembolic events.

CONCLUSION

The use of systemic cancer treatment includes drugs that are directly cytotoxic to tumor cells, or affect tumor cell proliferation, by a wide variety of different mechanisms, as well as compounds that may affect the hormonal milieu in which the tumor proliferates. The use of each of these classes of systemic therapies provides curative treatment options for patients with several forms of disseminated hematological malignancies as well as postsurgical adjunctive therapy that improves the cure rate for early stages of breast, ovarian, and colorectal cancer; and effective palliative treatment for all of the common solid tumors in man. Systemic cancer treatments can best be understood through an appreciation of several critical concepts in tumor biology that form the foundation of medical oncology as well as an understanding of the clinical and molecular pharmacology of the specific drugs currently in use.

FURTHER READING

Chabner BA, Longo DL (eds.) (2001) *Cancer Chemotherapy and Biotherapy: Principles and Practice*, 3rd edition. Lippincott, Williams, and Wilkins, Philadelphia.

Doroshow JH (1999) Pharmacological basis for high-dose chemotherapy. In *Hematopoietic Cell Transplantation*, 2nd edition. Thomas ED, Blume KG, Forman SJ (eds.) Blackwell Science, Inc., Malden, MA, pp. 103–122.

Goldie JH, Coldman AJ, Gudanskas GA (1982) Rationale for the use of alternating non-cross-resistant chemotherapy. *Cancer Treat Rep* 66:439–449.

Grochow LB, Ames MM (eds.) (1998) *A Clinician's Guide to Chemotherapy, Pharmacokinetics, and Pharmacodynamics*. Williams and Wilkins, Baltimore.

Mendelsohn J, Howley PM, Israel MA, Liotta LA (eds.) (2001) *The Molecular Basis of Cancer*, 2nd edition. WB Saunders, Philadelphia.

Ratain MJ, Schilsky RL, Conley BA, Egorin MJ (1990) Pharmacodynamics in cancer therapy. *J Clin Oncol* 8: 1739–1753.

Reed JC (1999) Dysregulation of apoptosis in cancer. *J Clin Oncol* 17:2941–2953.

Schilsky RL, Ratain MJ, Milano GA (eds.) (1996) *Principles of Antineoplastic Drug Development and Pharmacology*. Marcel Dekker, New York.

CHAPTER 11

Principles of Tumor Immunotherapy

JOSHUA D. I. ELLENHORN

City of Hope National Medical Center, Department of General and Oncology Surgery, Duarte, California

KIM MARGOLIN

City of Hope National Medical Center, Departments of Medical Oncology and Therapeutics Research and Hematology and Bone Marrow Transplant, Duarte, California

In this chapter, humoral and cellular immunity are reviewed as well as the role of the dendritic cell in immune responses. The discussion of immunotherapeutic interventions begins with antibodies, as unmodified immunoglobulins, as modified or conjugated structures and as targets for vaccines. Advances in cytokine therapy using interleukin-2 and interferon are summarized. The identification and categorization of tumor associated antigens is then discussed. Cancer vaccine approaches targeting cellular immunity are reviewed. These include peptide vaccines; viral and DNA vaccines; dendritic cell therapy; and allogeneic, autologous, and gene therapy vaccines. Adoptive cellular immunotherapy is discussed in the context of lymphokine-activated killer, tumor-infiltrating lymphocytes, and allogeneic hematopoietic cell therapy.

There is considerable experimental data from preclinical models to support a prominent role for the immune system in the immunosurveillance and elimination of malignancy in animal model systems. The evidence for an effective antitumor immune response in humans is more elusive, but several "experiments of nature" suggest that the occurrence and behaviors of human malignancies may be influenced by the immune response to tumor antigens. The increased incidence of a number of malignancies in the immunocompromised patient probably results from a deficit in tumor antigen recognition and a failure to eliminate an otherwise immunogenic tumor. A number of additional mechanisms exist by which tumors "escape" from host immunologic control. The occasional spontaneous regression of melanoma, renal cell carcinoma, or other malignancies is also likely immune

UICC Manual of Clinical Oncology, Eighth Edition. Edited by Raphael E. Pollock
ISBN 0-471-22289-5 Copyright © 2004 John Wiley & Sons, Inc.

mediated. In addition, recent experience with allogeneic bone marrow and stem cell transplantation for hematologic malignancy has clearly implicated a role for the T-cell response in the prevention of recurrent malignancy.

TUMOR IMMUNOLOGY

The immune response is composed of humoral and cellular arms, both of which have broad implications with respect to tumor immunology. Humoral immunity is largely associated with B lymphocytes and the production of antibodies (Abs). Cellular immunity involves a number of cell types including T cells and natural killer (NK) cells.

B Lymphocytes

B lymphocytes or B cells are bone marrow–derived cells that recognize extra-cellular as well as cell-surface antigens through their membrane-anchored Ab. This antigen may be in the form of polysaccharides, nucleic acids, or proteins. Antigen binding to the cell surface Ab can stimulate the B cells to proliferate and differentiate into terminally differentiated plasma cells, which produce and release soluble antibodies into extracellular fluids. The binding of Abs to their cellular antigen target results in one or more forms of target damage, including (1) comp-lement fixation, leading to a multienzyme cascade resulting in the formation of lethal membrane pores; (2) the recruitment and binding to specialized receptors of cells that mediate Ab-dependent cellular cytotoxicity (ADCC), including phago-cytes and lymphocytes; and (3) direct binding to tumor cells with resulting negative proliferative signals or the induction of apoptosis.

The diversity of Ab specificities within an individual's repertoire is almost limitless. This heterogeneity results from a complex process of recombination of a number of immunoglobulin (Ig) germline genes during stem cell maturation into B cells in the bone marrow. Each resulting B cell expresses Ab of a single specificity. Immature B cells express IgM or IgD as their antigen receptor. Inappropriate activation of immature B cells by cross-linking surface IgM molecules with either high-affinity antigen or anti-IgM antibodies can result in cell deletion, a protective mechanism against autoreactive B cells but a potential tolerance-inducing escape mechanism in tumor immunity. Naïve B-cell recognition of antigen occurs in secondary lymphoid organs after the B cells have left the bone marrow. Recognition and activation for most nonmicrobial antigens commonly depends on an effective interaction between the B cell and a CD4 helper T cell. Appropriately stimulated B cells undergo Ig class switching, in which cells expressing IgM and IgD as their antigen receptors differentiate into cells expressing IgG, IgA, or IgE as their receptors for antigen. Because the cell's variable region identity never changes, Ab molecules resulting from a class switch express a new isotype that confers changes in the functional aspects of the Ab but retains its original antigen specificity (termed *idiotype*). Successfully stimulated B cells differentiate into Ab-secreting plasma cells or into memory cells that respond in an accelerated fashion to subsequent stimulation with the same antigen.

Monoclonal Antibodies

One widespread application of B-cell immunology has been the generation of monoclonal antibodies (Mabs). Cloned Ab-producing B cells can be immortalized by fusion between B lymphocytes of individuals immunized to a particular antigen and plasma cell clones that do not secrete their own idiotypic Ig but nevertheless are capable of supporting Ab synthesis and secretion based on the genetic material provided by the lymphocyte. The resulting "hybridoma" produces large amounts of homogeneous Ab with the antigen specificity of the immunized B lymphocyte.

T Lymphocytes

The T lymphocyte or T cell provides specificity to the cellular immune response. T cells recognize processed intracellular antigen expressed on the cell membrane of targeted cells by major histocompatibility complex (MHC) molecules otherwise known as human leukocyte antigen (HLA) molecules. The ability to recognize intracellular antigen underlies their primary function in protection against intracellular viral pathogens. In addition, they are the mediators of delayed type hypersensitivity (DTH) and rejection of grafts and tumors. These thymus-derived lymphocytes all express CD3 and recognize antigens via the T-cell receptor (TCR). This receptor has a diversity and specificity derived through gene rearrangements analogous to those of the immunoglobulins. T cells can be divided into two major types: CD8 cytotoxic T lymphocytes (CTLs), which are capable of direct cellular killing, and CD4 T helper (Th) lymphocytes, which produce cytokines. CD8 T cells interact with target cells expressing HLA class I molecules on their cell surface. The HLA class I molecule is ubiquitously expressed on all nucleated cells and presents antigen as short 8–10 amino acid peptides, termed *minimal cytotoxic epitopes*. These peptides derive from proteolysis of intracellular proteins in specialized proteasomes within the cytoplasm of all cells. The TCR/CD3 complex of a CD8 T cell specifically recognizes a single peptide/HLA complex and, along with secondary signals related to the interaction of an elaborate array of accessory molecules, is then triggered to destroy that cell. The principal mechanism of CTL-mediated killing is through the elaboration of perforin and granzymes (serine protease containing granules), which result in target cell cytolysis. An alternate pathway involves the expression of Fas ligand by the T cell. Interaction with a target cell expressing Fas results in apoptosis of the target cell.

The CD4 T cell interacts with specialized antigen-presenting cells (APCs) such as macrophages, dendritic cells (DC), and B lymphocytes that express HLA class II molecules. HLA class II molecules present longer 12–20 amino acid peptides derived from exogenous proteins that have been taken up and processed by the APC. When the specific TCR of a CD4 T cell has been activated, the cell begins to produce cytokines that enhance B-cell Ab production, support T-cell responses, and activate other immune cells.

Dendritic Cells

The central role in initiating the antitumor immune response is played by the DC. DC are a group of related cell types with differing precursor lineage, location, and stage of maturation. Myeloid-lineage DC, which include Langerhans cells, peripheral blood DC, veiled DC in the afferent lymphatics, and germinal center DC, are thought to derive from bone marrow precursors. Lymphoid DC, a less abundant subpopulation, appear to arise from "double-positive" (CD8$^+$/CD4$^+$) early thymocytes and to play a potential role in the phenotypic and functional development of helper T cells.

DC are large cells with stellate processes that abundantly express the antigen presentation molecules CD1 and MHC class I and II, the costimulatory molecules CD40, CD80/B7.1, and CD86/B7.2, and various adhesion molecules. They possess the ability to internalize extracellular material and migrate through the lymphatics into the T-cell-rich regions of lymph nodes and spleen. DC contain an efficient antigen-processing system that precisely coordinates the uptake, proteolysis, and presentation of antigenic peptides on HLA molecules. Antigenic peptides presented on the DC HLA in conjunction with membrane-bound costimulatory molecules, control the initiation of the immune response. DC are also the source of secreted cytokines that also influence all aspects of the cellular response to antigen. Full DC maturation is thought to occur following the formation of an immunologic "synapse" between the DC and a CD4$^+$ T cell recognizing a class II restricted epitope presented by the DC. This synapse is composed of MHC and TCR molecules, adhesion molecules and costimulatory molecules. If the interaction activates the CD4$^+$ T cell, it can in turn activate the DC through the coupling of CD40 ligand on the T cell with CD40 receptor on the DC. Alternatively, DC maturation can be triggered through exposure to one of several "danger signals," which include bacterial products like lipopolysaccharide (LPS) and bacterial DNA sequences (C$_p$G), necrotic cells, and viral infection.

DC possess the unique property to stimulate naïve T cells. CD4$^+$ T cells effectively activated through the immunologic synapse with the DC can, along with the DC, produce cytokines that can propagate the immune response. Type I cytokines (interferon [IFN]-γ, interleukin [IL]-2, and tumor necrosis factor [TNF]-α) produced by the CD4$^+$ T cell or DC can facilitate the development of CD8$^+$ CTL. CTL, the major effector cells of the antitumor immune response, are activated via Type I cytokine and MHC/peptide along with co-stimulatory signals on the DC to directly mediate tumor cell lysis (Fig. 11.1).

NK Cells

A distinct population of lymphocytes responsible for innate tumor immunity is the NK cell. These large granular lymphocytes tend to be toxic for tumor cells

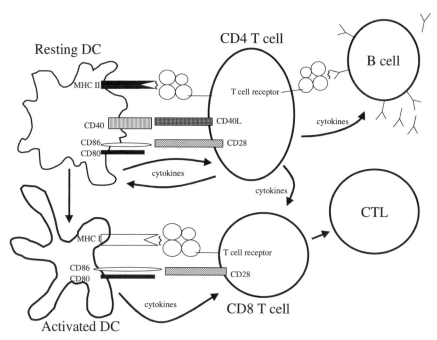

Figure 11.1   Interactions between DC and lymphocytes. DC engage TCR on CD4$^+$ T cells with peptide presented in the context of MHC class II molecules. Resting DC become activated following stimulation of CD40 by CD40 ligand on CD4 T cells. Following the interaction with DC, some CD4 T cells stimulate B cells to activate and produce Ab. Activated DC can also stimulate CD8 T cells through their TCR to become CTL. Co-stimulatory and adhesion molecule interactions, such as CD80/CD28 or CD86/CD28, and others prolong cell contact time, and enhance lymphocyte activation.

and virus-infected cells. NK cells express the receptor for immunoglobulins (FcR) and can participate in ADCC. They also express a number of cell surface inhibitory receptors that recognize MHC class I molecules expressed by target cells. When cross-linked, these receptors deliver a signal that inhibits triggering of cytotoxic activity and cytokine expression. Therefore, if tumor cells lose MHC class I expression and escape CTLs, they may become more susceptible to NK cells.

IMMUNOTHERAPUTIC INTERVENTIONS

Antibodies

The method for producing Mab in mice was first described by Georges Kohler and Cesar Milstein in 1975. In the years that followed, there were numerous phase I

TABLE 11.1. Therapeutic Antibodies in Tumor Immunotherapy

Antibody Structure	Modification	Rationale for Design/ Therapeutic Goal	Examples/Status
Native IgG	None	Antigen recognition complement fixation, ADCC, direct target cell toxicity	Chimeric anti-CD20 approved for B-cell lymphomas; Murine 17-1A available in Europe for adjuvant Rx of colorectal cancer
Radioimmuno conjugate	Radioisotope covalently bound to native Ab	Focused delivery of radiotherapy to tumor target, imaging antigen-expressing tumor	^{131}I-labeled anti-B1 ^{90}Y-labeled anti-CD20, both approved for B-cell malignancies; ^{111}In-labeled anti-CEA
Immunotoxins	Intracellular toxin covalently bound to native Ab	Focused delivery of potent intracellular toxin to tumor target	Calicheamycin conjugated to humanized anti-CD33 approved for myeloid leukemia
Immunocytokines	Mab linked to cytokine molecule	Recruit/stimulate effector cells in high concentration at target sites	Chimeric 14:18 against GD_2 ganglioside expressed on melanoma, neuro-blastoma conjugated with IL-2
Anti-idiotype "Ab2"	Ab1 = Ab specific for tumor antigen; Ab2 = Ab recognizing idiotype of Ab1 as antigen, possesses internal image of original tumor antigen; Ab3 = induced Ab against tumor antigen	Optimize structure/ function characteristics of anti-tumor Ab	Anti-ids under investigation include Ab2 for melanoma ganglioside GD2, Ab2 for CEA

trials involving the administration of murine Mabs reacting with melanoma, neuroblastoma, breast cancer, lymphoma, colon cancer, and other malignancies. Unfortunately, only limited and short-lasting responses were seen. There were numerous major drawbacks to these early antibodies. Because the Mabs were of mouse origin, there was a vigorous human anti-murine Mab (HAMA) response that rapidly cleared the murine Mabs. Antigen modulation or internalization and shedding resulted in limited Mab targeting and short Ab half-life. The early murine Mabs were unable to induce direct antitumor effects or enhance effector cell functions.

Many of the early limitations have been overcome by humanizing Mabs using recombinant techniques, and by better selection of antigenic targets. Numerous Mabs with potential antitumor efficacy have reached the clinical trial stage (Table 11.1). Not all of these Mabs mediate their effect through ADCC or complement fixation. For example, some Mabs block essential signal transduction pathways in malignant cells (e.g., C225, an inhibitor of epidermal growth factor receptor function) or proliferative stimuli in tumor neovasculature (e.g., Ab to vascular endothelial growth factor or integrin).

Three Mabs are currently in clinical use today. These include trastuzumab (Herceptin) for breast cancer, rituximab (Rituxan) for non-Hodgkin's lymphoma (NHL), and Mab 17-1A for colorectal cancer. Trastuzumab is a humanized Ab that recognizes the human epidermal growth factor receptor (EGFR) oncoprotein HER-2/neu or c-erbB-2, which is overexpressed on some breast cancers, particularly the more aggressive ones. An initial phase II study published by Baselga examined women with metastatic breast cancer and demonstrated an overall response rate of 11.6% in a group with progressive disease despite having been previously heavily pretreated with chemotherapy. A second, larger study of 222 women published by Cobleigh found an overall response rate of 15% with a median response duration of 8.4 months and a median survival time of 13 months. Based on these results, Slamon et al. performed a randomized trial on more than 469 breast cancer patients. In this study, trastuzumab was administered in combination with either doxorubicin/cyclophosphamide or paclitaxel chemotherapy or chemotherapy was administered alone for therapy of recurrent metastatic disease. The addition of trastuzumab to either chemotherapy regimen resulted in improved response rates and overall survival compared with chemotherapy alone. The efficacy of trastuzumab is thought to result from direct cell growth inhibition following binding to the EGFR.

Rituximab is a chimeric Mab (the original murine Ab partially "humanized" by grafting the murine antigen-combining site onto a human IgG framework) that binds to CD20, a differentiation antigen found exclusively on B cells and on more than 95% of B-cell NHL. CD20 does not modulate when bound with Ab and is not shed from the cell surface. The Mab fixes complement, mediates ADCC, and can cause apoptosis of NHL cell lines *in vitro*. A pivotal trial conducted by McLaughlin et al. on 166 patients with recurrent or refractory low-grade lymphoma produced an overall response rate of 48%. In a subsequent trial of 54 patients with recurrent or refractory intermediate or high-grade lymphoma, 31% demonstrated a response. In an attempt to improve upon the results with rituximab alone, Czuczman reported that the combination of rituximab with CHOP in patients with newly diagnosed and relapsed low grade lymphoma resulted in a 100% response rate (63% complete response [CR], 37% partial response [PR]) in 35 patients. A similar approach yielded responses in 32 of 33 patients with untreated intermediate or high-grade lymphoma. In a French randomized trial reported by Coiffier et al., 400 patients over the age of 60 with diffuse large B-cell NHL were randomized to CHOP or CHOP plus rituximab. The addition of rituximab improved both the CR rate and overall survival.

Murine Mab edrecolomab or 17-1A (Panorex) recognizes the nonsecreted molecular weight 40,000 glycoprotein CD17-1A, which is overexpressed by most epithelial tumors. Occasional clinical responses have been described in patients with metastatic gastrointestinal malignancies following infusion of unlabeled 17-1A Mab. The mechanism of action is thought to involve the initiation of ADCC or the activation of anti-idiotype responses. The most impressive clinical trial with 17-1A is a German trial reported by Riethmuller. A total of 189 Dukes' C patients were randomized to treatment with 17-1A or observation. After a median follow-up of 7 years, the Mab-treated group had a reduced mortality rate of 32% and reduced recurrence rate of 23%. This led to the approval of 17-1A for the adjuvant treatment of colon cancer in Germany. Confirmatory studies are presently underway in the United States and Europe.

Radioimmunotherapy

Radioactive isotopes coupled to monoclonal Mabs offer potential advantages over Mabs alone. These include more effective cytotoxicity even in the absence of a functional immune system and greater bystander effect on adjacent antigen-negative tumor cells. Radioimmunotherapy (RIT) has been the source of several promising clinical results, particularly in the treatment of chemotherapy-refractory lymphomas. In the past, most RIT studies used iodine 131, but improvements in chelation technology have enabled the study of yttrium 90 conjugates. ^{90}Y offers the benefit of a long path length of up to 12 mm, high-energy beta-emissions, lack of volatility, and the relative ease and safety of its conjugation to antibodies.

Although early studies of RIT demonstrated partial, short-lived clinical responses in some patients with advanced solid tumors, subsequent experience has been largely disappointing. The development of HAMA has been seen in 40–80% of patients, and dose-limiting hematologic toxicity was seen at radioactive isotope activities of 30–100 mCi/m^2. Recent studies in NHL patients have yielded more promising results. Trials using an ^{131}I-labeled murine anti-CD20 Mab showed response rates of ~80%. Y2B8 (Ibritumomab), which is the parental murine Mab of rituximab labeled with ^{90}Y, produced responses in 34 of 51 patients in a phase I/II NHL study. Particularly encouraging were the responses seen in rituximab-refractory patients. An area of intense clinical study is the use of radiolabeled anti-CD45 and anti-CD33 Mabs in myeloablative doses in preparation for bone marrow/stem cell transplants for leukemias.

Other Ab Applications

A number of other strategies have been used to take advantage of the exquisite antigen specificity conferred by Ab molecules. One such strategy is the creation of bispecific Abs, which are Ab constructs resulting from the combination of two separate Ab specificities. The combination of tumor antigen–specific Abs with Abs recognizing immune cells can result in bispecific Abs that accumulate and activate immune cells at the tumor site. Mabs can also be conjugated to various substances. In addition to the focused radiation conferred by the radioimmunoconjugates described above, additional conjugates include cytokines such as IL-2, which stimulate immune cells, and toxin molecules, which can be cytotoxic to tumor cells.

An approach that links the antigen specificity conferred by Ab with the powerful cytolytic properties of T cells is the genetic modification of *ex vivo* expanded CTL to express chimeric T cell receptors. The chimeric T-cell receptors include the antigen recognition elements of Mab linked to the intracellular components of the T-cell receptor responsible for effector function. The resulting CTL possesses the desired antigen-specificity and binding properties of the Ab with a fully functional T-cell receptor. Clinical trials of this "T-body" approach are in progress using T-cell receptors specific for anti-CD20 in B-cell malignancies, CE7 in neuroblastoma, and anti-HER-2/neu and anti-CEA in malignancies expressing these antigens.

One application of Mab therapy involves the stimulation of idiotype networks. Antigen on tumor cells is recognized by the antigen-combining site or idiotype of an antibody. This antibody, termed Ab1, can stimulate an anti-idiotype (Ab2) response directed against Ab1. Because the idiotype of Ab1 is a complementary image of the antigen and the anti-idiotype on Ab2 is a complementary image of Ab1, Ab2 contains a surrogate tumor epitope. Idiotype or antiidiotype Ab can be used to immunize patients, leading to the production of anti-antiidiotype Ab (i.e., Ab3) that in part bind to the tumor epitope against which the Ab1 was directed.

Ganglioside Vaccines

A number of vaccine approaches have been designed to stimulate a humoral response to tumor antigen. The most successful of these target gangliosides. Gangliosides are neuraminic acid-containing glycophospholipids and are over-expressed on melanomas, neuroblastomas, astrocytomas, sarcomas, and small-cell lung cancer. Livingston and colleagues performed a number of early studies using GM2 monosialoganglioside-based vaccines. A proportion of patients developed humoral responses to GM2, and the IgM Ab produced was able to lyse melanoma cells via a complement-mediated pathway. The development of a humoral response correlated with an improved clinical outcome even though no cytotoxic T cells were produced. These results were confirmed in a trial of 120 stage III melanoma patients who were randomized to combined GM2/BCG or BCG alone. Although the development of a humoral response correlated with improved survival in vaccinated subjects, there was no overall survival difference between the groups. To enhance the generation of cytotoxic Ab, GM2 has been conjugated to the hapten

KLH and administered with the adjuvant QS-21. Recently, a large multicenter phase III adjuvant trial was performed to compare GM2/KLH/QS21 "GMK" vaccine administered intermittently subcutaneously over 2 years versus high-dose IFN-α subcutaneously over 1 year, the standard adjuvant therapy (see below) for patients with high-risk melanoma (deep primary lesions and/or positive regional nodes). Eight hundred patients were randomized and started on treatment. The results of a planned interim analysis demonstrated that the relapse-free and overall survival were superior with IFN-α, and further therapy with GMK vaccine was not recommended. The future role of ganglioside-based tumor vaccination remains unknown, although melanoma gangiosides are currently the subject of investigation in the area of anti-idiotype Ab development.

Cytokine Therapy

Interleukin-2   IL-2 is the most extensively studied cytokine to date. A 15-kDa glycoprotein produced by T helper cells, IL-2 has numerous cellular regulatory effects, including stimulation and expansion of lymphocytes. Although IL-2 has no direct effect on tumor cells, at high doses it induces lymphokine activated killer (LAK) cells from NK precursors. LAK cells can nonspecifically lyse tumor. The administration of high-dose recombinant IL-2 to humans has been reported to mediate the regression of even bulky, invasive tumors in selected patients with metastatic melanoma, renal cancer and non-Hodgkin's lymphoma. A review of 409 consecutive patients with advanced melanoma (182 patients) or renal cancer (227 patients) treated with high-dose IL-2 at the National Cancer Institute demonstrated responses in up to 19% of patients. Seven percent of patients with melanoma had a complete response, and 9% had a partial response. In patients with renal cancer, the complete and partial response rates were 9% and 10%, respectively. Studies of 255 patients with metastatic kidney cancer and 270 patients with metastatic melanoma from 22 different institutions achieved similar results and provided the basis for the approval of this agent in the treatment of both advanced renal cancer and melanoma.

Interferon-α   IFN-α is a member of the pleiotropic IFN family of leukocyte-secreted protein cytokines. The precise mechanism of action of IFN-α in humans is unclear. IFN-α appears to possess direct antiproliferative effects on malignant cells. IFN-α also up-regulates HLA class I and tumor antigens in addition to enhancing NK, lymphocyte, and macrophage function. In patients with high-risk melanoma, defined as a primary lesion with a Breslow depth of greater than 4 mm or the presence of one or more lymph nodes, a randomized controlled trial of high-dose IFN-α versus observation following surgery was reported by the Eastern Cooperative Group (ECOG) in 1996. The results of this important study (E1684) demonstrated for the first time a statistically significant overall survival advantage to IFN-α given in the postoperative setting for high-risk melanoma. At five years, there was an 11% improvement in disease-free survival (26% *vs.* 37%) and an 8% improvement in overall survival (37% *vs.* 45%). The high-dose regimen, consisting of IFN-α, 20 mU/m^2 intravenously 5 days per week for 4 weeks followed by 10 mU/m^2 subcutaneously 3 days per week for 48 weeks, was associated with significant toxicity, mainly hepatic enzyme elevation, leukopenia, and thrombocytopenia, requiring dose-modifications or delays in about 50% of patients. This stimulated interest in reducing toxicity by reducing the dose of IFN-α. Unfortunately, two subsequent randomized trials, one by the World Health Organization (WHO-16) and the other by ECOG (E1690), failed to demonstrate efficacy for low-dose IFN-α, consistent with the results of many smaller studies that also showed no survival benefit and only occasional relapse-free survival benefit with low-intensity IFN-α regimens. E-1690 was a three-way randomization of patients between high- and low-dose IFN-α and control. This study also suggested less benefit for high-dose IFN-α than had been observed in E1684. The high rate of crossover to IFN-α following subsequent lymph node dissection in patients originally assigned to observation in this latter trial raised the likelihood that there was benefit to delayed IFN-α treatment administered at the time of recurrence. The survival advantage of high-dose IFN-α compared with GM2-KLH/QS-21 vaccine in Intergroup trial E1694, has established high-dose IFN-α as a standard therapy against which all new approaches must be compared for the adjuvant therapy of high-risk melanoma.

IFN-α as a single agent has been reported to yield responses in 12–15% of patients with metastatic renal cell cancer and complete responses in 2–5%. Based on observations of synergy between IFN-α and IL-2 in preclinical models and on the lack of fully overlapping clinical toxicities, the possibility of enhanced antitumor activity at a lower level of toxicity has been evaluated by combining the two agents in several clinical trials. The results of randomized trials comparing the combination of IFN-α with IL-2 revealed no superiority and no reduction in toxicity compared to high-dose IL-2 alone. Even when more intensive regimens were studied, such as the Cytokine Working Group trial of intravenous IL-2 plus IFN-α versus IL-2 alone in 99 patients with advanced renal cancer, there was no advantage seen with the combination. The French CRECY trial added IFN-α to a very aggressive IL-2 regimen and randomized 425 patients with renal cancer between each of the single agents or the combination. The superior response rate of the combination was associated with unacceptably high toxicities, including a high mortality rate, and the higher response rate of the combination did not lead to improved survival. In melanoma, combinations of IL-2 and IFN-α have also been disappointing, although the addition of both cytokines to combination chemotherapy is undergoing investigation in patients with advanced melanoma and in the adjuvant setting.

Tumor-Associated Antigens

Methods for Antigen Identification The identification of tumor-associated antigens (TAA) capable of being recognized by a cellular immune response has been progressing at an accelerated pace. Three general methods have been used to identify candidate TAA. The first requires the generation of tumor-specific CTL using established *in vitro* sensitization techniques. The CTL are then tested for their ability to recognize HLA-matched target cells that have been transfected with tumor-derived "libraries" of cDNA, the complementary DNA derived from reverse transcription of messenger RNA extracted from the cells of interest. This method, also known as expression cloning, ultimately results in the identification of one or more genes unique to the tumor that may act as TAA recognizable by CTL. Alternatively, peptides eluted from the surface of tumor cells can be pulsed onto HLA-matched APCs such as DC or virally immortalized B-lymphocytes. These APCs are tested for CTL recognition, which is generally assayed by the release of cytokines such as IFN-γ upon recognition by the T cell of a specific TAA. Those peptides, representing one or more portions of the antigen that are processed and presented on HLA molecules and recognized by CTL, are termed *cytotoxic* or *dominant epitopes*. In many cases, these antigens are shared among a variety of different tumor types, and among many different individuals, an advantage for the development of vaccines for general use.

The second general method of TAA identification is often referred to as "reverse immunology." This method involves identifying candidate tumor antigens by virtue of their aberrant- or over-expression on tumor cells. *In vitro* sensitization techniques are then used to detect and expand existing CTL responses, which identify the candidate protein as a TAA.

The third and newest method of tumor antigen recognition involves serologic analysis of recombinant cDNA expression libraries (SEREX). This method uses serum from cancer patients to screen for Ab against proteins encoded by tumor cell cDNA libraries expressed in target cells. The assumption is that the humoral response to TAA results from T helper cell recognition of the TAA.

Known Tumor-Associated Antigens Using these established methods, hundreds of TAA have been identified and each is a potential target for an immunotherapy approach to malignancy. The TAA, which can be recognized by CTL can be divided into several general categories, shown in Table 11.2. The first TAA was identified by Thierry Boon's group in 1991 by expression cloning using melanoma-specific CTL. The antigen was designated MAGE-1 (melanoma associated antigen). Later, a family of MAGE-1–related genes (MAGE-3, BAGE, GAGE, RAGE) were identified. These so-called cancer-testis genes encode antigens that are expressed in melanomas and some other tumors, but not in normal tissues except the testis. A second category of TAA derives from melanocyte differentiation antigens. These TAA are recognized by melanoma-specific CTL and are also expressed on normal melanocytes. Examples include the self-antigens MART-1/Melan A, tyrosinase, gp100/Pmel17, and gp75/TRP-1. A third category of TAA is true tumor-specific antigens that result from point mutations, translocations, or Ig gene rearrangements occurring as part of the oncogenic transformation and propagated by clonal expansion of the malignant cells. These TAA are the optimal immunotherapeutic targets, because their expression in cancer cells is unique. Examples include *p53* and *ras* point mutations found abundantly in lung cancer and other solid tumors, BCR/ABL

TABLE 11.2. Potential Tumor Antigens for Immunotherapy

Antigen Class	Antigen	Malignancy
Tumor-specific antigens	Immunoglobulin idiotype	B-cell non-Hodgkin's lymphoma, multiple myeloma
	TCR	T-cell non-Hodgkin's lymphoma
	Mutant p21/ras	Pancreatic, colon, lung cancer
	Mutant p53	Colorectal, lung, bladder, head and neck cancer
	p210/bcr-abl fusion product	Chronic myelogenous leukemia, acute lymphoblastic leukemia
Development antigens	MART-1/ Melan A	Melanoma
	MAGE-1, MAGE-3	Melanoma, colorectal, lung, gastric cancers
	GAGE family	Melanoma
	Telomerase	Various
Viral antigens	Human papilloma virus	Cervical, penile cancer
	Epstein Barr virus	Burkitt's lymphoma, nasopharyngeal carcinoma, post-transplant lymphoproliferative disorders
Tissue-specific self-antigens	Tyrosinase	Melanoma
	Gp100	Melanoma
	Prostatic acid phosphatase	Prostate cancer
	Prostate-specific antigen	Prostate cancer
	Prostate-specific membrane antigen	Prostate cancer
	Thyroglobulin	Thyroid cancer
	α-fetoprotein	Liver cancer
Overexpressed self-antigens	Her-2/neu	Breast and lung cancers
	Carcinoembryonic antigen	Colorectal, lung, breast cancer
	Muc-1	Colorectal, pancreatic, ovarian, lung cancer

fusion peptides in chronic myelogenous leukemia, and idiotype in the case of B-cell lymphomas and plasmacytomas. A fourth category of TAA is the overexpressed antigen. These TAA are expressed on a wide variety of normal cells but are expressed in abundance by tumor cells. Examples of these are wild-type epitopes of *p53*, HER-2/*neu*, Melan A, carcinoembryonic antigen (CEA), and prostate-specific antigen (PSA). A fifth category of TAA is viral antigens that are associated with some malignancies. Examples of these include Burkitt lymphoma and Epstein-Barr virus (EBV), hepatocellular carcinoma and hepatitis B and C, cervical and anal carcinoma and human papilloma virus, and human T lymphotrophic virus and T-cell leukemia.

Cancer Vaccines

The idea of immunizing patients against malignancy has intrigued physicians for over a hundred years. Success in vaccination programs for infectious disease has led to numerous reports of patients treated with crude tumor extracts. Unfortunately, most of the early studies were poorly controlled, and responses were rare to nonexistent. Better understanding of TAA and recent advances in immunology have led to promising new approaches to tumor vaccine development. In addition to whole tumor cells as vaccine agents, multiple vectors have been used to provide immunization, including peptides, proteins, DNA, and a variety of recombinant viruses such as adenovirus, avipox viruses, and vaccinia virus. A variety of adjuvants are available to enhance the immune response, including bacillus Calmette-Guerin (BCG), incomplete Freund's adjuvant (IFA), QS21, and others. Dendritic cells, with their efficient antigen-processing and presenting machinery and their rich array of accessory molecules and cytokine production, can also be used as a cellular form of immunologic adjuvant.

Peptide Vaccines The understanding that CTL recognize small peptide fragments presented by class I and the identification of shared TAA, particularly among the differentiation antigens of melanoma, has led to numerous peptide vaccine clinical trials, using immunodominant peptides. In the initial trials, peptides were injected alone without adjuvant. Marchand et al. vaccinated advanced melanoma patients with a MAGE-3 peptide epitope and reported four partial responses and three complete responses among 25 treated. The same investigators reported that in some patients with progressive disease, the growing tumors no longer expressed the antigen used for vaccination, implying that vaccination resulted in selection pressure and outgrowth of antigen-negative clones. In subsequent studies, patients with melanoma were immunized with MART-1 or gp100 peptides in IFA. Although immunological responses were seen, meaningful clinical responses were rare. Peptide-based vaccine approaches to renal cell, pancreatic, colon, breast, ovarian, and other cancers have also been disappointing.

One approach based on the use of differentiation antigens known to possess CTL epitopes common to most tumors of a particular histology involves the modification of peptide by chemical substitution of an amino acid that alters its affinity for either the MHC molecule or the T-cell receptor. An altered peptide may also be able to circumvent tolerance mechanisms that limit the immunogenicity of an autoantigen like gp100. Using altered gp100 peptide immunization, Rosenberg et al. were able to demonstrate enhanced gp100 and melanoma cell-specific CTL activity. When administered with systemic IL-2, 13 out of 31 (42%) patients achieved an objective tumor response. These data form the basis of two ongoing randomized clinical trials in patients with advanced melanoma. One of these trials is designed to assess the optimal sequencing of peptide vaccine and high-dose IL-2, and the other trial will assess the overall impact of adding peptide vaccine to IL-2.

Viral Vaccines and DNA The success of viral immunization for infectious disease has stimulated interest in genetically modified viruses as vectors for vaccine immunotherapy. The principal vectors used in successful tumor protection experiments in the mouse include adenoviruses and poxviruses including vaccinia and avipox viruses. Clinical trials with the same viruses modified to express melanoma antigens MART-1 and gp100, adenocarcinoma antigen CEA, and prostate cancer antigen PSA yielded few responses. This failure may be due to the presence of virus-specific inactivating antibodies or the inability to overcome tolerance to autoantigen.

Direct immunization with plasmid DNA can stimulate a response to the encoded protein. The responses tend to be less robust than those following recombinant viral immunization, but the avoidance of introducing viral sequences may provide a safer method and a more restricted immune response. Naked plasmid DNA injected alone is a relatively inefficient method of gene transfer. However, cationic lipids complexed to DNA are capable of mediating high gene-transfer efficiencies *in vitro* and *in vivo*. An alternative currently under investigation is the gene "gun" technology, which propels gold beads coated with antigen-encoding DNA through the skin and into associated antigen-presenting cells. Bacterial DNA sequences may provide immunologic adjuvant effects; those in commonly used plasmid vectors include CpG-oligodinucleotides with immunostimulatory properties. Unmethylated CpG-oligonucleotides are potent stimulators of DC and can activate an innate immune response in an antigen-independent manner, which may contribute in the early steps preceding the development of antigen-specific responses. The combined use of recombinant viral vaccines and plasmids expressing tumor antigens is a promising approach that will undergo further testing over the next several years.

Dendritic Cell Therapy One of the most exciting advances in immunotherapy is the discovery that DC can accumulate and process antigen and stimulate T-cell cytotoxicity against tumors. Experimental studies in the mouse have clearly demonstrated the ability of expanded DC pulsed with antigen to mediate tumor rejection. Over the past few years, there have been numerous phase I and II clinical trials designed to exploit the unique features of the DC in cancer patients. Various methods have been used to optimize the expression and/or presentation of tumor antigen by DC, including peptide pulsing, gene transfer, uptake of tumor cells treated with cytotoxic or apoptosis-inducing agents, and tumor cell-DC fusions. Successful stimulation of antitumor CTL responses using DC immunization in patients have been achieved for a wide variety of malignancies, including melanoma, renal cell cancer, colon cancer, prostate cancer, head and neck cancer, gynecologic cancers, and brain tumors.

Nestle treated 30 advanced melanoma patients with autologous DC pulsed with a variety of immunogenic peptides and observed partial response in five and complete response in three patients. Rosenberg immunized 31 melanoma patients with peptide-pulsed DC and achieved responses in 13. In other melanoma studies, the response rates have been around 10%. In recurrent prostate cancer patients, Murphy reported a 30% response rate (drop in PSA >50% or resolution of lesions on ProstaScint scans) to DC pulsed with peptides derived from prostate-specific membrane antigens. Reports of prostate cancer patients treated with DC loaded with prostatic acid phosphatase (PAP) linked to granulocyte-macrophage colony-stimulating factor (GM-CSF) reveal vigorous immune responses and occasional PSA responses. The latter observation provided the rationale for an ongoing phase III trial of DC loaded with the PAP-cytokine fusion molecule versus unmanipulated DC in patients with hormone-refractory prostate cancer. Another novel DC approach involves transfection of DC with mRNA encoding tumor antigens. Immunotherapy with DC transfected with the mRNA for PSA resulted in a decreasing PSA "slope" in the majority of patents.

The challenge of developing effective immunotherapy for tumors that do not express known common TAA is enormous. In this situation, it is necessary to design vaccine approaches that do not involve defined antigen. In one example, treatment with DC pulsed with peptides eluted from tumor cell culture have generated immune responses and T-cell infiltration of cranial glioblastoma and anaplastic astrocytoma lesions. DC transfected with tumor-derived mRNA have achieved similar results in experimental models. Another intriguing approach utilizes the unique antigen-presenting capabilities of the DC to compensate for relatively poor antigen presentation by tumors. The electrofusion product of autologous tumor cells and DC may enhance the immunogenicity by stimulating both helper and cytotoxic cell responses. This approach is currently undergoing investigation at several institutions in the United State.

Allogeneic Tumor Vaccines An early randomized trial of BCG plus an allogeneic melanoma cell vaccine demonstrated an improved disease-free survival but no improvement in overall survival for stage III melanoma patients. Several allogeneic melanoma cell vaccines are currently being tested. CancerVax is an allogeneic, viable melanoma vaccine composed of three melanoma cell lines that are irradiated prior to administration. Phase II trials of CancerVax in patients with metastatic melanoma suggested improved outcome compared with historical controls and a strong correlation between survival and cellular and humoral res ponses to the vaccine. Based on these data, a multicenter randomized phase III study was initiated in March 1998 comparing CancerVax plus BCG versus placebo plus BCG for patients with stage IV melanoma. Another randomized phase III study is currently comparing CancerVax plus BCG versus IFN-α for stage III melanoma.

Melacine is a lyophilized preparation from two melanoma cell lines. A phase II trial yielded response rates of 20%, with 5% CRs in metastatic melanoma patients. Unfortunately, a multicenter phase III trial comparing low-dose cyclophosphamide plus Melacine to standard four-drug chemotherapy for metastatic melanoma yielded no significant differences in response rates (less than 15% in both treatment arms) or survival. An ongoing multicenter trial compares Melacine plus IFN versus IFN alone for stage IV melanoma. The results of a recently published trial of 689 patients randomized to receive Melacine versus observation following surgical excision of early-stage, intermediate-risk melanoma demonstrated only a trend toward improved disease-free survival. However, a subsequent statistical analysis demonstrated that certain class I HLA types were associated with an improved outcome in patients randomized to receive vaccine. Further studies of the impact of HLA type and other genetic and immunologic characteristics on the immune and clinical response to tumor vaccines are ongoing.

Two vaccinia virus-based allogeneic melanoma vaccines, vaccinia melanoma oncolysate (VMO), and vaccinia melanoma cell lysate (VMCL), have been tested in clinical trials. Despite enthusiastic results from phase II trials, neither agent has demonstrated significant survival advantage over controls in phase III trials. A variation of the allogeneic cell vaccine is the use of antigens shed from allogeneic melanoma cell lines. This approach can yield both humoral and cellular immune responses. Initial results of a small clinical trial using a polyvalent vaccine prepared from material shed by viable melanoma cell lines have been encouraging, and larger trials are currently underway.

Autologous Tumor Vaccines   Active specific immunotherapy (ASI) involves immunization with irradiated autologous tumor cells mixed with viable BCG organisms, viruses or other bacteria as adjuvants. Three randomized trials with 98, 412, and 254 patients each examined the role of ASI as adjuvant therapy for stage II and III colorectal cancer. Although ASI treatment resulted in a trend toward improved disease-free survival, none of the studies provided an overall survival benefit to ASI. ASI for metastatic melanoma and renal cell carcinoma has also been disappointing, with responses in very few patients.

A variety of autologous tumor cell–based vaccine approaches have yielded promising results in small phase I and II trials. Recombinant human GM-CSF has been injected as an adjuvant to ASI for melanoma with promising initial results. GM-CSF acts as a local chemoattractant and stimulator of DC. Another approach to increase the immunogenicity of autologous vaccines is to hapten modify the tumor cells. A hapten is a molecule that itself is not immunogenic, but when combined with a native antigen yields a new immunogen. In a recent group of studies reported, the hapten dinitrophenol (DNP) was added to autologous melanoma cells administered with BCG. Intravenous cyclophosphamide was used to limit T-cell suppressor function. Durable responses were seen in about 25% of those with lung metastases. The DNP vaccine appeared to improve the survival of patients with involved lymph nodes following resection, compared with that reported in matched historical controls.

Heat-Shock Proteins   An efficient method for generating antitumor responses is to prepare heat-shock proteins for use as autologous vaccines. Heat-shock proteins (HSP) are a group of highly conserved proteins found in bacteria and eukaryotic cells that are expressed in the presence of various conditions of environmental stress pressures distinct from those associated with cell necrosis or the induction of apoptosis. HSP function as molecular chaperones, transporting various proteins around the cell. It has been shown in animals and in early human studies that HSP from tumor cells can be highly immunogenic. The immunogenicity derives, at least in part, from the processed intracellular proteins carried by the HSP. This area of investigation has led to the initiation of multicenter clinical vaccine trials of autologous HSP derived from renal cancer.

Gene Therapy   Advances in gene therapy have provided an array of new approaches to enhancing the efficacy of autologous tumor vaccines. In preclinical animal tumor models, introduction of cytokine genes, genes for alloantigen, or co-stimulatory molecules into autologous tumor cell vaccines have all augmented the cellular response and affected tumor regression. A number of gene immunotherapy approaches have reached the clinic. In phase I clinical trials, metastatic melanoma and renal cancer patients treated with irradiated autologous tumor cells engineered to secrete human GM-CSF developed vigorous cellular and humoral responses, but only rarely were objective clinical responses achieved. Gene transfer of IL-2 by direct intratumoral injection of IL-2 DNA in a lipid complex has yielded responses in melanoma and renal cancer in the injected tumor in less than 15%, with only rare responses outside the injected site. In a trial of intratumoral injection of IFN-α in a retroviral vector, there were no responses.

A novel gene immunotherapy approach to malignancy involves the direct intratumoral injection of a DNA plasmid, Allovectin, containing the human gene HLA-B7, which is found infrequently in the human population. The theory behind this approach is that an allogeneic response to the HLA-B7 results in the initiation of a rejection response to the tumor. Gonzales reported a series of 75 end-stage melanoma patients treated with intratumoral injections of HLA-B7 in a DNA/lipid complex, with response in almost 15% of lesions injected. Of 60 head and neck cancer patients treated in three trials, 6 patients achieved clinical responses.

Adoptive Cellular Immunotherapy

LAK Cell Therapy   Studies in the early 1980s revealed that lymphocytes incubated in the presence of high concentrations of IL-2 evolve into lymphokine activated killer (LAK) cells with non-MHC-restricted cytolytic activity against a broad range of tumor targets. In the mouse, administration of LAK cells and IL-2 could mediate the regression of established tumors. Although initial clinical studies were promising, subsequent randomized trials revealed no survival advantage for LAK/IL-2 therapy compared with IL-2 alone.

Tumor-Infiltrating Lymphocyte Cell Therapy   Lymphocyte infiltration of malignant tumors is a well recognized phenomenon. Prior to the era of identification of TAAs, attempts were made to exploit the antigen specificity of the tumor infiltrate for immunotherapy. Tumor infiltrating lymphocytes (TIL) expanded in the presence of IL-2 and autologous tumor cells were found to be 50 to 100 times as potent as LAK cells in mediating the regression of established metastases in mice. Initial clinical studies reported by Rosenberg revealed objective responses in 29

(34%) of 86 patients with metastatic melanoma. Figlin reported a response rate of 35%, with 9% CRs in a series of 55 patients with metastatic renal cell carcinoma. However, a subsequent phase III trial of TIL and IL-2 versus IL-2 alone following nephrectomy in 160 patients with metastatic disease demonstrated no survival advantage for the addition of TIL to IL-2 therapy post nephrectomy.

There are several potential explanations for the limited efficacy of TIL therapy relative to that of IL-2 alone. While some TIL demonstrate cytolytic specificity toward TAAs, many TIL precursor cells are bystander cells without TAA specificity. The resulting TIL are a heterogeneous population that may only include a minority with TAA specificity. The TIL may also lack the ability to propagate *in vivo*, and may lack strong cytolytic activity because of issues of tolerance to autoantigen. Advances over the past few years have enabled the expansion of large numbers of monoclonal or oligoclonal CTL with TAA specificity. This technology has been successfully used to treat post-transplant lymphoproliferative disease with EBV-specific CTL. Current investigation is aimed at enhancing the CTL by inserting genes encoding antitumor or chemokine receptors or genes encoding antitumor cytokines. While studies of monoclonal CTL therapy for solid tumors are progressing, recent reports suggest that efficacy is often hampered by the emergence of antigen loss tumor variants that evolve under the selective pressure of effective CTL therapy.

Allogeneic Hematopoietic Cell Transplant as Tumor Immunotherapy

Immunotherapies can be divided into active and passive treatments, based on whether they depend on an immunization of the tumor-bearing host and lead to a memory response or merely provide a temporary, nonimmunizing exogenous source of immune effectors. One novel approach that combines the properties of active and passive immunotherapy is that of the allogeneic hematopoietic cell transplant, a technique that allows the replacement of the patient's lymphohematopoietic elements with those of a healthy donor. This approach has recently shown promise in malignancies that are resistant to chemotherapy and radiotherapy, elements of the conditioning regimen for traditional transplants that also provide major cytoreduction. For immunogeneic hematologic malignancies such as the myeloid leukemias and lymphomas, it is well known that donor-derived cellular immunity (graft-versus-malignancy, GVM) contributes substantially to long-term disease control. For malignancies that are chemo- and radioresistant, the value of the intense conditioning regimen required for ablation of recipient marrow (and residual malignant clones) is minimal. Therefore, regimens that provide sufficient immunosuppression to allow donor engraftment and suppression of graft-versus-host attack on recipient tissues have been developed. This so-called nonmyeloablative allogeneic stem-cell transplantation is thus a form of allogeneic active immunotherapy in which activation and propagation of a GVM response is achieved during the post-transplantation period. The antigens responsible for durable immune-based control of malignancy are, in most cases, unknown. In selected malignancies, candidate antigens (e.g., minor histocompatibility antigens in myeloid leukemias) have been identified and can be the focus of additional immunologic interventions, including the use of *ex vivo* repetitively stimulated donor-derived T-cell clones. Intriguing methods to enhance the GVM response involve immunization of the donor or *in vitro* stimulation of donor cells with antigen-manipulated DC.

FURTHER READING

Atkins MB, Sparano J, Fisher RI, Weiss GR, Margolin KA, Fink KI, Rubinstein L, Louie A, Mier JW, Gucalp R (1993) Randomized phase II trial of high-dose interleukin-2 either alone or in combination with interferon alfa-2b in advanced renal cell carcinoma. *J Clin Oncol* 11:661–670.

Baselga J, Tripathy D, Mendelsohn J, Baughman S, Benz CC, Dantis L, Sklarin NT, Seidman AD, Hudis CA, Moore J, Rosen PP, Twaddell T, Henderson IC, Norton L (1999) Phase II study of weekly intravenous trastuzumab (Herceptin) in patients with HER2/neu-over-expressing metastatic breast cancer. *Semin Oncol* 26:78–83.

Berd D (2001) Autologous, hapten-modified vaccine as a treatment for human cancers. *Vaccine* 19:2565–2570.

Childs R, Chernoff A, Contentin N, Bahceci E, Schrump D, Leitman S, Read EJ, Tisdale J, Dunbar C, Linehan WM, Young NS, Barrett AJ (2000) Regression of metastatic renal-cell carcinoma after nonmyeloablative allogeneic peripheral-blood stem-cell transplantation. *N Engl J Med*, 343:750–758.

Cobleigh MA, Vogel CL, Tripathy D, Robert NJ, Scholl S, Fehrenbacher L, Wolter JM, Paton V, Shak S, Lieberman G, Slamon DJ (1999) Multinational study of the efficacy and safety of humanized anti-HER2 monoclonal antibody in women who have HER2-overexpressing metastatic breast cancer that has progressed after chemotherapy for metastatic disease. *J Clin Oncol* 17:2639–2648.

Coiffier B, Haioun C, Ketterer N, Engert A, Tilly H, Ma D, Johnson P, Lister A, Feuring-Buske M, Radford JA, Capdeville R, Diehl V, Reyes F (1998) Rituximab (anti-CD20 monoclonal antibody) for the treatment of patients with relapsing or refractory aggressive lymphoma: a multicenter phase II study. *Blood* 92:1927–1932.

Figlin RA, Thompson JA, Bukowski RM, Vogelzang NJ, Novick AC, Lange P, Steinberg GD, Belldegrun AS (1999) Multicenter, randomized, phase III trial of CD8(+) tumor-infiltrating lymphocytes in combination with recombinant interleukin-2 in metastatic renal cell carcinoma. *J Clin Oncol* 17:2521–2529.

Fyfe GA, Fisher RI, Rosenberg SA, Sznol M, Parkinson DR, Louie AC (1996) Long-term response data for 255 patients with metastatic renal cell carcinoma treated with high-dose recombinant interleukin-2 therapy. *J Clin Oncol* 14:2410–2411.

Gleich LL, Gluckman JL, Armstrong S, Biddinger PW, Miller MA, Balakrishnan K, Wilson KM, Saavedra HI, Stambrook PJ (1998) Alloantigen gene therapy for squamous cell carcinoma of the head and neck: results of a phase-1 trial. *Arch Otolaryngol Head Neck Surg* 124:1097–1104.

Hanna MG, Hoover HC, Vermorken JB, Harris JE, Pinedo HM (2001) Adjuvant active specific immunotherapy of stage II and stage III colon cancer with an autologous tumor cell vaccine: first randomized phase III trials show promise. *Vaccine* 19:2576–2582.

Hsueh EC, Gupta RK, Qi K, Morton DL (1998) Correlation of specific immune responses with survival in melanoma patients with distant metastases receiving polyvalent melanoma cell vaccine. *J Clin Oncol* 16:2913–2920.

Khayat D, Coeffic D, Antoine EC (2000) Overview of medical treatments of metastatic malignant melanoma. *ASCO 2000 Education Book*. ASCO, Alexandria, VA, pp. 414–427.

Kirkwood JM, Ibrahim JG, Sondak VK, Richards J, Flaherty LE, Ernstoff MS, Smith TJ, Rao U, Steele M, Blum RH (2000) High- and low-dose interferon alfa-2b in high-risk melanoma: first analysis of intergroup trial E1690/S9111/C9190. *J Clin Oncol*, 18:2444–2458.

Kirkwood JM, Ibrahim JG, Sosman JA, Sondak VK, Agarwala SS, Ernstoff MS, Rao U (2001) High-dose interferon alfa-2b significantly prolongs relapse-free and overall survival compared with the GM2-KLH/QS-21 vaccine in patients with resected stage IIB-III melanoma: results of intergroup trial E1694/S9512/C509801. *J Clin Oncol* 19:2370–2380.

Kirkwood JM, Strawderman MH, Ernstoff MS, Smith TJ, Borden EC, Blum RH (1996) Interferon alfa-2b adjuvant therapy of high-risk resected cutaneous melanoma: the Eastern Cooperative Oncology Group Trial EST 1684. *J Clin Oncol* 14:7–17.

Livingston PO, Wong GY, Adluri S, Tao Y, Padavan M, Parente R, Hanlon C, Calves MJ, Helling F, Ritter G (1994) Improved survival in stage III melanoma patients with GM2 antibodies: a randomized trial of adjuvant vaccination with GM2 ganglioside. *J Clin Oncol* 12:1036–1044.

Marchand M, Van Baren N, Weynants P, Brichard V, Dreno B, Tessier MH, Rankin E, Parmiani G, Arienti F, Humblet Y, Bourlond A, Vanwijck R, Lienard D, Beauduin M, Dietrich PY, Russo V, Kerger J, Masucci G, Jager E, De Greve J, Atzpodien J, Brasseur F, Coulie PG, van der BP, Boon T (1999) Tumor regressions observed in patients with metastatic melanoma treated with an antigenic peptide encoded by gene MAGE-3 and presented by HLA- A1. *Int J Cancer* 80:219–230.

Mitchell MS (1998) Perspective on allogeneic melanoma lysates in active specific immunotherapy. *Semin Oncol* 25:623–635.

Murphy GP, Tjoa BA, Simmons SJ, Ragde H, Rogers M, Elgamal A, Kenny GM, Troychak MJ, Salgaller ML, Boynton AL (1999) Phase II prostate cancer vaccine trial: report of a study involving 37 patients with disease recurrence following primary treatment. *Prostate* 39:54–59.

Negrier S, Escudier B, Lasset C, Douillard JY, Savary J, Chevreau C, Ravaud A, Mercatello A, Peny J, Mousseau M, Philip T, Tursz T (1998) Recombinant human interleukin-2, recombinant human interferon alfa-2a, or both in metastatic renal-cell carcinoma. Groupe Francais d'Immunotherapie. *N Engl J Med* 338:1272–1278.

Riethmuller G, Schneider-Gadicke E, Schlimok G, Schmiegel W, Raab R, Hoffken K, Gruber R, Pichlmaier H, Hirche H, Pichlmayr R (1994) Randomised trial of monoclonal antibody for adjuvant therapy of resected Dukes' C colorectal carcinoma. German Cancer Aid 17-1A Study Group. *Lancet* 343:1177–1183.

Rosenberg SA, Yang JC, Schwartzentruber DJ, Hwu P, Marincola FM, Topalian SL, Restifo NP, Dudley ME, Schwarz SL, Spiess PJ, Wunderlich JR, Parkhurst MR, Kawakami Y, Seipp CA, Einhorn JH, White DE (1998) Immunologic and therapeutic evaluation of a synthetic peptide vaccine for the treatment of patients with metastatic melanoma [see comments]. *Nat Med* 4:321–327.

Rosenberg SA, Yang JC, White DE, Steinberg SM (1998) Durability of complete responses in patients with metastatic cancer treated with high-dose interleukin-2: identification of the antigens mediating response. *Ann Surg* 228:307–319.

Schadendorf D, Nestle FO (2001) Autologous dendritic cells for treatment of advanced cancer—an update. *Recent Results Cancer Res* 158:236–248.

Slamon DJ, Leyland-Jones B, Shak S, Fuchs H, Paton V, Bajamonde A, Fleming T, Eiermann W, Wolter J, Pegram M, Baselga J, Norton L (2001) Use of chemotherapy plus a monoclonal antibody against HER2 for metastatic breast cancer that overexpresses HER2. *N Engl J Med* 344:783–792.

CHAPTER 12

Bone Marrow Transplantation

GEORGE SOMLO

City of Hope Comprehensive Cancer Center, Department of Medical Oncology, Duarte, California

Bone Marrow Transplantation (BMT) is a therapeutic procedure consisting of procurement of approximately 500–1,000 mL (2–3×10^8 nucleated marrow cells/kg of recipient body weight) of bone marrow followed by intravenous reinfusion into the recipient. Bone marrow is aspirated from the posterior iliac crests either under general or epidural anesthesia. The marrow suspension contains hematopoietic progenitor cells characterized by the presence of the CD34 surface antigen, as well as their committed progeny, stromal supportive elements, and other regulatory/facilitating components such as the T lymphocytes. After procurement, the marrow is placed in a container of tissue culture medium and heparin and is filtered through stainless steel screens. The bone marrow is usually reinfused shortly after procurement although it can be frozen for future use.

Allogeneic BMT most frequently involves removal of bone marrow from a human leukocyte antigen (HLA)-matched sibling donor. Two sets of HLA of the class I (A and B loci) and II (HLA-DR) group—three loci each inherited on chromosome 6 from each parent, totaling six loci—need to be identical in the donor and recipient for a perfect 6/6 histocompatible match. Serological testing and, more recently, molecular methods such as polymerase chain reaction (PCR) amplification of HLA genes and the use of allele-specific or sequence-specific oligonucleotides are available to define the suitability of an allogeneic related, or unrelated donor.

Syngeneic BMT implies BMT between an identical twin donor and recipient; partially matched (5/6, one HLA mismatch) donor marrow from a parent or other family members can also be used as the source of BMT. The probability of finding a matched related sibling donor within one's family depends on the number of siblings and may be as low as 25% (in the case of two siblings) and greater than 90% in families with five or more siblings.

With the availability of millions of potential volunteer donors in the International Donor Registry, candidates for BMT may find a suitable donor by searching

UICC Manual of Clinical Oncology, Eighth Edition. Edited by Raphael E. Pollock
ISBN 0-471-22289-5 Copyright © 2004 John Wiley & Sons, Inc.

the registry computer files. The feasibility of BMT from an unrelated donor is then verified by serological and molecular confirmation of a histocompatible 6/6 or 5/6 HLA-A, -B, and -DR match. Presently, the timely availability of a suitable unrelated donor depends greatly on the ethnicity and social background of the recipient. Efforts to expand the pool by including previously under-represented categories of donors are ongoing worldwide.

Hematopoietic progenitor cells are also present in peripheral blood, although their number is relatively low at 1%, compared with the 3–5% estimate in the bone marrow. The population of CD34 antigen-positive progenitors contains the very early hematopoietic progenitor cells—stem cells—capable of repopulating the ablated bone marrow as well as generating and maintaining long-term hematopoiesis. These peripheral blood progenitor stem cells (PBPC) can be collected by a cell separator. The procedure, leukapheresis, or apheresis, usually takes 3–4 hours and is repeated daily until the targeted number of cells (the recommended minimum is $\geq 2 \times 10^6$ CD34$^+$ cells/kg of recipient body weight) has been procured and cryopreserved. In order to improve the yield and quality of the PBPC product, the donor undergoes "priming" or "mobilization" by receiving subcutaneous or intravenous injections of the cytokines granulocyte colony-stimulating factor (G-CSF) or granulocyte-macrophage colony-stimulating factor (GM-CSF) for several days prior to, and during, the days of PBPC collection. Early data suggest that PBPC allows for faster hematopoietic recovery. However, longer follow-up and further studies are needed to assess the efficacy and safety of allogeneic PBPC in comparison to BMT from either related or unrelated donors.

Another promising and relatively rich source of allogeneic hematopoietic stem cells is umbilical cord blood. Cryopreserved cord blood from a fully or partially matched, related, or unrelated donor provides a potentially unlimited source of transplantable cells. Presently, the relatively small volume of cord blood makes this source available mostly for pediatric recipients. *Ex vivo* expansion may render this type of transplant more universally available in the future.

During autologous BMT or PBPC transplant, the patient's own bone marrow and/or PBPC are procured and are cryopreserved for future use. The target number of nucleated and CD34$^+$ cells/kg of patient body weight are the same as for patients undergoing allogeneic bone marrow or PBPC transplants. Priming/mobilization with the hematopoietic growth factors G-CSF or GM-CSF and with or without the addition of chemotherapeutic agents such as cyclophosphamide, improves the quality of PBPC products dramatically and accelerates granulocyte and platelet recovery following PBPC reinfusion in comparison to autologous BMT. To avoid reinfusion of potentially tumor-contaminated bone marrow or PBPC grafts, several methods of positive and/or negative selection have been undergoing clinical testing. Negative selection via chemical (4-HC), and chemical-immunological (removal of CD8 and or CD4 antigen-positive T lymphocytes by lectins covalently bound to the surface of a plastic chamber) methods, or positive selection of CD34 antigen-bearing hematopoietic progenitor cells by means of flow cytometric sorting, or by applying magnetic bead-bound, or avidin/biotin -bound anti-CD34 antibodies are aimed to both decrease the percentage of potentially clonogenic tumor cells and increase the CD34 antigen-positive progenitor cell content in the graft. Whether any of these purging methods will lead to improved outcome is still unknown.

INDICATIONS FOR BMT AND PBPC TRANSPLANT

Allogeneic BMT/PBPC Transplant

Allogeneic BMT could potentially benefit and possibly cure patients suffering from diseases of the following categories:

1. Either genetically determined or secondarily *diminished hematopoiesis* of single or multiple cell lineages. Diseases under such etiology include aplastic anemia, the thalassemias and other red cell disorders, and the myelodysplastic syndromes. Because the pathology is inherently caused by a malfunction in the patient's own hematopoietic system, presently only replacement of the entire bone marrow by an allogeneic transplant can be considered effective except for very special circumstances where immunosuppressive therapy alone may be sufficient (e.g., aplastic anemia).

2. Diseases consisting of predominantly genetically predetermined *deficiencies of specific enzymatic functions.* Severe combined immune deficiency syndrome (SCID) caused by adenosine deaminase deficiency, or Gaucher's disease fall into this category. An allogeneic source of replacement is curative in such conditions.

3. Development and *expansion of malignant clones* within the bone marrow. The bone marrow is either the primary source of disease, such as in the case of chronic myelogenous leukemia, acute myeloid and lymphocytic leukemias, and multiple myeloma, or is a prominent site involved in an otherwise systemic process, as in the case of non-Hodgkin's lymphomas and Hodgkin's disease. Hence, chemoradiotherapeutic elimination of the malignant clone with the concurrent ablation of normal bone marrow necessitates hematopoietic rescue (i.e., transplant).

An allogeneic transplant not only replaces the malfunctioning or ablated bone marrow compartment, but it may—through the graft-versus-tumor phenomena—inflict direct cytotoxic damage upon the targeted malignant elements.

The following hematological malignancies should be considered for treatment by allogeneic BMT in patients under age 60 or younger who are otherwise in good general condition. For patients < 55 years without the availability of a matched, related donor, BMT from an unrelated donor can also be considered for the same indications, inasmuch as the outcome is similar.

Acute Myeloid Leukemia (AML)

- First remission
  - Patients with poor risk cytogenetic features at diagnosis ($-5, -7, +8$, 11q23), or with multiple chromosomal abnormalities

○ Patients with intermediate risk leukemia with normal karyotype, or solitary, nonmyelodysplasia associated, cytogenetic abnormalities
● Induction failure, early relapse, or second remission

In two randomized trials of allogeneic BMT versus autologous BMT versus intensive chemotherapy of patients in first remission AML, results turned out to be somewhat contradictory. In the European Organization for Research and Treatment of Cancer (EORTC) trial, both autologous and allogeneic BMT yielded better survival, whereas in the Eastern Cooperative Oncology group/Southwest Oncology group (ECOG/SWOG) trial, no difference in outcome was observed accross the board among the three arms. However, in the group of patients with unfavorable cytogenetics, allogeneic transplant resulted in the best—5-year survival (40%), and among patients with favorable cytogenetics those treated on the two transplant arms experienced better outcome. Relapse-free survival is 20–30% in patients transplanted in second remission.

Acute Lymphocytic Leukemia (ALL)

● First remission
  ○ White cell count is $> 30,000/\mu L$ at diagnosis
  ○ Presence of Philadelphia chromosome, translocations (8, 14), (4, 11), (1,19)
  ○ Extramedullary disease
  ○ L3 phenotype
  ○ >4 weeks of induction therapy required to achieve remission
● Early relapse, or second remission

The probabilities of relapse-free and overall survival for high-risk patients at 5 years are 39% and 44% in first remission and approximately 20–30% in second remission.

Chronic Myeloid Leukemia (CML)   In the chronic phase, patients under age 40 should undergo BMT from a matched sibling donor, preferably within one year from diagnosis inasmuch as this is the only proven curative treatment for CML. Relapse-free survival rates following BMT are estimated at 60–70%. Older patients could undergo a trial of alpha interferon and could be considered for allogeneic BMT up to age 60 should they fail to achieve cytogenetic remission. More recently, cytogenetic remissions have been obtained after administration of Gleevac^{TM}, a specific tyrosine-kinase inhibitor of the BCR-ABL fusion protein. Whether complete cytogenetic response after Gleevac would lead to long-term survival or cure is unknown at this point, and this question needs to be answered in carefully designed clinical trials.

For patients with CML in accelerated phase or in blast crisis, allogeneic BMT or BMT from an unrelated donor yield relapse-free survival rates of 40% and 15%, respectively. Nonmyeloablative transplant (see below) could be considered for patients who are otherwise not candidates for a full transplant.

Non-Hodgkin's Lymphoma (NHL)   Carefully selected patients with high-grade lymphomas with evidence for bone marrow and peripheral blood involvement and patients with low-grade, therapy-resistant or relapsed disease are considered candidates for either allogeneic or nonmyeloablative BMT.

Multiple Myeloma (MM)   Patients with a suitable sibling donor can be considered candidates for allogeneic BMT. The projected progression-free survival is 30–40% at 3 years from BMT. The mortality rate following BMT is relatively high, approximately 30% in the first 12–16 months. The role of nonmyeloablative allogeneic transplant is currently being tested in order to reduce regimen-related toxicity.

Three Phases of Allogeneic BMT/PBPC Transplant

Pretransplant Phase   Patients with minimal residual neoplastic disease benefit the most from a transplant. To optimally utilize the allogeneic BMT/PBPC procedure, patients first undergo treatment with a preparatory regimen. The ideal preparatory regimen would eradicate all residual malignant elements and would provide sufficient immunosuppression to prevent graft rejection, in addition to inflicting only mild and reversible toxicities. The following preparatory regimens have been used most frequently in the largest series of allogeneic BMT: cyclophosphamide 120 mg/kg and fractionated total body irradiation (FTBI) with 8–14 Gy; etoposide 60 mg/kg and FTBI 12–13.2 Gy; melphalan 110 mg/m^2 and FTBI 9.5–14 Gy; cyclophosphamide 120 mg/kg with busulfan 14–16 mg/kg (more recently, the intravenous formulation at a somewhat lower but bioequivalent dose has been used with less toxicity), and BCNU 300–600 mg/m^2, cyclophosphamide 6 gm/m^2, and etoposide 600–2,400 mg/m^2. Newer regimens adding a third therapeutic drug to well-tested two-drug combinations, or incorporating radioactive iodine-or yttrium-chelated antitumor antibodies against a variety of target antigens such as the myeloid marker CD33 and the B lymphoid marker CD20 are presently being evaluated in the preclinical and clinical setting.

Regimen-related toxicities (RRT) vary depending on the specific and potentially additive side effects of the individual therapeutic agents. Acute and subacute toxicities include nausea, vomiting, mucositis, diarrhea (cyclophosphamide, etoposide, FTBI), seizure, mental status changes, headaches (busulfan, BCNU), rash, facial and salivary gland swelling, acidosis, hypotension (etoposide), hemorrhagic cystitis (cyclophosphamide), rash (FTBI), cardiac toxicity (cyclophosphamide), and veno-occlusive disease consisting of hepatomegaly, jaundice, and weight gain starting 10–25 days after administration of the preparatory regimen (busulfan, FTBI). Prophylactic use of antiemetics, intense hydration, and antiseizure medications aimed to prevent or ameliorate the specific side effects associated with the given preparatory regimen are necessary. Long-term toxicities include sterility; cataracts; osteoporosis; and renal, pulmonary, cardiac, hepatic, and central and peripheral nervous system abnormalities. Potentially fatal long-term side effects include the development of secondary malignancies, both solid tumors and hematologic malignancies.

To substantially reduce regimen-related toxicities, and to offer allogeneic transplant to patients who are too old or weak to withstand regimen-related toxicities of an allogeneic transplant, nonmyeloablative transplants have been evaluated by investigators. The preparatory regimen is administered primarily for the purpose of allowing engraftment, so a therapeutic graft-versus-tumor effect can then take place. The immunotherapeutic agents fludarabine or antithymocyte globulin together with either low-dose total body radiation, or chemotherapeutic agents (cyclophosphamide, busulfan, melphalan, and others) are well tolerated by older and more fragile patients. The immediate treatment-related morbidity/mortality is low, but the incidence of potentially life-threatening graft-versus-host disease (GVHD) remains high, hence immunosuppression (most frequently with a combination of cyclosporin and mycophenolate) is necessary. Follow-up times for most studies using this modality are quite short.

Transplant Phase ABO incompatibility between the donor and recipient could be the source of life-threatening hemolytic complications in up to 30% of allogeneic BMT. Incompatibility is not a contraindication in an otherwise well-matched transplant setting. In case of a major ABO mismatch, the recipient's plasma contains isoagglutinins against the donor red cell antigens (e.g., the recipient's blood type: O; donor type: B). The solution is removal of red cells from the donor graft prior to BMT via a variety of methods (e.g., by continuous flow cell separators) and plasma exchange from the recipient in case of high titers ($\geq 1 : 256$). The management of minor mismatch (e.g., group O donor, group B recipient) includes red cell exchange from the recipient and removal of plasma from the donor marrow if the isoagglutinine titer is ≥ 128.

To decrease the incidence of potentially life-threatening grade II–IV GVHD, several methods to deplete the number of T lymphocytes in the graft cells, thought to be primarily responsible for the development and severity of GVHD, have been applied prior to transplant. Methods of T-cell depletion include exposure of the graft to monoclonal antibodies and to complimentary physicochemical techniques of cell separation. The result is a decrease in the incidence and severity of GVHD. T-cell depletion unfortunately has been associated with an increased incidence of relapse due to the loss of the graft-versus-tumor effect thought to be caused by subsets of primarily T lymphocytes. Additional complications include the development of Epstein-Barr virus-associated B-cell lymphoproliferative disorders and increased incidence of graft failure. Therefore, shortly prior to BMT, instead of T depletion of the graft most transplant teams initiate administration of an immunosuppressant combination to prevent severe acute GVHD.

The actual reinfusion of BM or PBPC product usually takes place 1–3 days after completion of the preparatory phase to avoid any potential damage to the graft caused by circulating metabolites or parent compounds from the preparatory regimen.

Transfusion   Recipients with defective cell-mediated immunity are at risk of T-lymphocyte–mediated GVHD. Therefore, all products should be irradiated with 1.5–2 Gy to avoid engraftment of lymphocytes contained in the transfusion product. Transfusion products are also filtered to decrease the chance of febrile reactions caused by agglutinins. Patients who become refractory to random platelet transfusions may require single pheresis units, ABO-matched products, HLA-matched products, and occasionally IVIgG and plasma exchange to maintain acceptable levels of platelets at >5–$10,000/\mu L$ in patients without severe mucositis or bleeding.

Infectious Complications

Most centers prescribe prophylactic antibiotics to achieve bowel decontamination, as well as fungal prophylaxis, and for patients who are seropositive for herpes simplex, antiviral prophylaxis is routinely provided. Almost all patients undergoing allogeneic transplant develop neutropenic fever. Even if a specific organism is identified by culture, broad-spectrum antibiotics for suspected enteric organisms or skin contaminants are required through recovery from neutropenia.

Cytomegalovirus (CMV) pneumonia may occur in the first 4–10 weeks after BMT, predominantly in already seropositive, and subsequently blood-culture-positive, patients with GVHD. Hence, seronegative patients should be provided with CMV-negative blood products, although seropositive patients may also benefit from leukocyte-free blood transfusions. Monitoring for the potential CMV infection by radiographs, and by twice-a-week shell virus culture or PCR is mandatory in order to initiate gancyclovir therapy at the earliest sign of active disease, especially if prophylactic gancyclovir is not being used for all seropositive patients.

In the post-transplant phase, because of ongoing immune suppression, patients are susceptible to *Pneumocystis carinii*, hence trimethoprim-sulfamethoxazole, or pentamidine prophylaxis is necessary. Reactivation of herpes zoster may occur in 40% of patients after allogeneic BMT. Pre- and post-BMT vaccination strategies are currently being investigated to counteract this problem.

Veno-occlusive disease is a syndrome of hepatomegaly, jaundice, and fluid retention/weight gain due hepatocyte/endothelial damage caused by the preparatory regimen. The onset may vary from within one to several weeks of receiving a usually busulfan-containing preparatory regimen. Management is conservative, and in the most severe cases there are anecdotal reports of successful outcome following the use of thrombolytic agents.

GVHD

At least 50% of post-transplant (both related and unrelated) mortality is caused by GVHD. Therefore, all patients, except recipients of syngeneic BMT, receive GVHD prophylaxis for 6–12 months consisting of combinations of cyclosporin and methotrexate, cyclosporine and prednisone, or all three drugs.

GVHD is caused by transplanted lymphocytes targeting HLA-related antigens in the recipient. T-cell depletion of BM by a variety of methods will decrease the incidence and severity of GVHD but at the price of an increased incidence of graft failure and relapse in the case of leukemias. Because of the ablative effects of the preparatory regimens, host-versus-graft reaction and the resulting graft rejection are quite rare.

Acute GVHD is a syndrome occurring within the first 100 days post allogeneic BMT. HLA mismatch, unrelated donor BMT, sex mismatch between the donor and recipient, donor with multiple prior pregnancies, and older age of the recipient are all factors predicting higher incidence and possibly greater severity of GVHD. The incidence of GVHD varies from 20% in a recipient with fully matched BMT and no other adverse factors to a probability of greater than 80% for developing grade II–IV GVHD in a case of two to three loci mismatched BMT. Biopsy confirmation is recommended because a variety of pathological conditions arising in the post-BMT phase need to be distinguished in the differential diagnosis. The primary manifestations of GVHD include at least one and possibly all three entities of dermatitis, enteritis, and hepatitis. The overall grade of acute GVHD predicts the final outcome. Additional adverse prognostic features include thrombocytopenia and anemia. Patients suffering from grades III–IV GVHD have a greater than 80% probability of dying. Treatment options are limited and include increased doses of corticosteroids, antithymocyte globulin (ATG), daclizumab, and ultraviolet irradiation. Response to treatment is also a predictor of outcome.

Chronic GVHD can develop as the continuation of acute GVHD, or could manifest *de novo*. Under the second scenario, the clinical features are similar to certain autoimmune diseases. The incidence of chronic GVHD varies depending on the age of the recipient and the type of BMT; in younger patients following fully matched BMT, the incidence is under 20%; in recipients of unrelated donor BMT, the incidence is closer to 60%. The primary manifestations include lichen-like or scleroderma-like skin and oral GVHD, keratoconjunctivitis sicca, liver dysfunction, bronchiolitis obliterans, myositis, and occasionally cerebral and peripheral nervous system involvement. Treatment options include immunosuppression with corticosteroids, cyclosporine and azathioprine, thalidomide, mycophenolate, rapamycin, total lymphoid irradiation, and photophoresis. Patients with *de novo* chronic GVHD, without preexisting liver dysfunction and thrombocytopenia and with limited skin and liver function abnormalities, have a far better prognosis then those with extensive GVHD evolving from acute GVHD. The clinical staging system of acute GVHD is illustrated in Table 12.1. During the post-BMT period, patients with chronic GVHD may require long-term antibacterial prophylaxis with trimethoprim-sulfamethoxazole, or a penicillin compound.

Post-transplant strategies in the management of relapse include withdrawal of immunosuppression, administration of interferon α in the case of chronic myelogenous leukemia, and donor leukocyte infusion (DLI). These strategies are most effective in patients with CML and occasionally in patients with acute myeloid leukemia.

TABLE 12.1. Clinical Staging of Acute GVHD

Stage	Skin	Liver	Gut
1	Maculopapular rash on <25% of body surface	Bilirubin 2–3 mg/dL	Diarrhea 500–1,000 mL/day
2	Maculopapular rash on 25–50% of body surface	Bilirubin >3–6 mg/dL	Diarrhea >1,000–1,500 mL/day
3	Generalized erythroderma	Bilirubin >6–15 mg/dL	Diarrhea >1,500 mL/day
4	Desquamation and bullae	Bilirubin >15 mg/dL	Severe pain or ileus

	Stage		
Grade	Skin	Liver	Gut
I	1–2	0	0
II	1–3	1	1
III	2–3	2–3	2–3
IV	2–4	2–4	2–4

Secondary Malignancies The incidence of secondary malignancies (lymphoproliferative disorders, squamous-cell carcinomas, and tumors of the aerodigestive system) depends to a large extent on the underlying disease condition and preparatory regimen and is estimated at 6% 15 years from BMT. Patients treated with an FTBI-containing preparatory regimen seem to be at a higher risk.

Autologous BMT/PBPC Transplant

Of the three disease categories listed as indications for allogeneic BMT, treatment of genetically diminished/dysplastic hematopoiesis is not possible by autologous BMT at the present time, because the problem is inherent to the malfunction of the patient's own bone marrow. Hereditary deficiencies of specific enzymatic functions might be suitable targets for gene transfer. An autologous BMT/PBPC transplant of gene-transfected progenitor cells has the potential to supplement missing enzymatic functions and is an attractive—and possibly the only—option in view of the scarcity of suitable allogeneic donors. The feasibility of such approaches applying a variety of gene transfer methods/factors is presently under investigation.

Inadequate hematopoiesis secondary to the effects of high-dose chemo-/radio-therapy can be supplemented/supported by autologous bone marrow, or by growth factor primed/mobilized PBPC transplant, procured prior to therapy. Autologous BMT has been almost completely replaced by the use of growth factor (G-CSF or GM-CSF) primed/mobilized PBPC transplant in the treatment acute myeloid leukemia, multiple myeloma, and the lymphomas. In the treatment of solid tumors, especially breast, ovarian, and testicular carcinomas, the role of autologous PBPC transplant is primarily supportive following high-dose chemo-/radiotherapeutic consolidation at a time when the tumor load in the hematopoietic system is supposedly minimal, hence the risk of reinfusion of clonogenic tumor cells is thought to be the lowest.

Patients with the following hematologic and solid neoplasms should be considered candidates for autologous BMT/PBPC transplants:

Acute Myeloid Leukemia

- First remission

Earlier randomized trials demonstrated only borderline benefits when comparing autologous BMT with intense chemotherapy consolidation/maintenance. With the advance of PBPC transplants, the mortality rate associated with autologous BMT decreased from the previous 15% to approximately 5%. Accordingly, projected event-free and overall survival is approaching that of patients undergoing allogeneic BMT for intermediate risk AML, although further randomized trials are necessary to confirm this trend. Although methods to purge the harvested BM, especially by chemotherapeutic means (e.g., 4-HC), have been utilized in clinical trials, no clear benefit has been demonstrated in comparison to more intense *in vivo* depletion of potential tumor contamination by intravenous chemotherapy prior to procurement of the BM or PBPC graft.

Non-Hodgkin's Lymphoma

- First remission
- Sensitive and resistant relapse
- Primary resistant NHL

Patients with high-risk disease (age <60, elevated lactate dehydrogenase [LDH], poor performance status, ≥ 1 extranodal site and slow response to induction chemotherapy) and relapsed high-grade and intermediate grade lymphomas benefit from high-dose chemo-/radiation therapy and autologous PBPC transplant. Projected event-free survival for high-risk patients in first remission is 60–80% at 4 years. Patients with chemotherapy-sensitive relapse or resistant relapse experience event-free survival rates of 35–46% and 20%, respectively. In one randomized study of chemotherapy-sensitive NHL, relapse-free and overall survival rates at 5 years were 46% and 53% in the transplant group compared with 12% and 32% in the cohort of patients treated with chemotherapy only.

Patients with low-grade lymphomas may also benefit from PBPC transplant, or alternatively from undergoing high-dose chemotherapy and monoclonal antibody purged BMT. However, because of the long natural history of low-grade NHL, longer follow-up is necessary to definitely prove the benefits of BMT.

Clinical trials are currently ongoing to define the optimal timing and dosage of recently developed anti-CD20 antibodies and their contribution in the setting of an autologous transplant. Similarly, the potential role of radioimmunotherapy incorporating a variety of monoclonal antibodies chelated to radioactive isotopes is now under evaluation.

Hodgkin's Disease

- Induction failure
- Early (<12 months from induction therapy) relapse

The projected event-free survival rates are 60% for patients failing only one prior therapy and approximately 20% for those failing more than two regimens.

Multiple Myeloma

- Stage I–III disease with minimal bone marrow involvement in response

In a randomized trial of 200 patients treated first with induction chemotherapy, the probabilities of event-free and overall survival at 5 years were 28% and 52% for patients undergoing consolidation with BMT and alpha interferon. Event-free and overall survival were lower at 10% and 12% in the control group treated with chemotherapy/interferon only. More recently, tandem cycle peripheral blood progenitor cell supported autologous transplants resulted in higher complete response rates and possibly prolonged progression-free and overall survival.

Breast Cancer   For high-risk primary breast cancer, several phase II trials suggest that high-dose chemotherapy and PBPC transplant may improve relapse and progression-free survival for patients with stage II (>10 axillary lymph nodes involved with metastasis) and IIIA and B (locally advanced and inflammatory) breast cancer in comparison to historical controls. However, maturation of data from several already completed, prospective, randomized trials is necessary to clarify the degree of potential benefit associated with such treatment. The preparatory regimens include combinations of cyclophosphamide with either etoposide and cisplatin, cisplatin and BCNU (most toxic), or carboplatin and thiotepa. Newer regimens have been incorporating taxanes with combinations of cisplatin and cyclophosphamide, or doxorubicin and cyclophosphamide.

For stage IV responsive metastatic disease, pooled data from the international bone marrow registry project an approximately 35% 3-year survival, suggesting improved outcome in comparison to historical controls. Repeated cycles of primarily alkylator-based high-dose chemotherapeutic regimens are presently being tested in phase I–II clinical trials. A randomized trial suggested that a single cycle of high-dose therapy in patients with responding stage IV breast cancer was as effective as a median of eight cycles (range, 1–24 cycles) of standard therapy.

Other Solid Tumors   There are encouraging preliminary results with high-dose chemotherapy and BMT/PBPC transplant with phase II trials of ifosfamide, etoposide, and carboplatin, or cisplatin and cyclophosphamide based combinations for testicular carcinoma, with an estimated 20–25% salvage rate in therapy-resistant/relapsed patients.

Ovarian Carcinoma Several phase II/pilot studies (with preparatory regimens including high-dose carboplatin, melphalan, or anthracyclines) suggest an improved approximately 25–30% progression-free survival at 2–3 years from BMT. Data are currently being generated from recently completed prospective, randomized trials of high-dose therapy versus standard treatment.

Three Phases of Autologous BMT/PBPC Transplant

The preparatory regimens are similar to those used for allogeneic BMT, and need further improvements to improve efficacy. Although quite a few of the regimens are identical to those used in the allogeneic setting, because of the variety of diseases targeted with autologous BMT, the number of preparatory regimens are far greater. The toxicities associated with cyclophosphamide, etoposide, BCNU, FTBI, busulfan, and melphalan have been described earlier. Additional side effects include renal failure, electrolyte wasting, high-frequency hearing loss (cisplatin, carboplatin), confusion, seizure, hemorrhagic cystitis, renal failure (ifosfamide), myalgia, peripheral and central neuropathy (paclitaxel), and cerebellar toxicities (Ara-C).

Transplant Phase The side effects associated with the infusion of marrow or peripheral blood-derived stem cell product are usually minimal and include nausea, potential fluid overload, shortness of breath, and headache. Decreased oxygen saturation can be observed in up to 15% of patients because of fluid overload and the irritant effects of the cryopreservative DMSO.

Post-transplant Phase General support is similar to that described under allogeneic BMT, but there is rarely the need for pneumocystis or CMV prophylaxis.

Graft Failure Following G-CSF-or GM-CSF-primed PBPC transplant, graft failure is extremely unusual. Application of negative selection techniques (purging) or positive selection of CD34 antigen positive progenitor cells, however, may deprive the graft of sufficient numbers of facilitator cells, resulting in delayed neutrophil and platelet recovery.

Bacterial Infections The incidence and types of bacterial infections are similar to what has been observed following an allogeneic BMT, but the period of absolute neutropenia (average duration, 10 days) is shorter. Similarly, while antifungal and antiherpetic prophylaxis is useful, the threat of fatal viral and fungal infections is relatively small.

Secondary Malignancies Myelodysplastic syndrome and secondary leukemias have been reported following autologous BMT/PBPC transplants, and topoisomerase-inhibiting agents applied as part of the preparatory regimen have been implicated. The reported incidence of clonal karyotypic abnormalities can be as high as 9% by 9 years following PBPC transplant, making vigorous follow-up mandatory.

FUTURE DIRECTIONS

Allogeneic BMT

- Improved preparatory regimens with the possible incorporation of radio-immunotherapeutic agents
- Increased utilization of PBPC in order to accelerate engraftment
- Further expansion of the unrelated donor pool
- *Ex vivo* expansion of cord blood
- Further assessment of the role of nonmyeloablative transplants, including their potential benefit in the treatment of solid tumors such as renal cancer.
- Possible incorporation of disease-specific drugs, such as Gleevac, into the treatment regimen either as induction or maintenance
- Further development of specific agents interfering with GVHD.
- Separation of GVHD from the graft-versus-tumor effect by T depletion and subsequent selective reinfusion of tumor-specific, and if necessary graft-facilitating, elements of the negatively selected lymphocyte population
- Incorporation of more efficient antiviral and antifungal agents into the supportive care
- Fast reconstitution of immune competence via T-cell clone transfer from the recipient

Autologous BMT

- Improved preparatory regimens, with the possible incorporation of radio-immunotherapeutic agents and novel therapeutic agents/combinations
- Multiple cycles of BMT
- Incorporation of new growth factors (e.g., thrombopoietin) into the therapeutic schema as mobilizers of PBPC and as accelerators of post-transplant recovery
- *Ex vivo* expansion of purified hematopoietic progenitor cells
- *Ex vivo* expansion of autologous cytolytic tumor-specific lymphocytes and development of adaptive immune therapy through vaccine or antigen-presenting cell generation
- Anti-sense and other gene therapeutic approaches against fusion targets (e.g., bcr-abl)
- Possible incorporation of disease-specific drugs, such as Gleevac, into the treatment regimen either as induction, or maintenance

FURTHER READING

Bensinger WI, Martin P, Storer B, Clift R, Forman S, Negrin R et al. (2001) A prospective, randomized trial of transplantation of marrow versus peripheral blood cells from HLA-identical siblings in patients treated for hematologic malignancies. *N Engl J Med* 344: 175–181.

Burnett A, Goldstone AH, Stevens RMF, Hann IM, Rees JK, Gray RG, Wheatley K. (1998) Randomized comparison of addition of autologous bone-marrow transplantation to intensive chemotherapy for acute myeloid leukemia in first remission: results of MRC AML 10 trial. *Lancet* 351:700–708.

Childs R, Chernoff A, Contentin N, Bahceci E, Schrump D, Leitman S et al. (2000) Regression of metastatic renal-cell carcinoma after nonmyeloablative allogeneic peripheral-blood stem-cell transplantation. *N Engl J Med* 14:750–758.

Freedman AS, Neuberg D, Mauch P, Soiffer RJ, Anderson K, Fisher DC et al. (1999) Long-term follow-up of autologous bone marrow transplantation in patients with relapsed follicular lymphoma. *Blood* 94:3325–3333.

Michallet M, Bilger K, Garban F, Attal M, Huyn A, Blaise D et al. (2001) Allogeneic hematopoietic stem-cell transplantation after nonmyeloablative preparatory regimens: impact of pretransplantation and posttransplantation factors on outcome. *J Clin Oncol* 19:3340–3349.

Rocha V, Cornish J, Sievers E, Filipovich A, Locatelli F, Peters C et al. (2001) Comparison of outcomes of unrelated bone marrow and umbilical cord blood transplants in children with acute leukemia. *Blood* 15:2962–2971.

Thomas ED, Blume KG, Forman SJ (eds) (1999) *Hematopoietic Cell Tranplantation*, 2nd edition. Malden, Massachusetts, Blackwell Science.

Zittoun RA, Mandelli F, Willemze R, de Witte T, Labar B, Resegotti L et al. (1995) Autologous or allogeneic bone marrow transplantation compared with intensive chemotherapy in acute myelogenous leukemia. European Organization for Research and Treatment of Cancer (EORTC) and the GIMEMA Leukemia Cooperative Groups. *N Engl J Med* 332:217–223.

CHAPTER 13

Biostatistics and Clinical Trials

RICHARD SYLVESTER, PATRICK THERASSE,
MARTINE VAN GLABBEKE, and XAVIER PAOLETTI

European Organization for Research and Treatment of Cancer (EORTC),
Data Center, Brussels, Belgium

The rapid introduction of new treatments into daily clinical practice requires a co-ordinated research program going from basic research to the implementation of phase I, phase II, and phase III clinical trials. Changes in clinical practice are the logical consequence of conclusions drawn from clinical trials. It is therefore essential to use appropriate methodology to ensure that clinical trials produce robust and reliable results. This chapter reviews the basic principles involved in the design, conduct, analysis, and reporting of clinical trials.

Medical practice and medical research, including basic research, clinical research, and teaching, all depend on each other. Clinical research in cancer is not a luxury, but is essential in order to rapidly develop and identify new state-of-the-art treatments and to invalidate ineffective ones. In order to decrease the time needed to evaluate new therapeutic modalities and transfer laboratory discoveries into routine clinical practice, various partners in clinical research such as the pharmaceutical industry, academic centers, international research organizations, and regulatory authorities must all work together. A multinational, multicenter, and multidisciplinary team effort allows complex therapies to be evaluated even in rare cancers.

To have the most impact on day-to-day clinical practice, simple, large-scale, multicenter, randomized, phase III clinical trials with key endpoints are required. The role of biostatistics in the field of cancer research, clinical trials in particular, has undergone enormous changes since the first randomized clinical trial in acute lymphocytic leukemia, which was organized in 1954 by the U.S. National Cancer Institute (NCI). It is just within these past 40 years that the ground rules for

UICC Manual of Clinical Oncology, Eighth Edition. Edited by Raphael E. Pollock
ISBN 0-471-22289-5 Copyright © 2004 John Wiley & Sons, Inc.

conducting clinical trials on a scientific basis have been worked out and the appropriate statistical methodology developed.

A number of authorities have been actively involved in the development of statistical guidelines. Within the European Union, in 1990, the Committee for Proprietary Medicinal Products (CPMP) published an EEC Note for Guidance dealing with the subject of Good Clinical Practice. In 1995, the CPMP adopted a Note for Guidance dealing with biostatistical methodology in clinical trials, which was followed up by a Note for Guidance on the Evaluation of Anticancer Medicinal Products in Man. The International Conference on Harmonization (ICH), a joint effort of the United States, European Union, and Japan, has developed the ICH Harmonized Tripartite Guidelines ICH Topic E8, entitled General Considerations for Clinical Trials, and ICH Topic E9, entitled, Statistical Principles for Clinical Trials. This chapter will review some of the basic biostatistical and methodological principles involved in conduct of cancer clinical trials.

WHAT IS A CLINICAL TRIAL?

A clinical trial may be defined as a carefully designed, prospective medical study that attempts to answer a precisely defined set of questions with respect to the effects of a particular treatment or treatments. The results of a clinical trial, which are based on a limited sample of patients, are then used to make decisions about how a given patient population should be treated in the future.

A prerequisite for any clinical trial is a good idea that is worth testing. A clinical trial should attempt to answer the most important questions concerning the disease under study, obtain reliable results, and be able to convince others of the validity of the results. A clinical trial is a major undertaking that requires considerable money, personnel, facilities, time, and effort. Thus, the need for the study, its value, and its potential impact on the medical community must all be carefully considered to ensure that the interest of the question justifies, within the boundaries of accepted ethical standards, the time, and expense necessary to carry it out.

THE PROTOCOL

The most important document pertaining to any clinical trial is the protocol, a self-contained description of the rationale, objectives, and logistics of the study. The success or failure of the trial may depend on how well the protocol was written, because a poorly designed, ambiguous, or incompletely documented protocol will result in a trial that may not be able to answer the questions of interest. The protocol must be detailed and precisely worded so that the study is uniformly carried out by all participants.

A committee of researchers representing each of the different disciplines involved in the study should be appointed to plan, design, and write the protocol. Sufficient time must be allowed for the protocol to be designed, written, revised (one or more times), and eventually reviewed by external review boards before its implementation and the start of patient enrolment.

TYPES OF STUDIES

The testing of a new therapy is a long-term project, involving different types of trials during its development. The first step in planning a new trial is to precisely define its objectives and to determine the type of study to be carried out. Studies generally fall into one of three categories: phase I, phase II, or phase III. However, under certain conditions, some trials may be designed up front as phase I/II or phase II/III, consecutively addressing two different primary endpoints. In the same perspective, the development of certain new classes of anticancer agents may not need to go through the classical phase I, II, III development sequence to prove their efficacy. Under such circumstances, certain phases may sometimes be omitted. Trials within the pharmaceutical industry also go through phase IV or post-marketing surveillance studies. Phase IV trials will not be considered in this chapter.

Phase I Trials

Phase I trials are the first studies in humans after the completion of preclinical studies. They screen for toxicity as the dose is gradually escalated. The fundamental assumption is that both the antitumor effect and the toxicity increase as the dose is increased.

Objectives   The usual aims of a phase I study are to:

- establish the maximum tolerated dose (MTD) for the new drug for a given schedule via a given route of administration and propose a dose for phase II evaluation in man that is an acceptable trade-off between potential activity and toxicity
- identify the dose-limiting toxicity (DLT) and determine the qualitative (which organ system is involved) toxicity as well as the quantitative (predictability, extent, duration, and reversibility) toxicity of the drug
- determine the pharmacokinetic and the pharmacodynamic profile of the drug
- document possible antitumor activity.

Different definitions of the MTD have been used. In the Unites States, it is the highest dose at which one or no DLTs have been observed among six patients. It is then the MTD that is recommended for use in phase II trials. In Europe, the MTD is defined as the lowest dose that produces an unacceptable rate of DLTs, generally two out of three or two out of six patients. The recommended dose for phase II studies is then the dose level just below the MTD.

Patient Selection Criteria The following general eligibility criteria are applicable for phase I trials of anticancer drugs:

- all patients must have microscopically confirmed advanced disease that is no longer amenable to established forms of treatment
- a reasonable performance status (World Health Organization [WHO] ≤ 2)
- in general, patients should not have received chemo-, immuno-, or radio-therapy within the last 4 weeks prior to entry in the trial
- patients should have a normal bone marrow function and no major impairment of hepatic, renal, and cardiac functions
- all patients must give their written informed consent

Further eligibility criteria will depend on the drug under study.

Statistical Design Various methods for selecting a safe starting dose are used. For example, in EORTC studies, one-tenth of the LD10 (lethal dose) in mice, expressed as milligrams per meter squared, is used as the starting dose for phase I trials, provided that this dose is not toxic in a second species (normally the rat).

The successive dose levels to be investigated are based on a sequence of incremental increases that are generally independent of the design used to allocate patients to the various dose levels. For example, a classical method of dose escalation (called Fibonacci increments) specifies that successive dose levels are increased by 100%, 67%, 50%, 40%, 33%, 33%, 33%, and so on above the preceding dose level. Another possibility is to base the next higher dose level on the toxicity observed at previous levels, for example, to increase by 100% when mild toxicity has been reported but by only 50% in case of moderate toxicity.

The Fibonacci search scheme (also called the Up and Down or 3 + 3 scheme) is the most widely used because it does not require statistical expertise. An initial cohort of three patients is given the new compound at the starting dose level and the toxic effects are carefully observed. If no DLT is observed after a predetermined period of observation, the dose is escalated in another cohort of three patients and toxicity is again documented. If one DLT is reported among the three patients, another three patients are treated at that dose level. The dose escalation procedure is continued until two out of three or two out of six patients experience DLTs at a given dose, a level of toxicity that is usually considered to be unacceptable. Generally, it is requested that a minimum of six patients are treated at the dose level to be recommended for phase II studies and kept on treatment to determine chronic or cumulative toxicity.

The two main criticisms of this design are the high number of patients included at very low dose levels that have little or no antitumor effect and the poor accuracy of the final recommended dose level when only six patients have been included at that dose.

Alternative designs have been explored in an attempt to improve the efficiency of the dose finding process. A method that is increasingly used is the Continual

Reassessment Method (CRM). The successive dose levels to be tested are determined as explained above, for example, using a Fibonacci sequence or even increments based on toxicity data from previous levels. However, the design itself is radically different. The MTD is now precisely defined as the dose level associated with a predefined percent of DLTs (generally 20%). The MTD is the dose recommended for use in phase II trials. The general idea is to include patients at the best current estimate of the MTD. The design is divided into two stages, an initial escalation stage until the first DLT is observed, and then a second, model-guided stage.

The escalation stage is model free and designed by the statistician in collaboration with the investigator. One possible rule is to escalate the dose level after each patient has been treated as long as only mild toxicity has been observed. When the first moderate (not DLT) toxicity occurs, cohorts of three patients are then treated before continuing to the next dose level.

After the first DLT, the model comes into play. The dose for the next patient is now recommended based on estimates of the probability of toxicity at each dose level. A dose-toxicity curve is fit to the data after each new patient has been assessed. This curve provides updated estimates of the probability of a DLT at each dose level. Among the set of available doses, the one whose probability of a DLT is the closest to the target is allocated to the next patient. Not only are we assured that each patient is treated at the best current estimate of the MTD given all previous data, but, in addition, the accuracy of the estimate of the MTD improves as the sample size increases.

The main advantage of the CRM is to decrease the number of patients included at very low dose levels and to concentrate most of the dose levels actually used around the MTD. A confidence interval for the final estimate can also be calculated.

Other designs have also been proposed to consider particular situations such as phase I trials of combinations of well-known agents, trials based on both activity and toxicity, and pharmacokinetically guided dose escalation. So far, none of these methods have really been applied in practice. More recently, the U.S. NCI has opened new perspectives for phase I trials with the accelerated titration method that empirically permits intrapatient dose escalation in successive cohorts of single patients. This method also has the advantage of providing more information on cumulative toxicity.

Phase II Trials

Phase II trials are carried out following the phase I assessment of a new agent, but before large-scale comparative studies are launched in the framework of randomized phase III trials.

The term *phase II* encompasses clinical studies of widely differing intentions. A major distinction should be made between single-agent phase II trials, assessing the activity and toxicity of a new agent in a defined tumor type, and feasibility studies, exploring the therapeutic effect of a new agent or of an established active agent in combination with other drugs or other treatment modalities.

Single-Agent Phase II Trials Within the category of single-agent phase II trials, a further distinction should be made between early phase II trials and late phase II trials, which differ in both their goals and the need for intensive monitoring.

Objectives. Early (single-agent) phase II trials are designed to identify antitumor activity in a representative sample of tumor types, usually selected on the basis of the targets used for drug development and the results of both preclinical studies and phase I trials. A further aim of early phase II trials is to obtain a more detailed description of the drug's toxicity, particularly cumulative toxicity (which is easier to study in a phase II patient population than in phase I) and to study ways to manage toxicity (e.g., by preventive measures, concomitant medication, etc.). Early phase II trials may also study the pharmacokinetics/pharmacodynamics relationship. At the conclusion of an early phase II trial, a decision is made whether to stop the further research and development of a new agent or to continue its clinical development.

Once early phase II trials have been successfully conducted in an initial sample of tumor types, late (single-agent) phase II trials may be conducted to document antitumor activity in other types of tumors. Further documentation of the toxicity profile is also a goal in late phase II trials, but at this stage the principal toxicities have generally already been identified. At the conclusion of a late phase II trial, a decision is made whether to further evaluate the drug in a specific tumor type.

Endpoints. The primary endpoint for both early and late single-agent phase II trials is antitumor activity, expressed in terms of response to therapy. Toxicity is often a secondary endpoint.

Response to therapy is assessed on the basis of objective criteria that measure the decrease in size of prospectively selected target lesions. International standards are available for measuring response in phase II trials, the most common being RECIST (http://www3.oup.co.uk/jnci/extra/920205.pdf). It should be underlined that response to therapy is not an appropriate surrogate for therapeutic benefit but only an indicator of antitumor activity. Toxicity is graded according to standard scales based on objective parameters. The Common Toxicity Criteria (CTC) has been the most widely used criteria. In October 2003, this was replaced by the Common Terminology Criteria for Adverse Events v3.0 (CTCAE) (http://ctep. info.nih.gov/reporting/ctc.html). In single-drug phase II studies, toxicity should be separately assessed for each cycle of therapy in order to evaluate potential cumulative side effects.

Pharmacokinetic parameters are generally secondary endpoints in early phase II trials.

Patient Selection Criteria. Essential patient selection criteria for both types of single-agent phase II trials are:

- histological confirmation of the tumor type specified in the trial
- presence of objectively measurable disease

Furthermore, patients selected for these studies should have a reasonable potential for responding to an active compound and should not have any extra risk of experiencing toxicity. The remaining selection criteria therefore concern the prior therapy that the patient has received and ensure that the patient is fit to receive an investigational drug:

- patients should not be candidates for standard therapy or they should have progressed under those therapies
- patients should have a reasonable performance status (WHO ≤ 2)
- bone marrow, hepatic, renal, and cardiac function must be normal (impaired hepatic or renal function may result in abnormally elevated serum drug levels that could induce unexpected or more severe side effects)
- written informed consent must always be obtained from the patient

Further specification of the targeted population for late phase II trials may require more restrictive patient selection criteria (i.e., in terms of histology and/or prior therapy)

Statistical Design. Single-agent phase II trials enrol as few patients as possible and can only demonstrate whether a new agent has antitumor activity or not. They are generally nonrandomized with all patients receiving the same treatment.

For ethical reasons, some type of sequential approach is necessary so that inactive drugs and drugs for which the toxicity has been underestimated in phase I studies are rejected from further study as quickly as possible.

When deciding on the future of a new agent, two types of errors can be made: a false-positive or type I error (recommending an inactive agent for further study) and a false-negative or type II error (declaring an active agent to be inactive). The false negative is the more serious error of the two because, once rejected, the drug will generally have no further chance to show its activity, whereas an inactive drug can still be rejected if its activity is not validated at a later stage. Thus, most designs employed in this type of trial try to minimize the probability of a false-negative result.

A number of two-stage statistical designs have been developed that allow the drug to be rejected at the end of the first stage if there is insufficient activity to warrant further testing. Otherwise, the second stage continues to the full sample size allowing a more precise evaluation of the response rate (Gehan 1961) or a decision rule for further investigation of the agent (Fleming 1982, Simon 1989).

The Gehan design is generally preferred for early phase II trials because it minimizes the number of patients treated during the first stage if the drug is totally inactive. Its major drawback is that it does not provide a clear statistical decision rule concerning the further development of the drug. Therefore, the Simon or the Fleming designs are generally preferred for late single-agent phase II trials because they provide such a decision rule.

Randomized phase II trials are of potential interest in the following situations:

- if different schedules of the same drug are to be tested
- if two or more drugs are ready for testing at the same time
- if an analogue of an active compound is to be screened.

A randomized phase II trial should be viewed as a simultaneous screening of several compounds and *not* as a comparative trial. The principal purpose of randomization is to eliminate conscious or unconscious bias on the part of the investigator in assigning treatments, that is, to balance the treatment groups with respect to all prognostic factors, both known and unknown, which may affect a patient's response to treatment.

When screening analogues, it may be useful to carry out a randomized phase II trial including the parent compound as a control arm in order to reduce the incidence of false negatives. That is, if the analogue is found to be inactive but the parent compound is also found to be inactive in a patient population for which it is normally active, then the negative results with the analogue may be due to the patient population studied and does not necessarily mean that the analogue is inactive.

In randomized phase II studies, the sample size for each arm is computed using one of the previously described classical phase II designs.

Feasibility Trials

Objectives. Although a phase II trial might demonstrate that a potential new therapy has some activity, it can never conclude that it would be of therapeutic benefit to patients. This is the goal of phase III trials. In most situations, the information provided by phase I and single-agent phase II trials is not sufficient to justify the treatment of a large number of patients with the new drug in a randomized phase III trial. Particularly when a new agent is incorporated in a combined therapy, the feasibility of the new therapeutic approach is unknown.

Feasibility studies aim at providing the justification for a subsequent large randomized phase III trial that will assess the potential therapeutic value of a new treatment. It must be underlined that a nonrandomized feasibility study will never provide evidence of a possible therapeutic benefit.

Endpoints. The choice of an appropriate endpoint(s) that reflects the feasibility of a new therapeutic approach is delicate. The toxicity profile of the complete projected plan of therapy is an obvious index of the treatment's feasibility. If possible, it may also be desirable to study the treatment's long-term side effects. The proportion of patients completing therapy may also be used as an index of its feasibility.

Response to therapy is not necessarily an endpoint in these trials: indeed, antitumor activity of all agents should have been previously documented in single-agent trials and response to treatment is not an appropriate surrogate for therapeutic benefit. However, a minimum response rate is sometimes used as a criteria for continuing investigation of the treatment.

The interest of the investigators and the potential of the group to conduct the phase III trial may also need to be evaluated in the framework of a feasibility study. The recruitment rate may be used to assess these factors.

Patient Selection Criteria. Patients selected for a feasibility study should be those that would be included in the following randomized trial. Therefore, inclusion and exclusion criteria should be as close as possible to those that will be used in the future phase III trial.

Statistical Design. The diversity of possible endpoints explains the diversity of statistical designs proposed for feasibility studies.

For trials where toxicity and response rate have been chosen as principal endpoints, Bryant and Day (1995) have proposed a two stage design based on predefined "acceptable" and "unacceptable" levels of toxicity and response rate. This design provides a decision rule based on the number of responses and the number of cases with unacceptable toxicity observed during the first and second stages of the trial. Both the Simon optimal design and the Bryant and Day design can be calculated at http://www.biostats.upci.pitt.edu/biostats/ClinicalStudyDesign/.

If feasibility trials are not randomized, they will then provide the temptation of making conscious or unconscious comparisons based on "historical" controls. This attitude carries a high risk of the medical community adopting overly toxic or overly aggressive therapies despite the lack of scientific evidence of a real therapeutic benefit. In this situation, large-scale randomized trials may become extremely difficult to conduct.

It is therefore recommended in feasibility studies to randomize the new treatment versus the standard therapy that would serve as the control arm in the future phase III trial. Patients randomized in the feasibility trial might then be included in the phase III trial reducing the total number of patients needed to complete both studies.

Therapeutic Approaches Other than Cytotoxic Drugs The methods described above have been developed for the investigation of cytotoxic drugs. They are based on the assumption of an increasing dose-effect relationship, both for efficacy and adverse events. They should not be blindly applied in other situations, for example, when investigating:

- a drug for which a maximum in its dose response curve has been attained
- a drug designed to enhance the activity of another agent
- a drug designed to reduce the side effects of another agent
- an investigational radiotherapy schedule
- a radiosensitizer.
- a biological response modifier
- a cytostatic drug

In these cases, the whole policy of early development may need to be redefined because standard guidelines are inadequate.

Phase III Trials

After a drug has been found to have at least some predefined minimal amount of activity in phase II trials, the next step is to determine its relative efficacy in a randomized phase III trial. Phase III trials are thus comparative in nature, that is the experience of a group of patients receiving a new treatment is compared either with a group of patients receiving a standard treatment or to an untreated control group.

The possible goals of a phase III trial are:

- to determine the effectiveness of a treatment relative to the (treated) natural history of the disease; in this case, the trial has a no treatment or a placebo control arm
- to determine the effectiveness of the new treatment as compared with the best current standard therapy
- to determine if a new treatment is as effective as the standard therapy but is associated with less severe toxicity (equivalence or noninferiority study).

Phase III clinical trials should be planned to reliably detect small to moderate treatment differences, not to identify major breakthroughs. The minimum treatment benefit that is considered to be clinically worthwhile depends on the severity of the disease and on the side effects of the treatment. While a large survival improvement may be demanded of an aggressive therapy for a fatal condition, it is self-defeating to hope for more than a small survival improvement with an adjuvant therapy in good prognosis patients.

Preference should be given to large simple studies that compare two treatments that are as different as possible. Crossover trials are generally to be avoided because the underlying assumptions for carrying out such trials are almost never valid in cancer studies.

Patient Selection   In randomized trials the entry of patients should be guided by the uncertainty principle. That is, only if there is substantial uncertainty over the best treatment should the patient be randomized.

Two diverging attitudes may be adopted in defining eligibility criteria: they can be very precisely and narrowly defined so that only a small fraction of the available patients are eligible, or at the other extreme they can be left as loose as possible so that most available patients can be entered into the trial.

Narrow eligibility criteria make the patient sample as homogeneous as possible. This may be desirable to unequivocally identify treatment benefits in a subgroup of patients with well-defined prognostic features. All future patients in the same group may then be offered the treatment should it prove to be effective in the clinical trial. Narrow eligibility criteria are preferable to broad ones when there are good *a priori* reasons to believe that the treatment will be beneficial only to a subgroup of patients, an assumption that is rarely true in practice. Patient accrual may suffer, however, if the patient eligibility criteria are too restrictive.

Broad eligibility criteria result in a faster patient accrual into the trial, therefore reducing the total duration of the study. They also yield a sample of patients that is more closely representative of the total patient population. Their results can therefore be more readily extrapolated to all future patients outside the trial. Broad eligibility criteria are preferable to narrow ones when little is known at the time of designing the trial concerning the possible benefit that may be expected from the treatment under investigation in different subgroups of patients. In this (common) situation, the most plausible hypothesis is that the treatment effect will be similar in different subgroups of patients and that the best strategy is to then choose eligibility criteria that are as broad as possible.

Randomization and Stratification   Treatment allocation by a random process is the method of choice in phase III trials. Randomization ensures that the decision of treating a patient with one of the treatments being tested does not depend on the patient's characteristics. Therefore, if a difference in outcome is observed, it can reasonably be attributed to a difference in treatment effect and not to differences in the prognosis of the groups of patients being treated. Randomization is the single most important technique to prevent selection bias.

Randomization does not only guarantee the validity of the statistical tests used to compare treatments, but also balances, on the average, the distribution of both known and unknown prognostic factors in the treatment groups. To reduce the possibility of bias, a central randomization via the Internet or by telephone is recommended.

Especially in small to moderate size trials, random allocation does not assure that an equal number of patients will receive each treatment or that all the prognostic factors will be equally distributed in the treatment groups. Consequently, the randomization should be stratified for a small number of factors of known prognostic importance.

With stratified randomization, patients are stratified prospectively at the time of entry into the trial in order to obtain an approximately equal balance of patients and important prognostic factors in the treatment groups. Two different techniques may be used: static methods, for example, based on randomized blocks, or dynamic methods such as the minimization technique.

With the system of randomized blocks, a separate randomization list (set of treatment assignments) for each possible cross-classification of the prognostic factors to stratify for is required. Within each block the treatments are ordered at random. If there are only a few patients within a block, balance within the block and hence within the trial is not assured. Stratification by too many factors may, by chance, be worse than no stratification at all.

Dynamic methods use the actual treatment assignments and the baseline characteristics of patients who have already been entered to determine the treatment assignment for each new patient. The minimization technique's goal is to ensure a balance within each level of each stratification factor separately, but not necessarily within all the possible combinations of the different factors.

Multicenter trials should be stratified by institution. If the minimization technique is used to allocate treatments, a larger number of stratification factors may eventually be taken into account. It is recommended, however, that the randomization procedure be kept simple by stratifying only by the one or two most important prognostic variables in addition to institution.

Endpoints

Adjuvant Trials. Adjuvant therapy is given to patients treated by a potentially curative primary therapy, but for whom there is a substantial risk of recurrence. The primary therapy is usually surgery, but may also include radiotherapy, chemotherapy, or a combination of these. Adjuvant trials thus study treatments given to patients who are clinically disease free after a "curative" primary treatment.

The goal of an adjuvant trial is generally to compare the duration of survival, disease-free survival, or disease-free interval in two or more treatment groups. Another characteristic of adjuvant trials is the necessity for large sample sizes and long-term follow up. Large sample sizes are needed because the power to detect differences in survival and disease-free interval depends on the number of events (deaths or recurrences) in each group rather than on the total number of patients entered.

Advanced Disease Trials. Advanced disease includes all patients for whom local treatment is no longer curative. There are two types of advanced disease: recurrent or locally advanced disease, in which the disease is still confined to the region of the primary tumor, as opposed to metastatic disease, where the disease has spread to distant sites.

When studying the effects of a new agent in patients with advanced disease, the CPMP recommends the following endpoints: progression-free survival, overall survival, and response rate. Late side effects may also be important in phase III trials. The "time to event" approach is preferred for the analysis of these endpoints.

To assess the symptomatic effect of a treatment, an additional efficacy endpoint that may be used is symptom control that is supported by quality of life data. In recent years, much interest has focused on integrating both quality of life endpoints and economic evaluations in randomized phase III trials. In both adjuvant and advanced disease trials, these may play an important role and may be among the endpoints studied. Quality of life assessment is the subject of another chapter in this book.

Definition of Endpoints. When comparing two treatments, the starting point in most time to event analyses is the date of randomization. Use of the date of surgery (or start of treatment) as the starting point may be biased if not all patients are operated on at the same point in time. If the event has not yet been observed at the time of the last available information, then the patient is censored at this date.

In the definitions that follow, disease "progression" will be understood to mean progression, relapse, or recurrence as appropriate. Thus, no distinction will be made between progression, relapse, or recurrence when defining the following time intervals.

- *Response to treatment*: to be assessed in accordance with RECIST recommendations. As a general rule, the denominator of the response rate must include all eligible patients.

- *Duration of complete response (complete responders only)*: the time interval between the date of complete response and the date of disease progression after complete response.
- *Duration of response (complete and partial responders taken together)*: the time interval between the date of first response and the date of disease progression.
- *Time to progression*: the time interval between the date of randomization and the date of disease progression.

Note: for these last three endpoints, in the case that progression has not yet been observed, the patient is censored at the date of the last examination.

- *Disease-free interval (adjuvant trials)*: the time interval between the date of randomization and the date of first disease progression (the period during which there is no evidence of disease activity). For patients who die prior to progression (for any reason other than malignant disease), their follow-up is censored at the date of death. Otherwise, it is censored at the date of the last follow-up examination if no progression has been observed.
- *Disease-free survival (adjuvant trials)*: the time interval between the date of randomization and the date of disease progression or death, whichever comes first. If neither event has been observed, then the patient is censored at the date of the last follow-up examination.
- *Duration of survival*: the time interval between the date of randomization and the date of death. Patients who were still alive when last traced are censored at the date of last follow-up. While a separate analysis of death due to malignant disease may be carried out (deaths due to other causes are censored at the date of death), the main analysis should always include deaths due to any cause.
- Any other *time to event* endpoint should be precisely defined in the protocol and include the starting date (generally the randomization date), an exhaustive list of events considered to be a failure and a definition of the date of censoring.

Number of Patients Required   In order to obtain the correct results and to be able to convince others of their validity, large randomized trials are required to have a high power to detect small but medically important differences: randomized in order to reduce the possibility of systematic bias and large in order to reduce the risk of random errors.

To ensure the feasibility of a phase III trial, the design should be kept as simple as possible. In most cases, a simple randomization between just two treatments is recommended. Trials with more than two treatment arms require proportionately more patients and are generally more difficult to recruit because patients must agree to receive any of the possible treatments.

A distinction should be made between trials attempting to show a difference in therapeutic effect (superiority trials) and trials designed to show noninferiority (one sided) or equivalence (two sided). In noninferiority trials, one considers a more conservative treatment to be noninferior to the standard when it is not worse than the standard by some given amount.

In both situations, the null hypothesis is the "opposite" of what you are trying to prove. In trials attempting to show a difference, one attempts to reject the null hypothesis of no difference in treatment efficacy, whereas in trials attempting to show the noninferiority of a new more conservative treatment, the null hypothesis is that the new treatment is less effective than the standard treatment by some given amount.

Using the primary endpoint of interest, the determination of the sample size depends on the following factors when planning a clinical trial:

- A realistic prior estimate for the endpoint of interest in the control group.
- Realistic estimates of the size of the plausible treatment effect and/or the medically worthwhile treatment effect.
- The size of the type I error α (false-positive rate; ≤ 0.05; generally two-sided except for noninferiority trials, where it is recommended to take a one-sided $\alpha = 0.025$) and type II error β (false-negative rate; ≤ 0.20). $1 - \beta$ is called the power.
- Realistic estimates of the expected accrual rate and duration of patient entry. In general, the expected duration of patient entry should not exceed 5 years.
- The duration of follow-up after closing the trial to patient entry.

Based on this information, the total number of events (in case of a time to event endpoint) and patients needed can be calculated in order to ensure a high power of detecting a postulated treatment difference at a prespecified significance level (α).

The number of patients sharply increases when the size of the treatment benefit of interest decreases. For example, the total number of deaths required in a phase III study may vary from 192 for a simple two-arm study trying to detect a 50% increase in the median duration of survival to more than 1,500 trying to detect a 5% difference in absolute survival. Enough patients must be entered so that the required number of events can be observed within a given follow-up period.

To detect a difference in response rate, assuming a response rate of 50% in the control arm, the number of patients required on each arm for a two-sided test, with type I and type II errors of 5% and 20% respectively, is approximately:

Number of Patients Per Arm	Difference
1400	5%
360	10%
160	15%
90	20%
60	25%

Noninferiority trials and equivalence studies require considerably more patients than superiority trials since the hypothesized difference in such trials should be no more than one-third to one-half of the difference sought in superiority studies.

It may be possible to use a two-by-two factorial design to answer two questions for the price of one. An example of such a trial is a study with the following treatment groups:

1. surgery
2. surgery + radiotherapy
3. surgery + chemotherapy
4. surgery + radiotherapy + chemotherapy

Through the proper use of retrospective stratification, each treatment group can be used twice, once to study the benefit of radiotherapy and once to study the effect of chemotherapy. For example, the effect of radiotherapy is assessed by comparing radiotherapy to no radiotherapy (2 and 4 versus 1 and 3) with a retrospective stratification for whether or not patients received chemotherapy. The number of patients required for this study will be similar to that needed for a two arm trial if there is no radiotherapy/chemotherapy interaction.

Statistical Analyses   The time to an event should be estimated using the Kaplan-Meier technique. In general, univariate time to event comparisons are based on the log-rank test, whether testing for a difference (two sided), equivalence (two sided), or noninferiority (one sided). For response data, chi-square tests are to be employed.

The main prognostic factors should be taken into account in a multivariate analysis. The Cox model for time-to-event analyses and logistic regression for binary endpoints are to be recommended. Retrospective stratification or multi-variate models may be employed in order to adjust the treatment comparison for the possible effect of prognostic factors.

As a general rule, no subgroup analyses (comparing treatments in only a subgroup of patients) should be performed unless they were specified *a priori* in the protocol. Any subgroup analyses that are carried out should be considered to be hypothesis generating and must be interpreted with extreme caution.

Interim Analyses   If one or more interim analyses are performed, the following information should be clearly stated in the protocol:

1. The intention to perform interim analyses, their number and the timing of analyses.
2. The statistical stopping guidelines that will be used, whether it be to prematurely close the trial to patient entry or to decide whether to publish the results of the trial before observing the required number of events. Stopping guidelines based on an alpha-spending function with an O'Brien-Fleming boundary are generally to be recommended for efficacy endpoints.

While a trial is still open to patient entry, the results of the interim analysis must not be presented to trial participants. The report should be submitted to an Independent Data Monitoring Committee (IDMC) composed of at least one statistician and two medical doctors who are not participating in the trial. The IDMC will take into account not only the statistical stopping guidelines but also all other available information, for example, adverse events, quality of life and results from other similar trials in making their recommendations.

Inclusion/Exclusion of Patients from Analyses

Patient Eligibility. A patient is eligible if he or she satisfies all the patient inclusion criteria as defined in the protocol. Eligibility is based only on the patient's status at the time of entry into the trial and cannot be based on something that happens to the patient after registration or randomization.

All patients, including ineligible ones, should be treated and followed in accordance with the protocol whenever possible. If the cause of ineligibility is such that a patient cannot be kept in the protocol, then the patient must at least be followed for the duration of survival. Patients who are randomized and refuse all treatment and examinations should also be followed for the duration of survival. Thus, all randomized patients, including ineligible ones, should be followed for survival.

Patients who do not meet the entry criteria based on histological review (or the review of any other material that is taken prior to entry in the trial, but for which the conclusions are known only after the patient has been entered) should continue in the protocol whenever possible and at least be followed for the duration of survival.

Intent to Treat Principle. For efficacy comparisons in phase III trials, patients should be analyzed according to the "intent to treat" principle (all conclusions are based on all randomized patients according to the treatment group assigned by randomization).

Additional supportive "per protocol" analyses may be carried out, for example, analyses that are restricted to the eligible patients or eligible patients who started their treatment, especially in noninferiority or equivalence studies where an intent to treat analysis may dilute the size of the treatment effect. Toxicity analyses should be based on all randomized patients who started their assigned treatment.

Meta-Analyses Probably the biggest flaw in most clinical trials is that too few patients have been entered and an insufficient number of events have been observed to have a high probability of detecting a medically plausible difference in treatment efficacy should it exist. Meta-analysis (overview) is the process of using formal statistical methods to combine together the quantitative results of separate but similar studies in order to

1. increase the statistical power to detect differences in treatment efficacy
2. increase the precision of the estimated treatment effect

Although meta-analyses can play a very important role in the overall scientific assessment of a treatment's efficacy, they are not a panacea or a cure all. In particular, they should not be a replacement for large-scale randomized clinical trials.

QUALITY ASSURANCE

With clinical trials becoming more and more complex, necessary quality assurance systems must be established to ensure that the trial is performed and the data are generated in compliance with the standards of Good Clinical Practice. It is important that all observations and findings are verifiable. In multicenter trials quality control procedures may include:

- on-site monitoring of the participating institutions to ensure protocol compliance and data quality
- verification of data transfer to a central data center
- establishment of external review committees: treatment modality, response to treatment, pathology
- review and quality control of data by a central data center

REPORTING RESULTS

All patients entered in a trial must be accounted for when reporting results. The data presented per treatment group should include:

- Accrual per center.
- Patient eligibility: the reasons for being ineligible should be presented in detail.
- Patient characteristics at randomization.
- Treatment data based on all patients who started their treatment. For chemotherapy, this should include the number of cycles delivered, dose intensity, dose reductions and delays, premature interruption of treatment, reasons for the discontinuation of treatment, and side effects. For other modalities, corresponding data should be presented. Special attention should be paid to serious adverse events. Detailed case descriptions should be provided for each toxic or early death. A standardized toxicity grading system such as the Common Terminology Criteria for Adverse Events should be used.
- Efficacy results, generally including data on the duration of survival, cause of death, time to progression, and so on, for all randomized patients. While the trial is still open to patient entry, efficacy data *must not* be presented by treatment arm in order to avoid premature conclusions. Rather than just reporting P values, which give no information about the possible size of the treatment effect, it is important to provide an estimate of the size of the treatment effect along with its 95% confidence interval.

Guidelines (CONSORT) have recently been published in an attempt to standardize the format for the reporting of clinical trials and to improve the quality of published reports.

FURTHER READING

American Society of Clinical Oncology (1997) Critical role of phase I clinical trials in cancer treatment. *J Clin Oncol* 15:853–859.

Begg C, Cho M, Eastwood S et al (1996) Improving the quality of reporting of randomized controlled trials: the CONSORT Statement. *JAMA* 276:637–639.

Blackwelder W (1982) Proving the null hypothesis in clinical trials. *Control Clin Trials* 3: 345–353.

Bryant J, Day R (1995) Incorporating toxicity considerations into the design of two-stage phase II clinical trials. *Biometrics* 51:1372–1383.

Committee for Proprietary Medicinal Products (CPMP) (1999) Points to Consider on Biostatistical/Methodological Issues Arising from Recent CPMP Discussions on Licensing Applications: Choice of Delta. *CPMP/EWP/2158/99.*

Committee for Proprietary Medicinal Products (CPMP) (2000) Note for Guidance on Evaluation of Anticancer Medicinal Products in Man. *CPMP/EWP/205/95 rev. 1.*

Committee for Proprietary Medicinal Products (CPMP) (2000) Points to Consider on Switching Between Superiority and Non-Inferiority. *CPMP/EWP/482/9.*

CPMP Working Party on Efficacy of Medicinal Products (1990) EEC Note for Guidance: Good Clinical Practice for Trials on Medicinal Products in the European Community. *Pharmacol Toxicol* 67:361–372.

CPMP Working Party on Efficacy of Medicinal Products (1995) Note for Guidance III/3630/92-EN, Biostatistical Methodology in Clinical Trials in Applications for Marketing Authorizations for Medicinal Products. *Stat Med* 14:1659–1682.

Eisenhauer EA, Dwyer PJ, Christian M, Humphrey JS (2000) Phase I clinical trial design in cancer drug development. *J Clin Oncol* 18:684–692.

Fleming T (1982) One sample multiple testing procedure for phase II clinical trials. *Biometrics* 38:143–151.

Fleming T, DeMets D (1993) Monitoring of clinical trials: issues and recommendations. *Control Clin Trials* 14:183–197.

Gehan E (1961) The determination of the number of patients required in a preliminary and a follow-up trial of a new chemotherapeutic agent. *J Chronic Dis* 13:346–353.

Gelber R, Goldhirsch A (1991) Meta-analysis: the fashion of summing-up evidence. *Ann Oncol* 2:461–468.

ICH Topic E8 (1997) General Considerations for Clinical Trials. *CPMP/ICH/291/95.*

ICH Topic E9 (1998) Statistical Principles for Clinical Trials. *CPMP/ICH/363/96.*

Machin D, Campbell M, Fayers P, Pinol A (1997) *Sample Size Tables for Clinical Studies.* Blackwell Science Ltd, Oxford.

Moher D, Schultz KF, Altman DG for the CONSORT Group (2001) The CONSORT Statement: Revised Recommendations for Improving the Quality of Reports of Parallel-Group Randomised Trials. *Lancet* 357:1191–1194.

O'Quigley J, Shen LZ (1996) Continual reassessment method: a likelihood approach. *Biometrics* 52:673–684.

Parmar M, Machin D (1995) *Survival Analysis: A Practical Approach.* John Wiley and Sons, Chichester.

Perry KT (1997) From mouse to man: the early clinical testings. *Drug Info J* 31:729–736.

Pocock S (1979) Allocation of patients to treatment in clinical trials. *Biometrics* 35:183–197.

Simon R (1989) Optimal two-stage designs for phase II clinical trials. *Control Clin Trials* 10:1–10.

Simon R, Freidlin B, Rubinstein L, Arbuck S, Collins J, Christian M (1997) Accelerated titration designs for phase I clinical trials in oncology. *J Natl Cancer Inst* 89:1138–1147.

Smith MA, Ungerleider RS, Korn EL, Rubinstein L, Simon R (1997) Role of independent data-monitoring committees in randomized clinical trials sponsored by the National Cancer Institute. *J Clin Oncol* 15:2736–2743.

Sylvester R (1984) Planning cancer clinical trials. In *Cancer Clinical Trials, Methods and Practice.* Buyse M, Staquet M, Sylvester R, (eds.) Oxford University Press, Oxford.

Sylvester R, Collette L, Duchateau L (2000) The role of meta-analyses in assessing cancer treatments. *Eur J Cancer* 36:1351–1358.

Therasse P, Arbuck SG, Eisenhauer EA, Wanders J, Kaplan RS, Rubinstein L, Verweij J, van Glabbeke M, van Oosterom AT, Christian MC, Gwyther SG (2000) New guidelines to evaluate the response to treatment in solid tumors. *J Natl Cancer Inst* 92:205–216.

CHAPTER 14

Skin and Melanoma Cancer

B.H. BURMEISTER, B.M. SMITHERS, and M.G. POULSEN

Princess Alexandra Hospital, Department of Radiation Oncology, South Brisbane, Queensland, Australia

Skin and melanoma cancers are common in white populations, especially within the tropics. True incidences of nonmelanomatous skin cancers are difficult to assess due to poor reporting by the physician and patient. A large proportion of skin cancers are, in fact, never biopsied and therefore never registered. Melanomas, however, are carefully registered and incidences are known in most countries. Although cure rates are high, it is important to remember that deaths still occur despite widespread public awareness of the importance of early diagnosis. Clinicians practicing in tropical areas or where sun exposure is common should be able to identify both melanomatous and nonmelanomatous skin cancers. Education of the patient in identifying lesions is also extremely important. Management of skin cancer is extremely complex and in this chapter some basic guidelines regarding management are outlined.

EPIDEMIOLOGY AND ETIOLOGY

Skin cancers are diseases of fair skin populations. The incidence of skin cancer rises steadily the closer one gets to the equator. More than 90% of skin cancers develop in exposed areas such as the head, neck, and limbs. Basal cell carcinomas (BCC) are the most commonly diagnosed nonmelanomatous skin cancers. Squamous cell carcinomas (SCC) are less common, and Merkel cell carcinomas are rare. The median age for BCCs and SCCs is 68 years. It is, however, common to see nonmelanomatous skin cancers in young people as a result of both recreational and occupational exposures. The male to female ratio is 4 to 1. Factors other than sunlight that may be related to the incidence of skin cancer include some genetic

UICC Manual of Clinical Oncology, Eighth Edition. Edited by Raphael E. Pollock
ISBN 0-471-22289-5 Copyright © 2004 John Wiley & Sons, Inc.

conditions such as xeroderma pigmentosum and Gorlin's syndrome. Prolonged immunosuppression associated with organ transplantation or low-grade lymphomas may result in a 20-fold increase in nonmelanomatous skin cancer. Rarer predisposing factors include exposure to chemicals such as arsenic, tar, nitrogen mustard, and ionizing radiation. Sites of trauma from burns or small pox vaccination scars may also be associated with skin cancers.

The incidence of melanoma varies, but the annual increase is between 2–5% in the white populations worldwide. In Australia, the mortality trends have stabilized recently, but in general the mortality trends have increased. In Europe, there is a higher rate of melanoma in the Scandinavian countries as compared with France and Italy. This may relate to behavioral patterns and a natural protection from increased pigmentation in the skin in the southern European countries. The incidence rises after 50 years of age. The incidence is similar between males and females within a population.

Pale skin, a tendency to sunburn, fair or red hair, large numbers of melanocytic nevi, and multiple dysplastic nevi have been shown to be independent risk factors for the development of melanoma. Sun exposure, in particular, exposure to UVB radiation has been shown to be an important risk factor. Melanoma is rare in black populations and has a lower frequency in populations with increased skin pigmentation, where the most common form of melanoma tends to be the subungual form and melanoma on the palms of the hands and soles of the feet.

SCREENING

Skin cancer prevention has been mainly in the form of education programs aimed at altering attitudes about sunlight and suntans. In Australia, this has resulted in increased wearing of hats, avoidance of the sun around the middle of the day, and the increased use of sunscreens. Recent data have suggested that the regular use of sunscreens certainly can prevent the development of new solar keratoses. The main purpose of screening is to detect tumors at an early stage and, in doing so, to reduce costs and morbidity of treatment. The American Academy of Dermatologists initiated a national melanoma/skin cancer prevention program in 1985 that has reached over 600,000 people. As a result of this program, there were more than 35,000 nonmelanomatous skin cancers diagnosed and 3,500 melanomas identified.

Screening high-risk individuals will detect melanoma at an early stage. Population screening has not been proven cost effective. People with a strong family history, especially in first-degree relatives, and those with more than 100 melanocytic nevi and multiple dysplastic nevi should be monitored by general skin examination and given advice relating to the appropriate measures of sun protection. Prophylactic excision of dysplastic nevi and other benign nevi does not reduce the melanoma risk because a melanoma may develop as a new lesion rather than from a pre-existing nevus.

DIAGNOSTIC MEASURES INCLUDING PATHOLOGY

BCCs and SCCs commonly present on sun-exposed areas. The most common sites to be affected occur in the head and neck area, forearms, and hands. BCCs usually present as a slow-growing well circumscribed papule, often with a pearly surface and telangectasiae visible. Larger lesions may have central ulceration. Sometimes central regression may occur. Melanin deposits can be seen in pigmented varieties of BCC, which may make the lesion difficult to distinguish from a melanoma. Less common varieties of BCC include the superficial multicentric, morphaeic, cystic, basosquamous, and fibroepitheliomatous variants. SCCs may have a variety of clinical appearances and may appear as a hyperkeratosis, an ulcer, or a scaly patch that bleeds. SCCs are commonly associated with actinic keratoses, which are flat scaly pink lesions. Only rarely do keratoses progress to become SCC, and they are common in sun-exposed populations. Some may resemble a proliferative lesion such as a keratoacanthoma, although they do not regress spontaneously. Merkel cell carcinomas do not have a classic appearance and typically arise in the head and neck region of an elderly person. Commonly, they present as a rapidly growing nodule that is painless and has a bluish-red color. Many patients may present initially with nodal disease and no obvious primary.

Clinical evaluation of all sun-exposed areas in the patient with skin cancer is essential. Examination of regional lymph nodes close to a documented lesion should also be performed. Suspicious lesions may be biopsied with a shave excision or punch biopsy. Advanced lesions may need further investigations to establish their true extent. Lesions on the face and scalp may be associated with bone or neural invasion. Computed tomography (CT) scan or magnetic resonance imaging (MRI) in this setting may be indicated. Merkel cell tumors have a high metastatic potential and may require a routine systemic baseline workup.

The pathology of nonmelanomatous skin cancers is well recognized. BCCs are characterized by nests of palisading small basal type cells with relatively large, basophilic nuclei. Mitoses are common. Several morphologic types are known, the commonest being solid, cystic, pigmented, and multifocal superficial varieties.

BCCs are generally not invasive during the first five to ten years of the growth cycle. Once invasive, however, extensive local destruction can occur. Nodal spread is exceptionally rare. SCCs arise from epidermal keratinocytes and are typified by keratinization and horn pearl formation. Most tumors are well differentiated, although if they occur in association with immunosuppression (e.g, renal transplant recipient or low-grade lymphoma), they may be very aggressive. In general, SCCs are more aggressive than BCCs, with a tendency to local recurrence and lymph node spread. Perineural invasion is also common, particularly around the face. Merkel cell carcinomas are of neuroendocrine origin and are composed of sheets of small cells that stain for neurone-specific enolase. The presumed cell of origin lies in the basal layer of the epithelium, particularly around hair follicles. Merkel cell carcinomas are commonly mistaken for BCCs or lymphomas of the skin. They are highly malignant, with a propensity for local recurrence, nodal spread, and distant metastases. Spontaneous regression has been documented.

The diagnosis of melanoma should be considered for any change in a pigmented lesion on the skin. The requirements to make the diagnosis of melanoma are understanding the variance of melanoma, the history relating to the lesion, a good light, and magnification. A melanotic melanoma is more difficult to diagnose but should be considered where there is any unusual nonpigmented lesion of the skin. The ABCDE mnemonic is useful.

A = Asymmetry in shape

B = Border notably irregular

C = Color variation, often with a number of different shades of black, brown, blue, or progressive pallor within a pigmented lesion

D = Diameter often greater than 5 mm

E = Elevation

Recently, the use of skin-surface microscopy (dermatoscopy, dermoscopy, epiluminescence microscopy) has been advocated to improve the diagnosis of pigmented lesions. This technique uses a high-quality light with magnification in combination with immersion oil at the skin microscope interface, allowing improved recognition of pigment patterns by making the epidermis translucent.

Melanoma is a cancer of the melanocytes and thus arises in the basal layer of the epidermis. Where the melanoma is confined to the epidermis, it is *in situ* and thus curable by local excision. Once it has invaded the basement membrane, there is the potential for metastases. The growth of a melanoma may be radial (horizontal) or vertical within the epidermis or dermis. The potential for metastasis relates to the depth of invasion, in particular the thickness of the melanoma at the time of diagnosis. The clinicopathologic classification of melanoma is into four categories:

1. *Superficial spreading melanoma* (50–60%)—Lateral growth phase predominates with subsequent vertical growth phase.
2. *Nodular melanoma* (10–15%)—Vertical growth phase predominates and thus melanomas tend to be thicker at the time of diagnosis.
3. *Lentigomaligna melanoma* (10–15%)—Slow-growing and commonly found in UV-exposed regions, particularly the head and neck.
4. *Acral lentiginous melanoma* (1–10%)—Occur on the palms, soles and nail beds and are not related to sun exposure.

Desmoplastic or neurotropic melanomas are variants of nodular or superficial spreading melanomas, having a propensity for local recurrence and spread along superficial nerves. Seventy percent of these tumors present in the head and neck region and are slightly more common in males.

Increasing number of nodes involved is associated with decreasing survival. The presence of extracapsular invasion of a lymph node may be associated with higher rate of local recurrence within a dissected lymph node basin as well as decreased overall survival.

TABLE 14.1. Survival According to Depth of Invasion

	10-Year Survival (%)
Melanoma *in situ*	100
<0.75 mm	97–98
0.75–1.5 mm	90
1.5–3.0 mm	75
>3.0 mm	55

The prognosis of melanoma is dependent on the depth of invasion (Table 14.1). Other indicators of a poor prognosis include male gender, ulceration, and a high mitotic rate.

STAGING

The stage at presentation of skin cancer and particularly melanoma is the most important factor influencing outcome. The following is the staging of according to the UICC 6th Edition (2002) TNM pretreatment clinical classification.

T—Primary tumor (nonmelanomatous skin cancer)

TX Primary tumor cannot be assessed
T0 No evidence of primary tumor
Tis Carcinoma *in situ*
T1 Tumor < 2 cm in greatest dimension
T2 Tumor > 2 cm but ≤ 5 cm in its greatest dimension
T3 Tumor > 5 cm in its greatest dimension
T4 Tumor invades deep extradermal structure, e.g, cartilage, skeleton, muscle, or bone

N—Regional lymph nodes (nonmelanomatous skin cancer)

NX Regional lymph nodes cannot be assessed
N0 No regional node metastasis
N1 Regional lymph node metastasis

M—Distant metastasis

MX Distant metastasis cannot be assessed
M0 No distant metastasis
M1 Distant metastasis

Stage grouping—Nonmelanomatous Skin Cancer

Stage 0	Tis	N0	M0
Stage I	T1	N0	M0
Stage II	T2	N0	M0
	T3	N0	M0

Stage III	T4	N0	M0
	Any T	N1	M0
Stage IV	Any T	Any N	M1

The staging system for melanoma is in evolution. The American Joint Committee on Cancer (AJCC), from a large combined database of patient data, has advocated a system reflecting the influence of thickness, ulceration, and lymph node status. The lymph node staging can be based on microscopic disease (sentinel node biopsy) or on macroscopic assessment. For metastatic disease, the number of involved nodes, the site of the visceral metastases, and the presence or absence of an elevated serum lactic dehydrogenase have also been shown to be markers of outcome and have been included in the AJCC staging system.

pT—Primary tumor (melanoma)
pTX Primary tumor cannot be assessed

pT0 No evidence of primary tumor

pTis Melanoma *in situ*

pT1 Tumor < 1.0 mm in thickness, a = without ulceration, b = with ulceration

pT2 Tumor > 1.0 mm but ≤ 2.0 mm in thickness, a = without ulceration, b = with ulceration

pT3 Tumor > 2.0 mm but ≤ 4.0 mm in thickness, a = without ulceration, b = with ulceration

pT4 Tumor > 4.0 mm in thickness, a = without ulceration, b = with ulceration

N—Regional lymph nodes (melanoma)
NX Regional lymph nodes cannot be assessed

N0 No regional lymph node metastasis

N1 One node, a = micrometstasis, b = macrometastasis

N2 Two or three nodes, a = micrometstasis, b = macrometastasis, c = in transit metastasis/satellite(s) without metastatic nodes

N3 Four or more nodes, matted nodes, in transit disease, satellite(s), and metastatic node(s) and/or in transit metastasis

M—Distant metastasis
MX Distant metastasis cannot be assessed

M0 No distant metastasis

M1a Distant skin subcutaneous or nodal metastasis

M1b Lung metastasis

M1c All other visceral metastasis or any distant metastasis with an elevated serum lactic dehydrogenase

Proposed stage groupings—Melanoma (clinical or pathological)

Stage 0	pTis	N0	M0
Stage IA	pT1a	N0	M0

Stage IIA	pT2b	N0	M0
	pT3a		
Stage IIB	pT3b	N0	M0
	pT4a		
Stage IIC	pT4b	N0	M0
Stage III	Any pT	N positive	M0
Stage IV	Any pT	Any N	Any M1

Pathological staging

Stage 0	pTis	N0	M0
Stage 1A	pT1a	N0	M0
Stage 1B	pT1b	N0	M0
	pT2a		

SURGERY

Surgical excision offers a high rate of cure for BCC and SCC and produces a specimen that can be analyzed for completeness of excision and subtype. Histological features are in turn predictive of the future behavior of the tumor where a recurrence would be destructive (e.g., adjacent to an eyelid, lip, or nasal margin) or in danger of becoming seriously invasive (e.g., inner canthus, nasal base, or postauricular areas). Maximum information about the tumor behavior is desirable. Surgical excision of primary BCCs offers a 4.8% recurrence at 5 years and 2.9% recurrence if the lesion is less than 5 mm. Curettage and electrocautery (C & E) can be effectively and efficiently used to treat small, peripheral BCCs, with a 9.5% recurrence rate at 5 years. Large lesions (> 1 cm) have a 22.7% 5-year recurrence rate, and lesions on critical features such as nose, lip, eyelid, and so on can recur without any obvious surface signs after C & E, thus delaying appropriate treatment and allowing added destruction. C & E is not considered complete treatment for SCC. Special problems attend recurrent lesions, infiltrative lesions, and lesions showing invasion along nerves. Generally, a wider margin of clearance and a more comprehensive pathology assessment is indicated. Recurrences are more likely with the infiltrative type of BCC, the poorly differentiated SCC, and certain positions. Clinically involved nodes should be treated at the time of surgery by means of a lymphadenectomy. In particular, mucocutaneous SCC, large SCCs, peripheral SCCs, and SCCs arising in burn scars will show a higher rate of metastasis.

With view to margins, BCCs can be cleared histologically with a 2–5 mm margin when of solid or circumscribed variety. SCCs generally require a 5–10 mm margin, depending on the size and aggressive nature of the tumor. Between 5 and 8 mm is required when BCCs are infiltrative. Incomplete deep margins involving BCCs should be re-excised, but incomplete lateral margins can be considered for observation. All incompletely excised SCCs should be re-excised where possible. Completeness of excision is enhanced by careful preoperative markings before the local anesthesia is infiltrated. Adequate lighting and good surgical technique increase the rate of complete excision. Moh's micrographic surgery can produce a 98% cure rate for BCCs but is tedious and slow. It should be reserved for difficult BCCs in critical sites because the operator maps out the entire cut surface histologically.

Lesions suspicious of being melanoma should be treated by *complete* excisional biopsy. Punch biopsy or incisional biopsy should be reserved for large lesions where complete excision is not reasonable as the initial diagnostic manoeuvre. The margin of diagnostic excisional biopsies should be a minimum of 2 mm.

The minimum margin for definitive therapy of an invasive melanoma is 1 cm. For melanomas greater than 4 mm and desmoplastic variants, the potential for local recurrence is greater and thus some experts would recommend margins of 2–3 cm. There is no evidence that this will offer a survival benefit and will only improve local control. The depth of excision should at least equal the excision margin. There is no need to excise the deep fascia. Re-excision is recommended if the margins of excisional biopsy were less than those recommended for a definitive lesion. At the time of definitive excision, a primary melanoma should be manipulated minimally to decrease the potential for implantation of the wound. Flap repair or skin graft may be required at certain sites to obtain satisfactory skin coverage. Melanoma *in situ* (level I melanoma) should be excised with a minimum margin of 5 mm.

Subungual melanomas are removed by amputation, usually proximal to the interphalangeal joint of the thumb or the distal phalangeal joint of a finger or toe. Tumors of the sole of the foot should be excised appropriately but with an aim to preserve weight-bearing skin. The use of specialized plastic surgical flap repairs may assist in coverage over weight-bearing areas at this site.

Elective lymph node dissection is not recommended for the majority of patients with melanoma. There may be some subgroups who benefit, but this is yet to be defined. The advent of sentinel node biopsy has further reduced the need for elective node dissection. It may be reasonable to perform an elective lymph node dissection where an advanced primary tumor is in reasonable proximity to a well-defined lymph node drainage site and sentinel node biopsy is not available. Clinical evidence of lymph node involvement should be confirmed with fine-needle aspiration cytology if this is available. If open biopsy is absolutely necessary, the biopsy excision should be removed in continuity with the lymphatic field on block dissection. Confirmed lymph node involvement indicates the need for a full therapeutic lymph node dissection. Removal of single nodes is not satisfactory because of the potential for multiple nodal involvement. There is a risk of local recurrence within a dissected lymph node field in patients who have positive lymph nodes, notably if there are multiple nodes involved or if there is the presence of extracapsular invasion.

Recently, lymphatic mapping, sentinel lymph node biopsy, and selective lymphadenectomy have been reported. In patients with a melanoma greater than 1 mm in thickness, the lymphatic drainage and the specific sentinel node is defined with lymphoscintigraphy. A blue dye that also contains a radioisotope is injected around the primary site. The lymph node is identified and removed. If positive for metastatic melanoma, the patient then proceeds to a prophylactic lymph node dissection. There is clear evidence of the prognostic value of the sentinel node biopsy. The effect of this technique on patient survival is being evaluated in randomized trials.

Metastases localized to a limb may be treated using a technique of limb vascular isolation with chemotherapy (typically melphalan). It is recommended that local recurrences or in transit metastases localized to a limb first be excised. Further recurrences should be considered for isolated limb therapy. The technique of isolated limb perfusion was developed as a means of ensuring high doses of regional chemotherapy accompanied by moderate hyperthermia as a way of dealing with regional melanoma. That technique requires a major operative procedure and can be associated with significant morbidity. In Australia, isolated limb perfusion has been replaced with the technique of isolated limb infusion. This technique is simpler and does not require the sophisticated equipment of isolated limb perfusion. It is performed using manual syringing of melphalan through the effected limb via radiologically placed catheters within the main vessels. The morbidity of the technique is far less than with isolated limb perfusion. The response rates of up to 80% have been reported, with 40% being complete responses. This group of patients may develop further local limb recurrences as well as distant disease. Eventually, 70% of these patients will fail because of the presence of distant metastases that were not evident at the initial presentation.

Surgery should be considered for patients with isolated distant metastases. A small percentage of these patients will have long-term survival. This is notably the case in solitary lung and cerebral metastases. Symptomatic resectable metastatic disease may be managed by surgical excision to offer a better quality of palliation in selected patients.

RADIATION THERAPY

Radiation therapy has been used in the treatment of skin cancer for more than 100 years. Approaches have evolved over this time from the early use of radium molds through to superficial therapy with photons and more recently electron beam therapy. Brachytherapy using molds with isotopes such as radon-222 and gold-198 is now uncommonly used for skin cancers but can provide good cosmetic results over stable areas such as the forehead, nose, and ear. Interstitial therapy can also be used to place radioactive wires directly into the tumor in sites such as the nasal vestibule, columella, or eyelid. In experienced hands, high local control rates can be achieved. The availability of electrons has provided a great deal more scope in delivery of radiation to a variety of treatment depths and field sizes. There are situations where radiation will be effective where other modalities are contra-indicated or cosmetically inferior.

In therapy with radiation, the size of the skin cancer is a strong prognostic variable. For tumors less than 1 cm in diameter, the local control with radiation therapy is 97% for BCC and 91% for SCC. For tumours 1—5 cm, the local control was 87% and 76%, respectively, and for lesions >5 cm the local control was 87%

and 56%, respectively. Other adverse features are the presence of perineural spread in the specimen, the histologic subtype (micronodular BCC, spindle cell BCC), the differentiation of the tumor (poorly differentiated do worse), the site (worse on the ear and lip), and the presence of positive margins after excision and previous treatment.

For early nonmelanomatous lesions, radiation therapy offers cure rates approaching 100%. Ashby summarizes the results of 19 publications reporting the use of radiation in nonmelanomatous skin cancer and noted that the cure rate varied from 86 to 97%. To maximize the effect on the tumor and minimize the effect on normal tissues, treatment is fractionated. For small lesions, a dose such as 40 Gy in 10 fractions is often sufficient. Larger tumors require higher doses and more fractions (e.g., a 10 cm tumour on the scalp could be treated with a dose of 60 Gy in 30 fractions, especially if it is invading bone). In some more elderly or frailer patients, shorter schedules (24 Gy in three fractions treating once a week) may be used, but they do result in more late effects in the skin and subcutaneous tissue.

Extensive infiltrating tumors are best managed in combination with surgery. Radiation combined with surgery may be used to minimize the morbidity of surgery and may limit the extent to which a radical surgical procedure needs to be performed. Radiation may also be used in association with simple excisions where margins are involved and a re-excision would result in cosmetic deformity. Radiation is still, however, recommended as the sole modality in the following situations:

1. Treatment in the elderly or frail
2. Where surgery will result in major cosmetic deformity (lower eyelids, nose and ears)
3. Treatment of advanced inoperable lesions where relief from bleeding, infection, odor, and pain may be required

Radiation should be avoided in areas of poor blood supply and areas that would be exposed to friction, trauma, or excessive sunlight. This is particularly applicable with lesions on the lower limb. It should also be avoided where there is exposed cartilage or bone, as control rates with radiation in this setting are poor. Good cosmesis and preservation of function may be an advantage around the nose, ears, and eyes. Elective nodal radiation is not required for BCCs and SCCs as the incidence of nodal spread is low. Clinically involved lymph nodes, however, should be therapeutically dissected after confirmation with cytology. Postoperative irradiation to the nodal basin is indicated if there are multiple nodes involved, extracapsular extension, or perineural spread. Metastatic involvement of the parotid nodes is not uncommon and is best managed with a superficial parotidectomy followed by postoperative irradiation to the parotid and ipsilateral neck. Recurrences usually occur within the first 2 years and 97% will occur by 5 years.

Merkel cell carcinoma is a most aggressive skin cancer with a propensity for local dermal recurrence, nodal metastases, and distant spread. Primary tumors should be resected if practical, but wide clearance is not required. Surgery should, however, always be followed by wide-field radiation therapy to the primary site and relevant nodal areas with the coverage of in-transit tissue. Gross tumor can be controlled with radiation alone. A dose of 50 Gy in 25 fractions over 5 weeks is recommended. The role of adjuvant chemotherapy remains unproven but is useful for the palliation of metastases.

Radiation for primary melanoma has been used on the face, but most melanomas are treated by primary excision. It may, however, be considered where a melanoma is close to an eye in an elderly frail patient. Alternatively, radiation can be used for recurrences following surgery where further surgery may be difficult or cosmetically deforming. The major role of radiation therapy for melanomas is for metastatic disease, where, contrary to popular belief, significant responses occur. Radiation may be used as an adjuvant following nodal dissection, although this area remains controversial. The policy at the Queensland Melanoma Project at Princess Alexandra Hospital in Queensland is to offer all patients adjuvant radiation therapy for the following situations:

1. Multiple nodal involvement
2. Extracapsular spread of disease
3. Tumor spill at surgery
4. Recurrences

Patients having these criteria are at high risk of local recurrence and retrospective evidence suggests that radiation reduces this risk, although this hypothesis has never been proven in a randomized trial. In addition, some patients with limited surgery for desmoplastic melanoma on the head and neck area are considered for postoperative irradiation to reduce the incidence of local recurrence. There is, however, no proven benefit in overall survival. Typical doses used are 48 Gy in 20 fractions. Shorter schedules such as 30 Gy in five or six fractions may also be used but may be associated with an increased incidence of late effects. Contrary to popular belief, there is only a very slight increase in the incidence of major side effects following surgery, with lymphedema of a breast or limb being the most common effect. In many instances, however the lymphedema is of low grade and not particularly troublesome. Moderate to severe lymphedema can occur in up to 15% of patients after inguinal node basin irradiation and 8% of those having the axilla treated. Bulky inoperable nodal disease in the absence of metastases is also amenable to high-dose radiation treatment. Doses of the order of 50 Gy in 20 fractions may be used, although hypofractionated regimes such as 21 Gy in 3 fractions or 30 Gy in 6 fractions may be used if the tumor is not close to the spinal cord or a major nerve. Although it is widely believed that radiation in large fractions is more effective in controlling bulky disease, there are no randomized trials to confirm this. Radiation may also be used extensively in the palliation of metastatic disease. Melanoma commonly spreads to the brain, bone, and subcutaneous tissues.

In these sites it can cause troublesome symptoms that may be rapidly relieved with the use of radiation therapy. For brain metastases, a dose of 30 Gy in 10 fractions is appropriate, although at other sites such as bone and subcutaneous tissues hypofractionated regimes may again be used.

CHEMOTHERAPY/IMMUNOTHERAPY

Topical 5-fluorouracil is useful for the management of solar keratoses and basal cell carcinomas but may allow deep progression of underlying BCC while the surface clinically regresses. Intralesional recombinant interferon alpha can control local BCCs but surgical approaches are preferred. Photodynamic therapy is associated with a significant risk of any sun exposure for many days, a problem in warm climates. There is no standard chemotherapy for metastatic BCC or SCC of the skin and the literature is sparse. However, drugs such as cisplatin, 5-fluorouracil, methotrexate, and bleomycin have recorded activity although there are no large-scale trials. One of the more commonly used regimes is one of cisplatin and infusional 5-fluorouracil, similar to that used in head and neck cancer. It is well tolerated and has a reasonable response rate. Toxicity of such treatments must be balanced against clinical improvement. There are major difficulties in managing metastatic skin cancer in transplant recipients with renal impairment. Merkel cell carcinomas respond well to a number of drugs, including regimens such as CHOP (cyclophosphamide, adriamycin, vincristine, prednisone) or carboplatin and etoposide. Response rates are variable but complete responses regularly occur.

In patients with high-risk melanoma (pT4 and N1b or greater), the only phase III randomized trials of adjuvant therapy showing a positive benefit have been with high-dose recombinate interferon alpha. The initial study by the Eastern Cooperative Oncology Group showed an improvement in both disease-free survival and overall survival, but a second confirmatory study showed only a benefit in disease-free survival. Toxicity is severe, with more than 50% of patients requiring significant dose reductions both during the first month of induction and the subsequent 11 months of maintenance. A further study by the same group has reported high-dose interferon to be better than a peptide-based vaccine. High-dose interferon, therefore, clearly has an effect on some patients with micrometastatic melanoma, but it is not clear which of the stage subgroups will benefit most, and its use needs to be balanced with potential toxicity and effect on quality of life. Although some phase II trials show promising activity of peptide-based vaccines, there are no randomized data reported as yet to support the use of other adjuvant immunotherapy strategies outside of a clinical trial.

For metastatic disease (stage IV), there is no standard therapy. Systemic chemotherapy has a low activity, with regular agents such as dacarbazine, lomustine, and cisplatin all having response rates of less than 17%. Fotemustine has a response rate of 24%. The duration of response is usually less than 6 months and complete responses are in less than 5% of cases. Systemic recombinant interferon alpha also has a response rate of 17% but is, however, associated with significant toxicity. Combinations of interferon and/or tamoxifen with chemotherapy are not superior to chemotherapy alone. interleukin 2 was shown to have activity against metastatic melanoma similar to the interferons. The addition of interferons or interleukin 2 to combination chemotherapy or biochemotherapy appear to result in higher partial and complete response rates when compared with single-agent or multiple-agent standard chemotherapy regimens. Biochemotherapy, however, is significantly more toxic and there are no randomized, trials to indicate a survival benefit with this form of therapy. Most centers would employ a standard therapy such as dacarbazine given once every 3 weeks, either as a single dose or over 5 days. With the use of serotonin inhibitors and dexamethasone, nausea and vomiting are uncommonly seen. There are many strategies under trial for patients with systemic disease. These include the use of new chemotherapeutic agents, new combinations, autologous vaccines, and dendritic cell–based therapies. All cases of metastatic melanoma should be considered for clinical trials of new agents and combinations.

FOLLOW-UP

Patients with both nonmelanomatous and melanomatous skin cancers require extremely close follow-up by the treating physician. It is extremely common for patients with skin cancers to develop second malignancies of both types, particularly in sun-exposed areas. Recurrences of the primary tumor may also occur. Most recurrences for BCCs and SCCs occur within the first 2 years. Patients with advanced nonmelanomatous tumors and melanomas may develop spread to the lymph nodes. Examination of regional lymph node areas is mandatory at follow-up examination. It is recommended that a 3-monthly follow-up visit be conducted during the first 2 years and 6-monthly after that period. Patients with melanoma having unusual symptoms such as headache, vomiting, abdominal pain, bone pain, or breathlessness should be investigated for the presence of metastases in the brain, abdomen, liver, or lungs.

REHABILITATION

Surgery or radiation therapy for skin cancers seldom requires extensive rehabilitation. After nodal dissection with or without postoperative irradiation, some rehabilitation may be required to maximize movement at a specific joint (e.g., shoulder). Patients having cosmetic surgery around the face area with removal or reconstruction of an important anatomical part may require appropriate rehabilitation to maximize function. Patients with metastatic disease require rehabilitation in accordance with their outlook.

PREVENTION

In most instances, skin cancer is preventable. Whites living in climates of high sun exposure should wear protective sunscreens with minimum sun protection factor

(SPF) of 15 on all sun-exposed areas. Where possible, parts of the body such as the head should be shielded with the use of hats and light clothing should be worn to cover other areas. Where possible, activities outdoors should be restricted to the early and late parts of the day, with avoidance of full sun between 10 a.m. and 2 p.m. Patients with a family history of melanoma or with the dysplastic nevus syndrome should be closely followed by clinicians with the object of detecting early melanomatous change of an existing nevus.

FURTHER READING

Ashby MA, McEwan, L (1990) Treatment of non-melanomatous skin cancer: A review of recent trends with special reference to the Australian scene. *Clin Oncol* 2:284–289.

Australian Cancer Network (1997) *Guidelines for the Management of Cutaneous Melanoma.* The Stone Press, Sydney.

Boyle F, Pendlebury S, Bell, D (1995) Further insight into the natural history and management of primary cutaneous neuroendocrine (merkel cell) carcinoma. *Int J Radiat Oncol Biol Phys* 31:315–232.

Balch CM, Urist MM, Karakousis CP et al. (1993) Efficacy of 2 cm surgical margins for intermediate-thickness melanomas (1 to 4 mm). Results of a multi-institutional randomized surgical trial. *Ann Surg* 218:262–269.

Burmeister BH, Smithers BM, Poulsen M et al. (1995) Radiation therapy for nodal disease in malignant melanoma. *World J Surg* 19:369–371.

Calabro A, Singletary SE, Balch CM (1989) Patterns of relapse in 1001 consecutive patients with melanoma nodal metastases. *Arch Surg* 124:1051–1055.

Emmett AJJ (1990) Surgical analysis and biological behaviour of 2277 basal cell carcinomas. *Aust N Z J Surg* 60:855–863.

Fleming ID, Amonette R, Monaghan T, Fleming, MD (1995). Principles of management of basal and squamous cell carcinoma of the skin. *Cancer* 75:699–704.

Fuhrmann D, Lippold A, Borrosch F et al. (2001) Should adjuvant radiotherapy be recommended following resection of regional lymph node metastases of malignant melanomas? *Br J Dermatol* 144:66–70.

Giles G, Armstrong B, Burton R et al. (1996) Has mortality from melanoma stopped rising in Australia? Analysis of trends between 1931 and 1994. *Br Med J* 312:121–125.

Huncharek M, Caubet JF, McGarry R (2001) Single agent DTIC versus combination chemotherapy with or without immunotherapy in metastatic melanoma: a metaanalysis of 3273 patients from 20 randomized trials. *Melanoma Res* 11:75–81.

Kirkwood JM, Strawderman MH, Ernstoff MS et al. (1997) Interferon alfa-2b adjuvant therapy of high-risk resected cutaneous melanoma: the Eastern Co-operative Oncology Group Trial EST 1684. *J Clin Oncol* 14:7–17.

Kirkwood JM, Ibrahim JG, Sondak VK et al. (2000) High and low dose interferon alfa-2b in high risk melanoma: first analysis of intergroup trial E1690/S9111/C9190. *J Clin Oncol* 18:2444–2458.

Marks R (1995) An overview of skin cancer. *Cancer* 75:607–612.

McDonald C (1995) Status of screening for skin cancer. *Cancer* 72:1066–1070.

McMasters KM, Reintgen DS, Ross MI et al. (2001) Sentinel node biopsy for melanoma: controversy despite widespread agreement. *J Clin Oncol* 19:2851–2855.

Morton DL, Wen DR, Cochran AJ (1992) Management of early-stage melanoma by intraoperative lymphatic mapping and selective lymphadenectomy. *Surg Oncol Clin North Am* 1:247–259.

Philip PA, Flaherty LE (2000) Biochemotherapy of melanoma. *Curr Oncol Rep* 2:314–321.

Ridge JA (2000) Adjuvant radiation after lymph node dissection for melanoma. *Ann Surg Oncol* 7:550–551.

Thompson JF, Waugh RC, Saw, RPM et al. (1994) Isolated limb infusion with melphalan for recurrent limb melanoma: a simple alternative to isolated limb perfusion. *Regional Cancer Treatment* 7:188–192.

CHAPTER 15

Head and Neck Cancer

JONATHAN IRISH

University of Toronto, Princess Margaret Hospital, Department of Surgical Oncology, Toronto, Ontario, Canada

BRIAN O'SULLIVAN

University of Toronto, Princess Margaret Hospital, Department of Radiation Oncology, Toronto, Ontario, Canada

LILLIAN SIU

University of Toronto, Princess Margaret Hospital, Department of Medical Oncology, Toronto, Ontario, Canada

ANNE LEE

Pamela Youde Nethersole Eastern Hospital, Clinical Oncology Department, Hong Kong

The rubric "head and neck cancer" covers a wide variety of cancers arising from the mucosal lining of the upper aerodigestive tract. Updates from the seventh edition of this text emphasize the technical developments in radiation therapy (intensity-modulated radiotherapy, stereotactic radiation treatment) and advances in treatment as a result of altered fractionation treatments (accelerated fractionation treatment, hyperfractionation treatment). Other advances include higher control rates with concurrent chemoradiation in head and neck cancers in general, including enhanced organ preservation in larynx cancer and survival advantages in patients with locally advanced nasopharyngeal cancer. Advances in the surgical treatment of head and neck cancer continue to be directed toward reducing morbidity. The general philosophy of treatment of this group of cancers maintains the need for multidisciplinary care in treatment and rehabilitation. Local and regional failure remain the paramount concern, although distant failure rates may increase as local and regional control rates improve. The challenge in the treatment is compounded by the fact that this patient population carries a significant risk of

UICC Manual of Clinical Oncology, Eighth Edition. Edited by Raphael E. Pollock
ISBN 0-471-22289-5 Copyright © 2004 John Wiley & Sons, Inc.

medical co-morbidity and risk of development of second primary cancers, both related to chronic exposure to tobacco and alcohol.

ETIOLOGY AND EPIDEMIOLOGY

Cancers of the head and neck comprise approximately 5% of all new cancer diagnoses. With the exception of the postcricoid subsite in hypopharyngeal carcinoma, where the male to female ratio is nearly equal, this is predominantly a disease of men. However, increased tobacco use by women over the last 20 years has led to an increase in incidence among women. Patients have usually attained their sixth decade of life.

The major etiological factor in the development of mucosal head and neck cancer is the use of tobacco, which confers a relative risk of cancer occurrence of two- to three-fold. In combination with alcohol, tobacco reacts synergistically, leading to a 10- to 15-fold increase in head and cancer risk. Human papillomavirus (HPV) has been identified in squamous cell carcinomas of the oral cavity and larynx but direct causation remains unconfirmed. Lip cancer is associated with sun exposure, whereas nasal and sinus squamous cell carcinomas have been linked to nickel exposure and to woodworking. Dietary deficiency of some vitamins (A, E, and C), elements (iron) and foods (fruit, vegetables, dairy products) have also been associated. In particular, the iron deficiency found in Plummer-Vinson syndrome is associated with cancer of the postcricoid hypopharynx and proximal esophagus. Poor oral hygiene and chronic mucosal inflammatory conditions such as lichen planus could also be etiological factors in oral cancer.

Two regions of the world merit special comment. In India, the custom of inverse smoking and the prevalent use of areca nut ("betel" nut) chewing has resulted in one-third of all cancers originating in the head and neck, with a high predilection to the oral cavity. There is also a high incidence of oral submucous fibrosis of the oral cavity in the Indian population, a condition related to areca nut chewing that is considered a premalignant condition.

Nasopharyngeal carcinoma (NPC) also manifests a particular geographic and ethnic distribution. The risk is highest among Chinese populations in Southeast Asia, intermediate for Greenland Eskimos and Maghrebin Arabs in North Africa, and lowest for Caucasian populations. More than 90% of NPC in endemic areas are the nonkeratinizing type, and patients are generally of a younger age (the peak being those in their fourth decade of life). Study of Chinese who had migrated to the United States showed that subsequent generations had progressively lower incidence, but their risk was still substantially higher than other races born in the same locality, suggesting that both genetic predisposition and environmental factors are important. Epstein-Barr virus (EBV) and high dietary intake of salted fish and preserved vegetable products have been incriminated in endemic areas.

SCREENING

Because head and neck cancer predominantly affects population groups that can be easily identified, there is a significant opportunity for early detection of

TABLE 15.1. Typical Symptoms by Common Sites of Origin in Head and Neck Cancer

Site of Origin	Symptoms
Nasopharynx	*Early*: Hearing loss, tinnitus, epistaxis, nasal obstruction, single lymph node
	Late: Headache, cranial nerve abnormalities, trismus, multiple lymph nodes, weight loss
Oral cavity	*Early*: Superficial mucosal pain, denture malposition, mouth bleeding
	Late: Pain from bone invasion, cranial nerve abnormalities, tongue tethering, trismus, palpaple lymph nodes, weight loss, skin infiltration
Glottic larynx	*Early*: Hoarseness (glottic)
	Late: Dyspnoea (airway obstruction), cartilage penetration (neck mass)
Supraglottis/oropharynx	*Early*: Dysphagia or otalgia (supraglottic)
Hypopharynx	*Late*: Dyspnoea (airway obstruction), odynophagia, palpable lymph nodes, weight loss

precancerous lesions and conditions and cancerous lesions. Despite this, in many parts of the world, patients present with advanced disease. Patient awareness about the adverse effects of tobacco use and the inability to access rural populations in many parts of the world probably contribute to this. In India, implementation of sentinel screening has yielded much of our knowledge of oral cancer and its premalignant conditions and illustrates the merits of such programs in the developing world.

As 90% of NPC patients in endemic areas have elevated serum level of immunoglobulin A against viral capsid antigen of EBV, this marker is a useful aid in early detection. Analyses of the cost-effectiveness of massive population screening are still lacking. However, regular screening including examination of the nasopharynx is advisable at least for those with a positive family history, as NPC shows a strong tendency of familial aggregation.

Populations at risk for head and neck cancer must be taught the early warning signs or symptoms of possible malignancy so that early presentation is possible. The typical symptoms are described by the common sites of origin (Table 15.1).

DIAGNOSIS

Pathology

The epithelial-lined tract of the upper aerodigestive tract gives rise to most of the malignancies of the head and neck and, in particular, squamous cell carcinoma, which is the most common and, therefore, the focus of this chapter. Tumors may also arise from other tissue, including connective tissues (sarcomas of bone and soft tissue), lymphoid tissue (lymphoma and plasmacytoma), skin (melanoma, squamous, and basal cell carcinoma), and major (parotid, submandibular, and sublingual glands) and minor salivary glands. The latter are distributed throughout the mucous membranes of the oral cavity, paranasal sinuses, and nasal cavity. Mucoepidermoid and adenoid cystic carcinomas comprise the majority of salivary gland malignancies. Lymphomas in this region have a particular prediliction to Waldeyer's ring.

The pathologic predictors of poor outcome for most typical squamous carcinomas include the presence of perineural spread (predictive of invasion along nerves), angiolymphatic invasion, high grade of tumor, and the presence of ulceration.

The 1991 World Health Organization (WHO) classification is used by the majority of centers for histological grading of NPC and recognizes two histological types: keratinizing squamous carcinoma (type I) and nonkeratinizing carcinoma (type II). The nonkeratinizing carcinomas are further divided into differentiated and undifferentiated subtypes. There is increasing evidence that the histological type 1 carcinomas, which occur mostly in nonendemic areas, is least radiosensitive and associated with a more unfavorable prognosis.

Natural History

The behavior of head and neck cancers is relevant to diagnosis because certain patterns exist and should be understood. Local spread is usually orderly to contiguous sites. However, submucosal spread is common and tumor may remain in the oral tongue and base of tongue until quite large with eventual ulceration, invasion of musculature, and fixation. Posterior pharyngeal wall lesions enlarge submucosally and may present as skip lesions. They tend to remain on the posterior wall and spread up and down with posterior tethering and painful ulceration when advanced. Extension into the nasopharynx superiorly, or inferiorly to the distal hypopharyngeal region may be unexpected in a lesion with its epicenter in the posterior oropharynx and should be looked for.

Tumors may penetrate potential spaces such as the pre-epiglottic space in base of tongue or supraglottic cancers. In many sites, a pattern of orderly infiltration provides common presentations for the different tumors at their various stages (e.g., orbit and facial skin in advanced paranasal sinus disease, mandibular invasion in advanced floor of mouth, and pterygoid muscle invasion when tumors gain access to the pterygo-maxillary region).

NPC often shows highly malignant behavior with extensive local infiltration. Tumor may penetrate through the sinus of Morgani, a defect in the muscular wall of the superior pharynx, to reach the parapharyngeal space. Presentation with skull base erosion and/or cranial nerves is evident in more than 30% of patients and relates to their proximity to the primary tumor. Lymphatic invasion to lymph nodes is also generally orderly and usually involves the upper and mid jugular chain (levels II and III—see definitions below). Anterior oral cavity characteristically may skip to levels III or IV in approximately 15% of cases without involvement of the upper neck. In general, lateral lesions of the tongue, tonsillar region, and floor of mouth tend to spread to the ipsilateral neck, whereas in midline lesions, for example, in the larynx, hypopharynx and nasopharynx, if treatment is required it should encompass both sides of the neck.

In NPC, 70% present with gross nodal enlargement and another 10% have occult lymphatic deposits. Bilateral cervical lymphatics, both anterior and posterior chains, are at risk. Lymphatic spread is generally orderly, commonly involving the retropharyngeal node (of Rouvière) and the jugulo-digastric node. Nodes of Rouvière can only be appreciated radiologically when early, although grossly enlarged nodes can displace the soft palate inferomedially and be palpable. NPC not infreqently involves any part of level V, although the upper portion is most common.

Distant metastates are uncommon in head and neck cancer, excepting NPC, and are usually associated with advanced N-categories. The most common sites are the lungs, followed by liver and bone. In NPC, the risk of distant failure also varies with extensiveness of disease (especially extensive regional lymph node diease) and success of locoregional control. Even for patients with sustained locoregional control, 30% of node-positive patients die of distant metastases.

Diagnostic Work-up

Every head and neck cancer case requires a complete history and physical examination with particular attention to the primary and neck disease extent for staging purposes. Examination with the patient awake is essential for some sites (e.g., tongue tethering denoting deep muscle extension of an oral cancer or glottic fixation in a laryngeal cancer require dynamic assessment). Examination under anesthesia (nasopharyngoscopy, laryngoscopy, esophagoscopy, and bronchoscopy) is important to assess the extent of primary disease and to exclude the presence of a synchronous primary cancer (5–15% risk) in another head and neck site or the esophagus or lung. If the presentation is with a metastatic lymph node in the neck from an unknown primary, the patient must also undergo endoscopy with guided biopsies of the nasopharynx, tongue base, and pyriform sinus and tonsillectomy to detect possible occult disease at these sites. If no primary disease is confirmed, an open biopsy of the lymph node is recommended to confirm histopathology. The presence of EBV genome on polymerase chain reaction of metastatic lymph node tissue can be highly suggestive of a nasopharyngeal primary.

Radiological investigations include a chest X ray to rule out metastatic disease or a second primary malignancy of the lung. Computerized tomography (CT) scan, with its ability to delineate soft tissue anatomy is particularly helpful in assessing the nasopharynx (especially retropharyngeal lymph nodes and invasion of the parapharyngeal space), and in oral and base of tongue lesions. In many cases, magnetic resonance imaging (MRI) and CT are complementary, especially in the vicinity of the skull base or where inflammatory changes are present around tumor (e.g., nasal cavity and sinuses). Signal changes on MRI scanning indicative of marrow replacement also help in early recognition of bony involvement at the skull base.

Panelipse and dental occlusive X rays can also assess mandible involvement in oral cancer. Coronal plane laryngeal tomograms in combination with CT imaging may facilitate assessment of subglottic involvement in laryngeal cancer. Although esophagoscopy is essential to assess proximal esophageal involvement in hypopharyngeal carcinoma and to rule out a second primary tumor of the esophagus, some authors prefer a barium swallow screening test.

Fine-needle aspiration (FNA) for cytological diagnosis may be useful in the investigation of patients with cervical lymphadenopathy or salivary gland tumors. Although the accuracy of cytology can vary from center to center, in salivary gland it can reach 75%.

STAGING

The TNM staging system is the only widely accepted staging classification. The sixth edition of the International Union Against Cancer (UICC) TNM classification reflects relevant assessment and management strategies and knowledge about outcome (Tables 15.2 and 15.3). In the head and neck, a major change has included a revision of the nasopharyngeal classification. The T classifications differ in specific details for each site because of anatomic considerations. A conspicuous feature of the change in NPC classification relates to the presence of parapharyngeal extension in the classification. It should be noted that even "early" disease that involves the parapharyngeal space should be classified as T2b, whether or not it involves the nasal fossa or oropharynx (L. Sobin, personal communication). The N classification for cervical lymph node metastasis is uniform for all mucosal sites except nasopharynx.

TABLE 15.2. TNM Classification (Sixth Edition) for Head and Neck Cancers

T Category—Primary Tumor

All sites	
TX	Primary tumor cannot be assessed
T0	No evidence of primary tumor
Tis	Carcinoma *in situ*
Lip, oral cavity, oropharynx	
T1	Tumor ≤ 2 cm in greatest dimension
T2	Tumor >2 cm but <4 cm in greatest dimension
T3	Tumor >4 cm in greatest dimension
T4a[a]	
Lip	Tumor invades through cortical bone, inferior alveolar nerve, floor of mouth, or skin (chin or nose)
Oral cavity	Tumor invades through cortical bone, into deep/extrinsic muscle of tongue (genioglossus, hyoglossus, palatoglossus, and styloglossus), maxillary sinus, or skin of face
Oropharynx	Tumor invades any of the following: larynx, deep/extrinsic muscle of tongue (genioglossus, hyoglossus, palatoglossus, and styloglossus), medial pterygoid, hard palate, and mandible

TABLE 15.2 (*Continued*)

T4b	
Lip and oral cavity	Tumor invades masticator space, pterygoid plates, or skull base, or encases internal carotid artery
Oropharynx	Tumor invades any of the following: lateral pterygoid muscle, pterygoid plates, lateral nasopharynx, skull base; or encases the carotid artery
Nasopharynx	
T1	Tumor confined to the nasopharynx
T2	Tumor extends to soft tissues
T2a	Tumor extends to oropharynx and/or nasal cavity without parapharyngeal extension[b]
T2b	Tumor with parapharyngeal extension[b]
T3	Tumor invades bony structures and/or paranasal sinuses
T4	Tumor with intracranial extension and/or involvement of cranial nerves, infratemporal fossa, hypopharynx, orbit, or masticator space
Hypopharynx	
T1	Tumor limited to one subsite of hypopharynx and ≤2 cm in greatest dimension
T2	Tumor invades more than one subsite of hypopharynx or an adjacent site, or measures >2 cm but <4 cm in greatest dimension, *without* fixation of the hemilarynx
T3	Tumor >4 cm in greatest dimension, or *with* fixation of hemilarynx
T4a	Tumor invades any of the following: thyroid/cricoid cartilage, hyoid bone, thyroid gland, esophagus, central compartment soft tissue[c]
T4b	Tumor invades prevertebral fascia, encases carotid artery, or invades mediastinal structures
Supraglottis	
T1	Tumor limited to one subsite of the supraglottis with normal vocal cord mobility
T2	Tumor invades mucosa of more than one adjacent subsite of supraglottis or glottis or region outside the supraglottis (e.g., mucosa of base of tongue, vallecula, medial wall of pyriform sinus) without fixation of the larynx
T3	Tumor limited to larynx with vocal cord fixation and/or invades any of the following: postcricoid area, pre-epiglottic tissues, paraglottic space, and/or with minor thyroid cartilage erosion (e.g., inner cortex)
T4a	Tumor extends through the thyroid cartilage, and/or invades tissues beyond the larynx (e.g., trachea); soft tissues of neck, including deep/extrinsic muscle of tongue (genioglossus, hyoglossus, palatoglossus, and styloglossus), strap muscles, thyroid, esophagus
T4b	Tumor invades prevertebral space, mediastinal structures, or encases carotid artery

TABLE 15.2 (*Continued*)

Glottis	
T1	Tumor limited to the vocal cord(s) (may involve anterior or posterior commissure) with normal mobility
T1a	Tumor limited to one vocal cord
T1b	Tumor involves both vocal cords
T2	Tumor extends to the supraglottis and/or subglottis, and/or with impaired vocal cord mobility
T3	Tumor limited to larynx with vocal cord fixation and/or invades paraglottic space, and/or with minor thyroid cartilage erosion (e.g., inner cortex)
T4a	Tumor invades through the thyroid cartilage, or invades tissues beyond the larynx (e.g., trachea); soft tissues of neck including deep/extrinsic muscle of tongue (genioglossus, hyoglossus, palatoglossus, and styloglossus), strap muscles, thyroid esophagus
T4b	Tumor invades prevertebral space, mediastinal structures, or encases carotid artery
Subglottis	
T1	Tumor limited to subglottis
T2	Tumor extends to vocal cord(s) with normal or impaired mobility
T3	Tumor limited to larynx with vocal cord fixation
T4a	Tumor invades through the cricoid or thyroid cartilage and/or invades tissues beyond the larynx (e.g., trachea); soft tissues of neck, including deep/extrinsic muscle of tongue (genioglossus, hyoglossus, palatoglossus, and styloglossus), strap muscles, thyroid, esophagus
T4b	Tumor invades prevertebral space, mediastinal structures, or encases carotid artery
Maxillary sinus	
T1	Tumor limited to the mucosa with no erosion or destruction of bone
T2	Tumor causing bone erosion or destruction, including extension into hard palate and/or middle nasal meatus, except extension to posterior wall of maxillary sinus and pterygoid plates
T3	Tumor invades any of the following: bone of posterior wall of maxillary sinus, subcutaneous tissues, floor or medial wall of orbit, pterygoid fossa, ethmoid sinuses
T4a	Tumor invades any of the following: orbital contents beyond the floor or medial wall including any of the following: anterior orbital contents, skin of cheek, pterygoid plates, infratemporal fossa, cribriform plate, sphenoid or frontal sinuses
T4b	Tumor invades any of the following: orbital apex, dura, brain, middle cranial fossa, cranial nerves other than maxillary division of trigeminal nerve V2, nasopharynx, clivus
Nasal cavity and ethmoid sinus	
T1	Tumor restricted to one subsite of nasal cavity or ethmoid sinus, with or without bony invasion

TABLE 15.2 (*Continued*)

T2	Tumor involves two subsites in a single site or extends to involve an adjacent site within the nasoethmoidal complex, with or without bony invasion
T3	Tumor extends to invade the medial wall or floor of the orbit, maxillary sinus, palate, or cribriform plate
T4a	Tumor invades any of the following: anterior orbital contents, skin of nose or cheek, minimal extension to anterior cranial fossa, pterygoid plates, sphenoid or frontal sinuses
T4b	Tumor invades any of the following: orbital apex, dura, brain, middle cranial fossa, cranial nerves other than V2, nasopharynx, clivus

Salivary glands—parotid, submandibular, and sublingual

TX	Primary tumor cannot be assessed
T0	No evidence of primary tumor
T1	Tumor $\leq$2 cm in greatest dimension without extraparenchymal extension[d]
T2	Tumor >2 cm but <4 cm in greatest dimension without extraparenchymal extension[d]
T3	Tumor >4 cm and/or tumor with extraparenchymal extension[d]
T4a	Tumor invades skin, mandible, ear canal, or facial nerve
T4b	Tumor invades base of skull, pterygoid plates, or encases carotid artery

N Category—Regional Lymph Nodes

All sites except nasopharynx[e]

NX	Regional lymph nodes cannot be assessed
N0	No regional lymph node metastasis
N1	Metastasis in a single ipsilateral lymph node, $\leq$3 cm in greatest dimension
N2	Metastasis in a single ipsilateral lymph node, >3 cm but <6 cm in greatest dimension; or in multiple ipsilateral lymph nodes, none >6 cm in greatest dimension; or in bilateral or contralateral lymph nodes, none >6 cm in greatest dimension
N2a	Metastasis in a single ipsilateral lymph node, >3 cm but <6 cm in greatest dimension
N2b	Metastasis in multiple ipsilateral lymph nodes, none >6 cm in greatest dimension
N2c	Metastasis in bilateral or contralateral lymph nodes, none >6 cm in greatest dimension
N3	Metastasis in a lymph node >6 cm in greatest dimension

Nasopharynx

NX	Regional lymph nodes cannot be assessed
N0	No regional lymph node metastasis
N1	Unilateral metastasis in lymph node(s), $\leq$6 cm in greatest dimension, above the supraclavicular fossa

TABLE 15.2 (*Continued*)

N2	Bilateral metastasis in lymph node(s), ≤6 cm in greatest dimension, above the supraclavicular fossa
N3	Metastasis in a lymph node(s) >6 cm in dimension or in the supraclavicular fossa
N3a	>6 cm in dimension
N3b	In the supraclavicular fossa

M Category—Distant Metastasis

All sites	
MX	Distant metastasis cannot be assessed
M0	No distant metastasis
M1	Distant metastasis

[a]Superficial erosion alone of bone/tooth socket by gingival primary is not sufficient to classify a tumor as T4.
[b]Parapharyngeal extension denotes posterolateral infiltration of tumor beyond the pharyngobasilar fascia.
[c]Central compartment soft tissue includes prelaryngeal strap muscles and subcutaneous fat.
[d]Extraparenchymal extension is clinical or macroscopic evidence of invasion of soft tissues or nerve, except those listed under T4a and T4b. Microscopic evidence alone does not constitute extraparenchymal extension for classification purposes.
[e]Midline nodes are considered ipsilateral nodes.

Any diagnostic information that contributes to overall accuracy of the pretreatment assessment should be considered in clinical staging and treatment planning. Cancer of the head and neck can be staged (pathologic stage: pTNM) using all information from the clinical assessment as well as from the pathologic study of the resected specimen. The pathologic stage does not replace the clinical stage, which

TABLE 15.3. TNM Sixth Edition Stage Groupings: Head and Neck Cancers

Stage—Excluding Nasopharynx				Stage—Nasopharynx			
0	Tis	N0	M0	0	Tis	N0	M0
I	T1	N0	M0	I	T1	N0	M0
II	T2	N0	M0	IIA	T2a	N0	M0
				IIB	T1	N1	M0
					T2a	N1	M0
					T2b	N0, N1	M0
III	T1	N1	M0	III	T1	N2	M0
	T2	N1	M0		T2a, T2b	N2	M0
	T3	N0, N1	M0		T3	N0, N1, N2	M0
IVA	T1, T2, T3	N2	M0	IVA	T4	N0, N1, N2	M0
	T4a	N0, N1, N2	M0				
IVB	T4b	Any N	M0	IVB	Any T	N3	M0
	Any T	N3	M0	IVC	Any T	Any N	M1
IVC	Any T	Any N	M1				

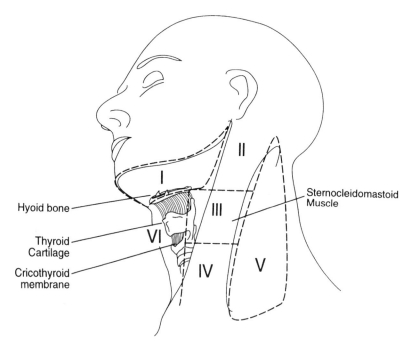

Figure 15.1 Schematic diagram indicating the location of the lymph node levels in the neck as described in the text (reproduced with permission of the AJCC, 1997).

must be reported because not every patient is treated with surgery. Thus, valid comparisons between groups of patients must rely on the clinical stage that can be recorded in every patient.

In addition to the N categories, an additional component of the description of neck node involvement concerns the localization of lymph nodes to levels in the neck (Fig. 15.1).

Level I   Contains the submental and submandibular triangles bounded by the posterior belly of the digastric muscle, the hyoid bone inferiorly, and the body of the mandible superiorly.

Level II   Extends from the level of the hyoid bone inferiorly to the skull base superiorly.

Level III   Extends from the hyoid bone superiorly to the cricothyroid membrane inferiorly.

Level IV   Extends from the cricothyroid membranes superiorly to the clavicle inferiorly.

Level V   Is the posterior triangle bounded by the anterior border of the trapezius posteriorly, the posterior border of the sternocleidomastoid muscle anteriorly, and the clavicle inferiorly.

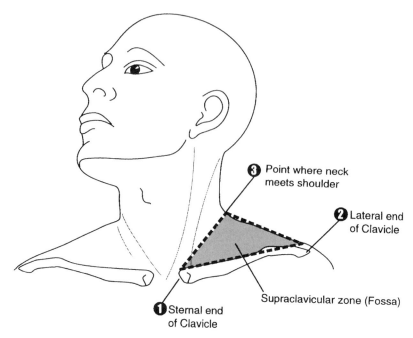

Figure 15.2 Shaded triangular area corresponds to the supraclavicular fossa used in the staging of nasopharyngeal carcinoma (reproduced with permission of the AJCC, 1997).

Level VI   Contains anterior neck compartment from the hyoid bone superiorly to the suprasternal notch inferiorly. On each side, the lateral border is formed by the medial border of the carotid sheath.

Level VII Contains the lymph nodes inferior to the suprasternal notch in the upper mediastinum.

In NPC, the neck description also requires an appreciation of the triangular supraclavicular fossa or zone described by Ho (Fig. 15.2) which includes caudal portions of levels IV and V. Nodes (whole or part) in the fossa are considered N3b.

MULTIMODALITY TREATMENT

Philosophy of Management

Although the definitive treatment of head and neck cancer has been an area of controversy, there is increasing evidence that organ preservation strategies are effective. In part, controversy has been fueled by the existence of two valid curative treatment options for many presentations of these diseases. Evidence exists that much of what is recommended as "best therapy" is determined as much by "accidents of geography and pattern of referral" and not only knowledge of the cancer or an impartial representation of the available treatment options. In general, treatment should be offered with several objectives and with attention to the ability to access medical care, the economics of therapy delivery, and available resources. Achievement of cure should be paramount, while also maximizing best functional and cosmetic outcomes.

However, patients who are unlikely to attend for regular follow-up are not ideal candidates for approaches requiring viligant surveillance for early salvage, most usually for radiation treatment failure.

NPC differs from other head and neck cancer because the standard treatment for locoregional NPC is radiotherapy and surgery is reserved for salvage of persistent or recurrent disease, especially if failure is confined to cervical nodes.

In general, standard therapy for most head and neck cancers consists of surgery or radiotherapy for early disease (T1 and T2 categories), whereas combined treatment may be used in the more advanced presentations (T3 and T4 categories). For advanced high-volume (node diameter >3 cm) regional disease, planned combined treatment is generally advocated. Combined treatment may consist of elective combined radiotherapy as a pre- or postsurgical adjuvant, or in a delayed combined approach with surgery following radiotherapy if planned surveillance does not confirm an adequate response (e.g., histologically proven disease three months after radiotherapy). The advantage of the latter is that surgery may not be needed, a major dividend where loss of function is of grave concern. More recent strategies for organ conservation promote the use of chemotherapy with response assessment and are discussed below.

Surgery

The main principle in the surgical management of head and neck cancer regardless of site is tumor-free margin resection of the disease. Adjuvant radiotherapy should be considered if there is concern about resection margins on the primary tumor or infiltration beyond the surgery field, as may occur with perineural invasion. Surgical options in the treatment of the primary lesion include the use of formal scalpel resection, electrodessication, or laser resection. Regardless of the modality of ablation, intraoperative pathology consultation to ensure disease-free margins is essential. In addition to surgical ablation, the head and neck surgical oncologist faces the challenge of reconstruction for acceptable cosmetic result and maintenance of function.

Primary surgical treatment is recognized as a mainstay of therapy for malignancies of the oral cavity. Surgical approaches include transoral for small tumors, mandibulotomy for larger tumors without bone involvement, and mandibulectomy for tumors with bone invasion. Reconstruction of the oral cavity is dedicated to reconstitution of the mandibular arch for contour and cosmesis, often using free fibular flaps. Soft tissue reconstruction necessitates use of low-bulk, pliable tissue with potential for re-innervation as afforded by the radial forearm flap.

Pharyngeal and laryngeal malignancies are treated in many centers with primary radiation, with surgery for residual or recurrent disease. The exception to this general philosophy is in T4 laryngeal and hypopharyngeal cancer, where combined modality treatment with surgery as primary therapy may be recommended. Surgery for pharyngeal cancer adheres to the concept of margin-free resection. Primary closure is employed for partial pharyngectomy and regional myocutaneous flaps are used for more extensive ablation. However, where a total circumferential resection is performed, free jejunal interposition or gastric pullup is employed depending on the length of pharyngo-esophageal segment that is ablated.

Surgical management of laryngeal cancer can include endoscopic resection, external conservation surgery, and total laryngectomy. Endoscopic resection may be performed with the microdissection technique or can employ the CO_2 laser. Generally, endoscopic resection can be used for superficial tumors limited to the mid-cord with no involvement of the anterior commissure. Recent reports from European and North American centers suggest high rates of local disease control in selected patients, with more advanced laryngeal disease treated with CO_2 laser endoscopy. However, long-term survival analysis needs to be reviewed carefully, and detailed swallowing and voice outcome measures using these techniques needs to be reported on in larger numbers of patients. External conservation surgery, where indicated, can preserve voice and deglutition and maintain airway. Although, in most cases, patients will regain normal swallowing function after conservative laryngeal surgery, most patients will have significant aspiration in the postoperative period. It is essential, therefore, to ensure that the patient has acceptable pulmonary reserve (forced expiratory volume in 1 second [FEV_1] >60% of predicted) to tolerate aspiration in the recovery period.

Conservative laryngeal surgery can include laryngofissure with cordectomy, hemilaryngectomy, extended or frontolateral vertical partial laryngectomy, and near total laryngectomy. For supraglottic cancer, a horizontal supraglottic laryngectomy may be employed. More extended resections with resection of glottic and supraglottic structures can be performed with supracricoid laryngectomy with cricohyoidopexy (SCL-CHP) or cricohyoidoepiglottopexy (SCL-CHEP), depending on the extent of resection and required reconstruction. Innovative reconstructive techniques applying free vascular tissue transfer to reconstruct and reinforce the proximal tracheal airway have allowed consideration of cricoid cartilage resection with thyrotracheal anastomoses. All patients considered for conservative options of local laryngeal disease control need to be selected carefully, as postoperative aspiration, dysphagia, and dysphonia remain as major obstacles during the rehabilitation of the postsurgical patient. In addition, all forms of conservation laryngeal surgery in early stage disease remain alternatives to radiotherapy, which continues to provide the highest level of tumor control and voice quality when case selection is accounted for.

Treatment of the neck is considered if the risk of occult spread is greater than 15–25%. The rate of occult regional disease is largely dependent on the site and T category of the primary disease. It has become standard to recommend conservative regional disease management for the N0 neck. This includes functional neck dissection (levels I–V), and selective neck dissection (e.g., supraomohyoid neck dissection of levels I–III, and anterolateral neck dissection of levels II–IV). The advantages include preservation of the sternocleidomastoid muscle, internal jugular vein, and accessory nerve. Radical neck dissection is employed for advanced regional disease where the risk of extracapsular extension of nodal metastases is high, necessitating sacrifice of muscle, vein, and nerve. Adjuvant radiotherapy should be considered for large metastatic lymph nodes (>3 cm), multiple nodes, or when extracapsular disease is present. In patients undergoing surgery with post-operative radiation therapy, consideration to submandibular gland transfer to the submental space thereby removing some of the functioning salivary gland tissue from the radiation field may preserve some salivary function in selected patients.

Radiation Therapy

Radiation therapy has been a mainstay of curative treatment for head and neck cancer for decades. The modern era is characterized by superior technology permitting higher precision in treatment delivery. Better imaging techniques coupled with superior methods to conform irradiation planning volumes permit a greater volume of normal tissue to be spared. In turn, this has opened the door to dose escalation with radiotherapy alone or combined with concurrent chemotherapy.

Radiotherapy is administered over a period of time that permits repair of normal tissue to take place between fractions, recruitment of cells into radiosensitive phases of the cell cycle, and reoxygenation of resistant tumor cells during the treatment course. It must also be delivered in a sufficiently short time period that prevents excessive tumor proliferation. A wide range of daily fractionation protocols are used across the world, ranging from schemes delivering doses of 50 Gy in as short as three weeks at one extreme compared with 70 Gy in seven weeks at the other. Tumor control rates for these schedules appear similar, although the shorter courses are associated with more intense acute radiation reactions. However, clinical and laboratory studies have suggested that protocols associated with more prolonged treatment administration require higher total doses to counteract the effect of accelerated proliferation of tumor cells, believed to commence after a lapse of several weeks of radiotherapy. Strategies to spare normal tissues by exploiting the relatively less damaging long-term normal tissue effect of smaller dose per fraction schedules (hyperfractionation) or by offsetting tumor proliferation using shorter treatment time (accelerated fractionation) schemes are becoming widely used and provide further opportunity for improvement in outcome compared with traditional radiotherapy regimens. Both strategies generally employ more than once-daily fractionation and are intended to deliver a biologically more effective total dose to the tumor. They differ in that the fraction size is smaller in hyperfractionation but is usually unchanged in the accelerated regimens compared with conventional daily regimens. Much evidence now exists from a series of randomized controlled trials in head and neck cancer (other than nasopharynx) performed in the 1990s showing that altered fractionation strategies are more effective compared with conventional fractionation approaches. One particularly prominent report (Radiation Therapy Oncology Group [RTOG] 9003) describes the efficacy of hyperfractionation and two types of accelerated fractionation individually compared with standard fractionation. Patients treated with hyperfractionation and accelerated fractionation with concomitant boost had significantly better local-regional control ($p = 0.045$ and $p = 0.050$, respectively) than those treated with standard fractionation. There was also a trend toward improved disease-free survival ($p = 0.067$ and $p = 0.054$, respectively). The second accelerated regimen used a split in the course to minimize acute side effects. That approach had similar outcome to those treated with standard fractionation. Although all of these regimes demonstrate greater acute toxicity, as yet the long-term toxicity remains unknown. In addition, whereas the local control rates with radiotherapy alone show consistently improved results with the newer fractionation strategies, the results of control in the regional lymph nodes have not been as impressive. For advanced regional lymph node disease, the addition of a planned neck dissection should therefore be considered a component of therapy. Additional information about efficacy will soon be available from an individual patient data meta-analysis of radiotherapy in carcinomas of the head and neck (MARCH), focusing on fractionation trials by the same group that performed the chemoradiotherapy meta-analysis (J. Pignon, personal communication). Finally, these principles may also be applicable in nasopharyngeal carcinoma. Retrospective comparison with historic data suggests that further improvement of local control may be achieved by accelerated fractionation for T3-4 tumors and dose escalation (by brachytherapy boost) for T1-2 tumors. However, it must be cautioned that excessive late neurological damage may occur with rapid acceleration using more than one fraction per day, unless normal tissues could be shielded without risking marginal miss by appropriate technique.

As noted above, oxygen-depleted cells are less radiosensitive, which is one of the reasons for fractionating radiotherapy, because reoxygenation takes place in the interfraction interval. An alternative strategy is to target hypoxic cells directly. Optimization of radiation effect could be achieved by the use of a drug that is toxic only to hypoxic cells. Tirapazamine, a benzotriazine bioreductive compound, is differentially toxic to hypoxic cells and, furthermore, potentiates the cytotoxicity of cisplatin. Preliminary trials of these agents given concurrently with fractionated radiotherapy have reported dramatic responses in locally advanced tumors. Sequelae from this approach have included muscle cramping, diarrhea, and marrow suppression. Long-term efficacy data are awaited.

With the anatomical proximity of critical structures in the head and neck, meticulous treatment planning is important. Maximization of local control with minimal damage demands not only optimal fractionation and methods of combating hypoxia and proliferation but also adequate coverage of target, proper protection of normal tissues, reliable immobilization, and accurate set-up. Conformal techniques may be applicable in some circumstances, and further improvement of dosimetry by intensity-modulated radiotherapy (IMRT) considered where appropriate (see below). If resource constraint only allows a conventional two-dimensional technique, maximum refinement by customized shield and the shrinking-field technique should be attempted.

With the high incidence of lymphatic involvement in nasopharyngeal, hypopharyngeal, certain oropharyngeal, and supraglottic tumors, there is little controversy that bilateral neck irradiation is indicated irrespective of the lymph node status. Other sites are at less risk, but generally relate to the size of the primary tumor. In diseases where the neck is also to be treated, it is an almost universal practice to treat the primary lesion and upper neck *en bloc* with opposing lateral portals during the initial phase of treatment. Additional fields are junctioned to encompass the additional lymph node regions. When the spinal cord dose reaches 40–45 Gy at conventional daily fractionation of 1.8–2 Gy, different field arrangements are used by different centers to boost the primary and the lymphatics. The standard practice is to treat the gross tumor to a total of 65–70 Gy in 6.5–7.5 weeks, and the elective sites to 50 Gy. The shrinking-field technique should be used, and, as far as possible, the dose to critical structures should be limited to 50–55 Gy. These prescriptions will vary in the contemporary era, as the new altered fractionation approaches become more widely adopted, and depending on whether chemotherapy is used concurrently.

In addition to altered fractionation, further improvements by escalation of total dose (using brachytherapy or stereotactic radiotherapy) have been advocated in different sites. Although encouraging results have been reported in comparison with historic controls, data from randomized studies are still awaited.

Intensity modulated radiotherapy (IMRT) is an advanced form of three-dimensional conformal radiotherapy in which radiation beams are not only shaped at their perimeters, but also include variable intensity across the beam profiles. This technique allows exquisite conformation of dose to targets, while maintaining high-dose gradients between tumor and normal tissue. Numerous reports indicate that this modality will likely shape the future of radiation treatment where target coverage and toxicity issues (including salivary gland sparing) are paramount. Preliminary evidence suggests a particular benefit in nasopharyngeal carcinoma and other tumors in proximity to critical skull base anatomy. Future studies should focus on patterns of locoregional recurrence and toxicity because of the extreme precision required to deliver these treatments. Both tumor target coverage and critical normal tissue avoidance must be emphasized more than usual with these approaches.

Chemotherapy

Squamous Cell Cancer in General   The median duration of survival of head and neck cancer patients with recurrent or metastatic disease is about 6 months. Factors that are predictive of a better outcome to chemotherapy include a high performance status of the patient, lack of prior treatment with irradiation or surgery, and absence of fixed nodes. The issue of whether chemotherapy conveys increased therapeutic benefit compared with best supportive care alone has not been tested formally in a large study. Prospective quality-of-life data and functional assessments to address the palliative value of chemotherapy are lacking in this morbid disease, and are of critical importance because chemotherapy might relieve symptoms, even though current drugs do not improve survival.

Chemoradiation for Locally Advanced Head and Neck Squamous Cell Carcinoma A recently published patient-based meta-analysis of 63 trials (10,741 patients) of locoregional treatment with or without chemotherapy demonstrated an absolute benefit of 8% in survival at 5 years with concurrent chemoradiation, but no benefit was observed with neoadjuvant or adjuvant therapy. Several randomized trials not included in the meta-analysis also evaluated the value of concurrent chemotherapy, delivered with either conventional radiation or hyperfractionated radiation. Although statistically significant improvements in locoregional control are observed in all such studies, along with overall survival benefits in some studies, acute toxicity is increased with concurrent chemoradiation. Moreover, the effects on important long-term toxicities (e.g., swallowing, and neurological effects) are yet to be determined. Toxicity may be of even greater concern with intensified accelerated fractionation approaches. In addition, Staar et al. compared intensified hyperfractionated accelerated radiation therapy with and without concomitant chemotherapy in a randomized trial and found that the efficacy of the combined chemoradiation approach may be less obvious. Not surprisingly, acute toxicity was enhanced with chemoradiotherapy, but of greater concern is the preliminary observation by Starr and colleagues that a significantly greater proportion of patients (51% *vs.* 25%, $p = 0.02$) continue to experience major swallowing difficulties, including feeding tube dependence, and potentially other late sequelae in the group that received chemoradiotherapy compared with radiotherapy alone.

An Intergroup phase III study (R91-11) compared induction chemotherapy plus radiotherapy versus concurrent chemoradiotherapy versus radiotherapy alone in laryngeal cancer. Concurrent chemoradiation with cisplatin resulted in a higher laryngeal preservation rate, whereas induction chemotherapy plus radiation had no advantage over radiation alone. No differences in overall survival were observed.

Chemoradiation for Locally Advanced Nasopharyngeal Carcinoma NPC exhibits greater chemosensitivity than squamous cell cancers in the other sites, and patients with NPC generally have a younger age and a better performance status. As discussed below, concurrent chemotherapy with radiotherapy appears to improve locoregional control. Although this is of paramount importance, the need for eradication of micrometastases in high-risk cases remains. The initial randomized trials for locally advanced NPC evaluated the role of induction chemotherapy given prior to radiotherapy. Unfortunately, these studies have not demonstrated any improvement in overall survival.

The Intergroup 0099 study randomized patients with stages III and IV NPC to radiotherapy alone versus concurrent cisplatin and radiotherapy with three subsequent cycles of adjuvant cisplatin and 5-fluorouracil. Statistically significant differences were noted in both three-year progression-free (24% *vs.* 69%, $p < 0.001$) and three-year overall survivals (47% *vs.* 78%, $p = 0.005$), favoring the combined modality arm. These differences have persisted at follow-up analysis at five years. Three concerns exist regarding the results of this study. First, the radiation-alone arm has fared worse than expected. Second, although acute toxicities such as nausea, vomiting, stomatitis, and myelosuppression were more severe in the chemoradiation arm, there is as yet no information available on the late toxicities of treatment. Finally, a substantial proportion of the patients had WHO type I squamous cell carcinoma. The natural history and the response to therapy of this histological type may be different from those of the more prevalent WHO type II and III tumors, and may thus limit the generalizability of the results from this study. Instead of adopting one strategy for all stage III–IV patients, treatment may need to be tailored in accordance with the different patterns of failure, depending on the status of the primary and regional disease. Thus, advanced local disease may require conformal radiotherapy techniques and/or altered fractionation, whereas advanced regional disease puts the patient at significant risk of distant metastasis. Randomized trials are in progress to identify the best option for different risk groups.

Organ Preservation

Organ preservation strategies have become widely studied in recent years, spurred by the results of two trials that randomized patients to either induction chemotherapy with response assessment (ICT), followed by radiotherapy if the chemoresponse was favorable (nonresponders receive ablative surgery), or to radical surgery. These trials were conducted by the VA Laryngeal Cancer Study Group in advanced laryngeal cancer and the European Organization for Research and Treatment of Cancer (EORTC) in hypopharyngeal cancer. While an alterative to ablative surgery, the goal of organ preservation can also be achieved with subtotal surgery with or without radiotherapy and by definitive radiotherapy, and not only by the ICT approach. Despite this, the ICT approach has been widely accepted by some practioners as synonymous with organ preservation, although the merits of induction chemotherapy are questioned in the RTOG 91-11 study in T3 larynx cancer, and have already been addressed without apparent benefit by French investigators. As already noted, a benefit for induction chemotherapy has not been upheld in meta-analyses of chemotherapy in head and neck cancer (four have been performed), and the concept is at odds with traditional outcomes of advanced disease, especially in larynx cancer where definitive radiotherapy without chemotherapy has been a standard practice in Canadian, European, and Australian centers. In the end, the major benefit to ICT will likely be that it opened the log-jam that existed in the discussion of the use of ablative surgery for advanced head and neck cancer, where the views were becoming entrenched.

Retreatment

For patients with recurrence following high-dose radiotherapy, the general principle is to salvage with surgery whenever feasible. However, for sites where complete resection is difficult (e.g., nasopharynx) or function preservation is important (e.g., larynx), aggressive re-irradiation may be considered in selected cases. Chance of success depends on the extensiveness of recurrence and the re-irradiation dose. The chance of local salvage ranges from 60% for rT1 to <10% for rT4 recurrence. A total re-irradiation dose of 60 Gy or above is needed for effective salvage. Late toxicity is a serious concern, and the risk is related to the total dose given during both courses (primary and retreatment) as well as the size of the dose per fraction. To avoid excessive complication, the total dose to normal structures should be kept to the minimum by using conformal techniques, and incorporating brachytherapy or stereotactic radiotherapy as boost. Avoidance of large dose per fraction radiotherapy should also reduce the complication rate.

Novel Targets in Head and Neck Squamous Cell Carcinoma

Recurrent squamous cell carcinoma of the head and neck not amenable to salvage radiation or surgery, or patients with metastatic disease, are incurable, with a median survival of about 6 months. Chemotherapy, whether given as single agents (e.g., methotrexate) or in combination (e.g., platinum-based combinations), has not been shown to prolong survival. The effects of chemotherapy on patients' overall quality of life are not well elucidated. Hence, there is strong rationale to develop novel agents for this patient population, with the potential of improving loco-regional control while minimizing toxicity and thereby improving the therapeutic index. The accessibility of tumoral tissues renders head and neck cancer an ideal disease site for the validation of drugs against specific molecular targets. Novel molecular targets currently under evaluation in recurrent or metastatic head and neck squamous cell carcinoma include p53 (e.g. ONYX-015, a selectively-replicating adenovirus), epidermal growth factor receptor (EGFR) (e.g. C225 antibody or Erbitux^{TM} [cetuximab], a chimerized monoclonal antibody against EGFR; Iressa$^{®}$ [gefinitib] and Tarceva^{TM} [erlotinib], EGFR tyrosine kinase inhibitors), angiogenesis (e.g., matrix metalloproteinase inhibitors; angiogenic factor inhibitors), apoptosis, and differentiation (e.g., retinoids, statins).

Supportive Treatment

It is essential to select those patients who may develop complications during treatment. The main systemic complications that arise during treatment are often related to airway compromise and nutritional depletion. Compromised airway usually requires a planned tracheotomy at the outset. Similarly, gastrostomy tube support is highly recommended early in the management to combat the catabolic and nutritionally depleted state commonly present in advanced cases. Dental care is required, as failure to extract or treat decayed or infected dentition carries an unnecessary risk of postradiation osteoradionecrosis, which can also be minimized by limiting the dose to the mandible and the amount treated. In addition, radiation-induced xerostomia will accelerate dental decay in the absence of preventative dental maintenance. Dental cleaning and topical fluoride to remaining teeth with fluoride trays should be encouraged.

During treatment, the acute side effects to the mucous membranes should be managed with pain relievers, oral hygiene by gargling with bicarbonate of soda, and topical applications of local anaesthesia (e.g., 2% viscous xylocaine). Hot and spicy foods and commercial mouthwashes must not be used as they may exacerbate radiation mucositis. Alcohol and tobacco should be avoided, because there is evidence that compromise in radiotherapy control of the cancer can result.

In the long term, patients should be monitored for laryngeal edema, which can present after radiotherapy and may represent a sign of tumor recurrence. Hypothyroidism and hypopituitarism can result from direct radiation to these structures and is readily managed with hormone replacement. Prospective randomized controlled study has shown that pilocarpine can relieve symptomatic oral dryness, and improve mouth comfort and speaking ability after radiation treatment. Adverse cholinergic side effects such as sweating, vasodilatation, and hypotension limit use in some patients. However, data from two recently presented randomized trials investigating the use of pilocarpine during radiation therapy for the amelioration of acute mucositis do not appear promising. An additional strategy is the use of amifostine (WR-2721) as a radioprotector to ameliorate the side effects of radiotherapy. Amifostine and its active metabolite, WR-1065, accumulate in high concentrations in the salivary glands. Evidence, including one large randomized trial, indicates that amifostine reduces acute and chronic xerostomia without apparently influencing the efficacy of the cancer treatment. That study did not reduce mucositis, although the strategy has been shown in another randomized trial to reduce the severity of mucositis resulting from very accelerated radiation therapy. The use of this medication is problematic due to the need of an infusion prior to each fraction of radiotherapy, the added expense of the medication, the possibility of tumor radioprotection, and the high incidence of side effects, including hypotension, nausea, and vomiting.

FOLLOW-UP

Excepting NPC and salivary gland tumors, the majority of recurrences of head and neck cancer occur during the first 2 to 3 years of follow-up, with the risk declining substantially thereafter. The high prevalence of tobacco and alcohol abuse among this patient population is also associated with a continuing threat of developing a second primary tumor of the upper aerodigestive tract, and with a multitude of comorbid illnesses. A reasonable schedule of follow-up is to assess patients several times per year for the first 2 to 3 years, and less frequently thereafter.

The approximate cure rates in head and neck cancer are related to the site and stage of disease. The presence of lymph node metastases does not mean cure is not achievable but generally halves the survival within a given T category. T1/T2 lesions should attain 70–95% probability of 5-year survival, whereas T3/T4 lesions do not fare as well (20–30% 5-year survival).

Unlike other head and neck cancers, delayed failure is not uncommon for nasopharyngeal carcinoma: although 80% of failures are detected within the first

3 years, 10% do not manifest until 5 years, and 1% manifest 10 years after initial treatment. Long-term follow-up is thus especially indicated.

PREVENTION

Lifestyle modifications following potentially curative treatment of a primary tumor may lead to a decreasing risk of second tumors with increasing time. In general, cessation of alcohol and tobacco, or areca nut exposure in India, may halt the multistep carcinogenic process, particularly in individuals who have never developed a malignancy.

Chemoprevention is an attempt to use agents to prevent, arrest, or reverse carcinogenesis before progression to invasive malignancy. A randomized, placebo-controlled trial has demonstrated that adjuvant isotretinoin (13-*cis*-retinoic acid) can reduce the incidence of second primary tumors, and confirmatory randomized trials are ongoing. Trials of other agents, such as alpha tocopherol (vitamin E), selenium, beta carotene, interferon alpha, DL-alpha-difluoromethylornithine (DFMO), and nonsteroidal anti-inflammatory drugs, are also underway to define chemoprevention activity.

The strong association between nasopharyngeal carcinoma and EBV has led to research on the possibility of prevention by antiviral vaccine, but, thus far, effective vaccines are still awaited.

FURTHER READING

Adelstein DJ, Lavertu P, Saxton JP, Secic M, Wood BG, Wanamaker JR, Eliachar I, Strome M, Larto MA (2000) Mature results of a phase III randomized trial comparing concurrent chemoradiotherapy with radiation therapy alone in patients with stage III and IV squamous cell carcinoma of the head and neck. *Cancer* 88:876–883.

Al-Sarraf M, LeBlanc M, Giri PGS, Fu KK, Cooper J, Vuong T, Forastiere AA, Adams G, Sakr WA, Schuller DE, Ensley JF (1998) Chemoradiotherapy versus radiotherapy in patients with advanced nasopharyngeal cancer: Phase III randomized Intergroup study 0099. *J Clin Oncol* 16:1310–1317.

Brizel DM, Albers ME, Fisher SR, Scher RL, Richtsmeier WJ, Hars V, George SL, Huang AT, Prosnitz LR (1998) Hyperfractionated irradiation with or without concurrent chemotherapy for locally advanced head and neck cancer. *N Engl J Med* 338:1798–1804.

Brizel DM, Wasserman TH, Henke M, Strnad V et al. (2000) Phase III randomized trial of amifostine as a radioprotector in head and neck cancer. *J Clin Oncol* 18:3339–3345.

Byers R, Weber R, Andrews T et al. (1997) Freqency and therapeutic implications of "skip metastases" in the neck from squamous carcinoma of the oral tongue. *Head Neck* 19: 14–19.

Calais G, Alfonsi M, Bardet E, Sire C, Germain T, Bergerot P, Rhein B, Tortochaux J, Oudinot P, Bertrand P (1999) Randomized trial of radiation therapy versus concomitant chemotherapy and radiation therapy for advanced-stage oropharynx carcinoma. *J Natl Cancer Inst* 91:2081–2086.

Chia K, Lee H (1997) Epidemiology. In *Nasopharyngeal Carcinoma.* Armour, Singapore, pp. 1–5.

Dawson LA, Anzai Y, March L, Martel M, Paulino A, Ship J, Eisbruch A (2000) Patterns of local-regional recurrence following parotid-sparing conformal and segmental intensity-modulated radiotherapy for head and neck cancer. *Int J Radiat Oncol Biol Phys* 46:1117–1126.

Eicher S, Weber R (1996) Surgical management of cervical lymph node metastases. *Curr Opin Oncol* 8:215–220.

Fleming I, Cooper J, Henson D et al. (eds) (1997) *AJCC Cancer Staging Manual.* Lippincott-Raven, Philadelphia,

Forastiere A, Koch W, Trotti A, Sidransky D (2001) Head and neck cancer. *N Engl J Med* 345:1890–1900.

Forastiere AA, Berkey B, Maor M, Weber R, Goepfert H, Morrison WH, Glisson BS, Trotti A, Ridge JA, Chao C, Peters G, Lee D, Leaf A, Ensley J (2001) Phase III trial to preserve the larynx: Induction chemotherapy and radiotherapy versus concomitant chemoradiotherapy versus radiotherapy alone. Intergroup trial R91-11. *Proc Am Soc Clin Oncol* 20:2a (abstract 4).

Fu KK, Pajak TF, Trotti A, Jones CU, Spencer SA, Phillips TL, Garden AS, Ridge JA, Cooper JS, Ang KK (2000) A Radiation Therapy Oncology Group (RTOG) phase III randomized study to compare hyperfractionation and two variants of accelerated fractionated to standard fractionation radiotherapy for head and neck squamous cell carcinomas: First report of RTOG 9003. *Int J Radiat Oncol Biol Phys* 48:7–16.

Gluckman J, Zitsch R (1995) Early detection and screening for head and neck cancer. *Cancer Treat Res* 74:141–157.

Harari P, Kinsella T (1995) Advances in radiation therapy for head and neck cancer. *Curr Opin Oncol* 7:248–254.

Ho J (1978) *Stage Classification of Nasopharyngeal Carcinoma, Etiology, and Control.* IARC Scientific Publications, Lyon, France, 20:99–113.

Jeremic B, Shibamoto Y, Milicic B, Nikolic N, Dagovic A, Aleksandrovic J, Vaskovic Z, Tadic L (2000) Hyperfractionated radiation therapy with or without concurrent low-dose daily cisplatin in locally advanced squamous cell carcinoma of the head and neck: a prospective randomized trial. *J Clin Oncol* 18:1458–1464.

Laccourreye H, Laccourreye O, Weinstein G, Meneud M, Brasnu D (1990) Supracricoid laryngectomy with cricohyoidopexy: A partial laryngeal procedure for selected supraglottic and transglottic carcinomas. *Laryngoscope* 100:735–741.

Lee A, Foo W, Law S et al. (1997) Re-irradiation for recurrent nasopharyngeal carcinoma: Factors affecting the therapeutic ratio and ways for improvement. *Int J Radiat Oncol Bio Phys* 38:43–52.

Lefebvre J, Bonneterre J (1996) Current status of laryngeal preservation trials. *Curr Opin Oncol* 8:209–214.

O'Sullivan B, Mackillop W, Gilbert R et al. (1994) Controversies in the management of laryngeal cancer: Results of an international survey of patterns of care. *Radiother Oncol* 31:23–32.

Pathmanathan R (1997) Pathology. In *Nasopharyngeal Carcinoma.* Armour, Singapore, pp. 6–13.

Pathmanathan R, Raab-Traub N (1997). Epstein-Barr virus. In *Nasopharyngeal Carcinoma.* Armour, Singapore, pp. 14–23.

Peters L, Ang K (1992) The role of altered fractionation in head and neck cancers. *Semin Radiat Oncol* 2:180–194.

Pignon JP, Bourhis J, Domenge C, Designe L, on behalf of the MACH-NC Collaborative Group. (2000) Chemotherapy added to locoregional treatment for head and neck squamous-cell carcinoma: Three meta-analyses of updated individual data. *Lancet* 355: 949–955.

Rao D, Ganesh B (1995) Epidemiological observations of head and neck cancers. In *Head and Neck Cancer: A Multidisciplinary Approach for Its Control and Cure.* UICC, Geneva, pp. 1–28.

Rieke JW, Hafermann MD, Johnson JT et al. (1995) Oral pilocarpne for radiation-induced xerostomia: Integrated efficacy and safety results from two propective randomized clinical trials. *Int J Radiat Oncol Biol Phys* 31:661–669.

Sanguineti G, Geara F, Garden A et al. (1997) Carcinoma of the nasopharynx treated by radiotherapy alone: Determinants of local and regional control. *Int J Radiat Oncol Biol Phys* 37:985–996.

Seikaly H, Jha N, McGaw T, Coulter L, Liu R, Oldring D (2001) Submandibular gland transfer: A new method of preventing radiation-induced xerostomia. *Laryngoscope* 111:347–342.

Sobin L, Wittekind C, Eds. (2002) *TNM Classification of Malignant Tumours*, 6th edition. Wiley-Liss, New York.

Staar S, Rudat V, Stuetzer (2001) Intensified hyperfractionated accelerated radiotherapy limits the additional benefit of simultaneous chemotherapy—results of a multicentric randomized German trial in advanced head and neck cancer. *Int J Radiat Oncol Biol Phys* 50:1161–1171.

Strong E, Karsdorf H, Henk J (1995) Squamous cell carcinoma of the head and neck. In *Prognostic Factors in Cancer.* UICC Geneva. Springer-Verlag, Berlin, pp. 23–27.

The Department of Veterans Affairs Laryngeal Cancer Study Group. (1991) Induction chemotherapy plus radiation compared with surgery plus radiation in patients with advanced laryngeal cancer. *N Eng J Med* 324:1685–1690.

Vokes EE, Weichselbaum RR, Lippman SM et al. (1993) Medical progress: Head and neck cancer. *N Eng J Med* 328:184–194.

CHAPTER 16

Endocrine Tumors

SANZIANA ROMAN and ROBERT UDELSMAN

Yale School of Medicine, Department of Surgery, New Haven, Connecticut

THYROID CANCER

Epidemiology

There are approximately 17,000 new cases of clinically significant thyroid cancer per year in the United States, or 2–4 new cases per 100,000 population, with a 1:2.7 male to female ratio. The annual mortality is 0.2–2.8 per 100,000 population, with a 1:2 male to female ratio. Microscopic carcinoma is extremely prevalent, reported at 35.6% in a series of 101 consecutive autopsies. It is the most common endocrine malignancy, also accounting for the most endocrine deaths per year. Most thyroid cancers are well-differentiated tumors with an excellent prognosis, although anaplastic carcinoma is one of the most aggressive human cancers. Risk factors for malignancy in a thyroid nodule are a history of neck irradiation, age <20 or >50, extremes of iodine dietary intake, and familial history such as multiple endocrine reoplasia (MEN) kindred, Pendred's syndrome, Gardner's syndrome, familial adenomatous polyposis, Cowden's syndrome, environmental exposures such as hexachlorobenzene and tetrachlorodibenzo-p-dioxin, or volcanic lava. There is a worldwide shift from follicular cancer (FTC) to papillary cancer (PTC), with a significant reduction in follicular and anaplastic cancers and an increase in PTC.

Radiation-induced thyroid cancer is predominantly PTC. Exposure to low- to medium-dose radiation such as 150–2,000 cGy increases the likelihood of thyroid cancer significantly and the risk increases with time. The prognosis is similar to sporadic PTC.

UICC Manual of Clinical Oncology, Eighth Edition. Edited by Raphael E. Pollock
ISBN 0-471-22289-5 Copyright © 2004 John Wiley & Sons, Inc.

Classification

The main framework for the classification of thyroid cancers was approved by the World Health Organization in 1988. It divides thyroid carcinomas into four general types: papillary, follicular, and anaplastic carcinomas, all of which arise from follicular cells, and medullary carcinoma, arising from the parafollicular C cells.

PTC is the most common thyroid malignancy, accounting for approximately 80% of cancers overall and 95% of radiation-induced cancers. Carcinomas that are less than 1 cm are known as micro- or occult carcinomas and are generally believed to be of small clinical significance. Twenty to thirty-five percent of people harbor them during their lifetime, and the microcarcinomas have 0.2% mortality. The presentation of well-differentiated PTC in adults is usually in an euthyroid patient with a palpable nodule that is either solid or mixed cystic-solid. The diagnosis of papillary carcinoma can be made by fine-needle aspiration (FNA), where typical cellular features such as enlarged nuclei with an "Orphan Annie eyes" pattern of nuclear clearing, grooves, and prominent nucleoli are pathognomonic. Macroscopically, papillary fronds and psammoma bodies can be seen. The follicular variant is devoid of papillae formation yet maintains the typical PTC cytologic features. These cancers have a similar clinical outcome as PTC.

Papillary cancer metastasizes mostly by lymphatic invasion. Intrathyroidal lymphatic spread occurs and is postulated to account for multicentricity. Concomitant lymph node involvement is common yet occult lymph node metastases do not appear to affect survival.

Papillary cancers with more aggressive behavior and moderate differentiation include the insular, tall cell, clear cell, and sclerosing variants.

In children, PTC is the predominant thyroid cancer and commonly presents with cervical metastases and bulky disease. With adequate treatment, the prognosis is good.

FTC is the most common thyroid malignancy in areas of iodine deficiency. In the United States it represents approximately 5–10% of all thyroid cancers. Hurthle cell carcinomas are derived from follicular cancers and are classified as such. The patients are usually euthyroid, with a palpable thyroid mass. The tumors are usually unifocal and encapsulated. The cytologic features of follicular cancers show varying degrees of follicular cell differentiation arranged in sheets or follicles. The Hurthle cell variant contains cells with acidophyllic, "ground glass" cytoplasm with abundant mitochondria. The criterion for diagnosing follicular or Hurthle cell carcinoma is the presence of capsular and/or vascular invasion. Vascular invasion carries a worse prognosis than pure capsular invasion. These features are seldomly seen on intraoperative frozen section. Distant metastases are more common with follicular cancers and they generally carry a slightly worse prognosis than PTC. Patients with minimally invasive follicular cancers have an excellent prognosis, with a long-term survival between 80 and 85%.

Medullary carcinoma of the thyroid (MTC) comprises 10% of all thyroid cancers. It arises in the calcitonin-producing parafollicular C cells. Twenty-five percent of all MTC are related to familial syndromes such as MEN 2a, MEN 2b, or familial MTC. In familial cases, the RET mutations are inherited in an autosomal dominant fashion. Genetic screening is routinely performed for patients from known kindreds because early diagnosis and treatment has a profound impact on survival and recurrence. Patients will have an elevation in the serum calcitonin level and may have an elevated serum carcinoembyonic antigen (CEA) level. Patients with sporadic MTC usually present with a solitary mass or enlarged thyroid. Cytologic features may show noncohesive cells with elongated nuclei and 75% will stain for amyloid. Calcitonin antibody stains are diagnostic. Surgical resection at an early stage remains the only potentially curative treatment. Other endocrinopathies associated with MEN 2, such as pheochromocytomas, need to be ruled out prior to surgery. Routine meticulous lymph node dissection is paramount as most early cancers will have occult lymph node metastases. Most patients with MTC will develop recurrences or metastases. Reoperation and palliative surgery is associated with prolonged survival.

Anaplastic carcinoma is one of the most aggressive human cancers and carries a dismal prognosis. It accounts for <1% of all thyroid cancers. The typical presentation is rapid growth and metastasis from a thyroid mass in an elderly patient. It can arise in a longstanding follicular carcinoma and is more common in iodine-deficient areas of the world. Cytologic examination will show poorly differentiated cells with significant pleomorphism, large nuclei, and increased number of mitoses. Two distinct types have been identified: spindle cell and giant cell variants. The role of the surgeon for patients with anaplastic thyroid cancer is mostly providing a tissue diagnosis either using a core biopsy needle or an open incisional biopsy. Tracheostomy for airway control may be needed. Aggressive protocols employing radical surgery, external beam radiation, and chemotherapy with doxorubicin have limited success. The median survival is 6 months to 2 years, with most deaths occurring from overwhelming local invasion.

Lymphoma can arise in the thyroid gland and generally presents as a rapidly expanding mass. It can be diagnosed on a FNA by performing flow cytometry demonstrating monoclonal lymphocytes.

Evaluation of the Thyroid Nodule

Thyroid nodules are common, occurring between 4 and 7% of individuals in the general population. They increase in incidence with age, especially in females, where over 50% of women develop a thyroid nodule by age 60. Only 5% of all nodules will prove to be malignant. Ten to twenty percent will be cystic. Eighty percent of all nodules are cold on thyroid scintigraphy, and, of these, 20% will be malignant. The first and most effective test in the evaluation of a nodule, following a carefully performed history and physical examination, is an FNA performed with a 22–25-gauge needle. Seventy percent will prove to be "benign," 5% will be "malignant," showing PTC, MTC, or anaplastic carcinoma and having a 99% probability of malignancy. Definitive surgery may be planned based on a "malignant" FNA diagnosis. Twenty-five percent of FNA specimens will be suspicious or indeterminate, with a probability of malignancy of 10–20%. An FNA diagnosis of follicular cells demonstrating a follicular neoplasm will usually require thyroid lobectomy because of the inability of FNA to discriminate between a follicular adenoma and an FTC.

Genetic Abnormalities

The study of oncogenes and tumor suppressor genes in human thyroid tumors has led to the discovery of several mutations that may help direct more selective preventive or clinical treatment in the future.

Tyrosine Kinase Activity Genes   The RET/PTC proto-oncogene located on chromosome 10q11-2 encodes a transmembrane receptor of a tyrosine kinase domain. It was first found exclusively in papillary thyroid cancer, hence the name. It is present in a rearranged form in 5–35% of spontaneous papillary cancers and in 60–85% of radiation-associated PTC. TRK proto-oncogene on chromosome 1 and MET proto-oncogene both encode transmembrane receptors with a tyrosine kinase domain. TRK rearrangements have been found exclusively in PTC and are present in up to 10% of cancers. Overexpression of MET is found in over 70% of PTC and seems to be associated with a better prognosis.

The RET proto-oncogene is seen also in medullary thyroid carcinoma. The familial syndromes such as MEN 2a and 2b and FMTC all harbor activating mutations of this gene on chromosome 10. Up to 8% of patients with sporadic medullary thyroid cancer will have *de novo* RET proto-oncogene mutations. Patients with medullary thyroid cancer should be offered genetic testing for the RET proto-oncogene.

Intracellular Signaling Pathways   RAS oncogene point mutations are more common in iodine deficient countries and are more commonly associated with follicular carcinomas.

Cyclic Adenosinemonophosphate (cAMP) Pathways   Thyroid-stimulating hormone receptor (TSH-r) belongs to receptor families coupled to G-proteins increasing intracellular cAMP levels, which stimulate follicular cell proliferation. Mutations in the TSH-r have been found in up to 80% of follicular adenomas, toxic adenomas, and FTC. There is still significant discrepancy in the types of mutations across populations.

Tumor Suppressor Genes—p53   Inactivating point mutations in the p53 gene have been seen in up to 80% of anaplastic carcinomas but not in well-differentiated carcinomas. This may suggest a key step in progression from differentiated to anaplastic carcinoma.

Treatment

The patients with cytologically proven well-differentiated thyroid cancer or those with suspicious cytology should undergo surgical resection of the thyroid. Total thyroidectomy or near total thyroidectomy is recommended for patients with papillary carcinoma with poor prognostic variables and patients with follicular and Hurthle cell carcinomas. There are no randomized prospective trials comparing total thyroidectomy with less than total thyroidectomy for well-differentiated thyroid cancers. The rationale for employing total thyroidectomy was outlined by Clark in 1982, citing the common occurrence of bilateral PTC, contralateral recurrence rates of 4.7–24%, lower recurrence rates after total thyroidectomy, survival improvement in lesions >1.5 cm, use of ^{131}I for diagnosis and treatment, use of thyroglobulin as a useful marker, and ability to minimize remedial operative procedures.

Total thyroidectomy should be performed by experienced endocrine surgeons whose complication rates, such as recurrent laryngeal nerve injury and hypoparathyroidism, do not exceed 1%.

Patients with MTC require a total thyroidectomy with a central lymph node dissection and, if palpable thyroid disease is present, an ipsilateral modified radical neck dissection is indicated. In patients with well-differentiated thyroid cancer, a modified radical neck dissection is indicated only for macroscopic lymphatic involvement.

Most patients will benefit from adjuvant therapy. A TSH-stimulated postoperative ^{131}I scan to rule out residual uptake in the thyroid bed or distant metastasis is indicated for patients with papillary or follicular thyroid cancers once the patient's serum TSH is greater than 50 UIU/mL. Therapeutic radioactive iodine ablation (RAI) can be performed, if needed, and subsequently, thyroid hormone replacement with L-thyroxin is maintained to suppress the serum TSH. Serum thyroglobulin levels can be followed as markers for recurrence.

Patients with MTC do not benefit from RAI, as MTC does not demonstrate adequate iodine uptake. Surgery is the only viable modality to cure disease. External beam radiotherapy has a limited role for isolated unresectable metastases. Palliative reoperative resection of symptomatic lesions can provide significant long-term relief, and this should be considered even in the presence of widespread metastatic disease. Serum calcitonin and CEA levels are useful for follow-up. Occult recurrences are common and imaging techniques are often inadequate. Remedial neck surgery is generally performed in patients who have not had an adequate initial neck exploration when there is no evidence of extracervical disease. Laparoscopy can be useful in assessing occult liver disease. Patients with medullary thyroid cancer generally have an 80% 5-year and 60% 10-year survival.

The prognosis for most patients with well-differentiated thyroid cancer is good. Risk factors for recurrence are older age, large tumors, extrathyroidal extension, and inadequate primary surgery. Lymphatic involvement is a risk factor for local recurrence. Patients with well-differentiated PTC have a 95% 5-year and a 90% 10-year survival. Patients with follicular carcinomas have a 90% 5-year and a 70% 10-year survival.

Anaplastic carcinoma most commonly presents as stage IV disease. Surgery is indicated in the few cases where complete resection of the tumor can be achieved.

TABLE 16.1. Thyroid Cancer Staging

TNM Classification

(T) Primary tumor

Tx	Primary tumor cannot be assessed
T0	No evidence of primary tumor
T1	Tumor $\leq$2 cm
T2	Tumor >2 cm and <4 cm
T3	Tumor >4 cm or minimal extension
T4a	Tumor extends beyond thyroid capsule and invades any of the following: subcutaneous soft tissues, larynx, trachea, esophagus, recurrent laryngeal nerve
T4b	Tumor invades prevertebral fascia, mediastinal vessels, or encases carotid artery
T4a*	Tumor (any size) limited to the thyroid (anaplastic carcinoma only)
T4b*	Tumor (any size) extends beyond the thyroid capsule (anaplastic carcinoma only)

(N) Lymph nodes

NX	Regional nodes cannot be assessed
N0	No nodal metastasis
N1	Regional nodal metastasis
N1a	Metastasis in level VI (pretracheal and paratracheal, including prelaryngeal and Delphian lymph nodes)
N1b	Metastasis in other unilateral, bilateral, or contralateral cervical or upper/superior mediastinal lymph nodes

(M) Distant metastasis

MX	Distant metastasis cannot be assessed
M0	No distant metastasis
M1	Distant metastasis

Staging

Papillary or follicular under 45 years

Stage I	Any T	Any N	M0
Stage II	Any T	Any N	M1

Papillary or follicular, 45 years and older and medullary

Stage I	T1	N0	M0
Stage II	T2	N0	M0
Stage III	T3	N0	M0
	T1,T2,T3	N1a	M0
Stage IV	T1,T2,T3	N1b	M0
	T4a	N0,N1	M0
Stage IVB	T4b	Any N	M0
Stage IVC	Any T	Any N	M1

Anaplastic/undifferentiated (all cases are stage IV)

Stage IVA	T4a	Any N	M0
Stage IVB	T4b	Any N	M0
Stage IVC	Any T	Any N	M1

*Anaplastic cancer.

Debulking is futile, as the tumor regrows rapidly. External beam radiation coupled with doxorubicin may provide local control. Table 16.1 provides the thyroid cancer staging.

PARATHYROID CARCINOMA

Epidemiology

Parathyroid carcinoma arises in the background of primary hyperparathyroidism. Primary hyperparathyroidism is a common condition, with an incidence of 27.7 per 100,000 population annually. Benign adenomas comprise 85% of all causes of primary hyperparathyroidism, multigland hyperplasia accounts for 13–14%, and parathyroid carcinoma is seen in 1–2% of patients. This rare condition accounts for approximately 1,000 new cases per year in the United States.

Diagnosis

Parathyroid carcinoma is usually seen in patients in their fourth to sixth decade of life. These patients usually have high serum calcium levels (>13 mg/dL) and high serum intact parathyroid hormone (iPTH). It should be suspected, especially if a neck mass is palpable, the patient has hoarseness, difficulty swallowing or signs of aspiration. Computed tomography (CT) scan of the neck may establish the presence of a mass. Occasionally, the diagnosis of carcinoma is made intraoperatively, where a tan/gray gland with a thick capsule, desmoplastic reaction, and local invasion into thyroid or other neck structures is found. Frozen section of such a gland is rarely helpful unless direct invasion into surrounding structures is demonstrated.

Pathology

The pathological findings of parathyoid carcinoma are not distinct. Identification of trabeculae, thick fibrous reaction, increased mitoses, and vascular or capsular invasion are taken into account with the clinical suspicion of the surgeon. Because of the histologic overlap between benign and malignant lesions, differential cell cycle regulatory protein expression is being studied. P27, a cyclin-dependent kinase inhibitor that helps regulate the transition from the G1 to the S phase of the cell cycle, has been observed to have decreased expression in parathyroid carcinoma, whereas Ki67, a proliferation marker antigen, can have three-fold overexpression in carcinoma versus adenomas.

Treatment

A high clinical suspicion is the best intraoperative guide. *En bloc* resection of the parathyroid, the ipsilateral thyroid lobe, involved neck structures, including the recurrent laryngeal nerve (if invaded), and ipsilateral lymph node neck dissection if nodes appear clinically involved is the preferred surgical approach. Inadequate local excision leads to aggressive local recurrence.

In patients with distant metastases at the time of diagnosis, surgery has a lesser role unless lesions are amenable to resection. Usually, parathyroid carcinoma metastasizes diffusely to the lungs, bone, and liver and surgery may not prolong survival in these cases.

Chemotherapy with dacarbazine-based regimens may provide some control. Radiotherapy is not useful. Other therapies such as pamidronate, calcitonin, calcitriol, and mithramycin may ameliorate hypercalcemia and long-term remissions are reported.

Overall, 5-year survival for parathyroid carcinoma ranges between 25 and 40%.

ADRENAL CANCER

Epidemology

Adrenal cancers can arise in the adrenal cortex and are referred to as adrenocortical carcinomas. They can also arise in the adrenal medulla, where they are classified as malignant pheochromocytomas. Adrenal cancer is a rare entity with an incidence of 0.6–2 cases per million population per year. It accounts for 0.2% of all cancer deaths per year. It is twice as common in women between the ages of 30 and 50 and in children younger than 5 years old. The Li Fraumeni hereditary syndrome is a risk factor associated with p53 mutations involving multiple cancers of the soft tissues, breast, lung, and adrenal glands.

Classification and Diagnosis

Patients may present with an endocrinopathy, most commonly glucocorticoid excess resulting in Cushing's syndrome. Virilization, feminization, and, rarely, hyperaldosteronism may also occur in decreasing order. It is not unusual for patients to present with a large retroperitoneal mass in the absence of a clinically apparent endocrinopathy. However, biochemical screening will reveal excess secretions of one or more adrenal hormones in the majority of patients. Patients usually present with large tumors, with local invasion into adjacent organs. Almost 40% of patients will have distant metastases to liver, lung, bone, and brain at the time of diagnosis (Table 16.2).

Endocrinopathies

Endogenous Cushing's syndrome is caused by excess secretion of glucocorticoids, which results in the typical features of moon facies, truncal obesity, hypertension, muscle wasting, type II diabetes, polydipsia and polyphagia, osteoporosis, menstrual irregularities, infertility, and easy bruising. When associated with an adrenal tumor, it is usually adrenocorticotropic hormone (ACTH) independent. In this situation, the patient will demonstrate elevated serum and urine glucocorticoids and

TABLE 16.2. Staging of Adrenocortical Carcinoma

TNM Classification

(T) Primary tumor

Tx	Primary tumor cannot be assessed
T1	Tumor <5 cm, no invasion
T2	Tumor >5 cm, no invasion
T3	Tumor invasion into retroperitoneal fat
T4	Tumor invasion into adjacent organs

(N) Lymph node metastasis

Nx	Nodal metastasis cannot be assessed
N0	No nodes
N1	Nodal metastasis

(M) Distant metastasis

Mx	Metastasis cannot be assessed
M0	No distant metastasis
M1	Distant metastasis

Staging

Stage I	T1, N0, M0
Stage II	T2, N0, M0
Stage III	T1 or T2, N1, M0; T3, N0, M0
Stage IV	Any T, any N, M1; T3 or T4, N1, M0

suppressed serum ACTH levels. It is important to note, however, that the majority of adrenal tumors causing Cushing's syndrome are benign adenomas.

The demonstration of elevated urinary free cortisol, low serum ACTH, loss of diurnal cortisol variation, and a dexamethasone suppression test that fails to suppress can establish the diagnosis of ACTH-independent Cushing's syndrome. Imaging with CT or magnetic resonance (MR) scans can identify the adrenal tumor and demonstrate local invasion.

Sex hormone excess with virilization may be seen in combination with hypercortisolism. Elevated plasma levels of testosterone or estrogen, and elevated urinary levels of 17-hydoxysteroids and ketosteroids will confirm the diagnosis. The presence of excess sex steroid production associated with an adrenal mass is highly suggestive of malignancy.

Hyperaldosteronism caused by an adrenal cancer is a rare entity. The vast majority of patients with aldosteronomas (Conn's syndrome) have small benign tumors. These patients present with long-standing hypertension, hypokalemia, polydipsia, and polyuria. Primary hyperaldosteronism is typically diagnosed by demonstrating a serum potassium (K) level, off diuretic medications, of <3.5 mEq/L (although up to 30% of patients may have serum K levels >3.8 mEq/L), a plasma aldosterone to renin ratio >30, and elevated serum levels of 18-OH-corticosterone (usually >100 ng/dL). CT scans can often identify the abnormal adrenal, although, in equivocal cases, selective adrenal venous sampling may be necessary to lateralize the tumor.

Pheochromocytoma is a neuroendocrine tumor of the adrenal medulla chromaffin cells. Ten percent are malignant, 10% are extraadrenal, 10% are multicentric, and 10% are associated with genetic syndromes such as MEN 2a, MEN 2b, Von Recklingshausen's disease, or Von Hipple Lindau disease type 2. The diagnosis of malignancy is made by demonstrating local invasion or distant metastases. Pheochromocytomas secrete a variety of compounds such as norepinephrine, epinephrine, dopamine, and, less commonly, ACTH or vasoactive intestinal polypeptide (VIP). Patients may be asymptomatic or have episodic attacks of headaches, palpitations, syncope, and diaphoresis. Elevated serum levels of metanephrines, normetanephrines, and catecholamines may be more sensitive than the traditional 24-hour urinary catechlolamines, metanephrines, and vanillymandelic acid (VMA) in confirming the diagnosis. The clonidine suppression test and the glucagon stimulation test are rarely required to establish the diagnosis.

CT and MR scans (with typical T2 enhancement) can be used without IV contrast to localize the tumor. Met-iodo-benzyl-guanidine (MIBG) scanning is useful in extraadrenal, recurrent, or metastatic disease.

Familial pheochromocytomas are usually benign. It is prudent to perform laparoscopic unilateral adrenalectomy in patients with solitary macroscopic tumors, as only 52% of patients develop a contralateral tumor at a mean of 12 years after initial surgery. Furthermore, 48% of patients who undergo unilateral adrenalectomy in this setting have normal adrenal function for at least 5 years. This approach avoids Addisonian crisis, which occurs in 23% of patients following bilateral adrenalectomy.

Incidentalomas are unsuspected adrenal masses found during work up for unrelated issues. They are present in up to 5% of CT scans. The question to be answered is whether they represent a functional tumor, a primary adrenal malignancy, or a metastatic lesion.

A hormone evaluation to rule out pheochromocytoma, Cushing's syndrome, or aldosteronoma should be undertaken, as virtually all hormonally active tumors should be excised.

If the tumor is hormonally silent, size criteria and appearance on imaging studies should guide one to either resect or observe. Lesions <4 cm, with CT Houndfields units <10, are unlikely to be malignant and may be followed at 6-month intervals for growth. If growth is observed, lesions should be excised. If no growth is seen over 1–2 years, it may be deemed a benign adenoma. Lesions >4 cm or those suspicious for local invasion should be excised. Fine-needle biopsy is indicated only in cases when either a metastatic or infectious lesion is suspected. Fine-needle adrenal biopsy should never be performed without first ruling out a pheochromocytoma. Cytology alone cannot distinguish between a benign or malignant adrenal tumor but may reveal other malignancies such as lung cancer or melanoma.

Treatment

Complete excision is the only potentially curative therapy for malignant adrenal tumors, including pheochromocytoma. In tumors without features of malignancy by imaging studies, laparoscopic adrenalectomy is recommended. Patients with pheochromocytomas are often volume-depleted due to the excess catecholamines and are usually treated with preoperative alpha blockade with phenoxybenzamine starting at 10–20 mg two to four times a day, increasing in dosage to achieve orthostatic hypotension. Fluid replacement is encouraged. Patients who do not tolerate phenoxybenzamine can be given metyrosine, a tyrosine hydroxylase inhibitor, doxazosin, or prazosin. Breakthrough tachycardia can be controlled after alpha blockade with beta adrenergic blockers. Uncontrolled malignant hypertension can occur if beta blockade is initiated in the absence of alpha blockade.

Long-term follow up is necessary for all patients with pheochromocytoma as recurrence or metastasis can occur even after resecting apparently benign primary lesions.

Patients with metastatic pheochromocytoma can have prolonged survival, with 5-year rates of 25–40%. Resection of recurrences or metastases is indicated when feasible for hormonal control. Bone metastases may be radiated with improvement if 40 cGy can be administered. Cyclosphosphamide, vincristine, and dacarbazine are moderately successful. Newer modalities such as ^{131}I-MIBG therapies are under investigation.

Adrenocortical Carcinoma   Open *en bloc* adrenalectomy is the procedure of choice for adrenal cortical carcinoma. This may require resection of adjacent organs, including the spleen, tail of pancreas, or kidney. Recurrences are also best treated surgically if feasible. This increases the mean survival significantly compared with nonresected recurrences (15.85 vs. 3.2 months).

The most effective chemotherapeutic agent in adrenal cortical cancer is mitotane. Toxicity is dose dependent and rate limiting. Neurologic and gastrointestinal side effects are common. Patients may become adrenal insufficient, requiring hormonal replacement. Doxorubicin, etoposide, and alkylating agents have limited success.

The overall prognosis for adrenal cortical cancer is poor, with mean survival rates of 22–45 months.

NEUROENDOCRINE TUMORS OF THE GASTROINTESTINAL TRACT: CARCINOID TUMORS

Epidemiology

Clinically significant carcinoid tumors are rare. The clinical incidence is approximately 10 cases per million population per year, although incidental findings at autopsy can be up to 1.2%. They may be found in 1 in 300 appendectomies and 1 in 2500 proctoscopic examinations. There is no race or sex predominance. The incidence is highest in the fifth and sixth decades of life. They may be seen in MEN 1 syndrome.

Classification

The term *carcinoid* describes tumors of neuroendocrine origin of both intestinal and extraintestinal type. Macroscopically, carcinoids are solid, tan lesions that may produce desmoplastic reactions in the body. Microscopically, they have trabeculae and may form rosettes and glandular patterns. The cells have round nuclei with few mitoses. They are part of the *a*mine *p*recursor *u*ptake and *d*ecarboxylation (APUD) cells. They may take up silver (argyrophyllic cells) and reduce it (argentaffin cells) or take up chrome (chromaffin cells). The hormonal content of their granules can be measured by immunohistochemistry, which confirms the diagnosis. Many hormonal products are associated with carcinoid tumors. The breakdown product 5-hydro-xyindole-acetic-acid (5HIAA) is generally associated with carcinoids, yet peptides such as prostaglandins, kinins, ACTH, chromogranins, substance P, somatostatin, gastrin, insulin, and glucagon may also be secreted. The latter peptides are associated with pancreatic neuroendocrine tumors, which will be discussed in the next section.

There is a 10–20% association of gastrointestinal carcinoids with synchronous adenocarcinoma of the gastroin testinal (GI) tract. There are even "collision" tumors, where carcinoid cells are juxtaposed with adenocarcinoma cells. Ninety percent of carcinoid tumors are found in the GI tract and are classified by their embryologic relationship to the foregut, midgut, or hindgut, which correlates with their clinical behavior.

The appendix is the most common site, accounting for 35–38% of carcinoids. These tumors are usually small and found incidentally. If they are <2 cm in size, they may be treated by appendectomy alone. Moertel followed 150 patients with these tumors and found no recurrence or metastasis at 26 years for tumors <2 cm. Tumors >2 cm necessitate colonic resection with lymph node sampling as they commonly metastasize to lymphatics.

The terminal ileum and small intestine harbor approximately 20% of carcinoid tumors. At autopsy, the incidence of small, most likely benign tumors is much more common. Tumors >2 cm, which also have lymphovascular invasion, may cause symptoms of local obstruction and are more likely to metastasize. Local obstruction is usually caused by the dense mesenteric desmoplastic reaction that is character-istic of these tumors. Their treatment is segmental bowel resection with lymph node sampling.

The rectum and the stomach each comprise approximately 10% of the locations of carcinoid tumors. Rectal tumors are usually found incidentally at proctoscopy. Unless the tumors are deeply invasive, local resection may be adequate. If more extensive rectal resection is required for tumors >2 cm, sphincter-preserving procedures are recommended if possible, otherwise an abdominal perineal resection may be necessary. Rectal carcinoids do not usually produce the "the carcinoid syndrome."

Gastric carcinoids can be divided into three types: Type I carcinoids, associated with atrophic gastritis type A, result from hypergastrinemia in a neutral gastric pH milieu leading to antral G cells hyperplasia. These are usually small, benign tumors and endoscopic resection is adequate treatment. Type II tumors are seen in patients with MEN 1 or Zollinger Ellison syndrome and may be somewhat more aggressive than type I carcinoids. Type III are sporadic, unrelated to gastrin production, and are the most aggressive. For type I or II carcinoids >2 cm related to gastrin production, local resection of the carcinoid and antrectomy is recommended. For the type III carcinoids, gastric resection with lymph node clearance is preferred.

Colonic carcinoids comprise approximately 5% of these tumors. They are found most commonly in the right colon and may have hepatic metastasis at diagnosis. If <2 cm, they may be resected by colonoscopic excision. If this is not possible or the tumor is >2 cm, oncologically sound surgical resection is indicated.

Although not of GI origin, bronchial carcinoids are very similar to the intestinal tumors. They comprise approximately 5% of all carcinoids and are not related to smoking. They may produce ectopic ACTH resulting in Cushing's syndrome. They may also secrete antidiuretic or growth hormone releasing hormone. The treatment of choice is surgical resection.

The Carcinoid Syndrome

The symptoms of flushing, diarrhea, abdominal pain and, less commonly, wheezing, right heart failure, and pellagra usually represent synergistic interactions of 5HIAA, kinins, prostaglandins, and nicotinic acid deficiency in the systemic circulation and paracrine secretion into the intestine. Usually, only when liver metastases are present do these systemic features become apparent. Patients with small localized gastrointestinal carcinoids do not manifest the syndrome due to the first-pass effect of the hepatoportal circulation.

A carcinoid crisis may be triggered by an anesthetic or interventional procedure. The release of large amounts of amines into the circulation may lead to hypotension or severe hypertension, tachycardia, arrhythmias, wheezing, and neurologic abnormalities. Intravenous octreotide given as a bolus and then continued as an infusion for 24–48 hours in association with intravenous antihistamine or hydrocortisone is usually required.

Diagnosis and Treatment

For hormonal diagnosis, measurement of 24-hour urinary 5HIAA is highly specific. Plasma level of chromogranin A, a protein made in the secretory granules, is elevated in 80% of cases. Neuron-specific enolase levels are elevated in 40% of cases. Other gut hormones can be measured to exclude other hormonally active tumors, including gastrin, substance P, glucagon, calcitonin, and vasoactive intestinal polypeptide.

Appropriate imaging studies include CT and endoscopy. Magnetic resonance imaging (MRI) adds little. Angiography is invasive and rarely indicated. Scintigraphic imaging with radiolabelled somatostatin, octreotide or MIBG can detect either primary or metastatic tumors. Image fusion between single-photon emission computed tomography (SPECT) and dual-isotope tomoscintigraphy with technetium−99-hydroxymethylene diphosphonate and indium-111-pentetreotide can provide accurate localization. Symptomatic control of the carcinoid syndrome can be achieved by diet modification, such as avoidance of trigger foods (alcohol or spices), as well as targeted medications.

5HIAA receptor antagonists have limited success. Methysergide has been abandoned due to its incidence of retroperitoneal fibrosis. Ondansetron seems to be moderately effective, as are ketanserin and cyproheptadine. 5HIAA release inhibitors can result in symptomatic control. Octeotide, a somatostatin analogue, reduces flushing and diarrhea in more than 60–70% of patients. Lanreotide and Sandostatin LAR® (octreotide acetate) are long-acting somatostatin analogues and may be given intramuscularly every 2 or 4 weeks, respectively.

Surgery is the only curative therapy for carcinoids. Local resection and lymph node clearance is the treatment of choice for localized tumors. Debulking tumors may improve survival, provide symptomatic relief, and improve the efficacy of targeted therapies.

Cytotoxic chemotherapy is modestly effective in widely metastatic disease unresponsive to other treatments. The combination of streptozotocin and fluorouracil or cyclophosphamide may yield a short-lived response.

Hepatic artery embolization and chemoembolization can effectively treat isolated hepatic metastases. The response rate with reduction in symptoms and even tumor burden is promising. Precipitation of a carcinoid crisis can be prevented by pre-procedural IV octreotide.

Receptor-targeted therapy is based on the expression of neuroendocrine peptide receptors on carcinoid tumors and their avid uptake of [111]indium-labeled octreotide, [131]iodine MIBG, or [90]yttrium-labeled octreotide. Size reduction of tumors and symptomatic improvement is seen in up to 60% of cases. This treatment is promising as it has low morbidity.

Hepatectomy and liver transplantation for unresectable liver metastases is controversial, although the actuarial survival rate for metastatic carcinoid tumors at 5 years is 69% as compared with 8% for noncarcinoid neuroendocrine tumors.

These rare tumors need a multidisciplinary neuroendocrine team to achieve optimal management.

PANCREATIC NEUROENDOCRINE TUMORS

Insulinoma

Insulinomas are the most common pancreatic islet cell tumor. They are generally small and benign. In the sporadic form, they are solitary, but in the setting of MEN 1, they can be multiple, with equal anatomic distribution throughout the pancreas. They appear as reddish-brown tumors up to 2 cm in size. Microscopic examination cannot distinguish benign from malignant tumors. The diagnosis of malignancy is made by the presence of lymphatic spread or metastases.

Most patients with insulinomas have hypoglycemic symptoms. As a response to hypoglycemia, catecholamines are released, resulting in neuroglycopenic symptoms. A delay in diagnosis of up to two years is not uncommon. These patients are often characterized as neurotic and often gain substantial amounts of weight as they attempt to maintain euglycemia. Measurement of severe hypoglycemia and inappropriately elevated levels of insulin is essential for the diagnosis. The diagnostic test of choice is a 72-hour in-hospital fast during which serum levels of glucose and insulin are measured every 6 hours. The fast is terminated when neuroglycopenic symptoms occur. Serum glucose, insulin, proinsulin, and C peptide levels are measured. An immunoreactive insulin to glucose ratio >0.3 and elevated levels of proinsulin are diagnostic.

Radiologic studies are usually inconclusive as most tumors are too small to be easily identified. A preoperative CT or MR scan can rule out large tumors or metastatic disease. Endoscopic ultrasound has a sensitivity of 80%. Some experts have recommended surgical exploration and use of the intraoperative ultrasound as the most cost-effective approach. Preoperative regional localization can help operative planning. The best approach is the intra-arterial calcium stimulation test (Immamura-Doppman test), which can regionalize 90–100% of tumors.

Gastrinoma

Gastrinomas are associated with the Zollinger Ellison syndrome. Sixty percent are malignant with distant metastasis at diagnosis. Eighty percent are found in the "gastrinoma triangle," comprised of the first, second, and third portion of the duodenum and the head of the pancreas. Pancreatic gastrinomas have a higher incidence of liver metastases and thus a relative decreased long-term survival. Patients present with gastric ulceration and ulcers in unusual locations, such as the distal duodenum or jejunum. The mean period to correct diagnosis is 6 years. Elevated fasting serum level of gastrin (>100 pg/mL) and elevated basal acid output (>15 mEq/h) while patients are off all antisecretory medications are diagnostic. Secretin stimulation with a serum gastrin elevation of 200 pg/mL is confirmatory. CT scan can identify lesions >3 cm. Octreotide scanning (Octreoscan) is now regarded as the imaging test of choice. Its specificity approaches 100%. It will not identify small duodenal gastrinomas. Endoscopic ultrasound is also an excellent localization study. Intraoperative ultrasound and intraoperative endoscopy with or without transillumination can also be useful.

Glucagonoma

This is a rare, mostly malignant tumor often presenting with a red, pruritic rash in the pretibial, perioral, and intertriginous areas called necrolytic migratory erythema. Patients also develop type II diabetes, weight loss, and venous thromboembolism. Elevated plasma levels of glucagon (>500 pg/mL) and decreased levels of plasma amino acids are diagnostic. At the time of diagnosis, most tumors are large and often metastatic. Surgery is seldom curative.

Somatostatinoma

These are very rare, mostly malignant tumors. Duodenal tumors can be associated with von Reckingshausen's disease. Patients present with steatorrhea, cholelithiasis, type II diabetes, and hypochlorhydria. Most patients have advanced disease at the time of diagnosis.

Vipoma (Vasoactive Intestinal Peptide Tumor)

The syndrome associated with this tumor is also referred to as WHDA (watery diarrhea, hypokalemia, and achlorhydria), Verner Morrison syndrome, or pancreatic cholera. Patients present with severe diarrhea (5–10 L of stool per day), abdominal cramping, flushing, hypokalemia, and hypercalcemia. Elevated serum levels of pancreatic polypeptide and VIP can diagnose pancreatic tumors (80–90%). Octreotide reduces serum VIP levels and improves the symptoms in more than 80% of patients. This is a malignant tumor in 50% of patients and surgery is often curative.

Pancreatic Polypeptide Tumors (PPOMA)

This is a rare, mostly malignant tumor without an associated syndrome. It may produce local symptoms due to mass effect. Most tumors are resectable with pancreaticoduodenectomy or subtotal pancreatectomy.

Other Tumors

Tumors producing ACTH, growth hormone releasing hormone, serotonin, neurotensinogen, and other hormones can also occur. They are usually larger and visible on CT scan or octreoscan. Table 16.3 provides a concise summary of the neuroendocrine tumors of the pancreas.

Treatment

Adequate treatment should be aimed at controlling the symptoms and signs of hormonal secretion and, if possible, extirpation of local disease. The only chance to cure is surgical resection of all disease. Resectable metastases should be removed as this mitigates the severity of symptoms and prolongs survival. Octreotide can be used to control hormonal symptoms in most neuroendocrine tumors. Thirty to forty percent of patients with metastastatic disease will respond to combination chemotherapy using adriamycin, streptozotocin, and fluorouracil. Liver embolization does not seem to prolong survival. Due to the indolent course of the disease, widely metastatic patients have a 20% 5-year survival. Patients with stable metastatic disease may be observed and chemotherapy instituted only when there is evidence of tumor growth.

TABLE 16.3. Neuroendocrine Tumors of the Pancreas and Duodenum

Tumor	Malignancy (%)	Location	Symptoms	Diagnosis
Insulinoma	5	Pancreas	Hypoglycemia, neuroglycopenia	72-hour fast insulin/ glucose ratio >0.3
Gastrinoma	>60	"Gastrinoma triangle," pancreas	Persistent ulcers, GI bleeding	Elevated gastrin and BAO
Glucagonoma	>70	Pancreas	DM, glossitis, NME, thrombo-embolism	Elevated serum glucagon
Somatostatinoma	>90	Pancreas	DM, steatorrhea, cholelithiasis	Elevated serum somatostatin, low serum Cl^-
VIPoma	50	Pancreas, duodenum	Severe diarrhea	Elevated serum VIP, low K^+, Cl^-
PPoma	>60	Pancreas	Local symptoms, bleeding	Elevated serum PP, mass

DM: diabetes mellitus; NME: necrolytic migratory erythema; BAO: basal acid output.

MULTIPLE ENDOCRINE NEOPLASIA

MEN 1

Genetics   The MEN 1 syndrome is an autosomal dominant disorder caused by multiple chromosomal deletions encompassing chromosome 11q13, in keeping with a "two-hit" model for inactivation of a tumor suppressor gene called menin. There are no specific genotype-phenotype correlations established. There is no precisely identified role of the menin protein in cell regulation as of yet but it seems to involve inhibition of JunD-activated transcription.

Individuals suspected of having this syndrome should have genetic screening beginning in the second decade of life. Serum levels of calcium, prolactin, gastrin, and pancreatic polypeptide should be screened. Individuals will likely develop primary hyperparathyroidism, neuroendocrine tumors of the pancreas and duodenum, and pituitary tumors (Table 16.4).

Clinical Features   Primary hyperparathyroidism (HPTH) develops in more than 95% of individuals with MEN 1. Affected individuals develop multigland parathyroid hyperplasia, although asymmetric gland enlargement is common. The average age of onset of hypercalcemia is 25 years and is highly uncommon before age 15. The cumulative age penetrance of HPTH is 52% by age 20 years and 87% by 30 years. The presentation is similar to sporadic primary HPTH, including asymptomatic hypercalcemia, dyspepsia, depression, fatigue, bone pain, osteoporosis, and nephrolithiasis. Elevated serum levels of calcium and intact

TABLE 16.4. Inherited Endocrine Neoplasia Syndromes

	MEN 1	MEN2A	MEN2B	FMTC
Inheritance	Autosomal dominant	Autosomal dominant	Autosomal dominant	Autosomal dominant
Gene defect	Menin 11q 12-13	RET 10	RET 10	RET 10
Associated Neoplasia	Pituitary(30–50%)[*] Parathyroid(100%) Islet cell(50–70%)	MTC(100%) Parathyroid(10–35%) Pheochromocytoma	MTC(100%) Ganglioneuromas Pheochromocytoma	MTC(100%)

[*]Percentages refer to chance of developing the associated disorder for affected persons.

parathyroid hormone (iPTH) are diagnostic in the setting of normal renal function. Because this represents multigland hyperplasia, the treatment of choice is either total cervical parathyroidectomy with immediate heterotopic parathyroid autotransplantation into the forearm or subtotal three and one-half gland resection, retaining approximately 40 mg of well-vascularized parathyroid tissue *in situ*.

MEN 1 patients with HPTH and synchronous Zollinger Ellison syndrome (ZE) usually benefit from parathyroidectomy first as this corrects the hypercalcemia and improves ZE symptoms.

Neuroendocrine tumors of the pancreas, intestinal tract, or bronchi (carcinoids) develop in 35–75% of patients with MEN 1. The pancreaticoduodenal tumors behave aggressively and may be highly malignant. Pancreatic polypeptide tumors (Ppoma) are the most common neuroendocrine tumors of the pancreas in MEN 1. Gastrinoma (ZE), insulinoma, glucagonoma, VIPoma, and carcinoid tumors can also occur and are often multiple. Almost 40% of patients with ZE will have advanced disease with metastases at the time of diagnosis.

Beginning at age 10, routine serological biochemical screening should be instituted, measuring endocrine pancreatic hormones after administration of standardized meal tests. Detection of pancreatic endocrine involvement up to two decades earlier can be achieved. Genetic screening for the menin gene is already available in select research institutes.

Surgical resection of the primary tumor with involved lymph nodes in advanced localized tumors is indicated and has better outcome than no resection. Major pancreatic procedures can be performed safely in most patients, including pancreaticoduodenectomy if indicated. Aggressive surgical approaches should be considered before malignant spread occurs. Because these tumors tend to be multicentric, some surgeons have recommended aggressive pancreatic resection even in the absence of malignant disease.

Long-term pharmacologic treatment with omeprazole in ZE syndrome is also indicated because even aggressive surgical resection may not fully resolve hypergastrinemia.

Pituitary adenomas occur in 16–65% of patients. The most common pituitary tumor in MEN 1 patients is a prolactinoma. These patients develop impotence or galactorrhea. Elevated serum levels of prolactin and MRI evaluation of the sella turcica can be diagnostic. Bromocriptine can control the symptoms although transsphenoidal anterior pituitary resection is often curative. Other pituitary tumors may produce adrenocorticotropic hormone (ACTH), resulting in Cushing's disease, growth hormone leading to acromegaly, or TSH with resulting hyperthyroidism. Surgical resection is preferred, but radiation may help in nonresectable tumors.

Other tumors such as intestinal or bronchial carcinoids, benign thyroid and adrenal adenomas, and lipomas can also be seen in MEN 1 patients.

MEN 2

Genetics There are three MEN 2 syndromes with phenotypic expressions of variants of activating mutations in the RET proto-oncogene, a tyrosine kinase receptor, transmitted in an autosomal dominant fashion on chromosome 10. All clinical manifestations of the MEN 2 syndromes reflect the inappropriate transmission of the RET signal in the neural crest-derived tissues that naturally express it. The divisions are MEN 2a, MEN 2b, and familial medullary thyroid cancer (FMTC) syndromes. RET gene analysis is now available and is a sensitive screening method. Six to eight percent of "sporadic" medullary thyroid cancer (MTC) patients will have RET gene mutations.

Clinical Features

MEN 2a consists of MTC, pheochromocytoma, and parathyroid hyperplasia. MEN 2b patients have the recognizable phenotype of multiple neuromas of the tongue and lips, Marfanoid body habitus, skeletal abnormalities, MTC, ganglioneuromas of the intestinal tract, colonic dysmotility, Hirschsprung's disease, and pheochromo-cytomas. They do not develop hyperparathyroidism. FMTC consists of development of MTC without other endocrinopathies.

Medullary thyroid carcinoma will eventually develop in virtually all patients with MEN 2 or FMTC. It is the least virulent in FMTC and tends to be clinically apparent by the fifth decade of life. MTC in MEN 2a is of intermediate aggressiveness and is usually clinically apparent by the second decade. In contrast, MTC in MEN 2b is extremely aggressive and, commonly, has already metastasized before the age of 10.

MTC arises in the parafollicular C cells in the thyroid, which are located in the upper third of the thyroid lobes. Calcitonin is a sensitive plasma marker for detection of MTC or its precursor C cell hyperplasia. Early detection and treatment are key. Patients from an MEN 2a kindred should have RET mutation testing and should have early total thyroidectomy while MTC is still organ confined and therefore curable. This should be done by age 5 or certainly in the first decade of life. Total thyroidectomy with central lymphadenectomy can be performed after genetic testing. Ipsilateral or bilateral modified radical neck microdissection are indicated for most patients who have progressed beyond C cell hyperplasia to invasive MTC. MEN 2b patients should have a thyroidectomy as soon as the syndrome is recognized due to the aggressive nature of their MTC.

Disseminated MTC may cause secretory diarrhea, which is generally not well controlled with octreotide.

Pheochromocytomas are seen in 50% of MEN 2 patients. They develop bilateral microscopic adrenal medullary hyperplasia, but not all patients develop bilateral clinical disease. There is some controversy about the treatment of empiric bilateral adrenalectomy once the individual has developed a unilateral tumor or selective resection and observation. Given that not all patients will develop bilaterally clinically significant disease, unilateral laparoscopic adrenalectomy for the macroscopically and physiologically active side is preferable. Preserving adrenal function avoids the potential for life-threatening Addisonian crisis.

Malignant pheochromocytomas are highly infrequent in MEN 2 syndromes.

Hyperparathyroidism also develops in MEN 2a. It has similar manifestations as primary hyperparathyroidism, with multigland parathyroid hyperplasia, which is often asymmetric. It is common for these patients to have enlargement of only one or two glands. Surgery usually consists of either total cervical parathyroidectomy with immediate heterotopic autotransplantation or three and one-half gland resection with retention of a 40 mg well-vascularized parathyroid remnant *in situ*. Some surgeons have advocated a less aggressive approach and have only recommended resection of clinically enlarged parathyroid glands. There is disagreement among surgeons regarding whether a total parathyroidectomy and parathyroid transplantation should be done at the time of initial thyroidectomy.

Gastrointestinal manifestations can be seen in MEN 2b. Intestinal ganglioneuromas are multiple and some may cause intestinal obstruction or pain, necessitating resection. They can also lead to abnormal gut motility and development of constipation. Hirschprung's disease can be found in children.

FURTHER READING

Brennan MD, Bergstralh EJ, van Heerden JA et al. (1991) Follicular thyroid cancer treated at the Mayo Clinic 1946–1970: Initial manifestations, pathology findings, therapy and outcome. *Mayo Clinic Proc* 66:11.

Cady B et al. (1979) Risk factor analysis in differentiated thyroid cancer. *Cancer* 43:810.

Clark OH (1982). Total thyroidectomy: The treatment of choice for patients with differentiated thyroid cancer. *Ann Surg* 196:361.

Clark OH, Noguchi S (2000) *Thyroid Cancer: Diagnosis and Treatment*. Quality Medical Publishing, Inc., St. Louis, Missouri.

Doppman JL, Miller DL, Chang R et al. (1991) Insulinomas: Localization with selective intraarterial injection of calcium. *Radiology* 178:237.

Gagner M, Pomp A, Heniford TB et al. (1997) Laparoscopic adrenalectomy: Lessons learned form 100 consecutive procedures. *Ann Surg* 226:238.

Hoefnagel CA. (1994) Metaiodobenzylguanidine and somatostatin in oncology: Role in the management of neural crest tumours. *Eur J Nucl Med* 21:561.

Hoff AO, Cote J, Gagel RF. (2000) Multiple endocrine neoplasias. *Annu Rev Physiol* 62:377.

Kulke, MH, Mayer RJ (1999) Medical progress: Carcinoid tumors. *N Engl J Med* 340:858.

Le HN, Norton JA (2001) Parathyroid. In *Surgery: Basic Science and Clinical Evidence.* Norton JA, Bollinger RR, Chang AE (eds.) Springer, New York.

Malone MJ, Liberetino JA, Tsapatsaris NS et al. (1989) Preoperative and surgical management of pheochromocytoma. *Urol Clin North Am* 6:567.

Mazzaferi EL, Jhiang SM (1994) Long-term impact of intial surgical and medical therapy on papillary and follicular thyroid cancer. *Am J Med* 97:418.

Meko JB, Norton JA (1994) Endocrine tumors of the pancreas. *Curr Opin Gen Surg* 2:186.

Modlin IM, Sandor A (1997) An analysis of 8305 cases of carcinoid tumors. *Cancer* 79:813.

Moley JF (1995) Medullary thyroid cancer. *Surg Clin North Am* 75:405.

Norton JA, Cromack DT, Shawker TH et al. (1988) Intraoperative ultrasonographic localization of the islet cell tumors. A prospective comparison to palpation. *Ann Surg* 207:160.

Orth DN (1995) Medical Progress: Cushing's Syndrome. *N Engl J Med* 332:791.

Prinz RA (1995) A comparison of laparoscopic and open adrenalectomies. *Arch Surg* 130:489.

Ross NS, Aron DC (1990) Hormonal evaluation of the patient with an incidentally discovered adrenal mass. *N Engl J Med* 323:1401.

Schlumberger M, Pacini F (1999) *Thyroid Tumors.* Nucleon Edition, Paris.

Thompson NW (1997) Multiple endocrine neoplasia type 1. Surgical therapy. *Cancer Treat Res* 89:407.

Van Heerden JA, Young WF, Grant CS (1995) Adrenal surgery for hypercortisolism—surgical aspects. *Surgery* 117:466.

Vetto JT, Brennan MF, Woodruf J et al. (1993) Parathyroid carcinoma: Diagnosis and clinical history. *Surgery* 114:882.

Wells SA Jr et al. (1975) The early diagnosis of medullary thyroid carcinoma of the thyroid gland in patients with multiple endocrine neoplasia type II. *Ann Surg* 182:362.

Wells SA Jr, Chi D, Toshima K et al. (1994) Predictive DNA testing and prophylactic thyroidectomy in patients at risk for multiple endocrine neoplasia type 2A. *Ann Surg* 220:237.

Young WF, Hogan MJ, Klee GG et al. (1990) Primary aldosteronism. Diagnosis and treatment. *Mayo Clin Proc* 65:96.

CHAPTER 17

Lung Cancer

DAVID PAYNE

University of Toronto, Princess Margaret Hospital, Department of Radiation Oncology, Toronto, Ontario, Canada

RON BURKES

University of Toronto, Princess Margaret Hospital, Department of Medical Oncology, Toronto, Ontario, Canada

ROBERT J. GINSBERG

University of Toronto, Princess Margaret Hospital, Department of Surgical Oncology, Toronto, Ontario, Canada

Lung cancer is the most common cause of cancer death in both sexes and is increasingly common throughout the world. Screening programs are improving but infrequently detect cancer early enough to alter the survival outcome. Prevention programs that effectively decrease the smoking rates in the population would save more lives than are cured by present methods.

The vast majority of malignant tumors are carcinomas arising from bronchial epithelium. Regional spread to mediastinal lymph nodes is frequent, and is predictive of systemic metastases. Clinical staging is based on tumor size, involvement of associated structures, the location of lymph node metastases, and the presence of metastasis in distant organs.

Surgery plays an essential role in diagnosis of all forms of lung cancer, and in the curative treatment of early forms (UICC stages I, II, and some IIIA). Radiotherapy is required in nonsurgical cases of early stage, either as exclusive treatment, or as part of combined modality therapy programs for locally advanced disease. Radiotherapy is also highly effective in the palliative treatment of local tumor or distant metastases. Chemotherapy using current agents produces symptomatic responses and often good systemic palliation, but its impact on overall survival rates is modest, as is that of radiotherapy.

UICC Manual of Clinical Oncology, Eighth Edition. Edited by Raphael E. Pollock
ISBN 0-471-22289-5 Copyright © 2004 John Wiley & Sons, Inc.

ETIOLOGY

Tobacco smoking is by far the most important risk factor for lung cancer, and is estimated to be the cause of 85% of lung cancer deaths. The extent of exposure to tobacco smoke (carcinogen "dose"), as reflected in numbers of years an individual has smoked, number of cigarettes smoked per day, and tar content of the cigarettes, is correlated with the risk of lung cancer. The carcinogens in tobacco smoke include the polynuclear aromatic hydrocarbons (PAHs), N-nitrosoamines, aromatic amines, other organic and nonorganic compounds, and polonium-210. After smoking cessation, an individual's risk of lung cancer slowly comes to approximate but not equal that of a nonsmoker. It is also suggested that, even among nonsmokers, the "passive" smokers who have been exposed to environmental tobacco smoke have a significantly increased risk of lung cancer.

Other carcinogens that play a role in the development of lung cancer include pollutants in the urban air, such as benzopyrenes, indoor radon, and various occupational respiratory toxic substances. Asbestos exposure is the most widely recognized environmental carcinogen; it acts synergistically with tobacco smoke for lung carcinogenesis, and is also closely associated with the development of mesothelioma. In countries such as China, an excess risk of lung cancer is attributed to indoor air pollution originating from cooking.

Some nutritional elements have long been suggested to act as chemoprotective factors against carcinogenesis. Beta-carotene has been the most widely investigated. However, two large-scale randomized clinical trials have demonstrated no effect of this chemoprevention in reducing the risk of cancer.

Genetic factors appear to be important in lung carcinogenesis in some cases. There are several reports that genetic polymorphisms of carcinogen-metabolizing enzyme systems are associated with the risk of lung cancer. These may determine the different cancer susceptibility seen in various individuals and families.

None of the above-mentioned "causes" of lung cancer satisfactorily explains the recent increase in incidence of adenocarcinoma, although the increased use of filter cigarettes has been implicated on the basis of more peripheral deposition of carcinogens in the airway. It is clear that human tumors result from a complex sequence of mutational events, and it is likely that still unknown factor(s) play important roles in lung carcinogenesis.

SCREENING AND DIAGNOSIS

The purpose of screening is to accomplish early detection and treatment of as many cancers as possible, especially among smokers, who are at greatest risk. Public awareness of the risk of lung cancer induction by smoking is important. Physicians may screen individuals by means of chest radiograph and sputum cytology for atypical or cancer cells. Suspicious findings should lead to a diagnostic evaluation along the lines of the schema (Fig. 17.1). Note that peripheral lung tumors (surrounded by lung parenchyma) typically produce few symptoms and are best found

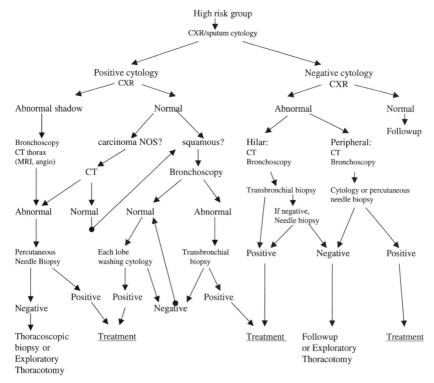

Figure 17.1 Diagnosis of lung cancer based on screening by chest radiograph and sputum cytology.

by chest radiography. The more common central tumors arise from the proximal airways and often attract attention because of cough hemoptysis or dyspnea.

If the screening process proves abnormal, the subsequent diagnostic evaluation depends on the original observation and the method of detection. Thus, while lung cancer screening typically includes chest radiograph and sputum cytology, the work-up may differ according to the particular finding and the location of the suspected lesion.

Because lung cancer at the time of presentation is frequently incurable, there is potential for screening of asymptomatic patients to discover cancers at an earlier stage, which may result in improved overall survival rates. Large scale screening programs must utilize simple techniques to be widely applicable. In the case of lung cancer, chest radiography and sputum cytology are the only practical methods currently available to screen large numbers of subjects. However, even these are expensive when applied to a population, and can only be justified if they yield significant numbers of early tumors and better long-term results.

The use of chest radiography and sputum cytology to screen high-risk patients for lung cancer was evaluated in the large scale, randomized controlled trials sponsored by the National Cancer Institute and conducted at Johns Hopkins Medical Institute, Memorial Sloan-Kettering Cancer Center, and Mayo Clinic. Patients, 45 years old and above, who were chronic heavy cigarette smokers, were screened every 4 months using chest radiography with or without sputum cytology. The trial detected more cancers, more resectable cancers, and more early stage cancers in the sputum-screened group than in the unscreened controls. The 5-year survival rate was higher for the screened groups than the controlled group, explainable by the effect of lead-time bias. However, the cancer-related mortality rates for the screened and control groups were virtually the same. Thus, the results did not justify recommending large-scale radiological or cytological screening for lung cancer.

These trials, done over 25 years ago, did not provide sufficient evidence to support large-scale screening by the methods used, even in the high-risk population studied. It should be noted, however, that modern technologies now permit greatly improved scrutiny of the airways and parenchyma, and spiral computed tomography (CT) can detect lesions under 3 mm. Nonrandomized trials in the United States and Japan have demonstrated higher yields of small peripheral cancers by this technique, but to impact overall survival rates a decrease in the prevalence of advanced stage tumors must occur. This has not been seen as yet. Newer methods of automated sputum cytology collection and immunoanalysis of samples may permit many molecular and genetic markers to be screened in a single specimen, and provide the capability for early diagnosis. These methods may result in a reappraisal of the need for lung cancer screening, but at present there is a need for large, well-conducted trials before screening can be recommended.

TECHNIQUES FOR DIAGNOSTIC EVALUATION

The investigation of patients with solitary pulmonary nodules should begin with the search for and examination of previous chest radiographs. Lesions that are new, radiologically suspicious for carcinoma, or increasing in size should be treated as pulmonary malignancies. Calcification is typically a sign of benign lesions, but may be seen in malignant tumors. Radiologic findings are not sufficient for pathologic diagnosis of lung cancer, much less for its subclassification.

The definitive diagnosis of a lung cancer requires histopathologic or cytologic confirmation. Among the four major subtypes of lung cancer (Table 17.1), small-cell carcinoma (SCLC) is distinguished from the other, non–small-cell lung carcinomas (NSCLC) because of its differences in biologic behavior and clinical course. These tumors exhibit different cellular characteristics, a pronounced tendency for metastasis to distant sites, and typically a marked response to chemotherapy. SCLC and NSCLC often require different treatment strategies. Physicians thus require pathologic information about the disease to perform therapeutic decision-making. In some cases, pathologists may require more tissue to determine whether an adenocarcinoma within the lung represents a primary lung cancer, or a metastatic focus from a metachronous or a synchronous cancer, be it

TABLE 17.1. Characteristics of Pathologic Cell Types of Lung Cancer

Cancer Type	Major Cell Type	Proportion of All Lung Cancers	Location	Histology	Volume Doubling Time (Days)	Cell of Origin
Non–small cell	Squamous cell	30–35%	Central large or medium bronchi	Intercellular bridges (desmosomes); keratin pearls	100	Multipotential epithelial cells
	Adeno carcinoma; subtype: bronchioloalveolar	25–30%	Peripheral	Gland formation; intracellular mucous	187	Goblet cells
	Large cell	10%	Peripheral	Undifferentiated large cells	100	—
Small cell	Small cell; subtypes: oat cell, intermediate cell	20–25%	Central		33	Kulchitsky's (K; neuroectodermal) cells
Others	Carcinoid; sarcomatoid salivary; etc	1%				

Based on WHO/IASLC Histologic Classification 1999.

from a source in the breast, colon, or a different part of the lung. An aggressive approach to diagnosis is usually justified, unless specifically contraindicated, to determine prognosis and a basis for management decisions. Multiple diagnostic procedures for a lung cancer are available, each with specific indications.

Sputum Cytology

Sputum cytology is positive in more than 15% of cases. Positive cytology is more likely when the suspected lesion is central in the thorax but has a negative prognostic significance when the cancer is located in the peripheral lung field. However, positive sputum cytology can result from a radiologically occult lesion such as a centrally located bronchogenic carcinoma or an upper airway cancer (e.g., from the larynx). Therefore, bronchoscopic examination is necessary before determining that a radiologically suspicious lesion is the source of the positive sputum cytology.

Bronchoscopy

Lung cancer patients are diagnosed by bronchoscopic biopsy or cytology. Hilar lesions such as centrally located squamous cell carcinomas often present as endobronchial tumors, diagnosed by biopsy, brush cytology, or wash cytology. Submucosal infiltration or an invasive nodal metastasis may be visible by bronchoscopy and the tumor diagnosed by biopsy or aspiration cytology. Even a bronchoscopically negative, peripherally located tumor may be diagnosed by fluoroscopy-guided transbronchial biopsy or cytology (taken by curettage, brush, lavage, or fine-needle aspiration). When a peripherally located tumor is too small or too faint in density to be detected by conventional x-ray fluoroscopy, transbronchial biopsy with CT fluoroscope guidance may be helpful. Major complications of transbronchial biopsy include hemorrhage, pneumothorax, and exacerbation of infection.

Transthoracic Needle Biopsy

Transthoracic needle biopsy can provide a definite diagnosis of lung cancer more easily than bronchoscopic examination when the suspicious lesion is peripherally located. It is usually performed with x-ray fluoroscopy guidance, but ultrasound guidance may be more appropriate when the lesion contacts the chest wall. CT-guided needle biopsy is helpful when the lesion is difficult to visualize on fluoroscopy or when it is located near vital organs such as major vessels. Pneumothorax is the most frequent complication of transthoracic needle biopsy.

Cytologic examination of other tissues such as pleural fluid, or biopsies of pleura, lymph nodes, liver, or bone marrow are sometimes the most appropriate way to make a diagnosis of lung cancer. A solitary mass in an adrenal gland or in the liver in a patient with otherwise potentially resectable lung cancer should be confirmed with needle biopsy before classifying it as a metastasis.

Mediastinoscopy

Mediastinoscopy is a surgical procedure in which superior mediastinal lymph nodes, which are often involved with metastases, can be evaluated and biopsied. It is performed under general anesthesia using a rigid scope through a suprasternal incision, providing access to pre- and paratracheal and subcarinal lymph nodes. Access to the aortopulmonary region requires a left parasternal incision, or extended mediastinoscopy. Although it can be diagnostic for a case in which no other lesions are available for biopsy, mediastinoscopy usually is a staging procedure for the evaluation of the N category (see below for TNM classification). Those with mediastinoscopy-proven nodal disease have a poorer prognosis, compared with cases where the nodal involvement was detected by postoperative pathologic examination only.

Anterior Mediastinotomy

Anterior mediastinotomy is used when aortopulmonary lymph nodes are enlarged, suggesting inoperability. A left second or third interspace incision provides access to the area in question.

Thoracoscopy

Thoracoscopy can be used as a staging procedure for the diagnosis of pleural dissemination or malignant effusion in a patient with lung cancer that otherwise may be suitable for curative resection or definitive radiotherapy. Thoracoscopy is also a useful tool when the diagnosis remains elusive after less invasive measures. It may suplant anterior mediastotomy as well. Video-assisted procedures allow examination of much of the pleural space, to identify and biopsy nodules or plaques of disease. In addition, wedge resection of peripheral nodules can be used for diagnosis. Thoracoscopy is more invasive than bronchoscopy, but can be done under local anesthesia and carries less risk than an open lung biopsy.

Open Lung Biopsy

Open lung biopsy is the most invasive diagnostic procedure but may be required when all other diagnostic procedures have failed. The "wait-and-see" attitude in an otherwise good-risk patient with a solitary pulmonary nodule is seldom justified unless radiologic or clinical evidence strongly suggests that it is benign. Even tumors with a diameter of less than 2 cm can metastasize to regional lymph nodes and spread systemically.

Search for Extrathoracic Metastases

A thorough systemic survey should be done as staging procedures in clinical trial patients (Table 17.2), and in most SCLC patients, since they frequently harbor

TABLE 17.2. Recommended Staging Procedures for Patients with Lung Cancer

Procedure	Standard Care	Patients on Clinical Trials
Complete physical examination	Yes	Yes
Hematology with differential, WBC, and platelet count	Yes	Yes
Biochemistry with electrolytes, liver function tests, lactate dehydrogenase	Yes	Yes
Chest radiograph	Yes	Yes
CT scan of thorax	Only for limited disease patients to facilitate radiotherapy planning	Yes
Ultrasound or CT scan of abdomen	Yes[*]	Yes
Radionuclide bone scan	Yes[*]	Yes
Skeletal radiographs	If bone scan is indeterminate	If bone scan is indeterminate
CT or MRI of brain	Yes[*]	Yes[*]
MRI of spine	Only if clinically indicated	Only if clinically indicated
Bone marrow aspiration and biopsies	Only if hematology is abnormal	Only for patients on trials of localized disease
Bronchoscopy	Only if needed for diagnosis	Baseline only necessary, unless post-treatment bronchoscopy is required to confirm complete response
Mediastinoscopy	Only if needed for diagnosis	Only if needed for diagnosis
Lumbar puncture	Only if clinically indicated	Only if clinically indicated
Liver biopsy	No	Only necessary if indeterminate results are obtained from CT or ultrasound of abdomen
Monoclonal antibody scans	No	No, unless the trial is specifically evaluating monoclonal antibodies
Biomarkers	No	No, unless the trial is specifically evaluating the role of biomarkers
Pulmonary function tests	Only if there is concern about the ability to deliver thoracic irradiation	Only if there is concern about the ability to deliver thoracic irradiation
Positron emission (PET) scan	No	No, unless the trial is specifically evaluating the role of PET

[*]If one of these studies is positive, further tests are not necessary because extensive disease will have been confirmed. The decision as to which scan should be done first should be guided by any abnormalities detected on the baseline history, physical examination, and blood work.

asymptomatic metastases. In NSCLC patients without clinical findings suggestive of extrathoracic cancer, a chest x-ray and chest CT scan are recommended to stage locoregional disease, with biopsy of mediastinal lymph nodes found on CT scan to be greater than 1 cm in shortest transverse diameter. Pretreatment bone scan and head CT scan are recommended only when signs or symptoms of disease are present, unless required by a specific research protocol.

PATHOLOGY AND NATURAL HISTORY

Lung cancers may arise from the epithelial or stromal tissues but the vast majority originate in the bronchial epithelium of the large to mid-size airways. This discussion will focus on these tumors, which form the overwhelming number of lung cancers. The major subtypes are listed in Table 17.1, according to the WHO/IASLC classification (World Health Organization/International Association for the Study of Lung Cancer). These subtypes identify carcinomas derived from cells with squamous or glandular features, or undifferentiated tumors that cannot be so classified. The "small-cell" subtype is distinguished by the presence of neurosecretory granules on electron microscopy and other clinicopathologic features. Its importance derives from its comparatively rapid growth rate, tendency to metastasize, and chemoreponsiveness. Its management is therefore somewhat different from the other carcinomas grouped under the designation "non–small cell." The vast majority of lung malignancies fall into one of these four categories. The bronchioloalveolar subtype of adenocarcinoma is thought to arise from the glandular epithelium of the small peripheral airways and alveoli. Malignant cells of this type have a tendency to spread in a superficial pattern along the epithelium of these structures. The relatively rare primary tumors of the trachea are predominantly squamous, although the glandular adenoid cystic carcinoma subtype is almost as frequent.

Lung tumors have been extensively studied by the methods of immunocytochemistry or molecular biology to identify proteins with functional significance or that may serve as tumor markers. These help to classify the tumor but have not so far led to significant treatment applications. Small-cell cancer has been linked to genetic changes in chromosome 3. Other gene abnormalities (*K-ras*, *HER-2/neu*, *p53*, *Rb*) have been identified to occur frequently in lung cancer, and in some cases (*K-ras*) to convey a poor outlook.

Bronchogenic carcinomas have a strong predilection for spread to the regional lymph nodes. Anatomically, these have been categorized as intralobar, hilar, and mediastinal (subcarinal, paratracheal, subaortic, and others). A standardized map and numerical nomenclature has been developed to facilitate accurate description of involved or uninvolved nodes (Fig 17.2). Some, but not all, of these nodes will be accessible at mediastinoscopy staging, while these and others may be visualized by CT or magnetic resonance imaging (MRI) staging. The risk that a node is involved with cancer increases dramatically as its diameter exceeds 1.5 cm; in the range of size 1–3 cm, however, many false negatives or false positives are possible.

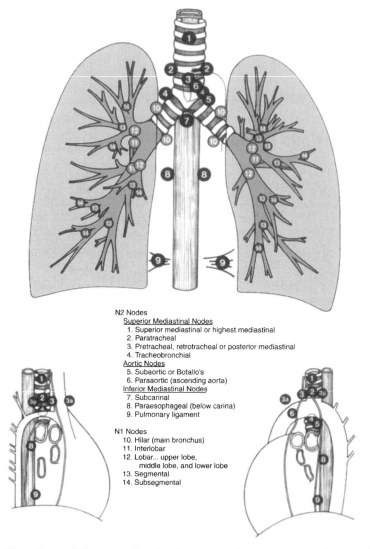

N2 Nodes
  Superior Mediastinal Nodes
    1. Superior mediastinal or highest mediastinal
    2. Paratracheal
    3. Pretracheal, retrotracheal or posterior mediastinal
    4. Tracheobronchial
  Aortic Nodes
    5. Subaortic or Botallo's
    6. Paraaortic (ascending aorta)
  Inferior Mediastinal Nodes
    7. Subcarinal
    8. Paraesophageal (below carina)
    9. Pulmonary ligament

N1 Nodes
    10. Hilar (main bronchus)
    11. Interlobar
    12. Lobar... upper lobe,
          middle lobe, and lower lobe
    13. Segmental
    14. Subsegmental

Figure 17.2 Regional lymph nodes for the staging for lung cancer. (Reprinted with permission from *TNM Atlas*, Fourth Edition, 1997, Springer, New York.)

Nodal involvement of lung cancer serves as an indicator of relative difficulty of achieving complete surgical removal, or of definite nonresectability. It also identifies disease for radiotherapy planning. More importantly, it serves as a marker of systemic metastatic spread. The risk of systemic metastases, whether clinical or occult, increases dramatically from the lymph node negative status (N0), through the hilar (N1), ipsilateral mediastinal (N2), or contralateral mediastinal (N3) lymph node involvement. Palpable disease in more distal lymph nodes (supraclavicular or cervical) signifies almost certain presence of distant metastases.

TABLE 17.3. TNM Staging for Lung Cancer

T—Primary tumor

TX   Primary tumor cannot be assessed, or tumor proven by the presence of malignant cells in sputum or bronchial washings but not visualized by imaging or bronchoscopy

T0   No evidence of primary tumor

Tis   Carcinoma *in situ*

T1   Tumor ≤3 cm in greatest dimension, surrounded by lung or visceral pleura, without bronchoscopic evidence of invasion more proximal than the lobar bronchus (i.e., not in the main bronchus)[a]

T2   Tumor with any of the following features of size or extent: >3 cm in greatest dimension; involves main bronchus, ≥2 cm distal to the carina; invades visceral pleura; associated with atelectasis or obstructive pneumonitis that extends to the hilar region but does not involve the entire lung

T3   Tumor of any size that directly invades any of the following: chest wall (including superior sulcus tumors), diaphragm, mediastinal pleura, parietal pericardium; or tumor in the main bronchus <2 cm distal to the carina[b] but without involvement of the carina; or associated atelectasis or obstructive pneumonitis of the entire lung

T4   Tumor of any size that invades any of the following: mediastinum, heart, great vessels, trachea, esophagus, vertebral body, carina; separate tumor nodule(s) in the same lobe; tumor with malignant pleural effusion[c]

N—Regional lymph nodes

NX   Regional lymph nodes cannot be assessed

N0   No regional lymph node metastasis

N1   Metastasis in ipsilateral peribronchial and/or ipsilateral hilar lymph nodes and intrapulmonary nodes, including involvement by direct extension

N2   Metastasis in ipsilateral mediastinal and/or subcarinal lymph node(s)

N3   Metastasis in contralateral mediastinal, contralateral hilar, ipsilateral or contralateral scalene, or supraclavicular lymph node(s)

M—Distant metastasis

MX   Distant metastasis cannot be assessed

M0   No distant metastasis

M1   Distant metastasis, includes separate tumor nodule(s) in a different lobe (ipsilateral or contralateral)

pTNM Pathological classification

The pT, pN, pM categories correspond to the T, N, and M categories.

pN0: Histological examination of hilar and mediastinal lymphadenectomy specimen(s) will ordinarily include six or more lymph nodes. If the lymph nodes are negative, but the number ordinarily examined is not met, classify as pN0.

---

[a] The uncommon superficial spreading tumor of any size with its invasive component limited to the bronchial wall, which may extend proximal to the main bronchus, is also classified as T1.

[b] Most pleural effusions with lung cancer are due to tumor. In a few patients, however, multiple cytopathological examinations of pleural fluid are negative for tumor, and the fluid is nonbloody and is not an exudate. Where these elements and clinical judgment dictate that the effusion is not related to the tumor, the effusion should be excluded as a staging element and the patient should be classified as T1, T2, or T3.

[c] Separate tumor nodule(s) in the same lobe is categorized as T4 and synchronous separate tumor nodule(s) in a different lobe (ipsilateral or contralateral) is categorized as M1.

TABLE 17.4. Lung Cancer Stage Grouping (Sixth Edition TNM)

Occult carcinoma	TX	N0	M0
Stage 0	Tis	N0	M0
Stage IA	T1	N0	M0
Stage IB	T2	N0	M0
Stage IIA	T1	N1	M0
Stage IIB	T2	N1	M0
	T3	N0	M0
Stage IIIA	T1	N2	M0
	T2	N2	M0
	T3	N1, N2	M0
Stage IIIB	Any T	N3	M0
	T4	Any N	M0
Stage IV	Any T	Any N	M1

Thus, the natural history of lung cancer is characterized by local, regional nodal, and systemic spread, with only modest differences attributable to histologic subtype or grade. Relatively few patients (15%) present with operable stage I disease. Most lung cancer patients will eventually develop distant metastases—typically in liver, brain and skeleton.

The TNM classification and stage grouping are given in Tables 17.3 and 17.4. The subsequent discussion will concentrate on clinical management based on stage. However lung cancer remains a disease with high overall mortality rates, and series based on selected patients and/or treatment techniques may not be representative of the overall clinical reality. To provide perspective, an overview of treatments and results may be considered (Table 17.5). The survival rates, while approximate, represent the current prognosis by stage when all patients are considered and

TABLE 17.5. Management and Survival in Lung Cancer

Stage	Cell Type	Principal Management	5-Year Survival (approximate)
I	NSCLC	S (some R)	65%
	SCLC	C + R ± S	50%
II	NSCLC	S (some ± R, ± C)	40%
	SCLC	C + R	25%
IIIA	NSCLC	C + R ± S	30%
	SCLC	C + R	20%
IIIB	NSCLC	R ± C	15%
	SCLC	C + R	5%
IV	NSCLC	C or R or C + R	2%
	SCLC	C ± R	2%
Overall	NSCLC		10%
	SCLC		5%

Abbreviations: S, surgery; R, radiotherapy; C, chemotherapy.

a reasonably wide range of modern treatments is available. It must be noted that the full spectrum of treatment options may not be available for all patients. In such circumstances, single-modality therapy with palliative intent may be all that is possible to offer them.

STAGING SYSTEM FOR LUNG CANCER AND PROGNOSIS

The International Union Against Cancer (UICC) staging system is based on anatomic routes of spread, and stage determination depends strongly on the type of diagnostic evaluations that are used. Staging classification does not determine treatment, but rather helps to assign prognosis to patients treated according to the standards and procedures that are current. In addition, staging assists in the comparison of treatment results between different centers. The current UICC and the identical American Joint Committee on Cancer (AJCC) criteria in lung cancer reflect the use of diagnostic techniques described above, but their application across regions and nations is highly variable. The 1997 system reflects the importance of local invasion by tumor, and of nodal metastases in the patient's prognosis. Important changes include the recognition of T3 tumors as relatively favorable provided that there is no lymph node invasion. Approximate survival rates anticipated are given by stage of disease in Table 17.5. There were no further revisions in the 2002 system.

Other prognostic factors include the performance status of the patient, significant weight loss prior to diagnosis, and the presence of associated hypercalcemia. Analyses of clinical data sets has identified other possible proliferation or biologic markers that may carry prognostic importance, but none are sufficiently well established to guide clinical treatment decisions.

PRINCIPLES OF MANAGEMENT BY STAGE OF DISEASE

Non–Small-Cell Lung Cancer

Stage I—Stage IA (T1N0M0) and Stage IB (T2N0M0)   Surgical resection is generally the choice of treatment, taking account of operability and the overall medical risk of the patient. The overall operative mortality is 3–4%, more for pneumonectomy and safer for lobectomy. Lesser resections, such as segmentectomy and wedge resection, carry less risk but a higher rate of recurrence. The post-resection 5-year survival rate in patients with T1N0M0 lesions is approximately 65–70%.

In T2N0M0 cases, lobectomy is generally preferred for lesions within the lung parenchyma or those with invasion of the visceral pleura. Lesions crossing the major fissure generally require pneumonectomy. T2 tumors arising in the lobar bronchus orifice or invading to the main bronchus require sleeve lobectomy or pneumonectomy.

Radiation therapy with curative intent is appropriate for the minority of patients with localized lung cancer who cannot undergo or will not accept surgery. This is usually given as a high total dose to the tumor with careful limitation of dose to nearby normal tissues. Radiation to the tumor is 70 Gy or more fractionated; pilot studies in selected patients with good lung function have delivered up to 100 Gy. Five-year survival rates of 15–25% reflect the fact that most are unfit for surgery.

Whether initial treatment is by surgery or radiation, there is no established role for subsequent adjuvant treatment such as chemotherapy, or radiotherapy after surgery.

Stage II—Stage IIA (T1N1M0) and Stage IIB (T2N1M0, T3N0M0)   In principle, a surgical operation is indicated for lesions even in the presence of lymph node metastases, provided a complete resection can be achieved. Curative operation is usually possible. Lymph node disease should be resected by systematic dissection of mediastinal nodes well beyond the involved ones. There is no evidence to suggest that "debulking" surgery (incomplete resection) is beneficial. The 5-year survival rate is 45–55% in T2N0M0 cases and 35–50% in T2N1M0 cases, respectively, following histologically confirmed complete resection. Given the frequent local recurrences and organ metastasis observed within these groups, some supplementary treatment may be considered. Postoperative irradiation may reduce the rate of mediastinal or local recurrence, while chemotherapy may reduce systemic relapse; however, neither strategy has been shown to significantly benefit overall survival in randomized trials.

The role of adjuvant therapy remains investigational only. Of six randomized trials in stage 2 and 3 patients, only two showed a benefit with adjuvant chemotherapy. Unfortunately, three recent trials using more up-to-date chemotherapeutic regimens also failed to show any benefit of adjuvant therapy. Most of these trials suffer from inadequate drug delivery, inadequate drugs, and few patients entered on study. The meta-analysis of eight randomized trials using cisplatin-based chemotherapy after surgery demonstrated a small incremental survival benefit associated with chemotherapy that did not quite reach statistical significance. Although adjuvant therapy may have a potential role, it is not yet considered standard practice. Present ongoing or just completed trials may hopefully shed further light on the role of adjuvant therapy.

The T3N0M0 group, due to its relatively favorable 5-year survival rate following complete resection, is now classified within stage II, according to the 1997 TNM classification. This group includes the superior sulcus tumor and its prognosis is the poorest of the IIB tumors. This presentation of lung cancer is due to tumor located at the thoracic inlet. Preoperative radiation has been advocated with the goal of tumor size reduction and an increased resectability rate, but combined modality (chemoradiotherapy) regimens prior to attempted resection are under investigation and may prove more effective. Patients with T3N0M0 due to chest wall invasion are usually treated with tumor and *en bloc* chest wall resection; the 5-year survival rates reported are approximately 35% in these generally fit patients. In cases where the adequacy of surgical margins is suspect, postoperative irradiation should be considered. Recently, induction chemoradiotherapy followed by surgical resection for superior sulcus tumors has demonstrated high pathological complete response rates, with improved resectability and overall survival compared with historical experience, especially for T4 tumors (see below). A combination of etoposide/cisplatin with concurrent radiotherapy (45 Gy) followed by surgery is now considered the standard practice for superior sulcus tumors.

A meta-analysis was performed of all nine available randomized trials of postoperative radiotherapy versus surgery alone for completely resected non–small-cell lung cancer. About two-thirds of the patients had stage I or II disease; there were 808 stage III patients analyzed. No patient group or subgroup was seen to benefit from postoperative radiotherapy in terms of overall survival or local recurrence-free survival. Indeed, radiotherapy was actually detrimental, especially in early-stage disease. This effect is almost certainly due to the adverse effect of irradiation on remaining normal lung tissue. Whether there is benefit for incompletely resected patients is not known. If postoperative radiotherapy is given in an effort to reduce the risk of local recurrence, the technique and dose should be chosen so as to avoid irradiating the remaining lung.

Stage III—Stage IIIA and IIIB

In general, patients are considered for both local and systemic components of therapy in light of their high risk of both types of relapse. The presence of mediastinal nodal disease is associated with a much increased risk of distant spread and ultimate relapse. On the other hand, many patients have significant co-morbid illness and cannot tolerate treatment by multiple modalities. Such patients should be offered treatment by palliative intent, minimizing associated morbidity.

Principles of surgical selection for stage III tumors are much discussed but general consensus has not been reached. Pneumonectomy may be required to completely resect the tumor mass but is appropriate only for patients with adequate pulmonary reserve. Bronchial sleeve resection in selected patients is an effective method for pulmonary preservation with mortality and survival rates comparable to those following pneumonectomy. Frequently, extended *en bloc* resections are required to effect complete removal of the tumor. The prognosis appears to be directly related to the extent of the N category. Surgery can sometimes be considered in T4 cases, but is of doubtful value if mediastinal nodes are involved. Surgery is usually appropriate only for highly selected T4 patients with tumors confined to the carina, or tracheobronchial angle; in such cases, carinal resection with lobectomy or sleeve pneumonectomy may be performed. If surgical resection is undertaken in these highly advanced cases, complete ipsilateral mediastinal lymph node resection is strongly recommended.

The ultimate value of surgical resection is greatly diminished by the fact that at this satge of disease patients have mediastinal lymph node involvement, frequently extensive and multinodal. The locations of each lymph node are identified using terminology of the lymph node map (Fig. 17.2), useful for assigning an N stage to the patient. Prognosis can differ depending on the nature of involvement. Generally, prognosis is less favorable when nodes are multiple rather than single; extranodal rather than intranodal; and distal rather than proximal to the primary tumor (with respect to lymphatic drainage pathways). Extensive surgical procedures, usually lobectomy or pneumonectomy with complete mediastinal lymph node dissection may produce 5-year survival rates of 20–30% when "minimal" disease is present. Many groups advocate preoperative chemotherapy but this experience is based on very small studies.

Radiotherapy as the sole modality is also limited by its inability to control systemic disease and the large population of clonogenic cells in bulky primary and nodal masses. Survival rates at 5 years may range from 5 to 20% but these results also depend on selection of patients, who usually are unfit for surgery. Newer approaches attempt to select smaller tumors, and employ modern three-dimensional shaped planning techniques, in order to escalate the dose delivered to the tumor without irradiating excessively the nearby normal tissues.

Combined modality regimens are frequently employed and adopt one of two strategies. Adjunctive therapies are administered following some form of local therapy. An example would be mediastinal radiotherapy and/or several cycles of chemotherapy administered after complete or incomplete resection. The second strategy associates the systemic therapy with the local one, according to a particular timing schema. The idea is to address multiple, possibly conflicting requirements, including (1) the need to control cells resistant to one modality that might be controlled by multiple non–cross-resistant agents; (2) the tendency for therapy to stimulate repopulation in surviving cells; (3) the presence of occult systemic disease; and (4) the problem of overlapping toxicities. Various timing protocols have been tried including prior chemotherapy (induction or neoadjuvant), concurrent chemoradiotherapy, or schemas in which chemo- and radiotherapy are interdigitated or "alternated."

Combined modality regimens are indicated because of the need to treat both local and systemic disease. Indeed, the randomized trials of chemotherapy and radiation therapy versus radiation therapy alone (formerly standard practice) have demonstrated a modest benefit in survival favoring the combined modality arm. The meta-analysis of these trials demonstrated a modest (2% at 5 years) increase in survival when cisplatin-based chemotherapy was added to a high-dose radiotherapy protocol. It should be noted that results with randomized trials concern patients with favorable prognostic factors (good performance status, minimal weight loss) and IIIA disease. These results may not apply to patients with poor prognostic factors, who may respond less well and suffer more toxicity than more favorable patients.

Even assuming combined modality therapy is given, many practical questions remain, including the role of radiation versus surgery, the sequencing of chemotherapy and radiation therapy (sequential versus concurrent radiotherapy), and the role of newer agents. A large randomized trial in North America in progress compares surgical resection to additional radiotherapy, immediately following a combined modality induction regimen. The influential Cancer and Leukemia group B (CALGB) trial showed the superiority in terms of survival at 5 years of induction chemotherapy prior to thoracic radiotherapy over radiotherapy alone. Two more recent trials comparing the induction sequence to a schema in which the chemo- and radiotherapy are given concurrently show an advantage to the concurrent regimen, though with somewhat enhanced toxicity. A Japanese trial comparing these two sequences illustrates the principle and clearly favored the concurrent approach (5-year survival, 16% vs. 9%). Clearly local control as well as systemic control of disease remains a problem and the role of the novel molecular approaches (targeted therapy) remains to be elucidated. On the other hand, prognosis is poor after all therapies and the impact of treatment on the patient's quality of life must always be considered.

Important advances in radiotherapy have established the biologic and clinical importance of the dose per fraction (on normal tissue effects), and the overall duration of therapy (on induced tumor repopulation). A British trial treating three times daily over 12 days showed a 2-year survival advantage of 30% versus 20% and an even larger effect in this squamous cell subgroup. This result is significant compared with survival benefits attributable to chemotherapy, has influenced practice, and encouraged ongoing testing of altered fractionation regimens. These protocols are also under testing in combination with chemo- therapy.

Technical advances in radiotherapy imaging, planning, and delivery now permit more precise targeting of intrathoracic tumors and sparing of critical normal tissues (lung, cord) using computerized three-dimensional shaped (conformal) techniques. Normal lung may sustain radiation injury at very modest doses, but this important new technique permits unwanted dose to regions of noncancerous lung to kept within acceptable limits.

The new century is likely to see steady progress in the application of new and established therapies, refined together with newer selection techniques (biomarkers, predictive assays, etc.) to supplement the anatomical TNM system.

Small Cell Lung Cancer

The mainstay of treatment for small-cell lung cancer (SCLC) is systemic combina- tion chemotherapy, which unquestionably prolongs survival, improves symptoms, and dramatically reduces tumor bulk in the majority of previously untreated cases. Chemotherapy alone, however, is rarely curative, with usual remission duration of less than a year, because of drug resistance. While the staging procedures for small cell carcinoma do not differ appreciably from other forms of lung cancer, for practical purposes the TNM stages are usually collapsed into a simple binary classification. There is no role for exclusive radiation and/or surgery in patients with extensive disease (ED)-SCLC, which has already spread beyond the hemi- thorax, mediastinum, and supraclavicular nodes. The limited disease (LD)-SCLC patients, whose disease is confined within these limits, are best treated with combination of systemic chemotherapy and thoracic radiotherapy, unless compli- cated by malignant effusion.

The role of surgery in the treatment of LD-SCLC is not established. Stage I patients (rare) are usually treated by surgical resection of the tumor followed by adjuvant chemotherapy of four to six courses, but its superiority to initial chemotherapy followed by surgery or chemoradiotherapy remains unproven. In stage II or III patients, surgical resection of tumor after induction chemotherapy has been shown to offer no additional benefit compared to thoracic radiotherapy in a randomized trial. Surgical salvage of the residual tumor after chemoradiotherapy might be beneficial in selected patients, but it is doubtful whether its merit surpasses its risk.

Thoracic irradiation associated with chemotherapy in limited disease improves both local control and overall survival according to multiple randomized trials and two meta-analyses. The dose of the thoracic radiotherapy should be at least 40–45 Gy. The clinical benefit of further dose escalation is not yet proven. Twice-daily radiotherapy of 1.5 Gy to 45 Gy/30 fractions/3 weeks appears to be superior to once-a-day 1.8 Gy to a total of 45 Gy/25 fractions/5 weeks in an American Intergroup randomized trial. However, this accelerated hyperfractionated schedule has never been compared with a standard (once-a-day) regimen with reduced toxicity.

The current chemotherapy standard includes cisplatin-etoposide (PE), carboplatin-etoposide, cyclophosphamide-doxorubicin-etoposide (CAE), and alternation of PE with cyclophosphamide-doxorubicin-vincristine (CAV), each for four to six cycles. Schedules containing platinum derivatives seem to be superior, especially combined with thoracic radiotherapy in LD cases.

The optimal timing of combining chemo- and radiotherapy in LD-SCLC remains controversial. Recent controlled trials have suggested that early concurrent combination, in which thoracic radiotherapy is given with the first or the second chemotherapy course, yields the most favorable results. It appears to be superior to other treatment schedules, such as alternating chemoradiotherapy or chemotherapy sequentially followed by radiation, although it also is more toxic to esophagus or bone marrow.

Prophylactic cranial irradiation (PCI) is shown to decrease the frequency of, or at least delay the emergence of, brain metastases. Its contribution to overall survival in SCLC patients is unclear, but is supported by a recent meta-analysis. At present, it is indicated only in LD patients who achieved complete remission (CR) or near CR after induction therapy. The recommended dose is 30 Gy/15 fractions or equivalent, but should be less than 3 Gy per fraction to minimize late toxicity. It is best administered shortly after the induction therapy. Concurrent chemotherapy with PCI should be avoided because of potential toxicity.

PALLIATIVE THERAPY IN LUNG CANCER

For the many lung cancer patients destined to relapse eventually, the availability of effective relief of cancer-induced symptoms is essential. Occasionally, there are surgical (e.g., orthopedic procedures for pathologic fractures or relief of visceral obstruction), but, more commonly, local palliation is given by radiotherapy. Patients usually respond to simple short courses of radiotherapy delivered in 1 to 10 fractions, usually with very little morbidity Common symptoms treated are hemoptysis, pain, cough, dyspnea due to airway obstruction and collapse, and visceral metastases in brain, bone, and soft tissue.

Randomized trials have demonstrated the effectiveness of short courses [one to three fractions, using relatively large fraction sizes (3–10 Gy)]. Although these regimens do not usually eradicate the tumors, they provide symptomatic relief in most circumstances (30–70% depending on the clinical syndrome). This benefit is usually quite durable in the context of the typical short survival experience of these relapsed patients. Short regimens offer many conveniences to the patient, and in almost all randomized trials have proven to be at least as effective as protracted ones. Current research aims to optimize response and quality-of-life outcomes. Airway obstruction may require endoscopic relief either by removal of the obstructing tumor or by stent insertion.

Severe or emergency complications of lung cancer include superior vena cava (SVC) obstruction and spinal cord compression. These are relatively common and can be devastating unless treated promptly by radiotherapy. Occasionally, laminectomy and decortication are required. The role of stents in the management of SVC obstruction has yet to be defined.

Systemic chemotherapy can provide useful palliation, especially for patients with systemic symptoms and visceral disease. The newer agents have a better side-effect profile and efficacy compared to the older regimens. Modern supportive agents such as the 5-HT3 antagonists (ondansetron, granisetron) can greatly reduce adverse affects such as nausea and vomiting. A number of recent randomized trials have attempted to sort out which of the new agent/cisplatin-based regimens is superior and to date none have been shown to be better than the other. Thus, vinorelbine/cisplatin, gemcitabine/cisplatin, paclitaxel/carboplatin, and docetaxel/cisplatin are all acceptable doublets with response rates of 30–35% and 1-year survival in the range of 38–40%. The decision as to which regimen to choose must be based upon efficacy (response rate, time to progression, survival), toxicity, convenience, and cost. More recently of interest is the clear benefit of second-line chemotherapy following cisplatin-based chemotherapy. Two recent trials have demonstrated a significant survival benefit in favor of docetaxol at 75 mg/m^2 given every 3 weeks, with improvement in several quality-of-life as well as clinical benefit parameters. Future directions will look at novel strategies incorporating new molecular targets with current chemotherapy approaches.

REHABILITATION

The goals of post-treatment rehabilitation are to prevent complications, improve respiratory function, reduce physical and mental pain, and assist the patient's readjustment to the community. The impact of all three treatment modalities must be addressed.

In those patients undergoing surgery, control of postoperative pain is essential to maintain thoracic movement and pulmonary expansion. Important techniques besides the use of analgesics include muscle relaxation and psychological support. Measures to improve lung function include early mobilization from bed; deep breathing exercises, preferably in an upright position; and activities to increase expectoration. Bronchoscopic suction may be required to prevent retention of mucous secretions and stasis pneumonia. Major chronic postoperative complications must sometimes be managed, such as bronchopleural fistula, or empyema requiring chronic drainage.

Although rehabilitation may not be a major concern after palliative radiotherapy using low to moderate doses, the aftercare of the patient treated with high-dose thoracic irradiation is concerned with maintaining function of the irradiated organs. Skin reactions are rarely troublesome but symptomatic esophagitis must be managed both during and for a few weeks after treatment, particularly if associated with chemotherapy. Lung tissue within the irradiated volume will be subject to an inflammatory reaction and slowly progressive fibrotic changes resulting in loss of some function, in normal as well as diseased lung. Exercise, mobilization, prompt treatment of infection, and counseling will help the patient adapt to these changes. Uncommonly, patients may develop a symptomatic pneumonitis outside of the limits of the irradiated volume, attributed to an immune response to radiation-induced humoral factors. It requires management with corticosteroids and other measures.

Protracted chemotherapy regimens can be debilitating and may exacerbate the adverse effects of radiation and surgery. However, with careful monitoring of blood and organ function, and the use of supportive agents (modern antiemetics, hematopoietics, etc.), major problems are uncommon. Drug protocols in general use take account of the particular organ sensitivities (hepatic, renal, cardiac, etc.) with dose precautions and criteria for dose adjustment.

Modern approaches seek to optimize the quality of life of patients by finding a balance between the effects of a debilitating and usually lethal disease, and the noxious impact of treatment on normal tissues. Many unresolved questions remain in this field.

FOLLOW-UP FOR LOCAL, REGIONAL, OR DISTANT RECURRENCE

Unfortunately, the majority of patients treated for lung cancer will experience a recurrence of their tumor, either locally, in the regional lymph nodes, or in distant organs. Relapses frequently occur at multiple sites. Very few of these clinical events are curable. In essence, the goal will usually be to determine the metastatic nature of the problem, and treat it with palliative intent and minimal treatment related morbidity

The goals of follow-up may be listed as follows:

1. Early recognition of potentially curable situations (e.g., small localized stump recurrence, early "second primary" lung cancer).
2. Distinguishing genuine metastatic events from other conditions that might simulate them, resulting in either palliative treatment or reassurance to the

patient. Examples include skeletal or nerve pain of various causes, and lobar collapse associated with radiation fibrosis or tumor recurrence.

3. Review and reporting of clinical outcomes.

Local recurrences are relatively infrequent when patients are carefully selected and completely resected with generous margins. However, they may arise at the bronchial stump, pleura, drain track, or thoracotomy scar. Mediastinal relapses are more serious and are associated with a high risk of distant metastasis. Both are usually treated with radiotherapy, especially if not previously irradiated. On occasion, surgery is worthwhile.

In nonresected patients local control remains a major problem. Even with modern chemoradiotherapy regimens, long-term control of the primary occurs in only 15–20%, taking account of the fact that many patients die of distant disease before the local relapse becomes clinically evident.

Distant organs that are frequently the target of symptomatic metastases are the brain, skeleton, liver, and lungs. There is little variation in the frequency and distribution of metastases among the histological subtypes. However, a degree of organ selectivity has been noted in some series, such as a higher frequency of brain metastases in small cell and adenocarcinomas. Some controversy exists over the management of the patient with a metastasis determined to be "solitary" after a thorough search for other lesions. Such situations in which the rigors of therapy with curative intent may be justified are quite rare. Autopsy series reveal a pattern of widespread invasion of many other tissues, which may remain clinically silent during life, except insofar as they contribute to the general deterioration of the patient. On the other hand, a superior quality of life likely to be achieved with resection and radiotherapy versus radiation therapy alone, especially with the newer surgical techniques. Patients with solitary brain metastases and a controlled primary tumor should be considered for this form of management.

Considering that most lung cancer patients are destined to relapse, follow-up should generally be the responsibility of the general physician with specialist support based on the treatment given, the sites of most likely, or actual relapse, or anticipated complications. Similarly, frequency of follow-up will depend on the clinical situation, though usually four times per year for the first 2 years following definitive therapy.

PREVENTION

Because interventions are not yet possible at the level of the cellular events involved in lung cancer induction, prevention efforts must therefore focus on the elimination of modifiable risk factors. These include environmental and workplace air pollution, but the overwhelmingly significant and well-documented risk factor is the inhalation of tobacco products. Lung cancer is very rare in nonsmokers, and even a modest reduction in rates of tobacco smoking would result in the prevention of a substantial number of cancers.

FURTHER READING

The Alpha-Tocopherol, Beta Carotene Cancer Prevention Study Group (1994) The effect of vitamin E and beta carotene on the incidence of lung cancer and other cancers in male smokers. *N Engl J Med* 330:1029.

American Society of Clinical Oncology (1997) Clinical practice guidelines for the treatment of unresectable non-small-cell lung cancer. *J Clin Oncol* 15:2996.

Brundage M, Mackillop WJ (2001) Lung cancer. In *Prognostic Factors in Cancer*, 2nd ed. Wiley-Liss, New York, pp. 351–369.

Dillman RO, Seagren SL, Propert KJ, Guerra J, Eaton WL, Perry MC, Carey, RW, Frei, EF, Green, MR (1990) A randomized trial of induction chemotherapy plus high-dose radiation versus radiation alone in stage III non-small-cell lung cancer. *N Engl J Med* 323: 940–945.

Friedland DM, Comis RL (1995) Perioperative therapy of non-small cell lung cancer: A review of adjuvant and neoadjuvant approaches. *Semin Oncol* 22:571.

Furuse K, Fukuoka M, Kawahara M et al. (1999) Phase III study of concurrent versus sequential thoracic radiotherapy in combination with mitomycin, vindesine, and cisplatin in unresectable stage III non-small-cell lung cancer. *J Clin Oncol* 17:2692–2699.

Goss G, Paszat L, Newman TE, Evans WK, Browman G, and the Provincial Lung Cancer Disease Site Group (1998) Use of preoperative chemotherapy with or without post-operative radiotherapy in technically resectable stage IIIA non-small cell lung cancer. *Cancer Prev Control* 2:32–39.

Ihde DC (ed.) (1995) Current perspectives in the treatment of small cell lung cancer. *Lung Cancer* 12 (suppl 3):S1–S95.

Medical Research Council Lung Cancer Working Party (1991) Inoperable non-small-cell lung cancer (NSCLC): A Medical Research Council randomised trial of palliative radiotherapy with two fractions or ten fractions. *Br J Cancer* 63:265–270.

Medical Research Council Lung Cancer Working Party, and Bleehen NM, Girling DJ, Machin D, Stephens RJ (1992) A Medical Research Council (MRC) randomised trial of palliative radiotherapy with two fractions or a single fraction in patients with inoperable non-small-cell lung cancer (NSCLC) and poor performance status. *Br J Cancer* 65:934–941.

Medical Research Council Lung Cancer Working Party, and Macbeth FR, Bolger JJ, Hopwood P, Bleehen NM, Cartmell J, Girling DJ, Machin D, Stephen RJ, Bailey AJ (1996) Randomized trial of palliative two-fraction versus more intensive 13-fraction radiotherapy for patients with inoperable non-small cell lung cancer and good performance status. *Clin Oncol* 8:167–175.

Naruke T, Goya T, Tsuchiya R et al. (1988) Prognosis and survival in resected lung carcinoma based on the new international staging system. *J Thorac Cardiovasc Surg* 96:440–447.

Non-small Cell Lung Cancer Collaborative Group (1995) Chemotherapy in non-small cell lung cancer: A meta-analysis using updated data on individual patients from 52 randomised clinical trials. *Br Med J* 311:899–909.

Okawara G, Rusthoven J, Newman T, Findlay B, Evans W, and the Provincial Lung Cancer Disease Site Group (1997) Unresected stage III non-small-cell lung cancer. *Cancer Prev Control* 1:249–259.

Parkin DM, Saxo AJ (1993) Lung cancer: worldwide variation in occurrence and proportion attributable to tobacco use. *Lung Cancer* 9(suppl):1–16.

Patz EF, Goodman PC, Bepler G (2001) Screening for lung cancer. *N Engl J Med* 343:1627.

Pignon JP, Arriagada R, Ihde DC et al. (1992) A meta-analysis of thoracic radiotherapy for small cell lung carcinoma. *N Engl J Med* 327:1618–1624.

PORT Meta-analysis Trialists Group (1998) Postoperative radiotherapy in non-small cell lung cancer: A systematic review and meta-analysis of individual patient data from nine randomised controlled trials. *Lancet* 352:257–263.

Saunders M, Dische S, Barrett A, Harvey A, Gibson D, Parmar M, CHART Steering Committee (1997) Continuous hyperfractionated accelerated radiotherapy (CHART) versus conventional radiotherapy in non-small-cell lung cancer: A randomised multicentre trial. *Lancet* 350:161–165.

Schottenfeld M (1996) Epidemiology of lung cancer. In *Lung Cancer: Principles and Practice*. Pass HI, Mitchell JB, Johnson DH, et al. (eds.) Lippincott-Raven, Philadelphia/New York, pp. 305–332.

Shaw GL, Mulshine JL (1996) General strategies for early detection: New ideas and future directions. In *Lung Cancer: Principles and Practice*. Pass HI, Mitchell JB, Johnson DH, et al. (eds.) Lippincott-Raven, Philadelphia/New York, pp. 329–340.

Sibley, GS (1998) Radiotherapy for patients with medically inoperable stage I non-small cell lung carcinoma. *Cancer* 82:433–438.

Stahel RA (1991) Diagnosis, staging and prognostic factors of small cell lung cancer. *Curr Opin Oncol* 3:306.

Travis WD, Colby TV, Corrin B et al. (1999) *Histological Typing of Lung and Pleural Tumors*, 3rd ed. Springer Verlag, Berlin.

CHAPTER 18

Liver Cancer

ZHAO-YOU TANG

Liver Cancer Institute of Fudan University (formerly Shanghai Medical University), Shanghai, China

STEVEN A. CURLEY

University of Texas, M. D. Anderson Cancer Center, Department of Surgical Oncology, Houston, Texas

Hepatocellular carcinoma (HCC), the major cell type of primary liver cancer, is one of the most frequent malignancies in eastern Asia, sub-Saharan Africa, and Melanesia. Owing to the difficulties in early detection and effective treatment, HCC has long been regarded as a hopeless disease. Fortunately, the identification of hepatitis B/C virus as an important background of HCC, and the detection of subclinical HCC using alpha fetoprotein and/or ultrasonography screening, have provided important clues to the primary and secondary prevention of HCC. The outcome of HCC has also been improved with advances in medical imaging, regional cancer therapy, and liver cancer surgery. Studies on the molecular biology of HCC have potential clinical implications, particularly in the control of recurrence and metastasis.

ETIOLOGY AND EPIDEMIOLOGY

Pisani et al. (1999) reported that the global number of liver cancer deaths in 1990 was 427,000. Liver cancer was the fourth most common cause of death from cancer and the third most common in men. The high fatality of this cancer gives it a much more prominent place than in the ranking of incidence (eighth overall and sixth in men). Liver cancer is predominantly a problem of developing countries, which contribute 81% of all deaths due to this cause. The highest age-standardized mortality rate was in China (estimated ASR $34.7/10^5$ for males and $11.1/10^5$ for females), which alone accounts for 53% of all liver cancer deaths worldwide. In

UICC Manual of Clinical Oncology, Eighth Edition. Edited by Raphael E. Pollock
ISBN 0-471-22289-5 Copyright © 2004 John Wiley & Sons, Inc.

China, HCC has become the second most fatal cancer since the 1990s. ASRs greater than $15/10^5$ are observed in all eastern Asia, sub-Saharan Africa, and Melanesia. Among developed countries, the risk of liver cancer is high only in Japan, where 56% of cases are due to infection with hepatitis C virus. Mozambique, Zimbabwe, Uganda, Malaysia, Indonesia, Singapore, Thailand, Philippines, China, and Japan were among the highest incidence areas. Low incidence areas included United States (excluding Alaska), Canada, northern Europe, and Australia. A trend of increasing incidence was observed in Japan, France, Italy, and so on.

The peak age at onset of HCC was around 30–39 years in Africa, 45–54 in China, 50–59 in Japan, and 55–64 in the United States. Generally, HCC is more predominant in males than in females; however, the male to female ratio is usually greater in high prevalence areas, such as in China, where it was 3:1.

The major etiological factors of HCC varied in different geographic areas, and included the following: (1) Viral hepatitis infection and cirrhosis. In Southeast Asia, hepatitis B virus (HBV) infection was more common as compared with hepatitis C virus (HCV) infection. In China, around 80% of HCC patients had an HBV infection background, and only 10–30% HCV infection, whereas in Japan, France, and Italy, HCV-related HCC accounted for around 60–80%. The relative risk of HCC in HBV carriers was reported to be 10 to 100 times higher than that of non-HBV carriers. The X gene of HBV was thought important in hepatocarcinogenesis. In high prevalence areas, cirrhosis accounted for around 60–80% of the HCC background, of which most are posthepatitic (B or C) cirrhosis, especially the macronodular type. HGV and TTV (transfusion-transmitted virus) might not play an important role in the development of HCC. (2) Chemical carcinogens, particularly the intake of aflatoxin B_1 (AFB_1)-containing food, such as peanut and corn. Epidemiologic data revealed a strong correlation between HCC mortality and intake of AFB_1, and AFB_1 has been proved a strong hepatocarcinogen in experimental animal. (3) Contamination of drinking water. In rural areas of China where HCC is endemic, a strong correlation was found between HCC mortality and contamination of drinking water. People drinking pond-ditch water had a much higher HCC mortality than people drinking deep well water. Recently, microcystin was found in the pond-ditch water, and verified to be a strong promotor of hepatocarcinogenesis. (4) Alcohol, smoking, genetics, and other factors. In Italy, for attributable risk (AR) of HCC, heavy alcohol intake ranked first (45%), HCV second (36%), and HBV third (22%). It is estimated that only 15% of HCC cases in North America are attributable to alcohol use, and 12% or less to cigarette smoking. Hemochromatosis has also been reported as a risk factor for HCC. All of these indicate a multifactorial and multistep development of HCC. Interaction among HBV/HCV, aflatoxin, alcohol, and genetic susceptibility might be important (Yu, 1995).

SCREENING

A screening program for early detection of HCC has been debated for decades. In China, screening a high-risk population using serum AFP assay and ultrasonography

(US) has led to detection of resectable small (5 cm) HCC. The 5-year survival associated with small HCC resection was double that of large HCC resection, being around 60% versus 30%. In the 1990s, a prospective, randomized, controlled screening trial was conducted in Shanghai urban residents, aged 35–55 years, with serum evidence of HBV infection. The study included a screening group ($n = 8,109$) and a control ($n = 9,711$). Subjects in the screening group were tested with serum AFP and US every 6 months, and HCC patients detected were treated adequately. Comparison between screening and control groups revealed that the number of HCC patients detected was 86 versus 51; small HCC being 45.3% versus 0%; resection rate 46.5% versus 7.8%; 5-year survival 52.7% versus 0%; HCC mortality rate $77.3/10^5$ versus $121.4/10^5$. The lead time was estimated at 0.45 years. It is suggested that screening in HBV carriers in China using AFP and US is of value in detecting HCC in the early stage, increasing resection rate, and prolonging survival (Tang and Yang, 1995). A similar result was reported in screening Alaska natives. Instead of AFP and US, only US was used for screening in areas where serum AFP level was low in patients with HCC.

DIAGNOSIS

Pathology

Gross classifications of HCC have been advocated by several authors. The traditional Eggel's (1901) classification included massive, nodular, and diffuse types. Okuda (1984) divided HCC into expanding, spreading, multifocal, and indeterminate types. Nakashima and Kojiro (1987) classified it as expansive, infiltrative, mixed infiltrative and expansive, and diffuse types. Gross types differed among geographic areas; the expanding type is common in Oriental patients, whereas infiltrative type is seen more in the United States.

According to Ishak et al. (1994), HCC was defined as, "A malignant tumor composed of cells resembling hepatocyte but abnormal in appearance. A platelike organization around sinusoids is common and nearly always present somewhere in the tumor." For differentiation, Edmondson and Steiner (1954) proposed HCC be graded from I to IV. Cells with different gradings could be found in one HCC nodule. HCC is hypervascular in the majority of cases; arterioportal shunt is frequently found in large tumor. Tumor thrombi are also common in the portal and hepatic veins. Fibrolamellar HCC, a variant of HCC more frequent in the West, is abundant with fibrous stroma arranged in parallel lamellae; tumor cells are large and polygonal with granular cytoplasm; and prognosis is better than for classic HCC.

Several methods have been employed for studies on the cellular origin of HCC, such as integration of HBV DNA, loss of heterozygosity (LOH) pattern on chromosome 16, p53 loss of heterozygosity, and so on. Most of these approaches indicated that both a unicentric and a multicentric origin existed in multiple nodules as well as recurrent HCC.

In most HCC cases associated with cirrhosis, the posthepatitic type accounted for the majority; the macronodular type (with cirrhotic nodule >3 mm) was predominant. Adenomatous hyperplasia has been identified as a precancerous lesion.

Tabor summarized molecular events in HBV related-HCC: p53 mutation was found in 30–50%, positivity of Rb was 20–25%, overexpression was also found in TGF, IGF-II, N-ras, c-myc, c-fos, and so on. Multiple genetic alterations, including 4q, 8p, and 17p, were also found with relation to hepatocarcinogenesis of HCC.

Clinical Findings

In patient with subclinical HCC detected by screening, usually no symptom or sign exists. In clinical patients, the first complaint is usually pain or palpable mass in the upper abdomen; radiating pain to the right shoulder is common when the tumor is located in the upper part of the right lobe. Acute pain is encountered when rupture of a tumor nodule occurs; subcapsular rupture of HCC nodule in the right lobe is often misdiagnosed as gallbladder disease or appendicitis. Most of the symptoms are nonspecific, originating from HCC or the coexisting hepatitis and cirrhosis, and include hepatomegaly, fullness, poor appetite, weakness, weight loss, and lower extremity edema. Unexplained fever or diarrhea is often the first complain of patient with HCC. Jaundice and ascites usually appear in advanced stages. Variceal bleeding is also encountered.

Physical signs include hepatomegaly with or without nodule, splenomegaly, elevated right diaphragm, jaundice, and ascites. Reddish liver palm is found in patients with coexisting advanced cirrhosis.

Paraneoplastic syndromes, such as erythrocytosis and hypoglycemia, present in some patients with HCC. Coexisting diabetes seems to have been increasing recently.

Metastases in lung, bone, lymph nodes, brain, adrenal gland, or other organs present corresponding symptoms and signs.

Complications include rupture of HCC nodule, gastrointestinal bleeding, liver dysfunction and liver failure, infection, ascites, right pleural effusion, and pulmonary infarct due to tumor thrombus.

The natural course of HCC was estimated to take at least 2 years based on the study of subclinical HCC.

Laboratory Findings

Alpha fetoprotein (AFP) is the best tumor marker for HCC. A serum AFP level >20 µg/L is found in 60–70% of HCC patients in the Southeast Asia. Although an AFP level >500 µg/L is acknowleged to be diagnostic, it is recommended that HCC diagnosis be considered and ultrasonography checked when AFP level <500 µg/L but >20 µg/L.

The des–carboxy prothrombin (DCP) also known as "protein induced by vitamin K absence, or antagonism-II" (PIVKA-II) test measured by the revised enzyme immunoassay (EIA) kit with increased sensitivity has a stronger correlation than

AFP with size and histologic differentiation of HCC. This sensitive DCP is a useful marker for HCC and should be used in combination with AFP (Okuda et al., 2000).

Liver function tests are needed both for diagnosis and selection of treatment modality. Postoperative hepatitic status with high ALT increases risk of recurrence.

Serum HBV and HCV markers are important diagnostic aids for HCC, and are very helpful for differential diagnosis between HCC and other benign/malignant space-occupying lesions in the liver where HBV/HCV are prevalent.

Thrombocytopenia due to hypersplenism is common. Immunostatus is progressively depressed with the advancement of disease.

Imaging

US is the most commonly used noninvasive procedure; a lesion as small as 1 cm can be detected. A hypoechoic space-occupying lesion (SOL) with a halo is the common picture for small HCC. In large HCC, hyperechoic, isoechoic, or mixed hyper- and hypoechoic lesions are found. Satellite nodules surrounding the major nodule are often encountered. Tumor thrombus in portal vein, hepatic vein, or inferior vena cava; tumor invasion to biliary tree; collateral circulation of portal hypertension; and lymphnode involvement can also be observed. Color Doppler US can help to identified the vascularity of the lesion. An arterial blood supply is often found in HCC. Preoperative US by a surgeon is extremely helpful in selecting treatment modality as well as to guide surgery. Intraoperative US can help to guide the surgical approach, judge the extent of resection, and avoid injury of important vessels and ducts. US can also guide biopsy.

Computed tomography (CT) has been a routine imaging procedure for HCC. Spiral CT shows accumulation of contrast medium in the arterial phase, and becomes a low-density area in the venous phase. Lipiodol CT can detect HCC as small as 0.5 cm. A strong accumulation of Lipiodol in the SOL is observed after 1–2 weeks, however, sensitivity was not high and false positives were found.

Magnetic resonance imaging (MRI) is similar to CT but uses no radiation. The resolution capacity for soft tissue is superior to that of CT, and it is good for differential diagnosis between small HCC and hemangioma.

Nuclide imaging is less sensitive. Blood pool scanning remains useful for differentiating between HCC and hemangioma; a strong uptake is usually found in hemangioma. ^{99}Tc-PMT (*N*-pyridoxyl-5-methyltryptophan) scanning, a hepatobiliary imaging agent, is helpful for diagnosis of hepatic adenoma in the delayed phase. Positive imaging can be found in 60% of well and moderately differentiated HCC, and ^{99}Tc-PMT whole-body scanning is of value in detecting a metastatic lesion from HCC. Radioimmunoimaging using radiolabeled monoclonal antibody, such as AFP-Scan, may be of potential value for diagnosis.

The value of positron emission tomography (PET) has yet to be explored. PET using fluorine-18-fluorodeoxyglucose is useful in assessment of the therapeutic effect, but the sensitivity for HCC imaging is low.

Arteriography remains useful despite its invasive nature. Tumor vessel and tumor stain are two major features for HCC.

Laparoscopy and Needle Biopsy

Laparoscopy, an invasive procedure, is less useful because of the rapid progress of medical imaging. US-guided percutaneous fine needle biopsy is useful when diagnosis is difficult; however, it is not suggested as a routine procedure.

Differential Diagnosis

When medical imaging shows a solid SOL in the liver, the following diseases should be excluded:

1. *Secondary liver cancer*—with a history of original cancer, usually no HBV/HCV/cirrhosis background, AFP level ≤ 20 µg/L (except for a few instances with liver metastasis from gastric or pancreatic cancer), multiple evenly distributed nodules.
2. *Hepatic hemangioma*—female predominant, usually no HBV/HCV/cirrhosis background, AFP level ≤ 20 µg/liter, no halo on US, filling of contrast medium beginning from the peripheral zone in CT, strong filling in blood pool scanning.
3. *Hepatic adenoma*—usually no HBV/HCV/cirrhosis background, with history of oral contraceptive use in some patients, AFP level ≤ 20 µg/L, strong imaging in delayed phase of [99]mTc-PMT scanning.
4. *Inflammatory pseudotumor*—usually no HBV/HCV/cirrhosis background, AFP level ≤ 20 µ/L, lobular and no halo on US, no arterial blood supply by color Doppler US or spiral CT.
5. *Focal nodular hyperplasia* (FNH) and *adenomatous hyperplasia* (AH)—difficult to differentiate from small HCC, usually no HBV/HCV/cirrhosis background, AFP level ≤ 20 µg/L, no halo on US, arterial blood supply can be found.
6. *Sarcoma*—usually no HBV/HCV/cirrhosis background, AFP level ≤ 20 µg/L.
7. Liver abscess—usually no HBV/HCV/cirrhosis background, AFP level ≤ 20 µg/L, difficult to differentiate when abscess has not yet liquefied.

STAGING

TNM is the essential classification system, and includes: tumor size, number of tumor nodules, involvement, vascular invasion, invasion of major branch of portal or hepatic veins, regional lymph node metastasis, and distant metastasis. The UICC-TNM classification (6th edition, 2002) for liver is summarized as follows.

The T, N and M categories are based on physical examination, imaging, and/or surgical exploration. pTNM pathological classification corresponds to the T, N, and M categories.

T—Primary tumor

    TX Primary Tumor cannot be assessed

    T0 No evidence of primary tumor

    T1 Solitary tumor without vascular invasion

    T2 Solitary tumor with vascular invasion or multiple tumours, none more than 5 cm in greatest dimension

    T3 Multiple tumors more than 5 cm or tumor involving a major branch of the portal or hepatic vein(s)

    T4 Tumor(s) with direct invasion of adjacent organs other than the gall-bladder or with perforation of visceral peritoneum

N—Regional lymph nodes

    NX Regional lymph nodes cannot be assessed

    N0 No regional lymph node metastasis

    N1 Regional lymph node metastasis

M—Distant metastasis

    MX Distant metastasis cannot be assessed

    M0 No distant metastasis

    M1 Distant metastasis

Stage grouping

Stage I	T1	N0	M0
Stage II	T2	N0	M0
Stage IIIA	T3	N0	M0
Stage IIIB	T4	N0	M0
Stage IIIC	Any T	N1	M0
Stage IV	Any T	Any N	M1

Okuda proposed a staging system in 1985, which includes 1) tumor size >50% of the liver areas measured by CT (+), <50% (−); 2) ascites: (+) and (−); 3) albumin: <3 g/dL (+) and >3 g/dL (−); and 4) bilirubin: >3 mg/dL (+) and <3 mg/dL (−).

Stage I:	all (−)
Stage II:	1 or 2 (+)
Stage III:	3 or 4 (+)

MULTIMODALITY TREATMENT

Selection of Treatment Modalities

Treatment modalities that resulted in prolonging survival include hepatic resection, regional cancer therapies (such as radiofrequency [RF], microwave [MW], cryosurgery, high intensive focused ultrasound [HIFU], percutaneous ethanol injection [PEI], and transcatheter arterial chemoembolization [TACE]). Liver transplantation has been demonstrated effective in treating small HCC. Systemic chemotherapy is less effective. Biotherapy provides hope as a future therapy.

Selection of treatment modality depends on

1. *Tumor status*—usually T1, T2, and part of T3 are candidates for surgery or regional cancer therapies; part of T3 and T4 are indicated for TACE.
2. *Liver function*—the Child-Pugh classification for cirrhosis is universally accepted.

Usually Child A (Child-Pugh's class A) with localized HCC is a good indication for surgery. Child A or B with localized small HCC is indicated for regional cancer therapies. TACE can be considered with multiple HCC in Child A and part of Child B, and conservative treatment is the choice for Child C. Indocyanine green retention rate at 15 minutes (ICG-R15) is commonly used in Japan to guide indication for surgery as well as extent of resection.

3. *General condition*—age, cardiac and pulmonary function, coexisting diseases.

For small HCC with Child A cirrhosis, resection is the first choice. Limited resection is suggested in a cirrhotic liver. For patients with Child B cirrhosis or with contraindications to resection, regional therapies such as RF, microwave ablation, cryosurgery and ethanol injection can be chosen. For patients with Child C cirrhosis, only conservative treatment is indicated.

For localized large HCC with Child A cirrhosis, resection is the best choice. For unresectable localized HCC with Child A cirrhosis, downstaging and followed by resection (cytoreduction and sequential resection) is a new approach. Intraoperative hepatic artery cannulation combined with hepatic artery ligation (maintains the patency of the catheter) is effective for cytoreduction. Regional radiotherapy can be added. A small proportion of unresectable HCC can be converted to resectable if remarkable tumor shrinkage occurs.

For patient with multiple HCC and Child A or B cirrhosis, TACE is the best therapy. TACE can still be tried in individual patients who have tumor thrombus in the main portal vein. For HCC with Child C cirrhosis, only symptomatic treatment is indicated.

The indication for orthotopic liver transplantation (OLT) will be described later.

Surgery

Surgical resection provides the best outcome for patients with HCC. Since 1950s, lobectomy of large HCC has benefited 5% to 10% of HCC patients. The operative mortality has decreased from 20% to less than 5% and 5-year survival increased from 10% to 30%. In the 1970s, the application of serum AFP screening resulted in early detection of resectable small HCC. The operative mortality was less than 2%, and 5-year survival 50% to 60%. In the 1980s, based on follow-up after curative resection using AFP and ultrasonography, subclinical recurrence can be detected, and reresection has resulted in increased 5-year survival, 10% to 15% greater after curative resection of HCC. In the 1990s, downstaging using multimodality treatment and followed by resection has become an approach to treat localized unresectable HCC in cirrhotic liver. The 5-year survival after sequential resection was around 50–60%. Liver transplantation was proved superior to resection for small HCC in Western countries. Palliative surgery other than resection, such as hepatic artery ligation/cannulation, cryosurgery, and microwave ablation, has also yielded an acceptable outcome. Recently, basic research in molecular biology has deepened, which is of potential value in further prolonging survival after surgery, particularly in the control of recurrence and metastasis.

Adequate preoperative preparation is extremely important. Preoperative ultrasonography performed by the chief surgeon is helpful to guide the operative position and incision, estimate the distance between the tumor nodule and major vessels/ducts, and plan the extent of resection. Preoperative treatment is needed in patients with Child B cirrhosis. Right subcostal incision is commonly used. A strong retractor is very helpful for exposure.

The extent of resection is one of the key issues in decreasing operative mortality particularly in patient with cirrhosis. Recently, the Brisbane 2000 Terminology of Liver Anatomy and Resections has been advocated by the Terminology Committee of the International Hepato-Pancreato-Biliary Association (Strasberg et al., 2000). The terms for surgical resection are listed as follows: Right hepatectomy/hemihepatectomy (Couinaud segments referred to Sg5-8, +/−Sg1), left hepatectomy/hemihepatectomy (Sg2-4, +/−Sg1), right anterior sectionectomy (Sg5,8), right posterior sectionectomy (Sg6,7), left medial sectionectomy (Sg4) or resection segment 4 or segmentectomy 4, left lateral sectionectomy (Sg2,3) or bisegmentectomy 2,3, right trisectionectomy (Sg4-8, +/−Sg1) or extended right hepatectomy or extend right hemihepatectomy, left trisectionectomy (Sg2-5,8, +/−Sg1) or extended left hepatectomy or extended left hemihepatectomy.

For patients without cirrhosis, segmentectomy, sectionectomy, hemihepatectomy, or trisectionectomy can be chosen depending on the extent of tumor. Up to 80–85% of the liver can be resected. However, in patients with cirrhosis, limited resection, subsegmentectomy, or segmentectomy is the choice. Intraoperative ultrasonography is extremely helpful during hepatic resection. Minimizing blood loss is another key issue for hepatic resection. Techniques for this purpose include good exposure, fresh blood transfusion, step-by-step resection and ligation of intrahepatic vessels and ducts, and temporal occlusion of hepatic hilum. The occlusion time should not exceed 10–15 minutes for patient with cirrhosis. Repeated occlusion is needed for complicated operations. The cut end should be closed by mattress suture, covered by falciform ligament or omentum, or spray with fibrin. Adequate drainage is also important.

The important elements to a low operative mortality after HCC resection are careful selection of patients, adequate pre- and postoperative care, careful determination of the extent of resection in cirrhotic livers, adequate exposure, limited blood loss, short duration or without occlusion of the hepatic hilum, transfusion with fresh blood, and avoidance of unnecessary surgical procedures in severely cirrhotic livers.

Postoperative complications after HCC resection include the following: (1) Hepatic dysfunction remains the leading issue after major hepatic resection in a cirrhotic liver. High pulse rate, rapid increase of serum bilirubin, marked prolongation of prothrombin time, and early appearance of ascites are poor prognostic findings. Early aggressive treatment is important. (2) Postoperative bleeding has been less frequently encountered in the recent years. Carefully closing of the cut end is a key point. Prolonged prothrombin time and massive bleeding during operation are usually the background. (3) Bile leakage is more often encountered after resection of HCC in the hepatic hilum, and adequate drainage is the treatment of choice. (4) Subdiaphragmatic abscess was less common in recent years because of adequate drainage after resection, and is not difficult to control with ultrasound guided aspiration. (5) Pleural effusion often appeared in the right side after right liver resection in a cirrhotic liver; aspiration is the treatment. (6) Ascites is common in patient with cirrhosis; albumin and diuretics are needed. (7) Varix or stress ulcer bleeding is also encountered.

Comparison between small HCC (≤ 5 cm) and large HCC revealed higher resectability, lower operative mortality, and higher 5-year survival (Zhou et al., 2001). Pathological studies on small HCC revealed well-differentiated, more diploid, single encapsulated tumor in the majority, which became progressively less differentiated, more aneuploid, with more multiple nodules and poor encapsulation during their development to large HCC. These findings strongly support the strategy for early detection and early treatment.

Wakabayashi et al. (1997) reported that resectability can be increased and major hepatectomy can be made safer by employing portal vein embolization (PVE) preoperatively, in view of the fact that major hepatectomy was not considered feasible without PVE in these patients. PVE results in hypertrophy of remnant liver and atrophy of resected liver volume.

In patients with unresectable HCC, hepatic artery ligation (HAL), hepatic artery cannulation with postoperative infusion chemotherapy (HAI), cryosurgery, or microwave ablation can produce significant reduction of tumor nodule in a small proportion of patients. It has been demonstrated that the combination of HAL and HAI was superior to each alone. This combined treatment is performed by inserting a catheter with implanted injection port through the right gastric epiploic artery to the proper right or left hepatic artery according to the location of the tumor. The accuracy of catheterization should be verified by injection of methylene blue. HAL is done to occlude the arterial blood flow to the HCC-affected liver section, and HAL plus HAI to occlude the arterial blood supply but maintain the patency of the inserted catheter. Chemotherapeutic agents commonly used are cisplatin, adriamycin (or epirubicin), 5-fluorouracil or fluorodeoxyuridine, and mitomycin C. Hepatic artery embolization is done by injecting Lipiodol. Cryosurgery using $-196°C$ liquid nitrogen is performed using a cryoprobe covered or inserted into the tumor for 15–20 minutes. If remarkable shrinkage of tumor appears, usually in a small part of localized unresectable HCC, sequential resection is suggested. With advances of regional and multimodality combination therapy, downstaging followed by resection has appeared in the recent years as a new approach for treatment of some localized unresectable HCC (Tang, 1997). TACE has also been reported as an effective procedure for downstaging of some of the unresectable HCC. The 5-year survival after this approach has been reported as high as 50–60%. Systemic chemotherapy combined with interferon alpha was also reported to convert unresectable to resectable HCC (Leung et al., 1999).

Intrahepatic recurrence is frequently encountered after curative resection. The 5-year recurrence rate is around 60–70% after curative HCC resection, and 40–50% for curative small HCC resection. For early detection of subclinical recurrence, monitoring AFP and ultrasonography every 2 to 3 months for more than 5 years after curative resection are emphasized. Reresection remained the treatment for subclinical recurrence in the liver or solitary lung metastasis. Limited resection is the choice for reresection. TACE is indicated for multiple recurrent lesions. RF or PEI is the choice for small recurrent lesion when surgery is contraindicated. A routine biomarker for prediction of metastasis and recurrence is not yet available, although many biomarkers have been tried, such as AFP mRNA, circulating VEGF and PD-ECGF, human macrophage metalloelastase gene, p27, p53 mutation, telomerase activity, and so on. For prevention of recurrence, both pre- and postoperative chemotherapy or chemoembolization have not adequately proved to be effective. Interestingly, a randomized trial revealed that oral polyprenoic acid prevents second primary HCC after surgical resection (Muto et al. 1996). Another randomized trial indicated that a single dose of intra-arterial ^{131}I-Lipiodol increased the 3-year overall survival from 46.3% in the control to 86.4% in the treatment group (Lau et al., 1999).

The molecular basis of "HCC invasiveness" is similar to that of other solid cancers. It has been found that p16 and p53 mutation, p21, c-erbB-2, mdm2, TGF, EGF-R, MMP-2 (matrix metalloproteinase), uPA (urokinase-type plasminogen activator), uPA-P, PAI-1 (inhibitor of uPA), ICAM-1 (intercellular adhesion molecule), PD-ECGF, and VEGF were positively related to invasiveness of HCC. Whereas nm23-H1, Kai-1, TIMP-2 (tissue inhibitor of metalloproteinase), E-cadherin, and integrin α5 were negatively related to invasiveness. Some of these parameters might have potential as prognostic indicators. To clarify the mechanism and to develop new treatment approach of recurrence and metastasis, a metastatic model of human HCC in nude mice (LCI-D20) has been established with high rate of intrahepatic metastasis as well as metastasis in lungs and lymph nodes. For experimental intervention, antisense H-ras, BB-94 (matrix metalloproteinase inhibitor), TNP470, endostatin, suramin, and interferon alpha have been demonstrated to inhibit tumor growth and lung metastasis in this (LCI-D20) model. Gene therapy and novel tumor vaccine are also hopeful.

Orthotopic Liver Transplantation

There are no prospective, randomized trials comparing orthotopic liver transplantation (OLT) and partial hepatic resection for HCC. It is unlikely that such a study will ever be performed because of organ donor shortages and increasing patient population sizes with nonmalignant end-stage liver disease as an indication for OLT. Thus, the results of retrospective, nonrandomized studies must be evaluated to determine the role of OLT in the treatment of HCC.

For partial hepatic resection for HCC, prognosis is related to both the extent and biologic aggressiveness of the malignant disease and to the functional hepatic reserve remaining following the resection. For example, resection is a reasonable treatment option for a Child A cirrhotic patient with a solitary, <5 cm tumor located in the periphery of the liver, but it may not be possible to resect the same tumor in a Child C cirrhotic because of the high probability of postoperative liver failure. Patients with HCC confined to the liver with cirrhosis too severe to permit survival after partial liver resection may be candidates for OLT. However, initial reports of OLT for HCC from the 1980s cast significant doubts on the wisdom of this radical therapy. Tumor recurrence rates after OLT were as high as 75%, and 5-year overall survival rates were less than 20%. However, analysis of patterns of failure and prognostic variables from these early studies permitted the development of more stringent selection criteria for patients likely to benefit from OLT. Table 18.1 lists risk factors for recurrence of HCC following hepatic resection and OLT.

Using selection criteria derived from earlier studies of OLT to treat HCC, reports from the last decade indicate an improved probability of long-term survival following OLT. The 1-year, 3-year, and 5-year overall survival rates following OLT for HCC range from 75 to 84%, 46 to 74%, and 40 to 60%, respectively, in recent series (Hussain et al., 2001). Tumor-free survival rates are significantly higher in studies that compare OLT and resection for HCC. The 1-year, 3-year, and 5-year disease-free survival rates following OLT range from 75 to 84%, 63 to 72%, and 54 to 60%, respectively, versus 62 to 70%, 24 to 44%, and 14 to 31%,

TABLE 18.1. Risk Factors for Recurrence After Resection or Transplantation for Hepatocellular Carcinoma

	Hepatic Resection	Liver Transplantation
Tumor size	+	+/−
Gross vascular invasion	+	+
Microvascular invasion	+	−
More than three tumors	+	+/−
Bilobar involvement	+	+/−
Resection margin <1 cm	+	−
Tumor staging	+	+/−
Lymph node metastases	+	+

respectively, following resection for HCC (Esquivel et al., 1999; Yamamoto et al., 1999). It is important to note that these survival figures for OLT exclude the 12–20% of patients who do not survive the first 90 days after OLT because of complications or graft rejection. When these early patient deaths from postoperative complications are included in survival analysis, the 1-year and 3-year survival rates are similar or slightly better following resection compared to OLT. It is not until 5-year survival rates are compared that OLT demonstrates a clear benefit compared with resection for HCC.

The long waiting period for donor organs has led many investigators to study hepatic arterial chemoembolization, percutaneous ethanol injection, cryoablation, radiofrequency ablation, or combinations of these techniques to provide local control of intrahepatic tumor as a bridge to OLT and as neoadjuvant therapy in an attempt to reduce the incidence of tumor recurrence. Unfortunately, these studies have provided conflicting results, with minimal or no improvement in tumor recurrence or long-term survival rates, but with some success in local tumor control prior to OLT. Whether such local tumor control methods are used or not, the potential survival benefit of OLT for HCC is lost in patients on the organ waiting list more than 9–10 months after diagnosis of HCC. The problem of increasing numbers of patients dying while on a waiting list for organ donation has produced an increased interest in living-related and nonrelated split organ OLT. The many ethical dilemmas in these living donors are still being addressed by transplant programs worldwide.

Chemotherapy

Single-agent chemotherapy has been studied extensively to treat advanced HCC. 5-Fluorouracil (5-FU) was the first drug investigated. Overall, the response rate was 6%, with a median duration of response of only 3 months. The initial reports using doxorubicin to treat HCC were encouraging, but subsequent studies failed to confirm an antitumor response rate of greater than 20%. Review of the published trials using doxorubicin or other single-agent chemotherapeutic drugs to treat HCC reveals a response rate of less than 20% and a median survival of 4 months in treated patients. It is clear that for cytotoxic chemotherapeutic agents, no single agent has a high response rate, and the brief nature of the response in most patients (1–3 months), indicates that no significant effect on survival is to be expected (Hussain et al., 2001; Watkins and Curley, 2000).

Dissatisfaction with the results obtained with single chemotherapeutic agents led to trials involving combinations of cytotoxic drugs. Doxorubicin and 5-FU have been the most widely used agents in combination with a large number of other drugs. The response rates with combination chemotherapeutic regimens have been only slightly higher than those with single drugs (Hussain et al., 2001; Watkins and Curley, 2000). Presently, there is no evidence to support the routine use of combination chemotherapy to treat advanced HCC outside of a controlled clinical trial. Furthermore, there is no proven survival benefit for adjuvant single- or multiple-agent chemotherapy following resection or ablation of HCC.

There have been numerous reports of various combinations of chemotherapeutic agents delivered by hepatic arterial infusion to treat HCC. Fluoropyrimidines, like 5-FU and floxuridine (FUDR), have high rates of hepatic extraction, but alone have not produced marked improvements in response rates in HCC. Despite having lower rates of hepatic extraction, doxorubicin, cisplatin, and mitomycin C have been shown to produce substantial objective response rates when administered regionally. Unfortunately, the vast majority or reports of hepatic arterial delivery of chemotherapy to treat HCC describe small groups of patients in nonrandomized studies that lack stratification of response or survival based on stage of disease or tumor burden. Furthermore, higher response rates may be related to concomitant injection of arterial embolizing agents in many of the studies. While higher objective tumor response rates are achieved following arterial administration of chemotherapeutic drugs, this has generally failed to result in an improved overall survival rate. A subset of patients with initially unresectable disease may have a dramatic enough reduction in tumor burden following hepatic arterial chemotherapy administration to become candidates for resection, and thus achieve an increased potential for long-term survival benefit (Hussain et al., 2001; Watkins and Curley, 2000).

Chemoradiation Therapy

The full liver does not tolerate radiation therapy at high doses because radiation-induced hepatitis occurs at doses above 25–30 Gy. Two alternative approaches to treat HCC with chemoradiation therapy have been performed successfully. The first involves external beam whole-liver irradiation to a total dose of 21–24 Gy with concurrent administration of systemic or regional radiation sensitizing chemotherapy with 5-FU, FUDR, or cisplatin. Further irradiation is delivered to the tumor using ^{131}I antiferritin antibodies, ^{131}I iodized oil, or ^{90}Y-microspheres (Dancey et al., 2000; Hargreaves et al., 2000; Hussain et al., 2001; Watkins and Curley, 2000). Some programs deliver cycles of systemic or regional chemotherapy after the radiation therapy, or combine irradiation with arterial chemoembolization. There are also descriptions of treatment of unresectable HCC with radioisotopes delivered with antibodies, iodized oil, microspheres, or embolic particles; and a report suggesting improved disease-free and overall survival in patients treated with ^{131}I iodized oil as an adjuvant after resection of HCC (Lau et al., 1999). Response rates of 40–62% have been reported with programs of this nature. Median survival is improved and some patients are downstaged sufficiently to undergo resection, but overall long-term survival is not improved in most patients.

The second approach involves the use of computer-based modeling to deliver an arc rotation, three-dimensional conformal technique of external beam irradiation (Dawson et al., 2000; Gunderson et al., 1999). Once again, radiation sensitizing systemic intravenous or regional arterial chemotherapy is delivered with fluoropyrimidines. Higher doses of radiation, in some reports greater than 70 Gy, are delivered to the tumor while sparing nonmalignant liver parenchyma from high-dose radiation by delivering the focused beams from different directions with each daily treatment. Once again, this technique has successfully resulted in higher tumor response rates with modest toxicity, but the technique requires very precise modeling and treatment planning that is not readily available in all centers. Response rates surpass 60% with improved local disease control rates and prolongation of medial survival by several months. Combined modality chemoradiation therapy has also been reported to convert a small subset of unresectable HCC patients to a resectable volume of disease.

Ablative Techniques

Percutaneous Ethanol Injection   Direct image-guided intratumoral injection of absolute ethanol has been used extensively around the world. Percutaneous ethanol injection (PEI) is usually performed with transabdominal ultrasonographic guidance with the tumor injected with 5–10 mL of ethanol twice a week. The volume of ethanol required to ablate the tumor is estimated based on the diameter of the HCC. For tumors less than 2 cm in size, three to five injection sessions are required, whereas five to eight sessions are necessary for tumors 2–3 cm in diameter. Survival rates after PEI range from 1-year rates of 46–96% and 5-year rates of 0–72% (Hargreaves et al., 2000). Survival depends on severity of cirrhosis and the number and size of HCC tumors treated. Survival rates in patients with a solitary HCC tumor <3.0 cm in size are high, but the survival probability drops dramatically in patients with more than one tumor nodule or a single large (>3–5 cm) tumor nodule treated with PEI.

Patient compliance with PEI has been a problem because of the multiple injections required and the pain associated with the treatment, but serious complications such as intraperitoneal hemorrhage, hepatic insufficiency, bile duct necrosis or biliary fistula, hepatic infarction, and hypotension occur in less than 5% of patients. Local recurrence rates have been reported infrequently in most studies of PEI. Most reports mention that local recurrence is common in tumors greater than 5 cm in diameter and recommend that PEI not be used to treat such large HCCs. Furthermore, a recent report of PEI in HCC patients with tumors less than 3 cm diameter found a local recurrence rate of 38%. After a 3-year follow-up of all patients, HCC had recurred locally or at other intrahepatic sites in 81% of the patients. Because PEI required multiple treatment sessions and was associated with a high local recurrence rate, the authors recommended that PEI only be considered for tumors less than 1.5 cm in diameter and that all other patients with small HCC be treated with resection or other definitive, single-treatment ablation techniques.

Percutaneous Acetic Acid Injection   Acetic acid in concentrations of 15–50% has been used for ultrasound-guided percutaneous acetic acid injection (PAI) into small HCC (Hargreaves et al., 2000). The 1-, 3-, and 5-year survival rates after PAI of a solitary HCC tumor <3.0 cm in diameter were 95%, 80%, and 49%, respectively. A prospective randomized trial comparing PEI with PAI in 60 HCC patients was performed. Local recurrence rate in the PEI-treated patients was 37% versus 8% in the PAI-treated group. The 1- and 2-year survival was also better after PAI (100% and 92%, respectively) compared with PEI (83% and 63%, respectively). The experience with PAI is limited at this time, but these results suggest that further investigation of this technique to treat small HCC is warranted.

Cryoablation Cryoablation has been used to treat otherwise unresectable primary liver cancers. Studies have demonstrated that liver tumors must be cooled to at least $-35°$ C throughout the entire tumor to achieve a reliable tumor cell kill. Tumor cell death is not a direct consequence of lowering tissue temperature, but rather is caused by ice crystal formation during rapid freezing with resultant destruction of normal cellular structures. To ensure adequate cryoablation, most tumors are treated with two freeze/thaw cycles to maximize this mechanical disruption of tumor cells. The low temperature necessary for tumor cell destruction with cryoablation is difficult to achieve at the periphery of tumors larger than 5–6 cm in diameter, when the tumor abuts a major intrahepatic branch of the portal or hepatic veins, or if it lies near the inferior vena cava.

Most information on local tumor recurrence and complications after cryotherapy come from patients treated for colorectal cancer liver metastases. In these patients, local recurrence in the cryoablated tumor has been reported to range from 2.5 to 44%. The largest published series using cryotherapy to treat HCC in 235 patients reported that there were no treatment-related deaths, but complications and local recurrence rates in the cryoablated tumors was not reported (Zhou and Tang, 1998). This study is also difficult to interpret because cryotherapy alone was used in only 78 patients (33.2%), the majority of patients were treated with cryotherapy plus hepatic artery ligation, transarterial chemoembolization, hepatic artery infusion chemotherapy, or resection of the frozen tumor.

Complications described after hepatic cryoablation include a mortality rate of 1.6%, significant intraoperative hemorrhage, cold injury in adjacent organs, biliary fistulae, coagulopathy, thrombocytopenia, myoglobinuria, acute renal failure, intrahepatic abscess in the cryolesion, and symptomatic pleural effusions. The overall reported complication rates after cryoablation range from 15 to 60%, with an average of 45%.

Radiofrequency Ablation The use of radiofrequency (RF) energy to produce thermal tissue destruction has been the focus of increasing research and practice for the past several years. During the application of RF energy, a high-frequency alternating current moves from the tip of an electrode into the tissue surrounding that electrode. As the ions within the tissue attempt to follow the change in the direction of the alternating current, their movement results in frictional heating of the tissue. As the temperature within the tissue becomes elevated beyond $60°$ C, cells begin to die, resulting in a region of necrosis surrounding the electrode. A typical RFA treatment results in local tissue temperatures that exceed $100°$ C, which produces coagulative necrosis of the tumor tissue and surrounding hepatic parenchyma. The tissue microvasculature is completely destroyed, and thrombosis of hepatic arterial, portal venous, or hepatic venous branches <3 mm in diameter occurs. Only tissue through which radiofrequency electrical current passes directly is heated above a cytotoxic temperature. The geometry of the radiofrequency current pathway around the ablation electrode creates a relatively uniform zone of radiant/conductive heat within the first few millimeters of electrode-tissue interface. The conductive heat emitted from the tissue radiates out from the electrode; and if the tissue impedance is relatively low, a dynamic expanding zone of ablated tissue is created. The final size of the region of heat-ablated tissue is proportional to the square of the radiofrequency current, also known as the radiofrequency power density. The radiofrequency power/current delivered via a monopolar electrode decreases in proportion to the square of the distance for the electrode. Therefore, the tissue temperature falls rapidly with increasing distance away from the electrode.

The decrease in tissue heating with increasing distance away from the electrode results in only 1.0–1.5 cm cylindrically shaped zones of coagulative necrosis of tissue when using monopolar simple needle electrodes. New needles (13–15 gauge diameter) have been developed with multiple array hook electrodes. The insulated needle electrode shaft is placed into the tumor with the array retracted. Using real-time ultrasound guidance, the array is then deployed from the needle tip into the tumor. These deployed multiple array hooks create a series of electrodes with a diameter of 2.0–5.0 cm, across which the radiofrequency current can be passed. The multiple array electrode is a technologic innovation that permits ablation of much larger zones of tissue compared to simple needle electrodes.

The use of radiofrequency ablation (RFA) to treat HCC has been reported recently (Curley et al., 2000). The sizes of HCC treated with RFA in the 110 cirrhotic patients ranged from 1 to 7 cm in their greatest dimension. All 110 HCC patients in this study were followed for a minimum of 12 months after RFA; the median follow-up was 19 months. Percutaneous or intraoperative RFA was performed in 76 (69%) and 34 patients (31%), respectively. A total of 149 discrete HCC tumor nodules were treated with RFA. Local tumor recurrence at the RFA site developed in four patients (3.6%); all four subsequently developed recurrent HCC in other areas of the liver. New liver tumors or extrahepatic metastases developed in 50 patients (45.5%), but 56 patients (50.9%) have no evidence of recurrence. The follow-up of HCC patients treated with RFA is not yet sufficient to determine long-term disease-free and overall survival rates.

Procedure-related complications after RFA were minimal in patients with HCC. There were no treatment-related deaths, but complications developed in 12.7% of the HCC patients. These complications included symptomatic pleural effusion, fever, pain, subcutaneous hematoma, subcapsular liver hematoma, and ventricular fibrillation. No patient developed thermal injury to adjacent organs or structures, hepatic insufficiency, renal insufficiency, or coagulopathy following the application of RF energy into the target tumors. The overall complication rate following RFA of HCC was low, which is particularly notable because there were 50 Child class A, 31 class B, and 29 class C cirrhotic patients treated.

Other Forms of Thermal Ablation   Heat ablation of liver tumors can also be performed using microwave coagulation therapy or laser-induced thermotherapy (Hargreaves et al., 2000; Ishikawa et al., 2000). Like RFA, these procedures can be performed during an open laparotomy, with laparoscopic or thoracoscopic guidance, or percutaneously. The effectiveness of these treatments is currently limited by the small zones of necrosis achieved with the rapid heating and desiccation of the tissue around the microwave or laser probes. Multiple insertions of the probes are required to treat tumors more than 1 cm in diameter with microwave coagulation therapy, or more than 2 cm in diameter with laser-induced thermal ablation. Currently, the treatment complexity of placing multiple intratumoral probes and the cost for these microwave or laser systems (at least 10 times higher than RF generators and needle electrodes) is limiting more widespread clinical acceptance of these alternative thermal ablation techniques.

Hepatic Artery Chemoembolization Hepatic artery occlusion has been used alone or in combination with intra-arterial chemotherapy. Hepatic artery occlusion may be permanent, accomplished by surgical ligation or by inert particle embolization, or it may be intermittent by using balloon occlusion or by chemoembolization using degradable microspheres.

Patients with an occluded portal vein are at particularly high risk for post-operative liver failure, emphasizing the need for preoperative assessment of portal vein patency prior to hepatic artery occlusion by whatever means. Selective embolization of tumor feeding vessels is possible in the presence of portal vein occlusion, though this must be approached with caution.

Attempts have been made to increase the activity of locoregionally administered treatments by prolonging the duration of contact between tumor tissue and the chemotherapeutic agent. Intra-arterially administered contrast media (Lipiodol, ethiodol) is deposited selectively within HCCs, in which it remains for several months. These substances also may act as carriers for chemotherapeutic agents or radioactive iodine (^{131}I). A variety of chemotherapeutic agents have been coadministered with Lipiodol, including doxorubicin, FUDR, mitomycin C, epirubicin, cisplatin, and styrene maleric acid neocarzinostatin (SMANCS). In most of the trials, 50–90% of the patients have a decrease in serum AFP levels, with median survival rates ranging from 2 to 14 months and 1- and 2-year survival rates ranging from 33% to 55%. In a randomized, controlled multicenter clinical trial, Lipiodol transcatheter arterial embolization in the presence versus the absence of doxorubicin was studied (Kawai et al., 1992). The 3-year survival values for each group were 33.6% and 34.9%. The serum AFP level decreased by a significantly greater extent in the group that received doxorubicin compared with the group that did not.

Gelfoam powder (40–50 μ) or particles (250–589 μ) occlude the hepatic arterial circulation transiently. After the particles are degraded and resorbed in the circulation, vascular flow resumes within 48–72 hours. Coadministered with doxorubicin, mitomycin C, and cisplatin, an objective response rate of 24% and a 68% decrease in the serum AFP level was observed. In a nonrandomized trial comparing the intra-arterial infusion (without embolization) of 5-FU, cytosine arabinoside, mitomycin C, and doxorubicin with a combination of Gelfoam embolic particles mixed with mitomycin C and doxorubicin, the 1-, 2-, and 3-year survival rates following arterial infusion were 22%, 9%, and 4%, respectively, compared with 67%, 37%, and 22%, respectively, for the Gelfoam chemoembolic combination (Hirai et al., 1989). Thus, vascular occlusion may potentiate the tumoricidal effects of chemotherapy, but further controlled trials are needed to define optimal interactions (Trevisani et al., 2001).

Hepatic arterial embolization has been compared with resection and alcohol injection as primary therapies to treat HCC. Both alcohol injection and resection were found to be superior to embolization when survival rates were the end point, but most studies failed to randomize to specific therapies and those receiving embolization may have had more advanced stage of disease and were not candidates for other local therapies. In a series from the United States, chemo-embolization was compared with conventional chemotherapy or no antitumor therapy (Bayraktar et al., 1996). Admission criteria for this study included inoperability, with tumors larger than 5 cm, acceptable performance status, and absence of portal vein occlusion. Twenty-eight patients received chemoembolization in the form of Lipiodol, mitomycin C, and Gelfoam embolization. The chemoembolization group had a significantly higher mean survival of 13 months over both the chemotherapy (7.2 months), and no antitumor therapy groups (6.9 months).

In summary, despite numerous studies, systemic therapy remains investigational and is of minimal benefit to the patient with unresectable HCC, or as adjuvant therapy following resection or ablation of HCC. Regional therapy, particularly hepatic arterial chemoembolization may have palliative potential, and a few patients may be downstaged from unresectable to resectable tumors. Hepatic arterial chemoembolization has also been proposed as an effective neoadjuvant therapy prior to resecting small HCC, but this recommendation was based on retrospective review of nonrandomized patients and must be confirmed in pro-spective, randomized studies (Zhang et al., 2000).

FOLLOW-UP

In the United States, the relative 5-year survival for liver cancer only increased from 4% (1974–1976) to 6% (1986–1993) in whites, and from 1% to 4% in blacks (Landis et al., 1998). In Shanghai, the relative 5-year survival of liver cancer in 1988–1991 was 4.4%. These indicate that there is still a long way to go in conquer-ing HCC. However, the long-term results in some centers were encouraging.

Factors that influencing prognosis can be grouped into four aspects: clinico-pathological features, treatment modalities, biological characteristics, and coexist-ing hepatitis and cirrhosis.

Clinicopathological Features

Analysis of the factors influencing the prognosis of HCC revealed that patients discovered by screening, with subclinical HCC, normal value of serum gamma-glutamyl transpeptidase (GGT), small HCC (≤ 5 cm), single tumor nodule, well-encapsulated tumor, nonhepatic hilum located tumor, and no cirrhosis or micronodular cirrhosis had better outcomes than patients discovered in the clinic, with symptomatic HCC, abnormal GGT, large HCC, multiple tumor nodules, poorly encapsulated tumor, hepatic hilum located tumor, and macronodular cirrhosis. TNM classification correlates well to prognosis (Nonami et al., 1997).

Treatment Modalities

The 5-year survival rates for patients treated with hepatic resection were around 30–50%, being 50–60% for small HCC resection, and 20–30% for large HCC resection. Palliative surgery other than resection such as hepatic artery ligation/ cannulation (HAL/HAI), cryosurgery, and so on, yielded 10–20% of 5-year survival. The 5-year survival for large series of TACE was around 7–10%, with better result for segmental/subsegmental TACE. Radiotherapy, or internal irradiation using ^{90}Y-microsphere or ^{131}I-Lipiodol achieved results comparable to those using TACE. Unfortunately, systemic chemotherapy remained disappointing. Recently, cytoreductive therapies using HAL/HAI or repeated TACE for unresectable HCC have led to remarkable tumor shrinkage in a small number of patients, and sequential resection yielded 50–60% of 5-year survival rates.

Biological Characteristics

Biological characteristics remains the major prognosis-influencing factors of HCC. It has been found that patients without intrahepatic venous tumor thrombus, with diploid cancer, low positivity of proliferating cell nucleus antigen (PCNA), with expression of antimetastatic gene nm23-H1/tissue inhibitor of metalloproteinase-2 (TIMP-2), and without expression of transforming growth factor (TGF)/epidermal growth factor receptor (EGF-R) in HCC had higher 5-year survival than did patients with tumor thrombi, aneuploid cancer, high positivity of PCNA, without expression of nm23-H1/TIMP-2, and with expression of TGF/EGF-R.

Coexisting Hepatitis and Cirrhosis

HCC patient with hepatitic status and Child C cirrhosis often have poor prognosis.

PREVENTION

Few approaches of HCC prevention have been emerged: (1) Prevention of HBV infection using hepatitis B vaccination in newborn babies. Result from a universal hepatitis B vaccination program indicated that the incidence of HCC in children with vaccination has declined. (2) Prevention of viral hepatitis B or C progressing to cirrhosis and HCC by interferon (IFN) therapy. IFN decreased HCC incidence in patients with HBV-related cirrhosis. The cumulative occurrence rates of HCC in the treated group and the untreated group were 17.0% and 30.8%, respectively, at the end of 10 years (Ikeda et al., 1998). IFN therapy also decreased the development of

HCV-related HCC. HCC rates in the IFN-treated and untreated groups were 7.6% and 12.4% at the 10th year, respectively. IFN therapy significantly reduces the risk for HCC, especially among virologic or biochemical responders of patients with chronic hepatitis C. Retreatment with IFN-alpha appeared to have the additional effect of suppressing the development of HCC in patients who had incomplete responses to the initial treatment, even when the HCV was not cleared with retreatment. 3) Avoiding exposure to hepatocarcinogens (such as AFB_1) and promoters (such as microcystin) by changing daily food from corn to rice and changing drinking water. In Qidong County of China, after people changed their source of drinking water from pond-ditch water (microcystin was found) to deep-well water, the mortality rate of HCC stabilized and even decreased slowly to a level comparable with that seen in control areas (Yu, 1995).

In addition to IFN therapy as a preventive, postoperative, or post-treatment adjuvant therapy, some other antiviral drugs, such as lamivudine against HBV or ribavirin against HCV, have been added, and provide a hope for further improve of the effect of prevention. However, randomized trials and long-term follow-up studies are needed for the final evaluation.

REFERENCES AND FURTHER READING

Bayraktar Y, Balkanci F, Kayhan B, Uzunalimoglu B, Gokoz A, Ozisik Y, Gurakar A, Van Thiel DH, Firat D (1996) A comparison of chemoembolization with conventional chemotherapy and symptomatic treatment in cirrhotic patients with hepatocellular carcinoma. *Hepato-Gastroenterology* 43:681–687

Curley SA, Izzo F, Ellis LM, Nicolas Vauthey J, Vallone P (2000) Radiofrequency ablation of hepatocellular cancer in 110 patients with cirrhosis. *Ann Surg* 232:381–391

Dancey JE, Shepherd FA, Paul K, Sniderman KW, Houle S, Gabrys J, Hendler AL, Goin JE (2000) Treatment of nonresectable hepatocellular carcinoma with intrahepatic 90Y-microspheres. *J Nucl Med* 41:1673–1681

Dawson LA, McGinn CJ, Normolle D, Ten Haken RK, Walker S, Ensminger W, Lawrence TS (2000) Escalated focal liver radiation and concurrent hepatic artery fluorodeoxyuridine for unresectable intrahepatic malignancies. *J Clin Oncol* 18:2210–2218

Edmondson H, Steiner PE (1954) Primary carcinoma of the liver: a study of 100 cases among 48,900 necropsies. *Cancer* 7:462–503

Eggel H (1901) Uber das primare carcinoma der leber. *Beitr Pathol Anat* 30:506

Esquivel CO, Keeffe EB, Garcia G, Imperial JC, Millan MT, Monge H, So SK (1999) Resection versus transplantation for hepatocellular carcinoma. *J Gastroenterol Hepatol* 14(Suppl):S37–41

Gunderson LL, Haddock MG, Foo ML, Todoroki T, Nagorney D (1999) Conformal irradiation for hepatobiliary malignancies. *Ann Oncol* 10(Suppl 4):221–225

Hargreaves GM, Adam R, Bismuth H (2000) Results after nonsurgical local treatment of primary liver malignancies. *Langenbecks Arch Surg* 385:185–193

Hirai K, Kawazoe Y, Yamashita K, Aoki Y, Fujimoto T, Sakai T, Majima Y, Abe M, Tanikawa K (1989) Arterial chemotherapy and transcatheter arterial embolization therapy for nonresectable hepatocellular carcinoma. *Cancer Chemother Pharmacol* 23(Suppl):S37–41

Hussain SA, Ferry DR, El-Gazzaz G, Mirza DF, James ND, McMaster P, Kerr DJ (2001) Hepatocellular carcinoma. *Ann Oncol* 12:161–172

Ikeda K, Saitoh S, Suzuki Y, Kobayashi M, Tsubota A, Fukuda M, Koida I, Arase Y, Chayama K, Murashima N, Kumada H (1998) Interferon decreases hepatocellular carcinogenesis in patients with cirrhosis caused by the hepatitis B virus: a pilot study. *Cancer* 82:827–835

Ikeda K, Saitoh S, Arase Y, Chayama K, Suzuki Y, Kobayashi M, Tsubota A, Nakamura I, Murashima N, Kumada H, Kawanishi M (1999) Effect of interferon therapy on hepatocellular carcinogenesis in patients with chronic hepatitis type C: A long-term observation study of 1,643 patients using statistical bias correction with proportional hazard analysis. *Hepatology* 29:1124–1130

Ishak KG, Anthony PP, Sobin LH (1994) *Histological Typing of Tumours of the Liver*, 2nd ed. WHO International Histological Classification of Tumours. Springer-Verlag, Berlin, p. 20

Ishikawa M, Ikeyama S, Sasaki K, Miyauchi T, Fukuda Y, Miyake H, Harada M, Terashima Y, Yogita S, Tashiro S (2000) Intraoperative microwave coagulation therapy for large hepatic tumors. *J Hepato-Biliary-Pancreatic Surg* 7:587–591

Kawai S, Okamura J, Ogawa M, Ohashi Y, Tani M, Inoue J, Kawarada Y, Kusano M, Kubo Y, Kuroda C, et al. (1992) Prospective and randomized clinical trial for the treatment of hepatocellular carcinoma–a comparison of Lipiodol-transcatheter arterial embolization with and without adriamycin (first cooperative study). The Cooperative Study Group for Liver Cancer Treatment of Japan. *Cancer Chemother Pharmacol* 31(Suppl):S1–6

Landis SH, Murray T, Bolden S, Wingo PA (1998) Cancer statistics, 1998. CA *Cancer J Clin* 48:6–29

Lau WY, Leung TW, Ho SK, Chan M, Machin D, Lau J, Chan AT, Yeo W, Mok TS, Yu SC, Leung NW, Johnson PJ (1999) Adjuvant intra-arterial iodine-131-labelled Lipiodol for resectable hepatocellular carcinoma: a prospective randomised trial. *Lancet* 353:797–801

Leung TW, Patt YZ, Lau WY, Ho SK, Yu SC, Chan AT, Mok TS, Yeo W, Liew CT, Leung NW, Tang AM, Johnson PJ (1999) Complete pathological remission is possible with systemic combination chemotherapy for inoperable hepatocellular carcinoma. *Clin Cancer Res* 5:1676–1681

Muto Y, Moriwaki H, Ninomiya M, Adachi S, Saito A, Takasaki KT, Tanaka T, Tsurumi K, Okuno M, Tomita E, Nakamura T, Kojima T (1996) Prevention of second primary tumors by an acyclic retinoid, polyprenoic acid, in patients with hepatocellular carcinoma. Hepatoma Prevention Study Group. *N Engl J Med* 334:1561–1567

Nonami T, Harada A, Kurokawa T, Nakao A, Takagi H (1997) Hepatic resection for hepatocellular carcinoma. *Am J Surg* 173:288–291

Okuda H, Nakanishi T, Takatsu K, Saito A, Hayashi N, Takasaki K, Takenami K, Yamamoto M, Nakano M (2000) Serum levels of des-gamma-carboxy prothrombin measured using the revised enzyme immunoassay kit with increased sensitivity in relation to clinicopathologic features of solitary hepatocellular carcinoma. *Cancer* 88:544–549

Pisani P, Parkin M, Bray F, Ferlay J (1999) Estimates of the worldwide mortality from 25 cancers in 1990. *Int J Cancer* 83:18–29

Strasberg SM, Belghiti J, Clavien P-A, Gadzijev E, Garden JO, Lau W-Y, Makuuchi M, Strong RW (2000) The Brisbane 2000 terminology of liver anatomy and resections. *HPB* 2:333–339

Tabor E (1994) Tumor suppressor genes, growth factor genes, and oncogenes in hepatitis B virus-associated hepatocellular carcinoma. *J Med Virol* 42:357–365

Tang ZY (1997) Treatment of unresectable hepatocellular carcinoma: cytoreduction by chemotherapy, hepatic artery ligation, radioimmunotherapy, and other methods. In *Liver Cancer.* Okuda K, Tabor E (eds.) Churchill Livingstone, New York, pp. 537–541

Tang ZY, Yang BH (1995) Secondary prevention of hepatocellular carcinoma. *J Gastroenterol Hepatol* 10:683–690

Trevisani F, De Notariis S, Rossi C, Bernardi M (2001) Randomized control trials on chemoembolization for hepatocellular carcinoma. *J Clin Gastroenterol* 32:383–389

Watkins KT, Curley SA (2000) Liver and bile ducts. In *Clinical Oncology.* Abeloff MD, Armitage JO, Lichter AS, Niederhuber JE (eds.). Churchill Livingstone, New York, pp. 1681–1748

Yamamoto J, Iwatsuki S, Kosuge T, Dvorchik I, Shimada K, Marsh JW, Yamasaki S, Starzl TE (1999) Should hepatomas be treated with hepatic resection or transplantation? *Cancer* 86:1151–1158

Yu SZ (1995) Primary prevention of hepatocellular carcinoma. *J Gastroenterol Hepatol* 10:674–682

Zhang Z, Liu Q, He J, Yang J, Yang G, Wu M. (2000) The effect of preoperative transcatheter hepatic arterial chemoembolization on disease-free survival after hepatectomy for hepatocellular carcinoma. *Cancer* 89:2606–2612

Zhou XD, Tang ZY (1998) Cryotherapy for primary liver cancer. *Semin Surg Oncol* 14:171–174

Zhou XD, Tang ZY, Yang BH, Lin ZY, Ma ZC, Ye SL, Wu ZQ, Fan J, Qin LX, Zheng BH (2001) Experience of 1000 patients who underwent hepatectomy for small hepatocellular carcinoma. *Cancer* 91:1479–1486

CHAPTER 19

Esophageal Carcinoma

LAWRENCE LEICHMAN, LISA M. BODNAR, and IJAZ I. ARSHAD

Albany Medical College, Division of Medical Oncology, Albany, New York

INTRODUCTION

Despite a changing epidemiology in the Western Hemisphere, a growing knowledge of the molecular changes that contribute to carcinogenesis, more advanced clinical staging methodologies, and multimodality clinical strategies, the outlook for patients with esophageal cancer (EC) remains grim. Less than 12% of all patients presenting with symptoms of dysphagia or odynophagia will survive five years. Less than 25% of patients judged clinically to have potential for cure (stages I–III) will survive five years.

Although EC patients, especially those with squamous cell cancers of the esophagus (SCCE), may share a similar demographic and clinical profile with head and neck cancer patients, esophageal tumors, regardless of histology, have a far greater propensity for early systemic spread than head and neck cancers. Thus, clinical trials that have sought to define the role of systemic therapy for EC patients are relevant, but their results have not been uniform. Consequently, an agreed upon paradigm for curative therapy has remained elusive.

EPIDEMIOLOGY AND ETIOLOGY

The overwhelming majority of patients presenting with EC in Asia and the Middle East have SCCE. In the West, however, the overall incidence SCCE has decreased while the incidence of adenocarcinoma of the esophagus (ACE) has dramatically increased over the past 25 years. ACE has increased by 9–16% per year in Scandinavian countries and by as much as 20% per year in the United States and Australia (a 350% increase since the 1970s). In the West, this dramatic increase has

UICC Manual of Clinical Oncology, Eighth Edition. Edited by Raphael E. Pollock
ISBN 0-471-22289-5 Copyright © 2004 John Wiley & Sons, Inc.

radically shifted the ratio of ACE to SCCE from 1:20 in the decade of the 1960s to 2:1 or 3:1 over the past decade. On a population basis, ACE will be diagnosed in 2.8/100,000 in Denmark, 3.7/100,000 in the United States and 5–8.7/100,000 in the United Kingdom. On the other hand, Eastern European countries have experienced only a minor rate of increase in the incidence of ACE (1).

In the Unites States, the increased incidence of ACE has been mainly noted in white males. Rates of ACE have also increased (but far less steeply) in women and African-American males. The large increase in the incidence of ACE has been associated with the increasing recognition of Barrett's esophagus. Barrett's eso-phagus, characterized by a columnar epithelium lining and intestinal metaplasia in the distal esophagus, is found in 10–20% of patients with esophageal reflux. Patients with Barrett's esophagus have 30- to 50-fold increase in the incidence of ACE. Patients with symptoms of gastric esophageal reflux disease also have an increased incidence of ACE (2). The underlying reasons for increasing reflux disease and Barrett's esophagus have not been elucidated.

The currently increasing rate of gastric cardia adenocarcinomas has lead to speculation that adenocarcinoma of the gastric cardia and the esophagus are etiologically related. In comparison to healthy controls and patients with SCCE, patients with ACE and gastric cardia have been found to have an increased body mass index (BMI) (3). Whether elevated intraabdominal pressure found in BMI patients leads to an increased incidence of Barrett's esophagus has not been determined. Both cigarette smoking and alcohol consumption, in a time- and dose-dependent manner are associated with an increased risk of SCCE and ACE.

Histamine-2 (H_2) blocking agents such as cimetidine and ranitidine are nitro-sated under acidic conditions. H_2 blocking agents also act on P450 enzymes that may inhibit the clearance of cytotoxic agents. The increased use of these agents has been linked with ACE, but, to date, proof of this association is lacking. The hypothesis that ACE is related to the increased use of drugs and foods that relax esophageal sphincter tone is currently under investigation. Thus, the role of diet in the dramatic increase in ACE remains unresolved.

SCCE is a major health problem in China, South Africa, and Iran. There is increasing evidence that viruses, fungi, and diet have an etiologic role in the development of SCCE in these endemic regions. A study from China found that DNA sequences from human papilloma virus (HPV) 16, 18, and 30 were found in 5.8% of squamous cell tumors (4). Moreover, there is a statistically greater risk for non-cancer patients in high-incidence areas of China to carry HPV 16 with the E-6 gene in the cytoplasm of the normal esophageal mucosa than in areas of lower incidence (5). Investigators from India have reported that the consumption of fermented betel nut plus tobacco increased the odds ratio for developing SCCE to 7.1 for men and 3.6 for women.

Western Hemisphere population-based studies have reported that, in addition to cigarette and alcohol use, risk factors for SCCE include infrequent consumption of raw fruits and vegetables and low socioeconomic class. Regardless of socio-economic background, there is a higher incidence of SCCE among the African American population in the United States than among the U.S. white population (6).

MOLECULAR GENETICS AND TUMORIGENESIS

Hypermethylation

Hypermethylation is an epigenetic mechanism resulting in suppression of gene expression, especially tumor suppressor genes such as adenomatous polyposis coli (*APC*). DNA methylation patterns are commonly altered early in tumorigenesis. Hypermethylation of the promoter region of the *APC* gene has been found in 92% of ACE tissues, 50% of SCCE, and 39.5% of patients with Barrett's metaplasia. *APC* hypermethylation was not found, however, in esophageal tissue matching normal esophageal tissue. Hypermethylation of *p16/CDKN2*, a growth suppressor gene located at chromosome 9p that produces a protein product controlling S phase entry from G, has been detected at relatively high levels as an early molecular event in both SCCE and ACE (7).

Not only is hypermethylation an early event in EC tumorigenesis, there appears to be a relationship among the number of hypermethylated genes, tumor stage, and histologic differentiation. In an analysis that searched through a panel of 20 genes using a high-throughput methylation assay, more advanced cancers and less well-differentiated esophageal cancers were found to have an increased number of hypermethylated genes than less advanced cancers. Moreover, patients with nonmalignant Barrett's esophagus displayed more hypermethylated genes if there was associated dysplasia. Hypermethylation was also found in normal esophageal mucosa from patients with Barrett's esophagus and cancer (8).

Molecular Progression to ACE

Elucidation of the molecular progression of benign Barrett's esophagus to cancer would enable clinicians to standardize surveillance programs. The progression of Barrett's esophagus from benign metaplasia to invasive cancer appears to take place under the influence of an accumulation of genetic changes within the esophageal mucosa. Characteristically, tumor progression is found when esophageal mucosal cells within the Barrett's esophagus are mobilized from G_0 to G_1, which results in an increase of the 4N or G_2/tetraploid number of cells. The nonrandom loss of heterozygosity (LOH) in chromosomes 5q, 9p, 13q, 17p, and 18q has been identified as the common accumulation of genetic events indicating the malignant progression of Barrett's esophageal mucosa. Unlike colonic tumors, the loss of 17p (the locus for p53) is a relatively early event in the malignant progression of Barrett's esophageal mucosa (9).

Molecular Progression to SCCE

Without the benefit of an identifiable benign precursor lesion, the charting of molecular progression from benign to malignant mucosa is not as advanced for SCCE. LOH and point mutations of the tumor suppressor genes, *p53* and *RB*, can be found in approximately 30–40% of SCCE. Phosphorylation of the *RB* gene protein product blocks its inhibitory function on the later stages of the cell cycle (10).

Amplification of the cyclin D-1 gene may be an important event in the multistage development of a subset of SCCE. The cyclin D-1 protein product accelerates S-phase entry from G1 phase by activating CDK-4–mediated phosphorylation of RB protein. The *cyclin D-1/PRAD-1* gene, mapped to chromosome 11q, is amplified in approximately 30% of SCCE.

The binding of epidermal growth factor (EGF) or transforming growth factor-alpha (TGF-α) to epidermal growth factor receptor (EGFR) results in increased DNA synthesis and cellular proliferation. EGFR overexpression and gene amplication of EGFR have been found in over 70% and 20% of SCCE, respectively. That EGFR overexpression is found most frequently in normal and dysplastic tissue surrounding malignant SCCE, suggests it may have a central role in the tumorigenesis of SCCE (11).

MOLECULAR BIOLOGY IN PROGNOSIS OF EC

Following a potentially curative operative procedure, staging by light microscopy has been the gold standard for determining prognosis of solid tumors. Nevertheless, intratumoral molecular markers and intratumoral genetic events now have an established role in refining prognosis within a specific tumor stage.

The HER-2/*neu* oncogene, localized to chromosome 17q, encodes a transmembrane tyrosine kinase growth factor receptor that has significant homology with EGFR. For ACE patients ($n = 475$), the HER-2/*neu* positive rate between ranged between 11% and 73%. In multivariate analysis from two reports, HER-2/*neu* overexpression had a statistically significant, stage-independent impact on survival. For SCCE patients ($n = 406$), HER-2/*neu* overexpression ranged from none (one study) to 52%. Although two SCCE studies reported HER-2/*neu* overexpression to be associated with poor chemotherapy response and extramucosal invasion, investigators have yet to link HER-2/*neu* overexpression to survival for patients with SCCE (12).

In a study of 111 primary SCCE, overexpression of cyclin D1 (25%) in the primary tumor was an independent variable in predicting survival ($p = 0.01$). Although the loss of p16 protein expression (50%), was associated with nodal metastases, it did not have independent power to predict survival (13). An analysis of 107 primary EC tumors found that EGFR gene amplification (12%) is associated with a poor survival ($p = 0.001$) (14). In one study, patients with tumors demonstrating allelic loss (LOH) of both 17p and 18q had a worse survival rate than either those without LOH or those with loss of one allele ($p = 0.002$) (9). Unfortunately, the methodologies for measuring molecular parameters within primary EC have not been uniform and, consequently, the results of these trials cannot, at this time, be used to make clinical decisions.

SURVEILLANCE FOR BARRETT'S ESOPHAGUS

Although recommendations have been made for surveillance endoscopy of Barrett's patients on a yearly or biannual basis, the cost-effectiveness of this policy may be questioned. Those favoring routine endoscopic surveillance for Barrett's esophagus note that invasive cancers appear to be discovered at an earlier stage if routine surveillance is maintained. Furthermore, published 5-year survivals for those with cancer enrolled in surveillance programs have been better than those presenting with symptoms of cancer (nonsurveillance). These data are, at best, observational and subject to bias. Less than 1% of all patients with Barrett's esophagus will develop invasive ACE. Moreover, it has been estimated that endoscopic surveillance for Barrett's patients adds approximately 0.1 "quality adjusted life years to an individual's survival." Thus, recent reports suggesting little gain or no gain from endoscopic surveillance merit attention (15).

Among the most important uses for molecular biology in EC will be in determining those patients most at risk for developing cancer after Barrett's esophagus has been diagnosed. A prospective study found that Barrett's patients with 17p LOH had relative risk to develop cancer 16-fold greater than those who did not have 17p LOH ($p < 0.001$). Moreover, those Barrett's patients with flow cytometric features showing increased 4N and aneuploidy carried relative risks of developing cancer of 6.1 ($p < 0.001$) and 7.5 ($p < 0.001$), respectively (16). These results need confirmation in a larger cohort, but they give good reason to believe that surveillance for patients with Barrett's esophagus can be made more efficient and effective with the use of molecular profiling.

SYMPTOMS AND SIGNS OF EC

Regardless of histology, the best chance for cure for patients with EC is detection prior to the common symptoms of dysphagia and/or odynophagia. Although screening cytology has been successfully employed in areas that are endemic for SCCE, for the most part, small, incidental, and asymptomatic tumors are discovered only when endoscopy is performed for unrelated reasons or when patients with Barrett's esophagus undergo surveillance endoscopy.

Because of the rich venous and lymphatic drainage through the upper, mid, and distal esophagus, primary tumors invading into the esophageal muscularis layer have a propensity for rapid regional and systemic spread. The elasticity of the esophageal smooth muscle allows most patients to be asymptomatic until the esophageal lumen is narrowed to one-half to one-third of normal. By the time symptoms are present, most tumors have passed through the esophageal muscular layer.

Dysphagia, present in 95% of symptomatic patients, has a characteristic pattern of progression, beginning with difficulty swallowing solid foods and progressing to liquids. Weight loss is present in 40–50% of patients. When weight loss and weakness are accompanied by dysphagia, there may be rapid improvement if local measures can be taken to improve swallowing. Weight loss without dysphagia is ominous as it may represent systemic spread of the cancer. In reports from clinical trials, patients who have lost more than 10 percent of their normal weight have a significantly poorer prognosis regardless of tumor histology or therapy.

Cough and odynophagia are present in 20–25% of patients. Cough induced by swallowing may suggest either local extension into the trachea with resultant tracheo-esophageal fistula or chronic aspiration. Odynophagia and pain radiating to the back may signify regional extraesophageal spread with nerve involvement.

EC patients may present with local symptoms as described above or with symptoms due to malignant pleural effusions, bone, liver, pericardia, retroperitoneal, and pelvic lymph nodal metastases. Some EC patients, especially those with ACE, may present with signs and symptoms of dissemination without reference to the primary tumor. Thus, ACE must be considered in the differential diagnosis of a patient presenting with an unknown primary adenocarcinoma or in the presentation of gastrointestinal bleeding.

As usual, a careful history and physical examination provide the best clues to the local effects of the primary tumor, possible signs (e.g., lymphadenopathy, hepatomegaly) and sites of metastasis, general nutritional status, and pulmonary complications such as aspiration or tracheo-esophageal fistula.

DIAGNOSIS

Histology

Although over 95% of all esophageal tumors will be histologically classified as epidermoid (squamous cell) or adenocarcinomas, other histologies such as small cell, leiomyosarcomas, melanomas, and lymphomas of the esophagus may be found. The staging and treatment of these rare esophageal tumors are dictated by their histology.

Endoscopy and Barium Series

Esophageal endoscopy is the most common, effective, and efficient method for diagnosis of EC. Upper gastrointestinal endoscopy should be performed in patients presenting with symptoms of dysphagia, odynophagia, or for those presenting with metastatic unknown primary tumors for whom noninvasive x-ray methods fail to make a diagnosis. Upper gastrointestinal (UGI) series with barium swallow will give a more accurate estimate of tumor infiltration than endoscopy. An UGI series will also be the test of choice to show evidence of tracheo-esophageal fistula and/or aspiration.

Endoscopic Ultrasonography (EUS)

By virtue of its ability to depict five ultrasonically defined layers of the esophagus, EUS is most accurate when assessing T status. The detail of the esophageal layers is obtained by alternating echogenicities. The superficial mucosa is hyperechoic, the deep mucosa and muscularis mucosa is hypoechoic, submucosa plus the interface with the submucosa and muscularis propria is hyperechoic, muscularis propria minus the interface with the submucosa hypoechoic and adventitia is hyperechoic. Irregular, hypoechoic disruption of the normal esophageal layers signifies esophageal cancer. The reported overall accuracy of primary tumor assessment is between 85% and 90%, with the modality being most accurate in determination of full-thickness involvement (T3–T4) as compared with discrimination of degrees of intramural involvement.

Local inflammation can cause false overstaging whereas microscopic invasion below the spatial resolution of EUS may result in understaging. Nevertheless, the major technical limitation of EUS is mechanical, as stenosis caused by tumor infiltration may inhibit the passing of the endoscope and ultrasound probe past the tumor. With the development of smaller caliber ultrasound probes, EUS staging of the primary tumor is now available for a larger number of patients.

The presence of lymphadenopathy diagnosed by EUS is prognostic for survival. Lymph node metastases are usually described as irregular, hypoechoic, and round. Inflammatory lymph nodes on the other hand are more homogeneous, echogenic, and less well defined. Recently, ultrasonagraphy equipment has been designed to allow for a fine-needle aspiration (FNA) through the esophagus into adjacent lymph nodes.

In combination with EUS, FNA allows for the best possible accuracy of staging without a formal operation such as laparoscopy or thoracoscopy. Nevertheless, EUS is a relatively invasive and expensive procedure. Unless therapeutic decisions rest on the outcome of EUS, its routine use cannot be recommended.

Computed Tomography (CT)

CT is the most frequently utilized noninvasive procedure providing information to stage patients with EC. Intravenous and oral contrast improves definition of the posterior mediastinal structures, vascular tissue planes, differentiation of adenopathy from normal surrounding structures, and detection of liver metastases. Scanning should include the chest and upper abdomen with extension into the neck or lower abdomen depending on tumor location or signs of more extensive disease. Primary malignant esophageal neoplasms are typically irregular and asymmetric soft tissue masses. On CT scan, the primary tumor site can be seen either as a focal area of wall thickening or more commonly as an area of circumferential involvement.

Preoperative underestimation of tumor stage by CT is a relatively common problem. Significant weight loss from dysphagia will cause loss of periesophageal fat planes that will not allow the radiologist to distinguish growth of tumor around mediastinal structures such as the aorta. In one prospective trial, CT scanning failed to detect T1 lesions found at surgery; and it diagnosed only 40% of documented T2 lesions. The CT sensitivity for diagnosing lymph node metastases was less than 60%. Thus, CT is a relatively insensitive instrument to detect early primary esophageal tumors and mediastinal/abdominal lymph node involvement. In contrast to its limitations in T and N staging, CT is sensitive and specific for detecting metastatic disease to the lung, liver, or adrenal glands.

Magnetic Resonance Imaging (MRI)

MRI has shown similar limitations in sensitivity and specificity as CT. Currently, MRI has a no more definitive role in the preoperative staging of esophageal carcinoma than CT. A careful review of the recent literature would suggest that the expertise of the radiologist should determine whether the clinician orders a CT or an MRI. It is appreciated, however, that MRI is far more specific and sensitive than CT in determining whether a mass in the adrenal gland represents a malignant or benign process.

Positron Emission Tomography (PET)

Limited tumor involvement in the normal-sized organ or lymph node poses difficulty in detection by CT or MRI. PET uses metabolic tracers such as FDG (18-fluoro-2-deoxyglucose) to assess regional metabolism noninvasively. FDG, a glucose analogue, is transported and phosphorylated like glucose in most tissues but is a poor substrate for further metabolism and therefore metabolically trapped within the cells. The rate of FDG accumulation is proportional to the local rate of glucose metabolism. Both SCCE and ACE avidly accumulate FDG.

In a recently reported trial, 53 patients with primary esophageal tumors were prospectively evaluated with PET and chest CT. Of these, 50 patients underwent curative esophagectomy and radical lymph node dissection. PET and CT findings were compared with pathology findings of nodal metastases in 108 of 436 dissected lymph node groups. PET detected 56 metastatic node groups (51.9% sensitivity, 94.2% specificity, 83.7% accuracy), compared with CT, which detected 16 (14.8% sensitivity, 96.7% specificity, 76.6% accuracy; sensitivity: $p < 0.005$). In assessing distant metastases, PET sensitivity is approximately 88%, specificity, approximately 93%, and accuracy, approximately 91%. PET has also been evaluated as a predictor of response to therapy: a reduction of FDG uptake after 14 days of therapy has been found when patients respond to treatment.

Minimally Invasive Surgical Staging

To more clearly define patients with potential for cure, there is interest in defining the role of minimally invasive studies such as thoracoscopy and laparoscopy. The accuracy of these procedures is being compared with that of EUS with FNA. To date, the only published prospective trial designed to assess thoracoscopy and/or laparoscopy in staging EC found the procedures both feasible and safe. Nevertheless, a true comparison with noninvasive staging has yet to be completed.

Bronchoscopy should be performed for all tumors in proximity to the airway, including all cervical and upper thoracic tumors abutting the trachea, carina, or main-stem bronchi. Indentation of the membranous wall by an underlying EC in the absence of mucosal involvement does not preclude resection. However, evidence of transluminal invasion or tracheoesophageal fistula is considered a contraindication to surgical resection.

STAGING

In 1997, the American Joint Committee on Cancer (AJCC) changed TNM staging system for esophageal cancer from clinical to one based on pathologic classification. This staging system was developed because of convincing data that demonstrated significant prognostic implications of depth of esophageal wall penetration. Currently, tumor stage and prognosis are determined by (1) location of tumor, (2) depth of tumor infiltration into or through the esophageal wall, (3) tumor invasion of adjacent structures (T4), for example, invasion of the aorta or tracheobronchial tree, (4) presence or absence of regional lymph node metastases, and (5) presence or absence of distant metastatic disease. There were no further revisions in the 2002 system (Tables 19.1 and 19.2).

TREATMENT

Although the United States National Comprehensive Cancer Network guidelines offer surgery alone or radiation plus chemotherapy as equal "standards of care,"

TABLE 19.1. 2002 TNM Staging System for Esophageal Cancer

Primary tumor (T)

TX	Primary tumor cannot be assessed
T0	No evidence of primary tumor
Tis	Carcinoma in situ
T1	Invades lamina propria or submucosa
T2	Invades muscularis propria
T3	Invades adventitia
T4	Invades adjacent structures

Regional lymph nodes (N)

NX	Regional lymph nodes cannot be assessed
N0	No regional lymph node metastasis
N1	Regional lymph node metastasis

Distant metastasis (M)

MX	Distant metastasis cannot be assessed
M0	No distant metastasis
M1	Distant metastasis

Tumors of the lower thoracic esophagus

M1a	Metastasis in coeliac lymph nodes
M1b	Other distant metastasis

Tumors of the mid thoracic esophagus

M1a	Not applicable
M1b	Nonregional lymph nodes or other distant metastasis

Tumors of the upper thoracic esophagus

M1a	Metastasis in cervical lymph nodes
M1b	Other distant metastasis

TABLE 19.2. 2002 TNM-Based Staging System for Esophageal Cancer

Stage 0	Tis	N0	M0
Stage I	T1	N0	M0
Stage IIa	T2	N0	M0
	T3	N0	M0
Stage IIb	T1	N1	M0
	T2	N1	M0
Stage III	T3	N1	M0
	T4	Any N	M0
Stage IV	Any T	Any N	M1
Stage IVa	Any T	Any N	M1a
Stage IVb	Any T	Any N	M1b

chemotherapy and radiation prior to surgery are frequently utilized in centers that treat large numbers of esophageal cancer patients. Moreover, as the cure rate for esophageal cancer has not changed in the past 20 years, the search for better treatments through clinical investigation is rational and ethical. Once an esophageal tumor invades the submucosa, there is little data to suggest that tumor histology (ACE or SCCE) should play a significant role in determining therapy. Even with control of the primary EC, both ACE and SCCE of the esophagus have a strong propensity to metastasize to distant sites through lymphatic and/or venous spread. We will review surgery, radiation therapy, and chemotherapy as curative therapeutic modalities singly and in combination.

Surgery

As a treatment modality, surgery may be utilized in either the setting of cure or symptom palliation. Although the specific surgical approach continues to be a matter of debate, the most commonly used procedure in the West is a transthoracic esophagectomy (TTE) that includes *en bloc* resection with two-field lymphadenectomy to achieve wide and clear surgical margins. By definition, this resection includes the involved esophagus, surrounding soft tissue, pleura, regional thoracic lymphatics, and perigastric lymph nodes to the level of the celiac axis. An Ivor-Lewis approach, the most common TTE, utilizes a laparotomy for gastric mobilization with a resultant anastomosis in the upper thorax via a right thoracotomy.

Among proponents of TTE, the optimal extent of lymphadenectomy is also a matter of debate. As the vast majority of nodal recurrences occur outside the area of original dissection, Japanese surgeons pioneered an esophagectomy with three-field lymphadenectomy. This procedure extends lymph node dissection to include the cervical and upper thoracic region. Although a Japanese nationwide survey reported a significant improvement in 5-year survival over historical controls, randomized trials are lacking to justify its use as a standard of operative care.

A transhiatal esophagectomy (THE) uses cervical and abdominal incisions to construct a cervical anastomosis. Advocates of THE cite fewer pulmonary complications from avoidance of a thoracotomy, a shorter operative time, decreased incidence of gastric reflux, decreased postoperative morbidity, and the ability to place the anastomosis in the cervical region where a longer resection margin could be obtained and anastomotic leakage is less often fatal.

Proponents of TTE believe this approach allows for complete visualization of all perigastric and paraesophageal lymph tissue (allowing for better staging via access to mediastinal lymph nodes) as well as the thoracic esophagus, thus eliminating possible serious damage to adjacent structures which can rarely occur with THE. Few prospective randomized trials designed to compare TTE with THE have been attempted or reported. However, a meta-analysis reviewing all studies published between 1990 and 1999 found no significant differences in risk of perioperative or postoperative complications were identified (17).

Over the past two decades, incidences of morbidity and mortality following esophageal surgery have markedly decreased, especially in centers that perform esophagectomies on a regular basis. Average hospital mortality has improved over the past two decades from 29% in the 1980s to 7.5% at present. In centers that specialize in esophageal resections, mortality appears to be significantly less ($\sim$5%) than in those that perform only an occasional esophageal resection.

Radiation Therapy

In a report of a randomized trial comparing chemotherapy plus radiation with radiation alone, no patient treated with single modality radiation was alive at three years, versus a 20% survival for those treated with the combination. Thus, radiation as a single modality is not recommended for EC patients for whom cure is a goal. As an adjunct to surgical therapy, radiation alone does not improve survival nor has radiation been shown to improve local control following surgery. In general, radiation as a single modality for patients with EC should be relegated to those patients for whom palliative, nonoperative therapy is most appropriate.

Chemotherapy

Although many systemic chemotherapeutic agents have modest activity against both primary SCCE and ACE, the positive impact of currently available single agents or combinations is quite modest. Although a list of reportedly active chemotherapeutic agents against esophageal cancer now includes bleomycin, cisplatin, doxorubicin, 5-fluorouracil (5-FU), gemcitabine, irinotecan, methotrexate, mitomycin-c, paclitaxel, vindesine, and vinorelbine, the measurement of tumor effect in these reports has not been uniform or reproducible. Complete pathologic responses of the primary tumor are rarely reported when single agent or combination chemotherapy is used.

The most frequently used and reported chemotherapy combination is cisplatin and 5-FU. Recently, the activity of paclitaxel, as a single agent, in the face of cisplatin and 5-FU resistance, has been confirmed. Paclitaxel, in combination with 5-FU and cisplatin, has been reported to have a 48% rate against primary EC. Combinations with gemcitabine and irinotecan are currently being tested against primary tumors of the esophagus, but before assuming a major role in therapy, these newer agents will have to be placed in combination with either surgery and/or radiation.

Neoadjuvant Treatments

As most EC patients die from distant metastases, preoperative or neoadjuvant systemic treatment has been used to begin treatment relatively quickly after the diagnosis is made. With the increasing use of laser surgery on the primary tumor, most patients tolerate cytotoxic therapy quite well and most will be less debilitated upon going to surgery. In addition, when the primary tumor responds, the surgeon has a less bulky primary tumor to remove. Despite two decades of studies with neoadjuvant therapy, investigations have been conducted with flawed designs, findings of marginal statistical significance, and contradictory results. Thus, the question of whether preoperative therapy improves survival for EC patients remains fiercely debated.

Neoadjuvant Chemotherapy Prior to Surgery

The efficacy of cisplatin-based chemotherapy regimens in the treatment of EC prompted trials assessing these in combination with surgery. A U.S. National Cancer Institute (NCI) intergroup randomized trial compared preoperative chemotherapy followed by surgery to surgery alone in stage I–III EC patients (cervical tumors excluded). Between 1990 and 1995, 467 patients from 123 institutions were enrolled. Patients randomized to chemotherapy received three cycles of cisplatin ($100 \ mg/m^2$) and 5-FU ($1000 \ mg/m^2 \times 5$ days) prior to surgery; surgery-alone patients proceeded directly to esophagectomy. For patients responsive to chemotherapy, an additional two cycles were to be administered postoperatively. In an intention to treat analysis, the median duration of survival for the combined modality arm was 14.9 months, whereas in the surgery-only arm it was 16.1 months (no significant change). Differences in 1-, 2-, and 3-year survivals between the two groups, irrespective of histology, were also not significant. An overall clinical response rate to chemotherapy was 19% (18).

Although the results of the NCI trial seemed to be rather definitive, the value of cisplatin-based preoperative chemotherapy remains unsettled, as a recent report (in abstract form) from the United Kingdom indicates that cisplatin and 5-FU prior to surgery improves survival over surgery. In this trial, 802 patients with primary EC were randomized to receive two cycles of cisplatin 80 mg/m^2 and 5-FU 1000 mg/m^2 over 96 hours followed by resection of the primary tumor or resection without chemotherapy. Approximately two-thirds of the patients randomized had ACE. Seventy-eight percent of the cohort receiving preoperative chemotherapy underwent a potentially curative resection versus 70% of those who received surgery alone ($p < 0.001$). In an intent-to-treat analysis, the overall survival for the neoadjuvant chemotherapy group was significantly better than the group who went to surgery without neoadjuvant chemotherapy ($p = 0.004$). The median survival for the neoadjuvant chemotherapy group was 16.8 months compared with the 13.3 months for nonneoadjuvant group (19). It is not yet possible to comment on the reason for the differences in the U.S. and U.K. trials. Suffice it to state, however, that, in the near future, the standard of care for EC patients in these two countries will be substantially different.

Neoadjuvant Chemoradiotherapy (Trimodality Therapy)

Because infusional 5-FU does not commonly cause bone marrow toxicity, this schedule allows the drug to be combined with other systemic agents (e.g., cisplatin or mitomycin-c) and/or radiation. Preoperative (neoadjuvant) chemotherapy plus radiation followed by surgery for EC has become known as trimodality therapy. The many nonrandomized trials using cisplatin and 5-FU plus radiation prior to surgery established the following: (1) between 20% and 40% of those taken to surgery following neoadjuvant chemotherapy and radiation have had a pathologic complete response (pCR); (2) the pCR patients have had the best overall survival; (3) the median survival for patients treated with preoperative chemotherapy and radiation is between 16 and 20 months; and (4) preoperative therapy has minimal effect on surgical complications.

Several randomized prospective trials testing trimodality therapy against surgery alone have now been reported. The two most frequently noted come from single institutions: the University of Michigan, and a single center in Dublin. As a result, these randomized trials are somewhat underpowered and have been open to differing interpretations. The trial reported from Dublin noted a statistically significant improvement in survival for patients with ACE who received cisplatin and 5-FU plus radiation prior to surgery. Because the group that had surgery alone fared poorly in terms of expected survival (median, 11 months), these results have not been uniformly accepted as valid (20). In a trial that included both SCCE and ACE patients, the University of Michigan group reported no statistically significant difference in median survival for trimodality patients versus surgery only patients. Nevertheless, at three years, 16% of the patients who received surgery were alive whereas 30% of those who received trimodality therapy were alive. This difference, for the 100 patients randomized, approached, but did not attain, statistical significance (21).

In fact, radiation and chemotherapy as definitive therapy or as part of a neoadjuvant program before surgery have been part of modern Western medical practice for over two decades. In a recent survey of the treatment for over 5,000 U.S. esophageal cancer patients, only 18% were treated with surgery alone (22). Thus, it not surprising that a recent U.S. trial designed to definitively test trimodality therapy versus surgery alone had to be closed because it failed to accrue enough patients to fulfill its major objectives.

Chemotherapy and Radiation as Definitive Therapy

Nonoperative trials for potentially curable EC patients were stimulated by the knowledge that between 20% and 40% of patients treated with neoadjuvant chemotherapy and radiation had a pCR. Among the major concerns regarding a nonoperative approach to EC is the rate of local recurrence. Coia et al. (23) reported a series analyzing recurrence and survival for stage I and stage II esophageal cancer patients (clinically staged) after definitive therapy with 5-FU and mitomycin-c with concurrent external beam radiation (6,000 cGy). They reported a local failure rate of 25% and a five-year actuarial survival of 30% in 57 patients with SCCE and ACE. Investigators at Wayne State University treated 24 EC patients with intent to cure without surgery by using 5-FU and cisplatin with concurrent external beam radiation (5,000 cGy). The local failure rate was also found to be 25%, with 50% of the patients alive at three years and 30% alive at five years.

In 1985, a randomized trial was designed by the RTOG to test the role of chemotherapy in addition to definitive radiation. Patients were randomized to receive external radiation (6,400 cGy) alone versus four cycles of infusional 5-FU (1000 mg/m^2 over 24 hours for 96 hours) and cisplatin (75 mg/m^2) plus radiation (5,000 cGy at 200 cGy/d). Although some patients had stage IV EC (supraclavicular lymph node involvement) or were patients who could not have surgery because of a pre-existing medical problem, the patients in the combined modality arm experienced a 14-month median survival versus a 9-month median survival for those patients who received only radiation (24). Moreover, at five years, 26% of the patients who received chemotherapy and radiation were alive whereas none of the radiation only patients survived five years. A recent report noted the long-term survival and overall toxicity for the randomized group (123 patients) and for the additional 69 patients treated on this protocol after randomization was discontinued: for the group randomized, the eight-year survival was 22%; the projected 10 year survival is 20%.

Additional support for adding chemotherapy to radiation in the definitive treatment of EC is found in the analysis of the Eastern Cooperative Oncology Group (ECOG) trial, EST 1282. In this protocol, patients with relatively limited SCCE were randomized to radiation alone versus radiation plus 5-FU and mitomycin-c. Although some patients in this trial received surgery and the five-year survival was the same for both groups, the investigators concluded that combined chemoradiotherapy statistically improved the median survival from 9.2 months to 14.8 months (25).

Conclusions Regarding Definitive Therapy

Although current therapy for EC patients will cure only a small percentage of patients, the various therapeutic options need to be carefully considered for each patient. With the recognition that reflux esophagitis and Barrett's esophagus are precursors to ACE, patients may soon be presenting at earlier stages. In the young patient presenting with early-stage disease, surgery eliminates the Barrett's esophagus and the need for endoscopic follow-up of the Barrett's. In the elderly or medically frail patient, treatment with definitive radiation and chemotherapy offers the same chance for cure as surgery but without the prospect surgical mortality and/ or morbidity. Also, in the elderly patient, the residual Barrett's esophagus poses less of a threat for a new esophageal tumor.

The opportunity to cure advanced T-stage or N-stage EC remains limited. As the tumor has a strong propensity to metastasize early, it is rational to consider systemic chemotherapy and/or radiation as an adjunct to surgery with the caveat that the data for such treatment remains controversial. It is imperative to continue the search for new and effective molecular targets that would allow for greater treatment efficiency and efficacy. Thus, patients with tumors harboring low TS levels and poor capacity for repair (low ERCC-1), will be more responsive to chemotherapy including 5-FU and cisplatin. Moreover, agents that will target molecular markers on the tumor itself, for example, EGFR and/or HER-2/*neu* need to be tested against EC.

Follow-Up After Definitive Therapy

Optimal follow-up of patients with EC after they have been treated with intent to cure is not well defined. The most common complaint following treatment is dysphagia. Within a year of therapy, dysphagia is as likely to be due to treatment as to recurrent tumor. Stricture of the esophagus is among the most common findings in patients treated with surgery alone or with chemotherapy and radiation as definitive therapy. CT scan evaluation usually shows thickening of the esophagus and periesophageal tissues. This finding is not specific for tumor recurrence and may be frequently found as a long-standing change following radiation. Thus, the etiology of the stricture must be documented with upper gastrointestinal endoscopy and biopsy. Patients with benign strictures are best treated with esophageal dilatation. Those with recurrent cancer may, for a short time, benefit from dilatation, but these patients frequently need a permanent feeding tube to maintain nutritional status.

In patients with a Barrett's adenocarcinoma, for whom definitive radiation and chemotherapy was administered, surveillance endoscopy is appropriate because the Barrett's esophagus does not disappear with tumor regression or cure of the cancer. Otherwise, there is little data to suggest that the patient without symptoms benefits from surveillance endoscopy.

Although 80% of all EC recurrences are diagnosed within two years of definitive therapy, recurrences may be found after five or six years of follow-up. Recurrences in bone (especially vertebrae) are relatively common. Back pain in a patient with a history of EC requires rapid and thorough evaluation to rule out the possibility of impending spinal cord compression. Nevertheless, in patients who have received radiation, osteoporosis and osteopenia may be a contributing factor to bone pain. MRI is generally the most sensitive and specific test to rule out pain from recurrent tumor versus pain from other causes. Occasionally, back pain may be secondary to retroperitoneal lymph node recurrences. These patients generally report pain associated with significant weight loss.

Although liver and adrenal recurrences of esophageal cancer are relatively common, they are frequently found as a result of workup for unexplained weight loss or loss of appetite. CT scanning is most useful for the detection of these recurrences. Because EC cannot be cured when systemic spread is found, the question of how often or whether to perform routine surveillance CT scans remains open.

Palliative Therapy

Patients with disseminated EC should be palliated by addressing their symptoms. The goal of all palliative care is to keep the patient functioning as normally as possible in their home environment for as long as feasible. Unfortunately, those patients with recurrent EC or those presenting with disseminated EC rarely survive beyond one year. However, for patients with incurable EC presenting with symptoms of dysphagia or odynophagia, it is appropriate to offer radiation to the esophagus plus chemotherapy because the treatment generally offers the best opportunity to palliate symptoms. Likewise, because response rates approach 30%, chemotherapy treatment with agents such as cisplatin, 5-FU, and paclitaxel is appropriate initial therapy for patients with symptomatic retroperitoneal lymphadenopathy or symptomatic liver metastases. Treatment of painful bone metastases is usually best approached with local radiation. As treatment of the primary tumor has improved, there are a larger number of patients with EC living to develop brain metastases. For this complication, whole brain irradiation is appropriate palliative therapy.

REFERENCES

1. Bollschweiler E, Wolfgarten E, Gutschow C, Holscher AH (2001) Demographic variations in the rising incidence of esophageal adenocarcinomas in white males. *Cancer* 92:549–555.
2. Chow WH, Finkle WD, McLaughlin JK, Frankle H, Ziel HK, Fraumeni JF Jr (1995) The relation of gastroesophageal reflux disease and its treatment to adenocarcinomas of the esophagus and gastric cardia. *JAMA* 274:474–477.
3. Chow WH, Blot WJ, Vaughan TL, Risch HA, Gammon MD, Stanford JL, Dubrow R, Schoenberg JB, Mayne ST, Farrow DC, Ahsan Habibul, West AB, Roterdam H, Niwa S, Fraumeni JF Jr. (1998) Body mass index and risk of adenocarcinomas of the esophagus and gastric cardia. *J Natl Cancer Inst* 90:15–155.
4. Fuju C, Syrjänen S, Shen Q, Cintorino M, Santopietro R, Tosi P, Syrjänen K (2001) Evaluation of HPV, CMV, HSV and EBV in esophageal squamous cell carcinomas from a high-incidence area of China. *Anticancer Res* 20:3935–3940.
5. Li Tao, Lu ZM, Chen KN, Guo M, Xing HP, Mei Qiang M, Yang HH, Lechner JF, Ke Y (2001) Human papillomavirus type 16 is an important infectious factor in the high incidence of eopsahgeal cancer in Anyang area of China. *Carcinogenesis* 22: 929–934.

6. Brown LM, Hoover R, Silverman D et al (2001) Excess incidence of squamous cell esophageal cancer among US black men: Role of social class and other risk factors. *Am J Epidemiol* 153:114–122.

7. Wong D, Barrett M, Stöger R, Emond MJ, Reid BJ (1997) $P16^{INK-4a}$ promoter is hypermethylated at a high frequency in esophageal adenocarcinomas. *Cancer Res* 57:2619–2622.

8. Kawakami K, Brabender J, Lord RV, Groshen S, Greenwald BD, Krasna MJ, Yin J, Fleisher AS, Abraham JM, Beer DG, Sidransky D, Huss HT, Demeester TR, Eads C, Laird PW, Ilson DH, Kelsen DP, Harpole D, Moore MB, Danenberg KD, Danenberg PV, Meltzer SJ (2000) Hypermethylated APC in plasma and prognosis of patients with esophageal adenocarcinoma. *J Natl Cancer Inst* 92:1805–1811.

9. Galipeau PC, Cowan DS, Sanchez CA et al. (1996) 17p (p53) allelic losses, 4N (G2/tetraploid) populations and progression toaneuploidy in Barrett's esophagus. *Proc Natl Acad Sci U S A* 93:7081–7084.

10. Weinberg RA (1991) Tumor suppressor genes. *Science* 254:1138–1146.

11. Itakura Y, Sasano H, Shiga C, Furukawa Y, Shia K, Mori S, Nagura H (1994) Epidermal growth factor receptor overexpression in esophageal carcinoma: An immunohisto-chemical study correlated with clinicopathologic findings and DNA amplification. *Cancer* 74:795–804.

12. Ross JS, McKenna BJ (2001) The HER2/*neu* oncogene in tumors of the gastrointestinal tract. *Cancer Invest* 19:554–568.

13. Tekeuchi H, Ozawa S, Ando N, Shih CH, Koyanagi K, Uedea M, Kitajima M (1997) Altered p16/MTS/CDKNw and cyclin D1/PRAD-1 gene expression is associated with the prognosis of squamous cell carcinoma of the esophagus. *Clin Cancer Res* 3: 2229–2236.

14. Kitagawa Y, Ueda M, Ando N, Ozawa S, Shimizu N, Kitajima M (1996) Further evidence for prognostic significance of epidermal growth factor rceptor gene amplification in patients with esophageal squamous cell carcinoma. *Clin Cancer Res 2:909–914.*

15. Shaheen NJ (2001) Does surveillance endoscopy improve life expectancy in those with Barrett's esophagus. *Gastroenterology* 121:1516–1522.

16. Reid BJ, Prevo LJ, Galipeau PC, Sanchez, Longton G, Levine DS, Blount PL, Rabinovitch PS (2001) Predictors of progression in Barrett's esophagus II: baseline 17p (p53) loss of heterozygosity identifies a patient subset at increased risk for neoplastic progression. *Am J Gastroenterol* 96:2839–2848.

17. Hulscher JBF, Tijssen JGP, Oertop H, Lanschot JB (2001) Transthoracic versus transhiatal resection for carcinoma of the esophagus: a meta-analysis. *Ann of Thorac Surg* 72:306–313.

18. Kelsen DP, Ginsberg R, Pajak TG et al. (1998) Chemotherapy followed by surgery for localized esophageal cancer. *N Engl J Med* 339:1979–1984.

19. Clark PI (2001) Neoadjuvant chemotherapy in oesophageal cancer. *Eur J Cancer* ECCO: 11. The European Cancer Conference Abstract Book, #518 S140 (abstr).

20. Walsh T, Noonan N, Hollywood D et al. (1996) A comparison of multimodal therapy and surgery for esophageal adenocarcinoma. *N Engl J Med* 335:462–467.

21. Urba SG, Orringer MB, Turris A et al. (2001) A randomized trial of preoperative chemoradiation versus surgery alone in patients with locoregional esophageal cancer. *J Clin Oncol* 19:303–313.

22. Daly JM, Karnell LH, Menck HR (1996) National cancer database report on esophageal cancer. *Cancer* 78:1820–1828.

23. Coia LR, Engstrom PF, Paul AR et al. (1991) Long-term results of infusional 5-FU and mitomycin-C and radiation as primary management of esophageal carcinoma. *Int J Radiat Oncol Biol Phys* 20:29–36.

24. Herskovic A, Martz LK, Al-Sarraf M et al. (1992) Combined chemotherapy and radiotherapy compared with radiotherapy alone in patients with cancer of the esophagus. *N Engl J Med* 326:1593–1598.

25. Smith TJ, Ryan LM, Douglass HO Jr (1998) Combined chemoradiotherapy vs. radiotherapy alone for early stage squamous cell carcinoma of the esophagus: A study of the Eastern Cooperative Oncology Group. *Int J Radiat Oncol Biol Phys* 42:269–276.

CHAPTER 20

Cancer of the Stomach

KEIICHI MARUYAMA

Department of Surgical Oncology, National Cancer Center Hospital, Tokyo, Japan

YASUHIRO KODERA and AKIMASA NAKAO

Department of Surgery II, Nagoya University, Graduate School of Medicine, Nagoya, Japan

Despite the decreasing incidence in the Western countries, gastric carcinoma remains the most common malignancy of the gastrointestinal tract worldwide. Early diagnosis and radical curative surgery have been the main factors contributing to higher cure rates in the East, where the disease remains overwhelmingly common. On the other hand, enthusiasm for aggressive management of this disease has waned in the West because of the relative rarity of the disease, along with the fact that a large percentage of patients present with advanced and incurable disease. Consequently, several differences in diagnostic principles and treatment strategies exist between the West and the East. This, along with possible differences in pathology and biologic behavior of the disease, leads to unique difficulties when designing a manual that is internationally applicable. Recent research suggests that a number of molecular biologic differences exist among patients with gastric cancer. Further investigation in this area may, in the future, be a clue to adequate prediction of outcome and selection of therapeutic alternatives.

EPIDEMIOLOGY AND ETIOLOGY

In the United States, it was estimated that 21,500 new cases of gastric cancer would be diagnosed in the year 2000 and that 13,000 patients would die from the disease. Despite significant rates of death, age-adjusted gastric cancer death rates have decreased dramatically since 1930, from approximately 28 in 100,000 to 2.0 in 100,000 in females and 38 to 4.4 in 100,000 in males (Fig. 20.1). The causes of the decline in the U.S. rates are incompletely understood, but environmental factors,

UICC Manual of Clinical Oncology, Eighth Edition. Edited by Raphael E. Pollock
ISBN 0-471-22289-5 Copyright © 2004 John Wiley & Sons, Inc.

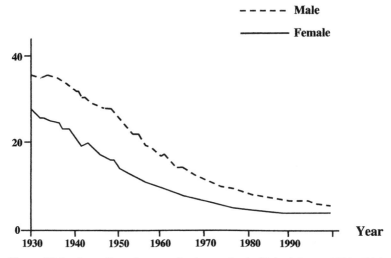

Figure 20.1   Age-adjusted cancer death rates in the United States, 1930–1996.

chiefly dietary, are suspected. Asian countries such as Japan, Korea, and China continue to have a high rate of death due to gastric carcinoma. In Latin America, Chile and Costa Rica have high incidences. The peak age incidence is the sixth decade, and about twice as many males suffer from gastric cancer as females.

Factors that have been associated with a higher incidence of gastric cancer include smoked or salted food, low intake of fruits and vegetables, and low socioeconomic status. Epidemiologic studies have consistently demonstrated an association between *Helicobacter pylori* infection and the risk of gastric cancer, but the role of this bacterium in the etiology of gastric cancer remains unknown. Precursor factors include pernicious anemia, achlorhydria, atrophic gastritis, gastric ulcers, and adenomatous polyps. Prior partial gastrectomy using Billroth II anastomosis for benign gastric or duodenal ulcer disease increases the risk of cancer in the gastric remnant, with latency periods of 15 to 20 years.

Molecular analysis of gastric tumor samples has been an active area of investigation. Multiple genetic alterations are involved in gastric carcinogenesis. Tahara proposed his hypothesis that there are two distinctive major genetic pathways for gastric carcinogenesis (Fig. 20.2). K-*ras* mutation, APC inactivation, loss of DCC, and amplification of *c-erb*B2 are preferentially found in well-differentiated gastric carcinomas, whereas gene mutations, loss of the cadherin-catenin system, and amplification of K-*sam* are frequently observed in poorly differentiated cancers. Early genetic changes, such as microsatellite instability, not only serve as good biological markers for screening precancerous lesions that have malignant potential but also for the possible development of secondary cancer. Alterations preferentially occurring at the point of malignant transformation, such as reactivation of telomerase and *p*53 inactivation, may provide a powerful tool for the evaluation of malignancy. The late changes, including amplification of *cyclin* E gene, *c-erb*B2 amplification, and 7qLOH, are good indicators for biological

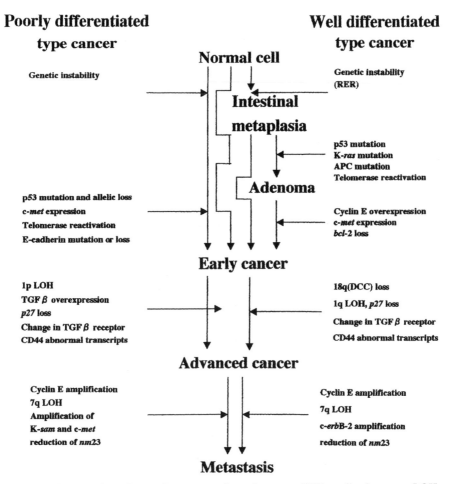

Figure 20.2   Genetic pathway of two types of gastric cancer. RER, replication error; LOH, loss of heterozygosity; TGF, transforminig growth factor. (From Molecular bases of human stomach carcinogenesis. In *Molecular Pathology of Gastroenterological Cancer*, Tahara E (ed.) Springer-Verlag, Tokyo, 1997, with permission.)

malignancy. The major remaining work on this field is identification of the specific gene(s) responsible for stomach carcinogenesis.

SCREENING

Early detection improves the prognosis of gastric cancer because surgery has high cure rates with lesions limited to the mucosa and submucosa—the lesions that have been defined by the Japanese Society for Gastric Cancer Study as early gastric

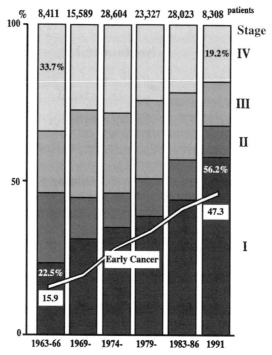

Figure 20.3 Increase of early stage cancer after introduction of mass-screening in Japan. Nationwide registry of gastric cancer, from 1963 to 1991.

carcinoma. However, the incidence of such early gastric cancers is less than 5% in the West. In Japan, where the incidence of early gastric carcinomas was only 3.8% in the period from 1955 to 1956, a mass screening system for early detection was established in the 1960s and has proved effective. By 1989, the incidence of early lesions had increased to 45% because of vigorous screening procedure primarily employing barium contrast x-ray studies, and the World Health Organization evaluated the Japanese system to be effective. Figure 20.3 shows a remarkable increase of early gastric carcinoma in Japan. However, benefits should outweigh risks and costs in order that a mass screening for cancer may be justified. Although the mass screening was found useful in Japan, defined high-risk populations do not exist in the United States and other Western countries to justify the expense of widespread screening. Individual physicians should use upper GI series and endoscopy to screen patients who have occupational or precursor risk factors or patients with persistent dyspepsia or gastroesophageal symptoms.

LOCATION AND PATHOLOGY

In the face of the overall decline in stomach cancer, a number of investigators in the West have reported rising incidence rates for cancer of the cardia, almost always in

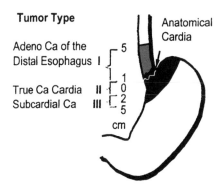

Figure 20.4 Classification of adenocarcinoma of the esophagogastric junction based on location of the tumor center or tumor mass. (From JR Siewert, HJ Stein (1996) Carcinoma of the cardia. In *Diseases of the Esophagus* Vol 9, Fig. 1 (pg 174), reproduced with permission from Blackwell Science Asia (www.blackwell science.com).)

conjunction with increases in oesophageal adenocarcinoma. There had been lack of a consensus definition of the cardia area, until classification by Siewert and Stein (Fig. 20.4) was approved at the consensus conference during the second International Gastric Cancer Congress in 1997. This classification defines carcinoma of the gastroesophageal junction as adenocarcinoma that has its center within 5 cm oral and aboral of the anatomic gastroesophageal junction. Carcinoma of the gastro-esophageal junction is classified further into three types according to the anatomical location, and true cancer of the cardia (type II of the three types) has its center located within 1 cm oral and 2 cm aboral of the junction. The histological classification and metastasis pattern suggest so far that cancer of the cardia should be treated as gastric carcinoma. Some postulate, however, that cancer of the cardia and esophageal adenocarcinoma (type I of the Siewert classification) are the same disease and propose to establish a new entity, which may emerge in future editions of the *Manual of Clinical Oncology*. This striking prevalence in proximal cancer has not been observed in Asia, where carcinoma in the gastric corpus, antrum, and pyloric regions are still commonly observed.

Macroscopic appearance of gastric carcinoma is classified according to the proposal of Borrmann in 1926 as type I (polypoid), type II (ulcerating), type III (ulceroinfiltrating), and type IV (diffuse linitis plastica). Types I and II that are resected have a considerably better prognosis than types III and IV. In addition, subtle lesions of early gastric carcinoma that by definition invades only as far as the submucosa have been defined as type 0 in recent years.

The UICC TNM Classification of Malignant Tumors provides histopathologic grading whereby gastric carcinomas are classified into well differentiated, moderately differentiated, poorly differentiated, and undifferentiated types. Well and moderately differentiated cancers typically present as solid ulcerating tumor and have inclination toward hepatic metastasis, whereas poorly differentiated cancer is often found as diffusely infiltrating lesion and is often accompanied with peritoneal

TABLE 20.1. Details of T, N, and M Categories for Gastric Carcinoma Defined in the TNM Classification

T—Primary tumor

TX	Primary tumor cannot be assessed
T0	No evidence of primary tumor
Tis	Carcinoma *in situ*: intraepithelial tumor without invasion of the lamina propria
T1	Tumor invades lamina propria or submucosa
T2a	Tumor invades muscularis propria
T2b	Tumor invades muscularis subserosa
T3	Tumor penetrates serosa (visceral peritoneum) without invasion of adjacent structures
T4	Tumor invades adjacent structures

Notes:

1. A tumor may penetrate muscularis propria with extension into the gastrocolic or gastrohepatic ligaments or the greater and lesser omentum without perforation of the visceral peritoneum covering these structures. In this case, the tumor is classified as T2. If there is perforation of the visceral peritoneum covering the gastric ligaments or omenta, the tumor is classified as T3.

2. The adjacent structures of the stomach are the spleen, transverse colon, liver, diaphragm, pancreas, abdominal wall, adrenal gland, kidney, small intestine, and retroperitoneum.

3. Intramural extension to the duodenum or esophagus is classified by the depth of greatest invasion in any of these sites, including stomach.

N—Regional lymph nodes

NX	Regional lymph nodes cannot be assessed
N0	No regional lymph node metastasis
N1	Metastasis in 1–6 regional lymph nodes
N2	Metastasis in 7–15 regional lymph nodes
N3	Metastasis in >15 regional lymph nodes

Notes:

1. The regional lymph nodes are the perigastric nodes along the lesser and greater curvatures and the nodes along the left gastric, common hepatic, hepatoduodenal, splenic, and coeliac arteries.

2. Involvement of other intra-abdominal lymph nodes such as retropancreatic, mesenteric, and para-aortic is classified as distant metastasis.

3. For pN classification, ≥ 15 nodes should be dissected from the regional lymph node stations and should be histologically examined.

M—Distant metastasis

MX	Distant metastasis cannot be assessed.
M0	No distant metastasis
M1	Distant metastasis

From Sobin LH, Wittekind Ch (eds.) (2002) *UICC TNM Classification of Malignant Tumours*, 6th edition.

dissemination at advanced stages. Gastric carcinoma is heterogeneous by nature, however, and a single lesion often comprises various histological types and, unfortunately, spreads through several metastatic pathways.

STAGING

The UICC/AJCC (American Joint Committee on Cancer) TNM Classification, revised in 2002, is the internationally accepted system for documentation and staging of gastric carcinoma among all other malignancies. This classification consists of grading systems for the three most important prognostic factors for gastric carcinoma; depth of invasion (T categories), extent of lymph node metastasis (N categories), and presence or absence of distant metastasis (M categories). Details of these grading systems are summarized in Table 20.1. Stage grouping is performed by combining the T, N, and M categories as summarized in Table 20.2. The three categories are evaluated on the basis of physical examination, imaging, endoscopy, and/or surgical exploration. A prefix "p" is attached when each category is confirmed histopathologically, and absence of node metastasis after microscopic examination of at least 15 lymph nodes, for example, is termed pN0. It has been reported already that the current TNM stage classification functions excellently in stratifying the patients according to the survival.

There are some concerns regarding the new system for classification of N categories, which is decided upon the number of metastatic lymph nodes regardless of their anatomical location. Although a recognized prognostic factor, incorporating the number of metastatic nodes as a key component in the stage classification has its

TABLE 20.2. Stage Grouping According to the TNM Classification

Stage 0	Tis	N0	M0
Stage IA	T1	N0	M0
Stage IB	T1	N1	M0
	T2a/b	N0	M0
Stage II	T1	N2	M0
	T2a/b	N1	M0
	T3	N0	M0
Stage IIIA	T2a/b	N2	M0
	T3	N1	M0
	T4	N0	M0
Stage IIIB	T3	N2	M0
Stage IV	T4	N1, N2, N3	M0
	T1, T2, T3	N3	M0
	Any T	Any N	M1

From Sobin LH, Wittekind Ch (eds.) (2002) *UICC TNM Classification of Malignant Tumours*, 6th edition.

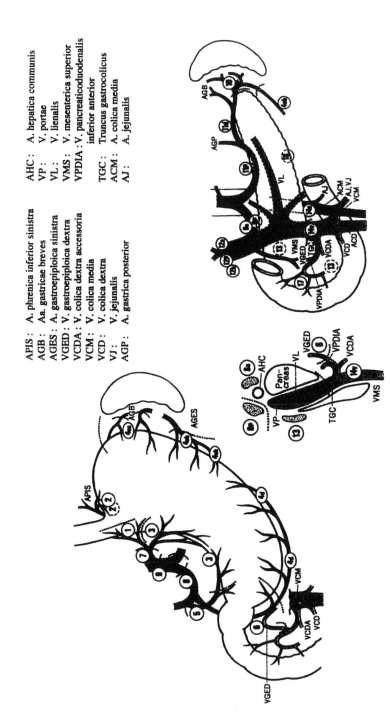

Figure 20.5 Lymph node station numbers defined in the Japanese Classification for Gastric Carcinoma. (From Japanese Classification for Gastric Carcinoma, 2nd Edition, *Gastric Cancer* Vol 1, Fig. 16 (pg 16), 1998, reproduced with permission from International and Japanese Gastric Cancer Association.)

APIS : A. phrenica inferior sinistra
AGB : Aa. gastricae breves
AGES : A. gastroepiploica sinistra
VGED : V. gastroepiploica dextra
VCDA : V. colica dextra accessoria
VCM : V. colica media
VCD : V. colica dextra
VJ : V. jejunalis
AGP : A. gastrica posterior

AHC : A. hepatica communis
VP : V. portae
VL : V. lienalis
VMS : V. mesenterica superior
VPDIA : V. pancreaticoduodenalis inferior anterior
TGC : Truncus gastrocolicus
ACM : A. colica media
AJ : A. jejunalis

own weaknesses. In the prior system of N categories based on the anatomical extent of node metastases, N staging had been possible with a few biopsies of the enlarged nodes. This will no longer be practical, given that at least 15 nodes will have to be examined and the number of metastatic nodes counted. For a similar reason, a significant proportion of resected specimens might still be classified as pNX due to the insufficient lymph node retrieval (with less than 15 nodes examined).

In the Japanese Classification for Gastric Carcinoma (JCGC), pN categories are still decided based on the anatomical extent of node metastasis. JCGC has categorized all regional lymph nodes into various topographic regions or stations identified by numbers (Fig. 20.5, Table 20.3). These lymph node stations are stratified into three compartments that correspond to location relative to the primary tumor and reflect also the likelihood of harboring of metastases. In brief, the perigastric nodes belong to compartment 1, whereas the nodes at the base of the left gastric artery, along the common hepatic and splenic arteries, and along the coeliac axis are defined as compartment 2 and the paraaortic nodes as compartment 3. The presence or absence of metastasis to each compartment is then reflected to the N categories. For instance, metastasis to any of the compartment 1 lymph nodes in the absence of metastases to more distant compartments would be staged as N1. This

TABLE 20.3. Nomenclature of the Regional Lymph Nodes According to the Japanese Classification for Gastric Carcinoma

Perigastric lymph nodes (LN)	
1	Right paracardial LN
2	Left paracardial LN
3	LN along the lesser curvature
4sa	LN along the short gastric vessels
4sb	LN along the left gastroepiploic vessels
4d	LN along the right gastroepiploic vessels
5	Suprapyloric LN
6	Infrapyloric LN
Retroperitoneal LN	
7	LN along the left gastric artery
8	LN along the common hepatic artery
9	LN around the coeliac artery
10	LN at the splenic hilum
11	LN along the splenic artery
12	LN in the hepatoduodenal ligament
13	LN on the posterior surface of the pancreas head
14a	LN along the superior mesenteric artery
14v	LN along the superior mesenteric vein
15	LN along the middle colic vessels
Paraaortic LN	
16	paraaortic LN

means that biopsy of a single paraaortic node could confirm the diagnosis of pN3, and could under certain circumstances facilitate the staging process.

Finally, it should be noted that the JCGC nomenclature of the regional lymph node stations by numbers as shown in Figure 20.5 continues to play an important role in numerous specialized centers outside of Japan, when documenting the findings at surgery or imaging studies.

DIAGNOSIS

Endoscopy performed on the symptomatic patients dominates the method of gastric cancer diagnosis in the West. In Japan where upper gastrointestinal series with barium contrast studies are performed as a mass screening procedure, gastric carcinoma is often diagnosed or suspected primarily with x-rays and the diagnosis confirmed with the endoscopic biopsies. Primary detection using the endoscopy, however, is becoming increasingly popular, and various new techniques have been introduced. Dye-spray method with Indigo-carmine has been employed to detect flat mucosal cancer, electronic endoscopy enabled several personnels to monitor the endoscopic procedure simultaneously, and stereoscopic endoscopy is used to magnify the fine mucosal changes. Besides detection or confirmation of the primary lesion, endoscopists should be aware that synchronous multiple cancer may exist at the rate of up to 10% and scrutinize the whole stomach. In addition, double-contrast x-rays may become a useful guide to surgery, especially when there is a possibility that a total gastrectomy might be avoided. It is worth noting that the x-rays indicate the location of the tumor (the distance between the esophagogastric junction and proximal tumor border, for instance) much more clearly than the endoscopic images.

Further imaging studies and diagnostic modalities are used for preoperative staging, which is mandatory for selecting rational treatment options that may range from surgical resection to best supportive care. Computerized tomography with contrast medium is useful for detection of hepatic and gross lymph node metastases. Endoscopic ultrasound in the experienced hands is useful for the evaluation both of T and N categories of the TNM classification. It is important to note, however, that not all node metastases can be detected by these imaging studies. Laparoscopy is the only method to sensitively detect the peritoneal deposits for accurate staging, and cytology examination of the peritoneal washes also provides useful prognostic information.

SURGICAL TREATMENT FOR RESECTABLE GASTRIC CARCINOMA

The primary curative treatment of gastric carcinoma is surgical resection. All patients with tumors that are considered potentially resectable should undergo surgery, provided that no distant metastasis has been found. Surgery requires complete removal of the tumor, preferrably with proximal and distal margins from gross tumor of 5 cm. The most widely practiced operations for gastric cancer have been distal gastrectomy for distal tumors (antral/pyloric lesions), high subtotal resection for smaller mid-gastric lesions, proximal gastrectomy for smaller tumors of the cardia, and total gastrectomies for the multicentric, larger mid-gastric, or proximal tumors. These operations include resection of the lesser and greater omenta and removal of the perigastric nodes along the lesser and greater curvatures for the extent of the gastric resection (D1 resection). Resection of perigastric nodes may lead to cure of a certain proportion of gastric carcinoma patients with metastases to these nodes. Co-resection of adjacent structures such as pancreas, transverse colon, and spleen are recommended in the event of contiguous involvement.

Although presence of distant metastasis or peritoneal dissemination precludes hopes for cure, gastric carcinoma with lymph node metastases limited to the regional nodes could be cured through meticulous co-resection of the metastatic lymph nodes. In this context, D1 resection as described previously has been commonly practiced throughout the Western Hemisphere. In theory, however, prophylactic removal of a wider range of lymphatic drainage may further increase the chance for cure. For this reason, resection of the retroperitoneal lymph nodes such as those along the common hepatic, splenic, and coeliac arteries *en bloc* with the perigastric lymph nodes, termed *D2 resection*, has been advocated and practiced by Japanese surgeons. Because regional lymph node metastasis is a critical prognostic factor, there is no doubt that D2 resection followed by microscopic examination of the resected lymph nodes contributes to accurate staging. In addition, Japanese surgeons for a number of years have actually reported superior results in terms of long-term survival with this type of surgical resection. Exemplary data from the National Cancer Center in Tokyo, for instance, has shown that five-year survival of the patients with metastasis to these retroperitoneal nodes ranges from 20 to 40%. Attempts to reproduce these in Western countries have been unrewarding, however, and no convincing survival advantage of D2 resection over the removal only of the perigastric nodes (D1 resection) has been demonstrated in two multi-institutional randomized trials independently performed in the Netherlands and Great Britain. This may be due in part to the extremely high surgical mortality observed in these studies. Mortality and morbidity were frequently associated with pancreatico-splenectomy, most of which had been performed not because of direct cancer invasion to these organs (T4 status), but as an integral part of systemic lymphadenectomy as defined by the Japanese Classification of Gastric Carcinoma. A feasibility study of pancreas-preserving D2 resection by Italian experts among others proved that D2 resection without resection of the pancreas and spleen can be performed without excessive mortality in specialized European centres. At the same time, a subset analysis of the British trial suggests that D2 surgery without pancreatico-splenectomy may carry better survival rates than D1 resection. Thus, debate regarding the value of extended lymphadenectomy continues. At this point, it should be emphasized that improved skills and better postoperative care are needed to accomplish D2 resection without excessive morbidity or mortality. This highlights the importance of adequate training in the procedure and justifies the restriction of this surgery to specialized centers.

Prediction of metastasis to each lymph node station has been made possible through use of a computer program, which contains data from over 3,000 treated patients at the National Cancer Center in Tokyo. Data contained in the program include gender, age, Borrmann classification, histology, depth of wall penetration, location, and diameter of the tumor together with details of node metastases to each station for each patient. This program enables surgeons to compile a group of patients with prognostic variables exactly matching those of an individual patient and calculate the metastatic rate to each lymph node station. The search result should be of value in making preoperative decisions concerning the extent of lymphadenectomies. Feasibility of this program has been tested in the Netherlands and Germany with success. In order that such database be of universal value, however, it is essential for investigators in each country to agree on a uniform system of data management based on uniform staging policies.

Treatment of T1 stage gastric carcinoma deserves special attention. For several years, Japanese surgeons have performed D2 resection as a routine procedure even with the patients with T1 stage disease. This led to precise staging for this subset and resulted in accumulation of extensive histopathologic data regarding the incidence and extent of lymph node metastasis. It is well documented that perigastric lymph nodes may contain cancer even in the patients with T1 tumor. However, agreement has been reached throughout Japan that mucosal cancer of the differentiated type with less than 2 cm diameter and without ulcer formation carry no node metastasis, and patients belonging to this small subgroup can be treated with endoscopic mucosal resection. The pretreatment diagnosis of the depth of cancer invasion can be made with reasonable accuracy using endoscopic ultra-sonography. Depth of invasion and absence of cancer at the resection margin must be confirmed histopathologically following the endoscopic resection, and those with massive submucosal invasion or cancer at the resection margin can be treated with salvage surgery. Whether the remaining majority of T1 disease should still be treated with gastrectomy plus systemic prophylactic lymphadenectomy is a matter of controversy, and the role of sentinel lymph node mapping in selecting candidates for more limited surgery (wedge resection) is currently under investigation.

MULTIMODALITY TREATMENT

The survival benefit of adjuvant postoperative chemotherapy, the traditional approach following potentially curative surgery for gastric carcinoma, has long been elusive. A well-known meta-analysis published in 1993 of past randomized trials comparing 5-FU-based postoperative chemotherapy versus surgery alone following curative resection suggests activity but without statistical significance. Recently, however, a significant survival advantage of this strategy over surgery alone was reported from two multi-institutional randomized trials conducted independently in Spain and Italy. The protocol for the Spanish study was a combination of intravenous mitomycin C (20 mg/m^2 on day 1) and oral tegafur

(400 mg per day, starting on day 30 and continued for 3 months) given to curatively resected stage III cancer. The strategy of the latter group was a combination of intravenous epirubicin (75 mg/m^2 on day 1) and 5-FU plus leucovorin (5-FU 450 mg/m^2 and leucovorin 200 mg/m^2 days 1–3, repeated every 3 weeks for 7 months) to curatively resected node-positive cancer. It seems now that the body of evidence is changing gradually, and adjuvant chemotherapy may, in the near future, be advocated for a selected group of patients with high risk of microscopic residual disease. The optimal regimen for use in this strategy has not been defined, although both of the successful studies investigated 5-FU–based regimens. Further studies assessing the value of this approach alone and in combination with neoadjuvant chemotherapy and/or radiation, and exploring also the role of newer generation cytotoxic drugs (such as docetaxel and irinotecan), are warranted in patients who undergo adequate surgery.

Data from modern postoperative adjuvant trials suggest a median survival of approximately 2 years for gastric carcinoma patients undergoing curative resection in the West. The poor prognosis by treatment either with surgery alone or with surgery plus postoperative adjuvant chemotherapy has prompted investigation of novel therapeutic strategies, of which current emphasis is on neoadjuvant chemotherapy owing to the favorable results seen in other tumors and for several oncologic principles. The application of this strategy, which had primarily been directed toward locally advanced unresectable tumors, has now been expanded to treat patients with potentially resectable disease. Experience with other tumor types suggests that drug combinations that are capable of achieving a significant rate ($>10\%$) of pathologic complete response are needed before significant improvements in long-term survival can be observed. There is now encouraging evidence from numerous phase II gastric cancer trials to provide confidence that efficacious drug combinations do exist, that toxicities are manageable, that the morbidity and mortality of surgery are not increased, and that survival appears to be enhanced. Random assignment phase III trial with drug combinations such as ECF (epirubicin, cisplatin, and 5-FU) and cisplatin plus 5-FU/leucovorin are now ongoing, and the results are awaited as critical next steps in evaluating the efficacy of this strategy.

Few studies have evaluated postoperative or neoadjuvant radiation without chemotherapy. Of these, a randomized trial from China revealed a significant survival benefit of preoperative external-beam radiation of 40 Gy over the control arm of surgery alone for the patients with adenocarcinoma of the cardia. The current trend in the radiation therapy for gastric carcinoma is toward the concurrent use of cytotoxic agents to enhance the effect of radiation. Recently, a treatment consisting of adjuvant postoperative radiation (45 Gy) with concurrent 5-FU/leucovorin, preceded and followed by further courses of intravenous 5-FU/leucovorin, was shown to improve both disease-free and overall survival in stages IB through IV gastric carcinoma patients who underwent potentially curative resection (Intergroup 0116 study, United States). Investigators claim that a new standard of care for patients with resectable gastric cancer has now been established through this study, but this conclusion has been subject to some criticism. Most patients who

were entered onto this trial had received gastrectomy without extended lymphadenectomy (54% of the patients underwent D0, 36% D1, and 10% D2 resection),
although D2 resection had been advocated in the study protocol. Chemoradiation
under such circumstances may have simply compensated for the suboptimal surgery
to achieve local control. D2 resection currently is not a standard practice in most
countries and institutions, however, and postoperative adjuvant chemoradiation may
indeed have a potential as a standard therapy following curative resection in these
institutions. It was made clear through this study along with others that radiotherapy is effective in decreasing the incidence of locoregional recurrence, while
the likelihood of developing distant metastasis cannot be reduced.

TREATMENT FOR UNRESECTABLE AND METASTATIC DISEASE

The prognosis of the patients who are not considered candidates for curative
surgery remains extremely poor. For gastric carcinoma with distant metastasis,
therefore, palliative resection is generally reserved for patients with continued
bleeding or obstruction. Current imaging studies, however, are notoriously useless
in detecting tiny peritoneal deposits that are not uncommonly observed in T3 ~ 4
cancer. More recently, laparoscopy has been recognized as a modality to carefully
identify candidates for potentially curative surgery, thus avoiding unnecessary
laparotomy for the remainders. Biopsy of the suspected tumor deposits and
cytology examination of the peritoneal washes can be performed under the
laparoscopy, along with meticulous observation of the peritoneal lining.

Treatment options for the patients who are not candidates for curative resection
remain a matter of controversy. Chemotherapy and radiation can be effective in
palliating the symptoms associated with gastric cancer, but have rather limited
value in improving survival. Past randomized trials comparing chemotherapy with
best supportive care have shown significant survival advantage of the chemotherapy
arm. In these studies, however, aggressive chemotherapy regimens such as FAMTX
(5-FU, doxorubicin, and high-dose methotrexate) were selected as a treatment arm,
indicating that the results of the trials apply only to the patients with good
performance status. Although various active drug combinations for advanced
gastric carcinoma now exist, optimal systemic therapy remains elusive. Generally
speaking, a regimen must overcome the established threshold of approximately
9 months for overall survival time and should probably confer close to 12 months in
a well-designed study to be considered a new standard of care for patients with
advanced gastric carcinoma. Commonly used regimens in the past trials had been
FAMTX, ECF, and a combination of protracted 5-FU and cisplatin. Again, numerous regimens that include new-generation cytotoxic drugs such as irinotecan,
docetaxel, and paclitaxel are under investigation. Combinations such as irinotecan
plus cisplatin, docetaxel plus cisplatin with or without 5-FU, and paclitaxel,
cisplatin plus 5-FU/leucovorin have recently shown promise with response rates
of over 50% and the median survival time extending beyond 10 months. These drug
combinations are toxic, however, and should only be given to the patients with good

performance status (ECOG performance score <2), preferably under the setting of clinial trials.

Moderate-dose external-beam radiation (35–50 Gy) as a single modality has minimal value in palliating unresectable gastric carcinoma and does not improve survival. When used concurrently with cytotoxic agents such as 5-FU and paclitaxel, however, it may provide palliation of various symptoms and local control in patients with locally advanced and metastatic gastric carcinoma.

FOLLOW-UP

Gastric cancer advances along several routes: lymphatic, hematogenous, by direct extension, and through peritoneal seeding. Unfortunately, it tends to disseminate simultaneously by several routes, creating a mixed pattern of treatment failure in a significant proportion of cases. This precludes the value of surgical resection in the vast majority of the recurrent disease, and the prognosis for this condition remains extremely poor. A rigorous follow-up program with intent to detect the recurrences early would therefore be rather unlikely to actually affect long-term survival. The majority of recurrences of gastric carcinoma occur within the first 2 years of curative resection, with the risk declining substantially thereafter, and this may be reflected in the postoperative follow-up program. An exemplary follow-up program has been published as a part of the National Comprehensive Cancer Network practice guidelines version 1.0. This is similar to the program at Aichi Cancer Centre, Japan, which consists of a complete history and physical examination every 3 months for the first 2 years and every 6 months for years 3 ~ 5, blood count, panels of biochemistry and tumor markers (CEA, CA19-9), chest x-rays every 6 months for 5 years, and computerized tomography every 6 ~ 12 months for 5 years. Because metachronous multiple cancer is not uncommon, annual endoscopic survey in search of remnant cancer may be recommended for those treated by distal or proximal gastrectomies, and is considered mandatory for the patients who were treated with endoscopic mucosal resection.

FURTHER READING

Boku N, Ohtsu A, Shimada Y, Shirao K, Seki S, Saito H, Sakata Y, Hyodo I (1999) Phase II study of a combination of irinotecan and cisplatin against metastatic gastric cancer. *J Clin Oncol* 17:319–323.

Bollschweiler E, Boettcher K, Hoelscher AH, Sasako M, Kinoshita T, Maruyama K, Siewert JR (1992) Preoperative assessment of lymph node metastases in patients with gastric cancer: Evaluation of the Maruyama computer program. *Br J Surg* 79:156–160.

Bonenkamp JJ, Hermans J, Sasako M, Van de Velde CJH for the Dutch Gastric Cancer Group (1999) Extended lymph-node dissection for gastric cancer. *N Engl J Med* 340: 908–914.

Cirera L, Balil A, Batiste-Alentorn E, Tusquets I, Cardona T, Arcusa A, Jolis L, Saigi E, Guasch I, Badia A et al. (1999) Randomized clinical trial of adjuvant mitomycin plus tegafur in patients with resected Stage III gastric cancer. *J Clin Oncol* 17:3810–3815.

Cushieri A, Weeden S, Fielding J, Bancewicz J, Craven J, Joypaul V, Sydes M, Fayer P for the Surgical Co-operative Group (1999) Patient survival after D1 and D2 resections for gastric cancer: long-term results of the MRC randomized surgical trial. *Br J Cancer* 79:1522–1530.

Degiuli M, Sasako M, Ponti A, Soldati T, Danese F, Calva F (1998) Morbidity and mortality after D2 gastrectomy for gastric cancer: results of the Italian Gastric Cancer Group prospective multicenter surgical study. *J Clin Oncol* 16:1490–1493.

Esophageal/Gastric Cancers Practice Guidelines Panel Members (1998) NCCN Practice Guidelines for Upper Gastrointestinal Carcinomas. *Oncology (Huntingt)* 12:179–223.

Greenlee RT, Murray T, Bolden S, Wingo PA (2000) Cancer statistics, 2000. *CA Cancer J Clin* 50:7–33.

Hermans J, Bonenkamp JJ, Boon MC, Bunt AMG, Ohyama S, Sasako M, Van de Velde CJH (1993) Adjuvant therapy after curative resection for gastric cancer: meta-analysis of randomized trials. *J Clin Oncol* 11:1441–1447.

Hisamichi S, Sugawara N, Fukao A (1988) Effectiveness of gastric mass screening in Japan. *Cancer Detect Prev* 11:323–329.

Japanese Gastric Cancer Association (1998) Japanese Classification for Gastric Carcinoma, 2nd English Edition. *Gastric Cancer* 1:10–24.

Karpeh MS, Leon L, Klimstra D, Brennan M (2000) Lymph node staging in gastric cancer: Is location more important than number? *Ann Surg* 232:362–371.

Kodera Y, Yamamura Y, Torii A, Uesaka K, Hirai T, Yasui K, Morimoto T, Kato T, Kito T (1995) Incidence, diagnosis, and significance of multiple gastric cancer. *Br J Surg* 82:1540–1543.

Macdonald JS, Smalley SR, Benedetti J, Hundahl SA, Estes NC, Stemmermann GN, Haller DG, Ajani JA, Gunderson LL, Jessup JM et al. (2001) Chemoradiotherapy after surgery compared with surgery alone for adenocarcinoma of the stomach or gastroesophageal junction. *N Engl J Med* 345:725–730.

Maruyama K, Gunven P, Okabayashi K, Sasako M, Kinoshita T (1989) Lymph node metastases of gastric cancer. General pattern in 1931 patients. *Ann Surg* 210:596–602.

Neri B, Cini G, Andreoli F, Boffi B, Francesconi D, Mazzanti R, Medi F, Mercatelli A, Romano S, Siliani L et al. (2001) Randomized trial of adjuvant chemotherapy versus control after curative resection for gastric cancer: 5-year follow-up. *Br J Cancer* 84:878–880.

Ono H, Kondo H, Gotoda T, Shirao K, Yamaguchi H, Saito D, Hosokawa K, Shimoda T, Yoshida S (2001) Endoscopic mucosal resection for treatment of early gastric cancer. *Gut* 48:225–229.

Sasako M, McCulloch P, Kinoshita T, Maruyama K (1995) New method to evaluate the therapeutic value of lymph node dissection for gastric cancer. *Br J Surg* 82:346–351, 1995.

Siewert JR, Stein HJ (1998) Classification of adenocarcinoma of the oesophagogastric junction. *Br J Surg* 85:1457–1459.

Smith JW, Brennan MF, Botet JF, Gerdes H, Lightdale CJ (1993) Preoperative endoscopic ultrasound can predict the risk of recurrence after operation for gastric carcinoma. *J Clin Oncol* 11:2380–2385.

Tahara E (1997) Molecular Pathology of Gastroenterological Cancer. Tokyo: Springer-Verlag.

Waters JS, Norman A, Cunningham D, Scarffe JH, Webb A, Harper P, Joffe JK, Mackean M, Mansi J, Leahy M et al. (1999) Long-term survival after epirubicin, cisplatin and fluorouracil for gastric cancer: Results of a randomized trial. *Br J Cancer* 80:269–272.

World Health Organization (1986) The use of quantitative methods in planning national cancer control programs. A WHO Meeting. *Bull World Health Organ* 64:683–693.

Zhang Z-X, Gu X-Z, Yin W-B, Huang G-J, Zhang D-W, Zhang R-G (1998) Randomized clinical trial on the combination of preoperative irradiation and surgery in the treatment of adenocarcinoma of gastric cardia (AGC): Report on 370 patients. *Int J Radiat Oncol Biol Phys* 42:929–934.

CHAPTER 21

Cancer of the Pancreas

DOUGLAS B. EVANS, ROBERT A. WOLFF, CHRISTOPHER H. CRANE, and PETER W. T. PISTERS

The University of Texas, M. D. Anderson Cancer Center, Houston, Texas

Cancer of the exocrine pancreas continues to be a major unsolved health problem, affecting over 185,000 people throughout the world each year. Pancreatic cancer is the fourth leading cause of cancer-related death for both men and women (following lung, colon, and breast cancers) and is responsible for 5% of all cancer-related deaths. In 2003, adenocarcinoma of the exocrine pancreas will account for approximately 30,000 deaths in the United States. Exocrine pancreatic cancer is characterized by early vascular and lymphatic dissemination to the liver, peritoneum, lungs, and regional lymph nodes. In fact, subclinical liver metastases are present in the majority of patients at the time of diagnosis, even when findings from imaging studies are normal. Because of difficulties in diagnosis, the aggressiveness of pancreatic cancers, and the lack of effective systemic therapies, only 1–4% of patients with adenocarcinoma of the pancreas will be alive five years after diagnosis. These humbling statistics have created a new wave of enthusiasm for basic research, more accurate diagnosis and staging, and improved clinical trial development in the fight against pancreatic cancer. All clinicians dealing with pancreatic adenocarcinoma should encourage patient participation in protoccol-based therapy when posssible.

ETIOLOGIC FACTORS

A number of important environmental risk factors have been investigated for their role in the etiology of pancreatic cancer. Cigarette smoking is the most firmly established risk factor associated with pancreatic cancer. Pancreatic malignancies can be induced in animals through long-term administration of tobacco-specific

UICC Manual of Clinical Oncology, Eighth Edition. Edited by Raphael E. Pollock
ISBN 0-471-22289-5 Copyright © 2004 John Wiley & Sons, Inc.

N-nitrosamines or by parenteral administration of other *N*-nitroso compounds. These carcinogens are metabolized to electrophiles that readily react with DNA, leading to miscoding and activation of specific oncogenes such as K-*ras*. Numerous case-control and cohort studies have reported an increased risk of pancreatic cancer for smokers in both the United States and Europe, and current estimates suggest that approximately 30% of pancreatic cancer cases are due to cigarette smoking. Recent studies that have explored the dose-response relationship have shown that the risk of pancreatic cancer increases as the amount and duration of smoking increases and that long-term smoking cessation (>10 years) reduces risk by approximately 30% relative to the risk of current smokers. Application of molecular epidemiologic techniques that are being developed for lung cancer may provide greater specificity in linking tobacco exposure with the development of pancreatic cancer and may facilitate the study of chemopreventive strategies.

Over the past 10 years, numerous dietary factors have been implicated in pancreatic cancer development. Generally, high intakes of fat or meat increase risk, and diets high in fruits and vegetables reduce risk. These clinical observations are supported by laboratory studies in animal models in which high-fat and high-cholesterol diets have been shown to promote pancreatic carcinogenesis. Decreased rates for pancreatic cancer have been associated with high consumption of vegetables, citrus fruits, fiber, and vitamin C. The association of diets high in citrus with a reduced risk of pancreatic cancer is particularly interesting given the recent observation that limonene, a natural product found in citrus fruits, is a potent inhibitor of the K-*ras* oncoprotein.

An association between pancreatitis and an increased risk of pancreatic cancer has long been suspected, although the magnitude of the risk remains uncertain. Clinical studies have suggested that chronic forms of pancreatitis, particularly those accompanied by pancreatic calcifications, were most closely associated with the subsequent development of pancreatic cancer. Calculation of a general estimate of population-attributable risk has suggested that chronic pancreatitis may explain as many as 5% of pancreatic cancer cases. However, the hereditary form of pancreatitis is associated with a much higher risk of pancreatic cancer; lifetime risk in affected individuals is 40% by age 70, or 50–60 times higher than expected. Hereditary pancreatitis has an autosomal dominant pattern of transmission with 80% penetrance. The onset of symptoms is usually by age 40 years but can occur before age 5 years. Recent pathologic and molecular biologic studies strongly suggest that mutations in the cationic trypsinogen gene play an important role in hereditary and possibly acquired forms of pancreatitis, thereby increasing the risk of pancreatic cancer. To prevent autodigestion, pancreatic enzymes are secreted as inactive proenzymes. Within the intestinal lumen, trypsinogen is hydrolyzed to (active) trypsin; trypsin then activates the remaining pancreatic enzymes. Multiple defense mechanisms are in place to prevent premature enzyme activation, including the presence of a cationic trypsin cleavage site within the trypsinogen molecule. If trypsin is activated within the pancreatic acinar cell, this feedback mechanism should inactivate wild-type trypsinogen. In hereditary pancreatitis, a single amino acid substitution inactivates the cationic trypsin cleavage site, causing uncontrolled trypsin activation and pancreatic autodigestion.

In addition to hereditary pancreatitis, an increased incidence of pancreatic cancer has been reported in various genetic syndromes. Up to 10% of patients with familial pancreatic cancer (two first-degree relatives affected) may have a germline mutation in the *BRCA2* gene. *BRCA2* is a tumor suppressor gene involved in the repair of DNA strand breaks. Germline mutations in *p16* are associated with the familial atypical multiple-mole melanoma (FAMMM) syndrome and individuals with this mutation may have a risk of pancreatic cancer up to 20 times higher than the general population. Hereditary nonpolyposis colon cancer (HNPCC) is caused by mutations in DNA mismatch repair genes including *hMSH2*, *hMLH1*, *hPMS1*, and *hMSH6*. It has been reported that families with HNPCC have an increased incidence of pancreatic cancer in addition to their known risk for colorectal and endometrial cancer. Peutz-Jeghers Syndrome may also be associated with an increased risk for pancreatic cancer. Peutz-Jeghers Syndrome is caused by mutations in the *LKB1/STK11* tumor suppressor gene on chromosome 19p13 and is characterized by hamartomatous polyps in the gastrointestinal tract and pigmented macules of the lips and digits. Finally, case reports and epidemiologic studies have suggested the possibility of familial aggregations of pancreatic cancer outside the context of these rare familial syndromes. One case-control study estimated that 3% of pancreatic cancers had a hereditary origin. A recent study of 150 families with presumed familial pancreatic cancer has suggested that relatives of patients with familial pancreatic cancer have a significantly increased risk of developing pancreatic cancer. Continued study of these patients and their families may provide insight into the critical molecular genetic abnormalities leading to familial pancreatic cancer. Such information is necessary to develop effective strategies for early detection and chemoprevention.

MOLECULAR PATHOGENESIS

Studies using archival human pancreatic tumor tissue and human pancreatic cancer cell lines have identified an increasing number of characteristic genetic abnormalities. These studies have revealed specific point mutations at condon 12 of the K-*ras* gene in 75–90% of pancreatic adenocarcinoma specimens. The K-*ras* gene on chromosome 12 is the most frequently activated oncogene in pancreatic cancers. Mutations alter the ability of the intrinsic GTPase to hydrolyze GTP to GDP, resulting in the Ras protein remaining in the constitutively active GTP-bound form. Ras proteins are essential to the transduction of growth-promoting signals from cell surface tyrosine kinase receptors to intracellular pathways involved in cellular differentiation and proliferation. Therefore, constitutive activation of these proteins results in uncontrolled cell growth.

Additional genetic alterations have been described in human pancreatic cancer, appropriately termed Deleted in Pancreatic Cancer (DPC). These candidate tumor suppressor genes include *DPC1/2* on chromosome 13q (the region of the *BRCA2* gene), *DPC3* (*p16/MTS-1*) on chromosome 9p, and *DPC4* on chromosome 18q. The p16 protein belongs to a class of cyclin-dependent kinase (CDK)-inhibitory proteins (including *p21/WAF1/Cip1*). The p16 protein inhibits CDK4 and CDK6, which normally act to phosphorylate the Rb1 protein. Phosphorylation of Rb1 results in the transcription of genes that promote cell cycle progression (G_1/S transition). Inactivation of *p16* therefore leads to unregulated cell growth. Inactivation of *p16* occurs in 95% of human pancreatic xenografts. *DPC4* (Smad4) is a tumor suppressor gene whose protein product functions as a transcription factor in the transforming growth factor-β (TGF-β) receptor-mediated signal transduction pathway. The TGF-β signaling pathway has been shown to be involved in the down-regulation of epithelial cell growth and in the promotion of differentiation of certain cell types. TGF-β is believed to exert its effects on cellular proliferation and differentiation through the induction of CDK inhibitors, specifically *p21/WAF1/CIP1* and *p15INK4*, which is thought to be mediated through *Smad4*. Based on the frequency with which mutations in K-*ras*, *p53*, *p16*, and *DPC-4* are found, a model of pancreatic carcinogenesis has been suggested whereby the malignant clone evolves from cells driven by a dominant oncogene (K-*ras*) with subsequent deregulation of cell growth precipitated by abnormal cell-cycle control resulting from mutations in p53, p16, and/or DPC-4.

CLINICAL SIGNS AND SYMPTOMS

The lack of obvious clinical signs and symptoms delays the diagnosis of pancreatic cancer in most patients. Jaundice, due to extrahepatic biliary obstruction, is present in approximately 50% of patients at diagnosis and is often associated with a less advanced stage of disease than are other signs or symptoms. Small tumors of the pancreatic head may obstruct the intrapancreatic portion of the bile duct and cause the patient to seek medical attention when the tumor is nonmetastatic and potentially resectable. In the absence of extrahepatic biliary obstruction, few patients present with localized, potentially resectable disease. The pain typical of locally advanced pancreatic cancer is a dull, fairly constant pain of visceral origin localized to the region of the middle and upper back. The pain is due to tumor invasion of the celiac and mesenteric plexus. Vague, intermittent epigastric pain occurs in some patients; its etiology is less clear. Fatigue, weight loss, and anorexia are common even in the absence of mechanical gastric outlet obstruction. Pancreatic exocrine insufficiency due to obstruction of the pancreatic duct may result in malabsorption and steatorrhea. Although malabsorption and mild changes in stool frequency are common, diarrhea occurs infrequently. Glucose intolerance is present in the majority of patients with pancreatic cancer. Although the exact mechanism of hyperglycemia remains unclear, both altered islet cell function and impaired tissue insulin sensitivity are present.

NATURAL HISTORY AND PATTERNS OF TUMOR PROGRESSION

Pancreatic cancer spreads early to regional lymph nodes, and subclinical liver metastases are present in the majority of patients at the time of diagnosis, even when findings from imaging studies are normal. Patient survival depends on the extent of disease and performance status at diagnosis. Extent of disease is best categorized as resectable, locally advanced, or metastatic. Patients who undergo surgical resection for localized nonmetastatic adenocarcinoma of the pancreatic head have a long-term survival rate of approximately 15–20% and a median survival of 15–24 months. However, disease recurrence following a potentially curative pancreaticoduodenectomy remains common. Local recurrence occurs in up to 85% of patients who undergo surgery alone owing to inaccurate preoperative staging, poor operative technique, and failure to deliver all components of multi-modality therapy. With improved local-regional disease control, liver metastases become the dominant form of tumor recurrence and occur in 50–70% of patients following potentially curative combined-modality treatment.

Patients with locally advanced, nonmetastatic disease have a median survival of 6–10 months. A survival advantage has been demonstrated for patients with locally advanced disease treated with 5-fluorouracil (5-FU)-based chemoradiation compared with no treatment or radiation therapy alone. Patients with metastatic disease have a short survival (3–6 months), the length of which depends on the extent of disease and performance status.

STAGING

The system published in the sixth edition of the International Union Against Cancer (UICC) and the American Joint Committee on Cancer (AJCC) TNM classifications appears in Table 21.1. Because a minority of patients with pancreatic cancer undergo surgical resection of the pancreas (and adjacent lymph nodes), a single TNM classification was developed to apply to both clinical and pathologic staging. The T classification was modified from the fifth edition to reflect a more clinically relevant system based upon both preoperative CT assessment of resectability and final pathologic evaluation of the resected specimen. Pancreatic tumors are judged unresectable (T4) when they cannot be separated (on high-quality CT images) from the adjacent large arterial structures (celiac axis or superior mesenteric artery). It would be unusual for an exocrine pancreatic cancer to exhibit local tumor extension to the retroperitoneum or adjacent organs, which would preclude surgical resection, in the absence of arterial involvement. Tumor involvement of the superior mesenteric or portal veins is classified as T3 in the new T classification; such tumors are considered resectable in some centers and there are few data on the prognostic value of venous invasion. The difference between T3 and T4 reflects the distinction between potentially resectable (T3) and locally advanced (T4) primary pancreatic tumors, both of which demonstrate radiographic or pathologic evidence of extrapancreatic tumor extension.

In the fifth edition of the UICC/AJCC classification, patients with unresectable T3 primary tumors were considered to have stage II disease (the lymph node status was unknown because no surgical resection was performed); in contrast, a patient

TABLE 21.1. UICC/AJCC TNM Staging System

Primary tumor (T)

TX	Primary tumor cannot be assessed
T0	No evidence of primary tumor
Tis	Carcinoma *in situ*
T1	Tumor limited to pancreas, ≤2 cm in greatest dimension[*]
T2	Tumor limited to pancreas, >2 cm in greatest dimension[*]
T3	Tumor extends beyond pancreas, but without involvement of celiac axis or superior mesenteric artery
T4	Tumor involves celiac axis or superior mesenteric artery

Regional lymph nodes (N)

NX	Regional lymph nodes cannot be assessed
N0	No regional lymph node metastasis
N1	Regional lymph node metastasis

Distant metastasis (M)

MX	Distant metastasis cannot be assessed
M0	No distant metastasis
M1	Distant metastasis

Stage grouping

Stage 0	Tis	N0	M0
Stage IA	T1	N0	M0
Stage IB	T2	N0	M0
Stage IIA	T3	N0	M0
Stage IIB	T1,T2,T3	N1	M0
Stage III	T4	Any N	M0
Stage IV	Any T	Any N	M1

[*]Measured by CT (largest transverse diameter) or by pathologic analysis of the resected specimen
From Sobin LH, Wittekind Ch (eds.) (2002) *UICC TNM Classification of Malignant Tumours*, 6th Edition.

with a 1-cm primary tumor and one positive regional lymph node who had undergone pancreaticoduodenectomy would be classified as having stage III disease. In general, patients with completely resected (R0 or R1) N1 pancreatic cancer have a superior survival duration compared with patients with locally advanced (unresectable) or metastatic disease. Therefore, in the sixth edition of the UICC/AJCC classification, stage III is reserved for patients with unresectable, locally advanced pancreatic cancer.

Similar standardized criteria are needed for the pathologic analysis of pancreaticoduodenectomy specimens to allow accurate interpretation of survival statistics. At The University of Texas M. D. Anderson Cancer Center (MDACC), the surgeon and pathologist evaluate each specimen first by frozen-section examination of the common bile duct transection margin and the pancreatic transection margin. A positive bile duct or pancreatic transection margin is treated with reresection. The retroperitoneal margin is defined as the soft-tissue margin directly adjacent to the proximal 3 to 4 cm of the superior mesenteric artery (SMA) (Fig 21.1), and is

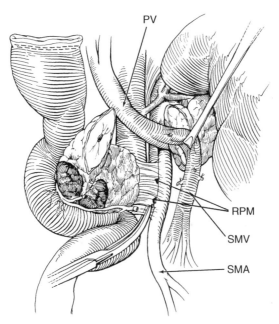

Figure 21.1 Illustration of the retroperitoneal margin as defined at the time of tumor resection. Medial retraction of the superior mesenteric vein (SMV) and superior mesenteric portal vein confluence facilitates dissection of the soft tissues adjacent to the lateral wall of the proximal superior mesenteric artery (SMA); this site represents the retroperitoneal margin (RPM). A grossly positive retroperitoneal margin should not occur if high-quality preoperative CT imaging is performed. A microscopically positive retroperitoneal margin occurs in 10–20% of cases. PV, portal vein.

evaluated by permanent-section examination of the margin (Fig. 21.2). The retroperitoneal margin must be inked at the time of gross evaluation of the specimen; identification of this margin of resection is not possible once the gross examination of the specimen has been completed. The retroperitoneal margin is the most frequent site of margin positivity following pancreaticoduodenectomy, and accurate analysis of this margin is critical when performing outcome studies using survival duration or local tumor control as primary study endpoints. Samples of multiple areas of each tumor, including the interface between tumor and adjacent uninvolved tissue, are submitted for paraffin-embedded histologic examination (5–10 blocks). Final pathologic evaluation of permanent sections includes a description of tumor histology and differentiation; gross and microscopic evaluation of the tissue of origin (pancreas, bile duct, ampulla of Vater, or duodenum); and assessments of maximal transverse tumor diameter, lymph node status, and the presence or absence of perineural, lymphatic, and vascular invasion.

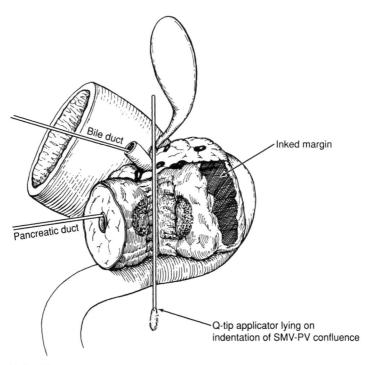

Figure 21.2 Illustration of a pancreaticoduodenectomy specimen; the retroperitoneal margin (tissue adjacent to the superior mesenteric artery) is inked for evaluation of margin status on permanent section histologic evaluation. The illustration shows a small probe placed in the bile duct and in the pancreatic duct. A Q-tip applicator stick lies over the indentation from the superior mesenteric-portal vein confluence. Complete permanent-section analysis of the pancreaticoduodenectomy specimen requires that it be oriented to enable the pathologist to accurately assess the retroperitoneal margin of excision and other standard pathologic variables.

THE IMPORTANCE OF PRETREATMENT DIAGNOSTIC STUDIES

If the primary tumor cannot be resected completely, surgery (pancreaticoduodenectomy) for pancreatic cancer offers no survival advantage. Therein lies the rationale for accurate preoperative radiographic imaging. Using conventional CT, less than 50% of patients who undergo operation for planned pancreaticoduodenectomy have their tumors successfully removed; the remaining patients are found to have unsuspected liver or peritoneal metastases or local tumor extension to the mesenteric vessels. Patients found to have unresectable disease at laparotomy receive no survival benefit from surgery; yet, the laparotomy results in a perioperative morbidity rate of 20–30%, a mean hospital stay of 14–20 days, and a median survival after surgery of only 6 months. Further, in patients whose tumors are resected with grossly positive margins, the survival duration is less than one year and no different from the survival duration achieved with palliative chemotherapy and irradiation in patients who have locally advanced, unresectable disease. Therefore, in contrast to the case for selected patients with colorectal or gastric cancer, there are no data in support of palliative (positive-margin) resection for adenocarcinoma of the pancreas.

Our recommended diagnostic schema, based on contrast-enhanced CT appears in Figure 21.3. A patient is deemed to have locally advanced, unresectable disease when there is clear evidence on CT scans of tumor extension to the SMA or celiac axis or occlusion of the superior mesenteric-portal vein (SMPV) confluence. The accuracy of CT in predicting unresectability is well established; current technology has eliminated the use of laparotomy to assess local tumor resectability. If a low-density mass is not seen on CT scans, patients undergo diagnostic endoscopic ultrasound (EUS) and, if necessary, therapeutic endoscopic retrograde cholangio-pancreatography (ERCP). A malignant obstruction of the intrapancreatic portion of the common bile dut is characterized by the double-duct sign (proximal obstruction of the common bile and pancreatic ducts), which can often be accurately differentiated from choledocholithiasis and the long, smooth tapering stricture seen with chronic pancreatitis. To prevent cholangitis in patients who undergo diagnostic cholangiography in the setting of extrahepatic biliary obstruction, endoscopic stents are routinely placed.

Accurate preoperative assessment of resectability will increase resectability rates and minimize positive-margin resections. A common misconception in pancreatic tumor surgery is that resectability is determined best at laparotomy. In fact, however, resectability is most accurately determined preoperatively by imaging studies, not at the time of "exploratory" laparotomy. Surgeons declare a tumor to be unresectable at the time of laparotomy when unsuspected liver metastases, peritoneal implants, or, most commonly, locally advanced disease is found. The term *locally advanced* is often poorly defined, leaving the patient, the medical oncologist, and the radiation oncologist without a clear understanding of why the primary tumor was not resected. Improved rates of resectability are achieved when high-quality, contrast-enhanced CT is combined with objective preoperative criteria for resectability. CT criteria for resectability include (1) the absence of extra-pancreatic disease, (2) a patent SMPV confluence, and (3) no direct tumor extension to the celiac axis or SMA. Patients whose tumors are deemed unresectable by these radiographic criteria are not considered candidates for potentially curative resection.

In patients with locally advanced or metastatic disease, operation for palliation is rarely needed. Multiple studies have attempted to compare operative biliary decompression and endoscopic stent placement in patients with jaundice due to obstruction of the intrapancreatic portion of the common bile duct. The higher initial morbidity and mortality rates and longer hospital stay associated with operative biliary bypass are countered by the higher frequency of hospital re-admission for recurrent stent occlusion and cholangitis with endoscopic stent placement. Patients with liver metastases or ascites have a median survival of

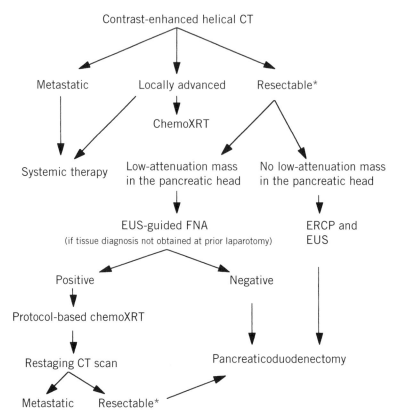

Figure 21.3   Management algorithm used at The University of Texas M.D. Anderson Cancer Center for patients with suspected or biopsy-proven (from previous laparotomy prior to referral) adenocarcinoma of the pancreatic head. Accurate radiographic imaging allows patients to be staged as having resectable, locally advanced, or metastatic disease. For patients with locally advanced or metastatic disease, biopsy confirmation of malignancy is mandatory before the initiation of specific anticancer therapy. Similarly, before initiation of neoadjuvant chemoradiation, cytologic confirmation of malignancy is required. The development of endoscopic ultrasonography (EUS)–guided fine-needle aspiration (FNA) has greatly simplified tissue acquisition for patients with localized, nonmetastatic pancreatic cancer. In patients without cytologic evidence of malignancy (negative biopsy) in whom clinical and radiographic evidence support the diagnosis of a pancreatic or periampullary cancer, we proceed directly to pancreaticoduodenectomy (followed by postoperative adjuvant therapy if indicated). CT, computed tomography; ERCP, endoscopic retrograde cholangiopancreato-graphy

less than 6 months, making endoscopic stent placement an obvious choice. Patients with locally advanced disease treated with chemoradiation have a median survival of 10–12 months, with 20% surviving 2 years. Patients with a superior performance status at diagnosis often survive longer, yet it is difficult in most patients to predict, at diagnosis, the tempo of disease progression. Clearly, one would like to avoid operation (with its morbidity and often lengthy recovery period) in patients with rapidly progressive disease. Similarly, one would like to have a durable means of biliary decompression in patients who are expected to survive longer than 6–9 months. Therefore, in patients with locally advanced, nonmetastatic disease, it is reasonable to proceed with endoscopic stent placement and reserve operative (open or laparoscopic) biliary bypass for patients who survive long enough to experience recurrent stent occlusion. Innovations in stent construction and the development of the expandable 10-mm metal stent have improved patency rates and are the cause for more widespread application of this technology.

Pancreatic Biopsy

In patients thought to have potentially resectable pancreatic or periampullary cancer, most experienced pancreatic surgeons believe that preoperative or intra-operative pancreatic biopsy is unnecessary. However, most pancreatic resections are not performed in regional referral centers or tertiary cancer centers. Indeed, a recent review of 24,926 patients undergoing pancreaticoduodenectomy in the United states revealed that 58% of patients underwent pancreaticoduodenectomy at rural or urban nonteaching hospitals where the operative mortality rate ranged from 10.6% (urban nonteaching) to 19.0% (rural). Because the majority of patients undergo pancrea-ticoduodenectomy with this risk for mortality, many physicians (including some surgeons) are not willing to proceed with pancreaticoduodenectomy in the absence of a tissue diagnosis of malignancy. Despite improvements in radiographic imaging, such diagnostic uncertainty often results in therapeutic indecision. Therapeutic indecision often leads to exploratory surgery at which time surgeons frequently attempt intraoperative biopsy (leading to unnecessary complications) or incorrectly judge a primary pancreatic tumor to be resectable or unresectable. The advent of EUS-FNA (combined with high-quality CT and endobiliary stent placement) allows the diagnostic phase to be separated from the treatment phase. Patients with suspected pancreatic or periampullary cancer can be accurately staged with contemporary CT imaging, biliary obstruction can be relieved with endobiliary decompression, and the diagnosis established endoscopically with EUS-FNA. Patients can then be counseled as to available treatment options and the established short- and long-term benefits of referral to a regional center with expertise in pancreatic surgery.

Pancreaticoduodenectomy

Current surgical treatment is based on the procedure of pancreaticoduodenectomy as described in 1935 by Whipple et al. In 1946, Waugh and Clagett from the Mayo clinic described their modification of the one-stage procedure to its current form. The goals of surgical therapy outlined by Waugh and Clagett have not changed in the past 50 years: (1) there should be reasonable opportunity for cure, (2) the risk of death should not outweigh the prospects for cure, and, (3) the patient should be left in as normal a condition as possible.

The 30-day in-hospital mortality rate is less than 2% for pancreaticoduodenectomy when performed at major referral centers by experienced surgeons. Recently reported mortality rates from other institutions, including university centers and the Department of Veterans Affairs hospitals, range from 7.8% to more than 10%. Data from Maryland, New York, and Ontario, Canada, have demonstrated that higher patient volume is associated with lower surgery-related mortality. The most compelling data on the relationship of hospital volume to perioperative mortality and long-term survival after pancreaticoduodenectomy come from Dartmouth Medical School. Birkmeyer and colleagues studied 7,229 Medicare patients older than 65 years who underwent pancreaticoduodenectomy at 1,772 hospitals from 1992 to 1995. The study population was divided into quartiles according to hospital volume; high-volume centers were defined as those that performed five pancreaticoduodenectomies per year. Forty high-volume hospitals (2%) performed 1,541 (21%) of the pancreaticoduodenectomies. The in-hospital mortality rate was 11% overall, 4% in high-volume hospitals, and 10–16% in medium-volume (two to five pancreaticoduodenectomies per year) and very-low-volume (zero or one pancreaticoduodenectomy/year) hospitals. These data suggest a linear relationship between surgical volume and outcome. Birkmeyer and colleagues suggested that the referral of pancreatic cancer patients to high-volume hospitals could potentially prevent more than 100 deaths per year.

Pancreaticoduodenectomy is performed using a six-step technique that emphasizes complete removal of all tissue to the right of the SMA and celiac axis. The technique advocated by the authors has been published (see selected references) and emphasizes complete mobilization of the superior mesenteric vein (SMV) and visual identification of the SMA. Exposure of the SMA avoids iatrogenic injury and ensures direct ligation of the inferior pancreaticoduodenal artery. The soft tissue adjacent to the proximal 3 to 4 cm of the SMA represents the retroperitoneal margin. Margin positivity can result from tumor spread along perineural sheaths and does not always result from direct extension of the primary tumor.

Segmental resection of the SMV or portal vein is performed when the tumor is inseparable from the lateral wall of the vein (Fig. 21.4). Recent data have confirmed that appropriately selected patients who require venous resection at the time of pancreaticoduodenectomy have a survival duration no different from that of patients who undergo pancreaticoduodenectomy without venous resection. Critical to a favorable outcome is the selection of patients (for pancreaticoduodenectomy) who do not have tumor extension to the SMA or celiac axis. Venous involvement in the absence of retroperitoneal tumor extension is a function of tumor location rather than an indicator of aggressive tumor biology. Because the need for venous resection is unexpected in many patients and is discovered only after gastric and pancreatic transection, when nonresectional procedures are no longer an option, surgeons who perform pancreaticoduodenectomies should be familiar with standard vascular techniques for resection and reconstruction of the SMV and/or portal vein.

After pancreaticoduodenectomy, pancreatic, biliary, and gastrointestinal reconstruction is performed (Fig. 21.5). The transected jejunum is brought through a small incision in the transverse mesocolon to the left of the middle colic vessels and

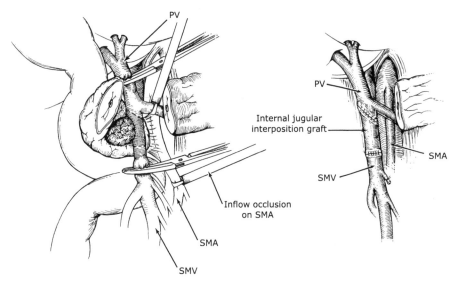

Figure 21.4 Illustration of segmental resection of the superior mesenteric vein (SMV) with preservation of the splenic vein confluence. The intact splenic vein tethers the portal vein (PV), making a primary anastomosis impossible in most cases. Our preferred method of reconstruction of the SMV is to use an internal jugular vein interposition graft. Segmental resection of the SMV with splenic vein preservation adds significant complexity to this operation. SMA, superior mesenteric artery.

a two-layer, end-to-side, duct-to-mucosa pancreaticojejunostomy is performed. A two-layer anastomosis that invaginates the cut end of the pancreas into the jejunum is occasionally performed when the pancreatic duct is too small for a primary duct-to-mucosa anastomosis. A single-layer biliary anastomosis is then completed, followed by an anticolic, end-to-side gastrojejunostomy constructed in two layers. A feeding jejunostomy tube is placed (in most patients) using the Witzel technique, and one or two closed-suction drains are placed in the majority of patients. Delayed gastric emptying is common after standard pancreaticoduodenectomy and may be more frequent with pylorus preservation. The cause is multifactorial but largely due to deinnervation of the upper gastrointestinal tract during resection of the pancreatic head and attached soft tissues and nerves to the right of the SMA. Symptoms of nausea, vomiting, and postprandial fullness resolve in two to four weeks in virtually all patients. The placement of a jejunostomy tube at the time of surgery allows patients to be discharged while receiving enteral feeding. In addition, such tube placement prevents the expense and potential complications associated with intravenous hyperalimentation in patients who require prolonged hospitalization because of perioperative or postoperative complications.

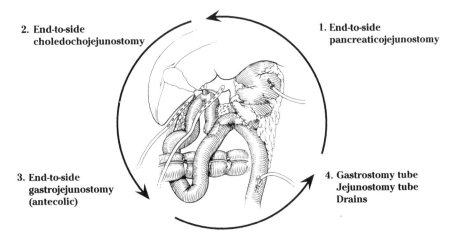

2. End-to-side
   choledochojejunostomy

1. End-to-side
   pancreaticojejunostomy

3. End-to-side
   gastrojejunostomy
   (antecolic)

4. Gastrostomy tube
   Jejunostomy tube
   Drains

Figure 21.5   Illustration demonstrating the pancreatic, biliary, and gastrointestinal reconstruction performed after pancreaticoduodenectomy. A two-layer, end-to-side, duct-to-mucosa pancreaticojejunostomy is followed by a single-layer hepaticojejunostomy and then a two-layer (anticolic, loop) gastrojejunostomy. When pylorus preservation is performed, a single-layer duodenojejunostomy completes the recostruction. A feeding jejunostomy tube is commonly placed to assist in postoperative management.

ADJUVANT THERAPY

Postoperative (Adjuvant) Chemoradiation

The largest single-institution experience with postoperative adjuvant chemoradiation has been reported by Sohn and colleagues from Johns Hopkins University. Of 498 evaluable patients who underwent pancreatectomy for adenocarcinoma of the pancreas, 366 (74%) received adjuvant chemoradiation and 132 (26%) declined adjuvant therapy for "various reasons." The successful delivery of adjuvant therapy was associated with a statistically significant improvement in survival duration (19 vs. 11 months; $p < 0.0001$). The very low mortality and morbidity for pancreatic surgery at Johns Hopkins University would suggest that 26% represents the minimum percentage of patients who will not receive adjuvant therapy if a postoperative strategy is used by other less experienced centers. It is noteworthy that in all previously reported and currently ongoing postoperative adjuvant trials (with the exception of the Hopkins data), patient enrollment occurs following recovery from surgery; the number of patients not referred for trial entry (due to delayed recovery from surgery) is not known.

Prospective data is available from both the Gastointestinal Tumor Study Group (GITSG) and the European Organization for Research and Treatment of Cancer (EORTC). The GITSG randomized study of adjuvant chemoradiation (5-FU 500 mg/m^2 for 6 days, and radiation 40 Gy) following pancreaticoduodenectomy demonstrated a survival advantage from multimodality therapy compared with resection alone.

However, 24% of the patients in the adjuvant chemoradiation arm could not begin chemoradiation until more than 10 weeks after pancreaticoduodenectomy because of a prolonged recovery time. Similar findings were recently reported by the EORTC. Between 1987 and 1995, 218 patients who had undergone pancreatico-duodenectomy for adenocarcinoma of either the pancreas or the periampullary region were randomized to receive either chemoradiation (40 Gy in a split course and 5-FU given as a continuous infusion at a dose of 25 mg/kg per day during EBRT) or no further treatment. Eleven patients were deemed ineligible for analysis due to incomplete resection in the setting of extensive local disease. As in the GITSG trial, patients in the EORTC trial were considered for enrollment after recovery from pancreaticoduodenectomy. Despite this selection bias, 21 (20%) of 104 evaluable patients assigned to receive chemoradiation did not receive the intended therapy because of patient refusal, medical comorbidities, or rapid tumor progression. Of the 207 eligible patients, 114 (55%) had pancreatic cancer; the median survival was 17.1 months for those who received adjuvant therapy and 12.6 months for those who received surgery alone ($p = .099$). Although these differences were not significant, the wide confidence interval (CI) for the subset of patients with pancreatic cancer (relative risk, 0.7; 95% CI, 0.5–1.1) preserves the possibility that the chemoradiation arm had a clinically meaningful improvement in survival that was obscured by the small sample size.

The recently reported results of the European Study Group of Pancreatic Cancer (ESPAC)-1 study suggest that chemotheray, not EBRT is the important component of adjuvant therapy following pancreatectomy for adenocarcinoma. The ESPAC-1 trial is a four-arm study with a 2×2 factorial design that compared the effects of adjuvant chemoradiation (5-FU and 40 Gy in a split course), adjuvant chemother-apy (5-FU and folinic acid), chemoradiation followed by chemotherapy, and observation alone following pancreaticoduodenectomy for pancreatic or periam-pullary carcinomas. Accrual for this study began in 1994, and medical centers in 11 countries have randomized 541 patients. Most patients were entered into the randomized 2×2 factorial design.

However, either because of lack of access to EBRT or because of specific ins-titutional bias, 188 patients were randomized to receive only chemotherapy or no chemotherapy, and 68 patients were randomized to receive either chemoradiation or no chemoradiation. In the latter two nonfactorial groups, patients could receive nonstandardized therapy at the discretion of their treating physicians. For example, patients who were randomized in the nonfactorial design to chemotherapy or no chemotherapy could receive EBRT. Importantly, nonrandomized treatments were not standardized. The preliminary analysis of the ESPAC-1 trial concluded that (1) adjuvant chemoradiation provides no survival benefit; and (2) adjuvant systemic chemotherapy consisting of 5-FU and leucovorin (which is largely ineffective in patients with measurable metastatic disease) increased survival duration. However, in the subset of 285 patients randomized by the 2×2 factorial design there was no benefit to chemotherapy.

The most recent report of adjuvant therapy in pancreatic cancer has combined 45–54 Gy of external-beam irradiation with 5-FU, cisplatin, and interferon-α

(IFN-α). Nukui et al. reported data from a series of 33 patients who successfully underwent pancreaticoduodenectomy, and then were assigned in a nonrandomized fashion to receive either external-beam irradiation (45–54 Gy) and concomitant 5-FU, or IFN-α–based chemoradiation (45–54Gy, and concomitant continuous infusion 5-FU [200 mg/m^2/day], bolus cisplatin [30 mg/m^2/day], and Subcutaneous IFN-α[3 million μ, qod]). Although the sample size was small, the 17 patients who received the IFN-α regimen had a significantly greater actuarial two-year survival when compared with those receiving EBRT and 5-FU alone (84% vs. 54%, $p = 0.04$). The two-year survival in the "control" arm compares favorably with other recently published series of adjuvant 5-FU and EBRT, which have generally been in the range of 40%. The strategy of combination chemoradiation utilizing IFN-α provides yet another treatment schema which may prove beneficial in the adjuvant or neoadjuvant setting.

Preoperative (Neoadjuvant) Chemoradiation

Several considerations support the preoperative use of chemoradiation: (1) positive gross or microscopic margins of resection along the right lateral border of the SMA are common following pancreaticoduodenectomy, suggesting that surgery alone may be an inadequate strategy for local tumor control; (2) because chemoradiation is given before surgery, delayed postoperative recovery does not affect the delivery of multimodality therapy; and (3) patients with disseminated disease evident on restaging studies after chemoradiation are spared an unnecessary laparotomy.

A standard-fractionation treatment schema was used in the first studies of preoperative chemoradiation and pancreaticoduodenectomy at MDACC. Radiation therapy was delivered 5 days/week over 5.5 weeks using a four-field technique. Patients received a total dose of 50.4 Gy at 1.8 Gy/fraction (28 fractions) combined with 5-FU given Monday through Friday by continuous infusion at a dosage of 300 mg/m^2 per day. The liver was the most frequent site of tumor recurrence, and liver metastases were a component of treatment failure in 69% of all patients who had recurrences. Isolated local or peritoneal recurrences were documented in only 11% of patients. In contrast, previous reports of pancreaticoduodenectomy alone for adenocarcinoma of the pancreas documented local recurrence in 50–80% of patients. However, this 5.5-week standard-fractionation chemoradiation program was associated with gastrointestinal toxicity (nausea, vomiting, and dehydration) that required hospital admission of one-third of patients. Similarly, the multicenter Eastern Cooperative Oncology Group trial documented the need for hospital admission of 51% of patients during or within four weeks after completing preoperative chemoradiation.

These findings prompted a change in the delivery of preoperative chemoradiation in favor of rapid-fractionation or short-course EBRT. Investigators at MDACC recently completed a prospective trial of rapid-fractionation chemoradiation (30 Gy; 3 Gy/fraction [10 fractions] 5 days/week combined with 5-FU given by continuous infusion at a dosage of 300 mg/m^2 per day, 5 days/week) in patients with potentially resectable pancreatic cancer. This chemoradiation program was designed to avoid the gastrointestinal toxicity seen with standard-fractionation chemoradiation while attempting to maintain the excellent local tumor control achieved with multimodality therapy. Rates of local tumor control and patient survival times achieved were equal to the results obtained with standard-fractionation (5.5 week) chemoradiation: local-regional recurrence developed in only 10% of patients who underwent resection, and the median survival for patients who received preoperative chemoradiation and pancreaticoduodenectomy was 25 months. These very encouraging results are likely due to accurate patient staging and a standardized surgical technique (emphasizing margin-negative resection), in addition to the use of preoperative chemoradiation.

The survival duration of patients with even early stage pancreatic cancer will only improve with the addition of more effective systemic therapy designed to destroy the occult micrometastatic disease, which is present in the majority of patients at the time of pancreaticoduodenectomy. In addition, systemic agents capable of more effective radiation sensitization may result in a greater cytotoxic effect on the primary tumor. Gemcitabine ($2',2'$-difluorodeoxycytidine, Gemzar) is a deoxycytidine analogue capable of inhibiting DNA replication and repair, and is a potent radiation sensitizer of human pancreatic cancer cells. Because of encouraging results in patients with locally advanced disease, gemcitabine-based chemoradiation is being studied in patients with potentially resectable pancreatic cancer. Hoffman and colleagues have reported a phase I study of preoperative standard-fractionation EBRT (50.4 Gy) and escalating weekly doses of gemcitabine (300 mg/m^2, 400 mg/m^2, and 500 mg/m^2). Investigators at MDACC recently completed a phase II study of gemcitabine-based chemoradiation in patients with potentially resectable pancreatic cancer. Over 80 patients have been entered into this treatment program; the histologic responses to induction therapy (in the resected specimen) appear to be superior to those obtained with previous regimens, survival analysis awaits additional patient follow-up.

Despite surgeons' ability to perform pancreaticoduodenectomy safely, the procedure is too extensive and complex to enable the consistent postoperative delivery of standard-fractionation adjuvant chemoradiation. In the absence of data demonstrating superior survival results with either a preoperative or postoperative treatment approach, all available information suggests that a greater proportion of patients receive potentially beneficial adjuvant therapy, with a reduced overall treatment time, when chemoradiation is administered prior to surgery. Further, preoperative chemoradiation treatment strategies will spare many patients the morbidity and mortality associated with laparotomy, as up to one-fourth of patients will show evidence of metastatic disease at the time of preoperative restaging following chemoradiation and thus would not benefit from surgery.

TREATMENT OF LOCALLY ADVANCED DISEASE

Patients with clear evidence of encasement of the celiac axis or SMA on contrast-enhanced CT do not require laparotomy to confirm that the tumor is unresectable;

cytologic confirmation of malignancy can be achieved with fine-needle aspiration performed under the guidance of either EUS or CT. This fundamental advance in pretreatment diagnosis for patients with pancreatic cancer will improve the quality of patient survival and reduce health care costs by avoiding the morbidity and prolonged recovery associated with palliative pancreatic cancer surgery.

A pilot trial of 5-FU and supervoltage radiation therapy in patients with locally advanced adenocarcinoma of the pancreas served as the foundation for a subsequent study of 5-FU–based chemoradiation by the GITSG. The GITSG randomized patients with locally advanced pancreatic cancer to receive 40 Gy of EBRT plus 5-FU, 60 Gy plus 5-FU, or 60 Gy without chemotherapy. The median survival was 10 months in each of the chemoradiation groups and 6 months for patients who received 60 Gy without 5-FU. Additional chemotherapy beyond 5-FU–based chemoradiation increased toxicity without apparent therapeutic benefit. All patients had undergone laparotomy and therefore had been surgically staged; only patients with disease confined to the pancreas and peripancreatic organs, regional lymph nodes, and regional peritoneum were eligible for the study. Thus, although surgical staging resulted in a more uniform study population, it also introduced significant selection bias: only rapidly recovering patients were considered for treatment. Comparisons of these data with the results of future studies must take account of this selection bias.

Current 5-FU–based chemoradiation schemas use prolonged, low-dose, continuous-infusion 5-FU during EBRT. Continuous-infusion 5-FU in doses of 250–300 mg/m^2/day for 5 or 7 days/week is combined with EBRT to doses of 50–55 Gy in 5.5 weeks (1.8 Gy/fraction). Treatment is administered in the outpatient setting and 5-FU is given through a portable pump attached to a percutaneous central venous catheter. Acute side effects are largely gastrointestinal (nausea, diarrhea, weight loss, fatigue), leukopenia is rarely encountered. Acute toxicity during 5-FU chemoradiation appears to be decreased by administering 5-FU for 5 days/week rather than 7 days/week. The late effects of combined-modality therapy do not appear to be increased compared with those seen with EBRT alone. Despite continued refinements of 5-FU–based chemoradiation strategies, median survival for patients with locally advanced pancreatic cancer remains 10–12 months from the time of diagnosis. Further, the available literature suggests that it is unlikely that 5-FU–based chemoradiation schemas can make unresectable lesions resectable and thereby increase the number of patients who can be cured with multimodality therapy.

In an effort to improve on the results obtained with 5-FU-based chemoradiation, investigators have combined EBRT with other radiation-sensitizing agents given before, during, and after EBRT. Such data from small pilot studies provide the basis for ongoing phase I and II studies of gemcitabine in combination with EBRT in patients with locally advanced pancreatic cancer. Gemcitabine is being given in escalating doses weekly as a single agent with EBRT, in combination with 5-FU and EBRT, in combination with cisplatin and EBRT, at a fixed dose with escalating doses of EBRT, and as a twice-weekly infusion with either standard-fractionation EBRT or split-course EBRT. These studies suggest that the combination of multiple, more effective radiosensitizers with EBRT may result in significant local tumor response. However, as the definition of locally advanced pancreatic cancer is broadened, results will appear more promising. Thus, all studies of novel chemoradiation regimens should adhere to a strict CT-based definition of locally advanced pancreatic cancer that includes arterial involvement (low-density tumor inseparable from the SMA or celiac axis on contrast-enhanced CT) or venous (SMV or SMPV confluence) occlusion.

The increased length of survival for patients treated with chemoradiation is limited largely to patients with higher performance status. Therefore, a program of chemoradiation is justified in fully ambulatory patients with locally advanced disease who have minimal symptoms. Systemic therapy with gemcitabine alone or in combination also represents a reasonable alternative in these patients. For patients with poor performance status, chemoradiation is probably not indicated. Current pharmacologic and interventional techniques for pain control, including percutaneous injection of alcohol into the celiac plexus, have proven highly successful in patients with pancreatic cancer. Further, adequate pain control improves performance status and quality of life, which may translate into increased length of life. The limited therapeutic options available for patients with locally advanced disease and the modest impact of current treatments on survival rates provide the rationale for the entry of patients into trials examining novel systemic agents.

TREATMENT OF METASTATIC AND RECURRENT DISEASE

Most studies of single-agent or combination chemotherapy in patients with advanced adenocarcinoma of the pancreas have documented low response rates and little reproducible impact on patient survival or quality of life. Response rates as high as 15–30% occasionally seen in pilot studies of novel agents or combinations have not been reproduced, suggesting that patient selection often accounts for apparent differences between study results. The inherent difficulty in accurately applying bidimensional measurements to pancreatic masses and the problem of interobserver variations in the measurement of metastatic disease may contribute to the poor reproducibility of clinical trials in patients with locally advanced metastatic pancreatic cancer. Gemcitabine is a deoxycytidine analogue that is rapidly becoming the first-line therapy for patients with metastatic pancreatic cancer. Following phase I study, gemcitabine was evaluated in a multicenter trial of 44 patients with advanced pancreatic cancer. Only five objective responses (11%) were documented, but the investigators reported frequent subjective symptomatic benefits, often in the absence of objective responses. Based on these observations, two subsequent trials of gemcitabine for advanced pancreatic cancer were completed. In one randomized trial, gemcitabine was compared with 5-FU in previously untreated patients. Patients treated with gemcitabine achieved modest but statistically significant improvements in response rate and median survival compared with those treated with 5-FU (5.65 versus 4.41 months, $p = 0.0025$). The one-year survival rate for patients treated with gemcitabine was 18%, whereas the rate was only 2% for those treated with 5-FU. Importantly, more clinically meaningful effects on disease-related symptoms were recorded with gemcitabine than with 5-FU (23.8% vs 4.8%, $p = 0.0022$). These clinical benefits were also documented in patients treated with gemcitabine after experiencing disease progression while receiving 5-FU. These results suggest that gemcitabine will become the accepted first-line therapy for patients with advanced pancreatic adenocarcinoma.

Additional studies of gemcitabine as a treatment for pancreatic cancer have focused on its dose and schedule of administration, both alone and in combination with other cytotoxic agents. A phase I study of gemcitabine was conducted in patients with advanced solid tumors whereby dose escalation was achieved by increasing the duration of the weekly gemcitabine infusions while maintaining the dose rate at 10 mg/m^2/minute. A subsequent randomized phase II trial in patients with metastatic pancreatic cancer suggested that short infusional schedules of gemcitabine (10 mg/m^2/minute) may be more effective than the standard 30-minute bolus technique. Preliminary results from this trial demonstrated that, compared with 2,300 mg/m^2 over 30 minutes, 1,500 mg/m^2 delivered over 150 minutes (10 mg/m^2/minute) led to a higher objective response rate (16.2% versus 2.7%) and a longer median survival (6.1 versus 4.7 months). Gemcitabine has also been investigated in combination with other cytotoxic agents. Recent data have suggested superior activity with gemcitabine doublets (gemcitabine/5-FU, gemcitabine/cisplatin, gemcitabine/irinotecan) compared with single-agent gemcitabine. Phase III trials are currently being conducted to compare gemcitabine alone with these doublets. A recently completed ECOG trial comparing gemcitabine plus 5-FU with gemcitabine alone failed to demonstrate any statistically significant survival advantage to combination therapy.

Despite the recent encouraging results with gemcitabine, however, median survival for patients with metastatic disease continues to be less than six months, with very few patients achieving long-term disease stabilization. Some of the effects attributed to chemotherapy may not be substantially different from what can be achieved with aggressive supportive care alone. This grim reality provides strong support for the study of novel chemotherapeutic agents based on our improved understanding of the pathobiology of pancreatic cancer represent exciting areas of research. A number of general areas of clinical investigation may yield favorable results, including interruption or modulation of growth factors and signal transduction pathways, blockade of epidermal growth factor receptor, matrix metalloproteinase inhibitors, antiangiogenic agents, and receptor tyrosine kinase inhibition. As our understanding of the molecular and biochemical basis of pancreatic cancer expands, we will enter a new era in which treatments are tailored to interact with the specific molecular and biochemical targets thought to be important in the development or maintenance of neoplasia.

For some patients with metastatic pancreatic cancer who present with a good performance status, treatment with systemic chemotherapy is appropriate. In view of the limited impact of the currently available agents on survival, continued enrollment of patients in phase II trials of new agents or combinations is essential. In the absence of access to a phase II trial, treatment with gemcitabine appears to be the evolving standard. However, it must be recognized that the primary impact of gemcitabine is on quality of life; therefore, continued evaluation of novel agents, especially those targeted against specific molecular events important in the pathogenesis of pancreatic cancer, is crucial.

FURTHER READING

Birkmeyer JD, Siewers AE, Finlayson EVA et al. (2002) Hospital volume and surgical mortality in the United States. *N Engl J Med* 346:1128–1137.

Breslin TM, Hess KR, Harbison DB et al. (2001) Neoadjuvant chemoradiation for adenocarcinoma of the pancreas: Treatment variables and survival duration. *Ann Surg Oncol* 8:123–132.

Burris HA, Moore MJ, Andersen J et al. (1997) Improvements in survival and clinical benefit with gemcitabine as first-line therapy for patients with advanced pancreas cancer: A randomized trial. *J Clin Ocol* 15:2403–2413.

Crane CH, Janjan NA, Evans DB et al. (2001) Toxicity and efficacy of concurrent gemcitabine and radiotherapy for locally advanced pancreatic cancer. *Int J Pancreatology* 29:9–18.

Evans DB, Erickson RA. (2001) Diagnosis and assessment of resectability for neoplasms of the pancreas and periampullary region. In *Operative Techniques in General Surgery*. Evans DB (guest editor), vanHeerden JA, Farley DR (eds.) W.B. Saunders, Philadelphia, 3:5–16.

Evans DB, Wolff RA, Crane CH, Pisters PWT (2004) Combined modality treatment for pancreatic cancer. In *Progress in Oncology*. DeVita VT, Hellman S, Rosenberg SA (eds.) Jones and Bartlett, Boston, pp. 250–276.

Evans DB, Wolff RA (2000). Neoplasms of the ampulla of Vater. In *Cancer Medicine*, Fifth Edition. Holland JF, Frei E, Bast RC, Kufe DW, Pollock RE, Weichelbaum RR (eds.) B.C. Decker, Ontario, pp. 1431–1435.

Evans DB, Lee JE, Pisters PWT (2001) Pancreaticoduodenectomy (Whipple operation) and total pancreatectomy for cancer. In *Mastery of Surgery*, Fourth Edition. Baker RJ, Fischer JF (eds.) Lippincott Williams & Wilkins, Philadelphia, pp. 1299–1318.

Foo M, Gunderson L, Nagorney D, McLlrath D, van Heerden J, Robinow J et al. (1993) Patterns of failure in grossly resected pancreatic ductal adenocarcinoma treated with adjuvant irradiation +/− 5 fluorouracil. *Int J Radiat Oncol Biol Phys* 26: 483.

Freeny PC (2001) Pancreatic carcinoma: Imaging update 2001. *Dig Dis* 19:37–46.

Gastrointestinal Tumor Study Group (1987) Further evidence of effective adjuvant combined radiation and chemotherapy following curative resection of pancreatic cancer. *Cancer* 59:2006.

Hoffman J, Lipsitz S, Pisansky T, Weese J, Solin L, Benson AB (1998) Phase II trial of preoperative radiation therapy and chemotherapy for patients with localized, resectable adenocarcinoma of the pancreas: An Eastern Cooperative Oncology Group study. *J Clin Oncol* 16:317–232.

Hruban RH, Goggins M, Parsons J et al. (2000) Progression model for pancreatic cancer. *Clin Cancer Res* 6:2969–2972.

Jean ME, Lowy AM, Chiao PJ, Evans DB (2002) The molecular biology of pancreatic cancer. In *Pancreatic Cancer*. Evans DB, Pisters PWT, Abbruzzese JL (eds). Springer-Verlag, New York, pp. 15–28.

Kalser M, Ellenberg S (1985) Pancreatic cancer. Adjuvant combined radiation and chemotherapy following curative resection. *Arch Surg* 120:899.

Klinkenbijl JH, Jeekel J, Sahmoud T et al. (1999) Adjuvant radiotherapy and 5-fluorouracil after curative resection of cancer of the pancreas and periampullary region. Phase III trial of the EORTC Gastrointestinal Tract Cancer Cooperative Group. *Ann Surg* 230: 776–784.

Leach SD, Lee JE, Charnsangavej C, Cleary KR, Lowy AM, Fenoglio CJ, Pisters PWT, Evans DB (1998) Survival following pancreaticoduodenectomy with resection of the superior mesenteric-portal vein confluence for adenocarcinoma of the pancreatic head. *Br J Surg* 85:611–617.

Neoptolemos JP, Dunn JA, Stocken DD et al. (2001) Adjuvant chemoradiotherapy and chemotherapy in resectable pancreatic cancer: A randomized controlled trial. *Lancet* 358:1576–1585.

Nukui Y, Picozzi VJ, Traverso LW (2000) Interferon-based adjuvant chemoradiation therapy improves survival after pancreaticoduodenectomy for pancreatic adenocarcinoma. *Am J Surg* 179:367–371.

Pisters PWT, Hudec WA, Hess KR et al. (2001) Effect of preoperative biliary decompression on pancreaticoduodenectomy-associated morbidity in 300 consecutive patients. *Ann Surg* 234:47–55.

Pisters PWT, Lee JE, Vauthey JN et al. (2001) Laparoscopy in the staging of pancreatic cancer. *Br J Surg* 88:325–337.

Porter GA, Pisters PWT, Mansyur C et al. (2000) Cost and utilization impact of a clinical pathway for patients undergoing pancreaticoduodenectomy. *Ann Surg Oncol*, 7:484–489.

Sohn TA, Yeo CJ, Cameron JL et al. (2000) Resected adenocarcinoma of the pancreas-616 patients: Results, outcomes, and prognostic indicators. *J Gastrointest Surg* 4:567–579.

Spitz FR, Abbruzzese JL, Lee JE et al. (1997) Preoperative and postoperative chemoradiation strategies in patients treated with pancreaticoduodenectomy for adenocarcinoma of the pancreas. *J Clin Oncol* 15:928–937.

Yeo CJ, Abrams RA, Grochow LB et al. (1997) Pancreaticoduodenectomy for pancreatic adenocarcinoma: Postoperative adjuvant chemoradiation improves survival. *Ann Surg* 225:621–636.

Wolff RA, Abbruzzese JL, Evans DB (2003) Neoplasms of the exocrine pancreas. In *Cancer Medicine*, Sixth Edition. Holland JF, Frei E, Bast RC, Kufe DW, Pollock RE, Weichelbaum RR (eds.) B.C. Decker, Inc., Ontario, pp. 1585–1614.

Wolff RA, Evans DB, Gravel DM et. al. (2001) Phase I trial of gemcitabine combined with radiation for the treatment of locally advanced pancreatic adenocarcinoma. *Clin Cancer Res* 7:2246–2253.

Yen TWF, Wolff RA, Evans DB (2003) Neoplasms of the ampulla of Vater. In *Cancer Medicine*, Sixth Edition. Holland JF, Frei E, Bast RC, Kufe DW, Pollock RE, Weichelbaum RR (eds.) B.C. Decker, Inc., Ontario, pp. 1615–1621.

CHAPTER 22

Cancer of the Colon and the Rectum

M.A. GIL-DELGADO and D. KHAYAT

Medical Oncology Department, Salpétrière Hospital, SOMPS, Paris, France

J. TAIEB

Department of Gastroenterology, Salpétrière Hospital, SOMPS, Paris, France

EPIDEMIOLOGY

Colorectal cancer is one of the main causes of death in the Western world. It was diagnosed in an estimated 130,200 people in the United States in 2000, and there are more than 800,000 newly cases diagnosed of colorectal cancer worldwide, with an overall mortality of more than 500,000 each year, according to the World Health Organization. The number of colorectal cancers over the world has been increasing rapidly since 1975. Colorectal cancer represents 9.4% and 10.1% of all incident cancer in men and women, respectively. There is a geographic variation in incidence rates, with high rates in Western countries and lower rates in Asia, Africa, and South America. However, studies on migrants suggest that environmental factors play a major part in the etiology of the disease. Sixty percent of patients are initially diagnosed with stage II or III disease, and approximately 40% and 35% will recur with locally invasive or metastatic disease, respectively. However, in the past two decades, there has been an improvement in survival for colorectal cancer, mainly because of improvements in surgical techniques, adjuvant chemotherapy, radiotherapy, and early detection. The emergence of new chemotherapeutic combination, in the last 10 years, has also transformed the prognosis of metastatic disease with improvements in survival and quality of life.

RISK FACTORS

There are different population groups who could be predisposed to develop colorectal cancer. The largest group, average risk, includes patients without an

UICC Manual of Clinical Oncology, Eighth Edition. Edited by Raphael E. Pollock
ISBN 0-471-22289-5 Copyright © 2004 John Wiley & Sons, Inc.

TABLE 22.1. Risk Factors for Colorectal Cancer

Age ≥50 years
High-fat, low-fiber diet
Excess caloric intake
History of colorectal cancer or adenomatous polyps
Family history of colorectal cancer or adenomatous polyps
Chronic inflammatory bowel disease (ulcerative colitis, Crohn's colitis)
Hereditary polyposis and nonpolyposis syndromes
   Hereditary nonpolyposis colorectal cancer (Lynch's syndrome)
   Familial adenomatous polyposis
   Gardner's syndrome
   Turcot's syndrome
   Peutz-Jeghers syndrome
   Familial juvenile polyposis

evident risk factor for colorectal cancer, and for this group, alimentary factors should be mainly considered. The second group, high risk, includes patients with a history of longstanding inflammatory bowel disease, personal or family history of colorectal cancer, or adenomatous polyps. The third group, very high risk, includes patients with a genetic predisposition such as hereditary polyposis or hereditary nonpolyposis syndrome (Table 22.1).

Age

Age is an important risk factor for colorectal adenocarcinoma. The mean age of colorectal cancer patients is around 67 years old. The incidence rate increases from 1.59 per 1,000 individuals at 65–69 years of age to 3.87 per 1,000 in those older than 84. Furthermore, the population is getting older, and the proportion of subjects over 75 years old with colorectal carcinoma increased from 38% to 42.5% between 1976 and 1995.

Diet

Epidemiological studies have suggested that dietary factors are involved in the promotion of colorectal cancer. Excessive caloric intake with high dietary fat and meat is positively related to risk of colorectal cancer, whereas intake of fruit, vegetables, and fiber may be protective. These dietary factors are useful in explaining differences in colorectal cancer rates between southern and western countries, but their beneficial or deleterious role is still under discussion. Other factors such as calcium supplementation are associated with a modest reduction in colorectal adenoma risk. There is a weak association between high iron exposure and colorectal polyps.

Previous Bowel Diseases

More than 60% of colorectal cancers (60–80%) occur in patients with preexisting lesions such as benign adenomas. Different steps and molecular pathways occur

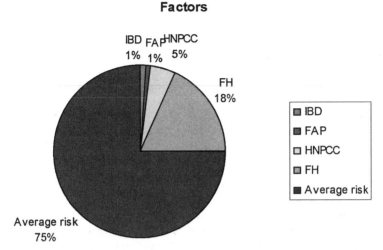

Figure 22.1 Factors associated with new cases of colorectal cancer. IBD, inflammatory bowel disease; FAP, familial adenomatous polyposis; HNPCC, hereditary nonpolyposis colorectal cancer; FH, family history. (From Schonoll-Sussman et al.)

from benign adenoma to invasive carcinoma. Chronic inflammatory diseases like sigmoiditis and Crohn's disease can predispose to colorectal carcinoma, as well (Fig. 22.1).

GENETICS

Major advances have been achieved recently in epidemiology and molecular biology of colorectal neoplasms that permit us to understand better the etiology of this disease. Understanding the roles of environmental exposures and host susceptibilities in molecular pathways has implications for screening, prevention, treatment, and surveillance. Several molecular pathways are found both in the two inherited autosomal dominant syndroms FAP (familial adenomatous polyposis) and HNPCC (hereditary nonpolyposis colorectal cancer), Sporadic cancer involves the *APC*-catenin-Tcf pathway and DNA mismatch repair. Expression of the key genes involved may be lost by inherited or acquired mutation.

Hereditary Syndromes

Familial Adenomatous Polyposis FAP is an autosomal dominant condition characterized by early development of multiple colorectal adenomas. It represent 1% of all cancer cases. This disease includes several extracolonic manifestations like upper gastrointestinal polyps, desmoid tumors, retinal pigmentation, and other malignancies (hepatoblastoma and thyroid carcinoma). Untreated patients with polyposis will develop colorectal carcinoma and will die in fourth decade of age (almost 100% risk). The identification of family risk in the early years offers the best method of prevention. The responsible *APC* gene is located at the long arm of chromosome 5 (5q21). The abnormalities of this gene are detected by molecular DNA analysis of blood samples. This process permits regular surveillance by periodic endoscopy and early colectomy resulting in an important reduction of colorectal cancers. Recently, it has been demonstrated that new Cox-2 inhibitors inhibit the growth of adenomas in the colon and possibly in the duodenum, that opens the possibility of pharmacological treatment instead surgery in the future for severe adenomatosis.

Hereditary Nonpolyposis Colorectal Cancer HNPCC (Lynch's syndrome) is an autosomal dominantly inherited disorder of cancer predisposition and it is responsible for 1–5% of all colorectal cancer cases. The risk of colorectal cancer in HNPCC patients begins to increase by age 20 and is very high after 45 years of age. The risk for colorectal cancer at age 60 is estimated to be 57–80%. Cancer lesions are frequently multiple, and are synchronous or metachronous in 35% of patients. The primary lesion is located in the proximal rather than the distal part of the colon. Adenoma usually precedes the carcinoma but sporadic neoplastic lesions without preexistent adenoma may also occur. The expression of disease may be limited to the colorectum or coexist with extracolonic tumors, typically endometrial cancer. Other associated malignancies include stomach, small intestine, hepatobiliary, pancreas, breast, ovary, brain, renal pelvis, ureter, and skin cancers.

The molecular genetic mutation of HNPCC is one of the sporadic cancer mismatch repair genes (MMR) proved to predispose to the disease. The MMR system inactivation results from a number of replication errors throughout the genome known as microsatellite instability (MSI). It has been shown that germline mutations in the following MMR genes cosegregate with HNPCC: hMSH2 on chromosome 2p16, MLH1 on chromosome 3p21, hPMS1 on chromosome 2q31-33, hPMS2 on chromosome 7p22, and hMSH6 on chromosome 2p16. Testing for these mutations allows the identification of mutation carriers prior to disease development.

Periodic endoscopic surveillance of the colon and removal of adenomas reduces the incidence of CRC ($p = 0.03$) and decreases the cancer related mortality ($p = 0.08$). Subtotal colectomy is the best surgical option for HNPCC patients with proximal carcinoma, and for females, subtotal colectomy and prophylactic hysterectomy (50–60% higher risk of gynecological tumors).

Other Hereditary Syndromes Gardner's syndrome, a variant of FAP, is characterized by colorectal adenomas and extraintestinal manifestations including osteomas, soft tissue tumors (lipomas, fibromas, etc.) desmoid tumors, mesenteric fibromatosis, and hypertrophy of the retinol pigmentation of epithelium. Turcot's syndrome is another variant of FAP, described as colorectal adenomas and brain tumors.

Personal and Family History of Colorectal Cancer or Adenoma

Individuals with prior family history of colorectal cancer or adenomas are at high risk of developing colorectal cancer by two- or threefold. The risk is increased if they have more than one first-degree relative (FDR) or the affected relative was diagnosed before 40 years of age. The possibility of an underlying hereditary syndrome should be considered. Subjects with prior colorectal cancer are at increased risk for developing synchronous (2–6%) or metachronous lesions (3–8%) and also for developing adenomas (25–40%).

SPORADIC COLON CANCER

Sporadic colon cancer is the most frequent type of colorectal cancer. This cancer appears in men and women older than 50 years of age without any family history of colon cancer or hereditary bowel diseases. Colorectal carcinoma originates from normal cells exposed to a series of insults resulting in the accumulation of mutations in a few key genes that result in clonal proliferation. The hypothesis that cancer is a multistep process that appears after a number of genetic errors that are accumulated in one cell has been illustrated for the first time in colon cancer (Fig. 22.2).

Methylation

Hypermethylation or hypomethylation is a mechanism of control of gene expression that also seems to be able to control oncogenesis in colon cancer by turning on the inappropriate expression of an oncogene or by turning off the appropriate expression. It is an early event in colon cancer.

Adenomatous Polyposis Coli

Mutations in the *APC* gene are responsible for the FAP syndrome. In sporadic colon cancer, such mutations or deletions also appear and are found in the beginning of the cascade in early adenoma formation.

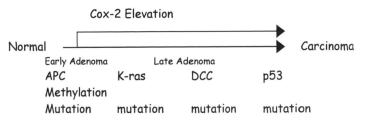

Figure 22.2 Working hypothesis for the potential role of cox-2 in colorectal carcinogenesis.

K-*ras*

K-*ras* is found in approximately 40% of colon cancer, after *APC* loss but before *DCC* (deletion colorectal cancer), and *p53* mutation. K-*ras* encodes a 21-KD guanosine triphosphate-binding protein that remains in its activated guanosine, triphosphate-bound state, thus activating a tyrosine kinase cascade, leading to *p21* activation and helping to maintain the transformed phenotype.

Deletion Colon Cancer (*DCC*) (18q)

The long arm of chromosome 18 is deleted in 70–80% of colon cancers. This deletion seems to appear later than *APC* and K-*ras*, but earlier than *p53*. Normal *DCC* seems to be able to stop cells in the G2/M phase of the cell cycle and induce apoptosis.

p53 Mutations in Chromosome 17 (17q)

Mutations of *p53*, which is a tumor suppressor gene, appear in 70% of most colon cancer tissues. However, *p53* mutations in early polyps or normal mucosa are not associated with a higher incidence of malignant evolution, which suggests that a *p53* mutation is only relevant if it appears in the right moment in the later stages of the cascade (late adenoma or early carcinoma).

SCREENING, EARLY DETECTION, AND PREVENTION

Screening involves testing asymptomatic individuals to assess the likelihood that they may have colorectal cancer or precursors. For a screening technique to be practical, it must be a risk-based approach to the assessment of asymptomatic patients. Periodic screening may lead to early detection of colon cancer at a curable stage or complete removal of precancerous lesions, such adenomatous polyps. The method for screening depends on the subject's condition.

Screening of Average Risk Subject Group

Subjects who are healthy and have an average risk of colon cancer represent the largest population appropriate for screening. Asymptomatic patients with no family history of colorectal cancer begin screening at 50 years of age with fecal occult blood assessment annually. This test has shown to be effective in reducing colorectal cancer mortality. Digital rectal examination is a complementary assessment, and flexible sigmoidoscopy every 5 years could be considered. Nevertheless, if a stool blood test is positive, the patient should undergo complete colon assessment by a more invasive techniques such as colonoscopy.

Screening of High-Risk Groups

High-risk patients are those older than 50 years with a personal or family history (FDR) of colorectal cancer or adenoma, longstanding inflammatory bowel disease, or a genetic predisposition (hereditary polyposis or hereditary nonpolyposis syndrome). For patients who have had colorectal adenoma, colonoscopy should be performed every 3 years after surgery. If the 3-year follow-up examination is negative, this surveillance can be performed every 5 years. In patients with a history of colorectal cancer, if the colonoscopy was incomplete or not performed before surgery, the first surveillance by colonoscopy should be performed within the year following resection. Subsequent follow-up surveillance by colonoscopy must be performed as described for patients with history of colorectal adenoma. People with a FDR who has had colorectal cancer or adenomatous polyps should be screened on a schedule similar to that for average-risk people, but starting at the fourth decade of age. Individuals who have a relative with early-onset disease should begin surveillance 3–10 years prior to the age of onset in the index individual. It is strongly recommended that a complete examination of the colon be performed for this group of subjects. In patients with inflammatory bowel diseases, colonoscopic surveillance should begin annually after 8 years of disease in patients with pancolitis or after 15 years of disease in those with colitis involving the left side of the colon.

These surveillance schedules should be continued at 1- to 2-year intervals and random biopsies should be routinely performed in order to detect dysplasia, which is a marker for the presence of colorectal cancer.

Screening of High-Risk Groups

In patients with FAP, Gardner's syndrome, or HNPCC, intensive follow-up must be done by a specialized gastroenterologist and genetic counseling should be provided. Gene tests must be performed in all members of these families.

PATHOLOGY AND LOCATION

Adenocarcinoma and mucinous adenocarcinoma account for 90–95% of colorectal carcinomas; all other types are uncommon. Mucinous adenocarcinoma are more often observed in the colon (15%) than in the rectum (10%). Colorectal carcinoma is located in the rectum in 45% of cases, in the sigmoid in 25%, and in the remaining parts of the colon in 30%. Some factors such blood and lymphatic vessel infiltration, poorly differentiated cells, and aneuploidy are associated with a poor prognosis of disease.

Spread

The natural history of colorectal cancer is summarized in Figure 22.3. The natural progression of colorectal cancer can be determined by three components: local invasion, lymphatic spread, and hematogenous spread. The knowledge of tumor spread is an important factor to establish the management of colorectal carcinoma.

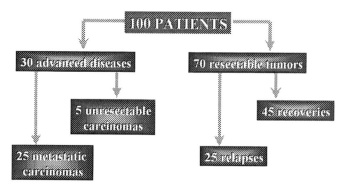

Figure 22.3   Natural history of colorectal cancer.

Different types of local spread will determine the extent of surgical resection, and will lead to the demand for avoidance of local tumor spillage.

Local growth of colorectal adenocarcinoma is characterized by the tumor expansion into the bowel wall, then a lateral progression occurs leading to circumferential growth. Mural invasion may result in local failure, peritoneal seeding, or both. Lymphatic spread is bidirectional for both flexures, right colon, and left third of transverse colon. It is unidirectional for other parts of the colon. The local and lymphatic spread status and T and N stages (Table. 22.2) allow prediction of the risk of developing disseminated disease.

The most frequent site of hematogenous spread of colorectal cancer is the liver, followed by the lung. The portal system represents the main venous drainage of the colon and upper rectum. However, isolated lung metastases can occur in patients with lower rectal tumors, because of tumor emboli circulating through the middle and inferior rectal veins, iliac vein, and the vena cava. Bone metastases in the sacrum and the vertebral bodies may also occur through the vertebral venous plexus.

Staging

Dukes developed the first practical system in the early 1930s. The initial Dukes' system was directed to rectal cancers and was remarkable for its simplicity and

TABLE 22.2. Prognostic Factors

Stage	TNM	5-Year Survival (%)
Stage 0	Tis, T1; N0; M0	>90
Stage I	T2; N0; M0	80–85
Stage II	T3, T4; N0; M0	70–75
Stage III	T2; N1-3; M0	70–75
Stage III	T3; N1-3; M0	50–65
Stage III	T4; N1-3; M0	25–45
Stage IV	M1	<3

ability to give adequate prognostic information. The tumors were classified from A to C, with stage A indicating penetration restricted to the bowel wall, stage B indicating penetration through the bowel wall, and stage C indicating lymph node involvement. Over the years, several authors have attempted to make improvements on the initial work by Dukes, and the system has been extended to include both colon and rectal cancers. Dukes himself made a few changes in his system. After different changes, the revision by Astler and Coller in 1954 altered the Dukes' classification substantially, introducing the concept of stages C1 and C2, which are used commonly today. One of the problems not addressed by any of the commonly used variations of the Dukes' system is its inability to classify patients based on the extent of their lymph node involvement. Positive nodes fared remarkably better

TABLE 22.3. TNM 2002 Classification in Colorectal Carcinoma

Primary tumor—T

Tx	Primary tumor cannot be assessed
T0	No evidence of tumor
Tis	Carcinoma *in situ*: intraepithelial or invasion of lamina propria
T1	Tumor invades submucosa
T2	Tumor invades muscularis propria
T3	Tumor invades through muscularis propria into subserose or into peritoneolized pericolic or perirectal tissues[a]
T4	Tumor directly invades other organs or structures and/or perforates visceral peritoneum[b]

Regional lymph nodes—N[c]

Nx	Regional lymph nodes cannot be assessed
N0	No regional lymph node metastasis
N1	Metastasis in 1–3 regional lymph nodes
N2	Metastasis in ≥4 regional lymph nodes

Distant metastasis—M

Mx	Distant metastasis cannot be assessed
M0	No distant metastasis
M1	Distant metastasis

pTNM pathological classification: The pT, pN, and pM categories correspond to the T, N, and M categories. PN0 histologic examination of a regional lymphadenectomy specimen will ordinarily include 12 or more lymph nodes

[a]With no extension through muscularis mucosae into submucosa.

[b]Includes invasion of other segments of the colorectum by way of the serosa. Tumor that is adherent to other organs or structures macroscopically is classified T4. However, if tumor is not present in the adhesion microscopically, the classification should be pT3.

[c]A tumor nodule in the pericolic/perirectal adipose tissue without histological evidence of residual lymph node in the nodule is classified in the pN category as regional lymph node metastasis if the nodule has the form and smooth contour of a lymph node. If the nodule has irregular contour, it should be classified in the T category and also coded as V1 (microscopic venous invasion) or V2, if it was grossly evident, because there is a strong likelihood that it represents venous invasion.

TABLE 22.4. UICC Stage Grouping in Colorectal Carcinoma

Stage	TNM[a]	Dukes	Astler & Coller	Repartition (%)	Surgery (%)	Adjuvant Chemotherapy (%)
0	Tis; N0 ; M0	A	A	—	—	—
I	T1, T2; N0; M0	A	B1	10	100	—
IIA	T3; N0; M0		B2	10		4
		B			100	
IIB	T4; N0; M0		B3	30		20
IIIA	T1, T2; N1; M0		C1			
IIIB	T3, T4; N1; M0	C	C2, C3	25	80–100	40
IIIC	Any T; N2; M0		C1,C2,C3			
IV	Any T; Any N; M1	D	D	25	80	—

[a]Summary: T1, submucosa; T2, muscularis propia; T3, subserosa, nonperitonealized pericolic/perirectal tissues; T4, other organs or structures/visceral peritoneum; N1, ≤ 3 regional; N2, >3 regional.

than did patients with larger numbers of involved nodes, and the number of positive nodes appeared to be the single most important prognostic factor. The newer classifications of colorectal cancer have incorporated the number of involved lymph nodes as an important prognostic factor. Even though the modified Dukes' staging still is commonly used worldwide, the number of applied variations makes correlation of different studies less than ideal.

The use of the TNM staging has been encouraged. At present, it is the preferred system for colorectal cancer patients. It is recommended that this staging system be used routinely. Starting in the late 1970s, and modified in 2000, both the American Joint Committee on Cancer (AJCC) and the Union Internationale Contre le Cancer (UICC) made attempts to unify the staging system for colorectal cancer with a simple classification similar to the TNM system used for most solid tumors. In 2002, this TNM classification was updated, as shown in Tables 22.3 and 22.4. The stage grouping of the TNM system and correspondences with the old Dukes' and Astler and Coller classifications are shown in Table 22.4.

DIAGNOSIS

Colorectal cancer may be diagnosed when a patient presents with symptoms or as the result of a screening program. Early colorectal cancer does not produce any symptoms. Often, most of the symptoms of colorectal cancer are nonspecific. Thus, efforts at detection through screening programs are essential.

Signs and Symptoms

Early symptoms of colorectal cancer such as intermittent abdominal pain, constipation or diarrhea, presence of mucus in stools, or iron deficiency are particularly unspecific. When the disease is more advanced, more alarming symptoms can occur such as weight loss, fatigue, obstruction, bleeding, or perforation. A palpable mass is possible in advanced disease, especially with right colon cancer. Bleeding may rarely be acute and most commonly appears as red blood mixed with stool. Occasionally, melena may be associated with right colon cancer. A lower degree of bleeding may be detected as part of a fecal occult blood test. Obstruction is, in most cases, secondary to cancer of the sigmoid. Acute perforation is associated with abdominal pain, fever, and palpable mass. Chronic perforation may also occur with a more insidious clinical presentation, often associated with a fistula into the bladder (pneumaturia, recurrent urinary tract infection) and, in women, the uterus and vagina.

Disease Assessment

Following are general guidelines for the assessment of patients with potentially curable colorectal cancer. Anamnesis and family history of all cancers and colorectal polyps should be obtained. A physical examination should be performed to check for hepatomegaly, ascites, and lymphadenopathy. Digital examination must be done to assess local extension of rectal tumor, and, in women, a complete pelvic examination. Blood count and liver chemistries must be performed. Testing for the carcinoembryonic antigen (CEA) provides independent prognostic information. Chest x-ray, ultrasound study of the liver, and abdominopelvic computed tomography (CT) scan, with contrast, is mandatory in order to detect possible metastases.

A complete colonoscopy is the most valuable diagnostic procedure for intraperitoneal colorectal cancer in order to histologically confirm adenocarcinoma through adequate biopsy. Colonoscopy is also useful to look for associated polyps or synchronous cancer in the other parts of the colon. In some patients, double-contrast barium enema is still performed because colonoscopy is not contributive or is technically impossible (because of tight stenosis, age greater than 85 years, or poor performance status).

For rectal cancer, endoscopic ultrasonography is required if possible, to determine the TNM stage of the tumor and help the physician in choosing among the different treatment modalities, especially for the use of adjuvant radiation or chemoradiation prior to surgery. Brain CT scan and bone scan are not routinely recommended but should be performed in cases with osteoarticular or neurologic symptoms. Magnetic resonance imaging and positron emission tomography are very useful in some equivocal situations such as dubious lesions in conventional imaging, preoperative staging before curative resection of recurrent disease, and high CEA levels in the absence of known tumor localization.

MANAGEMENT OF COLORECTAL CANCER

Surgery

Around 90% of patients with colon cancer and 84% of patients with rectal cancer are treated surgically, and, in most circumstances, with a curative intent. Surgery remains the primary modality of treatment for colorectal cancer, and standard resection is the only therapy required for early-stage cancer. A wide laparotomy, allowing complete abdominal assessment, is recommended, whereas laparoscopic colectomy has been confined to clinical trials. The surgical goals in the resection of a primary colorectal cancer are to achieve an *en bloc* removal comprising an adequate length of normal colon proximal and distal to the tumor. Adequate lateral margins are required by excision of all or a portion of adjacent structures when the primary tumor is adherent to them. Regional lymph nodes have to be removed primarily for the adequate evaluation of nodal invasion. The harvesting and examination of at least 12 nodes are required to allow a correct staging of the colorectal cancer, and to decide subsequent adjuvant chemotherapy.

Resection plus primary anastomosis is the surgical procedure of choice for intraperitoneal colorectal cancers. Radical resection should be performed as extended right hemicolectomy or extended left with extensive removal of the corresponding nodes in case of multidirectional lymphatic drainage (Fig. 22.4). For middle and low rectal carcinomas, two standard procedures are proposed:

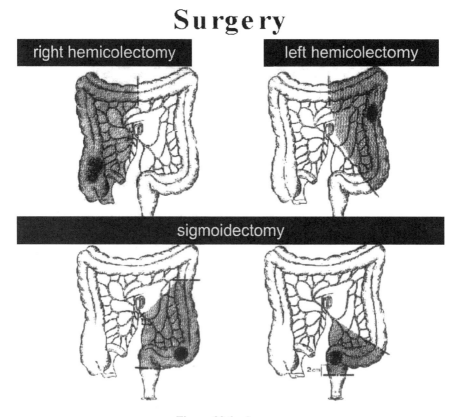

Figure 22.4   Surgery.

anterior resection or abdominoperineal resection. Sphincter-saving resections are increasingly used, but in about 30–40% of tumors of the lower third and 5–10% of tumors of the middle third of the rectum the anal sphincter can not be preserved. In these patients, abdominoperineal resection is performed, involving a wide excision of the rectum including the pelvic floor, the anal sphincter and the establishment of a permanent colostomy. When such type of surgery is performed, if postoperative radiotherapy is considered, care should be taken to keep the small bowel out of the pelvis (omentoplasty, prosthesis). In all cancers of the rectum, a total mesorectal excision is warranted to minimize the risk of local recurrence. New surgical therapies allow a decrease in damage to pelvic nerves governing bladder and sexual functions, without compromising chances for cure.

Temporary stoma is frequently used in the elective treatment of colorectal cancer in case of very low colorectal or coloanal anastomosis. In emergency situations of colorectal carcinoma (such as bowel perforation or acute bleeding), a temporary stoma is used either for a short period before the resection as to protect an anastomosis and then removed 3 to 6 months later, depending on the patient's condition. Other special surgical procedures such as liver or lung metastases resection could be also proposed to the patient if it is technically possible.

Chemotherapy

Adjuvant Chemotherapy   After curative surgery, 5-year overall survival rates vary between 75% and 80% for stage II colon cancer, and rarely exceed 60% for stage III disease. Therefore, there is an obvious need for adjuvant treatment in these cases. A large number of trials have been performed in the last 30 years to improve the outcome for operable patients.

Currently, the benefit of adjuvant chemotherapy is well established in stage III (Dukes' C) colon cancer after curative resection, reducing the risk of recurrence by 19–40% and death by 16–33%. The benefit of adjuvant chemotherapy for stage II patients (Dukes' B) is less clear. A number of clinicopathological features are now known to be associated with poor prognosis (perforated or obstructed tumors, T4 tumors, poorly differentiated, vascular invasion, and mucinuous differentiation) in addition to certain molecular prognostic markers such as loss of the DCC tumor suppressor gene, overexpression of thymidilate synthetase, and the presence of CEA mRNA, detectable by PCR (reverse-transcriptase polymerase chain reaction) in microscopically uninvolved lymph nodes.

Although 5-fluorouracil has been used for many years, results of studies optimizing its administration, particularly in combination with levamisol or leucovorin, have improved outcomes for patients treated with these regimens.

Fluorouracil and Levamisol   Levamisol is an anthelmintic agent that has immunomodulatory properties and mild toxicity when combined with 5-fluorouracil (5-FU). Fluorouracil is given in combination with levamisol for one year following surgery. Moertel et al. in 1990 showed a statistically significant survival advantage in patients treated with levamisol plus 5-FU compared with no treated patients after curative surgery (control vs. levamisol vs. 5-FU + levamisol). Results showed that 5-FU and levamisol significantly reduced recurrence rates ($p = 0.04$) and possibly increased survival in patients with stage III colon cancer. A 41% reduction in recurrence rates of the disease ($p < 0.0001$) and a reduction of mortality of 30% ($p = 0.006$) compared with surgery alone was achieved. A significant benefit could not be shown for patients with stage II disease. As a result, the 5-FU levamisol combination is one standard combination for adjuvant therapy in resected stage III colon cancer patients.

Fluorouracil and Leucovorin   The efficacy and safety of the modulation of 5-FU by leucovorin in advanced colorectal cancer is well known and has served as the rationale for the development of 5-FU leucovorin (5-FU/LV) regimens in the adjuvant setting. Different schedules of 5-FU/LV combinations with low or high doses of leucovorin have been used (Table 22.5) and shown to be superior to 5-FU alone.

A pooled analysis of various trials demonstrated a real advantage in terms of survival and disease-free survival. At 5 years, a 44% reduction in the risk of relapse ($p = 0.0016$) and 39% reduction of mortality ($p = 0.0025$) in patients with Dukes' C colon cancer was observed, versus no treatment after surgery. But no differences in terms of overall survival or DFS were observed with 12 months 5-FU/LV versus 6 months. On the other hand, 6 months of 5-FU/LV treatment is at least as effective as 1 year of 5-FU/levamisol. The National Surgical Adjuvant Breast and Bowel Program (NSABP C04 trial) comparing FU/LV over six cycles versus 5-FU/LV + levamisole over 1 year versus 5-FU/levamisol over 1 year showed an advantage in DFS (64% *vs.* 60%; $p = 0.06$) and overall survival (74% *vs.* 69%; $p = 0.05$) with the 5-FU/LV combination. Treatment with 5-FU/LV combination for 6 months appears to be the most effective combination for Dukes' C in terms of survival benefit.

TABLE 22.5. 5-Fluorouracil (5-FU)/Folinic Acid Schedules

Study	Drug	Dose	Schedule
Machover et al., France	Folinic acid	200 mg/m^2, IV	d1–5 every 28 d
	5-FU	375 to 400 mg/m^2, 2 h infusion	
Mayo Clinic, USA	Folinic acid	20 mg/m^2, IV	d1–5 every 28 d
	5-FU	375 mg/m^2, *bolus*, 2 h infusion	
De Gramont et al., France	Folinic acid	200 mg/m^2, IV, 2 h infusion	d1 and 2 every 2 weeks
	5-FU	400 mg/m^2, *bolus*, and 600 mg/m^2 22 h infusion	

Abbreviations: IV, intravenous; h, hour; d, day.

Monoclonal Antibodies (Edrecolomab: Monoclonal Antibody 17-1A of Murine Origins) Reithmuller et al., in Germany, studied edrecolomab monotherapy in an adjuvant setting for stage III colon cancer versus no treatment after surgery. Favorable overall and disease-free survival results were statistically significant for edrecolomab: $p < 0.01$ and $p = 0.02$, respectively. Recently, a large multicenter randomized trial comparing edrecolomab versus 5-FU/LV and 5-FU/LV plus edrecolomab demonstrated no advantage for edrecolomab or edrecolomab plus 5-FU/LV. Moreover, edrecolomab is statistically inferior to 5-FU/LV combination.

New Drugs The combination of CPT11 (irinotecan) plus oxaliplatin plus 5-FU/LV has been demonstrated to be superior to 5-FU/LV alone in recent phase III trials conducted in advanced disease. CPT11 and oxaliplatin are also active in 5-FU refractory patients, when there are reintroduced in combination with the same 5-FU/LV schedule in second line therapy. Recent trials are ongoing to compare the role of CPT11 and oxaliplatin in combination with 5-FU/LV to 5-FU/LV alone to establish their place in adjuvant setting.

Adjuvant Radiotherapy

Local recurrence is one of the first sites of failure for rectal cancer after curative resection, with equal distribution in the pelvis, liver, and lungs. Local recurrences are highly symptomatic and difficult to treat. Recurrence is low in stage I (5%) but varies from 20 to 40% for stage II and III. The metastatic evolution after local failure occurs in 25–50% of cases, representing a decrease in overall survival. Therefore, in addition to adjuvant chemotherapy to avoid distant spread, radiotherapy is necessary for local control.

In United States, the National Institutes of Health Consensus Conference stated that postoperative pelvic radiotherapy (45 Gy) and chemotherapy should be a standard treatment for stage II–III rectal cancer patients (4–5 weeks after surgery). Neoadjuvant radiotherapy has been evaluated in European trials in T3–T4 operable rectal cancer patients, evaluated by previous echoendoscopy. Results show a favorable trend for survival compared with surgery alone, and a statistically significant improvement for local recurrence ($p < 0.01$). Preoperative radiotherapy seems to be less toxic than postoperative radiotherapy because the irradiation area is smaller and the risk of post small bowel radiation decreases. In contrast, postoperative radiotherapy permits identification of small tumors that do not need radiotherapy (T1, T2 N-) and clip-marks at the time of surgery for more precise radiation application. In 1994, a national consensus conference held in Paris concluded that preoperative radiotherapy should be recommended for resectable T3–T4 rectal cancer patients.

MANAGEMENT OF METASTATIC DISEASE

Patients who have relapsed following surgery or who present with metastatic disease have a poor prognosis. Colorectal cancer patients are most likely to develop metastasis to the liver (30–40% have liver metastasis at the time of diagnosis, synchronous metastasis), the lung, or both. Although systemic treatment is possible, the effect is mainly palliative. For almost 40 years, fluorouracil has been the mainstay of treatment of patients with advanced colorectal cancer. Over the past 15 years, several attempts have been made to increase the efficacy of fluorouracil, either through modulation of its activity with compounds such as leucovorin, methotrexate, or interferon-α or through techniques that increase tumor exposure to the drugs by means of protracted continuous infusion. Although these methods have increased the efficacy of 5-FU by a factor of two to three in terms of response rate, survival of patients with advanced colorectal cancer remains relatively disappointing, rarely exceeding a median of 12 months. Treatment options for these patients remained limited until recently, when topoisomerase I inhibitor irinotecan and the diamino-cyclohexane (DACH) platinum derivative compound oxaliplatin were developed for use in advanced colorectal carcinoma. Both compounds proved their superiority against best supportive care. New combinations with these compounds have consistently increased response rate (by 35–55%), even in 5-FU refractory patients, and produced increases in time to progression and survival.

Hepatic metastases develop frequently. Unfortunately, the proportion of these patients with resectable disease is small. Oxaliplatin- and irinotecan-based therapies have significantly increased the resectability of inoperable patients, which offers the hope of cure for some.

Oxaliplatin and irinotecan in combination with 5-FU/folinic acid can now be considered standard therapy for the first-line treatment of advanced colorectal cancer patients. New combinations with other drugs are under investigation, such as mitomycin C or new thymidilate synthetase inhibitors like raltitrexed, oral fluoropyrimidines such as capecitabine, and UFT (ftorafur and uracil).

Hepatic Arterial Therapy

Liver metastases are infused almost exclusively by the hepatic artery, whereas normal hepatocytes derive their blood mainly from the portal vein. The drugs that should be most useful for hepatic arterial chemotherapy are the ones that are largely extracted on the first pass through the liver and that have short plasma half-lives and rapid body clearences, like 5-fluoro-2-deoxyuridine (floxuridine, FUDR).

FURTHER READING

Bonithon-Kopp C, Kronborg O, Giacosa A et al. (2000) Calcium and fibre supplementation in prevention of colorectal adenoma recurrence: a randomised intervention trial. European Cancer Prevention Organisation Study Group. *Lancet* 356:1300–1306.

Boyle P, Langman JS (2000) ABC of colorectal cancer: epidemiology. *BMJ* 321:805–808.

De Gramont A, Figer A, Seymour M, Homerin M et al. (2000) Leucovorin and fluorouracil with or without oxaliplatin as first-line treatment in advanced colorectal cancer. *J Clin Oncol* 18:2938–2947.

Dicato M, Van Cutsem E, Wils J (2000) Perspectives in colorectal cancer. *Semin Oncol.* 27 (5 suppl 10): 1–149.

Douillard JY, Cunningham D, Roth AD et al. (2000) Irinotecan combined with fluorouracil compared with fluorouracil alone as first-line treatment for metastatic colorectal cancer: a multicentre randomised trial. *Lancet* 355:1041–1047.

Compton C, Fenoglio-Preiser CM et al. (2000) American Joint Committee on Cancer Prognostic Factors Consensus Conference: Colorectal Cancer Working Group. *Cancer* 88: 1739–1757.

Eaden JA, Abrams KR, Mayberry JF (2001) The risk of colorectal cancer in ulcerative colitis: a meta analysis. *Gut* 48:526–535.

Gatta G, Sant M, Coebergh JW, Hakulinen T (1996) Substantial variation in therapy for colorectal cancer across Europe: EUROCARE analysis of cancer registry data for 1987. *Eur J Cancer* 32A:831–835.

Greenlee RT, Murray T, Bolden S, Wingo PA (2000) Cancer statistics, 2000. *CA Cancer J Clin* 50:7–33.

International Multicentre Pool Analysis of Colon Cancer Trials (IMPACT) (1995) Efficacy of adjuvant fluorouracil and folinic acid in colon cancer (IMPACT) investigators. *Lancet* 345:939–944.

Jatzko G, Lisborg P, Wette V (1992) Improving survival rates for patients with colorectal cancer. *Br J Surg* 79:588–591.

Kono S (2001) All epidemiological evidence is important in colorectal cancer. *Br Med J* 322:611.

Kronborg O, Fenger C, Olsen J et al. (1996) Randomised study of screening for colorectal cancer with faecal-occult-blood test. *Lancet* 348:1467–1471.

Levi F, Zidani R, Misset JL (1997) Randomised multicentre trial of chronotherapy with oxaliplatin, fluorouracil, and folinic acid in metastatic colorectal cancer. International Organization for Cancer Chronotherapy. *Lancet* 350:681–686.

Lynch PM, Kohlmann W, Ward PA (2000) Clinically oriented genetic counseling for familial colorectal cancer risk: familial polyposis, hereditary nonpolyposis colorectal cancer and "not otherwise specified"? In *Proceedings of the American Society of Clinical Oncology Clinical Practice Forum 2000*, pp. 44–51.

Mandel JS, Bond JH, Church TR et al. (1993) Reducing mortality from colorectal cancer by screening for fecal occult blood. Minnesota Colon Cancer Control Study. *N Engl J Med* 328:1365–1371.

Moertel CG, Fleming TR, Macdonald JS et al. (1990) Levamisole and fluorouracil for adjuvant therapy of resected colon carcinoma. *N Engl J Med* 322:352–358.

Moertel CG, Fleming TR, Macdonald JS et al. (1995) Fluorouracil plus levamisole as effective adjuvant therapy after resection of stage III colon carcinoma: a final report. *Ann Intern Med* 122:321–326.

Nelson H, Petrelli N, Carlin A et al. (2000) Guidelines 2000 for colon and rectal cancer surgery. *J Natl Cancer Inst* 18;93:583–596.

Nelson RL (2001) Iron and colorectal cancer risk: human studies. *Nutr Rev* 59:140–148.

National Institutes of Health Consensus Conference (1990) Adjuvant therapy for patients with colon and rectal cancer. *JAMA* 264:1444–1450.

O'Connell MJ, Mailliard JA, Kahn MJ et al. (1997) Controlled trial of fluorouracil and low-dose leucovorin given for 6 months aspostoperative adjuvant therapy for colon cancer. *J Clin Oncol* 15:246–250.

Popescu RA, Norman A, Ross PJ, Parikh B, Cunningham D (1999) Adjuvant or palliative chemotherapy for colorectal cancer in patients 70 years or older. *J Clin Oncol* 17:2412–2418.

Rougier P, Bugat R, Douillard JY, Culine S et al. (1997) Phase II study of irinotecan in the treatment of advanced colorectal cancer in chemotherapy-naive patients and patients pretreated with fluorouracil-based chemotherapy. *J Clin Oncol* 15:251–260.

Saltz LB, Douillard JY, Pirotta N et al. (2000) Combined analysis of two phase III randomized trials comparing irinotecan, fluorouracil (F), leucovorin (L) vs F alone as first-line therapy of previously untreated metastatic colorectal cancer (MCRC). *Proc Am Soc Clin Oncol* 19;242a.

Schnoll-Sussman F, Markowitz AJ, Winawer SJ (2001) Screening and surveillance for colorectal cancer. *Semin Oncol* 27(5 Suppl 10):10–21.

Sobin LH, Wittekind Ch, International Union Against Cancer (UICC) (2002) *TNM Classification of Malignant Tumors*, 6th Edition. Wiley-Liss, New York, pp. 72–75.

Vasen HFS, Wijnen JTh, Morreau H (2000) What does genetic testing tell and not tell in familial (nonpolyposis) colorectal cancer? In *The Proceedings of the American Society of Clinical Oncology Clinical Practice Forum 2000*, pp. 37–43.

Wolmark N, Rockette H, Mamounas EP et al. (1996) The relative efficacy of 5-FU + leucovorin (FU-LV), 5-FU + levamisole (FU-LEV), and 5-FU + leucovorin + levamisole (FU-LV-LEV) in patients with Dukes' B and C carcinoma of the colon: first report of NSABP C-04. *Proc Am Soc Clin Oncol* 15:205.

CHAPTER 23

Breast Cancer

CAROLINE LOHRISCH

British Columbia Cancer Agency, Vancouver, British Columbia, Canada

MARTINE PICCART

Institute Jules Bordet, Brussels, Belgium

Reducing breast cancer (BC) mortality requires several strategies. These include adequate identification of and effective preventative measures for high-risk individuals in addition to early diagnosis through screening and prompt evaluation of suspicious clinical and mammographic lesions. Finally, we also need local therapies that provide both sufficient prognostic information and risk reduction for recurrence, accurate assessment of the need for systemic adjuvant therapy according to recurrence risk, and identification and delivery of optimal adjuvant therapies. In metastatic disease, the goals are to enhance quality and duration of life by making use of the multiple therapies currently available and by exploring new target-specific therapies and factors predictive of response to these.

EPIDEMIOLOGY

BC is the most common cancer and the second leading cause of cancer death in western women. It is 100 times less common in men. The average lifetime risk for a woman in the western world is one in eight. The incidence is somewhat lower in other parts of the world and in non-Caucasians. Migrant populations assume a risk similar to the population risk in their new environment. The incidence of BC, especially of hormone receptor (HR)-positive disease, has risen in recent decades, in part due to increased detection of incidental cancers with screening. Screening mammography has changed the stage distribution of BCs, with more now being both smaller and of lower stage. Coupled with improved adjuvant therapeutic strategies, this has resulted in a modest overall reduction in BC mortality over the last 20 years.

UICC Manual of Clinical Oncology, Eighth Edition. Edited by Raphael E. Pollock
ISBN 0-471-22289-5 Copyright © 2004 John Wiley & Sons, Inc.

RISK FACTORS

The etiology of BC is multifactorial and the genetic evolution from malignant precursors to invasive disease is only partly understood. Risk factors include duration of uninterrupted estrogen exposure, nulliparity and late age at first parity, prior histologic breast abnormalities, genetic predisposition, and ill-defined environmental factors.

Estrogen

The duration of estrogen exposure is longer with early menarche, late menopause, and postmenopausal hormone replacement therapy (HRT). Estrogen levels are higher in obese postmenopausal women due to high levels of aromatase, an enzyme that converts androgens to estradiol in adipose tissue. Because of this, diets high in fat may slightly increase the risk of BC, although population studies are difficult to control for and their results are not conclusive. This may, however, in part explain the increased risk of Asian women in North America versus Asia. HRT prolongs exposure to estrogens beyond the natural menopause, and is associated with a hazard ratio for BC development of 1.3 compared with no HRT. Older oral contraceptive pills (OCPs) containing high levels of estrogen were associated with an increased risk of BC; however, this association has not been demonstrated with today's low dose estrogen OCPs.

Pregnancy

The influence of prolactin and human chorionic gonadotropin on the growth of ductal, lobular, and alveolar structures in the latter half of pregnancy is protective against future BC development. Therefore, nulliparous women who are of late age at first parity are at two-fold increased risk of developing BC. Breast feeding appears to be protective against BC development.

Prior Breast Pathology

A history of abnormal tissue in the breast also slightly increases the risk of developing BC. Such pathologies include ductal (DCIS), lobular (LCIS) carcinoma *in situ*, and atypical hyperplasia. Women who have had LCIS or DCIS have a 1% per year risk of developing BC, as compared with a 0.5% per year risk in the general population. A prior BC increases the risk of developing a contralateral malignancy by two- to fourfold. Finally, mammographically dense breasts are thought to be associated with increased BC risk, although this is inconclusive.

Family History and Genetic Factors

Having a first-degree relative with BC increases a woman's risk by twofold and two first-degree relatives (such as mother and sister) increases the risk further. A few well-characterized inherited gene disorders are associated with a high lifetime risk of breast and other cancers. Such inherited genetic syndromes usually result in a younger age of onset relative to the general BC population, and the tumors are often bilateral. Genetic mutations may result in loss of a tumor suppressor gene or activation of a tumor promoter gene and have variable penetrance. It is estimated that between 5 and 10% of BCs arise in women with such genetic mutations. Mutations of BRCA1 (chromosome 17) and BRCA2 (chromosome 11), found disproportionately in the Ashkenazi Jewish population, are associated with high lifetime risk of breast (80–90%) and ovarian cancer (20–30%) for BRCA1 mutations, and breast (40–60%), ovarian (40–50%), colon, and male breast and prostate cancers for BRCA2 mutations. Other less common genetic cancer syndromes associated with breast and other cancers include the Li Fraumeni (mutated p53), Cowden's (multiple hamartomas), Muir (Lynch II variant), Lynch II, and Ataxia Telangiectasia syndromes.

Environmental Factors

Putative but unproven environmental risk factors include high dietary fat, alcohol intake, smoking, and relative lack of exercise. Finally, previous local irradiation, such as mantle irradiation for Hodgkin's disease, increases the risk of future BC, in some series by up to 40%.

Risk Assessment

Several models exist that estimate an individual's lifetime risk of developing BC based on existing risk factors. The best known is the Gail model, which mathematically estimates the absolute risk of BC development over 20–30 years based on a woman's age, age at menarche and first parity, number of previous breast biopsies, first-degree family history of BC, and previous diagnosis of atypical hyperplasia. It has been used to select populations at risk for primary prevention trials and by some clinicians to guide prophylactic tamoxifen and mastectomy recommendations for women with higher than average risk.

PRIMARY PREVENTION

Several primary prevention strategies have been shown to reduce the incidence of invasive BC, particularly for women with high risk. Bilateral prophylactic mastectomy reduces the incidence of subsequent BC by 90%, although for many women this kind of surgery is not acceptable. Prophylactic oophorectomy is not recommended as a preventative strategy against BC development due to the associated premature osteoporosis and atherosclerosis risks. However, oophorectomy has been shown to reduce BC incidence and may be reasonably considered in women with a significant family history of ovarian and BCs and who have completed child bearing.

Adjuvant therapy trials of tamoxifen demonstrated a 47% lower incidence of contralateral BC in treated women compared with controls, leading to the speculation that it might be a useful preventative agent. Three primary prevention trials of tamoxifen versus placebo in women considered to be at high risk for BC development have been reported. The two smaller trials have reported no significant reduction in BC with tamoxifen, whereas the National Surgical Adjuvant Breast Project (NSABP) P-01 study, which randomized 13,000 women with an elevated BC risk, found a highly significant 49% reduction in the incidence of invasive and noninvasive hormone receptor (HR)-positive but not HR-negative BCs. Tamoxifen was associated with a higher incidence of endometrial cancer, thromboembolic events, and cataract surgery (1.5–2-fold) but fewer cardiovascular events and osteoporotic fractures. It is not clear whether tamoxifen provides a similar risk reduction for women with inherited BC syndromes. The ongoing STAR trial is exploring whether raloxifene, a tamoxifen analogue developed for osteoporosis prevention, is equivalent or superior in terms of both prevention and safety. Raloxifene has the potential advantage of less stimulation of endometrial proliferation compared with tamoxifen (and therefore lower risk of endometrial cancer), and was retrospectively observed to be protective against BC compared with placebo in osteoporosis trials. Prevention trials of aromatase inhibitors are also underway.

Surveillance

Increased surveillance with annual or bi-annual mammography with or without ultrasound and with bi-annual clinical forecast examinations is recommended for women with confirmed or suspected gene mutations that increase their BC risk. Because in these women BC often occurs at a younger age, screening from an earlier age than for the general population is also recommended. Several studies are addressing the value of MRI as a screen tool for this high-risk population.

GENETIC COUNSELING AND TESTING

Genetic counseling by an experienced professional is strongly recommended for individuals who are considering genetic testing for BC. Counseling addresses issues of who to share results with, including immediate and distant family members who may be at risk. Identification of an inherited gene can assist an individual in making decisions about prophylactic and surveillance measures that are available. However, it can also have negative consequences, including insurance discrimination, alienation of family members, guilt about possible transmission to one's children, and substantial anxiety. On the other hand, exclusion of the genetic mutation in question can be very reassuring. The possibility of an inconclusive test result must also be anticipated prior to proceeding with testing, and additional post-test counseling is advocated.

Genetic testing should be reserved for individuals with a clearly established family history. This increases the sensitivity and reduces the cost and waiting period of genetic testing. Probes are available to screen for the most common genetic mutations in BRCA1 and BRCA2 genes. Full gene sequencing is more time consuming, expensive, and not available everywhere. A tissue or blood sample from an affected family member, however, can substantially increase the probability of a conclusive test through comparative testing. Genetic testing is not available for all known gene mutations that increase BC development. In addition, there are some families with numerous affected members who do not have any of the known gene mutations. Genetic testing is an evolving field and one that can be expected to mushroom with the genetic discoveries accompanying the human genome project.

SCREENING

Mammography

Regular mammographic screening reduces BC mortality and can detect subclinical breast pathology. The institution of mammographic screening programs in many countries is partly responsible for the small rise in BC incidence and the large rise in the detection rate of DCIS. The rate of detection of invasive and noninvasive disease is estimated to be 8 per 1,000 among first screening mammograms and 2–3 per 1,000 for subsequent screens. Approximately 30% of the detected abnormalities are DCIS and more than 50% of the invasive cancers are <1 cm. Double reading of mammograms increases the BC detection rate by several percent and comparison with prior films aids in the evaluation of slowly evolving abnormalities. Multiple and magnification views also assist in the evaluation of a suspicious mammogram. Evidence shows a 25% reduction in BC mortality with screening for women aged 50–69. For women aged 40–49, the evidence is less solid. Based on the available evidence, most screening programs recommend bilateral mammograms once every year or every two years for women aged 50–69, and optional annual screening for women 40–49 and >69 years of age.

Although there is some overlap with benign lesions, there are several characteristic mammographic features of malignancy, including architectural distortions, certain calcification patterns (due to cellular necrosis), and multilobular or spiculated masses with irregular, ill-defined margins. Suspicious calcifications include those that appear in groups of at least five (either as clusters or in a branching pattern), and are heterogenous in shape and size, although are generally below 0.5 mm and almost always below 1 mm. Microcalcifications associated with *in situ* disease can only be distinguished from invasive disease on pathologic diagnosis.

Other Screening Tools

Ultrasound alone has not proven to be an effective screening tool, being both insufficiently specific and sensitive, and is more valuable in the investigation of known abnormalities. Evidence is lacking about whether careful regular breast self-examination facilitates earlier detection of cancer or reduces BC mortality. The results of a large cohort study involving more than 100,000 Russian women aged

40–64 are expected shortly and should help answer this question. Some BCs are detected during screening clinical breast exam, which underscores the importance of a thorough physical exam during routine health check-ups. Other putative, but as yet experimental, screening tools include ductal lavage, magnetic resonance imaging (MRI), and thermal imaging techniques.

DIAGNOSIS

Pathologic examination of a suspicious breast mass or mammographic abnormality is mandatory. When small and not clinically palpable, ultrasound-guided or stereotactic fine needle aspiration or biopsy will help adequately sample the lesion. However, excisional biopsy is the preferred definitive diagnostic procedure. If the lesion is small, a wire may be placed into the mammographic abnormality to assist the surgeon in precisely locating it. A positive fine-needle aspirate or biopsy should be followed by adequate surgical excision after exclusion of distant metastases. A chest x-ray, routine biochemistry and hematology analyses, bone scan, and liver imaging are a reasonable screen for distant metastases.

The diagnosis of a nonmetastatic invasive or *in situ* BC requires complete local staging, which includes tumor-free surgical margins and determination of axillary nodal status. Positive or close surgical margins should be re-excised or given "boost" radiotherapy. The axillary lymph nodes are generally recognized as the earliest detectable site of spread. Routine sampling or dissection of other regions into which the breast lymphatics drain, including the subclavicular and internal mammary nodes (IMN), has been largely abandoned with the advent of breast-conserving surgery.

Removal of the lymph nodes in axillary regions I and II but not III (those located lateral to and behind, but not those medial to the pectoralis minor) is considered to be the best balance between adequate prognostic information and morbidity. Acute postsurgical morbidity from axillary dissection includes seromas, hematomas, and wound infection. Restricted range of motion of the shoulder (due to subcutaneous scar tissue tethering), numbness of the axilla and lateral chest wall (due to injury of the intercostobrachial nerve), and lymphedema (due to disruption of the axillary drainage basin) may occur acutely, but are more likely to be late sequelae, and can become chronic.

The increasing diagnosis of *in situ* disease and tumors smaller than 1 cm and even 0.5 cm raises the question of whether the morbidity associated with axillary dissection is warranted, given the low incidence of axillary involvement (10–20% in tumors <1 cm) and favorable prognosis of small tumors. Sentinel node procedures, which use dye and/or a radioactive tracer to identify the most likely first node(s) of drainage of the breast tumor, seem to be a fortuitous solution to this quandary. Recent studies have shown low false-negative rates (<5%) for sentinel procedures. This is operator dependent, however: a minimum of 20–30 procedures with a demonstrably low false-negative rate is recommended before routine use of sentinel node biopsy without axillary dissection by an individual surgeon. Other factors that may increase the false-negative rate include increased patient age, single localization technique (dye or radioactive tracer alone), and upper outer quadrant location.

Many centers now routinely omit axillary dissection in patients with negative sentinel nodes. The goal of ongoing sentinel node studies is to determine whether axillary dissection and its associated morbidity can be safely avoided in women with negative sentinel nodes without compromising locoregional control or prognostic information. Others are exploring whether in the setting of a positive sentinel node, axillary radiotherapy provides the same regional control as, and morbidity similar to or lower than an axillary dissection. Until these studies are mature, axillary dissection is recommended for all women with pathologic evidence of spread to sentinel nodes. One disadvantage of replacing dissection with axillary radiotherapy in node-positive disease is loss of prognostic information from pathologic examination of the remainder of the axillary nodes. Benefits of sentinel node mapping, on the other hand, include reduced surgical morbidity, and potentially identification of tumors that drain medially to the internal mammary nodes (IMN), allowing targeted radiotherapy of this region in women at risk.

HISTOLOGY

Preinvasive Lesions

Ductal Carcinoma In Situ   Ductal carcinoma *in situ* (DCIS) can present as a palpable mass, with or without nipple discharge, or more commonly, a nonpalpable mammographic abnormality. DCIS represents a wide spectrum of noninvasive malignant epithelial cell growth within breast ducts, including comedo, cribriform, micropapillary, papillary, solid, and mixed types. DCIS is more frequently estrogen receptor (ER)-negative and is often associated with HER2 overexpression. There may be focal areas of microinvasion, and approximately 1% have axillary node metastases. Features associated with a high risk of recurrence include large size, high grade, necrosis (comedo-type), and inadequate surgical margins.

Lobular Carcinoma In Situ   Lobular carcinoma *in situ* (LCIS) is a marker and risk factor for subsequent ductal or lobular BC development in either breast. It is only detectable microscopically and thus is an incidental finding on investigation of other breast pathology, most commonly in younger women. The histologic appearance is fairly uniform: proliferation within the terminal duct-lobule of small cells with a round nucleus, low proliferative rate. LCIS is usually ER positive, but rarely HER2 (+).

Invasive Disease

The majority (>80%) of invasive BCs are of ductal or lobular histology. Although their relapse patterns and genetic profiles differ, they are often grouped together in terms of relapse risk and treatment recommendations, because node status and size are more relevant prognostic factors than ductal or lobular histology. Rare variants include medullary, tubular, mucinous, colloid, papillary, and adenoid cystic histologies. A tumor composed purely of these elements has a better prognosis than one of mixed, ductal, or lobular histology. Soft tissue and angiosarcomas of the breast are exceedingly rare, although radiotherapy coupled with lymphedema is a recognized risk factor for highly aggressive and uniformly fatal angiosarcoma and lymphangiosarcoma (Stewart-Treeves syndrome). Phylloides tumors of the breast are also rare, but associated with a good prognosis.

Lobular and ductal carcinomas are classified by nuclear and histologic grading. Nuclear grade compares nuclear structures of malignant cells with those of normal epithelial cell nuclei, and histologic grade examines growth pattern, including extent of tubule formation, nuclear hyperchromasia, and mitotic rate. The most common grading systems divide the nuclear and global architecture each into well, moderately, and poorly differentiated categories and give a composite score, from 1 to 3 (in essence, from the most to the least well differentiated).

STAGING AND PROGNOSIS

BCs are staged according to the size of the tumor, lymph node involvement, and presence or absence of distant metastates. The most commonly used staging system is the UICC TNM classification system (Table 23.1). The presence or absence of nodal metastases is the most important prognostic element in early BC, and recurrence risk increases with the number of involved nodes. Young age at diagnosis is also associated with a poorer prognosis. Other established prognostic factors include tumor size, the status of estrogen and progesterone receptors, and probably overexpression (or gene amplification) of HER2, an epidermal growth factor receptor with intracellular tyrosine kinase activity involved in cell growth and proliferation through intracellular signaling pathways.

Node-negative disease represents a spectrum of risk (Table 23.2). In node-negative disease particularly, several histologic features play a role in predicting the aggressiveness and recurrence risk of BC. There is an independent association between tumor differentiation and prognosis. In natural history studies, poor differentiation is also linked with a higher incidence of axillary nodal metastases and more frequent disease recurrence. In addition, the presence of tumor emboli in the specimen lymphatics or blood vessels may provide prognostic information: although unproven, the hypothesis is that lymphatic emboli predict for axillary metastases and vascular emboli for distant metastases.

Two-thirds of ductal and lobular carcinomas express the nuclear HRs, estrogen receptor (ER), progesterone receptor (PgR), or both. The absence of HRs is associated with a poorer prognosis and lack of benefit from hormone therapy. There is a gradient of responsiveness to hormone therapy that parallels the level of HR expression. HRs can be measured either by the older ligand-binding assay, or by immunohistochemistry (IHC), which detects lower levels of ER and PgR and more reliably predicts hormone responsiveness.

The identification of metastases within axillary lymph nodes has traditionally been achieved using hematoxylin and eosin (H&E) staining. More recent

TABLE 23.1. Risk Categories for Patients with Node-Negative Breast Cancer

Characteristic	Minimal/Low Risk	Average/High Risk[2]	
		Hormone Responsive[1]	Not Hormone Responsive
Hormone receptor status	ER and/or PgR positive must have all characteristics below:	ER and/or PgR positive And at least one of the following:	ER and/or PgR negative
Pathologic tumor size	≤ 2 cm	>2 cm	Any
Nuclear/histologic grade	1	2–3	Any
Age, years	≥ 35	<35	Any
Adjuvant therapy recommended	Premenopausal: Tam or none Postmenopausal: Tam or none	Premenopausal: OA + Tam [± CT][3] CT + Tam [± OA][3] Tam or OA Postmenopausal: Tam or CT[4] + Tam	Premenopausal: CT[5] Postmenopausal: CT[5]

Adapted from Goldhirsch A, Glick JH, Gelber RD, Coates AS, Senn H. Meeting Highlights: International Consensus Panel on the Treatment of Primary Breast Cancer. J Nat Cancer Inst 2001.

[1] Responsiveness to endocrine therapies is related to expression of estrogen and progesterone receptors in the tumor cells. The exact threshold of estrogen and/or progesterone receptor staining (with currently available immunohistochemical methods), which should be used to distinguish between endocrine responsive and endocrine nonresponsive tumor is unknown. Even a low number of cells stained positive (as low as 1% of tumor cells) identify a cohort of tumors having some responsiveness to endocrine therapies. Probably, as typical for biological systems, a precise threshold does not exist. However empirically chosen, about 10% positive staining of either receptor might be considered as a reasonable threshold, accepted by most. Furthermore, it is clear that the lack of staining for both receptors confers endocrine nonresponsiveness status.

[2] Some panel members recognize lymphatic and/or vascular invasion as a factor indicating greater risk than minimal or low.

[3] Brackets indicate an addition to the regimen that is being tested in current clinical trials.

[4] The addition of chemotherapy is considered an acceptable option based on evidence from clinical trials. Considerations about a low relative risk, age, toxic effects, socioeconomic implications, and information on the patient's preference might justify the use of tamoxifen alone.

[5] For patients with endocrine nonresponsive disease, questions of timing, duration, agent, dose, and schedules of chemotherapy are subjects for research studies.

Abbreviations: OA = ovarian ablation; Tam = tamoxifen; CT = chemotherapy.

TABLE 23.2. UICC TNM Staging of Invasive BC

		0	I	IIA	IIB	IIIA	IIIB	IV	Definitions
T	Tx						X	X	Primary tumor not assessable
	T0			X		X	X	X	No evidence of primary tumor
	Tis	**X**							*In situ* disease only (DCIS or LCIS)
	T1		**X**	X		X	X	X	Tumor ≤2 cm in largest diameter
	T1mic								Largest focus of invasion of ≤0.1 cm
	T1a								Largest area of invasion >0.1 cm to 0.5 cm
	T1b								Largest area of invasion >0.5 cm to 1.0 cm
	T1c								Largest area of invasion >1.0 cm to 2.0 cm
	T2			X	X	X	X	X	Tumor >2 cm to 5 cm in largest diameter
	T3				X	X	X	X	Tumor >5 cm in largest diameter
	T4						X	X	Tumor with chest wall and/or skin involvement
	T4a								Chest wall invasion
	T4b								Skin involvement (ulceration or peau d'orange)
	T4c								Chest wall and skin invasion
	T4d								Inflammatory (diffuse erythema and brawny induration of breast)
N	Nx						X	X	Nodal status not assessable
	N0	**X**	**X**	X	X		X	X	No involved nodes
	N1			X	X	X	X	X	Involved axillary nodes that are mobile
	PN1a								No focus of invasion >0.2 cm
	PN1b								Invasion of >0.2 cm invasion
	PN1bi								1–3 nodes involved, none with >2 cm invasion
	PN1bii								>3 nodes involved, none with >2 cm invasion
	PN1iii								Gross extracapsular spread
	PN1iv								Any involvement >2 cm
	N2					X	X	X	Involved nodes that are fixed or matted together
	N3						X	X	Involved ipsilateral internal mammary nodes
M	Mx								Presence of distant metastases not evaluable
	M0	**X**	**X**	**X**	**X**	**X**	**X**		No distant metastases
	M1							**X**	Distant metastases

A bold "X" indicates a mandatory condition to satisfy the stage. When an X is nonbold, any marked X within the category (T or N) can satisfy the stage criteria. Adapted from Sobin LH, Wittekind CH (eds): *TNM Classification of Malignant Tumors*, 5th edition, New York, Wiley and Sons, 1997, pp 121–130.

cytokeratin-based IHC techniques, combined with multiple section examination of sentinel nodes, have resulted in the detection of micrometastases (generally <2 mm foci) in nodes previously reported to be negative. The prognostic significance of micrometastases is unknown at present, but is being investigated prospectively.

Other putative prognostic factors include urokinase plasminogen-like activator (uPA) and plasminogen activation inhibitor 1 (PAI-1) in node-negative disease, markers of proliferation and mitotic activity (Mib1, ki67, S-phase fraction), regulators of apoptosis and cellular cycling (p53, bcl2), markers of angiogenic capacity (vascular endothelial growth factor [VEGF] levels, insulin-like growth factor [IGF-1], microvessel density), and others (cathepsin D, cell ploidy).

At present, patient age, menopausal status, pathologic nodal status, tumor size, HR status, and lymphatic and vascular invasion status provide adequate prognostic information to enable the clinician to make adjuvant treatment recommendations. With the development of target-specific therapies, other molecular markers, like HER2 status, are playing increasingly important roles as prognostic and/or predictive markers.

ADJUVANT THERAPY

Various nuances of adjuvant therapy are under clinical investigation in the continual search for improvements in survival/cure following early BC, however, it is possible to make several general statements about currently recommended adjuvant therapy (Table 23.3).

TABLE 23.3. Summary of the 15-Year Absolute Survival Benefits from Adjuvant Therapy

	Overall Survival		Breast Cancer Survival		
	%	p Value	%	p Value	Other Deaths
Ovarian ablation vs not[1]					
With no chemotherapy	9.4	0.00005	9.8	0.00003	
With chemotherapy	1.4	0.04	1.6	0.04	
Tamoxifen 5 years or not[2]		<0.00001			
All groups	5.8		9.0	<0.00001	0.2
Node negative	5.2				
Node positive	7.5				
<50 years old	4.9				
50–59 years old	4.5				
60–69 years old	7.9				
70+ years old	9.5				
No chemotherapy	5.9				
Chemotherapy	5.7				

[1] Women < 50 years only.
[2] ER poor excluded.

TABLE 23.4. Van Nuys Prognostic Index for Ductal Carcinoma *In Situ*

Points	1	2	3
Size, mm	<16	16–40	>40
Margin width, mm	>9	1–9	<1
Pathology	No high grade and no necrosis	No high grade, necrosis present	High grade with or without necrosis
	3–4 Points	5–7 Points	>7 Points
Recommended local therapy	Lumpectomy	Lumpectomy plus radiotherapy	Mastectomy plus level I axillary dissection

Noninvasive Disease

DCIS Randomized controlled trials in DCIS have shown a significant reduction in ipsilateral recurrence with the addition of radiotherapy to breast-conserving surgery. However, this approach may not be necessary for lesions that are of low recurrence risk and it may not be sufficient in reducing recurrence in high-risk DCIS. Several criteria have been explored to attempt to quantify recurrence risk, yielding assessment tools such as the Van Nuys Prognostic Index (Table 23.4). Using this index, it is estimated that breast-conserving surgery alone is sufficient for low-risk lesions, breast-conserving surgery followed by radiotherapy is preferable for intermediate-risk lesions, and for high-risk lesions, mastectomy with level I axillary dissection is recommended. Compared with placebo, 5 years of tamoxifen has been shown to reduce subsequent invasive and noninvasive breast malignancies by 49% after breast-conserving surgery and radiotherapy for DCIS. This adjunctive therapy has been widely adopted for the management of DCIS, although corroborative evidence from ongoing studies is desirable.

LCIS LCIS is associated with increased risk of BC in either breast. Options following a pathologic diagnosis of LCIS include surveillance and consideration of prevention strategies, including tamoxifen, and bilateral mastectomy. Alternatively, participation in a randomized trial addressing such controversies would be a reasonable management strategy. The NSABP P-01 primary prevention trial, which included women with prior LCIS, showed a 49% relative risk reduction for invasive and noninvasive BC for tamoxifen over placebo, suggesting that this may be an effective preventative strategy for this group of at risk women.

Invasive Disease: Local Therapy

The Breast Large randomized controlled trials have demonstrated equivalent local recurrence rates and overall survival for women with operable BC treated with either mastectomy alone or adequate local excision (partial mastectomy) followed by breast radiotherapy. Both approaches are considered standards of care. Recommended radiotherapy is 45–50 Gy given in fractions of 2–2.5 Gy to the breast, with or without an additional boost of 10–25 Gy to the tumor bed. Clinical situations where mastectomy (with or without reconstruction, using saline implants, transabdominal or latissimus dorsi muscles to form the new breast mound) is preferred include patient choice, large tumors (particularly if the breast is small), multicentric tumors, clinical evidence of dermal invasion (peau d'orange, tethering, ulceration, inflammatory disease), locally advanced disease (unless first cytoreduced by neoadjuvant therapy), and for anyone in whom radiotherapy is contraindicated (including inability to adequately abduct the arm, patient refusal, prior radiotherapy to the region, and connective tissue diseases such as scleroderma and systemic lupus). The highest recurrence risk occurs for tumors with four or more positive nodes, gross extracapsular extension, large primaries, and close or positive deep surgical margins, situations for which locoregional (supraclavicular, internal mammary node, and axillary regions) radiotherapy is recommended. In women with multiple node positive disease who have undergone mastectomy, chest wall radiation is also recommended based on evidence of survival benefit in several randomized controlled trials. Radiotherapy-associated morbidity from breast irradiation is low, particularly with modern radiation techniques that deliver less extraneous radiotherapy to the lung and heart. Nevertheless, accelerated atherosclerosis and increased late cardiac deaths have been associated with left-sided breast and chest wall radiotherapy, and breast angiosarcomas are a rare sequelae of radiation. Other rare side effects include radiation pneumonitis, arm edema (13–18%), and brachial plexopathy (1–6%). Hyperpigmentation and fine telangactasias are common, non-serious sequelae of radiation.

The Axilla and Other Nodal Areas   Adequate assessment of the axillary nodes is mandatory in the local management of invasive BC. The current standard of care, axillary node dissection, provides relevant prognostic information, and at least for women with axillary node metastases, significantly reduces the risk of axillary recurrence. Clinical assessment of axillary status is insensitive: studies in which women with clinically node negative disease had only a few or no nodes removed (and no axillary radiotherapy) had 10-year axillary recurrence rates of 18–37%.

Sentinel node biopsy alone may prove to be adequate for women with negative sentinel nodes, thus reducing the surgical morbidity of axillary dissection for this group of women. Whether axillary radiotherapy can safely replace dissection for women with positive sentinel nodes is under investigation. Routine biopsy of the IMN and subclavicular nodes has fallen out of fashion due to technical complexity (particularly when a breast-conserving surgery is performed) and lack of demonstrable enhancement of survival or local control.

Two randomized studies have shown reduction in distant recurrences and BC mortality in women with at least four positive lymph nodes who received radiotherapy inclusive of the axilla following mastectomy and adjuvant chemotherapy (CT). Evidence is not conclusive as to whether there is a survival benefit in women with one to three involved nodes. Whether incorporation of an IMN field provides additional benefit for women with node-positive disease is the subject of two ongoing large randomized controlled trials (NCIC and EORTC).

Invasive Disease: Systemic Therapy

Elderly Women The optimal treatment of women older than 69 represents a wide-open research opportunity, because most randomized trials to date have excluded this age group. Although compared with younger women, a greater proportion of tumors in older women are low grade and HR positive, a greater proportion are also stages III and IV, emphasizing the need to identify and provide adequate treatment for these women.

Elderly women with HR-positive, node-negative disease probably derive more harm (in terms of side effects) than benefit (in terms of recurrence risk reduction) from adjuvant CT. Adjuvant tamoxifen, on the other hand, has a low side effect profile and is recommended for both node-negative and node-positive HR-positive disease. Twenty-year follow-up of a trial in women >65 years old with ER-positive or unknown, node-positive BC treated with mastectomy showed a significantly better disease-free survival ($p = 0.002$) and time to relapse ($p < 0.001$) in the tamoxifen versus placebo-treated patients. Due primarily to death from other causes (40% of study population at 20 years), there was no overall survival advantage for tamoxifen, but there was a substantial reduction in BC-specific mortality (60% vs. 77%). The addition of CT requires careful consideration of individual absolute benefit and harm, which may be very different for 65- and 85-year-old women with similar tumors, and for women of the same age with different co-morbid illnesses and functional capacity.

CT remains a treatment option for fit elderly women with a reasonable life expectancy and HR-negative disease, based on extrapolation of risk and benefit in younger women. However, here again, the potential incidence and severity of side effects must be carefully weighed against the expected survival gain, recognizing that women are living longer than previously and that BC recurrences are generally incurable.

Other Age Groups

Hormone Therapy: Tamoxifen The proportional reduction in 10-year mortality in women of all ages with HR-positive BC treated with 5 years of tamoxifen versus no tamoxifen is 26% (absolute reductions in death of 5.6% and 10.9% for node-negative and node-positive BC, respectively). The 2000 Oxford Overview confirms a significant survival benefit for tamoxifen with 15 years of follow-up, with the most significant improvement starting after 5 years.

Adjuvant tamoxifen, 20 mg/day for 5 years, is therefore recommended for all women, both pre-and postmenopausal, with HR-positive BC. The estimate of benefit from tamoxifen is derived from a heterogenous group of trials and patients, making it impossible to approximate the benefit in particular risk subsets, such as women with very-low-risk node-negative BC. However, in general, it can be stated that the absolute benefit is proportional to the absolute risk. Because tamoxifen has a low level of serious side effects and has been shown to reduce HR-positive contralateral BC by 47%, secondary prevention may be a reason to consider tamoxifen even in women with very-low-risk HR-positive BC.

In postmenopausal women with HR-positive disease, tamoxifen should be offered if HRs are positive, regardless of whether CT is considered. The number of premenopausal women treated with adjuvant tamoxifen and with 10 or more years of follow-up is small, and several studies are still exploring the absolute magnitude of benefit in this population. Nevertheless, 5 years of tamoxifen is recommended for premenopausal women with HR-positive disease.

Additional benefits of tamoxifen include a reduction in low-density lipoprotein and total cholesterol, a probable reduction in the incidence of coronary artery disease–associated deaths, and protection against osteoporosis by stabilizing the rate of postmenopausal bone demineralization. The incidence of serious side effects with tamoxifen is low. There is a fourfold increase in endometrial cancer over the general population incidence of 0.1% (North America), and a 0.02% risk of endometrial cancer death. The risk of deep venous thrombosis (DVT) and its potential sequelae is in the order of 5%. The benefit risk ratio of tamoxifen must be carefully weighed for patients with a previous history of spontaneous DVT or pulmonary embolism, or with an inherited disorder of coagulation. The nonserious, but nevertheless potentially troublesome side effects include vaginal dryness, depression, cataract formation, and hot flushes, the latter being the most frequent.

Even tumors with very low expression of HRs derive benefit from tamoxifen. However tamoxifen provides no survival benefit and is not recommended for HR negative tumors.

The recently reported ATAC trial compared tamoxifen to anastrozole (an aromatose inhibitor) in postmenopausal women. A small but statistically significant improvement in disease-free survival was observed for anastrozole. In particular, anastrozole reduced the risk of contralateral BC buy a striking 60% compared with tamoxifen. There were fewer thrombotic events but greater risk of osteoporosis with anastrozole. Anastrozole is therefore a reasonable alternative to tamoxifen in women at high risk for DVT; however, bone density should be monitored. Longer followup will determine whether anastrozole also provides a survival benefit over tamoxifen.

Ovarian Ablation   In the absence of CT, ovarian ablation (OA) has been shown to improve survival (absolute improvement 9.8%) and reduce BC recurrence (absolute reduction 8.5%) in women <50 years compared with control. Ovarian suppression using a leutenizing hormone releasing hormone analog (LHRHa) is an alternative to surgical or irradiation-induced castration, with the added advantage of being reversible. The optimal duration of LHRHa suppression has not been established, although recent randomized trials have used between 2 and 5 years.

Whether OA is equivalent to adjuvant CT is still unclear, as many trials have reported only preliminary results or have important design limitations, such as no tamoxifen or suboptimal CT regimens. Results to date suggest equivalence in terms of relapse-free survival, but follow-up is too short to determine whether overall survival differences will emerge for one treatment or the other within the entire population or for particular subgroups. Several randomized trials comparing OA and CT are still accruing or are closed but unreported. A part of the benefit of adjuvant CT in premenopausal women is derived from the induction of amenorrhea. Thus, it seems logical that OA provides protection against relapse. However, it may be that OA is inferior to CT in some scenarios, such as tumors with aggressive features and in older premenopausal women. This is an area that requires further investigation.

Consideration of side effects and adverse sequelae of CT and OA must also enter the equation when assessing their relative benefits. Quality-of-life data from one large trial suggested better overall tolerance of LHRHa than CMF among premenopausal women with node-positive disease.

Finally, there is the question of whether the OA provides additional benefit when added to CT and tamoxifen in premenopausal women. The most recent Oxford Overview reported a nonsignificant decrease in recurrence rate and a nonsignificant increase in death with the addition of OA to CT. However, recent individual well-designed trials suggest that there may be a benefit. Two trials have reported increased disease-free survival (DFS) but equivalent overall survival for women randomized to CT followed by reversible ovarian suppression and tamoxifen for 5 years compared with either CT and OA or CT alone. It is possible that follow-up may insufficient to accurately reflect the effect of combined modality therapy on survival. Two additional studies reported in abstract form fail to show a survival improvement for the addition of OA to CT plus tamoxifen. A potential confounder in all these trials is the inclusion of premenopausal women who developed amenorrhea during CT, a group for which there is unlikely to be any added benefit of ovarian ablation. The ideal trial design, in which only women without CT-induced amneorrhea are randomized to ovarian ablation or not, is being planned by a large intergroup collaboration.

Predictive Factors for Hormone Responsiveness   Thus far, the presence of HRs is the only reliable predictor of hormone therapy sensitivity. Retrospective data suggest that overexpression of HER2 may be associated with tamoxifen resistance, but the quality of this evidence leaves us with indefinite conclusions. Women with tumors that overexpress HER2 and have positive HRs should not be denied tamoxifen; however, they should be followed carefully. Such tumors may be more sensitive to aromatase inhibitors. The relative sensitivity of HER2-positive tumors to tamoxifen and aromatase inhibitors requires prospective investigation.

Ongoing Investigations   Currently, active randomized controlled trials of adjuvant hormone therapy are examining whether more than 5 years of tamoxifen is superior to 5 years, based on the observation from Oxford Overviews that 5 years is better than 2 or 1 year. Although three randomized studies have thus far reported no benefit for prolonging tamoxifen, follow-up may be early, and the sample size too small to adequately test the hypothesis. Two large ongoing trials (the ATLAS and ATTOM trials) do have adequate size and power, however. The efficacy and adverse event rate (particularly endometrial proliferation and thromboembolic disease) of new aromatase inhibitors (letrozole, anastrozole, exemestane) and new selective estrogen receptor modulators are being explored in current adjuvant trials both on their own or in sequence with tamoxifen. Finally, whether the combination of OA with either tamoxifen or CT or both improves survival is under investigation.

Chemotherapy Recommendations for adjuvant CT are derived from the Oxford Overviews of polyCT, individual randomized trials, and the St. Gallen consensus on prognostic factors. Three to six months of adjuvant CMF or anthracycline-based polyCT is associated with highly significant 15-year absolute reductions in death for young women (<50 years) with node negative (7%) and positive (11%) BC, and older women (50–69 years) with node negative (2%) and positive (3%) BC, regardless of the added use of tamoxifen. Although not yet published, the Oxford 2000 overview confirms these figures.

CT is recommended for HR-negative BC, because hormone therapy is ineffective and relapse risk is higher than for HR-positive disease. However, the lower limit of size among HR-negative tumors that derive an absolute benefit from CT is unknown. This may be of particular relevance in older women, because both the tolerance to CT and the absolute benefit (due to competing causes of death) decrease with advancing age.

Premenopausal Women Premenopausal women with node-positive disease and with non–low-risk node-negative disease (Table 23.2) should be offered adjuvant CT, regardless of HR status. The relapse and death rates in women with very-high-risk disease, such as more than 10 positive lymph nodes, locally advanced and inflammatory disease remain unacceptably high, despite (neo) adjuvant CT and endocrine therapy. Whenever possible, women with very high risk of relapse should be offered participation in a randomized clinical trial exploring novel therapeutic strategies. At the other end of the risk spectrum are very small tumors that are node negative and have features suggestive of low aggressive potential. Here, the decision to offer CT must take into consideration a patient's willingness to accept the potential side effects associated with adjuvant regimens, for very low absolute gains in survival.

Postmenopausal Women The Oxford 2000 Overview suggests that the survival advantage of CT in women 50–69 years old endures to the 10-year follow-up mark, and is attenuated thereafter. Moreover, the benefit is greatest for women with ER negative and ER unknown disease. Subgroup analyses, such as by number of positive nodes and grade, are needed to determine the magnitude of benefit in different risk groups.

Whether the magnitude of benefit of CT in ER-positive, node-negative BC treated with tamoxifen warrants the associated side effects is debatable based on the latest Oxford Overview results. Given the worse prognosis, the presence of positive axillary nodes, particularly if multiple, merits the consideration of adding adjuvant CT to tamoxifen in ER-positive disease. A few randomized studies comparing CT plus tamoxifen to tamoxifen alone in node-positive disease suggest there is added benefit of CT, whereas others suggest there is none. Many of these trials have design flaws such as suboptimal CT regimens and less than 5 years of tamoxifen, making their results difficult to interpret. In general, however, studies that incorporated an anthracycline show a survival advantage for the combination, while incorporation of CMF did not. Most trials addressing the value of adding CT to tamoxifen in postmenopausal women have significant design flaws. However, one well designed radomized trial (intergroup 0100) reported a 25% reduction in mortality for the addition of CT (CAF) to tamoxifen in women with positive nodes.

The decision to offer CT to postmenopausal women with ER-positive BC who receive tamoxifen must be individualized, using clinical judgment and taking into account prognostic features of the tumor, including the number of involved nodes, tumor size and grade, and patient age, general health, and treatment preferences.

Anthracyclines versus CMF   The choice of CT regimen depends on recurrence risk, co-morbid illness, and patient preference. Anthracycline-based CT is associated with a 4% greater absolute risk reduction for recurrence and death than CMF at 10 years follow-up for node-positive disease and 1.7% for node-negative disease. A unique toxicity of anthracyclines is cardiomyopathy, with a risk of less than 5% when the maximum cumulative dose of doxorubicin does not exceed $450\,\text{mg/m}^2$. The risk increases with cumulative dose, preexisting cardiac dysfunction, and hypertension. Epirubicin has a wider therapeutic index with respect to cardiotoxicity (1.8 compared with doxorubicin).

Anthracycline-based CT should be considered for women with node-positive and high-risk node-negative disease, and CMF for women with either low-to-moderate relapse risk or high risk of cardiac failure. Anthracyclines are generally preferred for premenopausal women, given that young age is an independent negative prognostic factor. In postmenopausal women for whom CT is warranted, the benefit-harm ratio must be considered when choosing a regimen.

Taxanes versus No Taxanes   There is insufficient evidence to determine the value of adding taxanes to adjuvant polyCT. There are few ongoing large trials exploring their benefit in node-negative disease, and data is available for only about 8,000 (three trials) of the 24,000 women enrolled in adjuvant taxane trials for node-positive disease. The Cancer and Leukemia Group B (CALGB) 9344 trial of 4AC (doxorubicin and cyclophosphamide) followed or not by four cycles of paclitaxel showed a significant 2% ($p < 0.05$) survival advantage for paclitaxel, which may be greatest for patients with ER-negative disease. The extent to which this advantage is due to the additional 12 weeks of CT rather than the paclitaxel specifically, is not known. Two other trials (an M.D. Anderson trial and NSABP B-28), including one of similar size and design, have thus far reported equivalence for the addition or not of paclitaxel. A recently reported trial of anthracyclines plus docetaxel (TAC) versus FAC (BCIRG 001) showed superior disease free and overall survival for the taxane containing regimen. Confirmatory evidence of benefit is critical, particularly when adjuvant regimens of longer duration and potentially more toxicity are being considered for routine use.

Optimal Doses and Schedules

CMF   The classic Bonadonna CMF regimen is the most widely tested CMF schedule. Dose intensity is important, survival being better in women who receive at least 85% of the planned doses. Inferior survival was observed in the metastatic setting with alternate CMF schedules, which raises the hypothesis that the chief benefit of cyclophosphamide is in chronic continuous (oral) rather than bolus (intravenous [IV]) dosing. Although the various schedules have not been compared in the adjuvant setting, it is probably prudent to give the classic CMF regimen preferentially, reserving intravenous cyclophosphamide for women who are unable to tolerate oral cyclophosphamide.

One prospective study demonstrated that 6 cycles of CMF are as effective as 12. Trials comparing 3 cycles of CMF to 6 or 9 have insufficient follow-up to determine if fewer than 6 cycles is equally effective or if there are any subsets for which this is an adequate regimen. At least one trial (International BC Study Group IV), however, reported superiority for 6 versus 3 cycles, particularly for young women and women with HR-negative tumors. The majority of clinicians would advocate at least 6 cycles of CMF to achieve maximum benefit.

Anthracyclines   There are many anthracyline-containing adjuvant CT regimens in use worldwide. Doxorubicin (A) or epirubicin (E) and cyclophosphamide (C) (AC or EC) are commonly used, sometimes followed by several cycles of CMF in Europe. There are innumerable variations on the number of cycles, length of cycle, and dose per cycle of the drugs in the adjuvant combination 5-fluorouracil (F), E or A, and C (FEC/CEF, FAC/CAF), and the choice of schedule and number of cycles depends on clinician and center experience. However, it should be borne in mind that four cycles of AC or EC may be inferior to longer anthracycline regimens. This is based on the observation that more than four cycles but not four cycles of anthracyclines have shown superiority over CMF. Additionally, a few studies that directly compared anthracycline combinations that differed only in the dose per cycle or total number of cycles found that more cycles were better than fewer.

There appear to be two distinct risk profiles for BC, with recurrence rates peaking at either 2 and 5 years from diagnosis. The number of cycles may be of particular relevance for cancers that have a high risk of early recurrence, such as HR-negative or HER2-positive tumors. An additional reason for reduced efficacy of shorter anthracycline regimens may be a lower rate of CT induced-amenorrhea. Thus 4AC/EC may not be the optimal anthracycline regimen for young women and women with high-risk disease but may be reasonable in postmenopausal women and women with moderate relapse risk.

Dose Intensity   Although dose intensification of anthracyclines and cyclophosphamide have failed to show superiority over the doses in AC $60/600 \, mg/m^2$ or epirubicin $75–100 \, mg/m^2$, suboptimal dose intensity and/or cumulative doses are clearly linked with inferior survival. Thus, a concerted effort must be made to

TABLE 23.5. Adjuvant Trials of Herceptin in HER2 Overexpressing Breast Cancer

Group/Trial	Target Accrual	Design	Tamoxifen for 5 Years	HER2 Eligibility
NCCTG N9831	3,000	4 AC then T/weekly × 12 4 AC then T/weekly × 12 then H weekly × 12 m 4 AC then T+H/weekly × 12 then H weekly × 12 m	All ER (+) patients	3+ by IHC or FISH amplified with 2+
BCIRG	2,400	AC then 4D AC then 4D then H weekly × 12 m 6D/carbo/CDDP + H then H weekly × 12 m	All ER (+) patients	FISH amplified
NSABP B31	2,700	4AC then 4T 4AC then 4T + H/weekly then, H × 12 m	All patients except ER/PgR (−)	3+ by IHC or FISH amplified with 2+
BIG (HERA trial)	3,200	Any chemotherapy then H q3weeks × 12 m Any chemotherapy then H q3weeks × 24 m Any chemotherapy then observation	Not mandatory; each center to set a policy a priori	3+ by IHC or FISH amplified

Abbreviations: AC, doxorubicin and cyclophosphamide; BCIRG, Breast Cancer International Study Group; D, docetaxel; BIG, Breast International Group; carbo, carboplatinum; CDDP, cisplatin; FISH, fluorescence in situ hybridization; H, Herceptin or trastuzumab; IHC, immunohistochemistry; m, months; NCCTG, North Central Cancer Trials Group; NSABP, National Surgical Adjuvant Breast Project; T, paclitaxel;

deliver CT on time and at the planned doses, using colony growth-stimulating factors and/or prophylactic antibiotics after an episode of prolonged or febrile neutropenia that interferes with delivery of subsequent cycles. There is no evidence to support a survival advantage for high-dose CT with stem cell transplant after induction CT.

Toxicity The side-effect profile of individual drugs and drug classes differs and is covered in greater detail under the treatment for metastatic disease. Most women can expect to experience varying degrees of reversible alopecia, nausea, vomiting, temporary reductions in peripheral leucocyte and neutrophil counts, anemia, mucositis, and in premenopausal women, amenorrhea. Less frequent side effects include chemical cystitis (cyclophosphamide), diarrhea (5-fluorouracil), and peripheral neuropathy (taxanes). The incidence of febrile neutropenia is between 5–30%, depending on the regimen used. The permanence of amenorrhea, ovarian dysfunction, and infertility depends on the regimen duration and the patient's proximity to natural menopause. There is a small risk of anthracycline-induced cardiomyopathy that rises with cumulative dose. Both anthracyclines and CMF-based regimens are associated with a small risk (0.5–2.0%) of secondary leukemia. Cognitive dysfunction has been reported by many women having chemotherapy. However quantification of this side effect is only recently being prospectively evaluated.

Predictive Factors for Response to Chemotherapy There are no currently accepted definitive predictors of CT sensitivity or resistance. Putative predictors include overexpression of HER2, and p53 mutations, however, prospective confirmation is necessary. Retrospective observations suggest that HER2 overexpression may predict for relative sensitivity to anthracyclines and anthracycline dose intensity, however, the evidence is not rigorous. If HER2 status is available, preference for CT over none and for anthracyclines over CMF may be reasonable for women with HER2-positive tumors, based on evidence available today. HER2 overexpression, particularly at the 3+ level by IHC, or gene amplification, predicts for response to anti-HER2 therapy in metastatic disease and this strategy is being explored in ongoing adjuvant trials (Table 23.5).

Mutations of p53 predict for relative taxane sensitivity and anthracycline resistance in laboratory models. One prospective trial is examining its predictive value in patients with large operable and locally advanced BC. However, p53 status is not in common use in the clinical setting to aid the clinician in choosing a CT regimen. Other predictive factors for CT efficacy remain elusive. However, evolving expertise with molecular biology and DNA microarray analysis holds promise of identifying new genes or patterns of gene expression that can reliably predict responsiveness and thereby improve treatment individualization.

Ongoing Investigations Currently active randomized controlled trials are exploring the value of taxanes, bisphosphonates, and the anti-HER2 agent trastuzumab, in the adjuvant setting. Better risk assessment and refining the balance between toxicity and efficacy of polyCT are also being addressed.

LOCALLY ADVANCED BREAST CANCER

Locally advanced BC refers to any of clinically involved axillary nodes, a large and/or inoperable primary tumor, and inflammatory disease. Treatment of these high-risk breast cancers involves aggressive systemic therapy, radiotherapy, and surgery. Unfortunately, the recurrence and death rates following locally advanced and inflammatory disease remain high despite multimodality therapy. The 5-year overall survival after locally advanced disease is 20–30% and for inflammatory disease is 5–10%. Neoadjuvant CT, hormone therapy, and radiotherapy can reduce tumor volume, increasing the probability of being able to perform breast-conserving surgery. However, neoadjuvant therapy does not impact significantly on overall survival compared with adjuvant therapy. Pathologic complete response is an independent good prognostic factor. However, pathologic complete response rarely exceeds 20% for a given neoadjuvant regimen. New treatment strategies are needed for this high-risk BC population.

FOLLOW-UP

The goals of regular follow-up after and during adjuvant therapy include continuous monitoring of adjuvant therapy sequelae, early detection of operable locoregional recurrences, and surveillance for second primary BCs with annual mammograms. Although periodic follow-up visits provide reassurance for some patients, they induce anxiety in others. BC can have a profound effect on an individual's life and interpersonal relationships, and counseling is sometimes necessary to help a patient deal with altered body image, fear of death and illness, diminished libido, and other issues. Studies have failed to show a survival advantage for detection of asymptomatic distant metastases using periodic screening tests such as bone scans, chest x-rays, and liver imaging. Serial measurement of tumor markers has also not proven to impact on survival.

A rough guide for follow-up is every 3–4 months during the first 2 years, every 6 months thereafter to 5 years, and then yearly. A history and physical examination with or without routine blood tests are a minimum requirement at each visit. Annual mammograms are recommended to screen for second primary cancers. Patients with symptoms or signs suspicious for recurrence should have a full metastatic work-up, including symptom-directed exams. Premenopausal women with permanent amenorrhea should be assessed for osteoporosis risk. Routine endometrial ultrasound and biopsy for women on tamoxifen has not proved to be a cost-effective screen for endometrial cancer due to a high false-positive rate. Postmenopausal vaginal bleeding should be promptly investigated for women on tamoxifen.

Metastatic Breast Cancer

Metastatic breast cancer (MBC) is largely incurable. The exception is some isolated operable locoregional recurrences. Of note, future distant metastases occur in 85% of women (by 10 years) after such regional relapses and close surveillance is warranted. Although there are no sancturaries, the most frequent distant sites of recurrence are lung, liver, and bone. Lobular carcinomas can also recur with ovarian and peritoneal metastases. Less frequently, central nervous system metastases (single or multiple cerebral lesions and leptomeningeal carcinomatosis) can arise.

The goals of therapy include adequate symptom palliation, restoration/preservation of quality of life, and, whenever possible, prolongation of life of adequate quality. Given that therapy is not curative, the balance between toxicity, which can diminish quality of life, and expected benefit, is an important consideration, particularly for multiply pretreated patients. The median survival from diagnosis of metastatic disease is 18–24 months. However, the proportion of patients surviving 1, 2, and even more years may be slowly increasing as our armamentarium of active treatments increases. Of particular promise is the growing number of target-specific molecules that are in various stages of clinical trials that, alone or in combination with cytotoxic or hormonal therapies, may reduce tumor bulk and slow progression.

Hormone Therapy

Sequential hormone therapy can provide a substantial period of tumor shrinkage or stabilization with reduction in symptoms. However, the reduction in tumor volume tends to occur only after several months of therapy and, therefore, this treatment modality may be of limited value for patients with rapidly evolving disease or significant symptoms related to tumor bulk. Metastases from a HR-negative primary have an exceedingly low probability of response to hormone therapy and should be treated with other modalities.

The increasing use of adjuvant tamoxifen, eventual resistance in metastatic disease, and the high incidence of toxicity with early alternate hormone maneuvers (such as megace and aminoglutethimide) have led to the development of new hormone therapies. The nonsteroidal aromatase inhibitors anastrozole and letrozole are non-cross-resistant with tamoxifen and have proven to be more active and better tolerated than aminoglutethimide and megestrol acetate, quickly supplanting these drugs as second-line agents (Table 23.6). They effectively reduce circulating levels of estrogen by binding and reversibly inhibiting the activity of adipose and tumor tissue aromatase, which converts androgens to estrogens and provides the major source of estrogen following menopause. Letrozole has shown superiority in terms of time to progression (TTP) over tamoxifen in first-line therapy of postmenopausal women with hormone-sensitive disease. Interestingly, the study in question had a built in cross-over design at progression, so that it will be possible to conclude whether the order in which these two drugs is given is important in terms of survival. Anastrozole showed equivalent TTP and survival to tamoxifen in first-line therapy for postmenopausal women and a lower incidence of thromboembolic events. The steroidal irreversible aromatase inactivator, exemestane, is currently being compared in this setting in a randomized trial, and has already shown high activity and tolerability after tamoxifen and, to a modest extent, after nonsteroidal aromatase inhibitors.

For premenopausal women, tamoxifen and ovarian ablation are effective therapies in hormone-sensitive disease and are sometimes combined. At least one

TABLE 23.6. Randomized Trials of Third-Generation AIs Versus Standard Hormonal Therapy in MBC

Author, Year	AI	Control	Population	N	Endpt	AI	Control	p Value	Toxicity
			First-line Therapy						
Paridaens, 2000	Exemestane 25 mg/d	Tam 20 mg/d	MBC first line ER +/unk if DFI >2 y	100+	RR TTP	40.9 NA	13.6 NA	NA	N/A
Nabholtz and Bonneterre, two studies, and pooled results,* 1999	Anastrozole 1 mg/d	Tam 20 mg/d	Study 0027 Postmeno, ER or PgR + (44%) or unk	668	RR TTP CB	32% 8 m 56%	32% 8 m 55%	NS NS NS	Hot flushes: A 21% T 21% VTE: A 5% T 7% GI SE: A 23% T 28%
			Study 0030 Postmeno ER or PgR + (88%) or unk	353	RR TTP CB	21% 11 m 59%	17% 5.6 m 46%	0.005 0.009	Hot flushes: A 38% T 28% VTE: A 4% T 8% GI SE: A 54% T 57%
			Study 0027+0030	1021	RR TTP CB	29% 8.5 m 57%	27% 7.0 m 52%	NS 0.02 NS	VTE: A 4.5% T 7.6% p value not given
Mouridsen, 2003	Letrozole 2.5 mg	Tam 20 mg/d	MBC first line, postmeno ER or PgR + or unk		RR TTP CB	32% 9.4 m 50%	21% 6.0 m 38%	0.0002 0.0001 0.0004	Hot flushes: L 19% T 16%
			First and/or Second Line Therapy						
Buzdar and Jonat, two studies and pooled results,* 1996, 1997	Anastrozole 1 mg/d 10 mg/d	MA 160 mg/d	N. America (6 m fu)	386	RR CB	10/6% 37/30%	6% 36%	NS NS	A: GI SE MA: wt gain
			Europe/UK	378	CB	34/34%	33%	NS	A: GI SE MA: wt gain, edema, dyspnea
			Combined studies Postmeno, Tam failure	764	RR CB OS	10/9% 35/32% 26.7 m	8% 34% 22.5 m	NS NS 0.025	A: GI SE MA: wt gain

Study	Drug	Dose	Comparator/Dose	Population	N	Endpt	AI	Comparator	p	Side effects
Dombernowsky, 1998	Letrozole	0.5 mg/d 2.5 mg/d	MA 160 mg/d	Tam failure	551	RR TTP	12/24% 5.1/5.6 m	16% 5.5 m	0.004 (L2.5 v MA) 0.07	VTE: L0.5 mg L2.5 mg MA (n) 2 0 15
Gershanovich, 1998	Letrozole	0.5 mg 2.5 mg	AG 500 mg/d	Tam failure (first/second line MBC)	555	RR DR OS	17/20% 21/24 m 21/28 m	12% 15m 20 m	NS Trend 0.0002	Letrozole: nausea AG: rash
Kaufmann,[*] 1999	Exemestane	25 mg/d	MA 160 mg/d	Tam failures MBC	769	RR TTP OS	15% 4.7 m not reached	12% 3.8 m 28.4 m	NS 0.04 0.04	E: >5%: n, hot flashes, fatigue MA: >5%: fatigue, sweating, appetite, nausea, hot flashes

Abbreviations: AI, aromatase inhibitor; Endpt, endpoint; EORTC, European Organization for the Research and Treatment of Cancer; MBC, metastatic breast cancer; DFI, disease-free interval; postmeno, postmenopausal; TTP, time to progresssion; m, months; N/A not available; CB, clinical benefit (CR + PR + NC >6 months); VTE, venous thromboembolic disease; OS, overall survival; GI SE, gastrointestinal side effects; NS, not significant; MA, megestrol acetate; fu, follow-up; wt, weight; AG, aminoglutethimide; DR, duration of response.
[*]Significantly better OS for AI (for anastrozole 1 mg, only pooled studies showed OS advantage). OS was not the primary endpoint.
[**]Further development of the drug has been discontinued.

study and a meta-analysis suggest that the combination is superior to either alone. The reduction in estrogen levels achieved with aromatase inhibitors is insufficient to maximally suppress endogenous estrogen stimulation, and combination with oophorectomy or an LHRHa is recommended.

Several new selective estrogen receptor modulators and pure antiestrogens are in various stages of development. With higher specificity for the ER and less stimulatory effect on the endometrium, these drugs have the potential to provide superior efficacy and reduced toxicity compared with tamoxifen. One pure antiestrogen, faslodex, has demonstrated equivalence to anastrozole for response rate, TTP, and tolerability in first-line therapy. Survival data is not yet available.

Chemotherapy

HR-negative tumors and some HR-positive tumors are *de novo* insensitive to hormone therapy. In addition, hormone-sensitive disease eventually becomes resistant, possibly due to up-regulation of the ER and increased sensitivity to minute estrogen levels. CT must generally be employed in such cases. In addition, CT produces more rapid responses and is therefore preferred over hormone therapy for patients with threatening visceral disease, such as significant or impending perturbation in organ function, large-volume metastases or diffuse organ infiltration, large pericardial or pleural effusions, and disease that is significantly symptomatic or rapidly progressive.

Active Drugs   Numerous different cytotoxic drug classes are active in BC, including anthracyclines, alkylators, antimetabolites, and microtubule stabilizing agents. Because they have different mechanisms of action, they are often non-cross-resistant and can produce responses after resistance has developed to other drugs. In general, there is an inverse relationship between the probability of response to a drug and the number of prior therapies.

Anthracyclines are the most frequently used and arguably the most active cytotoxic drugs in MBC. A response rate (RR) of 40–60% has been consistently demonstrated using doxorubicin at doses of ≥ 60–75 mg/m^2 every 3 weeks. The combination anthracycline-cyclophosphamide (AC) is commonly used as first-line CT in MBC, with or without 5-fluorouracil (F) in patients who have not previously received anthracyclines. Recent data from phase III trials show RRs of 41–57% and median TTP ranging from 6 to 9 months for (F)AC type regimens.

Due to the relationship between cardiomyopathy and cumulative dose, there is a limit to the total safe dose of anthracyclines that can be given. Generally, the threshold cumulative dose is a little higher in the metastatic than in the adjuvant settings, particularly for a patient with good response. Anthracyclines are increasingly used in the adjuvant setting, and tumors that recur after a short disease-free interval (within 6 or 12 months from adjuvant CT completion) are less likely to respond to them a second time. The usual side effects include alopecia, nausea and vomiting, neutropenia, mucositis, and, with high cumulative doses, cardiomyopathy. Antiemetics and other supportive measures reduce the severity of some of these. Liposomal encapsulation of doxorubicin (caelyx and TLC-D-99)

TABLE 23.7. Randomized Trials of Taxanes in the Treatment of MBC

Author, Year	No.	Comparison Arms	% RR (p Value)	Median TTP, months (p Value)	Median OS, months (p Value)	Comments
		First Line CT				
Paridaens, 2000	331	1. Paclitaxel (P)	25	4.2	pNS	
		2. Doxorubicin (A)	41 (0.003)	7.5 (0.001)	pNS	
Sledge, 1997	739	1. Paclitaxel	33	5.9	pNS	Different toxicities, similar
		2. Doxorubicin	34	6.2		tolerability
		3. P + A	46 (<0.007)	8.0 (<0.009)	N/A	
Nabholtz, 1999	429	1. AC	47	8.0	N/A	A + tax more toxic
		2. A + Docetaxel	60 (0.01)	9.3 (0.01)		
Biganzoli, 2000	275	1. AC		Available at ASCO 2000		
		2. A + P				
Bishop, 1999	209	1. Paclitaxel	29	5.3	17.3	Adj CMF with 6m DFI eligible for
		2. CMF-pred	35 (0.037)	6.4 (0.025)	13.9 (0.06)	trial
Müller, 1999	505	1. E + P	Overall response rate 48%. Results per arm not yet available			
		2. E + C				
Pluzanska, 1999	267	1. A + P	68	8.3	N/A	
		2. 5FU + A + C	55 (0.03)	6.2 (0.03)		
		Second Line CT				
Chan, 1999	326	1. Docetaxel	47.8	6.5	15	Previous alkylator-based CT allowed
		2. Doxorubicin	33.3 (0.008)	5.3 (NS)	14	
Sjöström, 1998	199	1. Docetaxel	42	6.0	N/A	
		2. MTX + 5FU	19 (<0.001)	3.0 (0.006)		
Monnier, 1998	172	1. Docetaxel	33	6.0	N/A	
		2. Navelbine + 5FU	26 (NA)	5.0 (NA)		
Nabholtz, 1999	392	1. Docetaxel	30	4.8	11.4	
		2. Mitomycin + Vn	11.6 (<0.001)	2.8 (0.001)	8.7	
O'Reilly, 1998	44	1. Capecitabine	36	3.0	N/A	
		2. Paclitaxel	21 (N/A)	3.1 (NA)		

Abbreviations: MBC, metastatic breast cancer; RR, relative risk; TTP, time to progression; OS, overall survival; CT, chemotherapy.

substantially reduces the cardiac threat while maintaining efficacy and is being explored in several clinical trials.

Taxanes have gained widespread use in MBC over the last 15 years. Single-agent paclitaxel has been shown to be as or slightly less effective than anthracyclines, and superior to CMF in first-line therapy (Table 23.7). Docetaxel has shown superior response but similar long-term outcome as anthracyclines. The major side effects associated with this drug class are peripheral sensory neuropathy, alopecia, nail changes, myalgias and arthralgias (paclitaxel), and neutropenia. Toxic typhlitis is a rare but potentially fatal side effect of docetaxel that constitutes mandatory treatment discontinuation. Prophylactic corticosteroids dramatically reduced the incidence of hypersensitivity with paclitaxel and fluid retention syndrome observed with docetaxol. Weekly schedules minimize hematologic toxicity without compromising efficacy and are being used with increased regularity by many clinicians.

Vinca alkaloids, particularly vinorelbine, are another antimicrotubulin class with reasonable activity in BC. Vinorelbine is particularly favored for elderly patients due to its mild toxicity profile. The major limitation to its use is neutropenia, the severity of which varies depending on the amount of prior CT. Peripheral neuropathy and alopecia tend to be less severe than with taxanes.

Fluoropyrimidines, particularly when given continuously, such as infusional 5-fluoropyrimidine (5-FU) and oral capecitabine, are both active and relatively well tolerated. The incidence of severe side effects, primarily diarrhea, palmar plantar erythrodysesthesia, and mucositis, is low. Dose reduction or delay due to hematologic toxicity are rarely necessary, even in heavily pretreated patients. Deficiency of dihydropyrimidine dehydrogenase (DPD), involved in the metabolism of 5-FU to nontoxic molecules, can result in life-threatening diarrhea and mucositis. Happily, this is rare, although low levels of DPD may account for a relatively higher incidence of toxicity in elderly women. Other drugs with modest single-agent activity in MBC include cyclophosphamide, oxaliplatin, cisplatin, gemcitabine, raltitrexed, topotecan, and irinotecan.

Although the order in which CT drugs are given does not seem to alter long-term outcome, it may impact on patient quality of life and therefore bears mentioning. Patients with symptomatic disease are likely to derive more benefit from drugs with a high response rate (maximal tumor shrinkage), whereas elderly or poor performance status patients may be best treated with drugs whose toxicity profile is low. Patient preference must also be considered: the frequency of clinic visits may be more important to some patients, whereas the potential side effects or activity may be relatively more important to others. The duration of therapy must also be balanced between maximal antitumor effect and acceptable level of side effects. Continuous therapy has not conclusively proven to be superior to one or two cycles beyond maximal response, or a fixed number of cycles in the absence of progression and the strategy employed is highly dependent on clinician bias and individual patient benefit.

Monotherapy versus Combination Therapy The sum total of randomized trials would suggest that combination CT is not superior to monotherapy in terms of survival prolongation. Nevertheless, combination therapy is thought to produce a more rapid and greater reduction in tumor volume and may be preferable for patients with bulky symptomatic disease.

Combining anthracyclines and taxanes was examined as a strategy for improving overall survival given their high single-agent activity. A study that compared doxorubicin and paclitaxel monotherapy to the combination failed to show a survival difference despite improved response rate and time to progression for the combination. No significant differences were observed in response rate, time to progression, or overall survival for sequential docetaxel and doxorubicin versus the combination in a smaller trial. Anthracycline and paclitaxel combinations have not demonstrated improved efficacy compared with anthracycline and cyclophosphamide, despite greater hematologic toxicity with the former (Table 23.7). Comparisons of anthracycline plus docetaxel versus anthracycline plus cyclophosphamide show a little more promise for the former association, but mature results are not yet available. A recently reported study demonstrated a survival advantage for docetaxel plus capecitabine compared with docetaxel alone in first-line CT. One possible explanation is that the continuous exposure of a tumor to CT (capecitabine) up-regulates apoptosis.

Taxane and Anthracycline Failure Patients who have progressed after anthracyclines and taxanes represent an increasing population for which effective treatments are needed. In this population, capecitabine, docetaxel (after paclitaxel), vinorelbine, and caelyx (liposomal doxorubicin) have shown some activity. In the subgroup of patients with HER2-positive disease, trastuzumab (an antibody to HER2) also has activity after CT.

Combined Chemotherapy and Hormone Therapy There is insufficient evidence to suggest an advantage to concurrent hormone and CT in metastatic disease. However, at least one group is examining the role of maintenance hormone therapy after a response to CT, based on retrospective observation of benefit.

High-Dose Chemotherapy High-dose CT with autologous stem cell support following a response to conventional CT has proved to be a disappointing therapeutic strategy, with four randomized trials reporting equivalent survival to and higher treatment related mortality and morbidity than conventional polyCT. Ongoing randomized trials are exploring other biologically rational strategies using this treatment modality, including up-front high-dose CT (to minimize emergence of drug resistance), multiple high-dose cycles (to maximize cell kill), and refining patient selection. However, scientific enthusiasm for this avenue of research is rather diminished based on consistently negative studies to date.

Target-Specific Therapy

Increased knowledge of the molecular biology of cancer has enabled the development of molecules that target a specific protein or gene that imparts some survival advantage to the malignant cell. The most successful example of this strategy in BC is trastuzumab, a monoclonal antibody directed against the epidermal growth factor receptor, HER2. In addition to single-agent activity, trastuzumab has been shown to improve survival when added to first line paclitaxel and anthracycline plus cyclophosphamide (25.4 months) compared with CT alone (20.9 months) in HER2-positive disease ($p = 0.05$). Subsequent reports suggest that the benefit is almost exclusively in tumors with protein overexpression at the 3+ level (by IHC) or gene amplification. Ongoing trials are exploring other combinations (such as with vinorelbine and CMF) and schedules (such as three weekly trastuzumab). The unexpected finding of increased cardiomyopathy when trastuzumab and anthracyclines were given together highlights the importance of carefully controlled trials even for molecules with specific targets, for which the side effect incidence is expected to be low.

The HER2 and trastuzumab story provides a model for treatment individualization, which is becoming increasingly recognized as a strategy of high priority. Other therapeutic targets in various stages of clinical investigation include inhibition of key points in pathways of angiogenesis, invasion and metastasis formation, cell cycle regulation, and growth and proliferation. The potential of these target-specific molecules remains to be elucidated.

Supportive Care

Supportive care is a critical component of therapy for metastatic disease. Bisphosphonates, which inhibit the resorptive activity of osteoclasts, have dramatically altered the management of hypercalcemia, the incidence and severity of bone pain, pathologic fractures and their sequelae (including spinal cord compression and the need for surgery), and the evolution of bone metastases. Regular dosing effectively slows progression of bony disease and ameliorates related symptoms. Radiotherapy is also effective for localized problems, such as bone pain, cutaneous metastases, bronchial obstruction, and central nervous system metastases with or without surgery. Other important adjuncts include adequate pain medications, red cell transfusions and recombinant erythropoietin for symptomatic anemia, colony-stimulating growth factors for treatment limiting neutropenia, pleurodesis for recurrent pleural effusions, oxygen for disease related dyspnea, and emotional support to help patients and families cope with end-of-life issues.

CONCLUSIONS

BC develops as a result of numerous as yet poorly understood alterations in gene function. Phenotypic and genotypic expression varies from one BC to the other, and can evolve over time within a given cancer. These factors explain variable sensitivity to different treatment modalities and provide valuable potential therapeutic approaches. Although modest gains have been made in BC mortality, research aims at further improving risk assessment, primary prevention, and adjuvant therapies strategies to reduce this mortality rate. Major goals of therapy and supportive care research in metastatic disease are to improve quality and duration of life.

FURTHER READING

General References

Harris, Lippman, Morrow, and Hellman (eds) (1996) *Diseases of the Breast*. Philadelphia, Lippincott-Raven.

Sobin LH, Wittekind CH (eds) (1997) *TNM Classification of Malignant Tumors*, 5th edition. New York NY, Wiley and Sons, pp 121–130.

Nabholtz JM, Tonkin K, Aapro MS, Buzdar AU (eds) (2000) *Breast Cancer Management: Application of Evidence to Patient Care*. Martin Dunitz Ltd, London, 2000.

Breast cancer topics: http://www.cancernet.nci.nih.gov/cancer_types/breast_cancer.shtml.

Mammography

Fletcher SW, Black W, Harris R, Rimer BK, Shapiro S. (1993) Report of the International Workshop on Screening for Breast Cancer. *J Natl Cancer Inst* 85:1644–1656.

DCIS

Fisher B, Dignam J, Wolmark N et al. (1999) Tamoxifen in treatment of intraductal breast cancer: National Surgical Adjuvant Breast and Bowel Project B-24 randomized controlled trial. *Lancet* 353:1993–2000.

Silverstein MJ, Lagios MD, Craig PH et al. (1996) A prognostic index for ductal carcinoma in situ of the breast. *Cancer* 77:2267–2274.

Prevention

Fisher B, Costantino JP, Wickerham DL et al. (1998) Tamoxifen for prevention of BC: report of the National Surgical Adjuvant Breast and Bowel Project P-1 study. *J Natl Cancer Inst* 90:1371–1388.

Eeles RA, Powles TJ. (2000) Chemoprevention options for BRCA1 and BRCA2 mutation carriers. *J Clin Oncol* 18:93s–99s.

Hartmann LC, Schaid DJ, Woods JE et al. (1999) Efficacy of bilateral prophylactic mastectomy in women with a family history of breast cancer. *N Engl J Med* 340:77–84.

Radiotherapy

Early Breast Cancer Trialists' Collaborative Group (2000) Favourable and unfavourable effects on long-term survival of radiotherapy for early breast cancer: an overview of the randomized trials. *Lancet* 355:1757–1770.

Recht A, Edge SB, Solin LJ et al. (2001) Postmastectomy radiotherapy: guidelines of the American Society of Clinical Oncology, *J Clin Oncol* 19:1539–1569.

Bartelink H, Horiot J-C, Poortmans P et al. (2001) Recurrence rates after treatment of breast cancer with standard radiotherapy with or without additional radiation. *N Eng J Med* 345:1378–1387.

Sentinel Node Biopsy

Veronesi U, Paganelli G, Galimberti V et al. (1997) Sentinel-node biopsy to avoid axillary dissection in BC with clinically negative lymph-nodes. *Lancet* 349:1864–1867.

Prognostic Factors

Elston CW, Willis IO (1991) Pathological prognostic factors in BC. The value of histological grade in BC: experience from a large study with long-term follow-up. *Histopathology* 19:403–410.

Carter CL, Allen C, Henson DE (1989) Relation of tumor size, lymph node status, and survival in 24,740 BC cases. *Cancer* 63:181–187.

Perrone F, Carlomagno C, Lauria R et al. (1996) Selecting high-risk early BC patients: what to add to the number of metastatic nodes? *Eur J Cancer* 32A:41–46.

Slamon DJ, Clark GM, Wong SG et al. (1987) Human breast cancer: correlation of relapse and survival with amplification of the HER-2/neu oncogene. *Science* 9:177–182.

Adjuvant Therapy References

Early BC Trialists Collaborative Group (1998) Tamoxifen for early BC: an overview of the randomized trials. *Lancet* 351:1451–1467.

Early BC Trialists' Collaborative Group (2000) *2000 Analysis Overview Results*. Fifth Meeting of the Early BC Trialists' Collaborative Group. Oxford, UK, 21–23 September.

Early BC Trialists Collaborative Group (1998) PolyCT for early BC: an overview of the randomized trials. *Lancet* 352:930–942.

NIH consensus statement on adjuvant systemic therapy: http://odp.od.nih.gov/consensus/cons/114/114_intro.htm.

Metastatic Therapy

Hortobagyi G, Piccart M, Awada A, Hamilton A (1999) *Options for Treatment of Metastatic Breast Cancer*. Educational session, American Society of Clinical Oncology Spring Education Book. Alexandria, Virginia, pp 514–539.

Sledge GW, Neuberg D, Ingle J et al. (1997) Phase III trial of doxorubicin (A) vs paclitaxel (T) vs doxorubicin + paclitaxel (A + T) as first-line therapy for metastatic breast cancer (MBC): an intergroup trial. *Proc Am Soc Clin Oncol* 16:1a (abstr 2).

Vogel C, O'Rourke M, Winer E et al. (1999) Vinorelbine as first line CT for advanced BC in women 60 years of age or older. *Ann Oncol* 10:397–402.

Jassem J, Pienkowski T, Pluzanska A et al. (2001) Doxorubicin and paclitaxel versus fluorouracil, doxorubicin, and cyclophosphamide as first-line therapy for women with MBC: final results of a randomized phase III multicenter trial. *J Clin Oncol* 19:1707–1715.

Slamon D, Leyland-Jones B, Shak S et al. (2001) Use of chemotherapy plus a monoclonal antibody against HER2 for metastatic breast cancer that overexpresses HER2. *N Engl J Med* 344:783–792.

CHAPTER 24

Cancer and Precursor Lesions of the Uterine Cervix

MICHELE FOLLEN, GUILLERMO TORTOLERO-LUNA,
ANNE-THÉRÈSE VLASTOS, and DIANE C. BODURKA

The University of Texas, M. D. Anderson Cancer Center, Houston, Texas

The etiology of cervical cancer is multifactorial. Human papillomavirus (HPV) appears necessary, but not sufficient, as a causal agent. Screening in a systematic fashion has lowered the morbidity and mortality from cervical cancer in every country in which an organized screening program has been established. The diagnosis may begin with an abnormal Papanicolaou (Pap) smear; lesions visible to the naked eye are biopsied. The International Federation of Gynecology and Obstetrics (FIGO) staging system is used. The treatment for small stage I and stage II cancers is radical surgery; for larger stage I and stage IVA cancers, a combination of chemotherapy and radiation; and for stage IVB cancers, chemotherapy or palliation. Surveillance strategies concentrate on intense follow-up in the first 2–5 years after treatment. Rehabilitation after surgical and radiotherapeutic treatment is symptom based. Prevention currently consists of efforts to increase the number of women who are screened. Chemoprevention and an HPV vaccine may be preventive measures in the future.

ETIOLOGY

Cervical cancer, comprising 10% of all cancers in women, is the third most common cancer among women worldwide. It is estimated that about 500,000 women are diagnosed annually with cervical cancer and that almost half as many die of the disease. Up to 80% of cases are reported in developing countries, but economically disadvantaged women in both developing and developed countries are particularly affected. In the United States, cervical cancer is the third most

UICC Manual of Clinical Oncology, Eighth Edition. Edited by Raphael E. Pollock
ISBN 0-471-22289-5 Copyright © 2004 John Wiley & Sons, Inc.

common neoplasm of the female genital tract, with an estimated 12,900 new cases (6% of all cancers in women) and 4,400 deaths expected in 2001.

A continuous decline in incidence of and mortality from cervical cancer has been observed in most developed countries during the last 50 years. This decline is mainly attributed to early detection using the Pap smear. Despite this decline, cervical neoplasia continues to be an important health problem in women world-wide, particularly in underserved populations. Further, a shift in the declining trend of incidence and mortality has been observed in the United States and other developed countries since the mid-1980s. Since 1986, the incidence rate of cervical cancer in white American women under age 50 years has been increasing by about 3% annually, whereas rates have continued to decline in African-American women. In England and Wales, Canada, Italy, New Zealand, and Australia, similar trends have been reported. The reasons for this trend among young women are poorly understood, and should be interpreted with caution. Although the increase might be due to changes in the prevalence of risk factors, such as an increase in the prevalence of HPV infection or changes in sexual practices, childbearing patterns, and oral contraceptive use, other factors, such as changes in coding and registration procedures, screening coverage, hysterectomy rates, and the proportion of cases classified as "uterus not otherwise specified (NOS)," must be considered.

The overall 5-year relative survival rate has remained constant. In the United States, for the periods 1970–1973 and 1983–1989, the 5-year relative survival rates were both about 67%. Survival rates are higher for white women and women under 50 years of age. Survival rates are high ($\sim$90%) when the disease is diagnosed at early stages and poor ($\sim$13–14%) when diagnosed at advanced stages.

Epidemiologic evidence has long suggested that cervical neoplasia behaves like a sexually transmitted disease. In support of this hypothesis, several measures of sexual behavior are consistently associated with an increased risk of cervical neoplasia. Risk is higher among women with multiple partners, women whose sexual partners are more promiscuous, and women who first had sexual intercourse at an early age. In addition to sexual behavior, low socioeconomic status, reproductive history, smoking habits, oral and barrier contraceptive use, dietary factors, immunosuppression, frequency of obtaining Pap smears, and the character-istics of the male sexual partners have been implicated in the risk of cervical neoplasia.

Previous studies focused on the etiologic role of several sexually transmitted infections, including herpes simplex virus type 2, *Chlamydia trachomatis, Tricho-monas vaginalis,* cytomegalovirus, *Neisseria gonorrhoeae,* and *Treponema palli-dum.* Epidemiologic data obtained during the last 15 years support a strong role of HPV infection in the etiology of cervical neoplasia. This association seems to satisfy the criteria for causality in epidemiologic research: the association is strong, consistent, and specific; there are dose-response and temporal relationships, and the causal relationship is biologically plausible.

In a recent international collaborative study, HPV DNA was detected in 93% (range, 75–100%) of cervical cancer specimens collected in 22 countries and analyzed by the polymerise chain reaction. The percentages of cases of cervical cancer attributed to HPV infection have been estimated to be about 82% in developed countries and 91% in developing countries. Similarly, HPV has been reported in up to 94% of women with preinvasive cervical lesions and in up to 46% of women who are cytologically normal.

The association between HPV infection and cervical neoplasia is particularly strong with specific HPV types (16, 18, 31, 33, 35, and 45), increasing viral load, and infection with multiple HPV types. This association is consistent and independent of HPV assay method used and epidemiologic study design and appears to explain many of the previously established risk factors for cervical neoplasia, including sexual behavior and cigarette smoking, which are now thought to be confounding risks.

The difference between the high prevalence of HPV infection and the low incidence of cervical neoplasia in young healthy women, as well as the low rate of progression of untreated CIN lesions, suggests that HPV may be a necessary but not sufficient risk factor for cervical neoplasia. Although HPV is the most important risk factor, other cofactors seem to be necessary for the development of disease. The availability of more accurate and effective methods for detection of HPV infection will provide the opportunity to conduct epidemiologic studies to assess the role of previously established risk factors as independent factors or cofactors for the development of cervical neoplasia and to assess the effect of interaction between HPV and these factors, particularly smoking habits and hormonal and dietary factors. The role of HPV persistence in the progression of cervical neoplasia and the determinants of HPV persistence need further evaluation. Moreover, the impact of recent trends in risk factors on the occurrence of cervical neoplasia deserves future attention.

SCREENING FOR CERVICAL NEOPLASIAS

Cervical cancer meets the criteria for a disease to be considered for screening: (1) it is a frequent disease and an important health problem; (2) it has a long detectable precancerous stage; (3) there is a screening test, the Pap smear, that is quick, noninvasive, inexpensive, and widely accepted; and (4) there is treatment available, and the treatment of early-stage disease is more effective than the treatment of symptomatic disease.

The main purpose of the Pap smear, which was introduced in the mid-1940s in the United States, is the earliest possible detection of cervical cancer and its precursor lesions. Since the test's introduction, it has been shown to be an effective measure for the prevention of cervical cancer, and it has been credited with the decline in incidence and mortality in cervical cancer observed in most developed countries over the last 50 years. Mass screening with the Pap smear has been considered one of the most successful public health measures in the prevention of cancer and the best available method for the early detection of cancer.

Although the effectiveness of the Pap smear has never been evaluated in a randomized clinical trial, there is substantial evidence from many observational epidemiologic studies, including ecologic, case-comparison, and cohort studies, that the use of the screening is associated with a lower incidence of and mortality from cervical cancer. Cohort data from British Columbia and case-comparison studies from Geneva, Milan, and Toronto demonstrate the protective effect of the Pap smear. Ecologic studies from areas with screening programs, such as Scotland; British Columbia; Iceland; Manitoba; Maribo County, Denmark; Ostfold County, Norway; Sweden; and the United States, show sharp reductions in incidence and mortality after screening was introduced.

However, it is important to remember that the Pap smear is a screening, not a diagnostic, test and as such is not a perfect tool; in recent years, its accuracy has been questioned. Although there are not precise data on the accuracy of the Pap smear, primarily because of methodological problems (study design, study population, gold standard for comparison, etc.), most studies report a sensitivity between 60% and 85% and a specificity greater than 90%. In a recent meta-analysis of the accuracy of the test, Fahey et al. (1995) observed that in 59 studies published between 1984 and 1992 comparing results of Pap smears and histologic analysis, estimates of the sensitivity and specificity of the test ranged from 11 to 99% (median, 66%) and 14 to 97% (median, 67%), respectively. The large variation in the estimates of the sensitivity and specificity was mainly attributed to differences in the methodology and quality of the studies.

Several sources of error have been identified in the screening for cervical cancer, including sampling error, smearing technique, processing of the sample, visual screening of the smear, laboratory quality control, interpretation of the smear, and reporting errors. Of these sources of error, the two major contributors to the false-negative rate are poor specimen collection (sampling error), accounting for up to 60% of false-negatives, and interpretation error, accounting for approximately 40% of the false-negatives. Because of the potential significance of the adverse effects of both high false-negative and high false-positive rates, several methods, used alone or in conjunction with cytologic analysis, have been assessed to reduce the error rate, particularly the false-negative rate. Among these methods are targeted rescreening, colposcopy, cervicography, speculoscopy, HPV testing, monolayer cell preparations, and automated screening. All of these methods have been shown to increase the sensitivity of the Pap smear to 90% or more; however, most of these methods have the limitations of increasing screening cost and time and requiring highly trained personnel.

In addition to the accuracy of the test, there are several other unsolved issues regarding the Pap test: the ages at which screening should begin and end and the screening interval that will increase the cost-effectiveness of a screening program. In 1988, a consensus panel representing the American Cancer Society, the National Cancer Institute, the American College of Obstetricians and Gynecologists (ACOG), the American Medical Association, the American Nurses Association, the American Academy of Family Physicians, and the American Medical Women's

Association agreed on recommendations for Pap smear screening. They recommended annual Pap smears for all women who are or have been sexually active or have reached the age of 18 years. Low-risk women may be screened at 3- to 5-year intervals once two negative smears are obtained, whereas high-risk women (those with multiple sexual partners and those who commenced sexual activity at a young age) may be screened annually. The consensus panel did not recommend an age at which to discontinue the Pap smear.

Despite this recommendation, the most cost-effective screening interval is unknown. Data from case-comparison studies and mathematical modeling have shown a significant increase (from 64.2 to 83.9%) in the reduction in the risk of invasive cervical cancer by reducing the screening interval from 10 to 5 years, but less impact with shorter screening intervals. With screening at 3-year intervals, the risk of invasive cervical cancer is reduced by 91.4%; at 2-year intervals, 92.5%; and yearly, 93.3%. Therefore, based on these data, it is estimated that annual screening versus a 2- to 3-year screening interval has a very small impact on effectiveness at a two to three times higher cost. The preference for annual screening in the United States is based on the following rationale: (1) more frequent screening compensates for the high false-negative rate; (2) there is concern that long screening intervals may stretch longer, increasing the risk of losing contact with patients and forfeiting the opportunity to conduct screening during routine annual gynecologic examinations; (3) longer screening intervals may de-emphasize the importance of screening among high-risk women; and (4) longer screening intervals decrease the number of opportunities to detect rapidly progressing lesions early.

In developing countries, where most cases of cervical cancer occur but where cytologic screening services and medical services for further evaluation and treatment of cervical preinvasive lesions are unavailable or scarce, resources must be allocated in a cost-effective manner. Some of the recommended strategies for screening programs in developing countries include longer screening intervals (5–10 years); later age at first screening (>35 years old); "once in a lifetime" screening among women aged 35–40 years; screening of all women at least once before any woman is screened twice; downstaging; and the use of colposcopy, HPV testing, cervicography, and automated cytologic analysis.

Despite the long-term presence and recognition of the benefits of Pap smear screening for detecting cervical cancer, the need for further research remains. Some of the areas that deserve future research are: (1) identifying strategies to increase screening rates among socially disadvantaged and elderly women in both developed and developing countries; (2) determining the most cost-effective screening interval; (3) increasing the accuracy of the Pap smear by reducing sampling error; (4) assessing the role of monolayer smear techniques, automated screening devices, and HPV testing in the screening of cervical abnormalities; and (5) determining the most appropriate strategies for the evaluation and management of patients with abnormal cytologic results (considering cost, the emotional impact on women, criteria for referral, and the role of HPV testing in triage and follow-up).

DIAGNOSTIC MEASURES

Preinvasive Lesions

Abnormal Pap smears are classified according to the Bethesda system (Table 24.1). Once abnormal epithelial cell abnormalities are detected by Pap smear, the standard of care, where resources permit, is referral for a repeat Pap smear and colposcopically directed biopsies. This group usually includes patients with atypical cells of uncertain significance (ASCUS) and low-grade squamous intraepithelial lesions (LGSILs, those that show HPV and cervical intraepithelial neoplasia grade 1 [CIN 1]) although few cancers are found in these patients and most of these lesions regress. A triage strategy for lesions more likely to progress to higher grades and thus more likely to develop into invasive cancers is needed. Colposcopy, cervicography, and HPV DNA testing are being evaluated for identifying high-risk ASCUS

TABLE 24.1. The Bethesda System for the Classification of Abnormal Papanicolaou

Adequacy of specimen
  Satisfactory for evaluation
  Satisfactory for evaluation but limited by _____ (specify reason)
  Unsatisfactory for evaluation (specify reason)
General categorization (optional)
  Within normal limits
  Benign cellular changes: see descriptive diagnosis
  Epithelial cell abnormalities: see descriptive diagnosis
Descriptive diagnosis
  Benign cellular changes
    Infection
      Trichomonas vaginalis
      Fungal organisms morphologically consistent with *Candida* species
      Predominance of coccobacilli consistent with *Actinomyces* species
      Cellular changes associated with herpes simplex virus
      Other
   Reactive changes
    Reactive cellular changes associated with inflammation (atypical repair)
    Atrophy with inflammation (atrophic vaginitis)
    Changes due to radiation
    Changes due to intrauterine contraceptive device
    Other
Epithelial cell abnormalities
  Squamous cell abnormalities
    Atypical squamous cells of undetermined significance (qualify)
    Low-grade squamous intraepithelial lesion (encompassing HPV positivity, mild
      dysplasia, CIN I)
    High-grade squamous intraepithelial lesion (encompassing moderate and severe
      dysplasia, carcinoma in situ (CIS), CIN 2, and CIN 3)
    Squamous cell carcinoma

and LGSIL patients, but these tools are expensive. Triage strategies for ASCUS/ LGSIL may be a lower priority in developing countries.

At the first colposcopic visit, a complete history should be taken and a physical examination, pelvic examination, repeat Pap smear, and pan-colposcopic examination (including vulva, perineum, vagina, and cervix) should be performed. The colposcopic examination involves the application of 3–6% acetic acid, waiting 5 minutes to allow acetic acid to take effect, followed by a careful 3- to 6-minute examination of the cervix, identifying the endocervical canal, squamocolumnar junction, transformation zone, and lesions (which typically turn white in acetic acid). Lesions may or may not exhibit angiogenesis, for which a descriptive classification has been developed, including fine punctation, coarse punctation, mosaiform atypia, mosaic atypia, and atypical vessels. Atypical vessels are thought to be diagnostic of cancer. Mosaicism and coarse punctation are thought to be worse findings than fine punctation and mosaiform atypia. Abnormal areas of the ectocervix are biopsied, and an endocervical curettage is performed. Additional abnormal areas in the vagina, vulva, and perianal area are inspected and biopsied.

Several new approaches to diagnosis of preneoplastic lesions are being developed. They include targeted Pap smear rescreening, colposcopic screening, cervicography, HPV DNA testing (differentiating low- and high-risk viral types), speculoscopy (viewing the cervix under chemiluminescent illumination), digital-imaging colposcopy using computer assistance, fluorescent spectroscopy, reflectance spectroscopy, optical coherence tomography, confocal imaging, and computer-assisted automated image analysis of Pap smear readings. It is hoped that all of these will improve the performance of screening cytologic analysis or better diagnose high-grade lesions at the time of the initial visit. Currently, all of these modalities are expensive and the value they add must be carefully evaluated.

Cervical Cancer

In its early stages, cervical carcinoma tends to be asymptomatic. Early symptoms include vaginal discharge, vaginal odor, and abnormal vaginal bleeding. If the patient is sexually active, there may be postcoital bleeding.

When a gross cervical lesion is visible, a biopsy is indicated. Cervical cancers may be characterized by gross appearance as exophytic or endophytic. Exophytic lesions protrude from the cervical surface and can be easily visualized and measured. Endophytic lesions are more difficult to detect, often not visible on speculum examination. They may expand the endocervix considerably before being detected.

Cervical carcinoma has two predominant spread patterns: direct extension and lymphatic dissemination. Hematogenous spread occurs late in the natural history of the disease. In the first pattern, the cancer spreads from the cervix to adjacent tissues, especially to the upper vagina and the parametrial tissues (cardinal and uterosacral ligaments). These areas are best assessed by a careful pelvic examination. Following speculum examination with good visualization of the entire vagina, vaginal and rectovaginal palpation should be performed to evaluate vaginal or parametrial extension. In many countries, this examination is performed under general anesthesia for patient comfort. If a cytoscopy and proctosigmoidoscopy are planned, they can be performed at the same time.

The tumor may also involve the pelvic sidewall. Sidewall disease can be a result of direct lateral extension of the cervical tumor or medial growth of metastatic lymph node deposits. Direct extension is most common. Sidewall disease can result in pelvic pain, sometimes with associated radiculopathy in the lower extremity. Unilateral leg edema may be the result of lymphatic and venous outflow obstruction. Larger cervical cancers may cause an asymptomatic hydroureter, which may be diagnosed by intravenous pyelography (IVP) or computed tomography (CT) imaging. Uremia may be the presenting sign in a patient with bilateral ureteral obstruction. When the bladder or rectum is involved by direct extension, there may be hematuria, rectal bleeding, or rectal obstruction.

The lymphatic spread pattern of cervical cancer is thought to proceed in a stepwise fashion. It begins with cells spreading into paracervical lymphatic channels, then into the pelvic node chains associated with the obturator, internal iliac, and external iliac vessels. From there, the cells spread cephalad to the common iliac chain and the para-aortic lymph nodes. Finally, extension to the mediastinal and supraclavicular nodes may also be seen.

Hematogenous dissemination is most often seen in women who have been previously treated for cervical cancer and have had a recurrence. When it is seen at primary presentation, it is in patients with very advanced cancer or with early cancer of an aggressive histologic subtype, such as small cell carcinoma. Metastatic disease may involve the lungs, liver, bone, or peritoneal cavity.

STAGING

Preinvasive Lesions

Biopsies showing preinvasive lesions are being read in the United States in similar fashion as are Pap smears: as LGSILs and high-grade squamous intraepithelial lesions (HGSILs). Often the pathologist will further clarify whether the LGSIL is more consistent with HPV or CIN 1 and whether the HGSIL is more consistent with CIN 2, CIN 3, or CIS. Many cytologists worldwide have not yet embraced the Bethesda system and continue to use the classification Richart developed in the 1960s, in which Pap smears and biopsies are classified as atypias, HPV, CIN 1, CIN 2, CIN 3 (which includes CIS), or invasive cancer.

Cervical Cancer

Cervical cancer is staged by clinical evaluation, which enables comparison of treatment results around the world. The rules for staging cervical cancer have been established by the International Federation of Gynecology and Obstetrics (FIGO) and were revised in 1995 (Table 24.2). While the FIGO staging correlates well with survival, treatment planning often includes several other important prognostic

TABLE 24.2. FIGO Staging of Cervical Carcinoma

Preinvasive Carcinoma	
Stage 0	Carcinoma *in situ*; intraepithelial carcinoma
Invasive Carcinoma	
Stage I	Carcinoma confined to the cervix (extension to the corpus should be disregarded)
IA	Preclinical invasive carcinoma, diagnosed by microscopy only
IA1	Invasion up to 3 mm deep and 7 mm wide
IA2	Invasion between 3 and 5 mm deep and 7 mm wide
IB	Clinically apparent lesions confined to the cervix
IB1	Lesions no greater than 4 cm in diameter
IB2	Lesions greater than 4 cm in diameter
Stage II	Carcinoma extends beyond the cervix onto either the vagina or parametrium but not to the lower third of the vagina and not to the pelvic wall
IIA	No obvious parametrial involvement
IIB	Obvious parametrial involvement
Stage III	Carcinoma extends to either the lower third of the vagina or to the pelvic wall. Hydronephrosis or a nonfunctioning kidney, unless known to be due to another cause, necessitates classification as stage IIIB.
IIIA	Involvement of lower third of vagina. No extension to the pelvic wall
IIIB	Extension to the pelvic wall or hydronephrosis or a nonfunctioning kidney
Stage IV	Carcinoma extends beyond the true pelvis or involves the mucosa of the bladder or rectum. Bullous edema does not permit assignment to stage IV.
IVA	Spread to bladder or rectum
IVB	Spread to distant organs

variables, such as tumor volume and surgical or radiographic evidence of lymph node metastasis. Poor prognostic factors are advanced FIGO stage, large tumor volume, positive pelvic nodes, certain high-risk histologic types (adenosquamous, small cell), poorly differentiated squamous carcinoma or adenocarcinoma, and the presence of lymphatic or vascular space involvement.

All patients should undergo a thorough evaluation of medical history and a physical examination with attention to the supraclavicular, axillary, and inguinal lymph node chains. Pelvic examination, particularly inspection and palpation at the time of bimanual and rectovaginal examination, is important in determining the size of the lesion and the presence of vaginal or parametrial spread. The risk of complications from radiotherapy is increased if there is a history of prior abdominal surgery, pelvic inflammatory disease, hypertension, heart disease, or diabetes.

Chest radiography and IVP are mandatory. It is not unusual to find a unilateral or bilateral hydroureter that changes the stage and prognosis. The position of the kidneys prior to pelvic radiation is confirmed by the IVP.

Cystoscopy and sigmoidoscopy are used by FIGO for the evaluation of the bladder and rectum. Invasion must be ruled out before the initiation of therapy because of the proximity of these organs to the cervix. A biopsy specimen, not visual impression, is used to change the stage. Almost all patients, except those with the earliest and smallest lesions, should undergo these procedures.

The barium enema can be a useful procedure for patients who are older or who have glandular lesions. Asymptomatic polyps or diverticular disease may influence the choice of treatment. Most often, younger patients with smaller squamous lesions probably do not require a barium enema. Plain radiographs are permitted in the staging evaluation but have a low yield and are seldom performed.

Often, other radiologic tests are used to aid in the development of a management plan, but results of these tests do not alter the stage. Lymphangiography is extremely useful in determining the presence of pelvic or para-aortic node metastasis: because it can reveal the architecture of nodes, not the just the size, it can detect early lymph node metastasis. The CT scan is often used to evaluate nodal status but is not nearly as accurate as lymphangiography. Confirmation of a metastatic deposit should be obtained by fine-needle aspiration or surgical exploration. The use of magnetic resonance imaging (MRI) has been reported as helpful in determining the extent of cervical cancer. MRI can distinguish tissue density well, hence it may be useful in looking at the nodes, as well as in evaluating pelvic involvement.

Surgical staging of cervical cancer is widely performed around the world, despite the fact that it does not alter the FIGO stage. Surgical staging is used to gain additional prognostic information regarding the extent of disease and to tailor therapy. Transperitoneal approaches to the pelvic and para-aortic lymph nodes led to a significant increase in complications from radiotherapy, predominantly radiation bowel injury, so many surgeons have turned to extraperitoneal lymph node dissection. Surgical staging has the disadvantage of causing a 2- to 4-week delay in the initiation of radiotherapy. There is no evidence that patients who undergo pretreatment surgical staging have better survival rates than patients who have lymphangiography or MRI with fine-needle aspiration of positive nodes.

MULTIMODALITY TREATMENT

Preinvasive Lesions

High-grade intraepithelial lesions, once identified, are usually treated with ablative methods or cone biopsy; chemopreventive agents are being used experimentally. Cone biopsy, rather than ablation, is mandatory for HGSILs if there is suspicion of invasion on Pap smear, biopsy, or colposcopy; a positive endocervical curettage; a discrepancy between the Pap smear and biopsy (Pap smear suggesting a higher grade lesion than biopsy); an unsatisfactory colposcopy (entire lesion or squamo-columnar junction not entirely visualized); an adenomatous lesion (adenocarinoma *in situ* or adenocarcinoma); or if the patient is not compliant with follow-up. Low-grade intraepithelial lesions are treated similarly or simply followed every 6 months with repeat Pap smear and colposcopy. Biopsy-proven atypia, the histopathologic correlate of ASCUS, is usually followed without treatment.

The most popular techniques of ablation in the United States are cryotherapy, laser ablation, and the loop electrosurgical excision procedure (LEEP). Although the LEEP is excisional in nature, it removes as much tissue as is destroyed with cryotherapy and laser ablation and is therefore an equivalent therapy. All three techniques destroy a portion of the cervix for which the superior and deep margin is estimated at 6–8 mm in height around the endocervical canal and the inferior and ectocervical margin includes the transformation zone of the ectocervix. In nonrandomized series, the failure rates of all three therapies are 10–20% over 2 years. Randomized studies of laser ablation and cryotherapy show similar long-term cure rates and complications. A recent randomized trial of the three modalities, cryotherapy, laser ablation, and LEEP, with 31 months of follow-up showed failure rates of 15–20% for all three treatments and no significant differences in complications, either short or long term.

Cone biopsies remove the endocervical canal; specimens include a superior and deep margin 2–3 cm in height around the canal and an inferior and ectocervical margin including the transformation zone of the ectocervix. Because the endocervical canal is included, cone biopsies are diagnostic as well as therapeutic treatment. Cone biopsies in the United States are performed using the scalpel ("cold-knife" cone), electrocautery ("hot-knife" cone), laser, and LEEP. A LEEP cone removes the cervix in two to three specimens, whereas the other techniques remove the specimen in one piece. (The additional two specimens are portions of the endocervical canal removed with an endocervical loop that reaches up higher in the canal, giving a tissue specimen 3 cm in height like a cold knife cone.) The advantage of a LEEP cone is that it can be performed in the clinic under local anesthesia in less than 5 minutes, whereas the other techniques are typically performed under general anesthesia in the operating room. One randomized study of cold knife cone, laser cone, and LEEP cone showed many uninterpretable specimens using LEEP, but another randomized trial showed success rates and specimens for LEEP comparable with those for other types of cones.

Future treatment options may include chemoprevention, the use of micronutrients or pharmaceuticals to prevent or delay the development of cancer. Chemopreventives have the advantage of affecting the patient systemically and may be particularly advantageous in the patient who has multifocal vulvar, vaginal, and cervical disease or who is immunodepressed. Several chemoprevention trials have been carried out in the cervix with both micronutrients and pharmaceuticals. None of the micronutrient studies have demonstrated statistically significant regression of CIN lesions in randomized trials. Topical *trans*-retinoic acid caused significant regression of CIN 2, but not CIN 3, in a trial by Meyskens et al. Chemoprevention may become a treatment in the future but at present should be considered experimental.

Many interesting immunobiologic studies of HPV and patients' humoral and cell-mediated immunity have been published. All these studies suggest that patients who are able to mount an immune response to the virus are less likely to develop lesions or less likely to have a recurrence once a lesion has been treated. These results suggest that eventually initial cervical infections might be prevented by a humoral vaccine aimed at the capsid proteins, possibly administered before the onset of sexual activity in population-based vaccination programs. Once persistent infection has occurred or a lesion is present, efforts might eventually better be aimed at cell-mediated immunity using HPV type-specific peptides with the intention of causing regression of disease. This vaccine would be therapeutic and would be used in a well-defined group of women with disease.

Cervical Cancer

Careful choice of a primary therapy for cervical carcinoma is critical because recurrent disease is seldom curable. The primary approaches are surgery, radiotherapy, and multimodality therapy.

Microinvasive Cervical Carcinoma   The classification of microinvasive carcinoma of the uterine cervix is limited to squamous lesions. The distinction between adenocarcinoma *in situ* and microinvasive adenocarcinoma is not yet well defined. Invasive adenocarcinoma of the cervix should be treated by either radical surgery or radiotherapy. The diagnosis of microinvasion is made by cone biopsy.

For treatment planning, most clinicians in the United States use the functional definition of microinvasion described by the Society of Gynecologic Oncologists (SGO); this definition limits the depth of invasion to 3 mm and excludes patients with lymphatic or vascular space involvement. For patients with lesions with depths of invasion between 3 and 5 mm, options such as radiotherapy or radical surgery with either a type II (modified radical) or type III (radical) hysterectomy should be considered. Note that the FIGO definition of stage IA1 carcinoma, as modified in 1995, closely resembles the SGO definition of microinvasion.

For patients who have a depth of invasion of less than 3 mm and no lymphatic or vascular space involvement, hysterectomy by either the vaginal or abdominal route is appropriate. With this approach, the cure rate approaches 100%. Women of childbearing age who have a strong desire to maintain fertility and are compliant with follow-up can be treated with conization alone. Conization is acceptable only when the margins of the specimen are negative for invasive or preinvasive disease. Continued surveillance with colposcopy, cervical cytologic analysis, and endocervical curettage is indicated.

Invasive Cervical Carcinoma

Radical Hysterectomy.   Radical hysterectomy has long been the standard therapy for stage IB1 and small stage IIA cancers. Simple hysterectomy had been attempted with poor results; the spread pattern of cervical carcinoma showed that the uterine ligaments and pelvic lymphatics were at risk. When described in 1900 by Wertheim, the radical hysterectomy was successfully being used as a treatment for invasive cervical cancer; nodes were removed only if involvement was suspected. However, there was a high mortality rate from the procedure. During the same period, radiotherapy was being successfully used as well. Meigs modified the radical hysterectomy procedure in the late 1940s, taking a wider margin on the parametrial tissues and routinely dissecting the pelvic lymph nodes. With Meigs' approach and the use of blood transfusions and antibiotics, results of the surgical treatment of early cervical cancer soon equaled those of radiotherapy.

The radical hysterectomy begins with abdominal exploration, including careful inspection of the peritoneal surfaces, liver, bowel, ovaries, and other pelvic organs. Pelvic and para-aortic lymph nodes should be carefully palpated for clinically evident metastatic disease. The paravesical and pararectal spaces are then opened with careful palpation of the cardinal and uterosacral ligaments. Most surgeons will discontinue the surgery and treat the patient with radiation or multimodality therapy when extrauterine disease or parametrial extension is present.

Younger patients who are in good health and preferably not obese are the ideal candidates for radical hysterectomy. Cancer should be confined to the cervix, although some patients with upper vaginal involvement may be adequately treated with radical hysterectomy. The most important criterion is that the cervical lesions should not, in most cases, exceed 4 cm in size. Larger lesions are best treated by radiotherapy or multimodality therapy. Because ovarian metastases from early cervical cancer are exceedingly rare, the ovaries may remain in premenopausal patients.

Further prognostic and treatment planning information can be obtained by analysis of the surgical specimen. Most patients are treated with postoperative pelvic radiotherapy when lymph node metastases, close or positive surgical margins, or parametrial spread is detected. Results of radiotherapy after radical hysterectomy have been mixed. Although pelvic radiation following a radical dissection certainly adds morbidity, most gynecologic oncologists feel that the potential benefits outweigh the risks in these patients. Several prospective randomized trials evaluating the role of postoperative radiotherapy are underway.

The results for patients treated with radical hysterectomy are excellent, with 5-year survival rates ranging from 77 to 93%. A variety of authors have reported their experiences with laparoscopic lymphadenectomy, laparoscopic modified radical hysterectomy, and laparoscopy-assisted radical vaginal hysterectomy. To date, no large prospective randomized trials have compared abdominal radical hysterectomy with laparoscopic radical hysterectomy; these will be important to establish the value added by the laparoscopic approach.

Radiation and Chemotherapy. Ionizing radiation, combined with chemotherapy is most commonly prescribed for patients with stage IB2 to IVA disease, the majority of women who present with cervical carcinoma. Treatment involves delivery of radiotherapy in two separate phases, using an external beam and internal implants. Initially, external-beam radiotherapy (EBRT) is given to the pelvic area. The purpose of EBRT is twofold: it sterilizes microscopic disease that may exist in the pelvic lymph nodes, and it shrinks the central tumor in the cervix and paracervical tissues to provide better geometry for placement of the radiation implant. External therapy is given in a series of small fractions, most commonly

1.8 to 2.0 Gy daily for 4 to 5 weeks, for a total of 40 to 50 Gy. Delivery in multiple small fractions allows for maximal tumor cell kill with preservation of normal tissues.

Standard treatment areas measure 15 × 15 cm, and treatment fields may be divided between two separate fields (anterior and posterior) or four separate fields (anterior, posterior, and lateral fields). The lower border of the field is generally placed at the mid pubis or 4 cm below the lowest level of vaginal disease, which can be marked by placing silver pellets in the tumor that can be seen on x-ray examination. The upper border is placed at L4-L5 or L5-S1 unless the para-aortic nodes are believed to be at risk. The lateral borders are placed at least 1 cm lateral to the pelvic margins. The borders of the radiation field are tailored to the distribution of the tumor and the patient's anatomy.

The EBRT field is extended above the pelvis for patients who have known or suspected disease in the para-aortic nodes. When used for patients with surgically documented microscopic disease, extended-field EBRT has the potential to cure nearly 50% of patients. The results for patients with gross para-aortic metastases are very poor. Extended-field radiation exposes a greater volume of normal tissue to ionizing radiation, hence the risk of complications is significantly increased. More patients experience myelosuppression with extended-field therapy, and complications involving the small intestine are also more common. Chemotherapy is not always given in this scenario, due to the potential of significant side effects.

Following external radiation, patients usually receive two intracavitary radiation implants, also referred to as brachytherapy. A variety of applicator devices have been designed to give an intense dose of radiation to the central pelvis while sparing surrounding tissues. The most widely used applicator is the Fletcher-Suit-Delclos afterloading tandem and ovoid. This system is inserted about 1 week after the conclusion of EBRT and left in place for 48 hours; the sequence is repeated 2 weeks later. The system consists of a curved tandem that is placed within the uterine cavity and two ovoids that lie in the upper vaginal fornices. It produces a distribution of high-intensity radiation that treats the upper vagina, cervix, and uterine cavity. Shielding in the ovoids limits the dosage of radiation delivered to the bladder and rectum. The placement of the device by an experienced practitioner is of vital importance to ensure dose distribution that will improve local control of the cancer without increasing serious complications. In many places, hollow "afterloading" devices are used, which allow the radioactive source to be inserted in the patient's room following verification of proper placement by pelvic radiograph and transfer from the recovery room. This type of system minimizes the dose of radiation to hospital staff, a major improvement over the older "hot" systems.

The tandem and ovoids are loaded with radium or, more commonly, cesium. The major portion of the dose delivered by the implant is to the immediate surrounding tissues, as the energy from the radiation source decreases over distance. Treatment results with radiotherapy for stage IB disease are excellent and comparable to those achieved with radical surgery.

Intracavitary brachytherapy has traditionally been delivered at a low dose rate (LDR) of 0.4–0.8 Gy per hour. There has recently been a dramatic increase in interest, however, in high-dose-rate (HDR) brachytherapy. Although HDR is defined as a dose rate greater than 0.2 Gy per minute, 2–3 Gy per minute is usually administered, a rate similar to that of EBRT. Potential advantages of HDR include the outpatient nature of the procedure (each application lasts only 10–15 minutes), decreased cost, decreased anesthetic requirement, and minimization of applicator movement. Randomized trials will be needed to establish how the cure and morbidity rates with HDR compare with those of LDR.

Radiosensitizers potentiate the effect of radiation on tumors. The mechanism of action is not completely understood. Results from five randomized phase III trials reveal an overall survival advantage for cisplatin-based chemotherapy given concurrently with radiation therapy. The patient populations included women with FIGO stages IB_2-IVA cervical cancer treated with primary radiation therapy and women with FIGO stage I-IIA cervical cancer found to have poor prognostic factors at the time of primary surgery. These factors included parametrial disease, metastatic disease in the pelvic lymph nodes, and surgical margins positive for cancer. The dose of radiation, as well as the schedule and type of chemotherapy, varied somewhat from study to study.

All five trials demonstrated a significant survival benefit for the combination of radiation and chemotherapy. The risk of death from cervical cancer was decreased by 30–50% with the use of chemoradiation. This may be the most important breakthrough in the treatment of cervical cancer in the last 50 years. Based on these results, strong consideration should be given to the incorporation of concurrent cisplatin-based chemotherapy with radiation therapy in women who require radiation therapy for the treatment of cervical cancer. Cisplatin alone or a combination of cisplatin and 5-FU may be prescribed. No prospective, randomized trial has been performed to evaluate the efficacy or toxicity of weekly platinum and radiation versus a combination of platinum, 5-FU, and radiation. However, the standard of care has shifted to the combination of platinum-based chemotherapy with radiation for the treatment of cervical cancer.

Recurrent Cervical Cancer The great majority of patients with recurrent disease are incurable. Recurrent or metastatic cervical cancer may occur in one of four sites: the pelvic sidewall, para-aortic or other distal lymph nodes, lung, or bone (most commonly the vertebral bodies). A few patients will have a central pelvic recurrence. One reason for careful follow-up, after treatment, is to identify this last group of patients because they are candidates for curative therapy through a radical surgical procedure, exenteration.

The treatment of recurrent disease is based on the type of primary therapy delivered. Pelvic recurrence after radical hysterectomy can be treated with radiotherapy. For the patient who has already received pelvic radiation, additional radiotherapy is usually not possible. For disease outside the pelvis, radiation plays a palliative role in controlling the size and spread of metastatic deposits.

If a patient has a very small cervical recurrence after primary therapy with radiation, radical hysterectomy has been used as a less radical alternative to pelvic exenteration. Patients must be carefully selected for this approach, as the potential for complications is high. Most patients with a central pelvic recurrence of cervical cancer following radiotherapy should be considered for pelvic exenteration.

Pelvic Exenteration. Pelvic exenteration involves removal of the pelvic reproductive organs, including the uterus, tubes, ovaries, and vagina; the bladder and distal ureters; the rectum and anus; the pelvic floor, including the pelvic peritoneum and levator muscles; and usually the pelvic lymph nodes. Occasionally, a more limited procedure may be performed, such as an anterior exenteration (preserving the rectum and anus) or a posterior exenteration (preserving the bladder and ureters).

The initial experience with pelvic exenteration carried a very high mortality rate. In recent years, several technical advances (the continent conduit, vaginal reconstruction with muscle flap grafts, and distal rectal anastomosis) and refined patient selection have made pelvic exenteration a curative and well-tolerated operation for women with recurrent pelvic carcinomas. Other factors that have influenced the drop in mortality rate (from 13 to 4%) include the use of total parenteral nutrition in the postoperative setting, the use of antibiotics prophylactically and therapeuticaly, and intensive care unit monitoring in the postoperative setting.

The operative procedure itself can be broken down into three phases: the operative evaluation, surgical extirpation, and reconstruction. During the operative evaluation, a vertical midline incision is made with a thorough exploration of the abdominopelvic cavity. Washings are taken and sent for immediate evaluation to rule out the presence of peritoneal metastases. The liver, spleen, and other abdominal organs are carefully palpated and inspected and any suspicious areas are biopsied. If gross peritoneal disease is discovered or washings are positive for malignant cells, the procedure is abandoned. The para-aortic lymph nodes are selectively sampled and pelvic lymph nodes, if not previously removed, are excised. The paravesical and pararectal spaces are opened, and the surgeon ensures that there is adequate clearance of the tumor from the pelvic sidewall. It is estimated that about 20–30% of exploratory laparotomies performed in expectation of exenteration are abandoned because of adverse factors not detected preoperatively. If no adverse factors are found, surgical extirpation is then carried out with *en bloc* removal of the aforementioned organs. Anesthesia and blood bank support should be available; significant blood loss often occurs at this point. Surgery is most commonly performed with two teams, one working through the abdominal incision and the other working to excise the surgical specimen through the perineum. Many advances have been made in the reconstructive phase in recent years. A urinary conduit is constructed and can now be made to allow continence by catheterization. A low rectal anastomosis may be performed, sparing the anus and allowing rectal continence. The vaginal reconstruction can be performed with a variety of muscle flaps, often gracilis muscle flap grafts are used.

Acute complications of pelvic exenteration are the same as those associated with radical surgery, including cardiac decompensation, pulmonary embolism, deep vein thrombosis, and hemorrhage. Most patients require blood transfusion during and after the surgery. Infections are common, including necrosis of the myocutaneous graft with secondary infection, pyelonephritis, or sepsis. Complications involving the urinary conduit include obstruction at the ureteral conduit junction, fistula formation, and anastomotic leak. Long-term complications often involve the urinary diversion, such as recurring bouts of pyelonephritis. Psychosocial adjustments must also be considered after this surgery, and the patient's support system should include family and hospital staff. With the appropriate assistance, most women can resume an essentially normal lifestyle following pelvic exenteration. Following pelvic exenteration for a recurrent carcinoma of the cervix, 5-year survival, including death from all causes, is 44%.

Chemotherapy. Chemotherapy for recurrent cervical carcinoma should be regarded as a palliative treatment. The palliation is perhaps realized as decreased pain because of shrinkage of tumor mass. The opportunity for cure is very small and is limited to patients with a single lesion that can be resected. Even the best chemotherapeutic regimens have complete response rates of less than 10%.

The most active agent in the treatment of recurrent cervical cancer appears to be cisplatin. Used as a single agent, the expected response rate is about 30%. Other active agents include 5-fluorouracil, methotrexate, cyclophosphamide, melphalan, doxorubicin, mitomycin C, bleomycin, and carboplatin, with response rates of 10–23%.

Combination chemotherapy may provide an additional chance for response when compared with cisplatin alone. The use of cisplatin in combination with other agents has resulted in response rates that range from 30 to 50%. However, responses tend to be short lived, with median survival in the range of 7–10 months.

Palliative Therapy. Perhaps one of the most important roles of a physician with a patient with recurrent cervical cancer is delivering proper palliative treatment. The management of pelvic pain, renal failure, and infection are important aspects of the total care of the patient. Advanced cervical cancer often results in severe pelvic pain. A lesion on the pelvic sidewall may involve the sacral nerve roots or directly invade the bone. It is not uncommon for patients to have pain that radiates down the leg. The importance of adequate pain control with narcotics, antiinflammatories, and antidepressants and judicious use of radiation for bone metastases cannot be overemphasized. When local pain is resistant to these measures, patients may be helped by the use of epidural analgesia or ambulatory intravenous patient-controlled analgesia.

Recurrent or progressive cervical cancer may result in bilateral ureteral obstruction. This obstruction can cause infection, which can be treated with non-nephrotoxic antibiotics. In a patient who has not received radiotherapy, urinary diversion by percutaneous nephrostomy or ureteral stenting is indicated, which will allow the patient to proceed to radiation. In the patient with recurrent or progressive cancer after radiation, performing urinary diversion is controversial. Because there is no effective second-line therapy, saving a patient from death by uremia only to have her suffer with progressive pelvic pain may not be wise. The patient and her family must be counseled on the severity of the problem and the natural history of cervical carcinoma so that she can make an informed decision regarding urinary diversion and the use of chemotherapy.

FOLLOW-UP

It is estimated that 75% of cervical cancer recurrences occur within 2 years of therapy. Ninety-five percent of patients who will develop recurrent disease will have relapsed by the end of 5 years. Several studies suggest that for recurrences in early stages, survival is prolonged if recurrences are caught early and managed aggressively. Surveillance programs should focus on more visits (three or four per year) in the first 2 years and fewer (two per year) in the next 3 years. Yearly follow-up should occur thereafter. Each visit should include a thorough review and update of the patient's medical history, a review of systems, and a complete physical exam. Pap smears should be performed yearly. Chest x-ray films should be obtained at least yearly. Other studies can be ordered based on the review of systems.

REHABILITATION

Complications of Radical Hysterectomy

Many of the technical aspects of radical hysterectomy and pelvic lymphadenectomy have been refined in the last few decades, which has led to a reduction in the incidence of serious long-term complications. Great care is now taken in the handling of the ureters and their removal from the cardinal ligament, which leads to fewer ureteral fistulae. The patient who undergoes radical hysterectomy and pelvic lymphadenectomy is at risk for the typical acute postoperative complications from abdominal surgery, such as prolonged ileus and postoperative bowel obstruction. Particular to this procedure, however, is the long-term complication of an increase in constipation, which may be due to transection of the parasympathetic fibers in the uterosacral ligaments. Constipation, when present, may last for many years. The best management approach is to counsel the patient to begin a high-fiber diet, using laxatives only in resistant cases. The most common alteration in the urinary tract following radical hysterectomy involves the bladder, with women reporting an altered sensation of bladder fullness, with or without the urge to void. Urinary retention is a common problem during the postoperative period and sometimes longer. There are several management approaches, but a common one is using the technique of self-catheterization. Another complication can result from excision of up to half of the vaginal tube during radical hysterectomy; in some cases, the vaginal shortening may cause sexual dysfunction. Finally, as a result of the interruption of lymphatic channels in the pelvis, some patients develop a collection of lymphatic fluid, a lymphocyst. Patients with a lymphocyst may present postoperatively with pain, a pelvic mass, or ureteral obstruction. Some lymphocysts resolve spontaneously, but if patients are symptomatic or have signs of ureteral or intestinal obstruction because of mass effect, lymphocysts can be drained percutaneously.

Complications of Radiotherapy

Portions of the gastrointestinal tract will receive a significant radiation dose during the delivery of pelvic radiotherapy. The sigmoid colon is within the radiation field, and portions of the small intestine often enter the pelvis as well. With the intimate anatomic relationship of the sigmoid to the cervix, it is understandable how a tandem and ovoid system with a relatively posterior placement could result in a high dose of radiation to the sigmoid colon. The acute effects of radiation on the sigmoid colon are described as proctosigmoiditis. They include diarrhea, at times with passage of blood and mucus, and occasionally tenesmus. Patients with chronic narrowing of the rectosigmoid usually present with diarrhea alternating with constipation. Bloating, gaseousness, and crampy abdominal pain are not uncommon. As a result, patients will often have anorexia and weight loss. Patients with a high-grade obstruction require surgical intervention. Chronic radiation injury to the sigmoid colon may also result in progressive ischemia, leading to necrosis and perforation requiring aggressive surgical management.

The acute reaction of the small intestine to radiotherapy is often manifested as diarrhea and abdominal cramping, sometimes associated with nausea and vomiting. Often, this is a short-lived side effect that promptly disappears with the cessation of irradiation. As with rectosigmoid injury, however, chronic injury can take years to become manifest. The section of small bowel most prone to injury is the terminal ileum, although other small bowel segments can be involved, especially in patients who have had prior abdominal surgery. Patients who receive extended-field EBRT are at particular risk for small bowel complications. Patients who have mild to moderate symptoms can often be managed expectantly with a low-residue diet and careful observation. Patients with more severe symptoms, especially repeated episodes of partial obstruction, warrant surgical intervention.

During EBRT to the pelvis, patients will sometimes note urinary frequency, usually a short-lived side effect of treatment. A small percentage of patients, however, may develop chronic problems, such as a contracted fibrotic bladder, leading to frequent urination and, in some cases, incontinence. Hemorrhagic cystitis may also be present in some women. This may be an incidental microscopic finding, although occasional severe exacerbations with gross hematuria may occur. When the bleeding is significant enough to cause clot formation in the bladder, emergency intervention is indicated, with continuous irrigation and possibly even fulgurafion.

It is expected that patients who undergo a combination of EBRT and brachytherapy will have very high-dose radiation delivery to the superficial vaginal and cervical tissues. It is not uncommon to see some necrosis of these tissues in the weeks following completion of treatment. Treatment of cervicovaginal necrosis should be conservative, usually using cleansing douches and gentle debridement. The long-term sequelae are vaginal stenosis, vaginal dryness, and shortening of the vaginal vault. These defects can be treated with both systemic and local application of estrogen and the regular use of a vaginal dilator to maintain patency of the canal.

PREVENTION

There are many ways to strengthen efforts for prevention and early detection of cervical cancer. The most promising areas of research include those that focus on understanding and preventing HPV infections and understanding the process of cervical carcinogenesis and how it can be interrupted with chemopreventives. Preventing HPV infections with a humoral-based vaccine should eventually receive worldwide interest. Eventually, treating lesions with a cell-mediated-based vaccine would be exciting. Once the role of other cofactors (e.g., smoking, use of oral contraceptives, and diet) is assessed, specific behavioral interventions will be of interest. In general, the use of barrier contraception, delaying the onset of sexual activity, and limiting the number of partners should be encouraged as preventive behaviors. Early detection could be improved by increasing the use of the Pap smear in unscreened women, decreasing the false-negative rate of the Pap smear, automating the screening process to lower the cost, and better defining which patients need to be referred for colposcopy, which is expensive. Prompt evaluation and treatment of cervical cancer precursors should be encouraged, and technologies that automate or shorten the process should be vigorously developed.

FURTHER READING

American Cancer Society (2001) *Cancer Facts and Figures—2001*. American Cancer Society, Atlanta.

Coppleson M (ed) (1992) Carcinoma of cervix. In *Gynecologic Oncology: Fundamental Principles and Clinical Practice*. Churchill Livingstone, Edinburgh, pp. 543–728.

Clinical Announcement. Concurrent chemoradiation for cervical cancer. U.S. Department of Health and Human Services Public Health Service, National Institutes of Health, National Cancer Institute, February, 1999.

DiSaia PJ, Creasman WT (eds.) (1997) Invasive cervical cancer. In *Clinical Gynecologic Oncology*. Mosby-Year Book, St. Louis, pp. 51–106.

Eddy DM (1990) Screening for cervical cancer. *Ann Intern Med* 113:214–226.

Fahey MT, Irwig L, Macaskill P (1995) Meta-analysis of Pap test accuracy. *Am J Epidemiol* 141:680–689.

Follen M (2001) Preinvasive squamous lesions of the female lower genital tract. In *Operative Gynecology*. Gershenson DM, DeCherney AH, Stephen L, Brubaker L (eds.), WB Saunders, Philadelphia, pp. 273–299.

Follen M, Schottenfeld D (2001) Surrogate endpoint biomarkers: their modulation in cervical chemoprevention trials. *Cancer* 91:1758–1776.

Franco E, Monsonego J (1997) *New Developments in Cervical Cancer Screening and Prevention.* Blackwell, Malden, MA.

Hakama M, Miller AB, Day NE (1986) *Screening for Cancer of the Uterine Cervix.* IARC Scientific Publication No. 76.

International Agency for Research on Cancer Working Group on Evaluation of Cervical Cancer Screening Programs (1985) Screening for squamous cervical cancer: duration of low risk after negative results of cervical cytology and its implications for screening policies. *Br Med J (Clin Res Ed)* 293:659–664.

Kaufman RM, Henson DE, Herbst AL et al. (1994) Interim guidelines for management of abnormal cervical cytology. *JAMA* 271:1866–1869.

Lowy DR, Schiller JT (1998) Papillomaviruses and cervical cancer: pathogenesis and vaccine development. *Monogr Natl Cancer Inst* 23:27–30.

Meyskens FL, Surwit EA, Moon TE, Childers JM, Paris JR, Dorr RJ et al. (1994) Enhancement of regression of cervical intraepithelial neoplasia II (moderate dysplasia) with topically applied all trans-retinoic acid: a randomized trial. *J Natl Cancer Inst* 86:539–543.

Mitchell MF (1990) Diagnosis and treatment of preinvasive disease of the female lower genital tract. *Cancer Bull* 42:71–76.

Mitchell ME, Hittelman WN, Hong WK et al. (1994) Review: The natural history of cervical intraepithelial neoplasia: an argument for intermediate endpoint biomarkers. *Cancer Epidemiol Biomark Prev* 3:619–626.

Mitchell MF, Tortolero-Luna G, Wright T et al. (1996) Cervical human papillomavirus infection and intraepithelial neoplasia: a review. *J Natl Cancer Inst Monogr* 21:17–25.

Morris M, Burke TW (1983) Cervical cancer. In *Textbook of Gynecology.* Copeland LJ, Jarrell JF, McGregor JA (eds). WB Saunders, Philadelphia, pp. 989–1013.

Morris M, Tortolero-Luna G, Malpica A et al. (1996) Cervical intraepithelial neoplasia and cervical cancer. *Obstet Gynecol Clin North Am* 23:34710.

Morrow CP, Curtin JP, Townsend DE (eds) (1993) Tumors of the cervix. In *Synopsis of Gynecologic Oncology.* Churchill Livingstone, New York, pp. 111–152.

Munoz N, Bosch F, Shah KV, et al. (1992) *The Epidemiology of Human Papillomavirus and Cervical Cancer.* IARC Scientific Publication No. 119.

Murakami M, Gurski KJ, Steller MA (1999) Human papillomavirus vaccines for cervical cancer. *J Immunother* 22:212–218.

National Institutes of Health Consensus Conference on Cervical Cancer (1996) National Institutes of Health Consensus Conference on Cervical Cancer. Bethesda, Maryland, April 1–3, 1996. *J Natl Cancer Inst Monogr* 21:1–6.

Parkin DM, Pisani P, Ferlay J (1999) Estimates of the worldwide incidence of 25 major cancers in 1990. *Int J Cancer* 80:827–841.

Pisani P, Parkin DM, Munoz N et al. (1997) Cancer and infection: estimates of the attributable fraction in 1990. *Cancer Epidemiol Biomark Prev* 6:387–400.

Robin SC, Hoskins WJ (1996) *Cervical Cancer and Preinvasive Neoplasia.* Lippincott-Raven, Philadelphia.

Shingleton HM, Orr JW (1983) *Cancer of the Cervix: Diagnosis and Treatment,* 1st edition. Churchill Livingstone, New York.

Shingleton HM, Orr JW Jr (1987) *Cancer of the Cervix: Diagnosis and Treatment,* 2nd edition. Churchill Livingstone, New York.

Vlastos AT, Follen M (2004) Biomarkers and their use in cervical cancer chemoprevention trials. *Crit Rev Oncol Hematol* (in press).

Vlastos AT, Richards-Kortum R, Zuluaga A, Follen M (2002) New approaches to cervical cancer screening. *Contemp Ob Gyn* 5:87–103.

CHAPTER 25

Gynecological Cancer

J. L. BENEDET

British Columbia Cancer Agency, Division of Gynecologic Oncology, Vancouver, British Columbia, Canada

CANCER OF THE ENDOMETRIUM

Incidence

Endometrial cancer has become the most common gynecological cancer in many industrialized countries and is approximately three times as common as invasive cervical cancer. In both Canada and the United States, endometrial cancer ranks fourth in terms of incident cancers in women and approximately 8th or 10th in terms of death from malignancy. The estimated number of new cases in Canada for 2000 is approximately 3,500 cases with an estimate of 670 deaths. This gives a death to cases ratio of 0.19. Therefore, this malignancy has a very good prognosis in contrast to, say, lung cancer, where the death to case ratio is 0.83, reflecting its poor prognosis. The prominence of endometrial cancer in relationship to cervical cancer in industrialized countries is a reflection of the success of widespread screening programs for cervical neoplasia and its precursors. A longer life expectancy of women in industrialized countries is also a possible contributing factor to the increased frequency of this disorder.

Epidemiology and Etiology

Cancer of the endometrium is predominantly a disease of postmenopausal women, with the peak incidence occurring in women of approximately 60 years of age. Both hormonal and reproductive factors appear important in the etiology of this disorder. The basic mechanism that has been used to explain the development of endometrial cancer has been prolonged unopposed estrogen stimulation of the endometrium. A natural history model for this disease has been granulosa-theca cell tumors of the

UICC Manual of Clinical Oncology, Eighth Edition. Edited by Raphael E. Pollock
ISBN 0-471-22289-5 Copyright © 2004 John Wiley & Sons, Inc.

TABLE 25.1. Risk Factors for the Development of Endometrial Cancer

Endogenous	Exogenous	Demographic
Obesity	Hormone replacement	Higher social economic
Infertility	therapy with	status
Chronic anovulation	unopposed estrogen	Caucasian or Jewish
Nulliparity	Diet	Family history of
Polycystic ovarian		breast, colon, or
disease		endometrial cancer

ovary, which have an associated endometrial cancer at the time of diagnosis in approximately 5–10% of cases. Other conditions of altered hormone activity characterized by chronic anovulation such as seen in polycystic ovarian syndrome have also been associated with an increased frequency of endometrial cancer.

Obesity, diabetes, and hypertension increase the risk of endometrial cancer, possibly by indirect influences on estrogen levels, which in turn influence the level of stimulation of the target endometrial epithelium. Most studies have also demonstrated that early age of menarche, defined as before age 11 or 12 years, is associated with an increased risk for this disease, as is late menopause. Table 25.1 lists the risk factors for this disease. The most consistent factor identified with endometrial cancer is the use of estrogen replacement therapy after menopause. Increasing dosage or duration of estrogen therapy also raises the risk of endometrial cancer. Although the risk has been shown to decrease after cessation of estrogen therapy, an increased risk will persist for many years, with summary estimates suggesting that this risk is raised approximately twofold for 5 or more years after discontinuation of use. The addition of a cyclic progesterone would appear to counteract the continuous mitotic stimulation of the endometrium by unopposed estrogen therapy. The progesterone is thought to antagonize this stimulating effect by decreasing estrogen receptors and increasing the activity of enzymes that metabolize estradiol to less potent metabolites. The use of combined oral contraceptive medications has also been shown to reduce the risk of endometrial cancer, with long-term use thought to reduce the risk the most and its protective effect lasting for a long period after discontinuation. Reports from clinical trials in women treated for breast cancer with tamoxifen have shown an increase in endometrial cancer rates in these women. This risk also appears to be related to increasing duration treatment with tamoxifen as well as increasing cumulative dose.

Screening

In terms of population screening, the value of endometrial sampling as a screening test in asymptomatic women remains unproven. Both endometrial sampling and ultrasonography have been proposed as a screening modality for this cancer, but do not adequately satisfy the criteria for a good screening test. Given the low prevalence of this disease in asymptomatic women, it is difficult to justify routine screening with these techniques in such individuals. Women who are at high risk because of family history (Lynch syndrome type II) or who are on prolonged estrogen or tamoxifen therapy might benefit from endometrial sampling, and, in specific situations, transvaginal ultrasonographic assessment for endometrial thickness.

Pathology

The majority of endometrial cancers are well-differentiated lesions with an endometrioid pattern accounting for approximately 80% of cases. Papillary serous and clear cell carcinomas as well as adenosquamous cancers account for 10% of endometrial malignancies and are generally more aggressive lesions. Considerable controversy has existed over the significance of endometrial hyperplasia and its potential role as a cancer precursor. Lack of uniformity in the definition and classification of these lesions as well as differences among pathologists in classification and assessment have contributed to the problem. Currently, patterns that exhibit complex atypical hyperplasia are estimated to progress to endometrial cancer in approximately 20–25% of the cases if left untreated.

Most endometrial cancers are well-differentiated tumors with superficial myometrial invasion only. Tumor grade is also related to depth of invasion, with the more deeply invasive tumors usually being high grade. The most common site of origin for endometrial cancers is generally in the fundus, with subsequent spread by surface extension to the remainder of the endometrial surface as well as cervix, tubes, ovaries occasionally, and ultimately other peritoneal surfaces. Once these lesions invade the underlying myometrium they can also involve lymphatic or vascular spaces and in turn lead to pelvic and periaortic lymph node metastases. Periaortic lymph node metastases without pelvic node involvement can and do occur but would appear to be uncommon.

In general, papillary serous adenocarcinoma and clear cell lesions of the endometrium behave in an aggressive manner. However, some studies have shown that, if diagnosed as early superficial lesions, the prognosis may not be as poor for this histologic subtype. A problem in diagnosis and classification of these lesions is that there is no agreement among pathologists as to what percentage of an endometrial cancer needs to show clear cell or papillary serous features before being classified into one of these categories.

Diagnosis

Endometrial cancer has a classic presenting symptom, namely that of postmenopausal bleeding or spotting and, when present, this symptom should be regarded as endometrial cancer until proven otherwise. Although only 35% of such patients will be found to have endometrial cancer or other forms of pelvic malignancy, this disease remains the most important cause of this symptom. Prompt attention to this distinctive symptom by both patient and physician is undoubtedly responsible for the majority of cases being diagnosed in a stage I category resulting in a favorable outcome.

The diagnosis of endometrial cancer is determined by histopathological representative biopsy of tissue. Historically, these tissue samples were obtained by dilatation and curettage under general anesthesia, but more recently this has been largely replaced by outpatient investigation including endometrial biopsy, hysteroscopic evaluation and ultrasonography. Hysteroscopy has the advantage of providing visualization of the entire endometrial cavity and enabling a directed biopsy of any abnormal area. If endometrial biopsies fail to show endometrial cancer in patients with postmenopausal bleeding and, where the symptoms persist, hysteroscopy with dilatation and curettage would appear to be appropriate.

TABLE 25.2. Corpus Uteri: TNM Clinical Classification—Staging for Tumors and FIGO Surgical Staging

TNM Categories	FIGO Stages	Characteristic
TX		Primary tumor cannot be assessed
T0		No evidence of parimary tumor
Tis	0	Carcinoma *in situ*
T1	I	Tumor confined to corpus
T1a	IA	Tumor limited to endometrium
T1b	IB	Tumor invades up to or less than one-half of myometrium
T1c	IC	Tumor invades to more than one-half of myometrium
T2	II	Tumor invades cervix but does not extend beyond uterus
T2a	IIA	Endocervical glandular involvement only
T2b	IIB	Cervical stromal invasion
T3 and/or N1	III	Local and/or regional spread as specified in T3a, b, N1 and FIGO IIIA, B, C below
T3a	IIIA	Tumor involves serosa and/or adnexa (direct extension or metastasis) and/or cancer cells in ascites or peritoneal washings
T3b	IIIB	Vaginal involvement (direct extension or metastasis)
N1	IIIC	Metastasis to pelvic and/or para-aortic lymph nodes
T4	IVA	Tumor involves bladder mucosa and/or bowel mucosa
M1	IVB	Distant metastasis (excluding metastasis to vagina, pelvic serosa or adnexa; including metastasis to intra-abdominal lymph nodes other than para-aortic and/or inguinal lymph nodes)

Staging

Endometrial carcinoma staging is surgical and is presented in Table 25.2, with Figure 25.1 diagrammatically illustrating stage I disease. Though the staging system was changed to a surgical system in 1988, clinical staging is still important in assessing extent of disease and helping plan therapy. Clinical staging correlates well with surgical staging and prognosis. In the majority of cases, if the uterus is not enlarged and there is no evidence of extra uterine disease or cervical involvement, further assessment consisting of a chest x-ray and the usual preoperative blood work and chemistry is sufficient. More complex preoperative assessments such as magnetic resonance imaging (MRI) or computed tomography (CT) scans, barium enema, cystoscopy, and so on are indicated for patients whose disease suggests involvement of other organ systems or spread. MRI is the most accurate in assessing myometrial invasion or cervical involvement.

Approximately 10–15% of patients with clinical stage I disease will have evidence of more advanced disease underlying the importance of surgical staging. It is recommended that in patients with clinical stage I disease peritoneal washing should be obtained on entering the abdominal cavity. Careful exploration of the entire abdominal pelvic cavity should be carried out with biopsy of any suspicious areas including examination and removal of any enlarged para-aortic, iliac, or pelvic lymph nodes followed by total abdominal hysterectomy/bilateral and oophorectomy (TAH/BSO) cases in straightforward cases. Simple TAH and BSO is the preferred method of treatment for stage I endometrial cancer. Some have advocated that TAH/BSO be performed after washings are taken for clinical stage I patients with the removed uterus then immediately opened and carefully examined pathologically by frozen-section to assess depth of invasion and confirm grade and histologic type. If these findings show high-grade or deep (greater than 1/2) myometrial invasion, further staging with node dissection of the pelvic and para-aortic areas is then carried out.

Although surgical staging with pelvic and para-aortic removal clearly offers the most thorough assessment of disease it should be remembered that many of these patients are elderly, and often obese with complicating diseases including diabetes and hypertension. In these situations, clinical judgment should be used, as careful surgical-pathological assessment of the removed tissue can generally and accurately predict the likelihood of risk of recurrence and the need for adjunctive therapy. As yet, there are no studies clearly indicating improvement in survival from pelvic and/or para-aortic lymphadenectomy in patients with endometrial cancer.

Postsurgical Treatment

Once surgical staging has occurred and the resected tissue has been carefully assessed histologically, a decision is then made whether or not postoperative adjunctive therapy is needed. Cases can be classified as high or low risk for recurrence based on a variety of factors. High-risk patients are generally those with grade 2 or 3 disease, deep myometrial invasion (>50%) or where evidence of

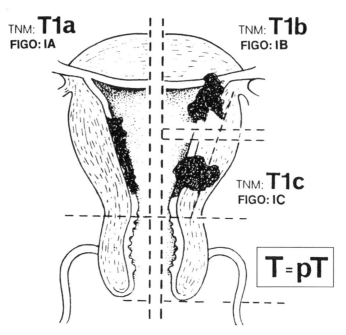

TNM: **T1a**
FIGO: IA

TNM: **T1b**
FIGO: IB

TNM: **T1c**
FIGO: IC

T = pT

Figure 25.1   Stage I carcinoma of the corpus uteri, depicting the three subcategories of T1.

lymphatic vascular space involvement is noted. Any extrauterine disease as well as nodal metastases are high-risk features. Papillary serous clear-cell and adenosquamous histologies are also considered high-risk. Individuals with well-differentiated grade 1 tumors confined to the inner one-third of the myometrium have an excellent prognosis with surgery alone and do not require adjunctive therapy.

A variety of hormonal and radiotherapeutic schemes have been used as adjunctive therapy in stage I cases with high-risk features. It is generally agreed that postoperative radiotherapy, either in the form of vault or pelvic irradiation, can help lower the incidence of local recurrence but does not appear to have any beneficial effect in terms of survival. Fortunately, the vast majority of cases are diagnosed with stage I low-risk disease and are successfully treated with simple hysterectomy.

Primary radiotherapy or preoperative intracavitary radiotherapy followed by hysterectomy is no longer commonly used. The present role of radiotherapy in endometrial cancer is in a state of flux largely as a result of increased use of surgical staging with better knowledge of prognostic factors, which has made routine radiotherapy less common and its overall use more selective.

Effective therapy for advanced stage disease or recurrent disease to date has proven to be elusive. Generally, a combination of radiotherapy and/or chemotherapy has been used in these situations. Currently, combinations of platinum and taxol chemotherapy are favored for recurrent or metastatic disease. These agents generally produce a good response but the duration of response, unfortunately, in most cases is short lived. Other medications with documented response in endometrial cancer have been adriamycin and 5-fluorouracil. Hormonal therapy with progestational agents can also lead to excellent responses in some patients with recurrent or advanced disease. Most often, individuals with better differentiated tumors are those most likely to respond to hormonal therapy.

Prognosis

The 5-year survival rate for stage I endometrial carcinoma is approximately 90%, with survival falling to 75% and 50% for stage II and III disease, respectively. Clearly identified prognostic factors for endometrial carcinoma consist of stage, grade, depth of myometrial invasion, lymphatic-vascular space involvement, and histologic type.

Summary

Endometrial adenocarcinoma is a common tumor, which fortunately most often presents with a distinctive symptom enabling a diagnosis to be made while the patient still has stage I disease. Generally, it has a favorable outcome and is usually treated with primary surgery with or without adjunctive radiotherapy depending on subsequent surgical pathologic findings.

CANCER OF THE VULVA

Vulvar cancer accounts for approximately 5% of all gynecologic cancers and is one of the least common of the major gynecologic tumors. Invasive carcinoma of the vulva is predominately a disease of older women although reports of the disease in younger reproductive age group women is becoming more common.

Epidemiology and Etiology

The etiology of this disease remains unknown. Factors that have been identified for other squamous cancers of the epithelium, such as exposure to sunlight and ultraviolet radiation, are not thought to be causative agents for these lesions. Recently, interest has focused on the possible role of prior human papilloma virus (HPV) infections as a potential agent or cofactor similar to that seen in squamous neoplasia of the cervix. The relationship to HPV has also been evoked to explain the not infrequent occurrence of lesions that involve the cervix, vagina, and vulva, either in a synchronous or metachronous fashion. Evidence also exists to suggest different etiologic mechanisms between young and older age group patients with lesions in the older age group being less likely to be related to prior HPV infections.

Pathology

Squamous cell carcinomas are the most common histologic types, followed in frequency by malignant melanoma, and much less commonly Paget's disease of the vulva and basal cell carcinoma. Carcinomas arising from Bartholin's gland itself is uncommon, and histologically show an adenocarcinoma cell type pattern. Lesions may also arise from Bartholin's duct and histologically these lesions will have either a squamous cell or uncommonly a transitional cell carcinoma pattern. Carcinoma *in situ* is considered to be a precursor lesion for invasive cancer of the vulva. This view is supported by the difference in age groups between the two types of lesions, a positive past history of carcinoma *in situ* in many patients, and also the presence of coexisting carcinoma *in situ* at the margins of many invasive lesions.

Diagnosis

The most common presenting symptoms of vulvar cancer are pruritus, irritation, discharge, or the presence of a lesion. Vulvar cancer can have a variety of clinical appearances based on duration, site, and histologic type. Lesions may be ulcerative, nodular, or exophytic and most often are located on the labia and lateral structures of the upper half of the vulva. Lesions arising in the perineum or clitoris are less common but clearly recognizable primary sites for vulvar cancer. It is recommended that all cases have a biopsy to confirm the diagnosis and histology of these lesions prior to any definitive therapy.

Vulvar cancer generally spreads by direct extension and via lymphatic channels to regional lymph nodes. Primary lymphatic drainage of the external vulvar structures is to the superficial inguinal femoral lymph nodes. The next nodal stations are the internal iliac and pelvic lymph nodes followed by the common iliac and para-aortic nodes. When vulvar carcinoma is suspected or diagnosed, careful palpitation of the inguinal-femoral areas should be carried out to assess for the possibility of clinically suspicious or enlarged nodes. Vulvar tumors, particularly neglected lesions, are often accompanied by superficial infection so the presence of groin lymphadenopathy is not uncommon and enlarged nodes are not necessarily indicative of metastatic disease but rather reaction to infection. On the other hand, lymph nodes that appear fixed to deeper groin structures or the overlying skin usually signify advanced stage disease with a poor prognosis.

Lesions that involve the clitoris or the perineum have the potential for spread directly to deeper pelvic lymph nodes, but such primary spread is uncommon without first involving the groin nodes.

Staging

The current staging system for vulvar cancer is presented in Table 25.3. Figure 25.2 illustrates the features of a stage I tumor.

TABLE 25.3. FIGO Staging for Carcinoma of the Vulva

Stage 0	
TIS	Carcinoma *in situ*; intraepithelial carcinoma
Stage I	
T1 N0 M0	Tumor confined to the vulva and/or perineum, $\leq$2 cm in greatest dimensions, nodes are negative
Stage IA	Lesions $\leq$2 cm in size confined to the vulva or perineum with stromal invasion <1.0 mm.
	No nodal metastases. The depth of invasion is defined as the measurement of the tumor from the epithelial-stromal junction of the adjacent most superficial derma papilla to the deepest point of invasion
Stage IB	Lesions $\leq$2 cm in size confined to the vulva or perineum with stromal invasion >1.0 mm. No nodal metastases
Stage II	
T2 N0 M0	Tumor confined to the vulva and/or perineum, >2 cm in greatest dimension, nodes are negative
Stage III	
T3 N0 M0	Tumor of any size with
T3 N1 M0	(1) Adjacent spread to the lower urethra and/or the vagina, or the anus, and/or
T1 N1 M0	(2) Unilateral regional lymph node metastasis
T2 N1 M0	
Stage IV	
T1 N2 M0	Tumor invades any of the following:
T2 N2 M0	Upper urethra, bladder mucosa, rectal mucosa, pelvic bone, and/or bilateral regional node metastasis
T3 N2 M0	
T4 any N M0	
Stage IVB	
Any T	Any distant metastasis including pelvic lymph nodes
Any N, M1	
T—Primary tumor	
Tis	Preinvasive carcinoma (carcinoma *in situ*)
T1	Tumor confined to the vulva and/or perineum <2 cm in greatest dimension
	T1a—with stromal invasion $\leq$1.0 mm
	T2b—with stromal invasion >1.0 mm
T2	Tumor confined to the vulva and/or perineum >2 cm in greatest dimension
T3	Tumor of any size with adjacent spread to the urethra and/or vagina and/or the anus
T4	Tumor of any size infiltrating the bladder mucosa and/or the rectal mucosa, upper part of the urethral mucosa and/or fixed to the pubic bone
N—Regional lymph nodes	
N0	No lymph node metastasis
N1	Unilateral regional lymph node metastasis
N2	Bilateral regional lymph node metastasis

TABLE 25.3 (*Continued*)

M—Distant metastasis			
M0	No clinical metastasis		
M1	Distant metastasis (including pelvic lymph node metastasis)		

Stage			
0	Tis	N0	M0
I	T1	N0	M0
IA	T1a	N0	M0
IB	T1b	N0	M0
II	T2	N0	M0
III	T1	N0	M0
	T2	N1	M0
	T3	N0,N1	M0
IVA	T1	N2	M0
	T2	N2	M0
	T3	N2	M0
	T4	Any N	M0
IVB	T1	Any N	M1

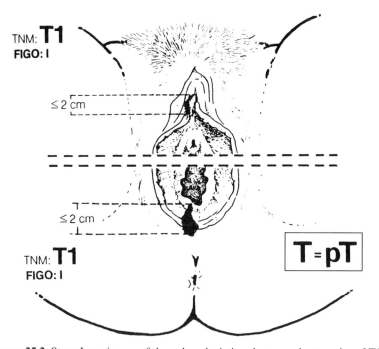

Figure 25.2 Stage I carcinoma of the vulva, depicting the two subcategories of T1.

Treatment

Treatment of vulvar carcinoma is primarily surgical with multiple modality therapy consisting of combined radiotherapy and surgery used in specialized situations. Radical vulvectomy with *en bloc* bilateral inguinal femoral lymphadenectomy has been the traditional treatment of choice for vulvar cancer but is used less frequently today as increased individualization of surgical resection has been shown to produce equally good results in terms of survival and outcome but with less morbidity. Radical vulvectomy and excision can be associated with significant psychosexual problems as well as physical complications from these operations. These complications may be classified as general surgical complications such as bleeding, infection, postoperative deep vein thrombosis, and also complications related specifically to either the groin dissections and/or vulvectomy. The complications specific to groin dissections can include such conditions as lymphedema of the lower extremities, hernia formation, and delayed wound healing. Complications specific to the vulvar surgery itself depend mainly on the extent and whether or not clitoral or other central structures were removed or altered. These complications include decreased sensation and sensitivity of the tissues, dyspareunia, introital stenosis, and stricture of the urethral meatus with voiding difficulties. Psychosexual identity and body image problems are not to be underestimated in women undergoing this type of surgery.

Currently, surgical management is individualized based on the size, site, depth of invasion, histologic type, age, patient general medical condition, and whether nor not lymphatic-vascular space invasion is noted. The most important prognostic factor in vulvar carcinoma is whether disease has spread to the regional lymph nodes. In addition, the number of positive nodes, whether bilateral or unilateral, the size of the nodal metastasis, and the presence of any extranodal disease are among the most important prognostic factors for vulvar cancer.

Tumor thickness also relates well to the incidence of nodal disease, particularly with smaller sized tumors.

Small, laterally located lesions can be managed with wide local excision with an attempt to obtain a 2-cm margin and a unilateral inguinal femoral node dissection. If the removed nodes are negative, no further surgery is usually needed and the prognosis is very good. Central lesions will require bilateral node dissection and unfortunately more radical vulvar excision. Surgery can be accomplished either through three separate incisions or in an en bloc fashion.

Radiotherapy is generally used to treat the pelvic nodal areas in those individuals found to have metastases in the inguinal femoral lymph nodes. Radiotherapy may also be used in patients with positive margins. Combined modality therapy with radiotherapy followed by surgery may be helpful in individuals with lesions that are close to or encroach on the anal sphincter. In such situations, radiotherapy may shrink these lesions and permit subsequent surgery to be less radical with preservation of the sphincter and anal continence thus avoiding the classic posterior exenteration or abdominal-peritoneal type resection for such lesions.

Late central recurrences do occur and many of these can be successfully managed by repeat wide local excision. This, in turn, seems to indicate that there are several variants to this disease that seem to behave as locally invasive lesions with little propensity for early distant spread. Nonetheless, the seriousness of this disease should never be underestimated as spread to extravulvar sites does occur and carries with it a poor prognosis.

Chemotherapy would appear to be of limited value in patients with vulvar cancer. It has been used not only as an adjunct in combined therapy but also as a radiosensitizer similar to its use in certain anal or rectal cancers.

In patients with malignant melanoma of the vulva, routine node dissection is no longer thought to have therapeutic value but any enlarged or suspicious nodes should be resected as a palliative measure.

Prognosis

Stage I and stage II tumors or tumors without nodal metastases have an extremely good 5-year disease-free survival approaching 90 to 95% in most series. Patients with only one positive lymph node without extranodal disease also appear to have an excellent prognosis similar to those without nodal disease. Clearly identified prognostic factors for nodal disease are (a) depth of invasion; (b) a number of positive nodes, whether or not bilateral nodal disease exists, or whether or not extranodal or extracapsular spread of disease is present; and (c) the size of deposits in nodes. Although regional lymph node involvement has been consistently shown to be the single most important prognostic factor for vulvar cancer, primary tumor size has also been shown in a number of studies to be a significant predictor for survival, local recurrence, but also for nodal metastasis itself.

Summary

In the past decade, a clearer understanding of the important prognostic for vulvar cancer has emerged. The presence of disease in regional lymph nodes is currently the single most important identifiable predictor for survival and recurrence. This understanding on the prognostic factors associated with vulvar cancer has led to more individualized and less radical treatment for individuals, particularly those with small, early stage, superficially invasive, laterally located lesions. In turn, this has resulted in less morbidity and better functional and cosmetic results without compromising the chance for cure for these women.

CANCER OF THE OVARY

The most common cause of death from gynecologic malignancy worldwide is from cervical cancer because of its frequent occurrence and poor outcomes, particularly in developing countries. However, in most industrialized countries, ovarian cancer is the leading cause of gynecological cancer deaths. Although our knowledge and approach to the management of ovarian cancer has changed in the past 25 years, the overall survival remains low and has improved little in this period of time. This has largely been attributed to the fact that the majority of patients diagnosed with epithelial ovarian cancer have stage III or IV disease at presentation.

Epidemiology and Etiology

Ovarian cancer is most common in women in their fifth to seventh decade, and an individual's lifetime risk for developing ovarian cancer is estimated to be 1 in 70. Fortunately, younger women are more likely to have tumors with low malignant potential. The etiology of ovarian malignancy remains unknown. Hereditary or genetic factors appear to play a role in approximately 5% of ovarian cancers. Some of the identifying risk factors for ovarian cancer are similar to breast cancer and include early menarche, delayed menopause, and nulliparity. High parity, breast-feeding, and prolonged use of oral contraceptive medications would seem to confer a degree of protection for ovarian cancer.

Individuals with a family history of ovarian cancer should have a careful assessment to determine their particular risk profile. In addition, individuals with a family history of breast, colon, endometrial, and prostate cancer also should have careful assessment of their pedigree to determine whether they have one of the recognized groups of either site-specific ovarian cancer or breast-ovarian cancer or breast-colon-endometrial-prostate cancer pedigrees, which would also place them at increased risk for ovarian malignancy. The risk for these latter two groups is not as high as for those with familial site-specific disease. However, as our ability to identify and test for specific gene mutations linked to this disease increases, such knowledge becomes important in the management in these individuals.

Pathology

Table 25.4 presents a modified World Health Organization (WHO) classification of ovarian tumors. This system basically classifies tumors into three major categories: those arising from the surface epithelium (the most common of all ovarian malignancies); tumors that arise from the ovarian stromal tissue, either the specialized ovarian stroma or the supportive stromal elements such as fibrous tissue, blood vessels, etc.; and tumors arising from germ cells. The common epithelial ovarian malignancies, serous mucinous and endometrioid and clear cell carcinoma, generally behave in a similar fashion on a stage-for-stage basis. Epithelial ovarian cancer has a propensity for spread along peritoneal surfaces following the pathway seen by the circulation of peritoneal fluid. Common sites of metastases are the pelvic peritoneum, pelvic organs, peritoneal surfaces of the abdomen, mesentery, omentum, and diaphragmatic surfaces. Lymphatic spread of ovarian cancer is also common.

It is important to differentiate between tumors of low malignant potential (borderline tumors) and frankly invasive epithelial ovarian cancers. The diagnosis of borderline tumors depends essentially on the presence or absence of stromal

TABLE 25.4. Modified WHO Classification of Ovarian Epithelial Tumors

I. *Common "epithelial" tumors*
    A. Serous
    B. Mucinous   (a) Benign
    C. Endometrioid   (b) Of borderline malignancy
    D. Clear cell (mesonephroid)   (c) Malignant
    E. Brenner
    F. Mixed epithelial
    G. Undifferentiated carcinoma
    H. Unclassified
II. *Sex cord stromal tumors*
    A. Granulosa—theca cell   (a) Benign
    B. Androblastoma (Sertoli-Leydig)   (b) Malignant
    C. Gynandroblastoma
    D. Unclassified
III. *Lipid cell tumors*
IV. *Germ cell tumors*
    A. Dysgerminoma
    B. Endodermal sinus tumor
    C. Embryonal carcinoma
    D. Polyembryoma
    E. Choriocarcinoma
    F. Teratomas: immature; mature (solid or cystic);
            monodermal (struma ovarii and/or
            carcinoid, others)

invasion in the primary ovarian tumor site, but does not consider the extraovarian spread of the disease. Most borderline tumors are diagnosed in early stages and represent approximately 5–10% of ovarian neoplasms with an overall 5-year survival rate ranging from 85 to 95%. Borderline tumors with a mucinous histology are the only group with a poor prognosis and are associated with pseudomyxoma peritonei. Currently, it is thought that most if not all ovarian mucinous tumors associated with pseudomyxoma peritonei are metastatic tumors of gastrointestinal origin mainly from the appendix and rarely from the colon itself. Of the true mucinous ovarian borderline tumors, those defined as endocervical mucinous type have a much better prognosis compared with those showing an intestinal mucinous pattern.

The overall clinical behavior of borderline tumors is much less aggressive than other epithelial ovarian lesions even when diagnosed with extraovarian spread. The extraovarian implants are generally assessed and can be further subdivided into those that are thought to have benign or noninvasive implants and those with invasive implants showing invasive patterns into the extraovarian fibrous tissue.

Germ cell tumors are the second most common group of ovarian malignancies with the majority of lesions occurring in women less than 40 years of age. In the past, with the exception of dysgerminomas, the overall prognosis was poor for these lesions, but with the advent of platinum-based chemotherapy utilizing multimodality regimens similar to that for testicular germ cell tumors, cure rates in excess of 80–85% have been obtained also with the preservation of menstrual and reproductive function. Currently, regimens containing BEP (bleomycin, etoposide, and cis-platinum) are the agents of choice.

In general, tumors that arise from the sex chord stroma tend to behave in a more indolent fashion with the exception of some granulosa-theca cell tumors. All these tumors may be hormonally active producing estrogen and/or androgen. The ovary is not an uncommon site for metastatic spread for tumors arising from the breast or gastrointestinal tract.

Screening and Diagnosis

Currently, there is no effective acceptable screening test for epithelial ovarian cancer. Tumor markers such as CA-125, although useful in monitoring disease states, unfortunately do not have sufficient sensitivity and specificity to be used as an effective screening test. Ultrasonography, either abdominal or transvaginal, has also been evaluated as a potential screening tool either in combination with CA-125 or alone, but has also not proven to be effective as a screening tool. However, individuals at risk for familiar ovarian cancer may benefit from assessment with ultrasound and tumor marker on a regular basis. Alpha-fetoprotein (AFP) and beta-human chorionic gonadotropin (BhCG) are tumor markers that are helpful in follow-up in patients with germ cell tumors.

Most women with early stage disease are asymptomatic and diagnosis at this stage is usually the result of incidental finding of an adnexal or ovarian mass either on the basis of some other pelvic examination or ultrasound scanning of the pelvis or abdomen for other problems. In such asymptomatic individuals, any adnexal enlargement greater than 5 cm on a routine pelvic exam should the suspicion of possible ovarian cancer, and, particularly if ultrasonography shows intracystic septations or papillary patterns. Prompt investigation with removal of such masses is generally indicated. Unfortunately, most patients diagnosed with epithelial ovarian cancer are diagnosed with stage III or IV disease. At this phase, patients most commonly present with vague gastrointestinal complaints often consisting of bloating, indigestion, and, ultimately, abdominal distention with ascites. Patients may also complain of increasing abdominal girth, decreased appetite, and a feeling of generally being tired and unwell.

Staging

Ovarian cancer is staged surgically and the currently used system is presented in Table 25.5. Figure 25.3 illustrates the features of a typical stage III cancer.

Treatment

The primary treatment of epithelial ovarian cancer is surgical with the intent of resecting all gross disease so that no tumor deposits or deposits less than 1 cm in

TABLE 25.5. Ovary TNM Clinical Classification: Staging for Tumors and FIGO Surgical Staging

TNM Categories	FIGO Stages	Characteristic
TX		Parimary tumor cannot be assessed
T0		No evidence of primary tumor
T1	I	Tumor limited to ovaries
T1a	IA	Tumor limited to one ovary; capsule intact; no tumor on ovarian surface; no malignant cells in ascites or peritoneal washings
T1b	IB	Tumor limited to both ovaries; capsules intact, no tumor on ovarian surface; no malignant cells in ascites or peritoneal washings
T1c	IC	Tumor limited to one or both ovaries with any of the following: capsule ruptured, tumor on ovarian surface, malignant cells in ascites or peritoneal washings
T2	II	Tumor involves one or both ovaries with pelvic extension
T2a	IIA	Extension and/or implants on uterus and/or tube(s); no malignant cells in ascites or peritoneal washings
T2b	IIB	Extension to other pelvic tissues; no malignant cells in ascites or peritoneal washings
T2c	IIC	Pelvic extension (2a or 2b) with malignant cells in ascites or peritoneal washings
T3 and/or N1	III	Tumor involves one or both ovaries with microscopically confirmed peritoneal metastasis outside the pelvis and/or regional lymph node metastasis
T3a	IIIA	Microscopic peritoneal metastasis beyond pelvis
T3b	IIIB	Macroscopic peritoneal metastasis beyond pelvis ≤ 2 cm in 35 greatest dimension
T3c and/or NI	IIIC	Peritoneal metastasis beyond pelvis >2 cm in greatest dimension and/or regional lymph node metastasis
M1	IV	Distant metastasis (excludes peritoneal metastasis)

Note: Liver capsule metastasis is T3/stage III, liver parenchymal metastasis M1/stage IV. Pleural effusion must have positive cytology for M1/stage IV.

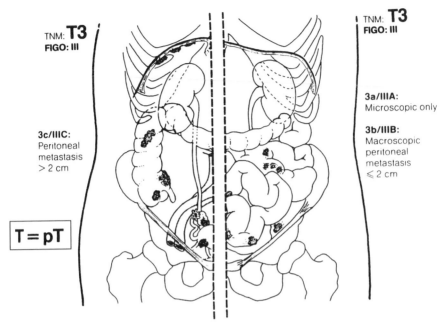

TNM: **T3**
FIGO: III

3c/IIIC:
Peritoneal
metastasis
> 2 cm

T = pT

TNM: **T3**
FIGO: III

3a/IIIA:
Microscopic only

3b/IIIB:
Macroscopic
peritoneal
metastasis
≤ 2 cm

Figure 25.3 Stage III carcinoma of the ovary, depicting the three subcategories of T3. In addition to the T3 category, N1 (regional lymph node metastasis) is included in the stage IIIC subgroup.

size are left at the completion of surgery. TAH/BSO and omentectomy are the main objectives of surgery, with some modifications for tumor distribution, patient medical condition, disease stage, and the patient's desire for fertility. Thorough surgical staging is important, particularly in younger patients with apparent stage I disease where fertility is desired. Careful attention and exploration of the retro-peritoneal lymphatic areas needs to be carried out with biopsy and removal of enlarged or suspicious nodes. Similarly, attention to diaphragmatic surfaces is mandatory to see whether unsuspected upper abdominal disease has occurred. Following surgery, patients are generally assigned into risk categories based on stage, residual disease, and grade of tumor, which appear to be the three most important factors with regards to prognosis and outcome. In general, the patients with stage Ia, grade I disease do not need any further adjuvant therapy postsurgery and have an excellent prognosis. Individuals with more advanced disease or with residual positive disease usually will receive combination chemotherapy. Currently, combination chemotherapy with platinum and taxol are those most favored for this condition. Carboplatinum has generally been substituted for cis-platinum because of less neurological and renal toxicity. Nonetheless, a large number of agents alone or in combination have been shown to be effective in epithelial ovarian cancer. The current concepts of interval debulking and neoadjuvant therapy are also gaining popularity, particularly for patients with advanced stage disease and in whom clinical and radiological findings suggest that the likelihood of achieving "zero residual" with initial surgery may be poor. Several studies have shown that many of these patients, if given three cycles of chemotherapy and followed by surgery, may do equally as well as patients treated with the more traditional primary surgery approach. The neoadjuvant and interval debulking approach for individuals who have obvious extensive intraabdominal disease may have the advantage of more quickly relieving symptoms of ascites, distention, and pressure. These approaches are also associated with an ultimate likelihood of achieving a high rate of zero residual postoperatively.

Multiple bowel loop resection at the time of primary surgery is generally not recommended. Often, such an approach still fails to result in zero residual disease and leads to delayed nutritional improvement and not infrequently complications related to this type of surgery in itself. Radiotherapy was used extensively to treat ovarian cancer in the past, but currently is used much less frequently. It is still useful in combination therapy in certain cases of low-residual, low-stage disease in an attempt to further consolidate response. Basic limitations to radiotherapy in ovarian cancer have been the large field size needed and the necessary shielding of kidneys and liver, which to a degree may also shield peritoneal tumor implants in these areas.

Prognosis

Prognosis of ovarian cancer is largely dependent on the stage at presentation and the effectiveness of surgical therapy and the response to chemotherapy. Table 25.6 presents the survival of patients by stage. Patients with no residual disease postsurgery have a much better survival rate than those with any residual disease following resection. Patients who ultimately succumb to this disease usually do so with extensive intra-abdominal disease resulting in malnutrition, cachexia, and ultimately bowel obstruction.

Summary

Ovarian cancer is relatively uncommon, which is fortunate because the majority of women afflicted present with stage III or IV disease. Unfortunately, the overall

TABLE 25.6. Survival Rates, Epithelial Ovarian Cancer by Stage

Stage	Survival Rate (%)
Ia	90
Ib	65
II	45
III	25
IV	5

survival rate remains low and has improved little over the past 25 years. Future strategies should focus on earlier diagnosis where possible and newer strategies for multimodality approaches.

GESTATIONAL TROPHOBLASTIC NEOPLASIA

Gestational trophoblastic disease (GTD) refers to a series of disorders that arise from the blastocyst and are characterized by an abnormal proliferation of trophoblastic tissue. Trophoblast is the ectodermal covering of the blastocyst that erodes into the uterine mucosa and through which the developing embryo receives nutrition from the maternal circulation. This tissue has metabolic, hormonal, and immunologic functions, which are all important in terms of the diagnosis of these disorders and their response to therapy. At present, it is thought that each of the specific forms GTD is related to discreet pathological aberrations, which occur at different stages of placentation or gametogenesis. This tissue is classified on the basis of the morphological features and anatomic location of its three cell types: the cytotrophoblast, the intermediate trophoblast, and syncytial trophoblast. Hydatidiform moles (complete partial and invasive) are thought to represent abnormally formed placentas with specific genetic abnormalities related to the villus trophoblast. In contrast, choriocarcinoma and placental site trophoblastic tumors are considered to be true neoplasms related to previllous and extravillous trophoblasts, respectively.

Epidemiology and Etiology

The frequency of this disease worldwide is quite varied with high rates noted in Asia and in Latin America as compared with Europe or North America. These rates range from a low of 1 in 2,000 pregnancies in North America to a high of 1 in 120 to 1 in 200 pregnancies in Asia. Specific etiologic mechanisms for this disease remain unknown. However, the one consistent factor that has been identified has been increasing maternal age. Dietary factors that have been implicated in this disorder with diets deficient in protein and poor in vitamin A as well as those low in calories are all thought to cause an increase risk for trophoblastic disease. Classification of GTD is presented in Table 25.7.

Complete Mole

A complete mole is characterized by the lack of a demonstrable fetus or embryo, and chromosomally these lesions have a diploid pattern, which is paternally derived. On occasion, a tetratoid or diploid pattern can be seen. Most of these patients will present with abnormal bleeding and a uterus that appears larger than its gestational age. Hyperemesis gravidarum and pregnancy-associated hypertension are common with the disorder. Complete moles also have generally markedly elevated levels of BhCG and often diagnosed by a classic ultrasound appearance,

TABLE 25.7. Classification of Gestational Trophoblastic Disease

1.	Hydatidiform mole:
	(a) complete
	(b) partial
2.	Invasive hydatidiform mole
3.	Choriocarcinoma
4.	Placental site trophoblastic tumor
5.	Other lesions

which has been described as a "snowstorm pattern." Data would indicate that 10–30% of complete moles may persist following evacuation and may require further therapy.

Partial Mole

Partial moles have a triploid chromosomal pattern with two sets being paternal and one set being maternal. Partial moles may have an accompanying fetus or embryo and the degree of partial mole can be minor or major. Often, the uterus will be small-for-date with hCG levels that are only slightly elevated or not at all. Approximately 5–10% of partial moles will persist after evacuation.

Invasive Moles

Invasive moles are characterized by the presence of hydropic villi in the myometrium or in vessels and are usually diagnosed from plateauing or persisting hCG titers following the evacuation of a complete or partial mole. Invasive moles may also regress spontaneously.

Placental Site Trophoblast Tumor

These are uncommon tumors characterized by proliferation of the intermediate cytotrophoblast tissue. These tumors generally do not produce high titers of hCG and may have elevated levels of human placental lactogen (HPL), which can be detected immunohistochemically on histological sections as well as in the serum. Approximately 95% of placental site trophoblast tumor follow a term delivery with a few arising after abortion or molar pregnancy. These tumors tend to be less sensitive to chemotherapy than the other forms of GTT and may require hysterectomy for treatment.

Choriocarcinoma

Choriocarcinoma is a malignant tumor of the trophoblast and can follow any type of gestational event including hydatidiform mole, spontaneous abortion, or ectopic or term pregnancy. The more abnormal the pregnancy, the more likely it is to be associated with choriocarcinoma. Approximately one-half of the cases with choriocarcinoma are preceded by hydatidiform mole, with 25% occurring after an abortion. Twenty-two percent generally occur after a normal pregnancy and the remaining 3% after an ectopic pregnancy. The most common method of presentation is abnormal uterine bleeding, but they may also present with symptoms related to metastatic lesions in the lung, vagina, brain, or liver.

Staging

The staging system for GTD is presented in Table 25.8. In 2000, the FIGO oncology committee recommended that the staging be changed to reflect prognostic factors for this disease.

Management or Treatment

Lesions are generally divided according to good or poor prognosis based on a variety of assessment schemes. Currently, the staging system incorporates the prognostic features from various classification schemes derived by the National Institutes of Health (NIH), WHO, and the experience of Bagshawe and co-workers at the Charing Cross Hospital in London. The scoring system is presented in

TABLE 25.8. FIGO Staging for Gestational Trophoblastic Tumors

Stage I	Disease confined to the uterus
Ia	Disease confined to the uterus with no risk factors
Ib	Disease confined to the uterus with one risk factor
Ic	Disease confined to the uterus with two risk factors
Stage II	GTT extends outside of the uterus but is limited to the genital structures (adnexa, vagina, broad ligament)
Iia	GTT involving genital structures without risk factors
Iib	GTT extends outside of the uterus but limited to genital structures with one risk factor
Iic	GTT extends outside of the uterus but limited to the genital structures with two risk factors
Stage III	GTT extends to the lungs with or without known genital tract involvement
IIIa	GTT extends to the lungs with or without genital tract involvement and with no risk factors
IIIb	GTT extends to the lungs with or without genital tract involvement and with one risk factor
IIIc	GTT extends to the lungs with or without genital tract involvement and has two risk factors
Stage IV	All other metastatic sites
Iva	All other metastatic sites without risk factors
Ivb	All other metastatic sites with one risk factor
Ivc	All other metastatic sites with two risk factors

Table 25.9. WHO Prognostic Index Score for GTD

Prognostic Factor	Score			
	0	1	2	4
Age (years)	≤ 39	>39	—	—
Antecedent pregnancy	Mole	Abortion	Term	—
Interval (months)	<4	4–6	7–12	>12
HCG (mIU/mL)	$<10^3$	10^3–10^4	10^4–10^5	$>10^5$
ABO groups	—	O or A	B or AB	—
Largest tumor, including uterine	—	3–5 cm	>5 cm	—
Site of metastases	Lung, pelvis, vagina	Spleen, kidney	GI tract, liver	Brain
Number of metastases	—	1–3	4–8	>8
Prior chemotherapy	—	—	Single	Multiple

Table 25.9 and enables cases to be divided into low- and high-risk cases. Low risk is defined as a score of 6 or less and high-risk as a score of 7 or greater.

In terms of molar pregnancies, suction evacuation of the uterine cavity is the treatment of choice. It should be performed by an experienced surgeon, as there is significant risk perforation and hemorrhage, particularly with an enlarged uterus. All resected tissue should be sent for histologic examination and confirmation of the diagnosis. Serial serum hCG monitoring should be carried out after an evacuation of a molar pregnancy and should be performed on a weekly basis until the serum hCG level has returned to normal for approximately 4 weeks. Subsequently, the interval can be increased to every 2–4 weeks and, following this, monthly hCG titres should be performed for a 6-month period. Patients should be advised to practice effective contraception for 6 months after evacuation of a hydatidiform mole to avoid the possibility of confusing a rising aberrant hCG titre with that of a normal pregnancy. Routine use of prophylactic chemotherapy is controversial, but some have advocated its use in patients where monitoring of serum hCG is not possible. A potential risk in such individuals would be that they would develop drug resistance if they then develop GTD and then require chemotherapy.

Choriocarcinoma was the first solid gynecologic tumor and one of the first solid tumors in humans to be cured with chemotherapy. Methotrexate and actinomycin have been the mainstays of treatment since the introduction of methotrexate for this disease in 1956. Choriocarcinoma generally follows an identifiable gestational event and, the more abnormal the pregnancy, the more likely it is to be associated with a choriocarcinoma. Approximately one-half of the cases of choriocarcinoma are preceded by a hydatidiform mole with the remainder almost equally divided between a preceding abortion or a normal pregnancy. Most often these lesions will present abnormal uterine bleeding with the lungs being the most frequent site of metastatic disease. Individuals with blood-born metastases may present with hemoptysis or presentations related to hemorrhagic events in the central nervous system, liver, and gastrointestinal tracts. Thyrotoxicosis has also been reported in patients with choriocarcinoma because of the thyrotrophic activity of hCG.

Most cases of choriocarcinoma are detected because of a rising hCG or plateauing serum hCG level in women who have had evacuation of a molar pregnancy. Patients are then generally divided into high- or low-risk groups based on the criteria mentioned above.

Low-risk GTD patients may be managed with single-agent chemotherapy using methotrexate with or without folinic acid rescue and actinomycin D (MAC chemotherapy). If single-agent chemotherapy is used and this therapy appears to not be succeeding more aggressive treatment is warranted to try and prevent the emergence of drug resistance. Such therapy may include a combination of methotrexate and actinomycin D as well as an alkylating agent. If complete response is not achieved with this regimen, it is recommended that patients switch to etoposide, methotrexate, and actinomycin D alternating with cyclophosphamide and vincristine (EMA-CO). Patients with high-risk GTD present a significant challenge because they comprise cases with brain metastases, liver and GI tract lesions, and there is an inherent risk of significant massive bleeding from these metastatic sites. Most centers would use combination chemotherapy, either EMA-CO or CHAMOCA and, once again, MAC chemotherapy.

Surgery is also a useful adjuvant in cases where persisting molar pregnancy is present and where reproductive function is no longer important. Urgent radio-therapy has also been advocated to prevent or control intracranial lesions.

FURTHER READING

Cancer of the Endometrium

Abeler VM, Vergote IB, Kjorstad KE, Trope CG (1996) Clear cell carcinoma of the endometrium. Prognosis and metastatic pattern. *Cancer* 78:1740–1747.

Bokhman JV, Chepick OF, Volkova AT, Vishnevsky AS (1985) Can primary endometrial carcinoma stage I be cured without surgery and radiation therapy? *Gynecol Oncol* 20:139–155.

Boronow RC (1997) Surgical staging of endometrial cancer: evolution, evaluation, and responsible challenge—A personal perspective. *Gynecol Oncol* 66:179–189.

Boronow RC, Morrow CP, Creasman WT , DiSaia PJ, Silverberg SG , Miller A, Blessing JA (1984) Surgical staging in endometrial cancer: Clinical-pathologic findings of a prospec-tive study. *Obstet Gynecol* 63:825–832.

Burke TW, Gershenson DM, Morris M, Stringer CA, Levenback C, Tortolero-Luna G, Baker VV (1994) Postoperative adjuvant cisplatin, doxorubicin, and cyclophosphamide (PAC) chemotherapy in women with high-risk endometrial carcinoma. *Gynecol Oncol* 55:47–50.

Creasman ST, Morrow CP, Bundy BN, Homesley HD, Graham JE, Heller PB (1987) Surgical pathologic spread patterns of endometrial cancer. *Cancer* 60:2035–2041.

Creasman WT, DeGeest K, DiSaia PJ, Zaino RJ (1999) Significance of true surgical pathologic staging: A Gynecologic Oncology Group Study. *Am J Obstet Gynecol* 181:31–34.

Granberg S, Wikland M, Karlsson B, Norstrom A, Friberg L (1991) Endometrial thickness as measured by endovaginal ultrasonography for identifying endometrial abnormality. *Am J Obstet Gynecol* 164:47–52.

Kadar N, Malfetano JH, Homesley HD (1993) Steroid receptor concentrations in endometrial carcinoma: Effect on survival in surgically staged patients. *Gynecol Oncol* 50(3):281–286.

Morrow CP, Bundy BN, Kurman RJ, Creasman WT, Heller P, Homesley HD, Graham JE (1991) Relationship between surgical-pathological risk factors and outcome in clinical stage I and II carcinoma of the endometrium. A Gynecologic Oncology Group Study. *Gynecol Oncol* 40:55–65.

Potish RA, Twiggs LB, Adcock LL, Savage JE, Levitt SH, Prem KA (1998) Paraaortic lymph node radiotherapy in cancer of the uterine corpus. *Obstet Gynecol* 65:251–256.

Randall TC, Kurman RJ (1997) Progestin treatment of atypical hyperplasia and well-differentiated carcinoma of the endometrium in women under age 40. *Obstet Gynecol* 90:434–440.

Trimble EL, Kosary C, Park RC (1998) Lymph node sampling and survival in endometrial cancer. *Gynecol Oncol* 71:340–343.

Cancer of the Ovary

Bristow RE, Lagasse LD, Karlan BY (1996) Secondary surgical cytoreduction for advanced epithelial ovarian cancer. Patient selection and review of literature. *Cancer* 78:2049–2062.

Bristow RE, Montz FJ, Lagasse LD et al. (1999) Survival impact of surgical cytoreduction in stage IV epithelial ovarian cancer. *Gynecol Oncol* 72:278.

DePriest PD, Gallion HH, Pavlik EJ, Kryscio RJ, van Nagell Jr. JR (1997) Transvaginal sonography as a screening method for the detection of early ovarian cancer. *Gynecol Oncol* 65:408–414.

Di Re F, Baiocchi G, Fontanelli R et al. (1996) Systemic pelvic and paraortic lymphadenectomy for advanced ovarian cancer: Prognostic significance of node metastases. *Gynecol Oncol* 62:360.

Gayther SA, Warren W, Mazoyer S, Russell PA, Harrington PA, Chiano M, Seal S, Hamoudi R, van Rensburg EJ, Dunning AM et al. (1995) Germline mutations of the BRCA1 gene in breast and ovarian cancer families provide evidence for a genotype-phenotype correlation. *Nat Genet* 11:428–433.

Gershenson DM (1994) Chemotherapy of ovarian germ cell tumors and sex cord stromal tumors. *Semin Surg Oncol* 10:290–298.

Heintz APM, Van Oosterom AT, Baptist J, Trimbos MC, Schaberg A, Van Der Velde EA, Nooy M (1988) The treatment of advanced ovarian carcinoma (I): Clinical variables associated with prognosis. *Gynecol Oncol* 30:347–358.

Hoskins WJ (1993) Surgical staging and cytoreductive surgery of epithelial ovarian cancer. *Cancer* 71:1534–1539.

McGuire WP, Hoskins WJ, Brady MF, Kucera PR, Partridge EE, Look K, Pearson DL, Davidson M (1996) Cyclophosphamide and cisplatin compared with paclitaxel and cisplatin in patients with stage III and stage IV ovarian Cancer. *N Engl J Med* 334:1–6.

NIH Consensus Development Conference on Ovarian Cancer. (1994) Screening, treatment and follow-up. *Gynecol Oncol* 55:S1–73.

Pecorelli S, Odicino F, Maisonneuve P et al. (1998) Carcinoma of the ovary. *J Epidemiol Biostat* 3:75.

Prat J (1999) Ovarian tumors of borderline malignancy (tumors of low malignant potential): a critical appraisal. *Adv Anat Pathol* 6:247.

Surwit E, Childers J, Atlas I, Nour M, Hatch K, Hallum A, Alberts D (1996) Neoadjuvant chemotherapy for advanced ovarian cancer. *Int J Gynecol Cancer* 6:356–361.

Cancer of the Ovary

Swenerton K, Jeffrey J, Stuart G, Roy M, Krepart G, Carmichael J, Drouin P, Stanimir R, O'Connell G, MacLean G, Kirk ME, Canetta R, Koski B, Shelley W, Zee B, Pater J (1992) Cisplatin-cyclophosphamide versus carboplatin-cyclophosphamide in advanced ovarian cancer: A randomized phase III study of the National Cancer Institute of Canada Clinical Trials Group. *J Clin Oncol* 10:718–726.

Van der Burg MEL, Van Lent M, Buyse M, Kobierska A, Colombo N, Favalli G, Lacave AJ, Nardi M, Renard J, Pecorelli S, for the Gynecological Cancer Cooperative Group of the European Organization for Research and Treatment of Cancer (1995) The effect of debulking surgery after induction chemotherapy on the prognosis in advanced epithelial ovarian cancer. *N Engl J Med* 332:629–634.

Cancer of the Vulva

Benedet JL, Shepard J, Sideri M et al. (1998) Carcinoma of the vulva. *J Epidemiol Biostat* 3:111–127.

Cunningham MJ, Goyer RP, Gibbons SK, Kredentser DC, Malfetano JH, Keys H (1997) Primary radiation, cisplatin and 5-fluorouracil for advanced squamous carcinoma of the vulva. *Gynecol Oncol* 66:258–261.

Grimshaw RN, Murdoch JB, Monaghan JM (1993) Radical vulvectomy and bilateral inguinal-femoral lymphadenopathy through separate incisions: Experience with 100 cases. *Int J Gynecol Cancer* 3:18–23.

Hacker NF, Berek JS, Lagasse LD et al. (1984) Individualization of treatment for stage I squamous cell vulvar cancer. A Gynecologic Oncology Group Study. *Obstet Gynecol* 63:155–162.

Homesley HD (1995) Management of vulvar cancer. *Cancer* 76:2159–2170.

Homesley HD, Bundy BN, Sedlis A, Adcock L (1986) Radiation therapy versus pelvic node resection for carcinoma of the vulva with positive groin nodes. *Obstet Gynecol* 68:733–740.

Homesley HD, Bundy BN, Sedlis A, Yordan E, Berek JS, Jahshan A, Morrel R (1993) Prognostic factors for groin node metastasis in squamous cell carcinoma of the vulva: A Gynecologic Oncology Group Study. *Gynecol Oncol* 49:279–283.

Iversen T, Aberler V, Aalders J (1981) Individualized treatment of stage I carcinoma of the vulva. *Obstet Gynecol* 57:85–89.

Smyczek-Gargya B, Volz B, Geppert M, Dietl J (1997) A multivariate analysis of clinical and morphological prognostic factors in squamous cell carcinoma of the vulva. *Gynecol Obstet Invest* 43:261–267.

Stehman PB, Bundy BN, Dvoretsky PM, Creasman WT (1992) Early stage I carcinoma of the vulva treated with ipsilateral superficial inguinal lymphadenectomy and modified radical hemivulvectomy: A prospective study of the Gynecologic Oncology Group. *Obstet Gynecol* 79:490–497.

Thomas G, Dembo A, DePetrillo A, Pringle J, Ackerman I, Bryson P et al. (1989) Concurrent radiation and chemotherapy in vulvar carcinoma. *Gynecol Oncol* 34:263–267.

Van der Velden J, Van Lindert AC, Lammes FB et al. (1995) Extracapsular growth of lymph node metastases in squamous cell carcinoma of the vulva. The impact on recurrence and survival. *Cancer* 75:2885–2890.

Gestational Trophoblastic Neoplasia

Bagshawe KD (1969) *Choriocarcinoma: The Clinical Biology of the Trophoblast and Its Tumors.* Williams & Wilkins, Baltimore.

Bagshawe KD, Lawler SD, Paradinas FJ et al. (1990) Gestational trophoblastic tumors following initial diagnosis of partial hydatidiform mole. *Lancet* 335:1074–1076.

Bagshawe KD (1976) Risk and prognostic factors in trophoblastic neoplasia. *Cancer* 38:1373–1385.

Berkowitz RS, Goldstein DP, Bernstein MR (1990) Methotrexate infusion and folinic acid in the primary therapy of nonmetastatic gestational trophoblastic tumors. *Gynecol Oncol* 36:56–59.

Berkowitz RS, Goldstein DP, Bernstein MR, Sablinska B (1987) Subsequent pregnancy outcome in patients with molar pregnancy and gestational trophoblastic tumors. *J Reprod Med* 32:680–684.

Cole LA, Kohorn EI, Kim GS (1994) Detecting and monitoring trophoblastic disease. New perspectives on measuring human chorionic gonadotropin levels. *J Reprod Med* 39:193–200 (1994).

DuBeshter B, Berkowitz RS, Goldstein DP, Cramer DW, Bernstein MR (1987) Metastatic gestational trophoblastic disease: Experience at the New England Trophoblastic Disease Centre, 1965 to 1985. *Obstet Gynecol* 69:390–395.

Finkler NJ, Berkowitz RS, Driscoll SG, Goldstein DP, Bernstein MR (1988) Clinical experience with placental site trophoblastic tumors at the New England Trophoblastic Disease Center. *Obstet Gynecol* 71:854–857.

Goldstein DP, Berkowitz RS (1995) Prophylactic chemotherapy of complete molar pregnancy. *Semin Oncol* 22:157–160.

Hammond CB, Weed Jr. JC, Currie JL (1980) The role of operation in the current therapy of gestational trophoblastic disease. *Am J Obstet Gynecol* 136:844–858.

Kohorn EI (1993) Evaluation of the criteria used to make the diagnosis of nonmetastatic gestational trophoblastic neoplasia. *Gynecol Oncol* 48:139–147.

Newlands ES, Bagshawe KD, Begent RHJ, Rustin GJS, Holden L (1991) Results with EMA/CO (etoposide, methotrexate, actinomycin D, cyclophosphamide, vincristine) regimen in high risk gestational trophoblastic tumours, 1979–1989. *Br J Obstet Gynaecol* 98:550–557.

Redline RW, Abdul-Karim FW (1995) Pathology of gestational trophoblastic disease. *Semin Oncol* 22:96–109.

Soper JT (1995) Identification and management of high-risk gestational trophoblastic disease. *Semin Oncol* 22:172–184.

CHAPTER 26

Cancer of the Prostate

LOUIS J. DENIS

Oncology Center Antwerp, 2000 Antwerp, Belgium

MARY K. GOSPODAROWICZ

University of Toronto, Princess Margaret Hospital, Department of Radiation Oncology, Toronto, Ontario, Canada

KEITH GRIFFITHS

University College of Medicine, Cardiff, Wales, United Kingdom

Cancer of the prostate has become a major health problem with significant morbidity, mortality, loss of quality of life, and, moreover, substantial costs to those societies in which there is an increased life expectancy. The essential issue is that cancer of the prostate is a disease of the elderly man, with a peak incidence and mortality around the seventh decade, but involving a slowly, but continuously growing heterogeneous tumor that takes 20 or more years to develop from a focal lesion to the malignant aggressive phenotype. The natural history therefore covers a wide range of disease developing through a considerable age range.

The impact of the introduction of prostate-specific antigen (PSA) for the detection of prostate cancer, almost simultaneously with the development of the biopsy gun that enables painless transrectal biopsies to be performed under the visual guidance of transrectal ultrasound, has been a shift to the diagnosis of cancer at earlier stages of the disease.

The clinical result is that in countries where PSA and subsequent biopsy are popular, one rarely sees a new patient with metastatic disease but an avalanche of patients without symptoms, where a positive biopsy for cancer creates the dilemma of treating prostate cancer in its preclinical stages. The resultant dramatic division between perceived localised disease, usually divided into minimal and clinical disease, and advanced disease has created heated controversy on population screening, diagnosis, and appropriate treatment schedules.

UICC Manual of Clinical Oncology, Eighth Edition. Edited by Raphael E. Pollock
ISBN 0-471-22289-5 Copyright © 2004 John Wiley & Sons, Inc.

The controversy focuses mainly in perceived localized disease between active, curative treatment, usually surgery or some type of radiotherapy, versus watchful waiting. In locally advanced disease, cure is still attempted by radiotherapy, usually following a course of neoadjuvant hormonal treatment. Systemic advanced disease calls for primary hormonal treatment and the controversy focuses on early or delayed hormonal treatment when symptoms appear. Clinical decisions should be taken in a multiprofessional setting based on the available prognostic factors, treatment facilities, and the informed choice of the patient.

The early diagnosis in the treated natural history of the disease results in an extended follow-up, confirming the traditional principle that prostate cancer needs 15 years of follow-up to judge the outcome results of any treatment given.

Metastatic disease, usually in the form of osteoblastic bone lesions, signals unquestionably incurable disease. Hormonal treatment may delay the progression of disease, but the endstage cancers are hormone resistant, resulting in debilitating disease and death in 1 to 2 years. Research is essentially focused on prevention of the clinical stage, the prevention of metastatic disease and the hormone independent phenotypes.

ETIOLOGY AND EPIDEMIOLOGY

Clinical prostate cancer is a disease of the aging man, with a peak incidence and mortality around 70 years of age. The disease accounts for 10–30% of the reported clinical tumors in men and moreover, 6% of all male cancer deaths. Although the incidence rate varies enormously between and within continents and their differing ethnic populations, there is evidence that the mortality rate does not correlate with the incidence rate. The incidence of, and mortality from clinical prostate cancer is low in Asia, high in northern Europe and North America, with Latin America and southern Europe assuming intermediate rates.

It is estimated that there are approximately 1.6 million patients alive with prostate cancer throughout the world, and this represents 16% of all 5-year prevalent cancer cases in males. Of these cases, approximately 900,000 originated in the developed countries of the world, the remainder in those which are developing. These figures will increase during the early part of the 21st century as a result of the increasing life expectancy of the involved populations.

With regard to the geographical differences in the incidence of, and mortality from prostate cancer, it is important to note that the small focal regions of the well-differentiated latent prostate cancer, the prostate cancer clinically unsuspected throughout life, and discovered only at autopsy or incidentally at surgery for benign prostatic hyperplasia, remains evenly distributed throughout the male population of the world. Of all men from different ethnic groups and from both east and west, 12–16% will have this early form of prostate cancer. In contrast, the larger latent cancer, with a volume over 0.5mm and less well differentiated, shows a geographic and national distribution, similar to that recognized for the clinical symptomatic cancer and with an increasing prevalence that is directly related to increasing age.

It has long been accepted that the development of clinical prostate cancer is a multistep process. The geographic differences in the distribution of the earlier stages of prostate cancer, the microscopic foci of the disease that appear to be influenced by external and possibly avoidable growth regulatory factors, emphasizes the potential for lifestyle causes and, thereby, the possibility of primary prevention.

The prostate gland grows and functions within a multihormonal environment, responding to a wide range of growth regulatory factors, the most important of which are the androgens. Steroid hormones, androgens, estrogens, and glucocorticoids modulate the production and action within the gland of a range of growth stimulatory and inhibitory factors that act in an autocrine or paracrine manner. Androgens influence many of these complex interactions that regulate prostate function, growth, and also programmed cell death or apoptosis. Essentially, testosterone is the principal circulating plasma androgen. This is converted within the prostate to 5_{α}-dihydrotestosterone (DHT), the intraprostatic androgenic hormone, which then associates specifically with the androgen receptors to regulate the genes that determine secretion, cell proliferation, and apoptosis. In the progression of prostate cancer, this complex growth control process is dysfunctional, such that the regulatory influence of DHT is lost and the cancer growth is dominated by the action of the growth factors acting in an autonomous manner. The ultimate result in the hormone-unresponsive independent prostate cancer is uncontrolled growth driven by growth stimulatory factors.

There is, at present, no evidence of any primary endocrine disturbance that would be considered a risk factor in the etiology of prostate cancer, nor one that could explain the geographic variability in the incidence of clinical cancer in the different populations. The hypothesis that the inhibition of the activity of the intraprostatic 5_{α}-reductase that converts testosterone to DHT would reduce the incidence of prostate cancer is being challenged in a randomized trial of 18,000 men over 55 years of age, who are being followed for 7 years and receiving a 5_{α}-reductase inhibitory drug.

Other explanations for the variability in the geographical distribution of prostate cancer rest with lifestyle differences in nutritional practices. Prostate cancer risk has been reported to be associated with an enhanced intake of saturated fat, with vitamins A and E, as well as with various carotenes such as lycopene, offering a potential growth restraining influence. Any differences in dietary fat intake alone can, however, account for only, at most, 10% of the variation between the reported incidence within a race and of the community. These factors have to be taken into account when considering the reported risk of prostate cancer in first-degree relatives of patients with prostate cancer, because any familial clustering may have a genetic etiology as well as cultural features. Thus, the genetic susceptibility factor appears to account for 13% of reported prostate cancers.

The concept that particular dietary factors related to Asian men that may restrain the development of clinical prostate cancer must be seriously considered and, furthermore, that such agents that could offer effective primary prevention in communities in the west with a high prevalence of the disease. Considerable interest at present is centered on the isoflavonoids and flavonoids, sometimes referred to as phytoestrogens, as restraining factors in the pathogenesis of prostate cancer. A great deal of compelling scientific evidence supports this concept and, particularly, the study of immigrants. Sons of Japanese immigrants to the United States show an incidence of prostate cancer between that of homeland Japan and that of the native American male population.

Also of particular direct clinical importance is the observation that transurethral resection of the prostate for benign prostatic hyperplasia (BPH), as well as the diagnosis of BPH and also vasectomy, are not related to prostate cancer. Clearly, however, further epidemiologic and etiologic studies related to the genetic factors of prostate cancer are considered a research priority.

SCREENING

Screening should be designed to find cancer in its early, curable stages of the disease, in an asymptomatic population. Screening is therefore totally different from case finding or early diagnosis in symptomatic patients. The clinical value of population-based screening for prostate cancer is still a controversial topic of debate at the moment, because any specific beneficial effects on mortality or improvement in the quality of life (QOL) as a result of prospective randomized trials have yet to be demonstrated by the current screening program established in selected populations. However, several large early detection studies in different parts of the world have contributed a substantial amount of information to indicate that procedures are available for suspected cases of cancer that can result in an early diagnosis. A few randomized screening trials are effectively accruing information and it is expected that these will ultimately provide the missing data. A specific improvement would be to increase the specificity of the histological analysis of the biopsy sample to more precisely determine cancer aggressiveness and thereby decrease possible overtreatment. Underdiagnosis in locally advanced disease and overtreatment for clinically insignificant cancers are the fallacies of any screening program.

DIAGNOSIS

The diagnosis of prostate cancer is mainly based on the suspicion of cancer determined by the use of three tests. The digital rectal examination (DRE) feels for zones of induration in the prostate, or asymmetry of the gland. The serum PSA test determines the concentration of a nonspecific marker for prostate cancer, but it does provide a measure of increase in prostate volume, or for disease progression. Transrectal ultrasound (TRUS) can demonstrate echo-poor lesions in the prostate sonogram. None of the three tests have a high sensitivity for the detection of early prostate cancer. The use of the DRE and PSA tests provides reliable combination that quite effectively defines the degree of risk and the need to obtain a biopsy to confirm the diagnosis. Case finding and screening to identify early prostate cancer became feasible with the clinical introduction of the serum PSA test and, simultaneously, the TRUS-guided and spring-loaded biopsy device. The latter

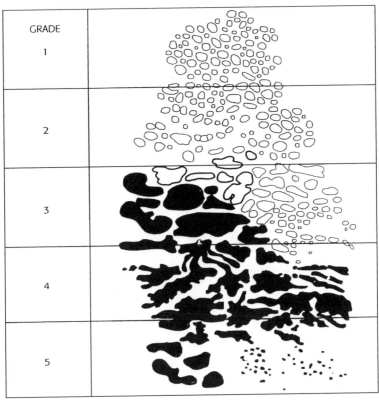

Figure 26.1 The Gleason score is based on the glandular and cellular characteristics and adding the grades. In grade 1 the glands look almost normal while in grade 5 sheets of undifferentiated cancer are present. The sum of the two most prominent grades is the score.

technique allows a number of biopsies of the prostate to be taken without an excessive burden to the patient.

The greater majority of prostate cancers are adenocarcinomas of a heterogeneous nature. The degree of differentiation, or grade of the tumor, is recognized as a dominating prognostic factor that predicts the outcome of the disease in both localized and metastatic disease, independently of the therapy that is applied. The Gleason grading score system is now widely accepted for the histologic assessment of the differentiation of prostate cancer (Fig. 26.1). The primary cancer may be unifocal or, in more, cases multifocal. The majority of the lesions are at the periphery of the gland, in the so-called peripheral zone, where they can be palpated by the examining finger on rectal examination. About 25% of the cancers arise in the transition zone. These transition zone tumors are reported to manifest a better prognostic pattern. Peripheral cancers are better situated for easier, early capsule invasion and extracapsular extension (ECE). PIN (prostate intraepithelial neoplasia) has been identified as a precursor lesion of prostate cancer, with high-grade PIN generally regarded as a potentially aggressive preclinical lesion.

Most of our preoperative clinical assessment of the local tumor relies on the histological analysis of these biopsies to assess the grade and extent of the tumor. The system is not perfect, but a definitive poor prognosis starts with a Gleason score of 7. Additional predictive markers such as PSA or tumor volume, when available, allow treatment selection for individual cases. The development of new markers of progression such as prostate-specific membrane antigen (PSMA) and cell proliferation and molecular genetic markers are a current clinical research priority.

The suspicion of advanced prostate cancer is determined by the DRE, rarely by superficial lymph node indurations, together with the rate of increase of serum PSA values (PSA velocity) over time, if available. The diagnosis of prostate cancer is of clinical value if the subsequent staging and evaluation of prognostic factors is properly performed.

STAGING AND PROGNOSIS

Clinical and pathologic staging attempts to determine the anatomic extent and tumor burden of the the primary tumor (T), the original lymph nodes (N), and the metastatic spread (M) as defined by the TNM system. The 2002 staging system is advocated by the Union Internationale Contre le Cancer (UICC) and the American Joint Committee on Cancer (AJCC). The details of the system are summarized in Table 26.1. The T-classification covers a wide variety of tumors, ranging from category T1a, which is a small, well-differentiated cancer with a median time of progression of 13.5 years, to T1b tumors, with higher volumes and less differentiation and where the median time to progression is 4.7 years. The category T1c classifies all tumors that are nonpalpable on DRE and not visible on TRUS, but are usually detected by the confirming biopsies after establishing an abnormal serum PSA level. It is now recognized that the T1c classification is mainly composed of several types of clinically significant tumors.

The staging is completed by determining the grading (G) of a positive biopsy. A serum PSA level above 10 ng/mL, with overlap for benign disease, may indicate metastatic disease. The tumor volume, a parameter that can be estimated through systematic biopsies, may improve the staging accuracy, which currently is characterized for a significant level of clinical understaging and overstaging.

There is no pathologic stage that is an equivalent for clinical stage T1c, and these cancers are usually upstaged after pathologic examination to pathologic stages pT2 or pT3. The prediction of an invasion of the regional lymph nodes (N), correlates with increasing tumor grade, tumor volume, and high serum PSA levels. Currently, this is generally achieved by the lymph node sampling of the obturator region. Clinical metastasis (M) is usually demonstrated on a positive radionuclide bone scan, computerized tomography (CT) scan, or a magnetic resonance imaging (MRI) scan of the abdomen. Recent literature surveys indicate that bone scans are rarely positive in newly diagnosed patients with a serum PSA level below 20 ng/mL. False-positive results are possible with a bone scan, owing to either metabolic activity within the bone, for example, or post-fracture, or arthritis, and the accuracy

TABLE 26.1. TNM Classification of Prostate Cancer (ICD-O C61) in Schematic Form

T		
	TX	Primary tumor cannot be assessed
	T0	No evidence of primary tumor
	T1	Clinically inapparent tumor not palpable or visible by imaging
	T1a	Tumor incidental histological finding in ≤5% or less of tissue resected
	T1b	Tumor incidental histological finding in >5% resected
	T1c	Tumor identified by needle biopsy (PSA directed)
	T2	Tumor confined within prostate[a]
	T2a	Tumor involves one-half of one lobe or less
	T2b	Tumor involves more than one-half of one lobe
	T2c	Tumor involves both lobes
	T3	Tumor extends through prostatic capsule[b]
	T3a	Extracapsular extension (unilateral or bilateral)
	T3b	Tumor invades seminal vesicle(s)
	T4	Tumor is fixed or invades adjacent structures other than seminal vesicles: bladder neck, external sphincter, rectum, levator muscles, pelvic wall
N		
	NX	Regional lymph nodes cannot be assessed
	N0	No regional lymph node metastasis
	N1	Regional lymph node(s) metastasis[c]
M		
	MX	Distant metastasis cannot be assessed
	M0	No distant metastasis
	M1	Distant metastasis
	M1a	Nonregional lymph node(s)
	M1b	Bone(s)
	M1c	Other site(s)

[a]Tumor found in one or both lobes by needle biopsy, but not palpable or visible by imaging, is classified as T1c.
[b]Invasion into the prostatic apex or into (but not beyond) the prostatic capsule is not classified as T3, but as T2.
[c]Metastasis no larger than 0.2 cm can be designated pN1 mi.

of the imaging procedure decreases for small lesions. Patients with a small metastatic tumor burden, survive longer than patients with extensive disease. Newer staging techniques include radioimmunoscintigraphy, positron emission tomography (PET), scan and forms of molecular staging as the reverse Transcriptase polymerase chain reaction (RT-PCR) assay and the determination of tissue markers such as the p53 or Bcl-2 proteins.

At the present time, there is no clear foolproof prognostic index that guarantees a specific prognosis for each individual patient, but evaluation of a prognostic index based on tumor grade, stage, volume, and a serum PSA level, provides enough accuracy to enable treatment decisions to be made. A current list of prognostic factors of possible importance in prostate cancer is listed in Table 26.2. A number

TABLE 26.2. Prognostic Factors Prostate Cancer

Essential	Tumor	$\longrightarrow$	Grade (Gleason)
			Stage
			PSA
			Volume
	Host	$\longrightarrow$	Age
			Co-morbidity
			Performance status
Additional	Tumor	$\longrightarrow$	Ploidy
			Transition zone
	Host	$\longrightarrow$	Previous transurethal resection of prostate
			Race
			Social
	Environment	$\longrightarrow$	Access
			Expertise
Promising	Proteomics	$\longrightarrow$	p53
			Bcl2
	Growth factors		
	Androgen/estrogen receptors		
	Microvessel density		
	Neuroendocrine		

of prognostic nomograms are also available for many clinical states and outcomes. Few nomograms have been compared for predictive superiority as well as clinical judgment alone. Artificial intelligence networks are used to try to improve the prognostic ability. These tables, once validated, are useful to counsel patients, but unfortunately, each individual patient has a 25% chance of being categorized into more than one group.

MULTIMODALITY TREATMENT

Localized Disease

There is a dramatic difference in the ultimate outcome of patients with prostate cancer between those with extraprostatic extension (EPE) and patients with disease limited to the prostate. Even high-grade confined tumors are curable, by either surgery, radiotherapy, brachytherapy, or other treatments based on freezing (cryo-surgery) or heat (high focused ultrasound [HFU]).

Surgery involves a total anatomic prostatectomy, usually with the elimination of all prostatic tissue, whereas radiation and the other procedures aim to destroy the tumor without eliminating all prostatic tissue. There may be a problem of over-treatment in that some insignificant tumors might be better followed, or further evaluated by watchful waiting programs. Another problem may be undertreatment after the demonstration of EPE in the surgical specimen, or after a PSA increase subsequent to the nadir PSA being reached after any form of therapy.

Radical prostatectomy involves the removal of the entire prostate, the seminal vesicles, and adjacent tissues. It is best employed in patients with localized disease (T1–T2), and with a life expectancy over 10 years, with no co-morbidity, and no other contraindications to surgery. Selection is the key to success and many series show survival curves that match the normal survival of a given age group. The co-morbidity involves urinary incontinence, erectile dysfunction, or impotence, urethral strictures, and a potential mortality of less than 0.3. The appeal is in the radical approach, which provides precise histologic pathologic information and definitive cure with the relief of the patient's anxiety. Of course, it also shows immediate persistent disease that requires secondary treatment if the surgical margins are positive and PSA remains detectable. Current innovations in technical nuances include nerve sparing and nerve grafting to prevent impotence, as well as laparoscopic and robot-assisted procedures to minimize trauma.

External-beam radiotherapy using new technology to focus the radiation more precisely, as well as brachytherapy, in which radioactive seeds are implanted in the prostate, offer valid alternatives to surgery. The morbidities associated with their use include rectal and bladder irritation and impotence, but rarely incontinence. These treatments also provide opportunities for treating regionally localized disease, but are contraindicated if colorectal co-morbidity is present. Increased disease-free survival and even increased survival have been reported in randomized trials by adding neoadjuvant and adjuvant hormonal treatment to the radiation dose. No treatment option can be selected as a best treatment, because, at present, a proper randomized trial of surgery or radiation is unavailable.

Cryoablation of the prostate uses freezing temperatures to destroy the prostatic tissue by means of cryogenic probes that are inserted, via the perineum under TRUS guidance, into the prostate. HIFU destroys the tissue by focused heat wells. Excellent results are reported with both techniques, but large series with long-term follow-up are awaited. At this moment, both techniques are developed outside the mainstream of therapeutic interventions for prostate cancer. Their future interest may lie with failed radiation-treated cancers or with pinpoint destruction of areas of the prostate.

A list of currently available treatment options with the intention to cure localized prostate cancer, is presented in Table 26.3. Our greater understanding of the natural

TABLE 26.3. Curative Treatment Options for Localized Prostate Cancer

Surgery	Retropubic
	Perineal
	Laparoscopic
Radiation	External beam
	Conformal three dimensional
	Brachytherapy (I-125/Pd-103)
	Protons/neutrons
Tissue destruction	Cryosurgery
	High intensive focused ultrasound (HIFU)

history of prostate cancer directs attention to the slow rate of growth of the tumor, with variable factors influencing the loss of differentiation and the progression of the latent cancer to the disseminating malignant phenotype that is incurable. In relation to this, the age at the time of diagnosis, together with the tumor volume and stage of the tumor, are of value in the controversy centered on whether watchful waiting may be acceptable in elderly patients with small, well-differentiated tumors, whereas active treatment is recommended for those elderly patients with less well-differentiated tumors and a volume greater than 0.5 mm.

Simply stated, decreasing differentiation and increasing size relate closely to the biological activity of the tumor, although care is needed in applying this concept to the individual patient, because we still lack the complete precise understanding of the growth potential of each diagnosed prostate cancer.

Watchful waiting is really deferred treatment and is appropriate in patients over 70 years of age with a minimal tumor volume, well-differentiated disease, and significant co-morbidity. In selected instances, this conservative approach provides disease-specific survival rates similar to those patients treated surgically, 10 years after treatment.

Advanced Disease

The term *advanced disease* encompasses minimal extraprostatic disease to widespread metastatic cancer. Both stages of the disease are incurable. Increased survival due to the lead-time is recognized and particularly so for these early stages of prostate cancer when treatment opinions are very divergent. It is evident that surgery alone, even with wide excision, is not ideal to offer cure for these patients and attempts to down-stage by introducing neoadjuvant hormonal treatment in the expectation of improving the outcome have failed so far in T3 cancers. The first results from combinations of external-beam radiotherapy, together with neoadjuvant and adjuvant hormonal therapy, offer more hope, but until the endpoints in some of the randomized trials are met, these treatment strategies should be regarded as investigational.

Even the option of watchful waiting can be proposed to patients with significant co-morbidity, although some form of androgen withdrawal therapy seems to improve the morbidity and to increase the time to progression. This was established in randomized trials of M0 patients, comparing early versus deferred endocrine treatment. The option of intermittent androgen suppression for locally advanced prostate cancer is under investigation. The essential basis of intermittent androgen therapy is that after a limited period of androgen suppression, treatment is withdrawn such that the cancer may assume some degree of androgen regulation, thereby sustaining its capacity to respond to endocrine treatment and hopefully restraining its progression to independent autonomous growth. Intermittent therapy minimizes the side effects of the treatment, an important issue, because it is not only the usual endpoints of time to progression and specific cause of death that are researched, but also the quality of life of the affected patients.

Metastatic Disease

There is a universal consensus that immediate endocrine treatment is indicated for patients with symptomatic metastatic disease. The case as to whether endocrine treatment should be offered to patients without symptoms is still debated, but there is a trend of opinion toward immediate treatment. A wide choice of options for endocrine treatment is available, the basis of which is to either lower the circulating levels of plasma testosterone, or the blockade of the action of DHT within the prostate cancer cells by using antiandrogens. Some advocate both, a treatment option referred to as maximal androgen blockade (MAB). The available array of options for endocrine treatment is listed in Table 26.4.

An immediate choice has to be made between a medical or surgical castration, if androgen withdrawal therapy is chosen as a first-line approach. Controversy remains as to whether MAB is superior to monotherapy. Information derived from a series of consensus meetings allowed a meta-analysis of the combined results of all available randomized treatments, including trials using MAB. The analysis of the data showed only a minimal benefit for use of MAB treatment, the advantage in clinical terms being most unclear and of little significance.

There was some agreement, however, that MAB was indicated for a limited time to prevent tumor flare when the initial surge in plasma testosterone that occurs when medical castration by luteinizing hormone-releasing hormone agonist (LHRH A) is used as the preferred option. There is also some agreement that clinical responses are quicker with the combination treatment. However, despite this confusion, we may conclude that, for the time being, surgical or medical castration remains the simple standard treatment when endocrine treatment is chosen as the first option. Deciding for quality of life by intermittent treatment to lower the side effects, or by promoting antiandrogens to retain potency remains an unanswered question. The bottom line is that endocrine treatment never cures cancer, that long-term treatment

TABLE 26.4. Array of Current First-Line Endocrine Treatments Utilized in Daily Praxis to Palliate Prostate Cancer

Androgen withdrawal	
Castration	Bilateral orchiectomy
	Subcapsular orchiectomy
	Subepididymal orchiectomy
Medical castration	Estrogens
	Depot preparations LHRH antiandrogen
	Progestagens
Androgen blockade	
Antiandrogens	Cyproterone acetate 300 mg/d
	Flutamide 750 mg/d
	Nilutamide 300 mg/d
	Bicalutamide 150 mg/d
Combination treatment	
Maximal androgen blockade	LHRH antiandrogen Castration-antiandrogen

carries serious side-effects even with the antiandrogens and, most important, that endocrine treatment should be tailored to the individual patient.

The use of estrogens such as diethylstilbestrol (DES) in association with drugs such as aspirin to cover cardiovascular problems and the possibility of introducing intermittent endocrine treatment to lessen the adverse effects of long-term androgen withdrawal in elderly men remain intriguing options. The use of a 5_α-reductase inhibitor together with an antiandrogen offers a potentially useful alternative form of androgen blockade of metastatic prostate cancer, one which would sustain the levels of plasma testosterone and estradiol-17β at normal physiological levels. Currently, there is some interest in the possibility that estrogens may exercise a more important role in the prostate than hitherto believed and may have a synergistic role in supporting prostate cancer progression from the indolent latent cancer to the disseminated disease. Research centers on recently identified receptors for estrogen in the prostate and on appropriate antiestrogen therapy.

Classically, chemotherapy is given when clinical prostate cancer, after responding to endocrine treatment, eventually relapses and autonomous tumor growth is unresponsive to androgen withdrawal. It is now generally accepted that approximately 20–30% of prostate cancers do not respond to first-line endocrine therapy, presumably because the tumor is composed of androgen-independent cell lines. Here, the prognosis is generally poor and a number of second-line treatments remain an option to delay the progression of symptoms.

Second-line treatments for relapsed prostate cancer include cytotoxic chemotherapy, chemohormonal therapy, treatment with agents to restrain the growth promoting action of growth factors, differentiation treatment, and biologic response modifiers with the inclusion of vaccine therapy.

A multitude of small phase II trials have been conducted, mainly demonstrating a small number of partial responses. This tends to question the relevance of the therapy in relation to the associated high toxicity. The median survival in these patients has been in the order of 6–12 months, which is comparable to the survival achieved by standard palliative treatment. Combinations are most widely used, involving vincristine or vinblastine, epirubicin, paclidaxil, and mithoxantrone. All these treatments have significant adverse side effects in these weakened patients that create the need to evaluate their quality of life and the cost of treatment as secondary endpoints in these trials.

FOLLOW-UP

All patients treated for prostate cancer enlist in a follow-up program where the number one test is serum PSA. The vagaries of this test are a psychological burden to most patients, especially when the PSA does not decrease to 0.1 ng/mL after surgery, or when the PSA starts rising after a nadir following some type of radiation or tissue destructive therapy. Second-line treatment is available and there is a choice, but patience and measuring PSA velocity on at least three separate occasions, provide useful information in making a clinical decision on treatment.

REHABILITATION, PALLIATIVE CARE, PREVENTION

The most serious side effects of treatment, especially after surgery, remain impotence and incontinence. Specialized treatments for erectile dysfunction by new drugs, revascularization, and nerve regeneration have made great progress while in the prevention of incontinence, perineal training and prostheses aim to solve this problem.

Bone pain and a general feelings of tiredness are the most crippling effects of terminal prostate cancer and specific treatment of the pain by use of biphosphonates and radioactive isotopes such as strontium 89 are modern forms of management of pain and are indicated in selected cases.

The correct use of analgesics, steroids, and other supportive treatments are vital in these stages of the disease where palliation and quality of life are most important endpoints of any study. Great attention should be paid to the nutritional and psychological states of the patients in these specific palliative care programs.

Prevention of invasion and the dissemination of prostatic cancer cells complete our therapeutic armementarium. The perception that nutritional supplements and lifestyle would seem to be implicated in the biological processes concerned in the progression from a latent to a clinical cancer is appreciated by patients with active and especially progressive disease. Most importantly, it provides a ray of hope in hopeless situations. Awareness programs, correct and fast information on therapeutic progress, and the support of patient groups play a major role in sustaining the quality of life of these patients.

FURTHER READING

Biomarkers Definitions Working Group Bethesda (2001). Biomarkers and surrogate endpoints: preferred definitions and conceptual framework. *Clin Pharmacol Ther* 69:89–95.

de Koning HJ, Auvinen A, Berenguer Sanchez A, Calais da Silva F, Ciatto S, Denis L, Gohagan J, Hakama M, Hugosson J, Kranse R, Nelen V, Prorok PC, Schröder FH (2002). Large-scale randomized prostate cancer screening trials; program performances in the ERSPC- and PLCO-trials (European Randomized Screening for Prostate Cancer and Prostate, Lung, Colorectal and Ovary cancer trials). *Int J Cancer* 97:237–244.

Denis LJ (2000). The role of active treatment in early prostate cancer. *Radiother Oncol* 57: 251–258.

Denis LJ, Murphy GP, Schroder FH (1995). Report of the Consensus Workshop on Screening and Global Strategy for Prostate cancer. *Cancer* 75:1187–1207.

Gleave MM, Bruchovsky N, Goldenberg SL, Rennie PS (1998). Intermittent androgen suppression for prostate cancer: rationale and clinical experience. *Eur Urol* 34:37–41.

Gospodarowicz MK, Henson DE, Hutter RVP, O'Sullivan B, Sobin LH, Wittekind CH (2001). *Prognostic Factors in Cancer*, 2nd edition. Wiley-Liss, New York.

Griffiths K, Denis L, Turkes A (2002). *Oestrogens, Phyto-oestrogens and the Pathogenesis of Prostatic Disease*. Martin Dunitz, London, p 420.

Harlan LC, Potosky A, Gilliland FD, Hoffman R, Albertsen PC, Hamilton AS, Eley JW, Stanford JL, Stephenson RA (2001). Factors associated with initial therapy for clinically localized prostate cancer: Prostate Cancer Outcomes Study. *J Natl Cancer Inst* 93:1864–1869.

Kaisary AV, Murphy GP, Denis L, Griffiths K (eds) (1999). *Textbook of Prostate Cancer. Pathology, Diagnosis and Treatment.* Martin Dunitz, London, p. 367.

Kirby RS, Brawer MK, Denis LJ (2001). *Fast Facts on Prostate Cancer.* Health Press, Oxford, England.

Lieberman R, Bermejo C, Akaza H, Greenwald P, Fair W, Thompson I (2001). Progress in prostate cancer chemoprevention: modulators of promotion and progression. *Urology* 58: 835–842.

The Medical Research Council Prostate Cancer Working Party Investigators Group (1997). Immediate versus deferred treatment for advanced prostate cancer: initial results of the Medical Research Trial. *Br J Urol* 79:235–246.

Murphy G, Khoury S, Partin A, Denis L (2000). Second International Consultation on Prostate Cancer, Paris, June 27–29, 1999. Plymbridge Distributors, Plymouth, p 544.

Parkin DM (2001). Global cancer statistics in the year 2000. *Lancet Oncol* 2:533–543.

Partin AW, Mangold LA, Lamm DM, Walsh PC, Epstein JI, Pearson JD (2001). Contemporary update of prostate cancer staging nomograms (Partin tables) for the new millenium. *Urology* 58:843–848.

Sakr WA (1998). High grade prostatic intraepithelial neoplasia: additional links to a potentially more aggressive prostate cancer. *J Natl Cancer Inst* 90:486–487.

The Prostate Cancer Trialist's Collaborative Group (2000). Maximal androgen blockade in prostate cancer: an overview of the randomized trials. *Lancet* 355:1491–1498.

Scher HI, Kolvenbag GJCM (1997). The antiandrogen withdrawal syndrome in relapsed prostate cancer. *Eur Urol* 31:3–7.

Sobin LH, Wittekind CH (2002). *TNM Classification of Malignant Tumors*, 6th edition. Wiley-Liss, New York.

Tannock IF (2002). Eradication of a disease: how we cured symptomless prostate cancer. *Lancet* 359:1341–1342.

Wilkinson BA, Hamdy FC (2001). State-of-the-art staging in prostate cancer. *BJU International* 87:423–430.

CHAPTER 27

Nonprostate Tumors— Genitourinary Cancer

ANDREW BAYLEY and MARY K. GOSPODAROWICZ

University of Toronto, Princess Margaret Hospital, Department of Radiation Oncology, Toronto, Ontario, Canada

The term *genitourinary cancer* covers a wide spectrum of cancers, which arise in the genital and urinary systems. By convention, cancers arising in the female genital tract are classified and discussed as gynecological cancers, and those arising in the male genital and urinary tract as genitourinary cancers. The etiology, pathology, and management of genitourinary cancers is so distinct to their type and location that they are discussed as separate entities. Prostate cancer, which is the most common genitourinary cancer, is discussed in a separate chapter. Cancer of the urinary bladder is the most common of the cancers discussed in this chapter; other urothelial cancers such as those arising in the renal pelvis and ureter are seen much less frequently. Kidney cancer is also much less common, but is an important disease because of its significant mortality. In contrast, although its incidence is very low, testis cancer is very important because it affects young men and appropriate therapy cures the majority of patients. Finally, cancer of the penis is associated with significant mortality in the underdeveloped countries of Africa and South America but is a very rare disease in the Western World.

CANCER OF THE KIDNEY

Cancer of the kidney is relatively uncommon, accounting for approximately 3% of all adult cancers. The incidence has been increasing due to increased detection of small incidental cancers found on abdominal ultrasound or computed tomography (CT) scans in asymptomatic patients. The histopathological classification is outlined in Table 27.1. Adenocarcinoma, or renal cell carcinomas, comprise

UICC Manual of Clinical Oncology, Eighth Edition. Edited by Raphael E. Pollock
ISBN 0-471-22289-5 Copyright © 2004 John Wiley & Sons, Inc.

TABLE 27.1. Pathological Classifications of Renal Cell Carcinomas

Benign Neoplasms	Malignant Neoplasms
Papillary adenoma	Conventional (clear cell) renal carcinoma
Renal oncocytoma	Papillary renal carcinoma
	Chromophobe renal carcinoma
	Collecting duct carcinoma
	Renal cell carcinoma, unclassified

approximately 85% of these tumors. The median age at diagnosis is 65 years of age, with most tumors occurring in the fifth to seventh decade of life. Men are affected two to three times as often as women.

Etiology

The etiology of renal cell carcinoma remains uncertain. Epidemiological studies have suggested a correlation between tobacco use and renal cell carcinoma. Urban living and thorotrast exposure are also reported risk factors. Previous case control studies have implicated obesity and hypertension as risk factors. In a recent case control study from Sweden, consumption of fruit and vegetables were protective, whereas a diet of fried or sauteed meat or poultry was associated with an increased risk of renal cell carcinoma. The rare familial form of renal cell carcinoma has been associated with the specific chromosomal abnormality t(3:8 translocation). About 75% of sporadic kidney cancers will show chromosomal 3p deletions. The autosomal dominant Von Hippel-Lindau disease is frequently associated with renal cell carcinoma associated with the Von Hippel-Lindau tumor suppressor gene on chromosome 3p25. Hereditary papillary renal cell carcinoma seems to arise from abnormalities in chromosome 7 and 17.

Screening

Currently, there are no accepted screening programs for the general population. Some centers have conducted screening in high-risk populations such as those with familial cancers or the Von Hippel-Lindau syndrome.

Presentation

The primary renal lesion rarely produces early symptoms, with one-fourth of patients presenting with advanced disease. Early lesions are usually detected by chance on abdominal imaging for other health reasons. Progression may be by direct extension, regional lymphatics, and hematogeneously. The most common sites of metastases at presentation include the regional nodes, lungs, bone, and skin. The liver, adrenal, and contralateral kidney are often affected as the disease progresses.

There is a wide variety of clinical presentations of kidney cancer. Flank and back pain, anemia, hematuria, fatigue, and weight loss are the most common presenting symptoms. The classic triad of hematuria, flank pain, and palpable mass is found in only 10% of presentations; however, over 40% of patients will have one or more of these symptoms at presentation. With the absence of local signs or symptoms, 20–30% of cases of kidney cancers present with metastatic disease. Approximately 30% of patients present with a paraneoplastic syndrome, the occurrence of which is not necessarily indicative of distant metastatic disease. An uncommon presentation (2–3%) of adenocarcinoma of the left kidney is the sudden onset of left-sided varicocele. Tumor-related overproductions of renin, eryrthropoietin, prostaglandins, insulin, glucagon, enteroglucagon, β human chorionic gonadotropin (HCG), ferritin, ectopic adrenocorticotropin hormone (ACTH), and parathormone have been reported. Renal cell carcinoma may produce hypertension by a variety of mechanisms, including hyperreninemia, renal arteriovenous fistulae, polycythemia, ureteral obstruction, hypercalcemia, and raised intracranial pressure secondary to intracranial metastases. The finding of abnormal liver function tests can be present in the absence of liver metastases in kidney cancer patients (Stauffer's syndrome). The presence of paraneoplastic syndromes does not invariably indicate metastatic disease and therefore should not preclude curative management.

Pathology

Renal cell carcinomas arise from the epithelium of the proximal convoluted tubule. The local growth is well defined and the tumor is encompassed by renal parenchyma or perinephric fibrous tissue. Renal vein invasion by tumor is common. There is a direct correlation between both size and differentiation and the propensity for metastatic spread. The sarcomatoid histological type has been found to be associated with poorer survival, whereas clear cell and papillary growth pattern infers a better survival. Although many clear-cell tumors, both sporadic and hereditary share the loss of the Von Hippel-Lindau tumor suppressor gene on the short-arm chromosome 3 (3p25), it appears that papillary renal cell carcinomas arise by a different cytological mechanism, with trisomies and tetrasomies of chromosome 7 and 17 being the initiating event.

Diagnostic Measures

Whereas CT scan is currently the method of choice for detection and staging of kidney cancer, magnetic resonance imaging (MRI) is superior in determining extent of disease in cases of suspected renal vein or vena cava involvement. Staging investigations include a complete blood count, renal function tests, liver function tests, and a chest x-ray (CXR). Radioisotope bone scan is appropriate in patients with bone pain. The current UICC TNM staging classification is based on the size of the primary tumor, the presence of extrarenal extension, renal vein invasion, and nodal or distant metastases (Table 27.2).

TABLE 27.2. TNM Classification of Renal Cell Carcinoma

T—Primary tumor

TX	Primary tumor cannot be assessed
T0	No evidence of primary tumor
T1	Tumor ≤7 cm in greatest dimension, limited to the kidney
T1a	Tumor ≤4 cm
T1b	Tumor >4 cm but ≤7 cm
T2	Tumor >7 cm in greatest dimension, limited to the kidney
T3	Tumor extends into major veins or invades adrenal gland or perinephric tissues but not beyond Gerota's fascia
T3a	Tumor directly invades adrenal gland or perinephric tissues[*] but not beyond Gerota fascia
T3b	Tumor grossly extends into renal vein(s)[†] or vena cava or its wall below diaphragm
T3c	Tumor grossly extends into vena cava or its wall above diaphragm
T4	Tumor directly invades beyond Gerota fascia

N—Regional lymph nodes

NX	Regional lymph nodes cannot be assessed
N0	No regional lymph node metastasis
N1	Metastasis in a single regional lymph node
N2	Metastasis in more than one regional lymph node

M—Distant metastases

MX	Distant metastasis cannot be assessed
M0	No distant metastasis
M1	Distant metastasis

Stage groupings

I	T1	N0	M0
II	T2	N0	M0
III	T3	N0	M0
	T1,T2,T3	N1	M0
IV	T4	N0,N1	M0
	Any T	N2	M0
	Any T	Any N	M1

[*]Includes renal sinus (peripelvic) fat.
[†]Includes segmental (muscle-containing) branches.
Sobin LH, Wittekind Ch (eds.) (2002) International Union Against Cancer (UICC) *TNM Classification of Malignant Tumors*, 6th Edition. Wiley-Liss, NY.

Prognostic Factors

The overall 5-year survival for patients with stage I disease ranges from 60 to 85%, 45–80% for stage II, 30–50% for stage III, and 5–10% for stage IV. Approximately 20% of patients with metastatic disease at presentation have slowly progressive disease and remain relatively asymptomatic for several years. Renal cell cancer is one of the few tumors for which well-documented cases of spontaneous regression in the absence of therapy have been described, but this is exceedingly rare and is not always associated with long-term survival. The only therapy for renal cell carcinoma with curative potential is radical surgery for patients with localized disease. There is no evidence that any treatment affects the overall survival of patients with surgically unresectable disease. Thus, stage, which reflects the anatomic extent of the disease, is the most important factor predicting survival. Histological grade and DNA diploidy measurements are also important prognostic factors, with well-differentiated and diploid tumors having a better outcome. Anemia and elevated erythrocyte sedimentation rate suggest poor prognosis in all stages, whereas poor performance status and weight loss indicate poor prognosis in patients with metastatic disease. Given the variable clinical course of renal cell carcinoma and recent responses to immunotherapy, there has been an increase in the interest in immunohistochemical prognostic factors. Some factors that have shown some promise include epidermal growth factor receptor (EGF-r), Ki-67, cellular proteins nm23-h1 and nm23-h2, vascular endothelial growth factor, and silver staining for nucleolar organizing regions (AgNOR).

Multimodality Treatment

Management Philosophy   Surgery is the only curative treatment of renal cell carcinoma. Therefore, radical surgery is recommended in the majority of patients with locally extensive disease and minimal metastatic disease such as those with limited lymph node involvement and those with solitary distant metastases.

Surgery   The principles of the surgical management of localized renal cell carcinoma are well established. Radical nephrectomy includes the *en bloc* removal of Gerota's fascia and its contents, including the kidney and the adrenal gland. Gerota's fascia is an excellent barrier to local tumor spread and is only rarely involved. Perinephric fat is involved in approximately 30% of cases. Regional lymphadenectomy is performed at the time of radical nephrectomy to assess the status of lymph nodes, although its role in prolonging survival has not been demonstrated. Complete excision of localized lesions gives a greater than 70% chance of 5-year survival. Preoperative angioinfarction has been used to decrease operative complications brought about by large renal cell carcinomas, which may be very vascular at diagnosis and make excision difficult. Roughly 15% of patients with renal cell carcinoma will have vena cava involvement and extension to the level of the diaphragm and even into the right atrium. Fifty percent of those with involvement of vena cava will have concommitant metastases and have a life expectancy between 6 and 18 months. For the others, extensive surgical procedures using techniques of cardiopulmonary bypass and circulatory arrest have made removal of large thrombi and extension of disease into the right atrium surgically feasible. Cure rates for those who undergo complete resection of renal vein or vena cava involvement have been reported to be 30–60%, justifying the extensive surgery. The role of nephrectomy in patients with metastatic disease is evolving. Two recent, large, randomized phase III trials have demonstrated survival advantage for patients with good performance status. In addition, palliative nephrectomy may offer significant relief of severe local symptoms and should be considered in patients with poor performance status due to local disease, or those with the only symptoms due to local tumor, and a resectable tumor has been identified on imaging studies. The resection of metastatic lesions may occasionally be undertaken to improve quality of life and survival. Resection of solitary lesions of the brain or lung have occasionally been reported to provide prolonged survival.

Organ Preservation Although radical nephrectomy is the procedure of choice for localized disease, no randomized studies have shown a survival advantage over less-aggressive surgical management. A number of studies with short-term follow-up suggest that nephron sparing or partial nephrectomy may be equivalent to radical nephrectomy in terms of survival and local recurrences, particularly for tumors less than 4 cm in size. Currently, consideration of parenchyma sparing surgery is only indicated in patients with bilateral tumors, tumors of a solitary kidney, Von Hippel-Lindau disease or familial renal cell carcinoma, and whose remaining kidney is compromised by significant medical illness.

Radiation Therapy Radiation therapy has no role in the curative treatment of early stage renal cancer. Preoperative and postoperative radiation therapy has been used in the past as adjuvant treatment in patients with extrarenal involvement but there is no definite evidence that such treatment improves survival. Palliative radiotherapy may be used to control the bleeding from the primary tumor or palliate symptoms from metastases to the brain, bone, and soft tissues. Palliative radiotherapy produces symptomatic relief in 50% of patients with bone or soft tissue metastases. The newer development in the treatment of renal cell carcinoma brain metastases is stereotactic radiosurgery. Preliminary reports suggest that it may be as effective as surgical resection with a lower morbidity and mortality.

Chemotherapy and Immunotherapy Appropriate systemic management of renal cell carcinoma requires a detailed understanding of the unusual natural history of the disease. Progestins have been used in the treatment of metastatic disease, but responses are reported in fewer than 15% of patients. The reason that chemotherapy is ineffective is, in part, the presence of MDR-1 gene and its product p-glycoprotein. The recent advances in immunology and molecular biology have opened up new therapeutic avenues of research and treatment. Interferon and interleukin have been used as single agents or combined together. The toxicities of these treatments are not trivial. Combinations of interferon and interleukin have response rates between 13% and 31%. Trials of lymphokine-activated killer cells in combination with interleukin are underway. The trials of tumor-infiltrating lymphocytes have been disappointing to date.

Renal Cancer Follow-Up

Other than after partial nephrectomy, the risk of recurrence is related to the stage of the disease and the completeness of the surgical resection. As there are few effective treatments for relapse, the role of routine follow-up investigations is controversial. Regular clinic visits with abdominal ultrasound may allow the detection of retroperitoneal recurrence that may occasionally be treated with further surgery and the detection of contralateral primary tumors. Chest x-rays are used to detect resectable solitary pulmonary metastases.

Future

Clinical studies are actively researching immunotherapy, immune-stimulating agents, and gene therapy. Experimental agents including antiangiogenesis compounds and cyclin-dependent kinase are being actively investigated.

CANCER OF THE URINARY BLADDER

Bladder cancer is the most common malignancy of the urinary tract, excluding prostate cancer, and one of the most common cancers in men. The male to female ratio is 2.5; it most often occurs in the sixth and seventh decade of life. The management and prognosis of bladder cancer is related to the depth of bladder wall invasion. The risk of lymph node and distant metastases increases with the depth of invasion. Tumors limited to the bladder mucosa and submucosa can be managed by local therapies, whereas those that invade the detrusor muscle require more extensive therapy. The fact that 80% of bladder tumors are superficial at presentation accounts for the overall low mortality of bladder cancer.

Etiology

The current thinking suggests genetic alterations of normal bladder mucosa predispose to bladder cancer. The exact nature, location, and mechanism of these changes is not known. A number of environmental factors that predispose to bladder cancer have been identified. Approximately one-half of bladder cancers are associated with tobacco exposure, and, previously, a quarter with occupational exposures, which is less common now in developed countries. The latency period for occupational exposures is often very long in excess of 15 years. The link between aromatic amines and bladder cancer development is very strong. The use of aniline dyes in the textile, rubber, and cable industries is also a known industrial factor associated with bladder cancer. *Schistosoma haematobium* infection is strongly associated with squamous cell carcinoma, particularly in the developing world. The pathogenesis of the association is not understood. Squamous carcinoma occurs at a younger age and represents 70% of bladder cancer in Egypt, where the prevalence of *Schistosoma* infection is as high as 45%. Urinary stasis and recurrent urinary tract infection are associated with both squamous carcinoma and transitional cell carcinomas (TCC). The pathogenesis of this association is uncertain but may be due to bacterial nitrate production. Cyclophosphamide administration may also predispose to bladder cancer. Most chemical-induced bladder cancers are TCC.

Although the association between excessive phenacetin use and TCC of the renal pelvis and ureter is well established, the association with bladder cancer is unclear. The association between dietary factors, artificial sweetners, coffee consumption, and the development of bladder cancer is controversial and unclear.

Screening

No prospective randomized trials have documented that routine screening for bladder cancer improves survival. Some studies suggest that screening men age 50 years and older with home hematuria tests decrease bladder cancer morbidity and is cost effective. The use of urine cytology to screen those with industrial exposure may also be valuable. Recently, the use of molecular and cellular markers as noninvasive adjuncts to traditional diagnostic tests to detect bladder cancer has been an area of active research. Tests for bladder tumor antigen (BTA), bladder telomerase activity, telomeric repeat amplicatification assay protocol (TRAP), NMP22, fibrin degradation products, and ImmunoCyt® are commercially available. These tests will need to be prospectively evaluated prior to their addition to widespread clinical practice for surveillance or diagnosis of bladder cancer. Two questions are under investigation currently: (1) can these markers be used as surrogates for traditional cytology and cystoscopy, and (2) will these markers provide more accurate or earlier cost effective screening for cancer?

Presentation and Natural History

Approximately 70–80% of patients with newly diagnosed bladder cancer have tumors that are superficial and confined to the epithelium or underlying lamina propria. Lymph node or distant metastases are exceedingly rare in patients with superficial disease. These tumors are usually curable by local means. However, the likelihood of nodal or distant metastases rises sharply once the tumor invades the muscle wall of the bladder. Only a small proportion of patients presenting with extensive perivesical disease survive more than 2 years, although a third or more of patients with limited pelvic lymph node involvement and disease limited to the bladder survive more than 5 years. Almost 75% of patients with bladder cancer present with gross or microscopic hematuria. Hematuria associated with bladder cancer may be intermittent, and the degree of hematuria is generally not related to the seriousness of the underlying cause. Some patients present with urine infections. Urinary frequency, bladder irritability, and dysuria occur in one-third of patients at presentation. Patients may present with urinary tract obstruction in the later stages of disease. Fever occurs in up to 20% of patients but other systemic symptoms are rare.

Pathology

TCC derived from the uroepithelium make up more than 90% of bladder cancers in Europe and North America. Six to 8% are squamous carcinomas (SCC) and 2% are adenocarcinomas. Adenocarcinomas may be urachal or nonurachal in origin. The nonurachal type is thought to arise as a result of chronic irritation of transitional epithelium causing metaplasia. SCC predominate in Egypt and other areas where *Schistosoma* is endemic. SCC follow two distinct clinical courses. Those associated with *Schistosoma* grow to be large masses with central necrosis and tend not to metastasize, which contrasts distinctly with SCC occuring in North America. Many tumors show a mixed pattern with TCC with squamous or adenomatous hyperplasia. Tumors most commonly arise from the trigone or lateral walls. Cellular atypia, nuclear abnormalities, and number of mitotic figures form the basis of pathological grade, which is of prognostic significance. Carcinoma *in situ* (CIS), a cytological malignant epithelium, may exist as a distinct entity or coexist with other TCC. CIS is typically a flat, reddish lesion with a granular surface when cystoscopy is carried out. Macroscopic tumors may be exophytic (papillary) or solid (nodular). The former configuration is more common in low-grade disease, whereas the latter is usually associated with muscle invasive disease.

Diagnosis

Ultrasound, urine cytology, and cystoscopy have traditionally been the most common examinations for diagnostic evaluation. Currently, pelvic ultrasound and urine cytology are frequently the first tests performed. Once a bladder tumor has been identified, an attempt should be made to resect it in its entirety. This resection is therapeutic and provides important information about staging and grading of the tumor. Urine cytology is more sensitive for high-grade tumors, with between 50% and 80% of these lesions being detected. Meanwhile, only 20% of low grade lesions are detected by urine cytology.

Staging and Prognostic Factors

The most important prognostic factor in bladder cancer is the depth of bladder wall invasion. Other clinical and pathological prognostic factors described include tumor size, multiplicity, tumor configuration, grade, vascular invasion, positive urine cytology, or coexistent CIS. Although these clinical and pathological factors have been defined, the fundamental molecular and biological factors are less well known. There is now evidence that tumors with p53 mutations exhibit more aggressive behavior independent of other clinical and pathological factors.

The depth of invasion determines the stage of bladder cancer. The determination of stage requires an examination under anesthesia (EUA), cystoscopy with transurethral resection (TUR), biopsy and imaging with CT and MRI. Clinical staging often underestimates the microscopic tumor extent, even when CT or MRI are utilized. However, staging of tumors that do not invade muscle is usually quite accurate as nodal or distant metastasis are rare. The risk of nodal and distant metastases rises sharply with muscle invasion, and so a chest x-ray, bone scan, and CT scan of the abdomen and pelvis are indicated. MRI is very useful in assessing the local extent of bladder tumors because imaging in both the sagittal and coronal planes gives excellent definition of the bladder wall.

Bladder Multimodality Therapy

TUR, with or without intravesical therapy, prolongs survival in most patients with superficial disease. Recurrence is common for superficial disease but in less than 20% of cases does progression to muscle invasive or metastatic disease occur. In contrast, fewer than 50% of patients with muscle-invasive tumors are cured, even when radical locoregional therapy is applied.

Superficial Disease

The majority of bladder tumors are diagnosed as superficial papillary lesions, stage 0. Stage 0 bladder tumors are cured by a variety of treatments, but in over 50% disease will recur or new tumors develop. Tumors can occur synchronously or metachronously throughout the urothelium, suggesting that the recurrences may be secondary primary events in a urotherlium with a field defect. The alternate hypothesis suggests the recurrences are a result of tumor implants secondary to the initial resection. The majority of patients who develop recurrence do so within the first year. In a series of patients followed for at least 20 years (or until death), tumor recurrence occurred in 80%. Predictive factors for recurrence include multifocality of presentation, positive cytology, stage, grade, large size, solid configuration, and a history of smoking. The two strongest predictors are multifocality and positive cytology. Newer prognostic factors, including *p53*, are under investigation. Grade and stage correlate well among superficial tumors, with most Ta tumors being grade 1 and most grade 2 and 3 in T1 category. Ten to 20% of patients with superficial disease progress to muscle invasive or metastatic disease. The progression rate depends on the primary tumor character. CIS, particularly when diffuse, is associated with a rapid progression to muscle invasive disease. Transurethral resection and fulguration of the tumor is the most widely used form of therapy for superficial disease. Once the patient is disease free after primary therapy, close surveillance is essential due to high relapse rate. Typically, periodic cystoscopies with simultaneous urine cytology are used. The long-term disease free survival for patients with Ta–T1 disease ranges from 75 to 85%.

Other therapies utilized in superficial disease include intravesical chemotherapy, immunotherapy with bacille Calmette-Guérin (BCG), segmental cystectomy, or radical cystectomy in selected patients. Patients who recur after initial TUR are usually treated with repeat TUR and then intravesical chemotherapy with thiotepa, doxorubicin, or BCG prior to more radical therapies. BCG is effective in treating CIS with a 70% complete response rate (CR). However, 50% of patients with CIS who achieve CR will relapse. BCG delays tumor recurrence and progression. Newer therapies, include photodynamic therapy after hematophorphyrin-derivative administration, the use of intravesical interferon 2a, and the use of electrical current during instillation of BCG or mitomycin C.

Muscle Invasive Disease (T2, T3, T4, N1–N3)

Potentially curative forms of treatment for muscle invasive disease (T2–T4a) include radical cystectomy, with or without preoperative radiotherapy and chemotherapy and external beam radiation therapy with or without concurrent chemotherapy.

Surgery

Selected T2 lesions can be managed by TUR and intravesical chemotherapy or immunotherapy but, often, more aggressive treatment is required for recurrent tumors, tumor with large size, multiple foci, or undifferentiated grade. Radical cystectomy involves removal of the bladder, perivesical tissues, prostate, seminal vesicles in men, and the uterus, fallopian tubes, ovaries, and anterior vaginal wall and urethra in women. Pelvic lymph node dissection is often carried out with radical cystectomy. Recent advances in surgical technique allow for preservation of sexual function in men, and new forms of continent urinary diversion, like a neobladder, obviate the need for external devices. Acceptance of cystectomy has been poor prior to the continent diversion era. Retrospective studies suggest that early cystectomy may occur in patients who are candidates for a continent diversion. A survival advantage was found for these patients, perhaps due to earlier cystectomy or perhaps because of medical co-morbidities, which also prevented neobladder formation. Radical cystectomy is very effective treatment for patients with T2 disease, with a 60–75% 5-year survival. Unfortunately, it results in a cure for a small proportion of patients with extensive extravesical disease, with only 20–30% surviving 5 years. Early evidence from a prospective, randomized trial suggest that the addition of neoadjuvant chemotherapy may improve survival for patients with T2a–T4NOMO disease. A large, randomized trial utilizing CMV (cisplatin, methotrexate, vinblastine) revealed no significant survival benefit. A combination of gemcitabine and platinum has been shown to be as effective as MVAC (methotrexate, vinblastine, adriamycin, and cisplatin), with a better safety profile and tolerability in patients with locally advanced or metastatic disease. The role of routine postcystectomy chemotherapy remains controversial but some studies suggest a benefit in patients with pT3B disease, positive pelvic lymph nodes, or positive resection margins.

Radiation Therapy

Radiation therapy (RT) has been used in the management of transitional cell carcinoma of the bladder as definitive therapy or as an adjuvant treatment to cystectomy. The main advantage of RT is the opportunity to preserve normal bladder function and sexual function. In addition, RT remains a treatment option for those who are not medically fit for operation. Radical RT results in local tumor control in 50–70% of patients. The use of neoadjuvant chemotherapy and radiotherapy offers the opportunity for bladder preservation in selected patients, and preliminary results indicate that such an approach does not compromise survival. Selected reports document that radical RT with surgical salvage yield similar therapeutic results as radical cystectomy. The main goal of pre- or postoperative RT is to prevent local disease recurrence, but to date its benefit has not been confirmed in prospective clinical trials. Patterns of failure for muscle invasive disease include local bladder recurrence in patients treated with RT and pelvic recurrence in patients with extravesical extension treated with radical surgery or RT. The dominant pattern of failure is that of distant metastases, including pelvic and para-aortic lymph nodes, bone, lung, liver, and brain. As a result, it is estimated that local therapy will cure less than 50% of patients.

Metastatic Disease

Five to 10% of patients with bladder cancer will present with metastases at diagnosis. The majority develop metastases after treatment for muscle-invasive disease. The prognosis for patients who have recurrence after local treatment is poor. Effective systemic therapy is available and treatment with combination agents is superior to single-agent cisplatinum. More recently, a large, randomized clinical trial has shown that GC (gemcitabine and platinum) chemotherapy is equally efficacious as traditional MVAC or MVC chemotherapy, with a better side-effects profile. Survival for patients with metastatic disease ranges from 8 to 12 months. Chemotherapy is toxic and may not be appropriate for elderly patients with poor performance status. Other chemotherapeutic agents that show activity in bladder cancer continue to be evaluated, including gallium nitrate, the taxanes, and ifosfamide.

Organ Preservation

Organ preservation remains an important issue in bladder cancer, even with the advent of continent neobladders. Effective treatment of superficial disease with TUR and intravesical therapy has decreased the number of tumors that progress to muscle invasion. Despite the improvement in local disease progress, the treatment of locally advanced disease has been disappointing. Little effort has been made to improve the traditional bladder-preserving methods of radiotherapy with or without chemotherapy. Its use more recently has been restricted to the elderly and noncompliant patients, which makes critical evaluation of this treatment's efficacy difficult.

Follow-Up for Local and Distant Recurrences

Superficial bladder cancer is a chronic disease. As noted earlier, one study suggested that up to 80% of patients will develop a recurrence if they are followed for 20 years or more. Optimum follow-up scheduling has not been determined. Currently, periodic cystoscopies with simultaneous urine cytology have been used. The less invasive methods currently being investigated may play a large part in disease assessment in the future.

Prevention

Finally, more recently, the natural history of multiple recurrences is being addressed. There is no evidence that recurrence can uniformly be prevented, but several chemotherapeutic trials are ongoing using retinoids and megavitamins. Efforts to reduce industrial exposure and more importantly smoking should decrease the incidence of bladder cancer. Improved management of superficial disease has decreased the number who progress to muscle invasive disease.

TABLE 27.3. TNM Classification of Urinary Bladder Cancer

T—Primary tumor

TX	Primary tumor cannot be assessed
T0	No evidence of primary tumor
Ta	Noninvasive papillary carcinoma
Tis	Carcinoma *in situ*: "flat tumor"
T1	Tumor invades subepithelial connective tissue
T2	Tumor invades muscle
T2a	Tumor invades the superficial muscle (inner half)
T2b	Tumor invades the deep muscle (outer half)
T3	Tumor invades perivesical tissue
T3a	Microscopically
T3b	Macroscopically (extravesical mass)
T4	Tumor invades any of the following: prostate, uterus, vagina, pelvic wall, abdominal wall
T4a	Tumor invades prostate, uterus, vagina
T4b	Tumor invades pelvic wall, abdominal wall

N—Regional lymph nodes (Regional lymph nodes are those within the true pelvis; all others are distant lymph nodes.)

NX	Regional lymph nodes cannot be assessed
N0	No regional lymph node metastasis
N1	Metastasis in a single lymph node ≤ 2 cm in greatest dimension
N2	Metastasis in a single lymph node >2 cm but ≤ 5 cm in greatest dimension, or multiple lymph nodes, none >5 cm in greatest dimension
N3	Metastasis in a lymph node >5 cm in greatest dimension

M—Distant metastasis

MX	Distant metastasis cannot be assessed
M0	No distant metastasis
M1	Distant metastasis

Stage groupings

Oa	Ta	N0	M0
Ois	Tis	N0	M0
I	Tl	N0	M0
II	T2a	N0	M0
	T2b	N0	M0
III	T3a	N0	M0
	T3b	N0	M0
	T4a	N0	M0
IV	T4b	N0	M0
	Any T	Nl,N2,N3	M0
	Any T	Any N	Ml

Sobin LH, Wittekind Ch (eds.) (2002) International Union Against Cancer (UICC) *TNM Classification of Malignant Tumors*, 6th Edition. Wiley-Liss, NY.

CANCER OF THE RENAL PELVIS AND URETER

Upper urinary tract urothelial tumors are relatively uncommon. TCC represent 90% of these tumors. Renal pelvis tumors account for 5% of all urothelial tumors and 10% of all renal tumors. It occurs more frequently in men (male-to-female ratio: 2–3:1). Carcinoma of the ureter is even less common, representing 1% of malignancies of the upper genitourinary tract. Cigarette smoking is the strongest associated risk factor for upper tract tumors. Significant analgesic abuse has also been associated with renal pelvis tumors. Those areas endemic for Balkan nephropathy show a dramatically different incidence of upper urothelial tract tumors. The etiology of Balkan nephropathy remains unknown. The other etiological factors are similar to those for cancer of the urinary bladder. Molecular genetic studies suggest that abnormalities on chromosome 9, chromosome 17 near the *p53* locus, chromosome 17 near the retinoblastoma locus, and chromosome 3 near the kidney cancer gene locus are associated with upper urinary tract tumors. Upper urinary tract carcinomas are frequently multifocal. Bilateral involvement occurs in up to 10% of sporadic cases. Upper tract tumors also occur in 2–5% of patients with bladder cancer. Up to 75% of patients with an upper tract tumor will develop a bladder tumor when followed for some time. Ureteral tumors occur most commonly in the lower ureter. Hematuria is the presenting symptom in the majority of patients, but renal colic due to ureteric obstruction can also be present. Diagnosis is usually made on the basis of intravenous pyelogram or retrograde urography. CT is useful in assessing soft tissue extent of disease and to exclude metastases. Staging is based on the 2002 TNM Classification (Table 27.4).

Prognosis and treatment are based on stage and histologic grade. Carcinoma of the renal pelvis is treated with radical nephroureterectomy and removal of a cuff of bladder. Grade 1, low stage (Ta,T1) carcinomas of the ureter can be treated with partial ureterectomy. Patients with grade 2 and 3 disease are best managed with radical nephroureterectomy and removal of a cuff of bladder.

The 5-year survival rates are 85–95% for stage I disease, 40–60% for stage II disease, 20–30% for stage III, and less than 10% for stage IV disease. Adjuvant systemic chemotherapy with MVAC has been used in good performance status patients with a lymph node and distant metastases based on results with bladder TCC. There is no role for radiation therapy (RT) in stage I and II disease. RT may be useful as adjuvant therapy following incomplete tumor resection in stage III disease, but to date there is no definitive data to support its use.

CANCER OF THE URETHRA

Cancer of the Male Urethra

Carcinoma of the male urethra is exceedingly rare, with only 600 cases reported in the literature. Significant etiologic factors have not been identified, but chronic inflammation appears to play a role because many patients have history of prior

TABLE 27.4. TNM Classification of Renal Pelvis and Ureter Cancers

T—Primary tumor

TX	Primary tumor cannot be assessed
T0	No evidence of primary tumor
Ta	Noninvasive papillary carcinoma
Tis	Carcinoma *in situ*
T1	Tumor invades subepithelial connective tissue
T2	Tumor invades muscularis
T3	(Renal pelvis) Tumor invades beyond muscularis into peripelvic fat or renal parenchyma
T3	(Ureter) Tumor invades beyond muscularis into periureteric fat
T4	Tumor invades adjacent organs or through the kidney into perinephric fat

N—Regional lymph nodes[*]

X	Regional lymph nodes cannot be assessed
N0	No regional lymph node metastasis
N1	Metastasis in a single regional lymph node ≤ 2 cm in greatest dimension
N2	Metastasis in a single lymph node, >2 cm but not ≤ 5 cm in greatest dimension, or multiple lymph nodes, none >5 cm in greatest dimension
N3	Metastasis in a lymph node >5 cm in greatest dimension

M—Distant metastasis

MX	Distant metastasis cannot be assessed
M0	No distant metastasis
M1	Distant metastasis

Stage grouping

0a	TA	N0	M0
0is	Tis	N0	M0
I	T1	N0	M0
II	T2	N0	M0
III	T3	N0	M0
IV	T4	N0	M0
	Any T	N1,N2,N3	M0
	Any T	Any N	M1

[*]Laterality does not affect the N classification.

Sobin LH, Wittekind Ch (eds.) (2002) International Union Against Cancer (UICC) *TNM Classification of Malignant Tumors*, 6th Edition. Wiley-Liss, NY.

urethritis, stricture, or sexually transmitted disease. The most frequent site of the tumor is the bulbomembranous urethra, which is also the most frequent site of urethral stricture. Cancers occur in the bulbomembranous urethra in 60%, penile urethra in 30%, and prostatic urethra in 10%. Histologically, 80% are squamous cell cancers, 15% are transitional cell cancers, and 5% have other histology. The spread is usually by direct invasion and extension to the perineal tissues. Metastatic spread is to the inguinal and external iliac lymph nodes. The 2002 TNM classification is

TABLE 27.5. TNM Classification of Cancer of the Urethra

T—Primary tumor

| TX | Primary tumor cannot be assessed |
| T0 | No evidence of primary tumor |

Urethra (male and female)

Ta	Noninvasive papillary, polypoid, or verrucous carcinoma
Tis	Carcinoma *in situ*
Tl	Tumor invades subepithelial connective tissue
T2	Tumor invades any of the following: corpus spongiosum, prostate, or periurethral muscle
T3	Tumor invades any of the following: corpus cavernosum, beyond prostatic capsule, anterior vagina, or bladder neck
T4	Tumor invades other adjacent organs

Transitional cell carcinoma of the prostate (prostatic urethra)

Tis pu	Carcinoma *in situ* involvement of the prostatic urethra
Tis pd	Carcinoma *in situ*, involvement of the prostatic ducts
T1	Tumor invades subepithelial connective tissue
T2	Tumor invades any of the following: prostatic stroma, corpus spongiosum, periurethral muscle
T3	Tumor invades any of the following: corpus cavernosum, beyond prostatic capsule, bladder neck (extraprostatic extension)
T4	Tumor invades other adjacent organs (invasion of the bladder)

N—Regional lymph nodes

NX	Regional lymph nodes cannot be assessed
N0	No regional lymph node metastasis
Nl	Metastasis in a single regional lymph node ≤ 2 cm in greatest dimension
N2	Metastasis in a single lymph node, >2 cm in greatest dimension, or multiple lymph nodes

M—Distant metastasis

MX	Distant metastasis cannot be assessed
M0	No distant metastasis
M1	Distant metastasis

Stage grouping

0a	Ta	N0	M0
0is	Tis	N0	M0
	Tis pu	N0	M0
	Tis pd	N0	M0
I	Tl	N0	M0
II	T2	N0	M0
III	T1	N1	M0
	T2	N1	M0
	T3	N0,N1	M0
IV	T4	N0,N1	M0
	Any T	N2	M0
	Any T	Any N	M1

Sobin LH, Wittekind Ch (eds.) (2002) International Union Against Cancer (UICC) *TNM Classification of Malignant Tumors*, 6th Edition. Wiley-Liss, NY.

used for staging (Table 27.5). Investigations include urethroscopy, examination under anesthesia, and CT or MRI imaging to determine soft tissue extent.

The primary mode of treatment is surgical excision. The extent of surgery depends on the location and the stage of the tumor. Superficial tumors may be managed by transurethral resection, with high potential for cure. In rare cases that involve mucosa only, stage Ta, Tis, resection and fulguration are justified as initial therapy. Infiltrating lesions require penile amputation for cancers of anterior urethra. The role of RT for tumors of the anterior urethra is not well defined, but cure with RT has been reported. Most patients with bulbomembranous urethral tumors present with bulky infiltrative tumors, which require radical cystoprostatectomy and *en bloc* penectomy to achieve adequate margins of resection, minimize local recurrence, and achieve cure. There is little experience and data regarding the use of radiation therapy, but similar to the carcinoma of the female urethra, RT may be useful in achieving local disease control. Five-year survival can be expected in only 15–20% of patients with the latter tumors.

Cancer of the Female Urethra

Urethral carcinoma is an unusual genitourinary tract neoplasm as it is much more common in women than in men. Most patients are over the age of 50 years. The etiology is unknown, but similar to the relationship between male urethral cancer and chronic irritation, urinary tract infections have been reported. Most patients present with urinary frequency, obstruction, or palpable urethral lesion. Histology is that of squamous cell carcinoma in 60% of cases, transitional cell carcinoma in 30%, and adenocarcinoma in 10%. Other tumors, melanoma, or sarcoma are rare. Staging classification and assessment are similar to those described previously for male urethral cancer.

Significant prognostic factors for local control and survival are the anatomic location and extent of tumor. Histology does not seem to affect prognosis, and different histological types are often treated in a similar manner. Treatment may involve surgery or RT. For tumors of the anterior or distal urethra, local surgical excision or electroresection and fulguration may be sufficient for small distal tumors. Tumor destruction using Nd:YAG or CO_2 laser vaporization coagulation represents an alternative option. RT for larger and invasive tumors may be used with external-beam radiotherapy, often with brachytherapy boost using interstitial or intracavitary techniques. Treatment results for early stage disease are good (65–80% survival), but more extensive disease is associated with poor survival probability (20–30%). Combined modality approaches with concurrent chemotherapy and RT are currently being explored in an attempt to improve local disease control and survival. Tumors of the posterior female urethra or entire urethra are usually invasive and are associated with a high incidence of lymph node metastases. Treatment involves exenterative surgery and urinary diversion, with adjuvant RT. For smaller tumors, RT alone or in combination with local tumor excision may be sufficient. Five-year survival is 60% if lesions are less than 2 cm in diameter, and but only 10–20% if larger than 4–5 cm in diameter.

CANCER OF THE TESTIS

Testicular tumors are uncommon neoplasms but constitute the most common malignancies of men aged 15–35 years. The majority of these tumors are primary germ cell tumors (GCT). Epidemiological studies have shown a doubling of the incidence rate in the past 30 years, but mortality associated with them has markedly declined. The advent of tumor markers, CT imaging, and curative chemotherapy have contributed to these improved outcomes. The identification of prognostic factors has helped to re-evaluate treatment strategies and minimize treatment for those with favorable prognosis.

Etiology

Testicular cancer accounts for 1–2% of all cancers in men. Ethnic and geographic variation in the incidence of GCT is seen, with the highest incidence being reported from Denmark and Switzerland (6.2–8.84 per 100,000 per year). A history of testicular maldescent is the only factor that has been definitely associated with testicular cancer. Men with a history of cryptorchidism have an approximately fivefold increased chance of developing a testicular cancer. Familial clusters of testicular cancer have been reported, and patients with XY gonadal dysgenesis have an increased risk of developing testis cancer. Testicular cancer is not infrequently a bilateral disease. The cumulative risk of developing a contralateral testicular malignancy at 25 years after diagnosis is 5.2%. Controversy exists as to the relative importance of prenatal versus postnatal factors in the development of testicular cancers. Prenatal factors include threatened miscarriage, maternal nausea, and delivery by cesarean section. The prenatal theory proposes that excessive estrogen exposure *in utero* may affect the geminal epithelium, giving rise to subsequent cryptorchidism and risk of developing a testicular tumor. This theory remains unproven. Other reported postnatal factors included mumps orchitis, history of testicular trauma, exposure to pesticides and plastics, and electromagnetic radiation.

Screening

There is insufficient information to ascertain whether screening would result in a decrease in mortality from testicular cancer. Indeed, formal screening programs might not be cost effective given the exceptionally high cure rates for this disease. Most tumors are found by the patient either incidentally or by self-examination. No studies have been carried out to evaluate the value of testicular self-examination in reducing the mortality of this disease, which is an uncommon cause of death.

Diagnostic Measures

GCT are classified into two major groups: seminomas and nonseminomatous germ cell tumors (NSGCT). Approximately 45% of GCT are pure seminoma, 40% are

NSGCT, and 15% are mixed tumors. Carcinoma *in situ* (CIS) or intratubular germ cell neoplasia precedes the development of all cases of seminoma and NSGCT except spermatocytic seminoma. The incidence of CIS is very low (0.2–0.5%) in the general population, but it is somewhat higher in men with impaired fertility (0.5%) and in patients with cryptorchid testes (2–5%). Seminoma, the most common type of GCT, has a median age of onset of 35 years. NSGCT comprise 40% of germ cell testicular cancers and have a median age of onset at 25 years. In the World Health Organization classification system, NSGCT include embryonal carcinoma, teratoma (mature, immature, or with malignant differentiation), choriocarcinoma, yolk sac tumor, and mixed GCT (Table 27.6). Although some tumors are mixed, the association of seminoma within a histologically confirmed NSGCT has no major impact on the outcome.

Local or direct extension of tumor can occur into epididymis, through tunica vaginalis, into spermatic cord, and rarely into scrotum but has little prognostic impact. In GCT, lymphatic spread is the most common route of metastatic spread. NSGCT also spread hematogenously early in the course of the disease. The lymphatic drainage of the testis is directly to the paraaortic lymph nodes. Pelvic and inguinal lymph node involvement is rare (<3%). Factors predisposing to inguinal lymph node involvement include prior scrotal or inguinal surgery, scrotal orchiectomy with incision of the tunica albuginea, tumor invasion of the tunica vaginalis or lower third of the epididymis, and cryptorchid testis. The pulmonary parenchyma is the most common site of hematogenous spread in NSGCT but liver, bone, brain, kidney, and gastrointestinal metastases are also seen. The frequent finding of combinations of choriocarcinoma, embryonal carcinoma, and seminoma in a single tumor demonstrate that GCT have the capacity for totipotential differentiation. The finding of mature teratoma in residual post-treatment retroperitoneal masses reveals the GCT retain the ability to differentiate. Cytogenetic

TABLE 27.6. Histologic Classification of Germ Cell Testis Tumors

Intratubular germ cell neoplasia (carcinoma *in situ*)
Seminoma
Spermatocytic seminoma
Embryonal cell carcinoma
Teratoma
   Mature teratoma
   Immature teratoma
   Teratoma with malignant component
Yolk sac tumor
Choriocarcinoma
Mixed germ cell tumors
Polyembryoma

analysis of GCT has shown that chromosome numbers are more homogeneous in seminomas than in NSGCT. Triploid and tetraploid chromosomal patterns are common in seminomas, and hyperdiploid to hypertriploid counts are common in NSGCT. A characteristic chromosome anomaly in GCT of all histologic types is the presence of an isochromosome of the short arm of chromosome 12. It is present in more than 80% of cases, and in GCT without 12p isochromosome, extra copies of 12p segments are incorporated into other chromosomes. The 12p isochromosome is also found in testicular CIS. Isochromosome copies tend to be more numerous in NSGCT than in seminoma.

The most common presentation of testes tumor is painless testicular enlargement. Up to 45% of patients have testicular pain. Back pain and dyspnea are often presenting symptoms for those with metastatic disease. A radical inguinal orchiectomy is usually performed after the tumor is detected on physical examination, verified by ultrasonography and when serum tumor markers have been obtained. Serum tumor markers include α-fetoprotein (AFP), human chorionic gonadotropin (β-hCG), and lactate dehydrogenase (LDH). Preoperative measurement allows monitoring of decay with treatment. Staging investigations include chest x-ray film, CT of the abdomen and pelvis, CT of the thorax, and postoperative tumor markers for NSGCT. CT of the thorax is only carried out for those seminomas that have evidence of retroperitoneal lymph node involvement or symptoms or signs to suggest pulmonary disease. Measurements of AFP, β-hCG, and LDH are essential in the diagnosis and management of patients with GCT. β-hCG is a glycoprotein with a molecular weight of 45,000, composed of two subunits, of which the α-subunit is identical to that of luteinizing hormone (LH), follicle-stimulating hormone (FSH), and thyroid-stimulating hormone (TSH), and a distinct, β-subunit. The half-life of β-hCG in human serum is approximately 22 hours. AFP is a glycoprotein of molecular weight 70,000. It is a nonspecific marker and is also elevated in hepatocellular carcinomas, cirrhosis, hepatitis, and pregnancy. The half-life of AFP is approximately 5 days. AFP is not found in pure seminoma; its elevation in this setting implies the presence of NSGCT tumor elements. One or both of these markers are elevated in 85% of patients with NSGCT. LDH is an independent prognostic factor in patients with GCT, being elevated in up to 60% of patients with NSGCTs, and in a high proportion of patients with advanced seminoma. Placental alkaline phosphatase (PLAP) is an isoenzyme of alkaline phosphatase and is normally expressed by placental syncytiotrophoblasts. It is also expressed by testis tissue and has been used as a tumor marker in seminoma in the past. As a marker, PLAP has little value in routine clinical management even though it is often elevated in patients with seminoma.

Staging

The 2002 UICC classification in Table 27.7, which combines anatomic disease extent and tumor markers is the recommended staging system.

TABLE 27.7. TNM Classification of Testis Tumors

*T—Primary tumor**

pTX	Primary tumor cannot be assessed (If no radical orchiectomy has been performed, TX is used.)
PT0	No evidence of primary tumor (e.g., histologic scar in testis)
pTis	Intratubular germ cell neoplasia (carcinoma *in situ*)
pT1	Tumor is limited to testis and epididymis without vascular/lymphatic invasion; tumor may invade into tunica albuginea but not tunica vaginalis
pT2	Tumor is limited to testis and epididymis with vascular/lymphatic invasion, or tumor extends through tunica albuginea with involvement of tunica vaginalis
pT3	Tumor invades spermatic cord with or without vascular/lymphatic invasion
pT4	Tumor invades scrotum with or without vascular/lymphatic invasion

N—Regional lymph nodes, clinical

NX	Regional lymph nodes cannot be assessed
N0	No regional lymph node metastasis
N1	Metastasis with a lymph node mass ≤ 2 cm in greatest dimension; or multiple lymph nodes, none >2 cm in greatest dimension
N2	Metastasis with a lymph node mass >2 cm but not ≤ 5 cm in greatest dimension; or multiple lymph nodes, any one mass >2 cm but none >5 cm in greatest dimension
N3	Metastasis with a lymph node mass >5 cm in greatest dimension

pN—Pathologic lymph nodes

pNX	Regional lymph nodes cannot be assessed.
PN0	No regional lymph node metastasis
pN1	Metastasis with a lymph node mass ≤ 2 cm in greatest dimension and five or fewer positive lymph nodes, none >2 cm in greatest dimension
pN2	Metastasis with a lymph node mass, >2 cm but not ≤ 5 cm in greatest dimension; or more than more than five nodes positive, none >5 cm; or evidence of extranodal extension of tumor
pN3	Metastasis with a lymph node mass >5 cm in greatest dimension

M—Distant metastasis

MX	Distant metastasis cannot be assessed
M0	No distant metastasis
Ml	Distant metastasis
Mla	Nonregional lymph node(s) or lung
Mlb	Other sites

S—Serum tumor markers

	LDH		hCG (mIU/mL)		AFP (ng/mL)
SX	Marker studies not available or not performed				
S0	Marker study levels within normal limits				
Sl	$<1.5 \times N^{\dagger}$	and	$<5,000$	and	$<1,000$
S2	$1.5–10 \times N^{\dagger}$	or	$5,000–50,000$	or	$1,000–10,000$
S3	$>10 \times N^{\dagger}$	or	$>50,000$	or	$>10,000$

TABLE 27.7 *(Continued)*

Stage grouping

0	pTis	N0	M0	S0, SX
I	pT1–4	N0	M0	SX
IA	pT1	N0	M0	S0
IB	pT2	N0	M0	S0
	pT3	N0	M0	S0
	pT4	N0	M0	S0
IS	Any pT/TX	N0	M0	S1-3
II	Any pT/TX	N1–3	M0	SX
IIA	Any pT/TX	N1	M0	S0
	Any pT/TX	N1	M0	S1
IIB	Any pT/TX	N2	M0	S0
	Any pT/TX	N2	M0	S I
IIC	Any pT/TX	N3	M0	S0
	Any pT/TX	N3	M0	S I
III	Any pT/TX	Any N	Ml, M1a	SX
IIIA	Any pT/TX	Any N	Ml, Mla	S0
	Any pT/TX	Any N	Ml, Mla	S1
IIIB	Any pT/TX	N1–3	M0	S2
	Any pT/TX	Any N	M1,Mla	S2
IIIC	Any pT/TX	N1–3	M0	S3
	Any pT/TX	Any N	M1, Mla	S3
	Any pT/TX	Any N	Mlb	Any S

[*]Except for pTis and pT4, where radical orchiectomy is not always necessary for classification purposes, the extent of primary tumor is classified after radical orchiectomy.
[†]N indicates the upper limit of normal for the LDH assay.
Sobin LH, Wittekind Ch (eds.) (2002) International Union Against Cancer (UICC) *TNM Classification of Malignant Tumors*, 6th Edition. Wiley-Liss, NY.

Multimodality Treatment

The initial management of GCT involves a radical inguinal orchidectomy in almost all cases. Postorchidectomy management is based on the histology and stage of the tumor. The management policies for both seminomas and NSGCT have evolved separately.

Surgery

Orchidectomy is both diagnostic and therapeutic and offers cure in a high proportion (60–90%) of patients with stage I disease. The possibility of organ-sparing surgery with tumor enucleation, or partial orchidectomy with or without postoperative low-dose RT, has been proposed in patients with bilateral testis tumors more recently. Preservation of hormonal function was achieved in 10 of 14 cases managed by tumor excision with low-dose (18–20 Gy) postoperative RT to the residual testis.

SEMINOMA

The majority of patients with seminoma present with clinical stage I disease, 15–20% have infradiaphragmatic lymph node involvement, and less than 5% present with distant disease. Postorchidectomy treatment options in patients with stage I seminoma include adjuvant retroperitoneal RT, surveillance with treatment reserved for those who relapse, adjuvant chemotherapy, and retroperitoneal lymph node dissection (RPLND). The cause-specific survival with all these strategies approaches 100%. The overall survival for stage I seminoma following retroperitoneal RT ranges between 92% and 99% at 5–10 years, with most deaths being due to intercurrent illness. With moderate RT dose (25–30 Gy), infield disease control is almost 100%. Approximately 5% of patients will relapse outside the RT treatment volume, most commonly in supraclavicular lymph nodes, mediastinum, lung, or bone. The second treatment option is surveillance, with relapse rate in most studies approximately 20%. The predominant site of relapse in all surveillance studies is in the para-aortic lymph nodes (82–92%). The median time to relapse is 14–18 months, but late relapses have been observed with 25% of relapses occuring more than 4 years from the diagnosis. A recent pooled analysis from all surveillance studies show larger tumor size, invasion of rete testis, and small vessel involvement predict for relapse. At relapse, most patients are treated with retroperitoneal RT. Chemotherapy is very effective in advanced seminoma and is being investigated as an alternative to RT or surveillance in stage I seminoma. RPLND is another treatment option when patients are unwilling to comply with surveillance or those unable to be treated with RT.

In summary, almost 100% of patients with stage I testicular seminoma are cured regardless of the choice of treatment. Adjuvant RT remains the most common treatment approach. One of the most attractive features of surveillance is the ability to limit treatment to orchidectomy alone in the vast majority of patients. Although isolated occurrences of second nontesticular tumors following RT have been reported for decades, there is now convincing data indicating an increased risk of second malignancy.

Stage II and III Seminoma

The most common presentation is with stage IIA disease. Treatment with retroperitoneal RT carries only a 10% risk of relapse. Chemotherapy is also curative, but is associated with increased short- and long-term toxicity. Patients with stage IIC disease are at high risk of occult distant disease and should be treated with etoposide and cisplatin chemotherapy. The overall disease-specific survival of patients with stage II seminoma approaches 100%. Following treatment of stage II seminoma, especially stage IIC, patients may have a residual retroperitoneal mass after treatment and its management is controversial. Patients with residual mass less than 3 cm in diameter rarely had residual tumor (3%), whereas 27% of those with a mass >3 cm had viable tumor in the Memorial Hospital experience. Given this high proportion of persistent malignancy, resection or biopsy of masses of 3 cm or larger has been recommended. However, if residual retroperitoneal mass continues to decrease in size after treatment, observation is recommended. Periodic CT examinations are mandatory and treatment is indicated for residual masses that increase in size on follow-up. Stage III seminoma is uncommon (<5%) and has been shown to be exceptionally chemosensitive. In the International Germ Cell Cancers Collaborative Group study, two prognostic groups were identified in seminoma: a good prognosis group without nonpulmonary visceral metastases (NPVM) and a 5-year survival of 86%, and an intermediate prognosis group with NPVM and a 5-year survival of 72%. The Memorial Hospital results in 140 patients with advanced stage seminoma showed 93% complete response rate to chemotherapy and 88% 5-year survival. The current standard chemotherapy regimen is four courses of etoposide and cisplatin.

NONSEMINOMATOUS GERM CELL TUMORS

NSCGCT were associated with very poor survival and rarely were cured before the advent of cisplatin-based chemotherapy. With current chemotherapy regimens, complete responses to treatment are frequent and cures are apparent in patients with metastatic disease.

Stage I NSGCT

Current treatment strategies for these patients include either a modified bilateral RPLND or surveillance. RT has been recognized as ineffective in stage I NSGCT since the 1970s. The clinical factors associated with a high risk of occult distant disease include the presence of vascular invasion, embryonal carcinoma, and the size of the primary tumor. In the Medical Research Council UK study of 259 patients managed by orchidectomy, four factors (presence of embryonal carcinoma, absence of yolk sac elements, invasion of blood vessels, or lymphatics) were identified on multivariate analysis as predictive of relapse. Published studies of surveillance have shown a 30% risk of disease progression, with up to 95% of patients progressing within 12 months of diagnosis; progression more than 24 months from diagnosis is extremely rare. Approximately 60% of patients progress in the retroperitoneal lymph nodes, with or without other evidence of disease. The other common sites of progression are lung metastases or tumor marker elevation alone. The critical factors for successful surveillance include regular imaging of the retroperitoneal nodes and patient compliance. At the time of progression, patients are usually treated with chemotherapy, although RPLND is used in selected cases with small retroperitoneal lymph nodes. Most patients are cured at relapse and the cause-specific survival in most series is greater than 95%. RPLND is a recognized alternative to surveillance in clinical stage I disease. Surgical techniques have undergone considerable modification in the last 20 years. A modified unilateral infrahilar RPLND is now performed, with nerve-sparing techniques to preserve ejaculation. The relapse rate following surgery is approximately 10% for patients with clinical pathologic stage I disease. As with relapses on surveillance, most patients who relapse after RPLND are cured with subsequent chemotherapy. In some centers, patients with stage I NSGCT at high risk of relapse on surveillance are offered adjuvant chemotherapy. Because the outcomes of surgery, surveillance, and adjuvant chemotherapy are similar, some patients and physicians favor immediate treatment over a wait-and-see approach.

Stage II NSGCT

Treatment options include RPLND, chemotherapy, or a combination of both. Patients with retroperitoneal disease with nodes greater than 5 cm in diameter have a high relapse rate following RPLND and are usually approached with chemotherapy. The outcome is excellent. In North America, patients with solitary node mass less than 3 cm in size are treated with RPLND. Patients with retroperitoneal disease between 3 and 5 cm in size may be treated with initial surgery or primary chemotherapy. Published data suggest that 8–44% of patients will relapse following RPLND if lymph nodes less than 6 cm are involved, with no single node greater than 2 cm in diameter. The considerable treatment-related morbidity of adjuvant PVB chemotherapy prompted efforts to reduce toxicity. For this group of patients, surveillance, with chemotherapy reserved for relapse, is the recommended approach for compliant patients. Almost all patients who relapse can be salvaged with chemotherapy.

Stage III NSGCT

Many patients with metastatic NSGCT are cured, and this is one of the most remarkable advances in cancer therapy in the last 20 years. Initially, a lack of agreement on prognostic factors predictive for a favorable or unfavorable outcome caused difficulty in evaluating the various trials. Different prognostic groupings made comparison of trial results impossible. Stage migration and other similar factors could have accounted for observed differences, rather than different treatment protocols. Data from 5,168 patients with NSGCT were analyzed and independent prognostic variables included tumor markers AFP, β-hCG, LDH, and the presence or absence of NPVM, for example, metastases to the liver or gastrointestinal tract. Based on these factors, three prognostic groups have been recognized. The 5-year survival for the good prognosis group was 92%; for the intermediate group, 80%; and for the poor prognosis group, 48%. At present, patients with low-risk disease are routinely treated with four cycles of BEP (bleomycin, etoposide, cisplatin). Patients with high-risk disease have durable complete response (CR) rates of 28–63% with four courses of BEP, or with a similar cisplatin-based regimen. Patients with bulky retroperitoneal disease commonly have residual disease on CT scan after chemotherapy. Less frequently, residual mediastinal or pulmonary metastases may be seen. It is recommended that residual disease be resected. Approximately 85–90% of patients will have necrosis or mature teratoma, and 10% of patients will have active cancer. In the latter group, two additional cycles of a platinum-based chemotherapy are recommended.

Salvage Therapy

Approximately 30% of patients with high-risk GCT relapse or fail to achieve a CR with first-line chemotherapy regimens. Complete responses can be achieved with second- and third-line regimens in 25–35% of cases and 15–25% of patients treated in this way can be cured. Many of the currently used second-line salvage regimens include ifosfamide, often combined with cisplatin and etoposide or vinblastine. High-dose intensive therapy with peripheral blood stem cell support is being investigated, and preliminary reports indicate that up to 20% of heavily pretreated patients can achieve a durable complete response.

CNS Metastases

Approximately 2–3% of patients with stage III GCT will present with brain metastases, and up to 40% of patients who die of progressive disease will have brain metastases at autopsy. Approximately 25% of patients presenting with brain metastases, or who develop metastases after a favorable response to chemotherapy, can achieve long-term disease control. Whole-brain irradiation may be administered along with systemic chemotherapy. Patients who develop brain metastases during systemic chemotherapy have a very poor prognosis and should likely receive palliative RT only.

Toxicity

Testicular germinal epithelium is exquisitely sensitive to ionizing radiation. Although the contralateral testis is not located directly in the radiation field, scatter dose can be significant and may cause profound depression of spermatogenesis and compromise future fertility. A radiation dose between 20 and 50 cGy may produce temporary aspermia, and doses greater than 50 cGy may preclude recovery of spermatogenesis. The use of scrotal shielding reduces the scattered radiation dose to the testis, but cannot ensure protection of spermatogenesis in all patients. In men who recover spermatogenesis after RT for seminoma, there is no evidence of an increased incidence of genetic abnormalities among offspring. Limiting RT target volume to the para-aortic and common iliac area eliminates the concerns regarding RT-induced fertility.

Nausea and vomiting occur with chemotherapy, but are controlled effectively in most patients with 5-hydroxytryptamine3 (5-HT3) antagonists and steroids. Myelosuppression is frequent and febrile neutropenia is seen in about 10–15% of patients receiving etoposide and cisplatin, and such patients benefit from hematopoietic growth factors. Nephrotoxicity occurs with the use of cisplatin and ifosfamide. Raynaud phenomenon has been reported in 23–49% of patients.

Chronic peripheral neuropathy is well recognized after treatment with cisplatin, vinblastine, and etoposide. Pulmonary toxicity is seen with the use of bleomycin and is dose related. Impaired fertility, which may precede the use of chemotherapy, may also continue after its use. Although chemotherapy also produces infertility, recovery of sperm counts has been observed in the majority of patients.

Follow-Up

Follow-up is an integral part of the management of testis tumors. The patterns of failure are well defined, and follow-up investigations are focused on early detection of relapse, or treatment complications. Late relapse is rare, and its detection depends more on patient education than on close long-term follow-up in specialized centers.

CANCER OF THE PENIS

Penile cancer accounts for 0.4–0.6% of all malignancies in males in North America but accounts for up to 10% of male cancers in some African and South American countries. The incidence of penile cancer varies significantly with hygiene standards and cultural and religious practices. Neonatal circumcision offers significant protection against penile cancer, whereas adult circumcision offers little or no protection against development of this disease. Penile tumors usually present with a visible lesion confined to the glans (50%) and prepuce (20%). Histology is usually well-differentiated squamous cell carcinoma. Direct local invasion is the most common route of spread and spread to the inguinal lymph nodes. Stage is the strongest prognostic factor. The UICC TNM classification is used to describe the anatomic disease extent (Table 27.8).

CIS of the penis is referred to by urologists and dermatologists as erythroplasia of Queyrat if it involves the glans penis, prepuce, or penile shaft and as Bowen's disease if it involves the remainder of the genitalia or perineal region. CIS of the penis may be treated similarly to skin cancers with topical 5-fluorouracil, laser, or liquid nitrogen with excellent control and cosmetic outcome. Similarly, low-dose superficial radiotherapy (e.g., 20 Gy fractionated to the epidermis) is highly effective without adverse sequelae. For early lesions, conservative treatment with Mohs' micrographic surgery (MMS) has been used. MMS is a method of removing skin cancer by excising tissue in thin layers and includes color coding of excised specimens with tissue dyes and microscopic examination of excised layers with frozen-section techniques until all malignant tissues have been removed. Mohs reported excellent cure rates for tumors less than 1 cm in diameter.

For infiltrating tumors, the choice of treatments will depend on the tumor size, extent of infiltration, and degree of tumor destruction of normal tissue. The standard treatment involves total or partial penectomy. Patients with early tumors may be treated with RT using brachytherapy or external beam radiation therapy. The

TABLE 27.8. TMN Classification of Penis Tumors

T—Primary tumor

TX	Primary tumor cannot be assessed
T0	No evidence of primary tumor
Tis	Carcinoma *in situ*
Ta	Noninvasive verrucous carcinoma
T1	Tumor invades subepithelial connective tissue
T2	Tumor invades corpus spongiosum or cavernosum
T3	Tumor invades urethra or prostate
T4	Tumor invades other adjacent structures

N—Regional lymph nodes

NX	Regional lymph nodes cannot be assessed
N0	No regional lymph node metastasis
N1	Metastasis in a single, superficial inguinal lymph node
N2	Metastasis in multiple or bilateral superficial inguinal lymph nodes
N3	Metastasis in deep inguinal or pelvic lymph node(s), unilateral or bilateral

M—Distant metastasis

MX	Distant metastasis cannot be assessed
M0	No distant metastasis
M1	Distant metastasis

Stage grouping

0	Tis	N0	M0
	Ta	N0	M0
I	T1	N0	M0
II	T1	N1	M0
	T2	N0	M0
	T2	N1	M0
III	T1	N2	M0
	T2	N2	M0
	T3	N0,N1,N2	M0
IV	T4	Any N	M0
	Any T	N3	M0
	Any T	Any N	M1

Sobin LH, Wittekind Ch (eds.) (2002) International Union Against Cancer (UICC) *TNM Classification of Malignant Tumors*, 6th Edition. Wiley-Liss, NY.

former, with iridium implants, is very successful in early-stage lesions (80–90% local control) and offers the opportunity for organ preservation. Prophylactic or therapeutic inguinal lymph node dissection has been recommended for patients with Tl grade 2–3 tumors and T2–3 tumors. However, lymphadenectomy can carry significant morbidity, including infection, skin necrosis, wound breakdown, and chronic leg edema. Chemotherapy has not been particularly useful in the management of this disease, and has been used only for palliation. The active agents include bleomycin, methotrexate, and cisplatin.

FURTHER READING

Kidney Cancer

Bukowski RM (1997) Natural History and therapy of metastatic renal cell carcinomas: The role of interleukin-2. *Cancer* 80:1198–1220.

DeDernion JB, Hulland H (1990) The operable renal cell carcinoma: Summary and conclusions. *Eur Urol* 2:48–51.

Elson, PJ, Witte RS, Trump DL (1988) Prognostic factors for survival in patients with recurrent or metastatic renal cell carcinoma. *Cancer Res* 48:7310–7313.

Fyfe G, Fisher RI, Rosenberg, SA et al. (1995) Results of treatment of 225 patients with metastatic renal cell carcinoma who received high-dose recombinant interleukin-2 therapy. *J Clin Oncol* 13:688–696.

Godley PA, Stinchombe TE (1999) Renal cell carcinoma. *Curr Opin Oncol* 11:213–217.

Klotz L (2001) Back to nephrectomy for patients with metastatic renal cancer. *Lancet* 358(9286):966–970.

Montie J, El Ammar RR, Pontes J et al. (1991) Renal cell carcinoma with inferior vena cava tumor thrombi. *Surg Gynecol Obstet* 173:107–115.

Motzer RJ, Russo P, Nanus DM, Berg WJ (1997) Renal cell carcinoma. *Curr Prob Cancer* 21:185–232.

Ritchie A, deKernion J (1987) The natural history and clinical features of renal cell carcinoma. *Semin Nephrol* 7:131–139.

Schmid HP, Szabo J (1997) Renal cell carcinoma—a current review. *Schweiz Rundsch Med Prax* 86:837–843.

Sobin LH, Wittekind Ch (2002) International Union Against Cancer (UICC). *TNM Classification of Malignant Tumors*, 6th edition. Wiley-Liss, New York, pp. 193–195.

Storkel S, Thoenes W, Jacobi GH et al. (1990) Prognostic parameters of renal cell carcinoma. *Eur Urol* 2:36–37.

Cancer of the Urinary Bladder

Dalesio O, Schulman CC, Sylvester R et al. (1983) Prognostic factors in superficial bladder tumors. A study of the European Organization for Research on Treatment of Cancer: Genitourinary Tract Cancer Cooperative Group. *J Urol* 129:730–733.

Evans CP, Swanson DA (1996) What to do if the lymph nodes are positive. *Semin Urol Oncol* 14:96–102.

Gospodarowicz MK, Quilty PM, Scalliet P, Tsujii H, Fossa SD, Horenblas S, Isaka S, Prout GR, Shipley WU, Wijnmaalen AJ et al. (1995) The place of radiation therapy as definitive treatment of bladder cancer. *Int J Urol* 2:41–48.

Hautman RE, Paiss T (1998) Does the option of neobladder stimulate patient and physician decision towards earlier cystectomy. *J Urol* 159:1845–1850.

Heney NM (1992) Natural history of superficial bladder cancer. Prognostic features and long-term disease course. *Urol Clin North Am* 19:429–433.

Herr HW (1997) Natural history of superficial bladder tumors: 10- to 20-year follow-up of treated patients. *World J Urol* 15:84–88.

Hermann GG, Horn T, Seven K (1998) The influence of lamina propria invasion and the prevalence of level of p53 nuclear accumulation on survival in stage T1 transitional cell bladder carcinoma. *J Urol* 159:91–94.

Kantoff PW (1990) Bladder cancer. *Curr Prob Cancer* 14:235–291.

Kryger JV, Messing E (1996) Bladder cancer screening. *Semin Oncol* 23:585–597.

Kurth KH (1997) Diagnosis and treatment of superficial transitional cell carcinoma of the bladder: Facts and perspectives. *Eur Urol* 1:10–19.

Kurth KH, Schellhanumer PF, Okajima E, Akdas A, Jakse G. Herr HW, Calais da Silva F. Fukushima S, Nagayama T (1995) Current methods of assessing and treating carcinoma in situ of the bladder with or without involvement of the prostatic urethra. *Int J Urol* 2:8–22.

Lamm DL (1995) BCG in Perspective: Advances in the treatment of superficial bladder cancer. *Eur Urol* 1:2–8.

Lanum DL, Riggs DR, Shriver JS, vanGilder PF, Rach JF, DeHaven JI (1994) Megadose Vitamins in bladder cancer: A double blind clinical trial. *J Urol* 151:21–26.

Loehrer PS, Einhorn LH, Elson PJ et al. (1992) A randomized comparison of cisplatin alone or in combination with metbotrexate, vinblastine, and doxorubicin in patients with metastatic urothelial carcinoma: A cooperative group study. *J Clin Oncol* 10:1066–1073.

Martinez-Pineiro JA, Martinez-Pineiro L (1997) BCG update: Intravesical therapy. *Eur Urol* 1:31–41.

Natale RB, Grossman HB et al. (2001) SWOG 8710 (INT-0080): Randomized Phase III Trial of Neoadjuvant MVAC + Cystectomy Versus Cystectomy Alone in Patients with Locally Advanced Bladder Cancer. ASCO abstract available at http://www.asco.org/prof/me/html/ 01abstracts/0021/3.htm.

Paulson D, Denis L, Orikasa S. Bartolucci A, Bouffioux C, Hirao Y, Jewett MA, Pagano F, Pontes JE (1995) Optimal staging procedures, including imaging, to define prognosis of bladder cancer. *Int J Urol* 2:1–7.

Richie JP (1992) Surgery for invasive bladder cancer. *Hematol Oncol Clin North Am* 6: 129–145.

Roth BJ (1996) Chemotherapy for advanced bladder cancer. *Semin Oncol* 23:633-644.

Shipley WU, Prout GR, Kaufman DS (1990) Bladder cancer. Advances in laboratory innovations and clinical management, with emphasis on innovations allowing bladder-sparing approaches for patients with invasive tumors. *Cancer* 65:675–683.

Stadler WM, Kuzel TM, Raghavan D, Levine E, Vogelzang M, Roth B, Dorr FA (1997) Metastatic bladder cancer: Advances in treatment. *Eur J Cancer* 33:S23–26.

Sternberg CN (1996) Neoadjuvant and adjuvant chemotherapy in locally advanced bladder cancer. *Semin Oncol* 23:621–632.

Von der Masse H, Hansen SW et al. (2000) Gemcitabine and cisplatin versus methotrexate, vinblastine, doxorubicin and cisplatin in advanced or metastatic bladder cancer: results of a large randomized, multinational, multicentre, phase III study. *J Clin Oncol* 17:3068–3077.

Warde P, Gospodarowicz MK (1997) New approaches in the use of radiation therapy in the treatment of infiltrative transitional-cell cancer of the bladder. *World J Urol* 15:125–133.

Cancer of the Renal Pelvis and Ureter

Cozad S, Smalley S, Austenfeld M, Noble M, Jennings S, Reymond R (1995) Transitional cell carcinima of the renal pelvis or ureter: Patterns of failure. *Urology* 46:796–800.

Das A, Carson C, Bolick D, Paulson D (1990) Primary carcinoma of the upper urinary tract. Effect of primary and secondary therapy on survival. *Cancer* 66:1919–1923.

Krogh J. Kvist E, Rye B (1991) Transitional cell carcinoma of the upper urinary tract: Prognostic variables and post-operative recurrences. *Br J Urol* 67:32–36.

Nielson K, Ostri P (1988) Primary tumors of the renal pelvis: Evaluation of clinical and pathological features in a consecutive series of 10 years. *J Urol* 140:19- 21.

Raabe N, Fossa S, Bjerkhagen SB (1992) Carcinoma of the renal pelvis. Experience of 80 cases. *Scand J Urol Nephrol* 26:357–361.

Seaman E, Slawin K, Benson M (1993) Treatment options for upper tract transitional-cell carcinoma. *Urol Clin North Am* 20:349–354.

Cancer of the Urethra

Amin MB, Young RH (1997) Primary carcinomas of the urethra. *Semin Diagn Pathol* 14: 147–160.

Dinney CP, Johnson DE, Swanson DA, Babaian RJ, von Eschenbach AC (1994) Therapy and prognosis for male anterior urethral carcinoma: An update. *Urology* 43:506–514.

Grigsby PW, Corn BW (1992) Localized urethral tumors in women: Indications for conservative versus exenterative therapies. *J Urol* 147:1516–1520.

Linn R, Moskovitz B, Munichor M, Levin DR (1990) Transitional cell carcinoma of the distal female urethra. *Int Urol Nephrol* 22:275–277.

Micaily B, Dzeda MF, Miyamoto CT, Brady LW (1997) Brachytherapy for cancer of the female urethra. *Semin Surg Oncol* 13:208–214.

Ray B, Canto AR, Whitmore WF (1977) Experience with primary carcinoma of the male urethra. *J Urol* 117:591–594.

Sailer SL, Shipley WU, Wang CC (1988) Carcinoma of the female urethra: A review of results with radiation therapy. *J Urol* 140:1–5.

Zeidman EJ, Desmond P, Thompson IM (1992) Surgical treatment of carcinoma of the male urethra. *Urol Clin North Am* 19:359–372.

Cancer of the Testis

Bosl GJ, Motzer RJ (1997) Testicular germ-cell cancer. *N Engl J Med* 337:242–253.

Boyer M, Raghavan D (1992) Toxicity of treatment of germ cell tumors. *Semin Oncol* 19: 128–142.

Cullen M, James N (1996) Adjuvant therapy for stage I testicular cancer. *Cancer Treat Rev* 22:253–264.

Dieckmann KP, Krain J Kuster J et al. (1996) Adjuvant carboplatin treatment for seminoma clinical stage I. *J Cancer Res Clin Oncol* 122:63–66.

Doherty AP, Bower M, Christmas TJ (1997) The role of tumor markers in the diagnosis and treatment of testicular germ cell cancers. *Br J Urol* 79:247–252.

Giwercman A, von der Maase H, Rorth M, Skakkebaek NE (1994) Current concepts of radiation treatment of carcinoma in situ of the testis. *World J Urol* 12:125–130.

Herr HW, Sheinfeld J, Puc HS, Heelan R, Bajorin DF, Mencel P, Bosl GJ, Motzer RJ (1997) Surgery for a post-chemotherapy residual mass in seminoma. *J Urol* 157:860–862.

Horwich A, Dearnaley DP (1992) Treatment of seminoma. *Semin Oncol* 19:171–180.

Jewett MA, Incze P (1996) Retroperitoneal lymphadenectomy: The traditional treatment option. *Semin Urol Oncol* 14:24–29.

International Germ Cell Cancer Collaborative Group (1997) International Germ Cell Consensus Classification: A prognostic factor-based staging system for metastatic germ cell cancers. *J Clin Oncol* 15:594–603.

Mencel PJ, Motzer RJ, Mazumdar M et al. (1994) Advanced seminoma: Treatment results, survival, and prognostic factors in 142 patients. *J Clin Oncol* 12:120–126.

Motzer RJ (1996) Adjuvant chemotherapy for stage II nonseminamatous testicular cancer: What is its role? *Semin Urol Oncol* 14:30–33.

Sturgeon JF, Jewett MA, Alison RE et al. (1992) Surveillance after orchidectomy for patients with clinical stage I nonseminomatous testis tumors. *J Clin Oncol* 10:564–568.

Travis L, Curtis R, Storm H et al. (1997) Risk of second malignant neoplasms among long-term survivors of testicular cancer. *J Natl Cancer Inst* 89:1429–1439.

Warde P, Gospodarowicz MK, Panzarella T et al. (1995) Stage I testicular seminoma: Results of adjuvant irradiation and surveillance. *J Clin Oncol* 13:2255–2262.

Cancer of the Penis

Burgers JK, Badalament RA, Drago JR (1992) Penile cancer. Clinical presentation, diagnosis, and staging. *Urol Clin North Am* 19:247–255.

Delannes MN, Malavaud B, Douchez J, Bonnet J, Daly N (1992) Iridium 192 interstitial therapy for squamous cell carcinoma of the penis. *Int J Radiat Oncol Biol Phys* 21:178.

Gerbaulet A, Lambin P (1992) Radiation therapy of cancer of the penis: Indications, advantages, and pitfalls. *Urol Clin North Am* 19:325–332.

McDougal WS, Kirchner FK Jr, Edwards RH, Killion LT (1988) Treatment of carcinoma of the penis: The case of primary lymphadenectomy. *J Urol* 136:38–41.

Mohs F, Snow SN, Larson PO (1992) Mohs micrographic surgery for penile tumors. *Urol Clin North Am* 19:291–304.

Pizzocaro G, Piva L, Bandieramonte G, Tana S (1997) Up-to-date management of carcinoma of the penis. *Eur Urol* 32:5–15.

Sarin R, Norman AR, Steel GG, Horwich A (1997) Treatment results and prognostic factors in 101 men treated for squamous carcinoma of the penis. *Int J Radiat Oncol Biol Phys* 38:713–722.

Wiener JS, Walther PJ (1995) The association of oncogenic human papillomaviruses with urologic malignancy. The controversies and clinical implications. *Surg Oncol Clin North Am* 4:257–276.

CHAPTER 28

Central Nervous System Tumors

CHARLES J. VECHT

Department of Neurology, Medical Center, The Hague, The Netherlands

Primary brain tumors account for about 2% of cancer death. In children, they are the second most common type of cancer. Brain metastasis develops in more than 20% of all cancer patients. Primary brain tumors are diverse and can be distinguished in about some 20 main types. The spectrum is characterized by a wide variety in phenotype and a diversity of genotypic abnormalities in brain tumors. Hereditary factors may play a role, and about 5% of patients with brain tumors have a family history of cancer. Grossly, nervous system tumors can be divided into tumors of neuroepithelial tissue, of peripheral nerves, of the meninges, and lymphomas, germ cell tumors, tumors of the sellar region, and metastatic tumors (see Table 28.1 for the World Health Organization (WHO) classification of tumors of the nervous system).

EPIDEMIOLOGY

Compared with other types of cancer, brain tumors are relatively rare. In adults, the most frequent type is the non-pilocytic astrocytoma among which glioblastoma multiforme represents about half of all cases. The incidence varies between 2 and 10 per 100,000. Countries with a low incidence include Japan, India, and China and high frequencies occur in Sweden, New Zealand, and Israel. In many countries, an upward trend in frequency of brain tumors seems to be apparent.

Overall, with increasing age, the incidence of cancer goes up. The same trend seems true for brain tumors, showing an incidence in the younger population of 1.7 (<20 years of age) and going up as high as 15–19 between 60–79 years of age. In children, brain tumors constitute the second most frequent type of cancer after leukemia and lymphoma. Also, the type of brain tumors differs from adults. Patients under 20 years of age show a relatively high frequency of medulloblastomas, primitive

UICC Manual of Clinical Oncology, Eighth Edition. Edited by Raphael E. Pollock
ISBN 0-471-22289-5 Copyright © 2004 John Wiley & Sons, Inc.

TABLE 28.1. WHO Classification of Tumors of The Nervous System

Tumors of Neuroepithelal Tissue	*Tumors of Peripheral Nerves*
Astrocytic Tumors	Schwannoma
Diffuse astrocytoma	(Neurilemmoma, Neurinoma)
Anaplastic astrocytoma	Neurofibroma
Glioblastoma multiforme	Perineurioma
Pilocytic astrocytoma	Malignant peripheral nerve sheath tumors
Pleomorphic xantoastrocytoma	(MPNST)
Oligodendroglial tumors	Epitheloid
Oligodendroglioma	*Tumors of the Meninges*
Anaplastic oligodendroglioma	Tumors of meningothelial cells
Mixed gliomas	Meningioma
Oligoastrocytoma	Meningothelial
Anaplastic Oligoastrocytoma	Fibrous
Ependymal tumors	Transitional
Ependymoma	Psammomatous
Anaplastic ependymoma	Angiomatous
Myxopapillary ependymoma	Anaplastic meningioma
Subependymoma	Microcystic
Choroid plexus tumor	Clear cell
Choroid plexus papilloma	Mesenchymal, nonmeningothelial tumors
Choroid plexus carcinoma	Lipomas
Glial tumors of uncertain origin	Malignant chondrosarcoma
Astroblastoma	Rhabdomyosarcoma
Gliomatosis cerebri	Hemangiopericytoma
Chordoid glioma of 3rd ventricle	Primary melanocytic lesions
Neuronal and mixed neuronal-glial tumors	Melanocytoma
Gangliocytoma	Malignant melanoma
Central neurocytoma	Meningeal melanomatosis
Dysembryoblastic neuroepithelial tumor	Tumors of uncertain histogenesis
Neuroblastic tumors	Hemangioblastoma
Olfactory neuroblastoma	*Lymphomas and Hemopoietic Neoplasms*
Neuroblastoma of the adrenal gland	Malignant lymphomas
Pineal parenchymal tumors	Plasmacytoma
Pineocytoma	*Germ Cell Tumors*
Pineoblastoma	Germinoma
Embryonal tumors	Embryonal carcinoma
Medullepithelioma	Yolk sac tumors
Medulloblastoma	Choriocarcinoma
Neuroblastoma	Teratoma
Ependymoblastoma	Mature
Supratentorial primitive neuro-ectodermal	Immature
tumor (PNET)	Mixed germ cell tumor
Neuroblastoma	*Tumors of the Sellar Region*
Atypical teratoid/rhabdoid tumor	Craniopharyngioma
	Granular cell tumor
	Metastatic Tumors

Modified from Kleihues and Cavanee, 2000.

neuroectodermal tumors, pilocytic astrocytomas, and ependymomas. In young males of 20–39 years, brain tumors are the third or fourth most frequent cancer.

RISK FACTORS

Apart from genetic factors, exogenous influences, including carcinogenic factors like ionizing radiation, exposure to toxic agents, or use of specific nutrients, may contribute to the induction of CNS tumors.

Substances containing *N*-nitroso compounds (like some food products, smoke, cosmetics) may lead to increased risks on developing brain tumors (1,2). There is an increased risk of meningiomas occuring after nonserious head injury occurring >20 years previously (3). Despite initial suspicion, wireless communication systems like cell phones do not seem to confer a higher risk of primary brain tumors (4,5).

GENETIC FACTORS

Genetic defects in brain tumors include overexpression of oncogenes or deletion of tumor-suppressor genes. Frequently, loss of heterozygosity in hereditary and nonhereditary tumors results in inactivation of tumor-suppressor genes, which normally counteract the function of (proto-)oncogenes. In gliomas, genetic loss frequently occurs on chromosomes 1p, 9p, 10q, 17p, 19q, and 22q. Besides, overexpression of EGFR, PDGFR, MDM2, p53 mutation, and p16 deletion are associated with malignant transformation of gliomas. Primary malignant gliomas, which typically affect older patients and have a histologic grade of IV (glioblastoma multiforme) at diagnosis, commonly show loss of PTEN, CDKN2A deletions, and amplification of the epidermal growth factor receptor gene (EGFR), which encodes a tyrosine kinase involved in cell replication. Secondary malignant gliomas that evolve from low-grade lesions generally affect young adults, often have alterations in p53, platelet-derived growth factor (PDGF) and p16 (Fig. 28.1) (6,7).

In anaplastic astrocytoma, mutation of PTEN, amplification of EGFR (7–9) and loss of the q arm of chromosome 10 are less common than in glioblastoma multiforme, and mutations of p53 are more common (10). Overexpression of p53 in malignant gliomas during childhood is strongly associated with an adverse outcome, independently of clinical prognostic factors and histologic findings (11). Allelic losses of chromosomes 1p and 19q are the most common abnormalities in oligodendroglial tumors, together with an increased incidence of deletion of the p16 gene located on chromosomes 9p (9). In ependymomas, chromosome arm 22q has been the most frequent described region of genomic loss (8).

SIGNS AND SYMPTOMS

One feature of brain tumors is that neurological symptoms develop gradually over time in contrast to vascular (ischemic or hemorrhagic) lesions of the brain that arise

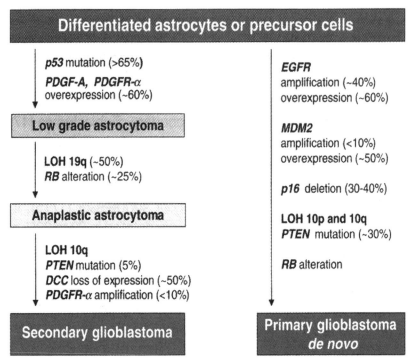

Figure 28.1   Genetic pathways in primary and secondary glioblastomas. (From Kleihues and Cavanee, 2000.)

acutely. Nevertheless, more than 25% of patients with brain tumors present instantaneously, often by seizures. In low-grade glioma, about two-thirds of patients present with epilepsy, often relatively refractory to antiepileptic agents. In high-grade glioma, the incidence of seizures is about 40%, and higher in anaplastic astrocytoma than in glioblastoma multiforme. Brain metastasis occurs about five times more frequent than gliomas, and seizures are the presenting symptom in about 20% of cases.

For that reason, the appearance of one or more seizures in an adult patient requires computed tomography (CT) or preferably magnetic resonance (MR) scan. Acute presentation may also possible be due to a bleeding in the tumor. Signs and symptoms of brain tumors can usually be explained by either the localization of the tumor within the brain, by the presence of increased intracranial pressure, or both. The actual location of a brain tumor defines the focal neurological signs caused by the tumor. A good working knowledge of neuroanatomy enables one to better understand and localize the appearance of neurological signs and symptoms within the CNS. Frontal tumors can lead to changes in personality, for example, loss of drive, poor social adaptation, indifference or loss of self-criticism, apathy, and occasionally by outbursts of aggression. Temporal tumors may lead to hemianopia and to aphasia if the left hemisphere is dominant. Parietal tumors lead to contralateral motor and sensory abnormalities and to apraxia. Occipital tumors lead to hemianopias and, if the tumor extends into the splenium to visual agnosia. In general, right-sided tumors (i.e., in the nondominant hemisphere), take more time to become symptomatic and may present with apraxia or visuoconstructive agnosias.

Cerebellar tumors (may give rise to ataxia, dysarthria), and early signs of increased intracranial pressure by obstructive hydrocephalus and direct compression of the brainstem. Focal brainstem signs may consist of cranial nerve signs including oculomotor signs, Bell's palsy (peripheral seventh nerve dysfunction), bilateral pyramidal weakness of the extremities, and sensory abnormalities.

Increased intracranial pressure is caused by a space-occupying lesion within the rigid boundaries of the skull. The presence of a tumor in one cerebral hemisphere can lead to a horizontal shift of midline structures, which can easily be seen on CT or MR (Fig. 28.2). Also, in particular with intraventricular or tumors in the brainstem or cerebellum, hydrocephalus by obstruction of cerebrospinal fluid (CSF) flow with signs of increased intracranial pressure may develop. Increased intracranial pressure with or without disturbance of CSF flow or direct compression of the brainstem may lead to herniation of the brainstem. This is indicated by disappearance of the mesencephalic and pontine cisterns around the brainstem. With gradual increasing volume of the tumor, an exponential or disproportional increase in intracranial pressure ensues. In physical terms, this phenomenon can be characterized by a shift to the right of the pressure-volume curve.

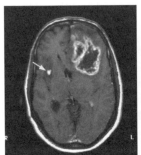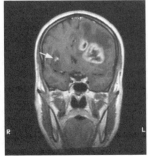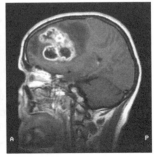

Figure 28.2   A 61-year-old man with a glioblastoma multiforme in the left frontal lobe. The MR (T1-weighted after administration of gadolineum) shows a large tumor of 6 cm diameter with cystic areas (black), representing necrosis, surrounded by thick and irregular gadolineum-enhancing zone and margins (white), indicating the presence of viable tumor with disturbed blood-brain barrier. Note the space-occupying behavior of the mass, with dark areas of edema around the gadolineum-enhancing mass with compression of the left ventricle and horizontal displacement of the falx cerebri to the right. Note also a second small gadolineum-enhancing lesion (*arrow*) surrounded by edema in the right temporal lobe (the area of the insula) also representing tumor, indicating the presence of a multifocal glioblastoma multiforme, which occurs in <10% of malignant gliomas.

The clinical signs of increased intracranial pressure are headache, nausea, and vomiting. Untreated, impaired consciousness begins as drowsiness and is followed by stupor and coma. Herniation of the brainstem is evidenced by ptosis and homolateral enlarged pupil (third nerve palsy) and flexor spasms of the arms with extension spasms of the legs and Cheyne-Stokes respiration (upper brainstem or diencephalic signs). This may evolve to fixed pupils, extension spasms of arms and legs, and hyperventilation (mid-brainstem or mesencefalic signs), followed by absent corneal and pupillary reflexes, pinpoint pupils, flaccid tetraparesis, hypoventilation (lower brainstem or pontine signs), and death.

IMAGING

Imaging of the brain has made great progress over the last 25 years. CT scanning of the brain can reliably delineate the contours of brain tumors located in the cerebral hemispheres. Use of iodinated contrast agents indicates the presence of blood-brain-barrier disturbances. MR scanning is more sensitive than CT, particularly following contrast administration, and is required for accurate delineation of lesions of the posterior fossa, the leptomeninges, and the spinal cord. In fact, the use of CT and MR has become indispensable for diagnosis and reliable follow-up of brain tumors. Probably, MR will completely replace CT for proper imaging of brain tumors.

Also, the response of brain tumors to therapy (complete or partial response, stabilization or progression) is mainly defined by radiological changes. Single photon emission computed tomography (SPECT) and positron emission tomography (PET) scanning can provide information about the grade of malignancy and may help in differentiating benign from malignant lesions, and recurrent tumors from radionecrosis.

GLIOMAS

The gliomas constitute of astrocytomas, oligodendrogliomas, and ependymomas and together they represent about 60% of all primary brain tumors with an incidence of ∼5 per 100,000. The astrocytomas can be graded as to their degree of malignancy. The most commonly used grading systems are those of the WHO and of the St. Anne/Mayo. Both systems use the presence of histological criteria like cell atypia, mitosis, endothelial cell proliferation, and necrosis as markers of malignancy. The WHO uses a three-tiered system dividing the astrocytomas in grade 2 (astrocytoma), grade 3 (anaplastic astrocytoma), and grade 4 (glioblastoma multiforme). The Daumas-Duport classification uses a four-tiered grading system: with one histological criterium an astrocytoma grade 2 is diagnosed, with two criteria grade 3, and with three or four criteria a grade 4 astrocytoma. Overall, in both systems the prognosis for grade 2, 3, and 4 astrocytomas corresponds well with each other (12,13). Of these, grade 4 tumor or glioblastomas are the most frequent type of primary brain tumors, constituting more than half of all gliomas.

Low-Grade Gliomas

The astrocytomas or low-grade gliomas can be divided in pilocytic and nonpilocytic astrocytomas. The pilocytic or juvenile astrocytoma is a benign tumor and represents more than half of all low-grade gliomas in childhood. Histologically, pilocytic astrocytomas are characterized by Rosenthal fibers and thin elongated astrocytes (pilocytes). Diagnosis is based on CT or MR showing an intensely enhancing mass with or without cyst formation or space occupying features. They are often located in the infratentorial compartment, usually the cerebellum. Presenting signs and symptoms are those of increased intracranial pressure (headache, nausea and vomiting, impaired consciousness with or without third or sixth nerve palsy as false localizing sign), secondary to obstructive hydrocephalus caused by compression of the sylvian duct. A unilateral cerebellar syndrome may be concomitantly present indicating the localization of the tumor. Supratentorially located pilocytic astrocytomas present themselves in the majority by epileptic seizures and in the remainder by neurogical signs depending on the localization of the tumor. The preferred treatment is surgery alone and when a gross tumor resection can be achieved 10-year survival is 80% or more.

Nonpilocytic low-grade gliomas are composed of diffuse, protoplasmatic, or fibrillary astrocytomas. They may occur anywhere in the brain, but characteristic localizations are the supratentorial compartment including optic pathways and the cerebellum and brainstem. About 60% of supratentorial tumors become manifest by epileptic seizures. The characteristic pattern on CT or MR is a nonenhancing lesion that can be space-occupying and often shows an infiltrating and irregular pattern in the white matter.

If the neuropathologist confirms a nonpilocytic low-grade glioma, the next question is whether these patients should have radiotherapy or not. One trial did not show a superior effect of 59 Gy radiation therapy over 45 Gy (14). Another trial has shown a longer progresion-free period following surgery and radiotherapy in a dose of 54 Gy but the overall survival was similar as patients treated by surgery alone were given radiotherapy at the time of recurrence (15). The outcome of these trials still complicates the question how individual patients with low-grade glioma should actually be treated. For a proper answer to this question, the influence of independent prognostic factors is important (16). Retrospective studies indicate that radiotherapy seems only effective in patients of 40 years and older. Thus, in patients with epilepsy only, <40 years of age and otherwise neurologically intact, a wait-and-see policy can be advocated. This would also pertain to the question of surgery or not. These patients may be followed by CT or MR as long as they have no symptoms or imminent signs.

However, if the tumor can be safely resected, this would in general be the preferred therapy, though subsequent radiotherapy can be withheld. In patients over 40 years of age, regardless of symptomatology, the combination of surgery and radiotherapy is advised. For symptoms other than epilepsy, irrespective of age, withholding treatment is in general not being advocated, and surgery followed by radiation therapy would be advocated. It is of note that nonenhancing lesions in patients over 40 years of age harbor high-grade gliomas in ~50% of patients.

High-Grade Gliomas

Anaplastic astrocytoma and glioblastoma multiforme (GBM) constitute together the high-grade or malignant gliomas of which the latter represent 80%. Following standard treatment, the median survival of anaplastic astrocytoma is 18 months and of GBM 9–11 months.

Prognostic Factors

The presence of favorable or unfavorable prognostic factors would determine the outcome of patients with malignant gliomas to a large extent. Prognosis depends on the presence of a number of independent prognostic factors (histology, age, performance status, mental status) and combination of these factors leads to six categories (recursive partitioning analysis) divided by age (younger or older than 50 years of age), histology (anaplastic astrocytom or glioblastoma multiforme), and mental status (normal or abnormal) for patients with anaplastic astrocytoma, and performance status for patients with glioblastoma multiforme. For patients aged 50 years or older, performance status is the most important variable, with normal or abnormal mental status creating the only significant split in the poorer performance status group. Median survival times vary from 5 to 60 months depending on the presence of independent prognostic factors (17). The standard therapy for malignant gliomas is surgery followed by radiation therapy. Extensive resection of the tumor, if possible and depending on the neuroanatomical localization of the tumor, leads to a longer survival and to a better postoperative condition than limited surgery or biopsy.

Postoperative conventional radiation therapy in a cumulative dose of 60 Gy leads to a median survival of malignant gliomas of about 9 months. With doses over 60 Gy, no addition in survival has been observed. Modifications in radiation therapy, including concomitant boost, hyperfractionation, accelerated hyperfractionation, or use of radiation sensitizers, have all been extensively tested in randomized trials and have not resulted in better outcome (18,19). Presently, whether application of stereotactic or conformal radiation therapy for malignant tumors of small volume would give better results is uncertain.

Chemotherapy

A number of randomized trials have been carried out on the efficacy of adjuvant chemotherapy in malignant gliomas. Most trials have concentrated on lipophilic agents that easily pass the blood-brain barrier. The alkylating agents lomustine (CCNU) and carmustine (BCNU) have shown a significant though very modest improvement in median survival of 9 months following surgery and radiation therapy up to 11 months following addition of BCNU or procarbazine. Meta-analysis of randomized trials on high-grade gliomas has revealed an absolute increase in 1-year survival of 6% (95% confidence intervals 3–9) from 40% to 46% with a 2-month increase in median survival time, and no evidence of effect depending on independent prognostic factor (20). There are some indications that adjuvant chemotherapy with temozolomide may give better results, and phase III trials with this agent are underway (21).

In contrast to anaplastic astrocytoma and GBM, the anaplastic oligodendrogliomas (AO) seem to be substantially more chemosensitive. A number of phase II trials in recurrent AO have shown response rates of 60–70 % with in the majority a response duration of 1 year or more (22,23). These results have been established by a combination of procarbazine, vincristine, and CCNU. Both in the United States and in Europe, two independent phase III trials are now carried out on the efficacy of adjuvant chemotherapy with this combination in AO following surgery and radiotherapy.

In recurrent tumors, following surgery and radiation therapy, useful reoperation of gliomas can be considered after a remission-free period of 6 months or more. Subsequently, systemic chemotherapy may be offered, preferably as part of phase II trials.

Meningiomas

These tumors arise from arachnoidal cells of the meninges and can be distinguished in diverse types including syncytial, transitional, and psammomatous meningiomas. They can be graded in four classes, but more than 80% are benign (grade 1). If feasible, the treatment exists of a surgical resection including the surrounding dura. For malignant, recurrent, or incompletely resected meningiomas, radiation therapy can be applied. Following surgical excision, the 20-year survival is ~80%. After partial resection, radiation therapy improves 10-year survival from ~50% to 80%.

Primary Brain Lymphomas

These tumors seem to appear with increasing frequency, either with or without the association with immunosuppression or HIV. Histologically, these are usually B-cell lymphomas and are purely restricted to the CNS, although they may occur simultaneously in the vitreous part of the eye (uveitis). Although the precise frequency is unknown, worldwide the incidence is rising. Apart from a diagnostic biopsy, preferably without preceding use of glucocorticoids, the treatment of choice is radiotherapy (45–50 Gy). In recent years, phase II studies have shown that intensive chemotherapy including high-dose systemic methotrexate followed by radiation therapy may prolong the median survival from about 12 months to 24–36 months. In patients over 60 years of age, this chemotherapeutic regimen may be given as the sole treatement followed by radiation on progression.

Germ Cell Tumors

These tumors can be distinguished in germinatous (germinomas) and nongermina-tous germ cell tumors (NGGCT). The NGGCT exist of teratomas, endodermal sinus tumors, embryonal, carcinomas, and choriocarcinomas. The presence of alfa-fetoprotein and beta-HCG in serum may help in the diagnosis of NGGCT. The majority of patients is between 10 and 21 years of age, and occurs mainly as midline tumor in the pineal or suprasellar area. As a rule, histological diagnosis is required for diagnosis, but may be difficult to obtain. As these tumors may spread through the leptomeninges, gadolineum-enhanced MR and CSF cytology should be included in the work-up.

For germinomas, radiation therapy is the standard treatment in a dose of ~50 Gy. For NGGCT, craniospinal axis radiation is usually advised, followed in some centers by systemic chemotherapy. Alternatively, systemic chemotherapy may also be given in a neoadjuvant setting, that is before the start of radiation therapy. The 5-year survival for germinomas is ~60% and for NGGCT less than 1 year.

Pituitary Adenomas

Pituitary adenomas arise from the anterior or posterior pituitary gland and can be divided into prolactin, growth hormone, or adrenocorticotropic producing tumors. Two-thirds of pituitary tumors are nonsecreting and the remainder produce pro-lactin (prolactinomas) or growth hormone causing acromegaly. The incidence is about 2 per 100,000. Treatment consists mainly of administration of dopamine agonists, which impair prolactin secretion, or drugs that inhibit either GH- or ACTH-secretion. If ineffective, surgery and radiation therapy can be employed.

Acoustic Schwannomas

These tumors are benign Schwannomas, which preferentially arise from the acoustic nerve and are located in the meatus acusticus internus or externus in the cerebello-pontine angle. Presenting signs are unilateral hearing loss with or without signs of vestibular dysfunction. The treatment of choice is surgical excision, although radiosurgical treatment with focused high-dose radiation in a single fraction can be used as well.

Spinal Cord Tumors

Tumors of the spinal cord are rare and mainly consist of astrocytomas and ependymomas. Patients present with signs of a myelopathy and initial diagnosis depends on MR. Often, these tumors cannot be surgically removed and final diagnosis is achieved by biopsy.

Astrocytomas of the spinal cord may be differentiated as low grade, anaplastic, or GBM. Radiotherapy is usually an indispensable part of the therapy. Ependymo-mas are usually low-grade tumors and are mostly confined to the lower part of the spine. Tumors located in the cauda equina can often be completely removed and, if so, do not require postoperative radiotherapy. Otherwise, following incomplete resection, radiotherapy is indicated. Extramedullary, intradural tumors of the spine are mainly meningiomas and neurinomas. Both may present with signs of radiculopathy, and diagnosis depends on MR. Complete resection, if possible, is the treatment of choice. Following incomplete resection or recurrence, radiation therapy may be indicated for meningiomas.

PEDIATRIC NEURO-ONCOLOGY

Ependymomas

Ependymomas are relatively frequent in children under 3 year of age and often arise in the posterior fossa around the fourth ventricle, although they may occur at any age and at any site in the CNS. The primary mode of therapy is surgery. Limited-field radiation is usually applied for well-differentiated ependymomas. For anaplastic tumors, particularly posterior fossa ependymomas, whole neuraxis radiation is often advised. The 5- and 10-year progression-free survival rate of ependymomas is 60% and 40%. Prognosis mainly is based on the extent of resection made at surgery and the amount of residual tumor on postoperative imaging as verified by centralized radiological review (24). Recurrence following surgery may necessitate reoperation, particularly when neurological signs become imminent. Occasionally, a positive response following chemotherapy has been reported.

Brainstem Tumors

These account for 10–20% of CNS tumors in childhood. Brainstem gliomas can be distinguished in focal brainstem tumors, which are often amenable to resection versus diffuse and large irresectable pontine gliomas. The latter have a median survival of less than 1 year, with 2-year survival of 10–20% following radiation therapy, and constitute the majority of brainstem tumors.

Primitive Neuroectodermal Tumors (PNET)

Medulloblastoma and other PNET are small-cell, highly cellular tumors that stain positively with S-100. If present in the posterior fossa, these tumors are designated as medulloblastomas. In the supratentorial compartment, they are in general labelled as PNET. Ependymoblastomas and pineoblastomas are other subtypes of the PNET. Medulloblastoma originate in the cerebellum or brainstem. This tumor mainly occurs in children under 15 years of age. Treatment consists of surgery followed by craniospinal axis radiation with a cumulative dose of 54 Gy to the posterior fossa and 36 Gy in 20 fractions to the remaining part of the CNS, resulting in a 5-year survival of 50–60%. Use of adjuvant chemotherapy (e.g., regimens employing CCNU, cisplatin, and vincristine) gives better results in high-risk patients—following an incomplete resection or in children younger than 3 years of age. In the latter group, radiation therapy is usually delayed until the age of 36 months to spare cognitive development and to prevent growth retardation. Treatment consists of extensive resection, if possible, followed by neuraxis radiation with a boost to the tumor bed. In children younger than 3 years of age, radiation thearapy is harmful to the developing CNS and, therefore surgery, plus adjuvant chemotherapy is favored in this age group.

Pediatric Malignant Gliomas

The 5-year median survival of childhood malignant gliomas is about 30–35%. A first randomized trial investigating CCNU, vincristine, and prednisone showed a benefit for progression-free survival and overall survival. A second trial comparing this regimen with the "8-in-1 drugs in 1 day" schedule did not show a difference in survival.

USE OF SURGERY AND RADIATION THERAPY IN NEURO-ONCOLOGY

In general, brain tumors often lead to changes in personality, cognitive abnormalities, severe handicap interfering with activities of daily life. In the early stages, prompt diagnosis and therapy are often necessary to prevent irreversible damage to the brain. The main options for therapy are surgery and radiotherapy, and for some tumors systemic chemotherapy can be applied.

Although radical surgery is often impossible with malignant brain tumors, as a rule, extensive resection of the tumor may have important benefits. It is virtually impossible to acquire prospective data on the influence of the extent of surgery in a randomized fashion, but most studies indicate that larger resections lead to longer periods of progression-free survival. The most reliable data show that the postoperative volume of the tumor strongly correlates with survival.

Although contrary to intuition, extensive surgery on patients with brain tumors and neurological deficit rather leads to improvement than to deterioration of postoperative neurological function. In general, lesions that are either deep-seated, or are located in eloquent areas, the motorstrip, or the brainstem are often difficult or impossible to excise and, under these circumstances, stereotactic or open biopsy can be the best approach.

Radiotherapy is of crucial importance for the control of brain tunors. The last decade has seen big advances in technique which enable more accurate radiation of the tumor with sparing of surrounding normal brain tissue. By the same reason, this has made it possible to deliver higher doses of radiation limited to the tumor with better chances on cure or longstanding progression-free survival.

One of these developments is application of brachytherapy. By this technique, one implants stereotactically placed radioactive iodine-125 or iridium-192 seeds in the tumor tissue. With computer software, one can calculate the number and precise locations of the radioactive seeds in order to deliver exactly the desired radiation dose. Another devopment is the application of radiosurgery or conformal radiation therapy. One is the gamma-unit or Leksell frame, which consists of multiple cobalt sources and a collimator that concentrates the gamma beams in a sphere. With this technique, tumor volumes of less than 30 mm diameter can be radiated with sparing of healthy surrounding brain tissue. Similar dose distributions can be achieved with a linear accelerator using a multiple beam technique by use of rotating arcs. This technique is also known as stereotactic or conformal radiation and it enables precise radiation of various tumor shapes and volumes.

BRAIN METASTASIS

A brain metastasis is the most frequent brain tumor and develops in about 20% of all cancer patients. The majority, over 80%, originate from lung and breast cancer. About one-third are single and two-thirds are multiple brain metastases. In patients with unknown cancer, surgery is required to obtain a tissue diagnosis. Occassionally, a diagnostic work-up may be indicated to see whether a space-occupying lesion in the brain rather represents a metastasis than a primary brain tumor. However, this may take too much time and, in the mean time, the patient may deteriotate neurologically. It has been shown that, in cancer patients, there is a $\sim$10% chance that the single enhancing lesion would not represent a metastasis, further substantiating the need for tissue diagnosis. As a rule, patients with brain metastasis cannot be cured, and the aim of treatment is preservation of a good quality of life for the remainder of a limited lifetime.

The prognosis of patients with brain metastasis is mainly determined by a number of independent prognostic factors. These are age (younger or older than 60 yrs), performance status (Karnofsky performance status over or under 70), and extent of systemic cancer (absent or controlled versus active extracranial cancer).

For a single brain metastasis, it has been shown that combined therapy of surgery and radiotherapy is useful in patients with no progression of systemic disease over the last 3 months. Otherwise, as in multiple brain metastasis, whole-brain radiation therapy is the treatment of choice. Instead of surgery, radiosurgery can be applied as well, producing similar results. For single brain metastasis with good prognostic factors, the 1-year survival is 40% and the 2-year survival 20%. For multiple brain metastasis and favorable prognostic factors, 1-year survival is 20% and 2-year survival 10%. In general, appearance of brain metastasis is a sign of progression of the tumor and, for that reason, the median survival of patients with multiple brain metastasis is overall about 3 months. Chemotherapy may be considered in patients with chemosensitive tumors (breast cancer, germ cell tumors).

LEPTOMENINGEAL METASTASIS

Leptomeningeal metastasis occurs as the consequence of spread of tumor cells to the leptomeninges surrounding the brain and spinal cord. For that reason, patients may show signs of increased intracranial pressure and multiple cranial nerve or nerve root dysfunction. For diagnosis, CSF cytology and gadolineum-enhanced MR is required. For chemoinsensitive tumors, radiotherapy only to the symptomatic part of the CNS is indicated. For leptomeningeal leukemias and lymfomas, intrathecal or intraventricular methotrexate and/or cytosine-arabinoside can be administered. Usually, after clearing the CSF from tumor cells, consolidation radiotherapy is applied.

In breast cancer with leptomeningeal spread, probably a regimen of systemic chemotherapy with involved radiation therapy (to symptomatic parts of the nervous system) would be as efficacious as addition of intrathecal or intraventricular methotrexate to this regimen.

METASTATIC SPINAL CORD COMPRESSION

Vertebral metastasis is the most common form of osseous metastasis. Symptoms consist of local pain and radiculopathy, and, when left untreated, may lead to epidural compression of the spinal cord. A complete transverse lesion of the spinal cord may develop rapidly and essentially manifests as painless weakness of both legs. This is a dreaded complication of cancer and impending spinal cord compression is an emergency. Diagnosis is made with MR. Therapy is initiated with high-dose dexamethasone, 10 mg intravenous bolus, followed by 16 mg/d. The standard therapy is radiotherapy to the involved part of the spine. Occasionally, when there is one metastatic vertebra and no systemic cancer elsewhere in the body, surgical resection of the tumor with implantation of artificial material and stabilization of the spine may be considered. Presently, a laminectomy for metastatic spinal cord compression is considered obsolete, although it may be applied for tissue diagnosis or occasionally for removal of a metastatic posterior arch of the spine.

SYMPTOMATIC CONTROL OF BRAIN EDEMA AND INCREASED INTRACRANIAL PRESSURE

Use of Glucocorticoids

Brain edema usually accompanies brain tumors because of damage to the blood-brain barrier and it is to a large extent responsible for the appearance of neurological symptoms. Glucocorticoids effectively counteract vasogenic brain edema and diminish the rate of transcapillary water and albumin flow into the peritumoral tissue. This is caused by a stabilizing effect on the endothelial cell membrane with an ensuing decrease in the permeability of the blood-brain barrier. The therapeutic effects become apparent within 24–48 hours and neurological symptoms generally resolve to a great extent.

Dexamethasone is often chosen because of lower mineralocorticoid activity and of lesser binding to albumin than prednisone. The generally prescribed dose is 16 mg/day, but if there is no increased intracranial pressure, doses of 4 mg/day are equally effective. In patients with impaired consciousness or impending herniation including posterior fossa tumors, a dose of 16 mg/d is usually recommended. Because radiation of the brain causes brain edema, one usually continues the use of dexamethasone until the end of the radiation in a dose of 4 mg/d.

Side-effects of glucocorticoids are dose and time dependent and, for that reason, one aims to prescribe the smallest effective dose. Apart from direct side effects, including Cushing face, steroid myopathy, or ankle edema, one should be well aware of adrenocortical insufficiency and of steroid withdrawal following disconti-nuation or tapering off glucocorticoids, particularly after long-term therapy in high dosage.

Mannitol can be given to counteract acutely raised intracranial pressure, before any other therapy, particularly surgery and glucocorticoids, can be instituted or becomes effective. The dose of mannitol is 1–1.5 g/kg intravenous bolus, followed by 0.5 g/kg every 4–6 h.

Glycerol can be given orally to control increased intracranial pressure when steroids are not tolerated or become insufficient. Glycerol is diluted with water or juice at a 50:50 ratio and administered at a dose of 0.25 g/kg every 6–8 h. Unpleasant side effects of glycerol are its taste and the marked diuresis.

Anticonvulsants

Seizures of partial-type epilepsy are frequent in patients with benign and malig-nant brain tumors. For that reason, in patients with one or more seizures due to brain tumors, one one often as anticonvulsant phenytoin, carbamazepine, or natriumvalproate. Phenytoin and carbamazepine lead to enzyme induction of the hepatic cytochrome P-450 system and may thus induce lower levels of con-comitantly administered chemotherapeutic agents, leading to potential ineffec-tive control of the underlying tumor. For these reasons, valproic acid, which shows no enzyme induction, and levetiracetam, which is a newer antiepileptic agent without interaction with the hepatic system, are to be the preferred anti-convulsants in patients with brain tumors. Prophylatic use of antiepileptics is not a common practice. Often, particularly with low-grade tumors located in the gray matter, surgical resection of the tumor results in disappearance of seizure activity. Another disadvantage of phenytoin is its small therapeutic window of efficacy.

Glucocorticoids also produce enzyme induction and may thus lead to ineffective serum levels of other enzyme-inducing anticonvulsants. A severe and not-infrequent side-effect is the Stevens-Johnson or erythema multiforme syndome. Occasionally, this may appear during or after the combined therapy of radiation, glucocorticoid, and fenytoin or carbamazepine. This dramatic drug toxicity results in severe swelling of the mucosa, with or without bullae, redness, and epidermolysis of the skin.

NEUROTOXICITY

Following radiation therapy and chemotherapy of brain tumors, toxicity of the nervous system may develop. Cerebral atrophy is commonly observed on neuroimaging following radiotherapy and chemotherapy, although this not necessarily implies neurological dysfunction. Brain necrosis in adults is rarely noted below 60 Gy in conventional radiation. However, neurocognitive effects can be observed at lower doses, especially in children. A more pronounced volume effect is believed to exist in the brain than in the spinal cord.

FURTHER READING

Berger MS, Wilson CB (eds) (1999) *The Gliomas*. WB Saunders, Philadelphia.

Kaye AH, Laws ER (eds) (2001) *Brain Tumors. An Encyclopedic Approach*, 2nd edition. Churchill Livingstone, Edinburgh.

Kleihues P, Cavenee WK (eds) (2000) *Tumors of the Nervous System: Pathology and Genetics*, 2nd edition. IARC Press, Lyon.

Levin VA (ed) (1996) *Cancer in the Nervous System*. Churchill Livingstone, Edinburgh.

Posner JB (1995) *Neurologic Complications of Cancer*. Davis Co, Philadelphia.

Vecht CJ (ed) (1997) Neuro-Oncology Parts 1 and 2: Primary tumors of brain and spinal cord. Part 3: Systemic cancer. In *Handbook of Clinical Neurology*, PJ Vinken and GW Bruyn. Volumes 67–69 (Rev. Series 23-25) Elsevier, Amsterdam.

REFERENCES

1. Lee M, Wrensch M, Miike R (1997) Dietary and tobacco risk factors for adult onset glioma in the San Francisco Bay Area (California, USA). *Cancer Causes Control* 8:13–24.

2. Giles GG, McNeil JJ, Donnan G et al. (1994) Dietary factors and the risk of glioma in adults: results of a case-control study in Melbourne, Australia. *Int J Cancer* 59:357–362.

3. Preston-Martin S, Pogoda JM, Schlehofer B et al. (1998) An international case-control study of adult glioma and meningioma: the role of head trauma. *Int J Epidemiol* 27:579–586.

4. Rodvall Y, Ahlbom A, Stenlund C, Preston-Martin S, Lindh T, Spannare B (1998) Occupational exposure to magnetic fields and brain tumors in central Sweden. *Eur J Epidemiol* 14:563–569.

5. Inskip PD, Tarone RE, Hatch EE et al. (2001) Cellular-telephone use and brain tumors. *N Engl J Med* 344:79–86.

6. Tortosa A, Ino Y, Odell N et al. (2000) Molecular genetics of radiographically defined de novo glioblastoma multiforme. *Neuropathol Appl Neurobiol* 26:544–552.

7. Louis DN (1997) A molecular genetic model of astrocytoma histopathology. *Brain Pathol* 7:755–764.

8. Ebert C, von Haken M, Meyer-Puttlitz B et al. (1999) Molecular genetic analysis of ependymal tumors. NF2 mutations and chromosome 22q loss occur preferentially in intramedullary spinal ependymomas. *Am J Pathol* 155:627–632.

9. Reifenberger J, Reifenberger G, Liu L, James CD, Wechsler W, Collins VP (1994) Molecular genetic analysis of oligodendroglial tumors shows preferential allelic deletions on 19q and 1p. *Am J Pathol* 145:1175–1190.

10. Smith JS, Tachibana I, Passe SM et al. (2001) PTEN mutation, EGFR amplification, and outcome in patients with anaplastic astrocytoma and glioblastoma multiforme. *J Natl Cancer Inst* 93:1246–1256.

11. Pollack IF, Finkelstein SD, Woods J et al. (2002) Expression of p53 and prognosis in children with malignant gliomas. *N Engl J Med* 346:420–427.

12. Daumas-Duport C, Beuvon F, Varlet P, Fallet-Bianco C (2000) [Gliomas: WHO and Sainte-Anne Hospital classifications]. *Ann Pathol* 20:413–428.

13. Kleihues P, Louis DN, Scheithauer BW et al. (2002) The WHO classification of tumors of the nervous system. *J Neuropathol Exp Neurol* 61:215–229.

14. Karim AB, Maat B, Hatlevoll R et al. (1996) A randomized trial on dose-response in radiation therapy of low-grade cerebral glioma: European Organization for Research and Treatment of Cancer (EORTC) Study 22844. *Int J Radiat Oncol Biol Phys* 36:549–556.

15. Karim AB, Afra D, Cornu P et al. (2002) Randomized trial on the efficacy of radiotherapy for cerebral low-grade glioma in the adult: European Organization for Research and Treatment of Cancer Study 22845 with the Medical Research Council study BRO4: an interim analysis. *Int J Radiat Oncol Biol Physiol* 52:316–324.

16. Pignatti F, van den Bent M, Curran D et al. (2002) Prognostic factors for survival in adult patients with cerebral low-grade glioma. *J Clin Oncol* 20:2076–2084.

17. Curran WJ Jr, Scott CB, Horton J et al. (1993) Recursive partitioning analysis of prognostic factors in three Radiation Therapy Oncology Group malignant glioma trials. *J Natl Cancer Inst* 85:704–710.

18. Walker MD, Alexander E Jr, Hunt WE et al. (1978) Evaluation of BCNU and/or radiotherapy in the treatment of anaplastic gliomas. A cooperative clinical trial. *J Neurosurg* 49:333–343.

19. Green SB, Byar DP, Walker MD et al. (1983) Comparisons of carmustine, procarbazine, and high-dose methylprednisolone as additions to surgery and radiotherapy for the treatment of malignant glioma. *Cancer Treat Rep* 67:121–132.

20. Stewart LA (2002) Chemotherapy in adult high-grade glioma: a systematic review and meta-analysis of individual patient data from 12 randomised trials. *Lancet* 359:1011–1018.

21. Stupp R, Dietrich PY, Ostermann Kraljevic S et al. (2002) Promising survival for patients with newly diagnosed glioblastoma multiforme treated with concomitant radiation plus temozolomide followed by adjuvant temozolomide. *J Clin Oncol* 20:1375–1382.

22. Cairncross JG, Macdonald DR (1988) Successful chemotherapy for recurrent malignant oligodendroglioma. *Ann Neurol* 23:360–364.

23. van den Bent MJ, Kros JM, Heimans JJ et al. (1998) Response rate and prognostic factors of recurrent oligodendroglioma treated with procarbazine, CCNU, and vincristine chemotherapy. Dutch Neuro-oncology Group. *Neurology* 51:1140–1145.

24. Robertson PL, Zeltzer PM, Boyett JM et al. (1998) Survival and prognostic factors following radiation therapy and chemotherapy for ependymomas in children: a report of the Children's Cancer Group. *J Neurosurg* 88:695–703.

CHAPTER 29

Soft Tissue Sarcomas

PETER W. T. PISTERS

University of Texas, M. D. Anderson Cancer Center, Department of Surgical Oncology, Houston, Texas

BRIAN O'SULLIVAN

University of Toronto, Princess Margaret Hospital, Department of Radiation Oncology, Toronto, Ontario, Canada

Soft tissue sarcomas are a group of rare, anatomically and histologically diverse malignant neoplasms. These tumors account for 1% of adult malignancies and 15% of pediatric malignancies. Although the overall mortality rate approaches 50%, a substantial proportion of patients can be cured with careful selection of single- or combined-modality treatment strategies.

ETIOLOGY

No specific etiologic agent is identified in the majority of patients with soft tissue sarcoma. There are, nevertheless, a number of recognized associations between environmental factors and the development of sarcoma. These factors include therapy with ionizing radiation; exposure to alkylating chemotherapeutic agents; occupational exposure to phenoxyacetic acids, chlorophenols, vinyl chloride, or arsenic; or exposure to the previously employed intravenous contrast agent Thorotrast. In addition, chronic lymphedema of congenital, infectious (filariasis), postsurgical, or postirradiation etiology has been implicated in the development of lymphangiosarcoma.

In clinical practice, the most commonly observed nongenetic predisposing factors are previous irradiation and chronic lymphedema. By definition, radiation-induced sarcomas arise no sooner than 3 years after completion of therapeutic radiation and often decades later. The vast majority of these sarcomas are of high grade, and the most common histology of radiation-induced sarcomas is

UICC Manual of Clinical Oncology, Eighth Edition. Edited by Raphael E. Pollock
ISBN 0-471-22289-5 Copyright © 2004 John Wiley & Sons, Inc.

osteosarcoma, possibly owing to the greater absorption of orthovoltage radiation by bone than by soft tissue prior to the era of megavoltage radiation. In women treated for breast cancer with radical mastectomy, chronic lymphedema of the arm may contribute to the development of lymphangiosarcoma.

A number of genetic conditions are also associated with an increased risk for development of soft tissue sarcoma. These conditions include neurofibromatosis, Li-Fraumeni syndrome, familial retinoblastoma, and Gardner's syndrome. Genetically associated soft tissue sarcomas occur most commonly in patients with neuro-fibromatosis or Gardner's syndrome. Patients with neurofibromatosis have a 7–10% lifetime risk of developing a malignant neurofibrosarcoma. Desmoid tumors occur in 8–12% of patients with Gardner's syndrome.

Apart from the diagnostic dilemma in distinguishing additional neurofibromas from primary or metastatic soft tissue sarcoma in patients with neurofibromatosis, the precise etiology of an individual sarcoma is of little clinical significance because it does not affect therapeutic decision-making beyond the obvious fact that patients who have sarcomas arising in a previously irradiated field usually cannot receive further external-beam radiotherapy.

PATHOLOGY

Anatomic Distribution

Soft tissue sarcomas have been found in virtually all anatomic sites. Approximately half of all soft tissue sarcomas occur in the extremities (lower, 38%; upper, 15%), where the most common histopathologies are liposarcoma (30%) and malignant fibrous histiocytoma (MFH) (22%). Retroperitoneal and intra-abdominal sarcomas constitute 15% of all soft tissue sarcomas, with liposarcoma being the predominant histologic subtype (41%). Visceral sarcomas account for 13% and head and neck sarcomas for approximately 5% of all soft tissue sarcomas.

Histopathologic Classification

The most common classification scheme for soft tissue sarcoma is based on histogenesis, as outlined in the recent World Health Organization (WHO) classi-fication of sarcomas (see "Further Reading"). This classification system is reproducible for the better differentiated tumors. However, as the degree of histologic differentiation declines, the determination of cellular origin becomes increasingly difficult. In particular, despite advanced immunohistochemical tech-niques and electron microscopy, determining the cellular origin for many spindle cell and round cell soft tissue tumors is difficult, occasionally arbitrary, and sometimes impossible.

Recent evidence suggests that MFH, a common specific diagnosis assigned during the 1980s and 1990s, is actually a more general diagnosis that can be subtyped by immunohistochemical and ultrastructural means in more than 80% of patients. The most common subclassifications are myxofibrosarcoma and leiomyo-sarcoma. MFH subtypes seem to have prognostic significance in that patients with

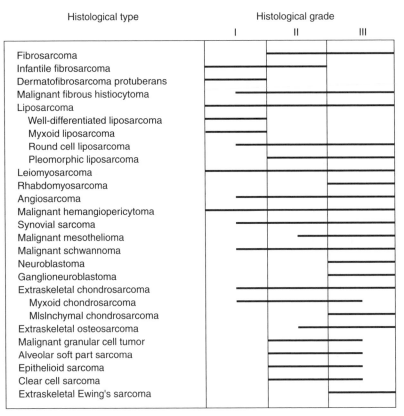

Figure 29.1 Spectrum of histologic grades observed among histologic subtypes of soft tissue sarcoma. (With permission from: Soft Tissue Sarcoma. In *Soft Tissue Tumors*, 3rd edition. Enzinger FM, Weiss SW (eds) Mosby-Year Book, St. Louis.)

MFH of myogenic origin (leiomyosarcoma, rhabdomyosarcoma, pleomorphic myogenic sarcoma, and myogenic spindle cell sarcoma) appear to be at greater risk for disease relapse than are patients with nonmyogenic subtypes of MFH.

Histologic Grading

Biologic aggressiveness can be best predicted by histologic grade. The spectrum of grades varies among histologic subtypes (Fig. 29.1). In comparative multivariate analyses, histologic grade is uniformly identified as the most important prognostic factor for distant metastasis and tumor-related death. Several grading systems have been proposed, but there is no consensus regarding the specific morphologic criteria that should be employed in the grading of soft tissue sarcomas. Two of the most commonly employed grading systems are the U.S. National Cancer Institute (NCI) system and the Federation Nationale des Centres de Lutte Contre le Cancer (FNCLCC) system developed by the French Federation of Cancer Centers Sarcoma Group. The NCI system is based on the tumor's histologic type or subtype, location, and amount of tumor necrosis, but cellularity, nuclear pleomorphism, and mitosis count are also considered in certain situations. The FNCLCC system employs a score generated by evaluation of three parameters: tumor differentiation, mitotic rate, and amount of tumor necrosis. Recent comparative evaluation of these grading systems suggests that the FNCLCC system may stratify patients more precisely for probability of overall and metastasis-free survival.

Molecular Pathology

The molecular characterization of specific types of soft tissue sarcoma has assumed increased importance. For example, most gastrointestinal stromal tumors (GIST) express a growth factor with tyrosine-kinase activity termed C-kit. C-kit can be detected by immunohistochemical staining for CD117; the presence of C-kit has become an important criterion for the diagnosis of GIST. The presence of C-kit also appears to have therapeutic implications in that recent reports demonstrate that a high proportion of patients with C-kit-positive GIST respond to the novel agent STI-571.

The analysis of fusion gene transcripts can also be helpful in the diagnosis of some forms of soft tissue sarcomas. Examples include the SYT-SSX2 fusion transcripts for the diagnosis of synovial sarcoma and the EWS-FLI1 fusion transcripts in the diagnosis and prognosis of Ewing's sarcomas.

CLINICAL PRESENTATION

The clinical presentation of patients with soft tissue sarcoma is highly variable. This reflects the anatomic heterogeneity of these lesions. The majority of patients with extremity sarcomas present with a painless soft tissue mass. Delay in diagnosis is common, with the most common misdiagnoses including intramuscular hematoma ("pulled muscle"), sebaceous cyst, and benign lipoma. Symptoms are often not experienced until these tumors grow large enough to press directly on nearby neurovascular structures, causing pain, numbness, or swelling.

Patients with intra-abdominal or retroperitoneal sarcomas commonly present with vague, nonspecific abdominal pain or a palpable abdominal mass. Retroperitoneal and intra-abdominal tumors can also produce symptoms of nausea, vomiting, abdominal distention, or early satiety. Sarcomas arising from specific viscera may produce symptoms or signs related to the organ involved. For example, patients with gastrointestinal or uterine leiomyosarcomas may present with symptoms related to gastrointestinal or uterine bleeding.

DIAGNOSTIC EVALUATION

The physical examination should include an assessment of the size and mobility of the mass. The relationship of the mass to the investing muscular fascia (superficial versus deep) and to nearby neurovascular and bony structures should be noted. A site-specific neurovascular examination and assessment of regional lymph nodes should also be performed.

The diagnostic evaluation of patients with suspected soft tissue sarcoma involves appropriate biopsy and imaging of the primary tumor together with complete staging evaluation. The following comments focus primarily on patients with extremity sarcomas because the extremities are the most common anatomic site.

Biopsy

Biopsy of the primary tumor is essential for most patients presenting with primary soft tissue masses. In general, any soft tissue mass in an adult that is asymptomatic or enlarging, is larger than 5 cm, or persists beyond 4–6 weeks should undergo biopsy. The preferred biopsy approach is generally the least invasive technique required to allow a definitive histologic diagnosis and assessment of grade. In most centers, core needle biopsy permits satisfactory tissue diagnosis. Biopsy of superficial lesions can commonly be guided by direct palpation, but less accessible sarcomas may require an imaging-guided (sonography or computed tomography [CT]) biopsy to safely sample the most heterogeneous component of the mass. In some centers, fine-needle aspiration may be an acceptable biopsy technique provided that an experienced sarcoma cytopathologist is available. However, because of the frequent difficulty in accurately diagnosing these lesions even when adequate tissue is available, the major utility of fine-needle aspiration in most centers is in the diagnosis of suspected recurrent sarcoma.

Incisional or excisional biopsy is rarely required but may be performed when a definitive diagnosis cannot be achieved by less invasive means. Several technical points merit comment. Relatively small, superficial masses that can easily be removed should be completely excised, with microscopic assessment of surgical margins. For extremity lesions, incisional and excisional biopsies should be performed with the incision oriented longitudinally to facilitate subsequent wide local excision and/or to permit radiation treatment volumes to adequately encompass the volume at risk while maximally sparing limb circumference. The incision should be centered over the mass at its most superficial point. Care should be taken not to raise tissue flaps. Meticulous hemostasis should be ensured to prevent dissemination of tumor cells into adjacent tissue planes by hematoma. All excisional biopsy specimens should be sent anatomically oriented for pathologic analysis. At definitive resection of a previously biopsied sarcoma, the biopsy scar should be excised *en bloc* with the tumor.

When radiologic assessment indicates that a presumed primary retroperitoneal (extravisceral) mass is resectable, fine-needle aspiration and core needle biopsy are not indicated. This is because the overall therapeutic plan is rarely altered by preoperative histologic diagnosis and the histologically heterogeneous nature of individual lesions precludes a plan of "observation" when biopsy findings are "benign" or indeterminate. Preoperative imaging-directed biopsy is invasive and expensive and rarely modifies treatment for patients in whom surgical exploration is planned. However, there are specific circumstances for which biopsy of primary retroperitoneal masses should be performed. These include (1) clinical suspicion of lymphoma or germ cell tumor, (2) tissue diagnosis for preoperative treatment, (3) tissue diagnosis of radiologically unresectable disease, and (4) suspected retroperitoneal or intra-abdominal metastasis from another primary tumor. Generally, however, for patients for whom exploratory laparotomy is planned, surgical resection is the best means of establishing a tissue diagnosis of a radiographically resectable retroperitoneal mass; intraoperative incisional biopsy is appropriate if the lesion proves to be unresectable. Given the poor long-term outcome for patients with retroperitoneal sarcoma (see "Treatment of Primary Soft Tissue Sarcoma of the Retroperitoneum"), preoperative evaluation and subsequent treatment may be best accomplished in a referral center involved in combined-modality therapy trials for these patients.

Radiologic Assessment

Optimal imaging of the primary tumor is dependent on anatomic site. Magnetic resonance imaging (MRI) has been regarded as the imaging modality of choice for soft tissue masses of the extremities. This is because MRI enhances the contrast between tumor and muscle and between tumor and adjacent blood vessel and provides multiplanar definition of the lesion. However, a study by the Radiation Diagnostic Oncology Group that compared MRI and CT showed no specific advantage of MRI over CT. On the other hand, although the diagnostic evaluation of extremity or superficial trunk lesion may be equally well served by both modalities, the treatment planning requirements (e.g., for both surgery and radiotherapy) may require additional information provided by the multiplanar capability of MRI and the ability to perform MRI/CT image fusion. For pelvic lesions, the multiplanar capability of MRI may provide superior single-modality imaging. In the retroperitoneum and abdomen, CT usually provides satisfactory anatomic definition of the lesion. Occasionally, MRI with gradient sequence imaging can delineate the relationship of the tumor to midline vascular structures, particularly the inferior vena cava and aorta. More invasive studies such as angiography or cavography are almost never required for evaluation of soft tissue sarcomas.

Cost-effective imaging to exclude the possibility of distant metastatic disease is dependent on the size, grade, and anatomic location of the primary tumor. In general, patients with low- and intermediate-grade tumors and patients with high-grade tumors 5 cm or smaller (T1) require only a chest x-ray for satisfactory evaluation for thoracic disease. This reflects the comparatively low risk for pulmonary metastases at presentation in these patients, and the fact that chest CT is not used to follow these patients after treatment. In contrast, patients with high-grade tumors larger than 5 cm should undergo more thorough staging by chest CT. Patients with retroperitoneal and intra-abdominal visceral sarcomas should undergo MRI or CT of the liver to exclude the possibility of synchronous hepatic metastases since the liver is a common site of first metastasis for these lesions.

STAGING

The relative rarity of soft tissue sarcomas, the anatomic heterogeneity of these lesions, and the presence of more than 30 recognized histologic subtypes of variable grade have made it difficult to establish a functional system that can accurately stage all forms of this disease. The sixth edition of the TNM staging system of the American Joint Committee on Cancer and UICC is the most widely employed staging system for soft tissue sarcomas. This TNM staging system is exceptional in that it incorporates histologic grade with the anatomic disease characteristics

TABLE 29.1. UICC/American Joint Committee on Cancer Staging System for Soft Tissue Sarcomas

T—Primary tumor

TX	Primary tumor cannot be assessed			
T0	No evidence of primary tumor			
T1	Tumor ≤5 cm in greatest dimension			
T1a	Superficial tumor[*]			
T1b	Deep tumor[*]			
T2	Tumor 5 cm in greatest dimension			
T2a	Superficial tumor[*]			
T2b	Deep tumor[*]			

N—Regional lymph nodes

NX	Regional lymph nodes cannot be assessed
N0	No regional lymph node metastasis
N1	Regional lymph node metastasis

M—Distant metastasis

MX	Distant metastasis cannot be assessed
M0	No distant metastasis
M1	Distant metastasis

Stage grouping

IA	T1a	N0, NX	M0	Low grade
	T1b	N0, NX	M0	Low grade
IB	T2a	N0, NX	M0	Low grade
	T2b	N0, NX	M0	Low grade
IIA	T1a	N0, NX	M0	High grade
	T1b	N0, NX	M0	High grade
IIB	T2a	N0, NX	M0	High grade
III	T2b	N0, NX	M0	High grade
IV	Any T	N1	M0	Any grade
	Any T	Any N	M1	Any grade

[*]Superficial tumor is located exclusively above the superficial fascia without invasion of the fascia; deep tumor is located either exclusively beneath the superficial fascia or superficial to the fascia with invasion of or through the fascia. Retroperitoneal, mediastinal, and pelvic sarcomas are classified as deep tumors. (Modified from UICC *TNM Classification of Malignant Tumors*, 6th edition. New York, John Wiley and Sons, 2002. With permission.)

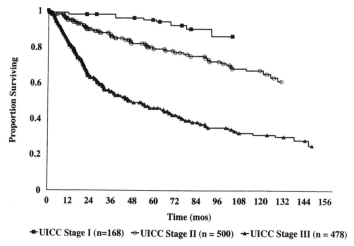

Figure 29.2 Overall survival by UICC stage in a population of 1,146 patients with primary extremity sarcoma treated at the Memorial Sloan-Kettering Cancer Center. (With permission from Pisters PWT and Brennan MF. (2000) Sarcomas of soft tissue. In *Clinical Oncology*, 2nd ed. Abeloff MD, Armitage JO, Lichter AS, Niederhuber JE, eds. New York, NY: Churchill Livingstone.)

(Table 29.1). All soft tissue sarcoma subtypes are included except dermatofibrosarcoma protuberans, a condition considered to have only borderline malignant potential. Four distinct histologic grades are recognized, ranging from well differentiated to undifferentiated. Histologic grade and tumor size are the primary determinants of clinical stage. Tumor size is further substaged as "a" (superficial tumor arising outside the investing fascia) or "b" (a deep tumor that arises beneath the fascia or invades the fascia). Stage-specific (UICC sixth edition) survival plots for patients with extremity sarcomas are shown in Figure 29.2.

A major limitation of the present staging system is that it does not take into account the anatomic and histologic heterogeneity of these lesions. The present staging system is optimally designed to stage extremity tumors but is also applicable to torso, head and neck, and retroperitoneal lesions. It should not be used for sarcomas of the gastrointestinal tract. Anatomic site, however, is an important determinant of outcome. Patients with retroperitoneal and visceral sarcomas have a worse overall prognosis than do patients with extremity tumors. Although site is not incorporated as a specific component of any present staging system, outcome data should be reported on a site-specific basis.

TREATMENT OF LOCALIZED PRIMARY SOFT TISSUE SARCOMA

A general stage-specific treatment algorithm for patients with primary sarcomas of the extremity and superficial trunk is outlined in Figure 29.3. The evidence

Biopsy/Radiographic Staging

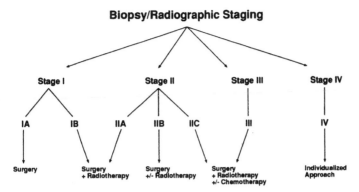

Figure 29.3 Treatment algorithm for patients with extremity or superficial trunk sarcomas based on UICC clinical stage. See Table 29.1 for staging system. Surgery consists of wide local resection with microscopic assessment of surgical margins. Radiotherapy consists of pre- or postoperative (50 or 65 Gy, respectively) external-beam radiation or brachytherapy (42–50 Gy) for eligible patients with G3/4 sarcomas. Chemotherapy consists of doxorubicin and/or ifosfamide pre- or postoperatively, optimally as part of a clinical trial. (With permission from Pisters PWT. (1998) Combined modality treatment of extremity soft tissue sarcomas. *Ann Surg Oncol* 5:464–472.)

supporting this stage-specific treatment approach is discussed below. The treatment of patients with retroperitoneal sarcomas is addressed separately.

Surgery

Surgical resection remains the cornerstone of therapy for localized disease. Over the past 20 years, there has been a marked decline in the rate of amputation as the primary therapy for extremity soft tissue sarcoma. With application of multimodality treatment strategies, less than 10% of patients presently undergo amputation. There is clear evidence that for patients for whom limb-sparing surgery is an option, a multimodality approach employing limb-sparing surgery combined with pre- or postoperative radiotherapy yields disease-related survival rates comparable to those of amputation while preserving a functional extremity.

Satisfactory local resection involves resection of the primary tumor with a margin of normal tissue around the lesion. Dissection along the tumor pseudocapsule (enucleation) is associated with local recurrence rates of at least 50%. In contrast, wide local excision that includes a margin of normal tissue around the lesion is associated with local recurrence rates in the range of 12–31%, as observed in the control arms (surgery alone) of randomized trials evaluating adjuvant radiotherapy. Unlike for other diseases such as malignant melanoma, there are no available randomized data to address what constitutes a satisfactory gross resection margin for a sarcoma.

Although the majority of patients with extremity soft tissue sarcoma should be treated with pre- or postoperative radiotherapy, there is evidence to suggest that radiotherapy may not be required for selected patients with completely resected, small primary soft tissue sarcomas. Surgical resection without radiotherapy may be considered for anatomically favorably located lesions that are 5 cm or smaller (T1). Patients considered for treatment by surgery alone should have sarcomas located superficially in a portion of the extremity or superficial trunk where it is not difficult to obtain a satisfactory gross surgical margin. The treatment of patients with category T2a and T2b (>5 cm) primary sarcomas by surgery alone is generally not recommended and should not be done outside a clinical trial.

Pre- or Postoperative Radiotherapy

Radiotherapy has been combined with conservative (limb-sparing) surgery to optimize local control for patients with localized soft tissue sarcoma. Radiation can be administered pre- or postoperatively by external-beam techniques or by interstitial techniques (brachytherapy). A randomized trial of postoperative brachytherapy (extremity or superficial trunk sarcomas) and a randomized trial of postoperative external-beam radiotherapy (extremity sarcomas) have confirmed several retrospective reports suggesting that surgery combined with radiotherapy results in superior local control compared to surgery alone (see "further Reading"). Although both randomized studies demonstrated an improvement in local control for patients treated with combined-modality therapy, this improvement did not translate into any detectable survival difference between the treatment (surgery plus radiotherapy) and control (surgery alone) arms.

Local failure rates with combined-modality regimens incorporating surgery and radiotherapy are generally less than 15% (Table 29.2). Despite theoretical advantages that may favor preoperative external-beam radiation, brachytherapy, or postoperative external-beam radiation, there does not appear to be a major difference in local control rates among these radiation techniques, although no presently available data directly compare the techniques. However, a phase III

TABLE 29.2. Local Control with Surgery and Radiotherapy for Localized Soft Tissue Sarcoma

Radiotherapy Approach	First Author	Radiation Dose (Gy)	Study Design	No. Patients	% Local Failure	
Preoperative EBRT	Suit	50–56	Retrospective	89	17	
	Barkley	50	Retrospective	110	10	
	Brant	50.4	Retrospective	58	9	
Brachytherapy	Pisters	42–45	Prospective (RCT)	119	9	(high grade)
				45	23	(low grade)
Postoperative EBRT	Lindberg	60–75	Retrospective	300	22	
	Karakousis	45–60	Retrospective	53	14	
	Suit	60–68	Retrospective	131	12	
	Yang	45 + 18	Prospective (RCT)	91	0	(high grade)
				50	5	(low grade)

EBRT, external-beam radiotherapy; RCT, randomized controlled trial.

prospective trial comparing preoperative external-beam radiotherapy with post-operative external-beam radiotherapy for patients with localized extremity soft tissue sarcoma (protocol SR-2) was recently completed by the National Cancer Institute of Canada Clinical Trials Group (NCIC CTG)/Canadian Sarcoma Group. This important study was designed to provide insight into the comparative efficacy, functional outcome, costs, and complication rates of these two options for external-beam radiotherapy. A recent abstract presentation (see "Further Reading") with a median of 3.3 years follow-up reported the following observations: acute wound complications were seen in 31 (35%) of 88 evaluable subjects treated preoperatively compared to 16 (17%) of 92 treated postoperatively ($p = 0.01$). Larger tumor size and lower limb site were adverse factors for wound complications on multivariate analysis. However, after 2 years, rates of grade 2 or greater fibrosis (56% vs. 28%, $p = 0.003$) and edema (24% vs. 7%, $p = 0.01$) were higher in the postoperative therapy group because of larger irradiation volumes and higher doses of radiotherapy with this approach. Local failure was identical in both arms (7%). An improvement in overall survival ($p = 0.0481$) in the preoperative therapy arm was partially explained by increased deaths in the postoperative therapy arm unrelated to sarcoma. Thus, while an increased risk of early wound complications with preoperative radiotherapy is confirmed by this multicenter trial, the higher late morbidity with postoperative radiotherapy suggests that the choice about radio-therapy approach should also consider other factors (e.g., tumor size and anatomic site).

Although external-beam radiotherapy is the most usual approach for local adjuvant therapy, another option is brachytherapy. With brachytherapy, the patient's entire local treatment (surgery plus radiation) can be completed within 10–14 days. Brachytherapy also has significant cost advantages and is more convenient for patients. In the absence of comparative data addressing the efficacy of the various radiotherapy techniques in achieving local control, such considerations assume increased importance. Until the final data from the NCIC CTG phase III compara-tive study are available, it appears reasonable to treat patients with either form of external-beam radiotherapy since local control rates are comparable. Where the necessary expertise is available for brachytherapy, this technique provides an excellent, cost-effective alternative for patients with appropriate high-grade lesions. Brachytherapy should not be used for patients with low-grade sarcomas, which are better treated with external-beam radiotherapy (Table 29.2).

Postoperative Chemotherapy

The role of postoperative chemotherapy in the management of localized soft tissue sarcoma remains controversial. The results of 12 randomized trials evaluating adjuvant chemotherapy in patients with extremity soft tissue sarcomas have been published. Each of these trials had a control arm that received no adjuvant therapy and a treatment group that received postoperative systemic therapy with doxo-rubicin alone or in combination with other drugs. Four of the trials reported improved relapse-free survival, but only 1 of the 12 trials found a statistically significant improvement in overall survival.

TABLE 29.3. Sarcoma Meta-Analysis Collaboration Group's Meta-Analysis of Randomized Studies of Doxorubicin-Based Postoperative Chemotherapy (vs. Local Therapy Alone) for Soft Tissue Sarcoma

Endpoint	Hazard Ratio	Absolute Benefit[*]	p Value
Local recurrence-free interval	0.74	6% (75% to 81%)	0.024
Distant recurrence-free interval	0.69	10% (60% to 70%)	0.0003
Recurrence-free interval	0.69	13% (45% to 58%)	0.000008
Recurrence-free survival	0.74	11% (40% to 51%)	0.00008
Overall survival rate	0.87	5% (50% to 55%)	0.087

[*]Numbers in parentheses represent 95% confidence interval. (Adapted from Tierney et al., (1997) *Lancet* 350:1647–1654. With permission.)

All of the published randomized trials of postoperative chemotherapy have recognized deficiencies in design and conduct. The most commonly cited deficiencies of these trials as a group relate to the relatively small sample size and to the fact that small differences in survival require relatively large numbers of patients to detect with sufficient statistical power. These deficiencies have been addressed to an extent in the Sarcoma Meta-Analysis Collaboration (SMAC) group's recent meta-analysis of the individual data in these randomized trials. This meta-analysis demonstrated statistically significantly higher local recurrence-free survival and disease-free survival rates in patients who received doxorubicin-containing postoperative chemotherapy (Table 29.3). However, there was no statistically significant improvement in overall survival rates. Because a significant improvement in survival with postoperative chemotherapy has not been detected with these advanced statistical techniques, it appears reasonable to conclude that if such a benefit exists, it must be quite small. Indeed, the meta-analysis suggests that if a survival benefit exists, it may be 5% or less (Table 29.3). Moreover, the local control rates in these trials fall short of the levels achieved in current outcome analyses evaluating the results of combined-modality treatment. This observation is confirmed in the NCIC CTG SR2 trial, which includes high-quality, real-time radiotherapy quality assurance.

Since publication of the SMAC meta-analysis, one other major study from Bologna has addressed the value of postoperative chemotherapy. One hundred four patients, ages 18–65 years, with high-risk (>5 cm, grade 3 or 4) STS of the extremities were randomized between no adjuvant therapy (control) and dose-intensive chemotherapy comprising five cycles of epirubicin (60 mg/m^2 on days 1 and 2), and ifosfamide (1.8 g/m^2 on days 1 to 5) plus mesna and granulocyte colony-stimulating factor, given every 3 weeks. The trial was stopped halfway through accrual because interim analysis showed a highly significant benefit for adjuvant chemotherapy. After a median follow-up of 59 months, 48 patients (46%) had died, 20 in the treatment and 28 in the control arm. The median disease-free survival was 16 months for the control group and 48 months for the treatment group ($p = 0.04$), and there was a survival difference favoring the chemotherapy arm ($p = 0.03$). Although a small survival advantage is evident, at 4 years the distant relapse rates are the same in the control and treatment arms (44% and 45%). Therefore, it is uncertain whether the chemotherapy is delaying or preventing recurrence.

At this time, given the overall results of the SMAC meta-analysis and the uncertain nature of the recent positive trial of adjuvant epirubicin and ifosfamide, postoperative chemotherapy cannot be considered standard therapy for patients with localized soft tissue sarcoma. Potentially toxic postoperative chemotherapy should be optimally provided within the context of a clinical trial and should be reserved for selected patients who present with adverse prognostic factors for overall survival. These factors include large tumor size, deep tumor location, and high histologic grade (TNM stage III, see Table 29.1).

Preoperative Chemotherapy

Proposed theoretical advantages to preoperative chemotherapy include (1) early treatment of occult micrometastatic disease, (2) *in vivo* evaluation of chemosensitivity, and (3) possible cytoreduction to an extent that less morbid local therapies might be applicable. There are only a few reports of long-term results with doxorubicin-based preoperative chemotherapy for patients with high-grade localized soft tissue sarcomas. These studies have revealed variable radiographic response rates ranging from 3 to 27%. The reasons for this variability are unknown but may include differences in patient populations, differences in chemotherapeutic drug dosing and number of cycles, and differences in the definition of major response. Long-term rates of local recurrence-free survival, distant metastasis-free survival, disease-free survival, and overall survival appear comparable to those reported for similarly staged patients treated with postoperative chemotherapy. At present, no studies have directly compared pre- versus postoperative chemotherapy.

Recently, ifosfamide-containing combinations have been used in the preoperative setting. Some patients treated with aggressive doxorubicin- and ifosfamide-based regimens have had major responses, and preliminary results suggest that radiographic response rates may be higher than in historical controls treated with non-ifosfamide-containing regimens.

A randomized trial of preoperative chemotherapy (50 mg/m^2 doxorubicin and 5 g/m^2 ifosfamide) and local therapy versus local therapy alone has recently been completed by the European Organization for the Research and Treatment of Cancer (EORTC) Bone and Soft Tissue Sarcoma Group (protocol 62874). The toxicity results of this trial have been presented, but data on event-free outcome have not yet been formally reported.

Combined Preoperative Chemotherapy and Radiotherapy

There has been recent interest in combined-modality preoperative treatment (sequential or concurrent chemotherapy and radiation) for patients with high-risk localized soft tissue sarcomas. The Radiation Therapy Oncology Group has completed a phase II trial of a preoperative combined-modality regimen consisting of three cycles of doxorubicin, ifosfamide, dacarbazine with Mesna (MAID), the first two of which were alternated with two 22-Gy courses of radiation (11 fractions each) for a total preoperative radiation dose of 44 Gy. This was followed by surgical resection with microscopic assessment of margins. An additional 16-Gy boost dose was delivered postoperatively for microscopically positive surgical margins. Observed toxicities were significant, with 27 (66%) of 41 patients and 12 (29%) of 41 patients experiencing grade 4 neutropenia and thrombocytopenia, respectively. Notwithstanding these toxicities, 88% of patients completed preoperative chemotherapy and 93% completed preoperative radiotherapy. The 2-year actuarial overall survival rate was 95%. These encouraging preliminary results will require longer follow-up and confirmation. Nonetheless, the preliminary survival data support additional studies evaluating preoperative combined-modality therapy for patients with localized high-risk sarcoma.

Concurrent doxorubicin-based chemoradiation has also been employed extensively by investigators at the University of California, Los Angeles. The treatment involved concurrent intra-arterial doxorubicin with unusually high dose per fraction radiotherapy (35 Gy of external-beam radiotherapy delivered in 10 daily fractions, which was reduced to 17.5 Gy in 5 daily fractions to minimize local toxicity). A subsequent prospective randomized trial compared preoperative intra-arterial doxorubicin to intravenous doxorubicin, both followed by 28 Gy of radiation in eight daily fractions followed by surgical resection. No differences in local recurrence or survival were noted, but there were increased local toxicities (largely vascular complications) in the intra-arterial therapy group. As a consequence, most groups that continue to investigate concurrent chemoradiation approaches have switched to the intravenous route for chemotherapy administration. Although the preliminary results of phase II studies appear encouraging, preoperative concurrent or sequential chemotherapy and radiotherapy regimens remain investigational and, given the significant risks for toxicity associated with them, should not be provided outside the context of a clinical trial.

TREATMENT OF PRIMARY SOFT TISSUE SARCOMA OF THE RETROPERITONEUM

Surgical resection with negative margins remains the primary treatment for patients with retroperitoneal sarcoma. Overall resectability rates in recent series combining patients with primary and recurrent retroperitoneal sarcomas range from 53 to 59%. Grossly complete resection may be possible in 80–90% of patients with primary retroperitoneal soft tissue sarcomas. The most common reasons for unresectability are the presence of major vascular involvement (aorta or vena cava), peritoneal implants, or distant metastases. In many cases, resection of adjacent retroperitoneal or intra-abdominal organs may be necessary to facilitate complete resection. Partial resections or debulking procedures have been performed, but there is no evidence that partial resection improves survival. In general, deliberate partial resection of retroperitoneal sarcomas should be reserved for relief of bowel obstruction or palliation of other critical manifestations of advanced disease. Results from recent series demonstrate 5-year actuarial survival rates in the range of 54–64% for patients with completely resected retroperitoneal sarcomas. Recurrent disease remains a significant problem, with local and/or distant recurrences developing in the majority of surgically treated patients (53–68%).

Although postoperative radiotherapy has been shown to reduce local recurrence rates for extremity and superficial trunk sarcomas, gastrointestinal and neurologic toxicities frequently limit the delivery of sufficient radiation doses to the retroperitoneum. Several retrospective reports have suggested that postoperative external-beam radiotherapy improves local control or at least prolongs the time to local failure after surgical resection of retroperitoneal sarcomas. No randomized trials have addressed this specific question. A randomized trial from the NCI demonstrated that surgical resection with intraoperative and subsequent postoperative external-beam radiotherapy resulted in improved local control versus resection and postoperative high-dose external-beam radiotherapy. However, intraoperative radiotherapy was associated with significant neurotoxicity (47% of patients). This technique remains investigational and is generally limited to specialty centers because of the need for a dedicated operating room.

Retrospective studies have not demonstrated any benefit to preoperative or postoperative doxorubicin-based chemotherapy for retroperitoneal sarcomas. Thus, at present, no data from randomized trials support pre- or postoperative chemotherapy as standard treatment for retroperitoneal sarcomas. Because of the disappointing results in these patients, they should be encouraged to enter clinical trials investigating novel multimodality treatment strategies and are probably best referred to centers participating in these trials.

TREATMENT OF MALIGNANT GASTROINTESTINAL STROMAL TUMORS

Malignant GIST are rare mesenchymal tumors originating in the wall of the gastrointestinal tract. There are no useful data from which to draw conclusions about optimal treatment. Much of the literature on these tumors comprises studies that have limited numbers of patients and that include malignant and benign cases from throughout the gastrointestinal tract. While malignant GIST may be localized at presentation, they are commonly locally advanced (invading adjacent organs or the peritoneum), with hollow viscus perforation in some patients. Distant metastases (usually to the liver) are evident at presentation in 10–15% of cases.

Unfortunately, GIST can be difficult to manage. Frequently causing obstructive symptoms, these tumors often require urgent surgery, and the preoperative staging workup may be incomplete. Resection is recommended but can be completed in only approximately 70% of patients. Resection of various intra-abdominal, pelvic, and retroperitoneal organs may be needed to obtain grossly clear margins. In some instances, resection of major vessels may be needed. The locoregional recurrence rate after resection is high (approximately 40%) and the distant metastasis rate even higher (at least 60%).

Radiotherapy is normally unrealistic owing to the mobility of these visceral tumors, especially those arising from the small bowel and intraperitoneal colon, the position of which changes throughout the day. Moreover, the radiation dose possible is often compromised by organ tolerance, especially small bowel tolerance. However, in rare situations, postoperative radiotherapy may be used if residual disease is present in the pelvic side wall regions, where radiotherapy fields can be localized. The adjuvant use of the tyrosine kinase inhibitor STI-571, which has significant activity against advanced GIST requires urgent study. (STI-571 is discussed further below: see "New Agents.")

TREATMENT OF LOCALLY RECURRENT SOFT TISSUE SARCOMA

Despite optimal multimodality therapy, local recurrence develops in a substantial number of patients with soft tissue sarcoma. Treatment approaches for locally recurrent soft tissue sarcoma need to be individualized based on local anatomic constraints and the limitations on present treatment options imposed by prior therapies. In general, all patients with local recurrences should be evaluated for re-resection. The results of such "salvage surgery" are good, with two-thirds of patients experiencing long-term survival. For patients who have not had prior radiotherapy to the area of recurrence, optimal treatment of the local recurrence includes surgery and pre- or postoperative radiotherapy. Few data have been published on the use of additional radiotherapy in patients who develop local recurrence in or at the margin of a previous external-beam radiation field. Brachytherapy may be an option for such patients. In addition, it may be reasonable to consider pre- or postoperative chemotherapy for patients with locally recurrent high-grade tumors because of the adverse prognostic significance of local recurrence and the fact that the SMAC meta-analysis of randomized postoperative chemotherapy trials suggests a local control advantage for patients receiving doxorubicin-based postoperative chemotherapy.

TREATMENT OF METASTATIC SOFT TISSUE SARCOMA

The most common site of metastasis from soft tissue sarcoma is the lungs. Primary visceral and gastrointestinal sarcomas also commonly metastasize to the liver. For most nongastrointestinal or visceral sarcomas, extrapulmonary metastases are uncommon forms of first metastasis and usually occur as a late manifestation of widely disseminated disease. The median survival from the time of development of metastatic disease is 8–12 months. Prospective studies have demonstrated an 11% 3-year survival rate among all soft tissue sarcoma patients presenting with pulmonary metastases. The optimal treatment of metastatic soft tissue sarcoma requires an understanding of the natural history of the disease and individualized selection of treatment options based on specific patient factors, disease factors, and limitations imposed by prior treatment.

Surgical Resection

Carefully selected patients may benefit from complete surgical resection of metastatic sarcoma. Unfortunately, this treatment approach benefits only a small fraction of patients with synchronous or metachronous pulmonary metastases. Among the subset of patients who are able to undergo complete resection of their pulmonary metastatic disease (approximately 50% of all patients with pulmonary metastases), the median survival from the time of complete resection is 18–27 months, and the 3-year survival rate is 23–54% (Table 29.4).

The rather disappointing overall treatment results for patients with metastatic disease underscore the importance of careful patient selection for resection of pulmonary metastases. The following criteria are generally agreed upon: (1) the primary tumor is controlled or is controllable; (2) there is no extrathoracic disease; (3) the patient is a medical candidate for thoracotomy and pulmonary resection; and (4) complete resection of all disease appears possible. With careful patient selection, the morbidity of thoracotomy can be limited to the subset of patients who are most likely to benefit from this aggressive treatment approach. The role of perioperative chemotherapy with complete resection of pulmonary metastases is unknown.

Chemotherapy

Systemic treatment remains the only therapeutic option for the majority of patients with metastatic soft tissue sarcoma. A detailed review of the single-agent and combination chemotherapeutic approaches for advanced sarcoma is beyond the scope of this text but is available in the general reviews referenced in the "further Reading" section. The combination of cyclophosphamide, vincristine, doxorubicin, and dacarbazine (CyVADIC) has been considered the standard of care for well over a decade. Complete and partial response rates on the order of 20–30% have been observed with this regimen. However, a randomized trial comparing CyVADIC to doxorubicin alone revealed no significant difference in response or survival rates. On the basis of these data, many investigators now consider single-agent doxorubicin to be the present standard of care against which new combinations should be evaluated.

Ifosfamide, an analogue of cyclophosphamide, has been reported to produce significant response rates, in the range of 30–40%, in patients with advanced soft tissue sarcoma. The most comprehensive comparative study performed to date was reported by the EORTC. In that study, 663 eligible patients were randomly assigned to receive doxorubicin (75 mg/m^2) (arm A); CyVADIC (arm B); or ifosfamide (5 g/m^2) plus doxorubicin (50 mg/m^2) (arm C). There was no statistically significant difference detected among the three study arms in terms of response rate (arm A, 23%; arm B, 24%; and arm C, 28%), remission duration, or overall survival (median, 52 weeks for arm A, 51 weeks for arm B, and 55 weeks for arm C). The

TABLE 29.4. Survival Following Complete Resection of Pulmonary Metastases from Soft Tissue Sarcoma in Adults

| First Author(s)/Institution (Year) | No. Patients | | | | Complete Resection (%) | Median Survival (mo) | % 3-Year Survival |
	Total	Pulmonary Metastases	Resection of Pulmonary Metastases				
Creagan/Mayo (1979)	112	112	112		64 (57%)	18	29
Putnam, Roth/NCI (1984, 1985)	487	93	68		51 (75%)	23	32
Jablons/NCI (1989)	74	57	57		49 (86%)	27	35
Casson/MDACC (1992)	68	68	68		58 (85%)	25	42
Verazin/Roswell (1992)	78	78	78		61 (78%)	21	21
							(5 yr)
Gadd/MSKCC (1993)	716	135	78		65 (83%)	19	23
van Geel/EORTC (1996)	255	255	255		255 (100%)	NR	54

Mayo, Mayo Clinic; Roswell, Roswell Park Cancer Institute; NCI, U.S. National Cancer Institute; MDACC, The University of Texas M. D. Anderson Cancer Center; MSKCC, Memorial Sloan-Kettering Cancer Center; EORTC, European Organization for the Research and Treatment of Cancer.

degree of myelosuppression was significantly greater for the combination of ifosfamide and doxorubicin than for the other two regimens. Cardiotoxicity was also more frequent in arm C. This study and others suggest that single-agent doxorubicin is still the standard against which more intensive or new drug treatments should be compared.

New Agents

ET-743 is a novel compound derived from the Caribbean marine tunicate *Ecteinascidia tuminata*. This agent is currently under intensive investigation as preliminary reports suggest that ET-743 has activity against advanced, highly pretreated soft tissue sarcomas.

STI-571 is an oral agent that inhibits the tyrosine kinase activity of C-kit. Preliminary results of phase I and II studies suggest that this agent has significant activity in patients with C-kit positive GIST. Further studies are under way to better define toxicities, response rates, and duration of responses in patients with both C-kit-positive and C-kit-negative soft tissue sarcomas. It is highly likely that STI-571 will play a central role in the overall therapeutic approach to patients with GIST.

FURTHER READING

General Reviews

Brennan MF, Alektiar K, Maki R (2001). Soft tissue sarcoma. In *Cancer: Principles and Practice of Oncology*, 6th ed. DeVita VT Jr, Hellman S, Rosenberg SA (eds). Philadelphia, PA: J.B. Lippincott; pp. 1841–1890.

Pisters PWT, Brennan MF (1999). Sarcomas of soft tissue. In *Clinical Oncology*. Abeloff M, Armitage J, Lichter A, Niederhuber J (eds). New York, NY: Churchill Livingstone, pp. 2273–2313.

Pisters PWT, Demetri G, O'Sullivan B (2000). Soft tissue sarcoma. In *Cancer Medicine*, 5th ed. Holland JF, Bast RC Jr, Pollock RE, Frei E III, Kufe DW, Weischselbaum RR (eds). Hamilton, ON: B.C. Decker, pp. 1903–1930.

Histopathology, Grading, and Biopsy

Enzinger FM, Weiss SW (1995). *Soft Tissue Sarcoma*, 3rd ed. St. Louis: Mosby-Year Book.

Fletcher CDM, Gustafson P, Rydholm A et al. (2001). Clinicopathologic re-evaluation of 100 malignant fibrous histiocytomas: prognostic relevance of subclassification. *J Clin Oncol* 19:3045–3050.

Guillou L, Coindre J, Bonichon F, Bonichon F, Nguyen BB, Terrier P, Collin F, Vilain MO, Mandard AM, Le Doussal V, Leroux A, Jacquemier J. Duplay H, Sastre-Garau X, Costa J (1997). Comparative study of the National Cancer Institute and French Federation of Cancer Centers Sarcoma Group grading systems in a population of 410 adult patients with soft tissue sarcoma. *J Clin Oncol* 15:350–362.

Heslin MJ, Lewis JJ, Woodruff JM, Brennan MF (1997). Core needle biopsy for diagnosis of extremity soft tissue sarcoma. *Ann Surg Oncol* 4:425–431.

Trojani M, Contesso G, Coindre JM et al. (1984). Soft-tissue sarcomas of adults: study of pathological prognostic variables and definition of a histopathological grading system. *Int J Cancer* 33–37.

Staging and Prognostic Factors

Coindre JM, Terrier P, Bui NB et al. (1996). Prognostic factors in adult patients with locally controlled soft tissue sarcoma: a study of 546 patients from the French Federation of Cancer Centers Sarcoma Group. *J Clin Oncol* 14:869–877.

Panicek DM, Gatsonis C, Rosenthal DI et al. (1997). CT and MR imaging in the local staging of primary malignant musculoskeletal neoplasms: report of the Radiology Diagnostic Oncology Group. *Radiology* 202:237–246.

Pisters PWT, Leung DHY, Woodruff J, Shi W, Brennan MF (1996). Analysis of prognostic factors in 1041 patients with localized soft tissue sarcomas of the extremities. *J Clin Oncol* 14:1679–1689.

Wunder JS, Healy JH, Davis AM, Brennan MF (2000). A comparison of staging systems for localized extremity soft tissue sarcoma. *Cancer* 88:2721–2730.

Surgical Treatment of Extremity Sarcoma

Rosenberg SA, Tepper J, Glatstein E et al. (1982). The treatment of soft-tissue sarcomas of the extremities: prospective randomized evaluations of (1) limb-sparing surgery plus radiation therapy compared with amputation and (2) the role of adjuvant chemotherapy. *Ann Surg* 196:305–315.

Williard WC, Collin C, Casper ES, Hajdu SI, Brennan MF (1992). The changing role of amputation for soft tissue sarcoma of the extremity in adults. *Surg Gynecol Obstet* 175: 389–396.

Pre- and Postoperative Radiotherapy

O'Sullivan B, Davis AM, Turcotte R, Bell R, Catton C, Chabot P, Wander J, Kandel R, Goddard K, Sadura A, Pater J, Zee B (2002). Preoperative versus postoperative radio-therapy in soft-tissue sarcoma of the limbs: a randomized trial. *Lancet* 359:2235–2241.

Pisters PWT, Harrison LB, Leung DHY, Woodruff JM, Casper ES (1996). Long-term results of a prospective randomized trial of adjuvant brachytherapy in soft tissue sarcoma. *J Clin Oncol* 14:859–868.

Yang JC, Chang AE, Baker AR et al. (1998). A randomized prospective study of the benefit of adjuvant radiation therapy in the treatment of soft tissue sarcomas of the extremity. *J Clin Oncol* 16:197–203.

Postoperative Chemotherapy

Bramwell VHC (2001). Adjuvant chemotherapy for adult soft tissue sarcoma: is there a standard of care? *J Clin Oncol* 19:1235–1237.

Frustaci S, Gherlinzoni F, De Paoli A et al. (2001). Adjuvant chemotherapy for adult soft tissue sarcomas of the extremities and girdles: results of the Italian randomized cooperative trial. *J Clin Oncol* 19:1238–1247.

Tierney JF (1997). Adjuvant chemotherapy for localized resectable soft-tissue sarcoma of adults: meta-analysis of individual data. *Lancet* 350:1647–1654.

Combined Preoperative Chemotherapy and Radiotherapy

Kraybill WG, Spiro I, Harris J, Ettinger D, Trotti A, Lucas D, Blum R, Eisenberg B (2001). Radiation Therapy Oncology Group (RTOG) 95-14: A phase II study of neoadjuvant chemotherapy (CT) and radiation therapy (RT) in high risk (HR), high grade, soft tissue sarcomas (STS) of the extremities and body wall: a preliminary report. *Proc Am Soc Clin Oncol* 20:1389.

Treatment of Metastatic Sarcoma

McCormack P (1990). Surgical resection of pulmonary metastases. *Semin Surg Oncol* 6: 297–302.

Santoro A, Tursz T, Mouridsen H et al. (1995). Doxorubicin versus CYVADIC versus doxorubicin plus ifosfamide in first-line treatment of advanced soft tissue sarcomas: a randomized study of the European Organization for Research and Treatment of Cancer Soft Tissue and Bone Sarcoma Group. *J Clin Oncol* 13:1537–1545.

Treatment of Retroperitoneal Sarcomas

Catton CN, O'Sullivan B, Kotwall C, Cummings B, Hao Y, Fornsier V (1994). Outcome and prognosis in retroperitoneal soft tissue sarcoma. *Int J Radiat Oncol Biol Phys* 29:1005–1010.

Lewis JJ, Leung DHY, Woodruff JM, Brennan MF (1998). Retroperitoneal soft-tissue sarcoma: analysis of 500 patients treated and followed at a single institution. *Ann Surg* 228: 355–365.

Sindelar WF, Kinsella TJ, Chen PW, Delaney TF, Tepper JE, Rosenberg SA, Glatstein E (1993). Intraoperative radiotherapy in retroperitoneal sarcomas. Final results of a prospective, randomized, clinical trial. *Arch Surg* 128:402–410.

Treatment of Gastrointestinal Stromal Tumors

Crosby JA, Catton CN, Davis A, Couture J, O'Sullivan B, Kandel R, Swallow CJ (2000). Malignant gastrointestinal stromal tumors of the small intestine: a review of 50 cases from a prospective database. *Ann Surg Oncol* 8:50–59.

DeMatteo RP, Lewis JJ, Leung D, Mudan SS, Woodruff JM, Brennan MF (2000). Two hundred gastrointestinal stromal tumors: recurrence patterns and prognostic factors for survival. *Ann Surg* 231:51–58.

New Agents

Delaloge S, Yovine A, Taamma A, Riofrio M, Brain E, Raymond E, Cottu P, Goldwasser F, Jimeno J, Misset JL, Marty M, Cvitkovic E (2001). Ecteinascidin-743: a marine-derived compound in advanced, pre-treated sarcoma patients—preliminary evidence of activity. *J Clin Oncol* 19:1248–1255.

Joensuu H, Roberts PJ, Sarlomo-Rikala M, Andersson LC, Tervahartiala P, Tuveson D, Silberman S, Capdeville R, Dimitrijevic S, Druker B, Demetri GD (2001). Effect of the tyrosine kinase inhibitor STI 571 in a patient with a metastatic gastrointestinal stromal tumor. *N Engl J Med* 344:1052–1056.

Taamma A, Misset JL, Riogrio M, Guzman C, Brain E, Lopez LL, Rosing H, Jimeno JM, Cvitkovic E (2001). Phase I and pharmacokinetic studies of ecteinascidin-743, a new marine compound, administered as a 24-hour continuous infusion in patients with solid tumors. *J Clin Oncol* 19:1256–1265.

CHAPTER 30

Lymphomas

M. A. GIL-DELGADO and D. KHAYAT

Medical Oncology Department, Salpétrière Hospital, SOMPS, Paris, France

S. A. N. JOHNSON

Taunton and Somerset Hospital, Department of Hematology, Taunton, Somerset, England

The malignant lymphomas are a highly complex group of neoplasms. Attempts to classify these disorders have tried to relate the malignant proliferation to the equivalent normal cells, and with the increasing sophistication of morphology, cytology, immunohistochemistry, and molecular biology it has become apparent that almost all non-Hodgkin's lymphomas are clonal proliferations in which all the cells arise from the same source. In contrast, although Hodgkin's Disease is a clonal proliferation of (in most cases) B cells, the broad morphological criteria used to establish the diagnosis may lead to problems in differentiating between Hodgkin's disease (HD), non-Hodgkin's lymphomas (NHL), and reactive lesions.

The wide distribution of lymphoid tissue within the body results in a range of clinical presentations and also produces a variety of sources for diagnostic material; lymph node biopsy may be replaced by or supplemented with tumor cells obtained from the blood, bone marrow, and a number of other extranodal sites that will together lead to accurate classification of the tumor.

NON-HODGKIN'S LYMPHOMAS

Epidemiology, Etiology, and Pathogenesis

The overall incidence of NHL is 10–15 cases per 100,000 population, with a male preponderance. However, there are very considerable geographical variations in prevalence of the specific subtypes.

UICC Manual of Clinical Oncology, Eighth Edition. Edited by Raphael E. Pollock
ISBN 0-471-22289-5 Copyright © 2004 John Wiley & Sons, Inc.

A viral etiology has been established for Burkitt's lymphoma (BL) by studies that emerged from its restricted geographical distribution; the high incidence of BL in tropical Africa and Papua New Guinea was shown to be associated with infection by the Epstein-Barr virus (EBV) at an early age. *In vitro* studies of EBV have shown that it is a potentially oncogenic virus that immortalizes B cells, and it is proposed that this is the initial event in a multistep model for the pathogenesis of African BL. Subsequent events consist of stimulation of the immortalized B cells to proliferate (by malarial infection or other immunosuppressive factors), then chromosomal translocation resulting in irreversible c-myc activation and true malignant transformation. EBV is thought also to play an etiological role in the causation of post-transplantation lymphoproliferative disorders (PTLD) in which it is proposed that the profound deficiency in cytotoxic T cells permits the outgrowth of EBV-transformed B cells. The pattern of lymphoma incidence in Japan is also dictated by the association between infection by human T-cell lymphotropic virus type I (HTLV-1) and a distinct form of T-cell lymphoma, adult T-cell lymphoma-leukemia (ATLL); the Caribbean basin is also an endemic area for HTLV-1. In recent years, acquired immunodeficiency syndrome (AIDS) following infection with human immunodeficiency virus (HIV) has resulted in a significant increase in the susceptibility to lymphoproliferative disorders, mostly of high or intermediate grade and B-cell origin although Hodgkin's disease may also occur. A recently described subset of AIDS-related NHL in which the tumor grows predominantly in the pleural, pericardial and abdominal cavities appears to be strongly associated with the presence of Kaposi's sarcoma-associated herpes virus (human-herpesvirus-8) in the malignant cells, implying a causative role for the virus in producing these "primary effusion lymphomas." The incidence of NHL, however, appears to have been increasing over the last 30 years independent of the rise in HIV-related cases, and the causative agents for most cases are not established.

A number of conditions that result in anomalies of the immune response are associated with an increased risk of developing NHL. Inherited conditions such as ataxia-telangiectasia and combined immunodeficiency syndrome are often accompanied by cytogenetic abnormalities, but the relationship between these changes and the nonrandom translocations involving genes responsible for immunoglobin synthesis are not clear. In the X-linked immunoproliferative syndrome, an expanded pool of immortalized cells is created as a result of EBV infection, and this may result in an unusual polyclonal malignant proliferation of B cells. Disease states that result in aberrant immunity as a secondary process, such as rheumatoid arthritis, celiac disease, immunosuppressive therapy, and hypogammaglobulinemia, are also associated with an increased incidence of NHL. Neither the mechanisms outlined above nor the involvement of specific viruses can account for the majority of cases of NHL; common subtypes such as follicular lymphoma (FL), although they are associated with well-defined nonrandom chromosomal translocation, do not appear to result from processes with an established sequence of steps leading to a malignant state.

The development of malignant lymphomas is assumed to result from the uncontrolled expansion of cells that have a normal counterpart in the immune system, and it is therefore not surprising that lymphoma cells share morphological and immunophenotypic characteristics with normal T and B cells in various states of activation and proliferation. The subsequent biological characteristics of the malignant cells may be governed by additional genetic "hits," which confer more aggressive behavior and independence from the normal control mechanisms that regulate the response to antigen and contribution to the immune response.

Lymphomas of mucosa-associated lymphoid tissue (MALT) are a particularly instructive example of the initiation of a malignant process from a reactive one. The association of MALT lymphoma with *Helicobacter pylori* infections of the stomach was followed by the observation that early-stage and low-grade disease could be induced to regress in response to anti-*Helicobacter* therapy (i.e., to withdrawal of antigenic stimulation) without the use of cytotoxic agents. It is models of disease behavior such as this that should encourage clinicians to treat each subtype of lymphoma as a different disease with its own distinctive genotypic and biological pattern of behavior and which will require its own specific approach to therapy.

The analysis of gene expression in lymphoma cells is a technique that is likely to further define the biological behavior of lymphoid malignancies. DNA microassay analysis has been used to subdivide diffuse large B-cell lymphoma into tumors derived from cells arising within the germinal center and those with postgerminal center origins; these two types are morphologically similar but have strikingly different prognoses.

Clinical Presentation, Investigation, and Staging

Although the majority of patients with NHL have generalized disease at presentation, it is important to identify those with only local involvement (20–30% of cases) who may be primarily managed with radiotherapy or where combined modality therapy is of value. The course of the disease, prognosis, and treatment are influenced by stage, histologic type, and bulk of the disease, so the most important initial management is designed to obtain an accurate tissue diagnosis and evaluation of disease extent.

Peripheral lymph node enlargement is present in 60–70% of patients, allowing an excision biopsy of a whole node to be taken so that both the nodal architecture and cytology can be assessed. If the lymphadenopathy is predominantly intra-abdominal, adequate tissue may be obtained by computed tomograph (CT)-guided needle biopsy, but representative material is not guaranteed by this approach. Other tissues may be the source of the primary site of NHL and so biopsy material from Waldeyer's ring, skin, gastrointestinal mucosa, liver, testis, and brain may prove to be involved by NHL. The incidence of bone-marrow involvement is high, especially in a number of indolent lymphomas; bone marrow aspiration may provide material for cytology, immunophenotyping, and molecular studies, whereas trephine biopsy has the advantage of demonstrating focal or patchy involvement and is generally recommended. It may be appropriate to retain part of the biopsy without fixation to permit immunocytochemical stains and extraction of DNA for

TABLE 30.1. Format for Documenting Palpable Disease

	Right	Left
Cervical	$a \times b$ cm	—
Axillary	—	$c \times d$ cm
Inguinal	—	—
Tonsil	Enlarged	—

Liver = cm below costal margin
Spleen = cm below costal margin

gene rearrangement studies, using the remainder for conventional histology as hematoxylin and eosin (H&E) and Giemsa-stained sections together with immunohistochemical techniques with antibodies suitable for use on paraffin-embedded tissue.

Assessment of the patient at presentation should document the anatomical extent of the disease by physical examination, and measurements by lymph nodes should be clearly recorded in the patient's records in a reproducible format such as that shown in Table 30.1.

The assessment should include radiological investigations including at least chest x-ray and abdominal CT scan; gallium isotope scanning may be a useful additional means of documenting involved areas. Magnetic resonance imaging (MRI) may be valuable in defining disease in areas such as the central nervous system, head and neck, and musculoskeletal system, whereas position emission tomography (PET) is proving to be a valuable technique for the interpretation of the residual mass still present after treatment. Initial laboratory tests should consist of a full blood count (FBC), erythrocyte sedimentation rate (ESR), measurement of renal and hepatic function, uric acid, serum lactate dehydrogenase (LDH), protein immunoelectrophoresis, and β_2 microglobulin.

Specific examination of extranodal sites is dictated by clinical signs, so although almost all patients will require bone marrow biopsy, fewer will need liver biopsy, gastrointestinal endoscopy, or detailed assessment of the CNS by lumbar puncture.

Although the Ann Arbor Staging System is used to help to define those patients who may be suitable for local therapy, treatment decisions are refined on the basis of risk stratification such as that proposed by the International Prognostic Index Project for patients with high-grade NHL (Table 30.2).

The problems of adequately staging extranodal lymphomas have resulted in alternative systems being proposed (Table 30.3). For gastrointestinal lymphomas, the definition of local disease by careful endoscopy is important, but extension of involvement into regional lymph nodes or distant sites must also be carefully assessed.

Cutaneous T-cell lymphoma is frequently managed by local treatment in its early stages, and a modified TNM system is used to define the extent of the disease (Table 30.4).

TABLE 30.2. International Index for Lymphoma

	0	1
Age (years)	< 60	>60
Performance status	0 or 1	2, 3, 4
Ann Arbor stage	I or II	III or IV
Extranodal involvement	< 2 sites	> 2 sites
LDH	Normal	High
Risk		
Low	0 or 1	
Low/intermediate	2	
High/intermediate	3	
High	4 or 5	

Classification and Diagnostic Methods

Since the 1970s, a number of different lymphoma classifications have been used in different parts of the world. The World Health Organization (WHO) classification for hematological malignancies has established an international consensus that takes into account current concepts of the biology of lymphomas.

The use of immunological reagents to assign lymphoma cells to either the B- or T-cell lineage and to a level of differentiation within the system has been extended by the realization that nonrandom chromosomal translocations are responsible for defining the biological features of many lymphomas (Table 30.5). Many of these translocations result in the alignment of an oncogene with the gene responsible for

TABLE 30.3. Modified Blackledge Staging System for Primary Gastrointestinal Lymphomas

Stage	Characteristic
I	Tumor confined to gastrointestinal (GI) tract; single primary site or multiple, noncontiguous lesions
II	Tumor extending into abdomen from primary GI site
II$_1$	Local nodal involvement (paragastric or paraintestinal)
II$_2$	Distant nodal involvement (mesenteric, retroperitoneal, pelvic, inguinal)
IIE	Penetration of serosa to involve adjacent organs or tissues (Enumerate actual sites of involvement, e.g., II$_E$ (pancreas), II$_E$ (post-abdominal wall.) Where there is both nodal involvement and penetration to involve adjacent organs, stage should be denoted using both a subscript ($_1$ or $_2$) and E, for example II$_{1E}$ (pancreas)
IV	Disseminated extranodal involvement or concomitant supradiaphragmatic nodal involvement

TABLE 30.4. TNM Classification of Cutaneous T-Cell Lymphoma

T—Skin

T0	Clinical/histologically suspicious lesions
T1	Plaques/eczematous lesions <10% skin surface
T2	Plaques/eczematous lesions >10% skin surface
T3	Tumors
T4	Erythroderma

N—Lymph nodes

N0	No clinically abnormal peripheral nodes
N1	Clinically abnormal peripheral nodes/pathology negative
N2	No clinically abnormal peripheral nodes/pathology positive
N3	Clinically abnormal peripheral nodes/pathology positive

B—Blood

B0	Atypical peripheral blood mononuclear cells <5%
B1	Atypical peripheral blood mononuclear cells >5%

M—Visceral organs

M0	No visceral organ involvement
M1	Confirmed histological visceral involvement

NP—Nodal pathology

NP0	Biopsy performed, not CTCL
NP1	Biopsy performed, CTCL

Treatment decisions are then based on the stage of the disease, which is derived from the following classification:

Stage classification of mycosis fungoides/Sézary syndrome

IA	T1, N0, NP0, M0
IB	T2, N0, NP0, M0
IIA	T1, 2, N1, NP0, M0
IIB	T3, N0, NP0, M0
III	T4, N0, NP0, M0
IVA	T1–4, N0, 1, NP1, M0
IVB	T1–4, N0, 1, NP0, 1, M1

either immunoglobin or T-cell receptor expression and produce specific abnormalities that favor the growth of the malignant clone. In addition to their use in establishing the diagnosis of an individual lymphoma, the detection of these translocations by sensitive polymerase chain reaction (PCR)-based assays may be utilized to monitor the presence of very low levels of "minimal residual disease" after treatment.

The WHO classification (Table 30.6) depends mainly on a combination of morphological (and cytological) criteria, combined with the use of immunological reagents to define cellular phenotype, a system that is aided by the availability of

TABLE 30.5. Chromosomal Tumor Translocations Associated with NHL

	Chromosomal Translocation	Proto-oncogene	Partner Gene
B-cell NHL			
LPL	t (9;14) (q13;q32)	PAX-5	IgH
FL, DLCL	t (14;18) (q32;q11)	BCL-2	IgH
	t (2;18) (q11;q11)	BCL-2	IgK
	t (18;22) (q11;q11)	BCL-2	Ig λ
DLCL	t (3;X) (q27;X)	BCL-6	IgH, IgL
BL	t (8;14) (q24;q32)	C-myc	IgH
	t (8;2) (p11;924)	C-myc	IgK
	t (8;22) (924;932)	C-myc	Ig λ
MCL	t (11;14) (q13;q32)	BCL-1	IgH
T-cell NHL			
CD30+ ALCL	t (2;5) (q23;q35)	ALK	—
CTCL	der (10) (924)	Lyt-10	X

Abbreviations: LPL, lymphoplasmacytoid lymphoma; MCL, mantle cell lymphoma; FL, follicular lymphoma; DLCL, diffuse large cell lymphoma; BL, Burkitt's lymphoma; ALCL, anaplastic large cell lymphoma; CTCL, cutaneous T-cell lymphoma

reliable reagents that can be used with paraffin-embedded tissue. Both lymphomas and lymphoid leukemias are included in this classification, because the distinction is an artificial one, and, in addition, Hodgkin's disease and plasma-cell myeloma are also included. The classification has been derived from experience in refining the reproducibility of morphological reporting based on the updated Kiel and REAL systems.

Although it would appear that the large number of disease entities defined by the WHO classification make clinical interpretation more difficult, it seems likely that real differences in the biology of lymphomas are being defined and, as a consequence, treatment decisions will be affected.

Treatment

A clinical schema can be derived from the WHO classification based on the clinical course of the respective entities and the results that can be expected from presently available treatment and modalities (Table 30.7). Although this allows a broad guide to therapy, there are considerable variations in treatment with respect to both individual disease and prognostic groupings.

The criteria for determining response in the treatment of NHL have been inconsistent between organizations and it has therefore proved difficult to make comparisons between trials conducted in different countries. Criteria for standardization have been published that establish important principles in the documentation of response (Table 30.8), although these currently address the recording of the anatomical extent of disease and do not take into account the use of flow-cytometric, cytogenetic, or molecular assays. The important standards established

TABLE 30.6. WHO Classification of Lymphoid Neoplasms

B-cell neoplasms

Precursor B-cell neoplasm

Precursor B-lymphoblastic leukemia/lymphoma (precursor B-cell acute lymphoblastic leukemia)

Mature (peripheral) B-cell neoplasms

B-cell chronic lymphocytic leukemia/small lymphocytic lymphoma

B-cell prolymphocytic leukemia

Lymphoplasmocytic lymphoma

Splenic marginal zone b-cell lymphoma (± villous lymphocytes)

Hairy cell leukemia

Plasma cell myeloma / plasmacytoma

Extranodal marginal zone B-cell lymphoma of MALT type

Nodal marginal zone B-cell lymphoma (± monocytoid B cells)

Follicular lymphoma

Mantle-cell lymphoma

Diffuse large B-cell lymphoma

Mediastinal large B-cell lymphoma

Primary effusion lymphoma

Burkitt's lymphoma / Burkitt cell leukemia

T-cell and NK-cell neoplasms

Precursor T-cell neoplasm

Precursor T-lymphoblastic lymphoma / leukemia (precursor T-cell acute lymphoblastic leukemia)

Mature (peripheral) T-cell neoplasms

T-cell prolymphocytic leukemia

T-cell granular lymphocytic leukemia

Aggressive NK-cell leukemia

Adult T-cell lymphoma / leukemia (HTLV1+)

Extranodal NK /T-cell lymphoma, nasal type

Enteropathy-type T-cell lymphoma

Hepatosplenic gamma-delta T-cell lymphoma

Subcutaneous panniculits-like T-cell lymphoma

Mycosis fungoides / Sézary syndrome

Anaplastic large-cell lymphoma, T/ null cell, primary cutaneous type

Peripheral T-cell lymphoma, not otherwise characterized

Angioimmunoblastic T-cell lymphoma

Anaplastic large-cell lymphoma, T / null cell, primary systemic type

Hodgkin's lymphoma (Hodgkin's disease)

Nodular lymphocyte-predominant Hodgkin's lymphoma

Classical Hodgkin's lymphoma

Nodular sclerosis Hodgkin's lymphoma (grades 1 and 2)

Lymphocyte-rich classical Hodgkin's lymphoma

Mixed cellularity Hodgkin's lymphoma

Lymphocyte depletion Hodgkin's lymphoma

Abbreviations: HTLV+, human T-cell leukemia virus; MALT, mucosa-associated lymphoid tissue; NK, natural killer;

Neoplasms are grouped according to major clinical presentations (predominantly disseminated/leukemic, primary extranodal, predominantly nodal)

The more common entities are expressed in boldface.

TABLE 30.7. Proposed Clinical Schema for Malignancies of the Lymphoid System

B-Cell Lineage	T-Cell Lineage
I. *Indolent lymphomas (low risk)*	**I. *Indolent lymphomas (low risk)***
Chronic lymphocytic leukemia/small lymphocytic lymphoma	Large granular lymphocytic leukemia, T and NK cell types
Lymphoplasmacytic lymphoma immunocytoma	Mycosis fungoides/Sézary syndrome
Waldenström's macroglobulinemia	Smoldering and chronic adult T-cell leukemia/lymphoma
Hairy cell leukemia	
Splenic marginal zone lymphoma	
Marginal zone B-cell lymphoma	
Extranodal (MALT-B-cell lymphoma)	
Nodal (monocytoid)	
Follicle center lymphoma/follicular (small cell)-grade 1	
Follicle center lymphoma/follicular (mixed small and large cell)-grade II	
II. *Aggressive lymphomas (intermediate risk)*	**II. *Aggressive lymphomas (intermediate risk)***
Prolymphocytic leukemia	Prolymphocytic leukemia
Plasmacytoma/multiple myeloma	Peripheral T-cell lymphoma, unspecified
Mantle cell lymphoma	Angioimmunoblastic lymphoma
Follicle center lymphoma/follicular, (large cell)-grade III	Angiocentric lymphoma
Diffuse large B-cell lymphoma (includes immunoblastic and diffuse large and centroblastic lymphoma)	Intestinal T-cell lymphoma
	Anaplastic large cell lymphoma (T- and null cell type)
Primary mediastinal (thymic) large B-cell lymphoma	
High grade B-cell lymphoma, Burkitt-like	
III. *Very aggressive lymphomas (high risk)*	**III. *Very aggressive lymphomas (high risk)***
Precursor B-lymphoblastic lymphoma/ leukemia	Precursor T-lymphoblastic lymphoma/leukemia
Burkitt's lymphoma/B-cell acute leukemia	Adult T-cell lymphoma/leukemia
Plasma cell leukemia	

by their publication include the fact that normal lymph node size is <1.5 cm in the greatest diameter on CT scan, whereas spleen size cannot be reliably graded so that it should be impalpable to examination with resolution of nodules on imaging; bone marrow involvement should be assessed by adequate trephine biopsy (≥ 20 mm core) with resolution of any infiltrate by morphological (but not other) criteria. The concept of complete response (CR)/unconfirmed (CRu) is defined as for CR but

TABLE 30.8. Response Criteria for Non-Hodgkin's Lymphoma

Response	Physical Examination	Lymph Nodes	Lymph Node Masses	Bone Marrow
CR	Normal	Normal	Normal	Normal
CRu	Normal	Normal	Normal	Indeterminate
	Normal	Normal	>75% decrease	Normal or indeterminate
PR	Normal	Normal	Normal	Positive
	Normal	≥ 50% decrease	≥ 50% decrease	Irrelevant
	Decrease in liver/spleen	≥ 50% decrease	≥ 50% decrease	Irrelevant
Relapse/ progression	Enlarging liver/ spleen; new sites	New or increased	New or increased	Reappearance

with a residual lymph node mass despite reduction >75% or an indeterminate marrow biopsy containing lymphoid aggregates that are not cytologically atypical.

INDOLENT (LOW RISK) LYMPHOMAS

Chronic Lymphocytic Leukemia/Small Lymphocytic Lymphoma

These conditions have been traditionally managed by observation only in the early stages or involved field radiotherapy. Alkylator (chlorambucil or cyclophosphamide) therapy is used for later stages, and anthracycline (CAP, CHOP, POACH) based combinations for advanced disease. There is strong evidence to suggest that purine analogues (fludarabine, cladribine) are more active as both second-line treatment and initial therapy, but they are contraindicated in patients with concurrent autoimmune hemolytic anemia. Combination purine analogue/alkylator therapy may be used as salvage therapy.

Waldenström's Macroglobulinemia

Purine analogues are considerably more active than alkylating agents in this condition.

Hairy Cell Leukemia

The use of α interferon has largely been supplanted by short courses of pentostatin or single 5–7 day infusions of cladribine.

Marginal Zone Lymphoma

Gastric MALT lymphoma at early/localized stages and with low-grade histology may regress with anti-*Helicobacter* therapy alone but requires close endoscopic surveillance; alkylator-based cytotoxic treatment may be needed for more extensive or unresponsive lesions. Of interest, involved-field radiotherapy is universally curative.

Follicle Center Lymphoma

The pattern of response to therapy followed by repeated relapse with an increasing risk of transformation to higher grade disease at each recurrence has resulted in the view that not all patients benefit from therapy immediately after they are diagnosed. When treatment is required, initial therapy usually consists of alkylator-based approaches, although patients with true stage I or II disease may be cured by involved-field radiotherapy. The duration of response may be increased by α interferon maintenance. Later recurrences associated with transformation to higher grade disease are usually managed by anthracycline-containing combinations (e.g., CHOP). Purine analogues are active as single agents and extremely active in combination therapy (e.g., FMD). The role of high-dose therapy with hemopoietic stem cell support is being evaluated in younger patients. There is evidence that active immunotherapeutic agents such as rituximab (anti-CD20) may have a role as single agents in chemorefractory disease or in combination with chemotherapy earlier in the course of the disorder. Radioimmunotherapeutic compounds in which a monoclonal antibody (such as 2B8 anti-CD20) is used to deliver a radioisotope (such as ^{131}I or ^{90}Y) are currently under evaluation.

Mycosis Fungoides/Sézary Syndrome (CTCL)

Localized disease is managed with topical therapy (steroids, mustine), whereas more extensive involvement may respond to PUVA (phototherapy plus UVA). In disease refractory to the above approaches but still localized, total skin electron beam irradiation (TSEB) may still be curative, however this does not apply to more extensive cutaneous involvement. Once the condition has progressed to tumor stage or erythrodermic forms, it is likely to require a combination of cytotoxic chemotherapy and either retinoids or interferon. Single agents with activity include methotrexate, chlorambucil, cyclophosphamide, fludarabine, cladribine, and pentostatin whereas conventional combinations such as CHOP have also been used. When the disease has progressed to the point where cells are found in the circulation (Sézary syndrome), responses may still be obtained by the use of extracorporeal photochemotherapy.

Smoldering/Chronic ATLL

Disease that is truly clinically unaggressive may be treated with a combination of zidovudine and α interferon while immunotherapeutic agents (anti-Tac) may also be active. The majority of patients treated in this way relapse and require more conventional cytotoxic therapy in conjunction with treatment to the CNS and aggressive control of hypercalcemia.

AGGRESSIVE (INTERMEDIATE RISK) LYMPHOMAS

Prolymphocytic Leukemias (B or T Cell)

These are generally refractory to alkylating agents but may respond to purine analogues. Immunotherapeutic agents such as alemtuzumab (Campath 1-H) (anti-CD52) appear promising.

Mantle Cell Lymphoma (MCL)

Even with modern therapy, MCL is probably the NHL that has the poorest survival. Most patients are initially managed with alkylator-based combinations, and the contribution of anthracyclines is uncertain. Trials are currently evaluating the early use of high-dose therapy with stem cell transplantation, although preliminary results do not demonstrate that this prevents relapse. Maintenance therapy with α interferon may prolong the duration of response.

Follicle Center Cell Lymphoma (Large Cell Type)

Study results suggesting that initial cyclophosphamide/anthracycline-based combination chemotherapy can achieve high response rates with long remission durations have not been confirmed by all investigators. The prognosis of these patients may prove to be more reliably predicted by the criteria of the International Prognostic Index than by histological selection alone.

Diffuse Large B-cell Lymphoma (DLCL)

A useful stratification can be made between patients whose condition is associated with a high rise of CNS disease (lymphoblastic lymphoma, Burkitt's lymphoma, aggressive HTLV1 + ATLL, and HIV-related lymphomas) who should be treated as having very aggressive lymphomas and other patients. For those with no strong risk of spread to the CNS, combination chemotherapy is the initial approach to treatment, and the large number of combinations promoted over the last 15 years have failed to produce results that are consistently better than those that can be achieved with CHOP for patients with low or low/intermediate risk disease. There are preliminary data to suggest that the results of chemotherapy can be improved by concurrent administration of therapeutic antibodies (rituximab).

Standard CHOP for High-Grade NHL

Patients with identifiably worse prognostic features, such as high-intermediate and high-risk IPI, have been evaluated to see whether they will benefit from intensified but conventional chemotherapy (Table 30.9) or high-dose therapy with stem-cell transplantation and in the younger patient population there is a survival advantage associated with early autotransplantation. Once a patient has failed initial

TABLE 30.9. Standard CHOP for High-Grade NHL

Cyclophosphamide	750 mg/m² i.v.		
Doxorubicin	50 mg/m² i.v.	Day 1	Repeated every 21 days
Vincristine	1.4 mg/m² (max 2 mg i.v.)		
Prednisolone	100 mg p.o. daily	Days 1–5	

chemotherapy, the outlook is poor; salvage therapy with etoposide or cisplatin-based combinations may be effective, but high-dose treatment is only likely to benefit those who are still at least partially sensitive to conventional-dose treatment.

Primary Mediastinal (Thymic) Large B-Cell Lymphoma

The initial management with conventional anthracycline-based combination chemotherapy commonly results in residual radiological abnormalities that may or may not represent active disease. Consolidation therapy with radiotherapy is frequently given.

Peripheral T-Cell Lymphoma/Angioimmunoblastic Lymphoma/ Angiocentric Lymphoma

These high-grade T-cell lymphomas are generally accepted to respond less well to conventional chemotherapy than the equivalent B-cell tumors.

Intestinal T-cell lymphoma

Conventional combination chemotherapy should be supplemented by gluten withdrawal for those patients whose disease arises on a background of celiac disease.

Anaplastic Large Cell Lymphoma (CD30⁺)

This was initially considered to be a very aggressive form of lymphoma, but this is not the case. Childhood disease has a better prognosis than that in adults and isolated cutaneous lesions are more responsive than nodal presentation. Lymphomatoid papulosis is a morphologically identifiable part of the spectrum of CD30⁺ cutaneous lymphoproliferative disorders, which characteristically undergo spontaneous resolution.

Primary CNS Lymphoma (HIV⁺)

The differential diagnosis of AIDS-related CNS lymphoma involves careful exclusion of infection (e.g., toxoplasmosis) and, even when biopsy material is available, the prognosis is poor. Good symptom control can be achieved with cranial irradiation, but survival is short; meningeal involvement may be treated with intrathecal methotrexate and/or cytosine arabinoside. Systemic cytotoxic agents with the capacity to cross the blood-brain barrier include idarubicin, high-dose methotrexate, high-dose cytosine arabinoside, nitrosoureas, and dexamethasone.

VERY AGGRESSIVE (HIGH RISK) LYMPHOMAS

Lymphoblastic Lymphomas (LL)/Acute Lymphoblastic Leukemia (ALL)/Burkitt's Lymphoma

These conditions are neoplasms arising from precursor cells at various stages of differentiation in both T- and B-cell lineages. Particular management problems at presentation may include anatomical complications of the presence of a large mediastinal mass or extensive intra-abdominal disease and metabolic consequences of uric acid nephropathy. Induction therapy tended to follow the pattern of treatment used for ALL, with full CNS prophylaxis involving intrathecal therapy and cranial irradiation but shortened courses of chemotherapy featuring dose-intensification, particularly by the inclusion of high-dose methotrexate, high-dose cytarabine, ifosfamide, and etoposide. With this therapy, adults have achieved results that are nearly as good as those seen in pediatric practice. Consolidation with autologous bone marrow transplantation has been widely used. The prognosis of disease associated with t(9;22) and t(4;11) is so poor that allogeneic transplantation is felt to offer the only chance of cure.

HODGKIN'S DISEASE

Epidemiology, Etiology, and Pathogenesis

Hodgkin's disease (HD) is an uncommon malignancy with incidence rates ranging between 1 and 4/100,000, except in Asian countries where it is much less common. There is an unusual age pattern, with a bimodal curve showing peaks at ages 15–40 and over 55 years. Overall, HD is more common in males than females, but there is little difference for the nodular sclerosing subtype, which also lacks the association with EBV infections of Reed-Sternberg cells—a feature of cases in children from lower socioeconomic groups. Considerable effort has gone into exploring an infectious etiology for HD, but, despite strong circumstantial evidence, a direct causative relationship has not been established.

Although HD classically has a low proportion of the clonal, malignant Reed-Sternberg (RS) cells, the immunophenotype of lymphocyte predominant (LP) HD is frequently associated with B-cell markers, and the RS cells may show rearrangements of the IgH locus, implying a B-cell germinal-center origin for these cases. The classical features of the other types of HD are variably associated with impaired immune response, sclerosis, T-cell activation and proliferation, plasmacytosis, and eosinophilia, all of which suggest a condition of abnormal cytokine production. There are proposals that the tissue eosinophilia may contribute to unregulated growth by providing ligands for CD30 and CD40, which can stimulate the RS cell.

Clinical Presentation, Investigation, and Staging

The diagnosis of HD is made after peripheral lymph node biopsy in over 90% of cases. The characteristic symptoms consist of weight loss, fever, sweats, and itching, but these are much less common in patients with localized disease (8% in stage I, 29% in stage II) than in extensive disease (41% in stage III, 71% in stage IV).

Investigations have been designed to define the anatomical extent of disease so that the appropriate treatment decision can be taken in relation to radiotherapy for localized disease or chemotherapy for more extensive disease. Although the detailed information provided by staging laparotomy has contributed greatly to knowledge of the natural history of HD, it is not now felt to be justified. Radiological investigation with lymphangiography has also been replaced by the use of CT imaging of the abdomen and thorax, although this approach may fail to detect splenic involvement. The yield of bone marrow biopsy in disease likely to be stage I and II is very low, but it is advisable in patients with extensive (stage III or IV) involvement by other criteria. Laboratory investigations are principally of use in following the response to treatment, where correction of abnormal erythrocyte sedimentation rate (ESR) or lactate dehydrogenase (LDH) may confirm resolution of disease whereas persistence of elevated levels may prompt a careful search for residual disease.

The well-established Ann Arbor system has been revised to clarify some aspects relating to the distribution of disease and the implications of large areas of involvement (Table 30.10).

Classification and Diagnostic Methods

It is now clear that HD is a clonal proliferation of (in most cases) B cells.

WHO Classification of Hodgkin's Disease

The WHO classifies HD as follows:

- Nodular lymphocyte predominance (LP)
- Classical HD
- Nodular sclerosis (grades 1 and 2)
- Lymphocyte-rich, classic disease
- Mixed cellularity
- Lymphocyte depletion (LD)

Although LP HD is a rare entity, its B-cell origin, high initial response rate, and occasional capacity for very late relapse are characteristic of the natural history.

TABLE 30.10. The Ann Arbor Staging System/Cotswold's Revision

Stage	Characteristics
I	Involvement of a single lymph node region or of a single extranodal organ or site (IE)
II	Involvement of two or more lymph node regions on the same side of the diaphragm or localized involvement of an extranodal organ or site (IIE) and one or more lymph node regions on the same side of the diaphragm. R and L hilum regarded as one area, each independent of mediastinum
III	Involvement of lymph node regions on both sides of the diaphragm, which may be accompanied by involvement of the spleen (IIIS) or by localized contignous involvement of only one extranodal organ site (IIIE) or both (IIIES)
III1	With involvement limited to spleen, hilar portal, or celiac nodes
III2	With involvement of para-aortic, iliac, or mesenteric nodes.
IV	Diffuse or disseminated involvement of one or more distant extranodal sites with or with or without associated lymph node involvement
Bulky disease	Mediastinum/thoracic ratio >1:3 at the T5-6 level; mass >10 cm
Subclassification	
A	No symptoms
B	Fever, night sweats, weight loss >10% of body weight over 6 months

The distinction from T-cell rich B-cell lymphoma (a form of NHL) may be very difficult. The natural history of LD HD is also established as being more aggressive than other types of HD, and differentiation between this subtype and anaplastic large cell lymphoma may cause problems unless the t(2;5) translocation characteristic of that form of NHL is detected. Nodular sclerosis histology is strongly correlated with young age, female gender, and clinical presentation with mediastinal involvement and has a favorable prognosis, especially in early-stage disease. Grading of the histological appearances according to the numbers of RS cells (few = grade 1, many = grade 2) has shown conflicting results, with some studies showing a poorer outcome for grade 2 disease and others showing no difference. Mixed cellularity is more frequently associated with extralymphatic spread and has a worse prognosis.

Treatment

The early experience of successful treatment of patients with HD by either radiotherapy or combination chemotherapy has been affected by the appreciation that increases in the aggressiveness of management were causing immediate and delayed toxicities that were not balanced by an improvement in survival. It also became clear that the efficacy of salvage therapy, especially in patients initially treated with radiotherapy alone, would achieve durable responses in many patients with relapsed disease.

TABLE 30.11. BEACOPP II for Hodgkin's Disease

Cyclophosphamide	650 mg/m^2	Day 1	
Doxorubicin	25 mg/m^2	Day 1	
Etoposide	100 mg/m^2	Days 1–3	Repeated every 21 days,
Procarbazine	100 mg/m^2	Days 1–7	with granuclocyte-colony-
Prednisone	40 mg/m^2	Days 1–14	stimulating factor
Vincristine	1.4 mg/m^2	Day 8	support if required
	(max 2 mg)		
Bleomycin	10 mg/m^2	Day 8	

Stage I and II patients without additional adverse prognostic factors (B symptoms, bulky disease including mediastinal involvement, large number of sites, age >50 years) have a low risk of occult abdominal disease and may be treated with radiotherapy to a mantle field alone. Although up to 40% of those staged clinically (i.e., without laparotomy) may relapse eventually, many of these patients will obtain further complete remissions with chemotherapy, whereas those continuing to be free of disease after radiotherapy alone will have preserved their fertility and have a low risk of secondary malignancy. Second solid tumors (e.g., lung, stomach, breast) are more common after extended-field radiotherapy.

Those patients with stage IA or IIA disease and adverse prognostic factors will require combined chemoradiotherapy, and, in a typical presentation such as a young woman with bulky mediastinal NS HD, treatment will consist of four cycles of combination chemotherapy followed by radiotherapy to 40 Gy to at least the area of bulky disease.

The nature of the chemotherapy administered to patients with either symptomatic or more extensive disease (IIB, III, IV) now generally reflects a compromise between effective eradication of HD and severe late toxicity. The association of older alkylator-based (MOPP type) chemotherapy with infertility and the induction of secondary acute leukemias has led to the wider use of anthracycline-containing single, alternating or "hybrid" combinations. Dose-and time-intensive schedules such as the German Study Group's BEACOPP (Table 3.11) regimen and the American Stanford V (Table 30.12) produce very high response rates but there are concerns about the rate of secondary leukemia or myelodysplasia. An analysis of the pattern of recurrence after chemotherapy has led many groups to follow chemotherapy by radiotherapy to initial sites of bulky disease.

Salvage therapy after failure of initial chemotherapy exploits the steep dose-response curve that HD has for many chemotherapeutic agents. Cytoreduction

TABLE 30.12. Standard ABVD for Hodgkin's Disease

Doxorubicin	25 mg/m^2	
Bleomycin	10 mg/m^2	Days 1 and 14, repeated every 28 days
Vinblastine	6 mg/m^2	
Dacarbazine	375 mg/m^2	

using non-cross-reactive agents (such as combinations with etoposide and/or vinorelbine) can be followed by high-dose chemotherapy (e.g., BEAM) supported by hemopoietic stem cells. As with the salvage of NHL, retention of some degree of response to conventional-dose chemotherapy is a prerequisite for achieving worthwhile responses.

FURTHER READING

The text has been prepared from a large number of published sources; the following list contains key papers that form a reading list for those wishing to extend their knowledge.

Alizaden A, Eisen M, Davis RE et al. (2000) Distinct types of diffuse B-cell lymphoma identified by gene expression profiling. *Nature* 403:503–511.

Bartlett NL, Rosenberg SA, Hoppe RT et al. (1995) Brief chemotherapy, Stanford V, and adjuvant radiotherapy for bulky or advanced-stage Hodgkin's disease: a preliminary report. *J Clin Oncol* 13:1080–1088.

Biti GP, Cimino G, Cartoni C et al. (1992) Extended-field radiotherapy is superior to MOPP chemotherapy for the treatment of pathological stage I-IIA Hodgkin's disease: eight-year update of an Italian prospective randomised study. *J Clin Oncol* 10:378–382.

Cheson BD, Horning SJ, Coiffier B et al. (1999) Report of an International Workshop to standardize response criteria for non-Hodgkin's lymphoma. *J Clin Oncol* 17:1244–1253.

Chopra R, McMillan AK, Linch DC et al. (1993) The place of high-dose BEAM therapy and autologous bone marrow transplantation in poor-risk Hodgkin's disease. A single-centre eight-year study of 155 patients. *Blood* 81:1137–1145.

Deangelis LM (1995) Current management of primary central nervous system lymphoma. *Oncology (Huntingt)* 9:63–71.

Diehl V, Sieber M, Ruffer V et al. (1997) BEACOPP: An intensified chemotherapy regimen in advanced Hodgkin's disease. *Ann Oncol* 8:143–148.

Fisher RI, Gaynor ER, Dahlberg S et al. (1993) Comparison of a standard regimen (CHOP) with three intensive chemotherapy regimens for advanced non-Hodgkin's lymphoma. *N Engl J Med* 328:1002–1006.

Gisselbrecht C, Gaulard P, LePage E et al. (1998) Prognostic significance of T-cell phenotype in aggressive non-Hodgkin's lymphomas. Groupe d'Etudes des Lymphomes de l'Adulte (GELA). *Blood* 92: 76–72.

Gribben JG, Saporito L, Barber M et al. (1992) Bone marrows of non-Hodgkin's lymphoma patients with a Bcl-2 translocation can be purged of polymerase chain reaction-detectable lymphoma cells using monoclonal antibodies and immunomagnetic bead depletion. *Blood* 80:1083–1089.

Haioun C, LePage E, Gisselbrecht C et al. (2000) Survival benefit of high-dose therapy in poor-risk aggressive non-Hodgkin's lymphoma: Final analysis of the prospective LNH 87-2 protocol – A Groupe d'Etudes des Lymphomes de l'Adulte study. *J Clin Oncol* 18:3025–3030.

Haluska FG, Brufsky AM, Cannellos GP (1994) The cellular biology of the Reed-Sternberg cell. *Blood* 84:1005–1019.

Harris NL, Jaffe ES, Diebold J et al. (1999) The World Health Organization Classification of neoplastic diseases of the hematopoietic and lymphoid tissues. Report of the Clinical

Advisory Committee meeting, Airlie House, Virginia, November 1997. *Ann Oncol* 10:1419–1432.

International Non-Hodgkin's Lymphomas Prognostic Factors Project (1993) A predictive model for aggressive non-Hodgkin's lymphoma. *N Engl J Med* 329:987–994.

Johnson SA (1996) Purine analogues in the management of lymphoproliferative diseases. *Clin Oncol* 8:289–296.

Jox A, Rohen C, Belge C et al. (1997) Integration of Epstein-Barr virus in Burkitt's lymphoma cells leads to a region of enchanced chromosome instability. *Ann Oncol* 8(suppl 2):S131–S135.

LeBlond V, Dhedin N, Mamzer Bruneel MF et al. (2001) Identification of prognostic factors in 61 patients with post-transplantation Lymphoproliferative disorders. *J Clin Oncol* 19:772–778.

Mac-Manus MP, Hoppe RT (1996) Is radiotherapy curative for stage I and II low-grade follicular lymphoma? Results of a long-term follow-up study of patients treated at Stanford University. *J Clin Oncol* 14:1282–1290.

Magrath I, Adde M, Shad A et al. (1996) Adults and children with small non-cleaved cell lymphoma have a similar excellent outcome when treated with the same chemotherapy regimen. *J Clin Oncol* 14:925–934.

Mauvieux L, MacIntyre EA (1996) Practical role of molecular diagnostics in non-Hodgkin's lymphomas. *Baillière's Clin Haematol* 9:653–667.

McLaughlin P, Grillo-López AJ, Link BK et al. (1998) Rituximab chimeric anti-CD20 monoclonal antibody therapy for relapsed indolent lymphoma: half of patients respond to a four-dose program. *J Clin Oncol* 16:2825–2833.

McLaughlin P, Hagemeister FB, Romaguera JE et al. (1996) Fludarabine, mitoxantrone and dexamethasone: an effective new regimen for indolent lymphoma. *J Clin Oncol* 14:1262–1268.

Morel P, Lepage E, Brice P et al. (1992) Prognosis and treatment of lymphoblastic lymphoma in adults: a report on 80 patients. *J Clin Oncol* 10:1078–1085.

Morgan G, Vornanen M, Puitinen J et al. (1997) Changing trends in the incidence of non-Hodgkin's lymphoma in Europe. *Ann Oncol* 8(suppl 2):S49–S54.

Nador RG, Cesarman E, Chadburn A et al. (1996) Primary effusion lymphoma: a distinct clincopathological entity associated with the Kaposi's sarcoma associated herpes virus. *Blood* 88:645–656.

Press OW, Eary JF, Appelbaum FR et al. (1995) Phase II trial of[131]I-B1 (anti-CD20) antibody therapy with autologous stem cell transplantation for relapsed B-cell lymphomas. *Lancet* 346:336–340.

Rohatiner A (1994) Report on a workshop convened to discuss the pathological and staging classifications of gastrointestinal tract lymphoma. *Ann Oncol* 5:397–400.

Siegel RS, Pandolfino T, Guitart J et al. (2000) Primary cutaneous T-cell lymphoma: review and current concepts. *J Clin Oncol* 18:2908–2925.

Velasquez WS, Cabanillas F, Salvador P et al. (1998) Effective salvage therapy for lymphoma with cisplatin in combination with high-dose ara-C and dexamethasone (DHAP). *Blood* 71:117–122.

Zucca E, Stein H, Coiffier B on behalf of the European Lymphoma Task Force (1994) Report on the workshop on Mantle cell lymphoma. *Ann Oncol* 5:507–511.

CHAPTER 31

The Leukemias

FREDERICK R. APPELBAUM

The Fred Hutchinson Cancer Research Center and the University of
Washington School of Medicine, Seattle, Washington

Normal hematopoiesis requires the controlled proliferation and orderly differentiation of pluripotent hematopoietic stem cells to become mature peripheral blood cells. Leukemia is the result of a genetic event or series of events occurring in a hematopoietic precursor causing the affected cell and its progeny to no longer proliferate and differentiate normally.

The leukemias are broadly categorized according to the normal cell population they most resemble (i.e., myeloid versus lymphoid) and according to their clinical aggressiveness (Table 31.1). In the case of the acute leukemias, the malignant event occurs in a very early hematopoietic precursor. The altered cells continue to proliferate but fail to differentiate, resulting in the rapid accumulation of immature myeloid (in acute myeloid leukemia) or lymphoid (in acute lymphoid leukemia) cells in the marrow. These cells replace normal bone marrow, resulting in the diminished production of normal red cells, white cells, and platelets, which, in turn, gives rise to the usual manifestations of acute leukemia, including anemia, infection, and bleeding. The leukemic cells also escape into the bloodstream and occupy the lymph nodes, spleen, and other vital organs. The acute leukemias are rapidly fatal if left untreated, with most patients dying within several months of diagnosis. The chronic leukemias are also clonal malignancies of hematopoietic cells but the malignant cells are able to differentiate in a more nearly normal manner. Accordingly, these disorders are characterized by the overproliferation of relatively mature cells, which resemble normal neutrophils (in chronic myeloid leukemia), normal lymphocytes (in chronic lymphocytic leukemia), normal red cells (in polycythemia vera), or normal platelets (in essential thrombocythemia).

This work is supported, in part, by grant number CA-18029 from the National Cancer Institute, National Institutes of Health, Department of Health and Humen Services.

UICC Manual of Clinical Oncology, Eighth Edition. Edited by Raphael E. Pollock
ISBN 0-471-22289-5 Copyright © 2004 John Wiley & Sons, Inc.

TABLE 31.1. The Leukemias

Acute leukemia
   Acute myeloid leukemia
   Acute lymphocytic leukemia
Chronic leukemia
   Chronic myeloid leukemia
   Chronic lymphocytic leukemia
Myelodysplastic syndromes
Chronic myeloproliferative disorders
   Polycythemia vera
   Essential thrombocythemia
   Agnogenic myeloid metaplasia
Hairy cell leukemia

Even untreated, patients can live for several years with these disorders. However, with time, the accumulation of abnormal cells results in lack of production of normal cells. In addition, the malignant clones are genetically unstable and accumulate additional genetic abnormalities, resulting in the eventual progression to a disorder that more closely resembles acute leukemia.

ETIOLOGY AND EPIDEMIOLOGY

Epidemiology

The annual incidence of leukemia is approximately 8–10 new cases per 100,000. The relative incidences of the four most common forms of leukemia are as follows: acute lymphocytic leukemia (ALL), 11%; chronic lymphocytic leukemia (CLL), 29%; acute myeloid leukemia (AML), 40%; and chronic myelogenous leukemia (CML), 14%. Males are more commonly affected than females. These incidence rates have been fairly stable over the last 30 years. ALL is the most common leukemia seen in childhood and shows the least increase in age. All other forms of leukemia are relatively uncommon in children and increase in incidence with age, particularly beyond age 50. In general, there are not marked variations in leukemic incidence among countries, although CLL is reported to be less frequent in the Asian population. In the large majority of cases, no cause of leukemia can be found, but in occasional cases, a likely reason can be identified.

Genetic Predisposition

There is an approximately one in five chance that a child will develop leukemia if they have an identical twin with leukemia diagnosed before age 10. Several rare familial syndromes with a high incidence of leukemia have been identified, including an autosomal dominant syndrome of thrombocytopenia and AML associated with mutations in the gene AML1. An increased incidence of leukemia exists in patients with autosomal recessive disorders associated with chromosomal instability, including Fanconi's anemia, Bloom's syndrome, and ataxic telangiectasia. Also, patients with congenital immunodeficiency disorders, including infantile X-linked agammaglobulinemia and Down's syndrome, have a higher than expected incidence of leukemia.

Viruses

An uncommon form of leukemia, adult T-cell leukemia (ATL), is associated with human T-cell lymphotrophic virus type 1 (HTLV-1). The virus is common in southwestern Japan, the Caribbean basin, and Africa and can be spread by sexual contact, blood transfusions, and from mother to fetus. Approximately, 1–2% of those infected with HTLV-1 will develop ATL, usually after a very long latency period of 10–30 years. Blood banks in the United States now routinely screen for HTLV-1. Rare cases of an unusual chronic lymphoid leukemia have been linked with a second human retrovirus, HTLV-2.

Radiation

Previous studies showed that the incidences of AML, ALL, and CML, but not CLL, were increased in patients given radiation therapy for ankylosing spondylitis, in radiologists practicing when shielding was inadequate and in survivors of the atomic bomb in Hiroshima and Nagasaki. The increased incidence of leukemia starts several years after exposure, appears to peak at 5–10 years, and then diminishes. A number of studies have asked whether exposure to low-frequency, nonionizing electromagnetic fields increases the risk of leukemia, and most have failed to find any association.

Chemicals and Drug Exposure

Heavy exposure to benzene and benzene-containing solvents such as kerosene can cause marrow damage leading to myelodysplasia or AML. There is a suggested link between heavy exposure to pesticides and an increased chance of developing CLL. Prior exposure to alkylating agents such as chlorambucil, nitrogen mustard, and melphalan increases the risk of developing AML. Such secondary leukemias often present initially as a myelodysplastic syndrome 4–7 years after exposure and are associated with abnormalities of chromosomes 5 and 7. Exposure to the epipodophyllotoxins teniposide or etoposide increases the risk for developing AML with abnormalities of 11q23. These cases develop after a shorter period, 2–3 years, lack a myelodysplastic prodrome, and often have a monocytic morphology.

ACUTE MYELOID LEUKEMIA

Biology

Pathophysiology AML, like all leukemias, is a clonal disorder with all leukemic cells developing from a single precursor. The precise molecular events causing malignant transformation in AML are not completely understood but result in the uncontrolled proliferation of immature hematopoietic cells that have lost the ability to differentiate. Several lines of evidence suggest that the development of overt leukemia is a multistep process, including the fact that, in many cases, AML is preceded by a prolonged myelodysplastic disorder, and the observation that, following chemotherapy, some patients enter a complete remission devoid of obvious malignant cells but with clonal hematopoiesis. Experiments in which selected AML cells are injected into immunodeficient mice suggest that, in most cases, the AML stem cell capable of engraftment is found in the relatively primitive $CD34^+$ $CD38^-$ cell fraction. The leukemic cells are often able to differentiate, albeit abnormally. As the malignant clone expands, normal hematopoiesis fails. The reasons for this are complex, but both actual physical replacement of normal precursors as well as release of soluble substances by leukemic cells that suppress normal hematopoiesis are thought to play important roles.

Classification AML is generally classified according to cell morphology but is also classified according to cell surface markers and cytogenetics. AML is usually classified according to the French-American-British (FAB) system, which subdivides AML into eight subtypes according to morphology and histochemistry (Table 31.2). AML cells are typically 12–15 μm in diameter with discreet nuclear chromatin, multiple nucleoli, and cytoplasmic azurophilic granules. Subtypes M0 through M3 reflect increasing degrees of maturation, M4 and M5 AML have some degree of monocytic differentiation, M6 leukemia has features of erythroid lineage, and M7 is acute megakaryocytic leukemia. FAB types M1–M4 contain myeloperoxidase whereas M4 and M5 have the monocytic enzyme, nonspecific esterase. These morphologic subtypes have some, but only limited, clinical relevance. The most distinct subgroup is M3 AML (also called acute promyelocytic leukemia), which is usually associated with the t(15;17) and responds well to all-*trans* retinoic acid or arsenic trioxide. Complete response rates and overall survival are best with M2, M3, and M4 AML. Patients with M6 AML may have a smoldering course. Antibodies reactive with cell-surface antigens can be used to help diagnose and classify AML. Most cases of AML react with antibodies specific for CD13, CD14, CD33, and CD34. M6 AML reacts with antibodies against glycophorin, whereas M7 AML cells react with antibodies against CD41, also known as GpIIb/IIIa.

AML can also be characterized by the clonal chromosomal abnormality seen in each case. Such abnormalities are the most powerful prognostic factors available in this disease, have provided insights into the mechanisms of leukemogenesis, and, in some cases, suggest specific therapeutic approaches. Favorable clinical outcomes have been associated with t(15;17), t(8;21), and inv(16). The t(15;17) abnormality associated with acute promyelocytic leukemia (APL) results in the fusion of a transcription factor (PML) on chromosome 15 with the alpha retinoic acid receptor gene (RARα) on chromosome 17. Patients with this disorder respond well to anthracyclines combined with all-*trans* retinoic acid. The t(8;21) abnormality and the inv(16) alteration both result in disruption of the normal formation of the heterodimeric transcription factor CBF, t(8;21) by altering CBFα and inv(16) by

TABLE 31.2. Classification of Acute Myeloid Leukemia (AML)

Subtype	Morphology	Histochemistry			Monoclonal Reactivity	Cytogenetic Abnormalities
		Myeloperoxidase	Nonspecific Esterase	PAS		
M0—Acute undifferentiated leukemia	Uniform, very undifferentiated	—	—	—	For subtypes M0-M5b, approximately 90% of cases will react with at least one of the following anti-myeloid antibodies: anti-CD13, anti-CD14, anti-CD33, anti-CD34	Various
M1—AML with minimal differentiation	Very undifferentiated, few azurophilic granules	+/−	+/−	—		Various
M2—AML with differentiation	Granulated blasts predominate; Auer rods may be seen	+++	+/−	+		Various
M3—Acute promyelocytic leukemia	Hypergranular promyelocytes predominate	+++	+	+		t(15;17)
M4—Acute myelomono-cytic leukemia M4a	Both monoblasts and myeloblasts present Like M4 but with eosinophils	++	+++	++		Various inv/del(16)
M5—Acute monocytic leukemia M5a M5b	Monoblasts predominate Type a >80% monoblasts Type b >20% promonocytes	+/−	+++	++		Various, including t(9;11)
M6—Acute erythroleukemia	Erythroblasts and megaloblastic red cell precursors seen	—	—	++	Antiglycophorin, antispectrin	Various
M7—Acute megakaryocytic leukemia	Undifferentiated blasts	—	+/−	+	Antiplatelet GpIIb/IIIa	Various

695

altering CBFβ. Both forms of leukemia appear to respond well to repeated exposures to high-dose cytarabine. The majority of cases of AML are associated with $+8$, $-y$, $+6$, del 12p or have normal karyotypes. Such leukemias fall into the intermediate-risk group. Patients with leukemias characterized by loss of part or all of chromosomes 5 or 7, or leukemias characterized by complex karyotypes with three or more abnormalities, have a poor prognosis. Conventional chemotherapy rarely results in long-term success and so early allogeneic marrow transplantation should be considered for such patients.

Clinical Features

The signs and symptoms of AML are the result of decreased production of normal blood cells and invasion of leukemic blasts into normal organs. Most patients are anemic and thrombocytopenic at diagnosis, resulting in fatigue and pallor and, in at least one-third of patients, clinically evident bleeding, usually in the form of petechiae, ecchymoses, and bleeding gums. Most patients are also granulocytopenic and approximately one-third will have a significant infection at diagnosis. Occasional patients will present with extramedullary leukemic masses, termed chloromas, which are rubbery and fast-growing. Also, cutaneous involvement (leukemia cutis) and central nervous system (CNS) involvement are occasionally seen.

Laboratory Manifestations

Anemia is seen in most patients at diagnosis as is thrombocytopenia. Approximately 25% of patients will have severe thrombocytopenia ($<20,000/mm^3$). Most will be granulocytopenic, but the total white count may be very high ($>50,000/mm^3$) in 25%, moderately elevated (between 5,000 and $50,000/mm^3$) in 50%, or low ($<5,000/mm^3$) in 25%. Blasts are usually present in peripheral blood. The bone marrow is usually hypercellular and contains from 30–100% blasts. Sometimes, other findings are also present, including marrow fibrosis (in M7 AML) or, rarely, marrow necrosis.

Differential Diagnosis

Although there are sometimes difficulties in subclassifying leukemia, usually the diagnosis is straightforward. Aplastic anemia and myelodysplasia can result in peripheral pancytopenia but in neither are large numbers of blasts seen on marrow exam. Other small round cell neoplasms can infiltrate the marrow and sometimes mimic leukemia, but immunologic and cytogenetic markers now make these distinctions usually relatively easy. Leukemoid reactions can be seen in certain infections including tuberculosis but, although young myeloid cells may be seen in the peripheral blood in some settings, they virtually never reach 30%.

Treatment

Remission Induction AML is a rapidly progressive disease and, without treatment, most patients will die within several months of diagnosis. With appropriate therapy, however, many patients can now be cured. The first goal of treatment is to achieve an initial remission. Treatment with a combination of an anthracycline (daunomycin or idarubicin) and cytarabine can induce complete remissions in 60–80% of patients. In randomized studies, use of additional drugs such as etoposide or high-dose instead of conventional dose cytarabine have failed to improve the complete response rate. Profound myelosuppression is always seen following induction chemotherapy. The period of myelosuppression can be shortened by several days with the use of myeloid growth factors but their use has not been found to improve overall complete response rates.

Postremission Chemotherapy If no therapy is given after induction, the duration of remission will be short and most patients will relapse within 6 months. If, after achieving a complete remission, patients are treated with two to four courses of consolidation chemotherapy using an anthracycline and cytarabine at doses similar to those used for initial induction, the median survival in AML can be extended to approximately 18 months and 15–20% of patients can be cured. The best results achieved to date with postremission chemotherapy involves treating patients with repeated cycles of high-dose cytarabine. In one large, randomized trial, approximately 40% of patients treated with four cycles of high-dose cytarabine, 1.5 g/m^2 every 12 hours on days 1, 3, and 5, were alive and disease-free at 3 years. In a second trial, approximately 35% of patients treated with two cycles of high-dose cytarabine, 1 gm/m^2 every 12 hours on days 1–6 were alive and disease-free at 3 years. If patients are treated with intensive postremission chemotherapy, there is no clear role for the addition of low-dose maintenance or late intensification chemotherapy, or central nervous system prophylaxis.

Risk Factors A number of factors correlate with the likelihood of achieving an initial complete remission and with remission duration (Table 31.3). Younger patients, those with a low white count at diagnosis, without a prior hematologic disorder, and with blasts with t(8;21), inv(16) or t(15;17) do relatively well. Older patients, patients with high white counts at diagnosis, a prior history of

TABLE 31.3. Prognosis in Acute Myeloid Leukemia

Unfavorable	Favorable
Advanced age	Younger age
High WBC at diagnosis	Low WBC at diagnosis
Prior myelodysplasia	No prior myelodysplasia
MDR1 positive	MDR1 negative
Cytogenetics	Cytogenetics
Abnormalities of 5,7	t(8;21)
Complex karyotypes	t(15;17)
	inv(16)

Abbreviations: WBC, white blood count; MDR1, multi-drug resistance gene 1.

myelodysplasia and with blasts that express the multidrug resistance gene 1 (MDR1), with abnormalities of chromosomes 5 or 7, or with complex abnormalities, do worse.

Chemotherapy for Relapsed Patients Patients who relapse following chemotherapy can, in approximately 30–50% of cases, achieve a second remission, but the duration of such remissions tends to be short, on average 6 months. The longer the initial remission, the better the chance of achieving a second complete remission (CR). Younger patients and those with leukemia characterized by favorable cytogenetics also tend to do better.

Bone Marrow Transplantation High-dose chemotherapy with or without total body irradiation (TBI) followed by matched sibling bone marrow transplantation is often used to treat AML in patients older than age 55. For patients who fail to achieve an initial CR, allogeneic marrow transplantation offers the only realistic chance for a cure. Prior studies have shown that approximately 15–20% of such patients can be saved. Similarly, patients who have relapsed after chemotherapy and have failed reinduction can be cured with allogeneic transplantation in 15–20% of cases. The results improve if transplantation is carried out earlier in the course of disease, with success in approximately 30–35% of patients transplanted in first relapse or second remission and with 50–60% cure rates with matched sibling transplantation in first remission. Only about one-third of patients have matched siblings. For those without such donors, the use of autologous transplantation has been studied. The results of autologous transplantation have generally been slightly inferior to those achieved with matched sibling transplantation owing to a considerably higher risk of posttransplant relapse, although the immediate risks with autologous transplantation are less. Several large prospective studies have been conducted attempting to define the relative roles of allogeneic transplantation, autologous transplantation, and conventional chemotherapy in the treatment of patients less than age 55 with AML. Perhaps because of differences in trial design and conduct, the results of these studies have not been consistent. In general, however, most of the evidence would suggest that patients with favorable risk cytogenetics can be treated with conventional chemotherapy with transplantation reserved as salvage therapy. Patients with poor risk cytogenetics should probably be treated with allogeneic transplantation, if possible. The results are less clear for patients with intermediate cytogenetics. Most studies show at least a trend toward improved disease-free survival and overall survival with allogeneic transplantation. Autologous transplantation also seems to improve survival if carried out after patients have received intensive consolidation chemotherapy.

Acute Promyelocytic Leukemia Acute promyelocytic leukemia deserves special mention because of its increased sensitivity to therapy with all-*trans* retinoic acid (ATRA). ATRA alone induces complete responses in 75% of patients with APL. Unlike conventional chemotherapy, ATRA appears to work, at least in part, by inducing terminal differentiation of leukemic blasts. Within several days of starting ATRA, the coagulation disorders associated with APL begin to improve and the number of both abnormal and normal granulocytes begins to increase. Morphologic analysis of bone marrow over the first weeks of ATRA therapy shows progressive differentiation of malignant cells without hypoplasia. Complete remissions using ATRA alone generally take 2–3 months. Although ATRA alone can induce complete responses, virtually all patients treated with ATRA as a single agent will subsequently relapse. The combination of ATRA with anthracycline-containing chemotherapy appears more effective in inducing CR than the use of either agent alone. The best form of postremission therapy in APL is not entirely defined. Studies suggest that APL is particularly sensitive to anthracycline treatment and, thus, most experts recommend its inclusion during consolidation, whereas the role of high-dose cytarabine is more questionable. Several randomized studies suggest that ATRA maintenance prolongs disease-free survival.

A potentially dangerous side effect of ATRA is the development of a syndrome characterized by pulmonary infiltrates and shortness of breath. This ATRA syndrome is more commonly seen in patients who develop leukocytosis on ATRA and can be fatal. Patients who develop evidence of the ATRA syndrome should have ATRA temporarily discontinued and should be treated with Decadron. In the majority of patients, the syndrome will resolve and ATRA can be restarted. Other adverse effects of ATRA include skin and mucosal membrane dryness, headache, and bone pain.

Although the inclusion of ATRA has remarkably improved the outcome of patients with APL, 20–30% will develop ATRA-resistant disease. Recently, arsenic trioxide has been found to be effective in inducing CR in the majority of such patients.

ACUTE LYMPHOCYTIC LEUKEMIA

Biology

Like AML, ALL is a clonal proliferation of an early hematopoietic progenitor, but in contrast to AML, the ALL blasts resemble very early lymphoid cells. The FAB schema classifies ALL cases as being L1, L2, or L3 (Table 31.4). L1 blasts are uniform in size with scanty cytoplasm, indistinct nucleoli, and few, in any, granules. L2 blasts are larger and more heterogenous in size and may have nucleoli. L3 blasts are quite distinct with deeply basophilic cytoplasm containing vacuoles and with prominent nucleoli. ALL cases can also be categorized according to cell surface antigens. Approximately 60% of cases express CD10, also known as the common ALL antigen or CALLA. Such cases usually co-express early B-cell antigens such as CD19 and, thus, are thought to represent a very early B-cell differentiation state (a pre-pre B cell). About 20% of CALLA-positive cases also have intracytoplasmic immunoglobulin, suggesting a slightly greater differentiative state (pre B cell). Approximately 5% of cases express surface immunoglobulin, thus representing a more differentiated state (B cell ALL). Approximately 20% of cases of ALL are of

TABLE 31.4. Classification of Acute Lymphocytic Leukemia (ALL)

Subtype	Morphology	Histochemistry			Monoclonal Reactivity	Cytogenetic Abnormalities
		Myeloperoxidase	Nonspecific Esterase	PAS		
L1—Acute lymphoid leukemia, childhood variant	Small, uniform blasts, nucleoli indistinct	—	—	+++	65% react with anti-CD10 (anti-CALLA)	Various
L2—Acute lymphoid leukemia, adult variant	Larger, more irregular nucleoli present	—	—	++	20% react with anti-CD5, 3, or 2 (anti-T cell)	Various, including t(1;19)
L3—Burkitt-like acute lymphoid leukemia	Large with strongly basophilic cytoplasm and vacuoles	—	—	—	Antisurface immunoglobulin, anti-CD19, anti-CD20	t(8;14)

T-cell origin and express CD5, CD3, or CD2. Finally, approximately 15% of cases express neither B-nor T-cell antigens and are termed null cell ALL. Myeloid antigens, such as CD13, CD14, or CD33, can be found on the surface of as many as 25% of ALL cases and in some but not all studies, the co-expression of myeloid markers on ALL blasts has been associated with a poor outcome.

The cytogenetic changes most often seen in adult ALL include t(9;22) (the Philadelphia chromosome) seen in 15–20% of cases; t(8;14), an abnormality associated with the L3 variant of ALL; and t(1;19), a translocation commonly seen in pre-B cell ALL. All of these abnormalities suggest a poor prognosis. In about 20% of cases, the leukemia cells gain chromosomes, often reaching more than 50 per cell. Patients with so-called hyperdiploid ALL tend to have a better prognosis. Some of the chromosomal abnormalities seen in ALL suggest their pathogenesis. For example, in ALL cases characterized by t(8;14), t(8;11), and t(8;22), the c-myc gene is translocated with the heavy or light chain immunoglobulin gene. In such cases, immature B cells could be driven to expand in an unregulated fashion by the presence of high and unregulated levels of the c-myc transcription regulatory protein.

Clinical Features

The clinical features of ALL, like AML, are usually the result of a diminished production of normal red cells, white cells, and platelets. Thus, signs of anemia, infection, and bleeding are common presenting symptoms. ALL tends to infiltrate normal organs more often than AML and, thus, enlargement of lymph nodes, liver, and spleen is common at diagnosis, being seen in approximately 50% of cases. Thymic enlargement is commonly seen in cases of T-cell leukemia. At the time of diagnosis, in approximately 5% of cases, ALL cells may infiltrate the leptomeninges, causing headache and nausea. In occasional cases, testicular involvement with leukemic cells may also be seen.

Laboratory Features

At the time of presentation, anemia is virtually always seen, most patients will have at least mild thrombocytopenia and most will also be granulocytopenic. The white count is elevated in approximately 50% of cases, usually due to presence of circulating leukemic blasts. The bone marrow is almost always hypercellular and largely replaced by leukemic blasts. Many patients will have an increased serum lactic dehydrogenase, and in some cases, serum uric acid is elevated. Lumbar puncture with cytocentrifuge evaluation will reveal leukemic cells in 5–10% of cases.

Differential Diagnosis

Clinically, the signs and symptoms of ALL may resemble those of any other marrow failure state. Infectious mononucleosis and other viral illnesses can sometimes resemble ALL, particularly when large numbers of atypical lymphocytes are present in the peripheral blood and when the disease is accompanied by hemolytic anemia or immune thrombocytopenia, but once a marrow exam is performed and current immunologic and molecular techniques are applied, the diagnosis is rarely in doubt.

Treatment

In childhood ALL, complete responses are achieved in better than 90% of cases and cures can be expected in 60–70% of children. Results in adults are not as favorable with complete response rates averaging 75% and cure rates closer to 30–40% in most studies.

Remission Induction   Standard remission induction usually includes vincristine, prednisone, an anthracycline, and often L-asparaginase. With such regimens, complete responses can be expected in 65–85% of cases. Other regimens, for example, the CVAD regimen, employing cyclophosphamide plus continuous infusion vincristine and anthracycline along with dexamethasone also yield high CR rates, but none have been shown to be superior to the more conventional regimens when tested in randomized trials. As in the case of AML, ALL induction therapy is followed by marked pancytopenia and, as in AML, the use of myeloid growth factors can shorten the period of myelosuppression, but doesn't improve overall complete response rates or survival.

Postremission Chemotherapy   If patients receive only induction chemotherapy, remissions are invariably short-lived, demonstrating the need for some form of postremission chemotherapy. The best results have been achieved using intensive consolidation chemotherapy, often using various combinations of cytarabine, cyclophosphamide, and an anthracycline followed by some form of maintenance chemotherapy using, for example, 6-mercaptopurine and methotrexate. Neither the optimal intensity nor duration of maintenance therapy has been precisely determined. Although CNS disease is less common in adults than in children, without CNS prophylaxis, at least 35% of adults will relapse with CNS disease. Patients with a very high white count at diagnosis or with an elevated serum LDH appear to be particularly at risk. With CNS prophylaxis using intrathecal methotrexate with or without CNS radiation, the incidence of CNS relapse can be reduced to less than 10%. With current chemotherapeutic regimens, 30–40% of adults can be cured.

Risk Factors   Younger patients, those with a low leukocyte count at diagnosis, with leukemic blasts with L1 morphology, with hyperdiploidy, and those who enter an initial remission early after induction appear to have the best prognosis. In contrast, older patients, those with a high white count at diagnosis, with an L2 morphology and those who require additional chemotherapy to achieve remission do worse (Table 31.5). In particular, patients with t(9;22), t(8;14), t(4;11), and t(1;19) have a poor prognosis. Patients with t(9;22) may respond, at least temporarily, to the tyrosine kinase inhibitor, STI-571. Patients with Burkitt-type

TABLE 31.5. Prognosis in Acute Lymphocytic Leukemia

Unfavorable	Favorable
Advanced age	Younger age
High WBC at diagnosis	Low WBC at diagnosis
Late achievement of CR	Early achievement of CR
Cytogenetics	Cytogenetics
t(9;22)	Hyperdiploidy
t(4;11)	
t(8;14)	
t(1;19)	

Abbreviations: WBC, white blood count; CR, complete remission.

ALL associated with t(8;14) appear to benefit from the inclusion of high-dose methotrexate and high-dose alkylating agents during consolidation. Whether similar intensification of therapy benefits patients with t(4;11) or t(1;19) is, as yet, unknown.

Bone Marrow Transplantation   Allogeneic transplantation is the only form of therapy that offers a realistic chance for cure to patients who fail to achieve an initial remission or who relapse with disease resistant to chemotherapy, curing approximately 10–20% of cases in both circumstances. If allogeneic transplantation is carried out earlier, while patients are in second remission, the results improve, with a 5-year disease-free survival of 35% being reported. The best results with allogeneic transplantation are seen in patients transplanted during first remission, with cure rates from 40 to 65% being reported. Whether these results are superior to what could be achieved adopting a strategy of first using chemotherapy and saving allogeneic transplantation for patients who relapse is untested in randomized trials. At present, there is general agreement that patients with ALL with unfavorable prognostic characteristics such as t(9;22) or t(4;11) should be transplanted in first remission if a matched sibling is available. Results with autologous transplantation are harder to evaluate. Patients with multiply relapsed disease rarely benefit, owing to a very high posttransplant relapse rate. Autologous transplantation in second remission results in long-term survival in 20–30% of cases that appears to represent a significant improvement over results achieved with conventional salvage chemotherapy. The role of autologous transplantation for patients in first remission is a subject currently being studied in prospective randomized trials. The use of matched unrelated donor transplantation is also currently under study.

CHRONIC MYELOGENOUS LEUKEMIA

Biology

Chronic myelogenous leukemia is characterized by the overproduction and accumulation of cells of the myeloid series, leading to marked splenomegaly and very high peripheral white blood cell counts. The circulating white cells are usually made up of normal appearing granulocytes or bands, some earlier appearing myeloid cells and occasional blasts. These cells retain most of their normal function and so patients can survive, often for several years, with active CML if treated with relatively nonspecific therapy such as busulfan or hydroxyurea in order to prevent the white count from reaching dangerously high levels. With time, however, the leukemic clone becomes less stable, and the disease progresses to a disorder which more closely resembles acute leukemia.

Studies of the biology of CML have found that the disease results from the clonal expansion of a very primitive pluripotent hematopoietic stem cell. Thus, although the clinical manifestation of the disease largely reflects overproduction of granulocytes, the erythrocytes, megakaryocytes, macrophages, and even B-lymphocytes in patients with CML derive from the malignant clone.

In greater than 90% of cases, the Ph chromosome is found in marrow cells from patients with CML. The Ph chromosome results from the balanced translocation between the long arm of chromosomes 9 and 22, and was the first chromosomal abnormality to be identified with a specific malignant disease. This translocation involves the movement of the majority of the *ABL* proto-oncogene from chromosome 9 to become contiguous with the 5′ portion of the *BCR* gene on chromosome 22. The breakpoint in the *BCR* gene occurs within one of two relatively short sequences. One sequence, the major breakpoint cluster region (M-*bcr*) is the one involved in all cases of CML and about half the cases of Ph+ ALL. The chimeric protein produced by this transcript is a hybrid p210 protein. The other sequence, the minor breakpoint cluster region (m-*bcr*), results in a p190 hybrid protein and is responsible for the other 50% of Ph+ ALL cases. In both situations, the translocation results in the constitutive expression of the *ABL*-specific tyrosine kinase. Recent studies have found a molecular *BCR/ABL* translocation in most of those cases with clinical evidence of CML but with normal conventional cytogenetics. It is now generally concluded that true *BCR/ABL*-negative CML does not exist. The *BCR/ABL* translocation is more than just a marker of CML. Insertion of a retrovirus that produces the p210 protein into hematopoietic cells of mice leads to the development of a syndrome resembling CML.

Clinical Features

CML is normally characterized as being in chronic phase, accelerated phase or blast crisis. More than 90% of cases are diagnosed while in chronic phase. As many as 25% of patients are diagnosed serendipitously when a routine blood count reveals an elevated granulocyte count. More often, however, patients present with fatigue, weight loss, night sweats, or complaints of fullness in the left upper abdomen due to splenomegaly. Rarely, bleeding associated with thrombocytosis is seen. Neutrophil function is usually normal, so infection as a presenting sign is uncommon. Leukostatic symptoms, such as dyspnea, drowsiness, confusion, or diminished visual acuity, which are due to sludging in the pulmonary, cerebral, or retinal vessels, are sometimes seen, especially when the presenting white count exceeds

400,000/mm^3. Splenomegaly is, by far, the most common physical sign of CML being present in more than 60% of cases and may be marked, extending down as far as the pelvic brim. Lymphadenopathy is uncommon during chronic phase. Rarely, patients with CML present in blast crisis at diagnosis. These patients have clinical manifestations similar to those seen in acute leukemia.

Laboratory Features

Virtually all patients have an elevated white count at diagnosis, with counts ranging from 10,000 to greater than 1,000,000/mm^3. The majority of cells are in the neutrophil series with cells ranging from myeloblasts to normal mature-appearing neutrophils. Eosinophilia is sometimes seen and basophilia is common. Platelets are often increased and mild anemia is sometimes present. Bone marrow examination shows marked myeloid hyperplasia and, occasionally, increased marrow fibrosis. Blasts usually make up less than 5% of the marrow cells in most cases. The peripheral blood neutrophils show a markedly decreased leukocyte alkaline phosphatase score. Vitamin B12 levels are often very high due to increased levels of transcobalamin I and III. Serum LDH and uric acid levels are sometimes increased. The diagnosis of CML is made by the finding of the Ph chromosome on cytogenetic analysis of marrow.

Differential Diagnosis

Usually, the diagnosis of CML is straightforward. Any patient with a sustained unexplained increase in the peripheral neutrophil count, particularly if splenomegaly is present, should be suspected of having CML. The diagnosis is generally made by bone marrow exam with cytogenetic analysis. In those cases where the clinical picture resembles CML but cytogenetics are read as normal, molecular studies looking for presence of the hybrid *BCR/ABL* gene product should be undertaken. Diseases that may resemble CML include the various myeloproliferative disorders (polycythemia vera [p-vera], agnogenic myeloid metaplasia and essential thrombocythemia) as well as chronic myelomonocytic leukemia.

Therapy

Patients usually tolerate the chronic phase of CML well but, over time, the clinical behavior of the disease changes. Approximately two-thirds of patients will transform into an accelerated phase characterized by an increase in blasts greater than 15% or basophils greater than 20% in blood or marrow, thrombocytopenia less than 100,000/mm^3 not due to therapy, documented extramedullary leukemia or the finding of a new chromosomal change in addition to the Ph chromosome. The other one-third of patients will abruptly develop blast crisis with more than 30% blasts in marrow or peripheral blood. Blast crisis in roughly two-thirds of patients resembles acute myeloid leukemia and in the remaining one-third more closely resembles acute lymphoblastic leukemia.

Conventional Therapy   The traditional therapy for newly diagnosed chronic phase CML consists of either busulfan starting at a dose of 2–4 mg/m^2 per day or hydroxyurea starting at a dose of 1–2 gm/m^2 per day. These agents are generally used to control patients' symptoms and keep the peripheral blood count under 20,000/mm^3. With these therapies, the duration of chronic phase is often quoted as 3.5 years and once blast crisis occurs, survival averages no more than 6 months. Sokol et al. studied 625 patients aged 5–50 and identified five variables that predicted survival for patients treated with conventional chemotherapy including sex, spleen size, platelet count, hematocrit, and percentage circulating blasts. Since the studies by Sokol, randomized trials comparing busulfan with hydroxyurea have documented that both the duration of chronic phase as well as overall survival are prolonged with the use of hydroxyurea.

Interferon   More recently, studies have found that interferon used either as a single agent or, more often, after counts are first controlled with hydroxyurea, can also control peripheral counts in CML. In addition, anywhere from 5 to 20% of patients will have a partial or complete cytogenetic response with interferon therapy, something that is rarely seen with hydroxyurea. The effectiveness of interferon is dose-dependent and best results are seen at doses of 5×10^6 units/m^2/day or above. Several randomized trials have now been completed comparing hydroxyurea with either interferon alone or interferon plus hydroxyurea. In most of these studies, the duration of chronic phase and overall survival was improved with interferon. A recent meta-analysis of these studies found a 15% improvement in 5-year survival (57% versus 42%) with the use of interferon-containing regimens. Those patients who achieve a complete cytogenetic response appear to do particularly well. More recently, randomized studies suggest that the addition of moderate dose cytarabine to interferon may increase hematologic and cytogenetic response rates, but it remains uncertain if survival is affected.

   Interferon is associated with considerably more toxicities than hydroxyurea, including fever, chills, malaise, anorexia, myalgia, and, rarely, autoimmune disorders. These complications can be lessened by increasing the dose slowly and adding acetaminophen. In most patients, these symptoms diminish after 2–3 months.

STI-571   STI-571 is a specific inhibitor of the *BCR-ABL* tyrosine kinase that is constitutively activated in virtually all cases of CML. In a recently completed dose finding study, patients with CML in blast crisis or Ph-positive ALL received 300–1,000 mg daily orally. Complete responses were seen in 4 of 21 CML patients and 14 of 20 ALL patients. Unfortunately, most of these responses were brief. More impressive results have been seen in patients with chronic phase CML where complete hematologic responses were seen in 53 of 54 patients and major cytogenetic responses were seen in 31%. The drug was generally well tolerated.

Bone Marrow Transplantation   Bone marrow transplantation is the only known cure for CML. Approximately 15% of patients transplanted from

HLA-matched siblings for CML in blast crisis can be cured. Results are improved if transplantation is carried out during accelerated phase where cure rates of approximately 40% are reported. The best results are seen if transplantation is carried out during chronic phase. Data from several thousand patients reported to the International Bone Marrow Transplant Registry, as well as large single institution experiences, such as those reported from Seattle, show that transplantation from an HLA-identical sibling can cure 65–75% of patients. The probability of relapse is approximately 15%, and 15% die from transplant-related complications.

In most studies of allogeneic transplantation for CML, age has been found to be an important prognostic factor. However, long-term survival in better than 50% of patients age 50–65 has recently been reported. In most studies, the interval from diagnosis to transplant has also influenced outcome with the best results seen in patients transplanted within 1 year of diagnosis. Most transplant studies have used either busulfan plus cyclophosphamide or cyclophosphamide plus total body irradiation as the preparative regimen, and in controlled randomized trials, the two appear equivalent. Graft-versus-host disease (GVHD) prophylaxis with cyclosporine and methotrexate is the most widely used approach.

The use of matched unrelated donor transplantation for patients with CML is being increasingly reported. Recent registry summaries report a 50% chance of long-term disease-free survival, while results from several large single institutions report outcomes as high as 75%. The somewhat worse outcome with matched unrelated donors is almost completely accounted for by an increase in GVHD and related infections. Several pilot studies of autologous transplantation for CML have been reported. As yet, there is no convincing evidence that autologous transplantation prolongs survival or cures patients with CML.

CHRONIC LYMPHOCYTIC LEUKEMIA

Biology

Chronic lymphocytic leukemia (CLL) defines a group of chronic B-cell diseases characterized by the abnormal proliferation and/or accumulation of mature-appearing lymphocytes. The clonality of CLL is best demonstrated by the finding of identical (i.e., clonal) rearrangements of the immunoglobulin gene in all malignant cells in individual cases of CLL. The fundamental abnormality in CLL is not well understood. Some investigators believe that CLL is the result of the overproliferation of mature B cells whereas others argue that CLL is more a disease of accumulation with CLL lymphocytes living for long periods. In either case, the end result is the existence of increased numbers of lymphocytes originating from the malignant clone with accumulation in blood, bone marrow, lymph nodes, and spleen, resulting in organomegaly and abnormal bone marrow function. In addition, the clonal expansion of one population of B cells is at the expense of other B-cell populations so that normal B-cell immunity is diminished. If untreated, CLL ultimately proves fatal in one of three general ways. In some patients, the relentless

TABLE 31.6. The Modified Rai Strategy System for Chronic Lymphocytic Leukemia

Rai Stage	Risk	Clinical Features	Median Survival (Years)
0	Low	Lymphocytosis only in blood and marrow	>10
I	Intermediate	Lymphocytosis and lymphadenopathy	7
II	Intermediate	As in stage I plus splenomegaly and/or hepatomegaly	
III	High	Lymphocytosis and anemia	1.5
IV	High	Lymphocytosis and thrombocytopenia	

accumulation of mature B cells leads to marrow failure and fatal granulocytopenia or thrombocytopenia. In some patients, there are further mutations in the CLL clone, leading to a more aggressive ALL-like disease, termed Richter's syndrome. In others, the diminished B cell function leads to fatal infectious complications.

The malignant B cell in CLL, in contrast to normal B cells, only weakly expresses surface immunoglobulin (sIg) and also expresses CD5, an antigen normally largely restricted to T cells or fetal lymphoid tissue. Otherwise, the B cells of CLL are similar to normal B cells expressing CD19, CD20, and CD24. CLL is usually staged according to the modified Rai system (Table 31.6). Patients with early stage disease have a median survival of better than 10 years whereas those with intermediate stage and advanced stage have median survivals of 5–7 and 1.5–3 years respectively. Other factors that influence survival include advanced age, diffuse marrow involvement, lymphocyte doubling time, and cytogenetic abnormalities. The most common cytogenetic abnormalities are trisomy 12, which is present in up to 40% of cases, 14q+ present in 25%, and abnormalities of the long arm of chromosomes 6 and 11. Patients with cytogenetic abnormalities seem to have a shorter survival than patients with a normal karyotype and those with a single cytogenetic abnormality appear to do better than those with complex chromosomal abnormalities.

Clinical Features

Many patients with CLL are asymptomatic and are diagnosed when an elevated lymphocyte count is noted during a routine examination or during evaluation for another unrelated problem. Some patients present with nonspecific symptoms including fatigue, lethargy, reduced exercise tolerance, or loss of appetite. Others present with enlarged lymph nodes, most often cervical, as their chief complaint. Infectious complications, including bacterial, fungal, and viral infections, although common during later stages of the disease, are uncommon at diagnosis. Occasionally, patients present with signs associated with immune thrombocytopenia or autoimmune hemolytic anemia and, on further evaluation, are found to have CLL.

The usual physical findings at diagnosis include lymphadenopathy, which is present in two-thirds of patients. Approximately 50% of patients will have splenomegaly, but hepatomegaly is much less common, seen in less than 10% of cases. Although massive adenopathy can cause dysfunction of other organs causing, for example, obstructive jaundice, obstructive uropathy, or partial bowel obstruction, these complications are rare at diagnosis and usually only seen late in the disease course. Similarly, unilateral or bilateral leg edema can occur, but is usually a late event.

Laboratory Features

The hallmark of CLL is a peripheral lymphocytosis, usually in the range of 40–150,000/mm^3. The lymphocytes are indistinguishable from normal small B lymphocytes on light microscopy but, as noted earlier, have abnormal immunophenotyping, including expressing CD5 on their surface and also are clonal and therefore exhibit either kappa or lambda light chain excess or a consistent immunoglobulin gene rearrangement. Also, as noted earlier, the cells may show a consistent cytogenetic abnormality. Bone marrow biopsy usually demonstrates a lymphocytic infiltrate, which amounts to more than 30% of cells and may be in a diffuse or nodular pattern. A diffuse pattern is felt to carry a somewhat worse prognosis. Anemia is present in approximately 20% of patients at diagnosis and thrombocytopenia in 10%. The anemia is usually mild and the direct cause uncertain but, in some patients, autoimmune hemolytic anemia, confirmed by a positive Coombs test, reticulocytosis, elevated bilirubin level, and low serum haptoglobin, is found. Similarly, autoimmune thrombocytopenia with antiplatelet antibodies is seen in some patients. The antibodies associated with red cell and platelet destruction are not a direct product of the malignant clone but both autoimmune hemolytic anemia and thrombocytopenia usually respond to treatment of the underlying CLL. Hypogammaglobulinemia is seen in 25% of newly diagnosed CLL patients and becomes a more frequent problem as the disease progresses, being seen in 50–70% of patients with more advanced disease.

Differential Diagnosis

The diagnosis of CLL is generally straightforward. Occasionally, lymphocytosis can be caused by an infection such as mononucleosis, cytomegalovirus, pertussis, or tuberculosis, but, in these cases, signs of the infection predominate and the lymphocytosis is not persistent. The more difficult problem is differentiating CLL from other indolent lymphoproliferative disorders including hairy cell leukemia, Waldenstrom's macroglobulinemia, large granular lymphocytosis, prolymphocytic leukemia, and the leukemic phase of nodular lymphomas. These distinctions are largely made by histopathology and cell surface immunophenotyping.

Treatment

Except for the uncommon application of allogeneic transplantation to treat the occasional patient, CLL is incurable with available therapies. Further, there is no evidence that treatment of early stage patients improves survival. Therefore, deciding when to initiate therapy in CLL is an important issue. Generally, treatment can be safely withheld until patients develop disease-related symptoms, progressive bone marrow failure, significant autoimmune anemia or thrombocytopenia, or recurrent infections. Radiation can be used to treat splenomegaly or bulky lymphoid masses in occasional cases, but chemotherapy is required for most patients. The greatest experience has been with chlorambucil, which is effective in controlling manifestations of the disease in most patients. Chlorambucil can be given at 6–8 mg daily, 15–20 mg/m^2 every 2 weeks, or 20–40 mg/m^2 monthly, with subsequent doses adjusted according to clinical response and myelotoxicity. Cyclophosphamide and combinations of cyclophosphamide with vincristine and prednisone (CVP) are approximately equivalent to chlorambucil with respect to response rates, time to progression, and survival. More intensive combinations, for example, CVP plus an anthracycline, appear to result in higher response rates than chlorambucil but it is less clear if survival is improved by their use.

The purine analogues, fludarabine, 2-chlorodeoxyadenosine (2-CDA), and 2-deoxycoformycin (DCF), have been found to have considerable activity in CLL. Fludarabine, at a dose of 25 mg/m^2 for 5 consecutive days each month for approximately 6 months, is often effective in patients who no longer are responding to alkylating agents, resulting in 15% complete responses and 45% partial responses. When compared with chlorambucil as initial therapy for CLL, fludarabine results in a significantly higher incidence of complete and partial remissions and a longer remission duration. Thus, although there is not yet evidence that use of fludarabine as initial therapy prolongs survival compared with a strategy of reserving it for salvage therapy, most experts recommend use of fludarabine as initial therapy in most patients. 2-CDA appears to produce response rates very similar to that achieved with fludarabine. Responses have also been seen with DCF, but the experience with this drug is limited. Unfortunately, there is little evidence for non-cross-resistance among the three purine analogues, and resistance of leukemic cells to one usually means resistance to the other two. All three purine analogues are myelosuppressive and immunosuppressive. The myelosuppression is short-lived but the immunosuppressive effects may be cumulative and render patients susceptible to opportunistic infections for considerable periods.

A humanized antibody against CD52, termed CAMPATH-1, has recently been found to result in partial responses in approximately one-third of patients who have recurred following fludarabine treatment. Similar response rates have been reported with use of rituximab. Current trials are evaluating combinations of fludarabine, alkylating agents, and monoclonal antibodies as initial treatment of CLL.

A major problem associated with CLL and its treatment is the risk of opportunistic infection. High-dose intravenous immunoglobulin therapy decreases the frequency of bacterial infections in patients with CLL. Although expensive, its use should be strongly considered for patients with documented recurrent bacterial infections. Use of purine analogues and CAMPATH-1 has increased the risk of infections with *Pneumocystis carinii*, candida, and other opportunistic agents, and so prophylaxis with trimethoprim-sulfamethoxazole and fluconazole might be considered during their use.

Long-term disease-free survival has been reported in a small number of patients with CLL treated with allogeneic marrow transplantation. The best preparative regimens and GVHD prophylaxis for this indication are uncertain. There does appear to be a potentially important role for a graft-versus-leukemia effect in this disease given the observation that following transplantation, it may take from months to years for the disease to entirely disappear, and that donor lymphocyte infusions are sometimes effective in reestablishing a complete response. This observation has spurred interest in the development of nonablative allogeneic transplantation for CLL.

The median survival of patients with CLL is 4–5 years following initiation of therapy but is heavily influenced by the stage of disease at diagnosis. Younger patients usually eventually die of progressive CLL with associated marrow failure and infectious complications. Older individuals often die of other intercurrent illnesses. In a small proportion of patients, CLL evolves into a more aggressive disease, commonly termed Richter's syndrome, which closely resembles a diffuse large cell lymphoma. In approximately half of the cases of Richter's syndrome, the malignant cells display the same cytogenetic and molecular features of the original CLL. Response to therapy is poor with a median survival of 4 months.

OTHER LEUKEMIA-LIKE DISORDERS

Myelodysplastic Syndromes

The myelodysplastic syndromes (MDS) describe a group of clonal hematopoietic disorders characterized by impaired maturation of hematopoietic precursors with the development of progressive peripheral cytopenias. MDS is the result of the neoplastic transformation of a cell at a level of differentiation close to that of the hematopoietic stem cell. Unlike the acute leukemias, the abnormal clone in MDS retains the ability to differentiate, albeit not entirely normally. With time, the abnormal clone suppresses all normal hematopoiesis and becomes increasingly abnormal. The final result is the development of either progressive severe pancytopenia or progression to an acute leukemia-like state. The cause of the defect in MDS is usually unknown but the disease is seen more often in patients with DNA repair deficiency syndromes, in those exposed to irradiation or other marrow toxins, and in patients previously exposed to alkylating agents. The disorder is much more common in the elderly, with a median age of onset of approximately 60 years. Symptoms are usually a direct result of impaired marrow function with the most common presenting complaints being fatigue, pallor, and, less commonly, recurrent infections. Occasionally, bruising or bleeding is the presenting symptom.

TABLE 31.7. FAB Classification of Myelodysplastic Syndromes

Classification	Marrow Blasts (%)	Peripheral Blood Blasts (%)	Ringed Sideroblasts >15% of Bone Marrow	Monocytes >1,000/μL
Refractory anemia	<5	≤1	−	−
Refractory anemia with ringed sideroblasts	<5	≤1	+	−
Refractory anemia with excess blasts	5–20	<5	−/+	−
Refractory anemia with excess blasts in transition	20–30	>5	−/+	−/+
Chronic myelomonocytic anemia	≤20	<5	−/+	+

The laboratory features of MDS include peripheral pancytopenia and marrow dysplasia including dyserythropoiesis, often with ringed sideroblasts, dysgranulo-poiesis with hypergranulation, and dysmegakaryocytopoiesis with micromegakar-yocytes. Five distinct forms of MDS have been defined by the French/American/ British Cooperative Group (Table 31.7). Clonal chromosomal abnormalities are found in 50–70% of MDS patients, most commonly loss of part or all of chromosome 7, trisomy 8, isochrone 17, 5q-, and 20q-. These abnormalities appear to carry independent prognostic significance, with abnormalities of chromosome 7 being particularly unfavorable. Even after FAB and cytogenetic classification, MDS remains a heterogeneous disease, particularly concerning prognosis. Accordingly, a number of scoring systems have been developed to help further categorize patients. Recently, a system based on an international study of 816 cases was published. This international prognostic scoring system uses marrow, blast percentage, cytogenetic data, and peripheral counts to categorize patients as being low, intermediate, or high risk (Table 31.8).

The category of MDS dictates the appropriate therapy. Except for allogeneic transplantation, there is no proven curative treatment for MDS. Patients with low-risk disease can generally be followed without treatment unless they have a single severe cytopenia requiring therapy. Erythropoietin has been studied in patients with low-risk MDS with anemia as their major problem and results in 20–30% of patients becoming red cell transfusion independent. Use of granulocyte macrophage colony-stimulating factor (GM-CSF) or granulocyte colony-stimulating factor (G-CSF) to treat granulocytopenia is associated with improved granulocyte counts in the majority of patients and should be considered in infected neutropenic patients. Whether long-term use of myeloid growth factors in MDS is warranted has not been determined. Differentiating agents, especially 13-*cis*-retinoic acid, have been tested in patients with MDS and were not found to improve progression-free or overall survival. Pilot studies of low-dose cytarabine suggested response rates of 15–20%,

TABLE 31.8. International Prognostic Scoring System for Myelodysplastic Syndromes

Characteristic	Individual Score
Good (normal, del 5q, del 20q and −y)	0
Intermediate	0.5
Poor (three or more abnormalities or abnormalities of 7)	1.0
Blasts (% in marrow)	
<5	0
5–10	0.5
11–20	2.0
Cytopenias (Hgb <10 g/dL, ANC <1,800/mm^3, platelets <100,000/mm^3)	
0–1	0
2–3	0.5
Risk groups	**Total score**
Low	0
Intermediate −1	0.5–1.0
Intermediate −2	1.5–2.0
High	>2.0

but randomized trials failed to show any improvement in overall survival. More recently, modest prolongation of survival has been suggested with the use of azacytidine. Occasional responses have been reported following treatment using ATG or other immunosuppressive agents. Intensive combination chemotherapy, similar to that used in AML, has been studied in younger patients with intermediate or high-risk disease and results in complete response rates of 40–60%. The highest complete response rates occur in younger patients. The average response duration is less than 12 months and few patients are cured, results that are inferior to that seen using similar chemotherapeutic approaches in patients with *de novo* AML.

The only curative therapy for MDS is allogeneic bone marrow transplantation, which results in long-term disease-free survival in 40–50% of transplanted patients. Results appear best for younger patients transplanted for early stage disease using human leukoayte antigen (HLA) matched sibling donors.

Chronic Myeloproliferative Diseases

The chronic myeloproliferative diseases are clonal disorders affecting cells of myeloid lineage, resulting in overproduction of relatively mature cells. These disorders are usually subdivided on the basis of the predominant phenotype of the abnormal cells population. Excess red cell production is categorized as "polycythemia vera" and platelet excess as "essential thrombocythemia." A third category of chronic myeloproliferative syndrome is "agnogenic myeloid metaplasia," a disease characterized by bone marrow fibrosis and extramedullary hematopoiesis. Chronic myeloid leukemia conceptually fits as a fourth syndrome, but because of its frequency and clinical uniformity, it is usually considered as a separate entity.

Polycythemia Vera Polycythemia vera (P-vera) is a clonal hematopoietic disorder resulting in an increased red cell mass. The disease has a peak incidence at age 60 and affects both genders equally. Patients are often asymptomatic, with the diagnosis initially being suspected following routine screening tests. Common symptoms include generalized pruritus, especially after showering or bathing, fatigue, paresthesias, headache, and epigastric distress. As many as one-third of patients present following thrombotic or hemorrhagic events. Patients often have a ruddy complexion and both splenomegaly and hepatomegaly are common. Most patients will have an elevated hematocrit but it is important to remember that a hematocrit may be elevated without an increase in red cell mass, for example, if the plasma volume is decreased and conversely, that the red cell mass can be increased without a marked increase in the hematocrit. The peripheral white cell count and platelet count are often mildly elevated and bone marrow examination usually shows trilineage hypercellularity. Iron stores are usually low whereas vitamin B_{12} levels are frequently elevated, in part due to an increase in B_{12} binding capacity.

The major concern in making a diagnosis of P-vera is distinguishing primary P-vera from secondary erythrocytosis. Secondary erythrocytosis is usually the result of increased erythropoietin levels that result from a physiologic demand, as in patients living at high altitudes, with chronic lung disease, or with arteriovenous shunts. Rarely, pathologic erythropoietin overproduction occurs from tumors, uterine fibroids, or as a result of renal disorders. Whereas in the past the diagnosis of P-vera required measurement of the red cell mass, currently, the easiest way to distinguish between primary and secondary erythrocytosis is to measure erythropoietin levels. An autonomous proliferation of erythrocytes, as in P-vera, is associated with low erythropoietin levels.

The cornerstone of therapy for P-vera is phlebotomy. Maintenance of a hematocrit of approximately 42% or less is recommended, which may require weekly phlebotomies of 500 mL. Therapy with phlebotomy alone is associated with an increased risk of thrombosis and so many experts recommend the use of hydroxyurea at 1–2 gm/day to keep the platelet count below 500,000/mm^3. Chlorambucil or radiophosphorus are not, in general, recommended for initial treatment of P-vera because of their leukogenic effects.

The average survival from diagnosis is greater than 10 years. Approximately 50% of patients will develop thrombotic or hemorrhagic complications, which can be generally controlled with therapy. In 5–10% of patients, the disease will evolve into an acute myeloid leukemia-like syndrome, whereas in another 20%, the disease transforms into a picture resembling that seen with agnogenic myeloid metaplasia.

Essential Thrombocythemia Essential thrombocythemia is a clonal hematopoietic disorder characterized by the autonomous overproduction of platelets and platelet precursors. Most patients are asymptomatic and the disease is generally diagnosed incidentally. However, approximately 25% of patients will present with either thrombotic or hemorrhagic events. Splenomegaly is present in 50% of patients but hepatomegaly and lymphadenopathy are rare. The platelet count is usually greater than 600,000/mm^3 but other peripheral counts are generally normal.

Marrow examination usually shows increased numbers of megakaryocytes, often appearing in clusters, and an increase in marrow reticulin fibrosis is sometimes seen.

Essential thrombocythemia is the least aggressive of the myeloproliferative syndromes and patients with this disease can have, on average, a nearly normal life expectancy. The disease rarely transforms into an acute leukemia. However, more than one-third of patients will suffer a major a thrombotic or hemorrhagic event. The risk of thrombotic events is increased with a previous history of a thrombotic event, with inadequate control of thrombocytosis and in patients with other cardiovascular risk factors. The risk for hemorrhage is increased when platelet counts exceed 2,000,000/mm^3 and in patients using nonsteroidal anti-inflammatory agents. Most experts recommend therapy to keep platelet counts less than 600,000/mm^3 for all patients over age 50 and in those with cardiovascular risk factors or a previous history of thrombosis. The appropriate management of younger patients without risk factors is unsettled, but some experts recommend treatment to keep the counts less than 600,000/mm^3 in these individuals, as well. The two most commonly used agents are anagrelide, 0.5 mg/four times per day, and hydroxyurea, 1 gm/day. Both are highly active, are administered orally, and are generally well tolerated.

Agnogenic Myeloid Metaplasia Agnogenic myeloid metaplasia (AMM) is characterized by substantial bone marrow fibrosis, peripheral blood leukoerythroblastosis, and marked splenomegaly. In this disorder, the marrow fibroblasts are polyclonal whereas a population of hematopoietic cells is clonal and, therefore, the marrow fibrosis is thought to be a reactive process caused by the clonal cell population. Current studies suggest that abnormally high levels of transforming growth factor-β (TGF-β) and, perhaps, platelet-derived growth factor produced by the clonal cell population are the predominant causes for the fibroblast proliferation.

Most patients with AMM present with symptoms related to anemia, approximately 25% present because of the mechanical effects of an enlarged spleen, although occasional patients have signs of bleeding or hypermetabolism (weight loss, night sweats) as their initial complaint. Usual laboratory findings include a peripheral leukoerythroblastosis with tear drop red cells and immature myeloid elements being present. Bone marrows are usually not aspirable and bone marrow biopsy shows bone marrow fibrosis and osteosclerosis. Large numbers of blasts are usually not seen in the marrow and, if present, suggest M7 acute myeloid leukemia. Other diseases sometimes confused with AMM are CML with marrow fibrosis and hairy cell leukemia.

Survival with AMM is quite varied, ranging from 1 to 30 years but averaging around 5 years. A poor prognosis is associated with increasingly severe anemia, thrombocytopenia, hepatomegaly, and B symptoms. AMM, in general, is considered incurable and therapy is aimed at treating the anemia and thrombocytopenia and the problems associated with an enlarged spleen, including pain, portal hypertension, and hypersplenism. Anemia is usually treated with transfusion therapy (with desferrioxamine if long-term support is anticipated) although some patients respond to androgens plus steroids and a few to erythropoietin. Treatment of thrombocytopenia is difficult, with platelet transfusion support the usual approach. Splenectomy should be considered for patients with splenic pain, portal hypertension, or hypermetabolic symptoms not responsive to hydroxyurea. Approximately 50% of patients with low blood counts will improve following splenectomy. Splenic irradiation (200–300 cGy delivered in 10–15 daily fractions) can provide transient benefit for patients with symptomatic splenomegaly but rarely improves peripheral blood counts. Recently, the use of allogeneic marrow transplantation has been reported in younger patients with AMM. Complete engraftment with evident eradication of the disease has been reported, with some patients remaining continuously disease-free for prolonged periods, suggesting that cure is possible.

Hairy Cell Leukemia

Hairy cell leukemia is an uncommon B-cell disorder, occurring in approximately 500 patients per year in the United States. The clinical picture is characterized by pancytopenia with an inaspirable bone marrow, splenomegaly, and often, lymphadenopathy. The malignant cells stain positively with tartrate resistant acid phosphatase. They also express pan-B-cell antigens such as CD19 and CD20 as well as the monocyte-related antigen CD11c. Hairy cell leukemia is an indolent disorder and as many as 10% of patients may never require treatment. Therapy is indicated for massive progressive splenomegaly, lymphadenopathy, worsening blood counts, or recurrent infections. Splenectomy, previously the traditional treatment, improves symptoms related to splenomegaly and, in most cases, peripheral blood counts, often for prolonged periods of time, but does not affect the disease itself. Because excellent results have been observed with interferon, 2-CDA, and DCF, splenectomy should be reserved for patients who do not respond to therapy with these agents. Therapy with interferon 2×10^6 units/m^2 per day or 3×10^6 units three times per week produces responses in 80% of splenectomized or unsplenectomized patients, however, only 10% of responses are complete. Responses generally occur within 3–4 months, although up to a year of therapy may be required. The disease invariably recurs after interferon therapy is discontinued but maintenance therapy is associated with excessive toxicity and expense. Therapy with DCF, 4 mg/m^2 intravenously every other week for 4–6 months, produces complete responses in 60–90% of previously treated or untreated patients, including those who failed to respond to interferon. Moreover, only 25% of patients relapse with more than 5 years of follow-up. Relapse is most often characterized by an increased number of hairy cells in the bone marrow without associated clinical indications for therapy. The drug is myelosuppressive and immunosuppressive with an increase in opportunistic infections even in the absence of neutropenia. However, the improved response rate makes DCF preferable to interferon as the initial therapy of hairy cell leukemia. A single 7-day continuous infusion of 2-CDA produces complete response rates of 65–85% and partial responses in another 10% of cases. Although follow-up is shorter than with DCF, the responses appear to be similar in their duration. Side effects of 2-CDA therapy include febrile neutropenia, immunosuppression, and myelosuppression with opportunistic infections as well as pulmonary, cutaneous, cardiac, and neurologic toxicity. Both DCF and 2-CDA provide excellent results in the treatment of hairy cell leukemia and there has not been a prospective randomized study comparing the two.

FURTHER READING

Appelbaum FR (2000) The acute leukemias. In *Cecil Textbook of Medicine*. Bennett JC, Plum F (eds), W.B. Saunders Company, Philadelphia p. 953.

Appelbaum FR, Anderson J (1998) Allogeneic bone marrow transplantation for myelodysplastic syndrome: outcomes analysis according to IPSS score. *Leukemia* 12(Suppl 1): S25–S29.

Bonnet D, Dick JE (1997) Human acute myeloid leukemia is organized as a hierarchy that originates from a primitive hematopoietic cell. *Nat Med* 3:730–737.

Burnett AK, Goldstone AH, Stevens RM, Hann IM, Rees JK, Gray RG, Wheatley K (1998) Randomised comparison of addition of autologous bone-marrow transplantation to intensive chemotherapy for acute myeloid leukaemia in first remission: results of MRC AML 10 trial. UK Medical Research Council Adult and Children's Leukaemia Working Parties. *Lancet* 351:700–708.

Byrd JC, Dodge RK, Carroll A, Baer MR, Edwards C, Stamberg J, Qumsiyeh M, Moore JO, Mayer RJ, Davey F, Schiffer CA, Bloomfield CD (1999) Patients with t(8;21)(q22;q22) and acute myeloid leukemia have superior failure-free and overall survival when repetitive cycles of high-dose cytarabine are administered. *J Clin Oncol* 17:3767–3775.

Cassileth PA, Harrington DP, Appelbaum FR, Lazarus HM, Rowe JM, Paietta E, Willman C, Hurd DD, Bennett JM, Blume KG, Head DR, Wiernik PH (1998) Chemotherapy compared with autologous or allogeneic bone marrow transplantation in the management of acute myeloid leukemia in first remission. *N Engl J Med* 339:1649–1656.

Copelan EA, McGuire EA (1995) The biology and treatment of acute lymphoblastic leukemia in adults [review]. *Blood* 85:1151–1168.

Degos L, Dombret H, Chomienne C, Daniel MT, Miclea JM, Chastang C, Castaigne S, Fenaux P (1995) All-trans-retinoic acid as a differentiating agent in the treatment of acute promyelocytic leukemia [review]. *Blood* 85:2643–2653.

Deininger MWN, Goldman JM, Melo JV (2000) The molecular biology of chronic myeloid leukemia. *Blood* 15:3343–3356.

Druker BJ, Sawyers CL, Kantarjian H, Resta DJ, Reese SF, Ford JM, Capdeville R, Talpaz M (2001) Activity of a specific inhibitor of the BCR-ABL tyrosine kinase in the blast crisis of chronic myeloid leukemia and acute lymphoblastic leukemia with the Philadelphia chromosome. *N Engl J Med* 344:1038–1042.

Druker BJ, Talpaz M, Resta DJ, Peng B, Buchdunger E, Ford JM, Lydon NB, Kantarjian H, Capdeville R, Ohno-Jones S, Sawyers CL (2001) Efficacy and safety of a specific inhibitor of the BCR-ABL tyrosine kinase in chronic myeloid leukemia. *N Engl J Med* 344:1084–1086.

Greenberg P, Cox C, LeBeau MM, Fenaux P, Morel P, Sanz G, Sanz M, Vallespi T, Hamblin T, Oscier D, Ohyashiki K, Toyama K, Aul C, Mufti G, Bennett J (1997) International scoring system for evaluating prognosis in myelodysplastic syndromes. *Blood* 89:2079.

Grimwade D, Walker H, Oliver F, Wheatley K, Harrison C, Harrison G, Rees J, Hann I, Stevens R, Burnett A, Goldstone A (1998) The importance of diagnostic cytogenetics on outcome in AML: analysis of 1,612 patients entered into the MRC AML 10 trial. The Medical Research Council Adult and Children's Leukaemia Working Parties. *Blood* 92:2322–2333.

Larson RA, Dodge RK, Burns CP, Lee EJ, Stone RM, Schulman P, Duggan D, Davey FR, Sobol RE, Frankel SR, et al. (1995) A five-drug remission induction regimen with intensive consolidation for adults with acute lymphoblastic leukemia: Cancer and Leukemia Group B study 8811. *Blood* 85:2025–2037.

Leith CP, Kopecky KJ, Godwin J, McConnell T, Slovak ML, Chen IM, Head DR, Appelbaum FR, Willman CL (1997) Acute myeloid leukemia in the elderly: assessment of multidrug resistance (MDR1) and cytogenetics distinguishes biologic subgroups with remarkably distinct responses to standard chemotherapy. A Southwest Oncology Group study. *Blood* 89:3323–3329.

Mayer RJ, Davis RB, Schiffer CA, Berg DT, Powell BL, Schulman P, Omura GA, Moore JO, McIntyre OR, Frei EI (1994) Intensive post-remission chemotherapy in adults with acute myeloid leukemia. *N Engl J Med* 331:896.

Rai KR, Peterson BL, Appelbaum FR, Kolitz J, Elias L, Sheperd L, Hines J, Threatte GA, Larson RA, Cheson BD, Schiffer CA (2000) Fludarabine compared with chlorambucil as primary therapy for chronic lymphocytic leukemia. *N Engl J Med* 343:1750–1757.

Tallman MS, Anderson JW, Schiffer CA, Appelbaum FR, Feusner JH, Ogden A, Shepherd L, Willman C, Bloomfield CD, Rowe JM, Wiernik PH (1997) All-trans-retinoic acid in acute promyelocytic leukemia. *N Engl J Med* 337:1021–1028.

Tefferi A (2000) Myelofibrosis with myeloid metaplasia [review]. *N Engl J Med* 342:1255–1265.

Zittoun RA, Mandelli F, Willemze R, De Witte T, Labar B, Resegotti L, Leoni F, Damasio E, Visani G, Papa G, Caronia F, Hayat M, Stryckmans P, Rotoli B, Leoni P, Peetermans ME, Dardenne M, Vegna ML, Petti MC, Solbu G, Suciu S (1995) Autologous or allogeneic bone marrow transplantation compared with intensive chemotherapy in acute myelogenous leukemia. *N Engl J Med* 332:217.

CHAPTER 32

Pediatric Malignancies

ALAN S. WAYNE and LEE J. HELMAN

National Cancer Institute, National Institutes of Health, Pediatric Oncology Branch,
Center for Cancer Research, Bethesda, Maryland

Approximately 1 in 8,000 children under 16 years of age will develop cancer. Although much less common than in adults, malignancy represents a leading cause of death from disease in pediatrics. There have been steady improvements in the treatment of childhood cancer such that the majority of patients are now cured. This has occurred in part due to widespread participation in pediatric cooperative group clinical trials, and in part as a result of advances in medical support, radiation therapy, and surgical techniques. Nonetheless, treatment of children and adolescents with cancer continues to pose great challenges, and thus should be undertaken in centers with multidisciplinary pediatric expertise. The most common pediatric malignancies (Fig 32.1) are reviewed in this chapter.

LEUKEMIA

Leukemia is the most common pediatric cancer, with an incidence of approximately 1 in 25,000 children. Acute lymphoblastic leukemia (ALL) accounts for about 80% and acute myelogenous leukemia (AML) about 15% of pediatric leukemia. Chronic myelogenous leukemia (CML) and juvenile myelomonocytic leukemia (JMML) occur with much lower frequency.

Etiology and Epidemiology

The majority of children with ALL present between the ages of 2 and 9 years. Infants and adolescents are more likely to have myeloid leukemia. There is a slight male predominance in ALL, an equal sex ratio in AML, and a strong male predominance in JMML. In the United States, Caucasians have a twofold increased

UICC Manual of Clinical Oncology, Eighth Edition. Edited by Raphael E. Pollock
ISBN 0-471-22289-5 Copyright © 2004 John Wiley & Sons, Inc.

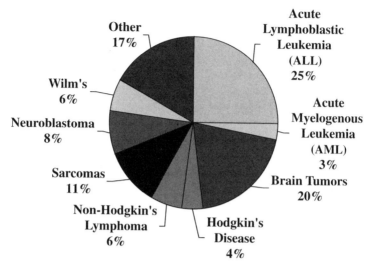

Figure 32.1   Distribution of childhood cancer. (Data from Reis LAG et al (eds). (1999) *Cancer Incidence and Survival among Children and Adolescents: United States SEER Program 1975–1995*, National Cancer Institute, SEER Program. NIH Pub. No. 99-4649, Bethesda, MD.)

risk of developing ALL compared with African Americans. There are a variety of conditions that predispose to leukemia (e.g., trisomy 21, immunodeficiency, chromosomal breakage syndromes), although most often no such underlying disorder is found. The majority of children with leukemia have chromosomal abnormalities in the malignant cells, including translocations and/or numeric alterations, which in some cases have been proven to be prenatal in origin. Notably, some translocations may not be apparent on routine cytogenetics, for example, t(12;21) or *TEL/AML1*, which represents the most common abnormality, occurring in 25% of childhood ALL. The genes involved in leukemogenesis are frequently transcription factors expressed in hematopoietic tissues.

Screening

There is little role for routine screening of healthy children, although those with underlying disorders that increase the risk of leukemia should be followed closely with serial physical exams and complete blood counts (CBC) with differential.

Diagnosis

The most common presenting signs and symptoms of leukemia include infiltration of the bone marrow (with resultant cytopenias and/or blasts in the peripheral blood), liver, spleen, and lymph nodes. Central nervous system (CNS) involvement manifested by blasts in the cerebrospinal fluid (CSF) and/or cranial neuropathies occurs in 5–20% of children with ALL and AML. Other sites of leukemic infiltration include testes, tonsils/adenoids, anterior mediastinum, skin, spine (epidural), eye, pericardium, and pleura. Diagnosis is readily confirmed by the demonstration of leukemic blasts in the blood, marrow, CSF, and/or pleural fluid. Routine hematopathological staining, immunohistochemistry, flow cytometry, and cytogenetics are used to define the diagnostic subtype. The majority of childhood ALL is of precursor B-cell phenotype, whereas T-cell ALL makes up 10–15% and mature B cell less than 5%. Molecular genetic testing should be performed for selected patients (e.g., *TEL/AML1* for those with ALL and normal karyotype).

Staging

By definition, patients with leukemia have bone marrow involvement. Those with ALL and AML should have lumbar punctures to evaluate for the possibility of meningeal leukemia.

Treatment

Approximately 75% of children with ALL are cured with combination chemotherapy. Treatment, which is stratified based on phenotype and prognostic factors (Table 32.1), consists of induction, consolidation, CNS sterilization, and maintenance for a total of 2–3 years. Those with mature B-cell phenotype should be treated as per Burkitt's lymphoma regimens (see below). About 40% of children with AML are cured with chemotherapy consisting of induction, consolidation, and CNS sterilization. Those with acute promyelocytic leukemia (M3-AML) have improved outcomes (~80% leukemia-free-survival) when all-*trans*-retinoic acid is included. In addition to routine CNS sterilization with intrathecal chemotherapy, patients with ALL and AML who have CNS involvement require craniospinal radiation. Allogeneic stem cell transplantation (BMT) is recommended for children with CML, JMML, and, when a matched sibling donor is available, for those with AML (excluding M3-AML) and Philadelphia chromosome–positive ALL in first remission.

TABLE 32.1. Prognostic Factors in Pre-B Acute Lymphoblastic Leukemia

	Lower Risk	Higher Risk
Age (years)	1–9	$<1, \geq 10$
WBC (per mm^3)	$<50,000$	$\geq 50,000$
CNS	Negative	Positive
Chromosomes	t(12;21), T-10, T-4	t(9;22), 11q23, t(1;19)
DNA index	>1.16	≤ 1.16
Response	Rapid	Slow

Abbreviations: WBC, white blood count; CNS, central nervous system; T, trisomy.

Management of Recurrence

Allogeneic BMT in second remission using a related or unrelated donor is usually recommended for those who sustain a bone marrow relapse, although curative salvage can sometimes be achieved with chemotherapy alone for individuals with ALL who have a long first remission duration (>12 months) or isolated extramedullary relapse.

LYMPHOMA

As in adults, lymphoma in children and adolescents can be classified as Hodgkin's and non-Hodgkin's. The diagnostic and therapeutic approach to Hodgkin's disease in pediatrics is similar to that in adult patients and will not be reviewed in this chapter. There are three predominant subtypes of non-Hodgkin's lymphoma (NHL) in pediatrics, each occurring with approximately equal frequency: lymphoblastic lymphoma (LBL), large cell (LCL), and small-non-cleaved cell (SNCL including Burkitt's and non-Burkitt's). The presentation and treatment are specific to each subtype.

Etiology and Epidemiology

The incidence of NHL in pediatric age groups is approximately nine per million. There is a male predominance ($\sim$2–3:1). The risk of developing NHL is increased up to 100-fold in certain congenital immunodeficiency syndromes, with a lifetime incidence as high as 15–25% in those with Wiskott-Aldrich syndrome, ataxia-telangiectasia, and common variable immunodeficiency. Patients with acquired immunodeficiency due to infection (e.g., HIV, HTLV) and medical treatment (e.g., post-transplant) are also at high risk. EBV infection serves as an important co-factor in the development of Burkitt's lymphoma, with EBV genome detected in 95% of endemic (i.e., African) and 20% of sporadic cases. There are a number of recurrent chromosomal translocations commonly associated with specific NHL subtypes. LBL represents the same cell of origin as T-cell ALL and translocations involving the T-cell receptor (TCR) genes (14q11, 7q34–q36) are seen in 30–50% of cases. Approximately 50% of children with LCL have a translocation, t(2;5), which involves the anaplastic lymphoma kinase gene (*ALK*) on chromosome 2. Finally, Burkitt's lymphomas are associated with translocations involving c-*myc* (8q24) and one of the immunoglobulin genes (14q32, 2p11, 22q11).

Screening

Children with immunodeficiency states should be followed closely with serial histories and physical exams to monitor for signs and symptoms of possible lymphoma. Appropriate laboratory testing (e.g., complete blood count, lactate dehydrogenase, chest x-ray) should be considered based on clinical findings.

Diagnosis

The presenting signs and symptoms of NHL are specific to each subtype. Notably, extranodal sites are common. Patients with LBL usually present with bulky lymphadenopathy. Common emergent presentations include airway obstruction due to anterior mediastinal mass and/or tonsilar enlargement, superior vena cava syndrome, and pleural and/or pericardial effusions. LCL commonly involves diffuse nodal and soft tissue sites including the head and neck, mediastinum, skin, and bone. Patients with sporadic Burkitt's present most often with abdominal involvement, including bulky masses, mesenteric and/or retroperitoneal lymphadenopathy, and/or intussusception. Patients with endemic Burkitt's present more commonly with jaw and/or orbital masses. Patients with Burkitt's lymphoma may present with signs of tumor lysis syndrome, which is a frequent and severe complication during the first days of treatment. Finally, bone marrow, and less frequently CNS involvement, are seen in LBL and Burkitt's and such patients should be approached as with ALL.

Routine hematopathological staining, immunohistochemistry, and flow cytometry are used to define the diagnostic subtype. LBL is characterized by a T-cell phenotype identical to T-ALL. Burkitt's lymphoma represents a late stage B-cell phenotype defined by surface-IgM expression. LCL may be B-, T-, or null phenotype. The 50% of LCL associated with t(2;5) are characterized by CD30 (Ki-1) expression. Cytogenetics and molecular analysis for TCR or immunoglobulin gene rearrangement can be used to confirm clonality in NHL. Notably, in contradistinction to adults, 90% of pediatric lymphomas are high-grade and approximately two-thirds are advanced stage (III, IV).

Staging

A variety of staging systems have been used in NHL, predominantly based on tumor volume. One of the most commonly employed is the St. Jude staging system (Table 32.2).

TABLE 32.2. Non-Hodgkin's Lymphoma Staging System

Stage	Characteristics
I	Single site (excluding abdomen or mediastinum)
II	Single extranodal site with regional nodes
	Two or more nodal sites, same side of diaphragm
	Two extranodal sites, same side of diaphragm
	Primary gastrointestinal, completely resected
III	Two extranodal sites, both sides of diaphragm
	Two or more nodal sites, both sides of diaphragm
	Primary thoracic
	Primary gastrointestinal, extensive
	Paraspinal, epidural
IV	CNS and/or bone marrow (<25%)

Treatment

Cure rates range from 70 to 100% for children with NHL depending on the subtype and stage. Treatment consists primarily of combination chemotherapy specific to the subtype and stage. LBL is managed like ALL and should include CNS prophylaxis. SNCL responds to short, intensive chemotherapy and also should include CNS prophylaxis. Patients with Burkitt's lymphoma require aggressive monitoring and prophylaxis against possible tumor lysis syndrome. The optimal approach to LCL is less clear, and both ALL and SNCL regimens have been used successfully.

Management of Recurrence

Although salvage can sometimes be achieved with chemotherapy and/or radiotherapy, allogeneic BMT in second remission using a related or unrelated donor is usually recommended for those with advanced stage disease who relapse.

OSTEOSARCOMA

Approximately half of pediatric bone tumors are malignant, the most common of which is osteosarcoma (OS). OS is a malignancy of primitive bone forming mesenchyme that is characterized by the production of osteoid.

Etiology and Epidemiology

Although OS can occur in any bone, it is most commonly seen in the metaphyses of long bones during periods of rapid growth. The peak age of presentation is 16 years in females and 18 years in males, corresponding with the pubertal growth spurt. There is a slight male predominance and patients are taller than age-matched peers. OS is rare in those of African heritage. Although OS most commonly develops *de novo*, there are a number of predisposing chronic bone diseases such as fibrous dysplasia and Paget's disease. OS also represents the most common second malignancy seen in prior radiation fields. Mutations in the retinoblastoma (RB) gene (13q14) are seen in around 50% of tumors, and patients with hereditary RB have a 100-fold increased risk of OS even without prior radiation. Alterations in *p53* can be detected in approximately 50% of tumors and germ-line mutations of this gene are associated with increased risk of OS, breast cancer, brain tumors, leukemia, and adrenocortical tumors (Li-Fraumeni syndrome). There are data to suggest that insulin-like growth factor-1 (IGF-1) serves as a growth and survival factor in OS.

Screening

Individuals at high risk, especially those with hereditary RB or with a history of radiation to bone, should be monitored closely for signs and symptoms of the development of OS. At a minimum, yearly history and physical examination and radiographs of areas of concern are recommended.

Diagnosis

OS most commonly presents with local pain, often of prolonged duration, with or without an associated soft-tissue mass. Some patients may come to medical attention with a pathologic fracture. Plain radiographs usually reveal characteristic findings of new bone or osteoid formation including sclerotic bone lesions, soft-tissue calcification, Codman's triangle, and a so-called "sunburst" pattern. Elevations in the serum alkaline phosphatase and lactate dehydrogenase (LDH) are common. Approximately 20% present with metastatic disease, usually to the lungs and/or other bones. Complete staging evaluation should include chest CT scan and total body bone scan. Diagnosis is confirmed by biopsy, which should be performed in such a manner that the entire biopsy tract can be excised during the final tumor resection. The most frequent histologic subtypes are osteoblastic, chondroblastic, and fibroblastic, less common is telangectatic, although all are high-grade and there is no impact on prognosis. The one exception is that of parosteal or juxtacortical OS, a low-grade tumor that arises from the cortex and does not invade marrow.

Staging

The staging system for OS is primitive and revision is planned (Table 32.3). By the old system, almost all cases were stage IIB or IV.

Treatment

The curative treatment of OS requires chemotherapy and surgical resection of the primary tumor by amputation or a limb-salvage procedure. Active chemotherapy agents include high-dose methotrexate, cisplatin, doxorubicin, and ifosfamide. Adjuvant or neoadjuvant chemotherapy has improved disease-free-survival (DFS)

TABLE 32.3. Osteosarcoma Staging System

Stage	Characteristics
I	Low grade
II	High grade
IIA	Intramedullary (old)
	$T_1 \leq 8$ cm (revised)
IIB	Extramedullary (old)
	$T_2 > 8$ cm (revised)
III	Not defined
IV	Metastatic disease
IVA	M_{1a} lung only
IVB	M_{1b} all other sites

from 20% to 65% in patients with localized disease. The response to pre-operative chemotherapy is prognostic; those with <95% tumor necrosis at the time of surgical resection fair poorly. The prognosis for those with metastatic disease is also poor, although long-term survival is possible if pulmonary lesions can be resected. Low-grade parosteal OS can be managed by surgery alone (to be distinguished from high-grade periosteal OS).

Management of Recurrence

The prognosis for those with recurrent OS is poor, with the occasional exception of those with isolated, resectable pulmonary nodules.

EWING'S SARCOMA FAMILY OF TUMORS

Ewing's sarcoma (EWS) represents a family of tumors of neuroectodermal origin including primitive neuroectodermal tumor (PNET), peripheral neuroepithelioma, and Askin tumor. It is the second most common malignant bone tumor in children.

Etiology and Epidemiology

EWS can arise in soft tissue or bone. Any bone can be affected, and EWS occurs with equal frequency in the axial skeleton and long bones of the extremities. EWS most commonly develops in the second decade of life, although approximately 25% of patients are diagnosed before age 10. Like osteosarcoma, there is a slight male predominance and EWS is rare in individuals of African heritage. The over-whelming majority of EWS family of tumors have recurrent chromosomal translocations involving the *EWS* gene on chromosome 22 and a gene from the ets family of transcription factors. EWS tumors display high levels of c-*myc* expression.

Screening

There is no known role for routine screening of healthy children in preventing this rare tumor.

Diagnosis

EWS usually presents with pain and/or swelling. Many patients will have had protracted symptoms as well as systemic signs such as fever. The pelvic bones are the most common primary site, and such tumors are frequently very large at diagnosis. Approximately 25% of patients present with metastatic disease, the most frequent sites being lungs, bone, and bone marrow. Plain radiographs usually reveal a lytic lesion, commonly in the diaphysis of bone, with soft tissue involvement and periosteal reaction giving a characteristic "onion skin" appearance. Staging evaluation should include chest CT scan, total body bone scan, and bone marrow biopsies. Serum LDH is commonly elevated, and bone marrow involvement may occasionally lead to cytopenias. Diagnosis is made by biopsy, which should be performed in such a manner that the entire biopsy tract can be excised in the event of subsequent tumor resection. EWS can be difficult to distinguish from the other "small round blue cell tumors of childhood," which include neuroblastoma, rhabdomyosarcoma, and lymphoma. Immunohistochemistry is positive for CD99 (Mic-2) and commonly markers of neural differentiation. Molecular cytogenetics are useful to confirm the diagnosis.

Staging

There is no standard staging system and EWS tumors are classified according to size and site.

Treatment

Curative treatment involves combination chemotherapy and local control with surgical resection and/or radiotherapy. The most common agents employed include vincristine, doxorubicin, cyclophosphamide, etoposide, and ifosfamide. Patients with localized disease have about 60–70% DFS, whereas those with metastatic disease have a very poor prognosis. Favorable prognostic factors include distal extremity sites, small tumor size or volume (<8 cm or 100 mL), young age, normal LDH, and good response to initial chemotherapy.

Management of Recurrence

No salvage regimens have been shown to be curative for patients who relapse after standard therapy. Pulmonary radiation may be effective for isolated lung metastases.

RHABDOMYOSARCOMA

Rhabdomyosarcoma (RMS) is the most common soft-tissue sarcoma of childhood, with an incidence of approximately five cases per million. RMS represents a malignancy of mesenchymal cells that would normally develop into skeletal muscle. There are a number of histologic subtypes, the two predominant ones being embryonal (ERMS) and alveolar (ARMS).

Etiology and Epidemiology

Two-thirds of cases occur in children under 6 years of age. There is a slight male predominance, and in the United States African American females have much lower rates than Caucasians. RMS is less common in Asian populations. The risk of

RMS appears to be increased in children whose parents used marijuana or cocaine in the year prior to the child's birth. A genetic predisposition can be found in 7–33% of cases. Notably, RMS was the index case in the Li-Fraumeni syndrome and germline *p53* mutations are found with increased incidence in children under 3 years of age with RMS. RMS has been associated with neurofibromatosis and Beckwith-Wiedemann syndrome due to paternal disomy/maternal deficiency of 11p15. Loss of heterozygosity (LOH) of 11p15 is associated with embryonal tumors, whereas approximately 85% of ARMS have one of two recurrent translocations. The t(2;13) fuses *Pax-3*, and the t(1;13) fuses *Pax-7*, with the *FKHR* gene on chromosome 13. Other described genetic modifications in RMS include *Ras* mutations, alterations in the p16-CDK4-RB pathway, and overexpression of *Met* (HGF receptor). Finally, there is ubiquitous over expression of IGF-2 in both ARMS and ERMS.

Screening

There is no known role for routine screening of healthy children in preventing RMS, although individuals with underlying predisposing conditions including Li-Fraumeni syndrome, neurofibromatosis, and Beckwith-Wiedemann syndrome should be monitored closely for signs and symptoms of malignancy. Screening for germline *p53* mutations is considered for children <3 years of age with RMS given the implications to family members.

Diagnosis

RMS can develop throughout the body with the most common sites in decreasing order of frequency being the head and neck, genitourinary system, and extremities. Symptoms often include pain, soft tissue mass, and signs specific to the tumor location such as cranial nerve palsies, nasal discharge, sinus congestion, headaches, hematuria, urinary obstruction, constipation, and vaginal discharge. Twenty percent of patients present with metastatic disease, most commonly to the lungs, bone marrow, bones, and/or lymph nodes. Staging evaluation should include radiographic imaging of the primary site, chest CT scan, total body bone scan, bone marrow biopsies, and, in cases of parameningeal RMS, lumbar puncture. Diagnosis is made by tumor biopsy, which reveals small round blue cells organized according to the histologic subtype: embryonal, botryoid, leiomyomatous, alveolar, or solid alveolar. Botryoid RMS most commonly occurs in the genitourinary region in young infants or in the nasopharynx of older children. Immunohistochemistry is positive for markers of skeletal myogenic lineage (e.g., desmin, muscle-specific actin, MyoD). Molecular cytogenetics can be used to confirm the diagnosis of ARMS, as the t(2;13) or t(1;13) are seen in most cases.

Staging

Historically, the most prevalent approach to staging has been the surgicopathologic Clinical Group system. More recently a tumor, nodes, metastasis (TNM)

TABLE 32.4. Rhabdomyosarcoma Staging System

Stage	Sites	T	Size	N	M
I	Orbit Head and neck (excluding parameningeal) Genitourinary (excluding bladder and prostate) Biliary tract	T_1 or T_2	a or b	N_0 N_1 or N_x	M_0
II	Bladder/prostate Extremity Cranial parameningeal Other (includes trunk, retroperitoneum, perineal/perianal, intrathoracic, gastrointestinal, liver, excluding biliary tract)	T_1 or T_2	a	N_0 or N_x	M_0
III	Bladder/prostate Extremity Cranial parameningeal Other (as in Stage II)	T_1 or T_2	a b	N_1 N_0 or N_1 or N_x	M_0
IV	All	T_1 or T_2	a or b	N_0 or N_1	M_1

Definitions
    Tumor

	T_1	Confined to anatomic site origin
	T_2	Extension and/or fixation to surrounding tissue
	a	≤ 5 cm in diameter in size
	b	>5 cm in diameter in size

    Nodes

	N_0	Regional nodes not clinically involved
	N_1	Regional nodes clinically involved
	N_x	Clinical status of regional nodes unknown

    Metastasis

	M_0	No distant metastasis
	M_1	Distant metastasis present

system that incorporates the primary tumor site and size has been employed (Table 32.4).

Treatment

Therapy is multimodal and is stratified according to tumor location, stage, and histology. Overall, 60–70% of patients with localized disease are cured, whereas less than 30% of those with metastatic disease achieve durable disease-free survival. Prognosis is better for botryoid, followed by embryonal, followed by alveolar histologies. Adolescents and infants have worse outcomes than children 1–10 years of age. Commonly employed active chemotherapy agents include vincristine, actinomycin-D, doxorubicin, cyclophosphamide, ifosfamide, etoposide, topotecan, and irinotecan. Local control is critical and complete surgical resection is recommended if feasible and not cosmetically damaging. Radiation is commonly employed with doses of 4,000–4,500 cGy for microscopic disease, 4,500–5,000 cGy for gross residual disease and tumors >5 cm, and 4,500–5,500 cGy for unresectable tumors.

Management of Recurrence

Complete surgical resection for localized recurrence followed by adjuvant radiation and chemotherapy can lead to long-term survival. For patients with disseminated recurrent disease, the outlook is poor, although many will respond to chemotherapy.

NEUROBLASTOMA

Neuroblastoma (NB) is the most common extracranial solid tumor in children. Derived from the primitive sympathetic cells of the neural crest, NB can be detected in the adrenal glands of normal fetuses. NB develops in approximately 1 per 7,000 live births and represents the most common malignancy in infants. The biologic behavior of NB is unique in that this otherwise highly malignant tumor commonly spontaneously regresses during the first year of life.

Etiology and Epidemiology

The median age at diagnosis is 22 months and most cases are diagnosed before 4 years of age. NB is extremely rare outside of childhood. There is a slight male predominance. A hereditary predisposition is apparent in a subset of patients. There are a number of recurrent genetic alterations that are associated with advanced stage disease, older age at diagnosis, and poor outcome. These include N-*myc* amplification with double minutes and homogeneously staining regions of 2p, gain of 17q21, and deletion of 1p. Of these, 17q gain is the most common finding (approximately 50% of tumor samples) and the most powerful independent prognostic risk factor. In contrast, expression of *TRK-A*, a tyrosine kinase receptor gene of the nerve growth factor family, is associated with low-stage disease, younger age, and improved outcome.

Screening

Given the concentration of NB in children under 4 years of age, a number of screening trials have been conducted. It has been demonstrated that urinary catecholamine screening can be used for early detection of NB, although this approach does not appear to impact on the incidence of advanced stage disease or survival.

Diagnosis

NB develops in sites of the sympathetic nervous system including the adrenal medulla and sympathetic ganglia. Two-thirds of NB arise in the abdomen, although infants are more likely to have thoracic or cervical tumors. Metastasis is common especially in older children and sites of involvement include the lymph nodes, bone, bone marrow, liver, and skin. Presenting symptoms vary depending on the sites of disease. Common presentations include pain, abdominal mass, proptosis, periorbital ecchymoses, skin nodules, spinal cord compression, systemic symptoms such as failure to thrive and fever, and paraneoplastic syndromes including opsoclonus-myoclonus and vasoactive intestinal peptide–induced secretory diarrhea. Staging evaluation should include CT scans of the chest, abdomen, and pelvis, total body bone scan, bone marrow biopsies, and urine catecholamines, vanillylmandelic acid (VMA) and homovanillic acid (HVA). Most NB is avid for meta-iodobenzylguanidine (MIBG), and a nuclear MIBG scan may be used to follow tumor response. Laboratory tests should include a CBC, chemistry panel, and serum ferritin, which is often elevated in NB. Diagnosis is confirmed by histopathology or the demonstration of metastatic involvement of the bone marrow in combination with elevated urine VMA and HVA. NB is characterized by small round blue cells with evidence for neural differentiation including positive staining for neuronal markers (e.g., NSE) on immunohistochemistry. The histopathology can include a range of benign to malignant features with mixed elements of ganglioneuroma, ganglioneuroblastoma, and neuroblastoma. The histology can be further classified as favorable or unfavorable based on the degree of differentiation, mitosis-karyorrhexis index, and patient age (the Shimada system). Tumor sample analysis for N-*myc* amplification, gain of 17q, and/or 1p deletion should be performed if possible due to prognostic value of these genetic markers.

Staging

Historically, a number of systems have been used. In recent years, a standard International Neuroblastoma Staging System (INSS) has been established (Table 32.5).

Treatment

Treatment is stratified according to stage and risk group. Spontaneous regression is frequent for those with IVS disease, although short-term therapy may be required to manage tumor-related symptoms. Surgery alone is adequate for stage I disease. For other stages, treatment is multimodal and should include chemotherapy, surgery, and radiation. Active chemotherapy agents commonly used include etoposide, cyclophosphamide, doxorubicin, cisplatin, carboplatin, and vincristine. Local control of bulky sites may require surgery and radiation. Second-look surgery is often helpful in removing residual disease and/or documenting tumor differentiation. DFS rates range from 85 to 90% for low-risk groups (stages I, IIA, IVS, and infants <1 year of age with stage III disease) to 10 to 25% for children >1 year of age with

TABLE 32.5. **Neuroblastoma Staging System**

Stage	Characterstics
I	Localized tumor confined to the area of origin
	Completely excised with no microscopic residual
	No lymph node involvement
IIA	Localized tumor
	Incomplete gross excision
	Negative lymph nodes
IIB	Localized tumor
	Complete or incomplete gross excision
	Positive ipsilateral lymph nodes
	Negative contralateral lymph nodes
III	Tumor crosses the midline, or
	Unilateral tumor, positive contralateral nodes, or
	Midline tumor, bilateral lymph node involvement
IV	Metastatic to distant lymph nodes or other organs
IVS	Stage I or II primary tumor
	Infant <1 year of age
	May be metastatic (excluding bone)

stage IV disease. High-dose chemotherapy with autologous stem cell rescue (ABMT) is recommended for this latter group after disease burden has been reduced to a minimal state. Recently, 13-*cis*-retinoic acid, which is known to induce NB differentiation *in vitro*, has been shown to improve disease-free-survival after ABMT.

Management of Recurrence

Cure after relapse has rarely been achieved, except for those with low-stage disease. A variety of novel therapies are currently undergoing clinical trials, including targeted immunotherapy, high-dose radiolabeled MIBG, retinoids, and new cytotoxic agents.

WILMS' TUMOR

Wilms' tumor (WT), or nephroblastoma, is the most common malignant renal tumor of childhood, with an incidence of approximately eight cases per million. WT is derived from primitive metanephric blastemal cells.

Etiology and Epidemiology

Diagnosis is made at a mean age of 3–4 years for those with unilateral tumors and 2–3 years for those with bilateral disease. There is a slight female predominance.

The incidence of WT is highest in those of African heritage, with a 3:1 ratio compared with Asians. Caucasian populations have an intermediate risk. Approximately 10% of patients with WT have an associated isolated anomaly such as hemihypertrophy, cryptorchidism, hypospadias, or aniridia. An additional 5–10% have a predisposing congenital syndrome such as WAGR (WT, aniridia, genitourinary malformations, mental retardation), Denys-Drash (renal disease, pseudohermaphroditism), chromosomal instability (e.g., Bloom), or a somatic overgrowth syndrome such as Beckwith-Wiedemann (hemihypertrophy, macroglossia, omphalocele, visceromegaly). It is estimated that 15–20% of WT is hereditary. There are a number of genetic alterations found in WT, the most common of which is loss of heterozygosity (LOH) of 11p, seen in 30–40% of tumors. Loss of the Wilms' tumor suppressor gene-1 (*WT-1*) located at 11p13 is associated with the WAGR and Denys-Drash syndromes, whereas loss of *WT-2* due to paternal disomy/maternal deficiency of 11p15 is associated with tumor development in the setting of the Beckwith-Wiedemann syndrome. Notably, the *IGF-2* gene is also paternally imprinted and located at 11p15. Thus, it is possible that overexpression of IGF-2 might play a role in the somatic overgrowth and tumorigenesis seen in that syndrome. Finally, although rare in WT overall, there is a strong association between *p53* mutations and anaplastic Wilms' histology.

Screening

The risk of developing WT is about 5% in Beckwith-Wiedemann syndrome and about 25–30% in those with aniridia or the WAGR syndrome. Thus, such children should be monitored closely for the development of WT by serial physical exams and urinalysis.

Diagnosis

Most commonly, WT presents with an asymptomatic abdominal or flank mass that is discovered by a parent. About 50% present with abdominal pain and/or vomiting, 25–50% have hypertension, and 10–25% have hematuria. Occasionally, children will present with rapid abdominal enlargement, anemia, hypertension, and/or fever due to subcapsular hemorrhage. This is often associated with an "eggshell" pattern of calcification on plain radiography. Approximately 20% of patients have metastases at diagnosis, most commonly isolated to the lungs, but also possibly involving the liver and/or lymph nodes. Staging should include ultrasonography and CT scan of the primary and chest. It is essential to evaluate for evidence of bilateral renal involvement and tumor extension into the renal vein and inferior vena cava. Laboratory studies should include a CBC, urinalysis, and chemistry panel including kidney function tests. Pathologic diagnosis can be confirmed by fine needle aspirate, although if the diagnosis is highly likely and complete tumor resection is possible, this may not be needed. Classic WT is composed of three cellular elements: blastemal, stromal, and epithelial, although mono- and biphasic tumors occur as well. WT is further classified as favorable or unfavorable (i.e., anaplastic) histology. Historically, clear cell sarcoma and rhabdoid tumor of the kidney were classified as unfavorable histologic Wilms' variants, although these are now considered and treated separately because they have unique patterns of spread and worse outcome. Finally, not all bilateral lesions are detected by radiographic imaging studies and the contralateral kidney should be manually inspected and suspicious lesions biopsied at the time of nephrectomy. Nephrogenic rests may represent Wilms' precursor lesions, and when found should be followed closely for possible progression.

Staging

The National Wilms' Tumor Study Group Staging System is widely used (Table 32.6).

Treatment

Great progress has been made in the treatment of WT and currently 85–90% of children are cured. Treatment is multimodal and involves surgery, chemotherapy, and, in some cases, radiation therapy, stratified according to stage and histology. Radical or modified nephrectomy is recommended whenever possible, except in cases of bilateral disease. Surgery should be performed via transperitoneal approach to allow for exploration of the contralateral kidney, liver, and regional lymph nodes. The chemotherapy agents employed include vincristine and actinomycin-D, with the addition of doxorubicin and cyclophosphamide for high-risk patients. Radiation may be used to treat the tumor bed, lungs, and/or sites of unresectable disease.

TABLE 32.6. Wilms' Tumor Staging System

Stage	Characteristic
I	Localized tumor confined to the kidney
	Completely excised with negative margins
	Intact renal capsule: no biopsy (except fine needle), rupture, or invasion
	No renal vessel involvement
II	Tumor extends beyond the kidney
	Completely excised with negative margins
	Renal capsule biopsied, ruptured, or invaded
	Disease extending into the inferior vena cava (IVC) is free floating and nonadherent
	Tumor spillage confined to flank without peritoneal involvement
III	Residual tumor in the abdomen (nonhematogenous) including
	lymph nodes, peritoneal implants, tumor spillage beyond the flank, adherent tumor thrombus in the IVC, incomplete resection
IV	Distant hematogenous metastasis
V	Bilateral renal disease

Management of Recurrence

Depending on the stage, histology, and prior treatment, curative salvage may be possible. As in primary therapy, treatment is multimodal. Chemotherapy agents commonly used include cyclophosphamide, ifosfamide, etoposide, doxorubicin, and carboplatin.

BRAIN TUMORS

As a group, brain tumors represent the second most common cancer in children, affecting approximately 3 per 100,000 children. Infratentorial lesions are much more common in pediatrics than in adults (Fig. 32.2). A complete review of pediatric brain tumors is beyond the scope of this chapter and only the most common diagnoses will be considered.

Etiology and Epidemiology

Brain tumors show a bimodal age incidence, with a peak in the first decade of life between 3 and 9 years and then another in adulthood. There is a slight male predominance and Caucasians have a higher incidence than those of African heritage. The brain tumor incidence rates in children have increased over the past 2 decades, although the explanation for this is unknown. The only environmental factor that has been clearly associated with brain tumor development is therapeutic ionizing radiation to the head and neck. A number of congenital and familial syndromes are associated with an increased risk of specific brain tumors including neurofibromatosis,

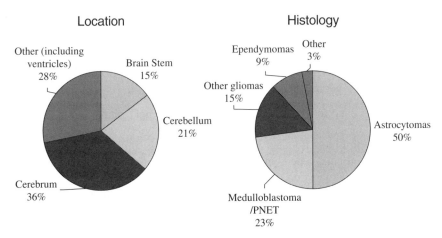

Figure 32.2   Distribution of pediatric brain tumors. (Data from Reis LAG et al. (eds). (1999) *Cancer Incidence and Survival among Children and Adolescents: United States SEER Program 1975–1995*, National Cancer Institute, SEER Program. NIH Pub. No. 99–4649, Bethesda, MD.)

tuberous sclerosis, von Hippel-Lindau, Li-Fraumeni, nevoid basal cell carcinoma, Turcot, ataxia-telangiectasia, and multiple endocrine neoplasia. A variety of chromosomal abnormalities occur in pediatric brain tumors, but few of these have been recurrent and characteristic. The most frequent cytogenetic abnormality is isochromosome 17q (with 17p loss and 17q gain) in medulloblastoma.

Screening

There is little role for routine screening of healthy children, although those with predisposing risk factors should be followed closely for signs and symptoms of neurologic deficits, increased intracranial pressure, and/or developmental delay.

Diagnosis

Brain tumors present with symptoms specific to the location. Cerebellar tumors commonly present with ataxia, dysmetria, nystagmus, cranial nerve palsies, and/or head tilt. Obstruction of the fourth ventricle by midline tumors frequently leads to signs of increased intracranial pressure including lethargy, early morning headache, and vomiting. Brainstem tumors may present with cranial neuropathy, bulbar palsy, long tract signs, and/or gait disturbances. Supratentorial lesions may present with headache, seizures, upper motor neuron deficits, and/or sensory loss. Brain imaging with CT and/or MRI scan should be performed on an emergent basis for a suspected brain tumor. Diagnostic confirmation is made by biopsy in most cases, with the exception of brainstem and optic chiasm tumors. For tumors with a high frequency of spread to the spinal column, such as medulloblastoma and ependymoma, spinal MRI and lumbar puncture should be performed.

Medulloblastoma, also known as primitive neuroectodermal tumor (PNET) of the cerebellum, is the most frequent malignant brain tumor in children. The most common location is the mid-line posterior fossa, typically in the area of the cerebellar vermis. The cell of origin is not known and histopathology reveals small round blue cells with variable degrees of glial or neuroblastic differentiation and characteristic Homer Wright rosettes and pseudorosettes. Extraneural spread to bone, bone marrow, lymph nodes, liver, and lung may occur. Cerebellar astrocytomas, the second most common posterior fossa tumor, are predominantly low-grade and pilocytic. Brain stem gliomas, approximately 80% of which arise in the pons, are the third most frequent infratentorial tumor in childhood. Ependymomas arise from ventricular ependymal cells and histopathology commonly shows pseudorosettes, calcification, hemorrhage, and cyst formation. Ependymomas typically occur in the floor of the fourth ventricle, although they may also arise in supratentorial locations. The majority of supratentorial tumors are cerebral astrocytomas, which may be high- or low-grade.

Staging

There is no uniform staging system used for brain tumors.

Treatment

Progress in the treatment of pediatric brain tumors has been slow, and outcome depends on histology, location, and extent of disease. Treatment may include surgery, radiation, and/or chemotherapy. Initial supportive care interventions that may be required include ventriculoperitoneal shunt placement for management of obstructive hydrocephalus, dexamethasone and/or mannitol to reduce cerebral edema, and anticonvulsants for seizure prophylaxis. When possible, surgical resection is usually the therapy of choice. Radiation therapy is the mainstay for unresectable lesions such as brainstem gliomas. Spinal radiation is also used for PNET and ependymoma due to their propensity for spinal metastasis. Chemotherapy has rarely been shown to improve survival, with the exception of PNET, where adjuvant treatment is beneficial in high-risk patients. Chemotherapy can also be used to delay the initiation of radiation therapy in infants and young children in an effort to decrease the risk of late neurocognitive dysfunction.

Management of Recurrence

In general, the same approach to primary treatment applies to patients with relapse. Cure may be possible for low-grade tumors if surgical resection can be achieved. Certain tumors, such as PNET, may respond to high-dose chemotherapy and autologous stem cell rescue. Finally, a variety of new chemotherapy agents that target the central nervous system and new methods of radiation therapy delivery are under study.

SUPPORTIVE CARE AND LONG-TERM FOLLOW-UP

Successful outcome for every child who develops cancer requires close attention to potential complications of the underlying malignancy and its treatment. Those with high tumor burden and rapid cell turnover, most notably acute leukemia and Burkitt's NHL, are at high risk of tumor lysis syndrome. During initiation of therapy, close monitoring of metabolic and renal function is required and prophylactic measures should include intravenous hydration, alkalinization, and allopurinol. Emergent, empiric therapy may be required to manage airway obstruction associated with an anterior mediastinal mass, common in T-ALL and LBL. Emergent diagnosis and intervention is required for spinal cord compression. To preserve neurologic function, immediate dexamethasone, radiation therapy, and/or laminectomy should be considered. Leukoreduction by apheresis may be required to manage symptomatic leukostasis due to hyperleukocytosis while preparing to initiate induction chemotherapy in ALL or AML. Cancer treatments are frequently myelosuppressive and many patients will develop anemia, thrombocytopenia, and/or neutropenia during the course of therapy. Appropriate transfusion support is essential and specialized products should be employed in attempt to minimize associated complications. Irradiated cellular blood products are required to prevent transfusion-associated graft-versus-host disease for those with Hodgkin's disease, after stem cell transplantation, and for others with severe immunosuppression. Leukodepletion is recommended to decrease the risks of platelet alloimmunization, febrile reactions, and CMV transmission. Single donor (i.e., apheresis) platelets are recommended when available to reduce donor exposure and associated risks of alloimmunization and septic reactions. To shorten the duration of neutropenia, myeloid growth factors (e.g., G-CSF, GM-CSF) are routinely employed with combination chemotherapy for solid tumors. All patients should be closely scrutinized for possible infections with bacterial, viral, fungal, and opportunistic organisms. Empiric, broad-spectrum parenteral antibiotics are life-saving for patients with neutropenic fever. Agents that have been proven beneficial in this setting include ceftazidime, imipenem, and the combination of an extended-spectrum penicillin with an aminoglycoside. Empiric amphotericin should be added for those with persistent neutropenic fever. Prophylaxis against *Pneumocystis carinii* pneumonia is essential for those undergoing treatment for acute leukemia and lymphoma, and for others with severe immunosuppression such as after stem cell transplantation. Patients should be monitored for coagulopathy associated with malignancy and infection. In particular, those with acute promyelocytic leukemia (M3-AML) are at high risk of disseminated intravascular consumptive coagulopathy (DIC) at presentation and during induction. Other components essential to the treatment of children with cancer include nutritional support, pain control, antiemesis, physical therapy/rehabilitation, and psychosocial support.

With the progress in achieving cure has come the realization that many survivors have substantial complications of therapy. Long-term follow-up is critical not only to monitor for disease recurrence, but also to manage toxicities such as hearing loss, renal dysfunction, avascular necrosis, pulmonary fibrosis, cardiomyopathy, neurodevelopmental deficits, and endocrinopathies. In addition, many patients are at risk of developing secondary malignancies. As in the case of primary treatment, the likelihood of success in managing such complications is improved with early recognition and intervention, as well as treatment at a center with multispecialty expertise.

FURTHER READING

Barrett AJ, Horowitz MM, Pollock BH et al. (1994) HLA identical sibling bone marrow transplants vs. chemotherapy for children with acute lymphoblastic leukemia. *N Engl J Med* 331:1253.

Brown N, Cotterill S, Lastowska M et al. (1999) Gain of chromosome arm 17q and adverse outcome in patients with neuroblastoma. *N Engl J Med* 340:1954–1961.

Matthay KM, Villablanca JG, Obert R et al. (1999) Treatment of high-risk neuroblastoma with intensive chemotherapy, radiotherapy, autologous bone marrow transplantation, and 13- cis-retinoic acid. *N Engl J Med* 341:1165–1173.

Pizzo PA, Poplack DG (eds.) (2002) *Pediatric Oncology*, 4th edition. JB Lippincott, Philadelphia.

Pui C-H (ed.) (1999) *Childhood Leukemias*, 1st edition. Cambridge University Press, New York.

Pui C-H, Evans WE (1998) Acute lymphoblastic leukemia. *N Engl J Med* 339:605–615.

Ravindrath Y, Yeager A, Chang MN et al. (1996) Autologous bone marrow transplantation versus intensive consolidation chemotherapy for acute myeloid leukemia in childhood. *N Engl J Med* 334:1428–1434.

Reis LAG, Smith MA, Gurney JG et al. (eds) (1999) *Cancer Incidence and Survival among Children and Adolescents: United States SEER Program 1975–1995*, National Cancer Institute, SEER Program. NIH Pub. No. 99-4649, Bethesda. (Available at: http://www-seer.ims.nci.nih.gov).

Sandlund JT, Downing JR, Crist WM (1996) Non-Hodgkin's lymphoma in childhood. *N Engl J Med* 334:1238–1248.

CHAPTER 33

AIDS-Related Neoplasms

DAVID T. SCADDEN

Massachusetts General Hospital, Dana-Farber/Harvard Cancer Center,
Harvard Medical School, Boston, Massachusetts

Immunodeficiencies in which T-cell function is compromised are associated with the development of opportunistic malignancies. The range of neoplasms is narrow and generally associated with secondary infectious agents. Whereas HIV-induced immunodeficiency is broad based, the tumor types that are associated with it are limited (Table 33.1) and notably absent are the epithelial neoplasms common in the general population. This chapter will focus on the most common neoplasms associated with HIV infection, non-Hodgkin's lymphoma (NHL) and Kaposi's sarcoma (KS).

EPIDEMIOLOGY

The incidence of tumors among individuals infected with HIV-1 infection is influenced by a number of factors, including the risk factor for HIV transmission, the presence of coincident oncogenic virus infection, host genotype, and use of combination, highly active antiretroviral therapy (HAART). The availability of HAART beginning in 1996 has dramatically altered the face of AIDS, markedly reducing most complications of HIV-1 infection, including malignancies. In particular, those with access to antiretroviral therapies have had an approximately one log reduction in the incidence of KS. This neoplasm was among the first recognized complications of HIV infection at the outset of the epidemic and had been present in approximately 20% of homosexual HIV-infected men. While the incidence of this tumor was declining prior to the advent of HAART, use of potent antiretrovirals has made this entity rare even in the high-risk population of men having sex with men.

There has also been a reduction in the incidence of AIDS-related lymphoma (ARL) with the use of HAART, but the effect has been most pronounced in the

UICC Manual of Clinical Oncology, Eighth Edition. Edited by Raphael E. Pollock
ISBN 0-471-22289-5 Copyright © 2004 John Wiley & Sons, Inc.

TABLE 33.1. Tumor Types with Increased Incidence in HIV Disease

Definite
Kaposi's sarcoma
Non-Hodgkin's lymphoma
Squamous cell neoplasia
Hodgkin's disease
Leiomyosarcoma (in children)
Plasmacytoma
Possible
Seminoma

subset of those patients presenting with primary Central nervous system (CNS) lymphoma. These patients have a tumor that is uniformly associated with Epstein-Barr virus (EBV) and expresses viral latent genes in a pattern similar to that of the lymphoproliferative disease seen in the post-transplantation setting (type III pattern expressing EBNA1-6 and LMP-1, -2,). Like that tumor, the primary CNS ARL requires severe immune incompetence potentially accounting for its reduced incidence among those whose immune function is preserved by HAART.

In contrast to primary CNS ARL, systemic lymphomas appear to be much more modestly affected by HAART. Although the data are conflicting, the weight of evidence indicates a reduction in incidence, but the extent of reduction is about two-fold, modest compared with the decline of KS. Among the types of systemic ARL, it is not yet clear whether particular subset are more profoundly affected than others, though one study has suggested that small noncleaved (Burkitt's and Burkitt's-like) lymphomas are disproportionately decreased. The discordant changes in systemic ARL compared with either KS or primary CNS ARL suggest a more complex pathophysiology in which simple control of an infectious pathogen may be insufficient to prevent malignant transformation of B lymphocytes.

NON-HODGKIN'S LYMPHOMA

Pathophysiology

EBV participates in all post-transplant lymphoproliferative disease and primary CNS ARL, but only a subfraction of the systemic ARL. Approximately one-third to two-thirds of systemic ARL are associated with EBV. The basis for transformation in those tumors expressing EBV latent genes in a type III pattern is thought related to LMP-2 altering the tumor necrosis factor (TNF) receptor signaling pathway leading to dysregulated proliferation. However, the type III pattern is not uniformly present and a number of other genetic abnormalities have been defined.

Other genetic alterations appear to be no more common in the EBV-associated ARL than in those tumors without EBV. Those patients with Burkitt's and Burkitt's-like histology commonly have c-*myc* rearrangements present, whereas the large-cell histologies are associated with *Bcl*-6 rearrangement, c-*myc* rearrangement and *p*53 mutations in approximately 33%, 40%, and 25%, respectively. The c-*myc* rearrangement that is observed in ARL indicates that the mutation arose late in the maturation of the B cell. The c-*myc* gene is juxtaposed with the immunoglobulin heavy chain switch region indicating that the rearrangement occurred at the time of immunoglobulin class switching. These data strongly argue for oncogenesis to have occurred after original rearrangement of the immunoglobulin locus and to be associated with a postgerminal center cell.

In the absence of EBV, the drive to B-cell proliferation that may contribute to the predisposition to lymphoma has been hypothesized to come from various sources. That B lineage cells behave abnormally in HIV disease is clear, not just from the excess risk of B-cell lymphoma in these patients, but also the extremely common hypergammaglobulinemia seen in HIV-infected individuals and the frequent lymphadenopathy seen throughout HIV disease. Each of these reflects disordered B-cell regulation that may have multiple underlying mechanisms. A distortion of $CD4^+$ T-cell subsets in addition to the overall decline in $CD4^+$ cells has been documented in HIV infection, leading to a relative excess of TH2 cells and a decline in TH1 $CD4^+$ cells. The TH2 subset is a population producing the cytokines interleukin (IL)-10 and IL-4, both known B-cell proliferative agents. Further, HIV products themselves may encourage B-cell proliferation. It has been noted that HIV envelope glycoprotein is capable of directly enhancing B-cell activation *in vitro*. HIV glycoprotein gp120 interacts with chemokines on the surface of B-cells. CXCR4 is a receptor for the B-cell growth factor, stroma-derived growth factor-1 (SDF-1), and has been shown to be activated by some HIV envelopes (those with R4 specificity). This association of chemokine receptors with ARL has been further supported by evidence that individuals with variant regulatory regions in the chemokine gene encoding the ligand for CXCR-4, SDF-1, have a higher risk of developing the Burkitt's lymphoma subtype of ARL. In addition, HIV-infected individuals heterozygous for a variant of CCR5 (CCR5delta32) have a three-fold decrease in their risk of lymphoma, possibly related to decreased sensitivity to the chemokine RANTES. Therefore, alteration in B-cell proliferation has multiple potentially contributing bases providing a background against which malignant transformation may occur.

Clinical Features

Systemic AIDS-related lymphomas present with a wide spectrum of clinical abnormalities due to the common extranodal location of the tumor. Lymphoma outside the confines of the lymphatic system is the rule rather than the exception in patients with ARL and has a predisposition for certain sites, including gastro intestinal (GI) tract, bone marrow, CNS, liver, and soft tissues. Although many also have nodal involvement, biopsy of extranodal tissue was the source of diagnosis in two-thirds of patients in one study, and evidence of extranodal tumor found in 95% of patients overall. There are certain tumor histologies that have been noted to be more closely associated with involvement of specific tissues such as large cell tumors preferentially involving the GI tract and small cell tumors preferentially found in the bone marrow and meninges. The clinical presentation of ARL in the HAART era compared with patients diagnosed prior to HAART availability has not been noted to be substantially different, but one report has indicated there may be a decrease in the small cell (Burkitt's and Burkitt's-like) histologic subtypes.

Among the systemic lymphomas, there is a unique subset that is distinct clinically, pathologically, and molecularly. Primary effusion lymphoma (PEL) is a rare tumor involving body cavities rather than solid tissues, although case reports of GI tract and other organs have appeared. The tumor is present in effusions from body cavities and histologically has large anaplastic- or immunoblastic-appearing cells that stain with antibodies to CD45 (common leukocyte antigen), but do not stain for markers of lymphocytes such as CD20 or CD19 (B-cell markers) or CD3 (T-cell specific marker). However, molecular analysis of the cells by Southern blotting of the immunoglobulin locus does reveal rearrangement of the immuno-globulin locus, defining a B-cell origin. Notably, the cells also uniformly have detectable genomic DNA for the gammaherpesvirus, human herpesvirus-8 (HHV-8), also known as KS herpes virus (KSHV). Many, but not all tumors also have evidence of coincident infection by EBV. The basis for KSHV participating in the transformation of these tumors is yet to be defined though a number of possible mechanisms have been raised as will be discussed below.

Patient Evaluation

Clinical assessment of ARL patients is guided by criteria for staging and evaluation defined for aggressive NHL outside the context of HIV infection. This should involve radiographic imaging including a chest x-ray and CT of the chest, abdomen, and pelvis. Further studies such as gallium or SPECT scanning may be particularly useful in patients with bulky disease who may be difficult to assess by CT scanning. Standard blood work including a complete blood count, differential and platelet count, liver and renal functional indices, uric acid, calcium, and lactate dehydro-genase (LDH). Bone marrow is also often performed and is particularly relevant for those patients with abnormal blood counts or cell morphology. The presence of "B" symptoms should be cautiously interpreted and vigilance maintained for a coincident secondary infection. Microbiologic assessment is particularly important for those who present with markedly suppressed CD4+ cell counts (<200 cells/ mm^3). Opportunistic infections such as *Pneumocystis carinaii*, cytomegalovirus, toxoplasmosis, mycobacterium, and fungal and parasitic pathogens should be considered.

Assessment of the CNS generally also accompanies staging of patients with ARL. CNS involvement in patients with systemic ARL lymphoma has been estimated to be as high as 20%, prompting imaging and cerebrospinal fluid (CSF) sampling. The frequency of involvement led to a practice of prophylactically treating all patients with intrathecal therapy. The necessity or efficacy of this practice has not been clearly defined and newer data has suggested that select patients may be a higher risk than others. The presence of EBV in the tumor sample for diagnosis was noted to be highly associated with a risk for CNS relapse in a study by Cingolani and colleagues ($p = 0.003$). Although only indirect, these data do suggest that it may be reasonable to selectively use CNS prophylaxis in those patients with EBV in the primary tumor. Other criteria for CNS prophylaxis that have been established outside the context of ARL, but may also apply to ARL, are lymphomatous involvement of the paranasal sinuses, bone marrow, and testis.

The prognosis in patients with ARL may be evolving in the era of HAART. Studies conducted prior to effective antiretroviral agents suggested a very poor prognosis despite tumor response rates that were comparable to patients with comparable histology tumors outside the setting of HIV infection. With improvement in the overall health of patients successfully controlling HIV replication with medication, tolerance of chemotherapy has improved and outlook is likely to substantially improve. Prognostic indicators defined prior to the advent of HAART have been examined in a number of studies. The largest to date involved 192 patients and identified CD4 count <100 cells/mm^3, age >35 years, intravenous drug use (IVDU), and stage III/IV disease as negative prognostic factors. The overall survival was 46 weeks when one of these was present, 44 weeks when two factors were present, and 18 weeks when three or four factors were present. Notably, histology, LDH, or bone marrow involvement have not been consistently identified as influencing outcome. The International Prognostic Index has been assessed in ARL with small scale studies indicating its usefulness.

Treatment

Prior to the availability of HAART, therapy for ARL was often compromised by limited tolerability and efforts were made to design regimens of minimal toxicity. This led to testing of half-dose regimens such as modified m-BACOD and demonstration in a phase III trial indicating equivalence in response rate and durability when compared with standard dose m-BACOD. Toxicity was improved as anticipated and suggested that using a half-dose regimen would be reasonable for patients with advanced HIV disease, particularly patients who have failed HAART. For patients responding to or yet to start HAART therapy, antitumor therapy may be used more aggressively. The equivalence of half-dose regimens was not in a HAART-treated group and concern about inadequate tumor sterilization has led to regimens of full or intensified dosing. The results of ARL treated with CHOP has indicated a response rate of approximately 50%. Efforts to improve this outcome have included infusional regimens and adding rituxan to CHOP. The latter trial was a multi-institutional phase III and did not indicate any benefit from adding rituxan to CHOP. CDE was defined by Sparano and colleagues to have a favorable response profile. A dose-adjusted EPOCH regimen has been tested at the U.S. National Cancer Institute (NCI) with impressive response rates and no evidence of relapse at greater than 2 years. The regimen is now being tested through the AIDS Malignancy Consortium and, if verified, may set a new standard of potent therapy for ARL.

Patients who fail initial therapy for ARL have traditionally had very few options and tolerated second-line therapies poorly. HAART appears to also be making a dramatic impact on this setting where it is increasingly clear that high-dose regimens with stem cell support are feasible and without undue toxicity. In addition, miniallogeneic transplants are being undertaken. The potential for these therapies in the setting of the altered immune state of HIV disease remains to be determined, but the use of stem cell therapies in AIDS presents an opportunity to also test stem cell manipulation strategies. For example, several trials using stem cell products modified to express HIV resistance genes have been undertaken in the context of ARL. Intensive immunologic, virologic, and tumor monitoring will be required in these early trials to better understand the complex physiology of the intensive, acute immunosuppression superimposed on a background of chronic, diverse immune dysregulation.

An issue of ongoing debate is the handling of antiretroviral therapy during the course of antitumor therapy. Two distinct approaches have been tested in clinical trials. The AIDS Malignancy Consortium used a fixed regimen of antiretroviral drugs (stavudine, lamivudine, and indinivir) in combination with CHOP chemotherapy, measuring pharmacokinetic and pharmacodynamic outcomes. The results indicated that the regimens could safely be combined and no alterations in serum levels of adriamycin or indinivir were evident. However, a delayed clearance of cyclophosphamide was noted, though this was without adverse clinical effect. An alternative approach was taken by the U.S. NCI in a trial testing EPOCH. In that trial, all antiretrovirals were discontinued resulting in a prompt increase in HIV RNA and a decrease in CD4 count. When the antitumor regimen was completed, the same antiretrovirals were reinstituted with prompt declines in viral load and gradual improvement in CD4 counts, both to levels comparable to those at baseline. The two distinct approaches provide alternative strategies and which tact to take depends on the agents involved, the relative tolerance to the medications and the psychological impact on patients taking antiretrovirals they legitimately regard as a lifeline. Regardless of the approach taken, the important issue to avoid is reduced dose antiretrovirals or intermittent use of antiretrovirals as these raise the risk of resistant HIV emerging.

The impact of chemotherapy on underlying immune function is not well defined, but the presumption that immunocompetence is diminished is a prudent tact that we and others take and begin all ARL patients on anti-PCP prophylaxis regardless of the starting CD4 count. Trimethoprim/sulfamethoxazole is agent of choice for those who can tolerate it, though dapsone, atovoquone, and aerosolized pentamadine are reasonable alternatives. In addition, patients may experience enhanced sensitivity to the myelotoxic effects of cytotoxic chemotherapy and often require growth factor support. At least one study has shown that granulocyte macrophage colony-stimulating factor (GM-CSF) provides statistically significant improvement in days of neutropenia, incidence of fever, and days of hospitalization in the setting of chemotherapy for ARL. Other studies have suggested utility for granulocyte colony-stimulating factor (G-CSF) as well.

KAPOSI'S SARCOMA

Epidemiology

The epidemiology of KS has been unique among complications of HIV in that risk for it was highly inhomogeneous among HIV-infected individuals. The risk of this tumor was extremely low among those contracting HIV from medical transfusion of a blood product, yet as high as 20% among HIV-infected homosexual men. The suspicion of second, sexually transmitted pathogen inducing this disease was born out by molecular analysis of tumor tissue compared with noninvolved tissue by Cheng and Moore in 1994. They documented a consistent presence of DNA with homology to gammaherpesviruses that has since defined HHV-8 or KSHV. This unique virus is a 165 kb double-stranded DNA virus with closest homology to Herpesvirsu saimiri and EBV, two viruses capable of transforming human cells. The link of KSHV as a causative agent for KS is based on the high seroprevalence for the virus among those with a high incidence of KS, the presence of the virus in the cells composing the tumors and evidence that viral infection uniformly precedes development of the tumor.

Assays for KSHV infection have yet to be standardized, but assaying for antibodies to the ORF 73 gene product has been shown to be highly specific if only sensitive to the 80% level. With the use of this method, the prevalence of KSHV infection has been estimated to be at least 1–2% in the U.S. blood donor population, compared with 2% of hemophiliacs, 3–4% of HIV-positive women, and 25–30% of HIV-positive homosexual men. An alternative, highly sensitive whole virus lysate assay has revealed viral reactivity in 92% of patients with KS regardless of HIV status and 11% of healthy blood donors. Overall, the prevalence of KSHV is more reminiscent of Herpes simplex infections than the more ubiquitous EBV infection in North American and European populations. In the Mediterranean basin and in parts of sub-Saharan Africa, prevalence rates may exceed 40%.

The presence of KSHV broadly in populations including children has suggested that multiple modes of transmission may exist. Following homosexual men over a 10 year interval in San Francisco demonstrated that seroconversion to KSHV was directly associated with the frequency of sexual contact. Men who had in excess of 250 sexual partners in the preceding 2 years had a seropositivity rate of 65%. However, other behaviors are also associated with risk of transmission and KSHV has been demonstrated in saliva and oral mucosa with risk of infection related to oral contamination.

Pathophysiology

KSHV is found in all variants of KS including those with HIV, after organ transplant, or in the elderly. How KSHV induces KS lesions remains unclear, however, as regions of homology do not exist with EBV genes known to cause transformation. Numerous KSHV genes have been implicated in altering cell function including those with homology to cellular cytokines, chemokines, an activated chemokine receptor, antiapoptosis, and genes capable of affecting cell cycle. A number of KSHV gene products such as K1, the constitutively activated chemokine receptor homologue, ORF74, the interferon regulatory factor family member, K9, and the unique K12 gene are all capable of transforming cells when ectopically expressed in cells. Mice that express the chemokine receptor develop lesions histologically highly similar to human KS. However, each of the candidate genes above are expressed in the lytic phase of the virus life cycle, not intuitively a phase of the virus that should permit cell survival, no less transformation. However, a new paradigm of viral oncogenesis may be active, where lytic genes are capable of having potent secondary effects at a distance. The potential for lytic phase KSHV having a role in KS is further indicated by the association of antilytic phase herpesvirus inhibitory drugs (foscarnet and ganciclovir) associated with a reduced incidence of developing KS. Defining the precise basis for the effects of the virus are impaired currently by the lack of robust virus replication *in vitro*, but as such methods are developed, improved molecular and virologic studies will likely yield the mechanisms for KS induction.

Clinical Evaluation

KS is usually evident on mucocutaneous surfaces inducing a hyperpigmented macule of purple or salmon color. The tumors often appear as solitary lesions, but may be clustered and are frequently confused with a bad bruise. The lesions are generally thickened, may become nodular, and are often plaque like. They do occur in an orderly manner and multiple lesions may emerge simultaneously at distinct sites. In addition to mucocutaneous locations, KS commonly involves the lymph nodes or lymphatic themselves and may be found in virtually any organ apart from the CNS. Common sites are GI or bronchial mucosa resulting in pain or cough, respectively, and bleeding. Pleural based lesions frequently induce pleural effusions that may be hemorrhagic and for which no studies short of bronchoscopic biopsy are definitive.

The invasive potential of KS is minimal. It rarely destroys adjacent tissue and often induces its worst clinical effects by alteration in lymphatic flow. The aberrant blood vessels that constitute the KS lesion are very leaky and cells within the lesion elaborate vascular endothelial growth factor, which is a permeability factor for normal adjacent vessels. The demand on local lymphatics is therefore great and local swelling is common from interstitial fluid. In addition, the lymphatics are often involved with KS, resulting in edema that may be extreme and highly debilitating.

The appearance of KS can be so characteristic to an experienced observer that histologic confirmation can seem superfluous, yet among immunosuppressed individuals, pigmented skin lesions may be due to other agents such as *Bartonella*, requiring a very different clinical approach using antibiotics. Only through biopsy and silver staining can bacillary angiomatosis due to *Bartonella* species be excluded and KS defined. Once histologic confirmation is obtained, it is important to measure blood CD4 and count and plasma HIV RNA levels and

TABLE 33.2. Secondary Virus Infections Associated with AIDS-Related Malignancies

Virus	Tumor
EBV	NHL (PCNS, some systematic ARL, oropharyngeal T-cell)
	HD
	Leiomyosarcoma (children)
KSHV	KS
	NHL (PEL)
HPV	Squamous cell neoplasia

ARL, AIDS-related lymphoma; EBV, Epstein-Barr virus; HD, Hodgkin's disease; HPV, human papillomavirus; KS, Kaposi's sarcoma; KSHV, Kaposi's sarcoma herpesvirus; NHL, non-Hodgkin's lymphoma; PCNS, primary central nervous system; PEL, primary effusion lymphoma.

obtain a history of antiretroviral therapy. Examination for adenopathy, edema, and definition of the number, size, and palpability (raised or not) of KS lesions are helpful gauges of extent of involvement and useful parameters to follow. Imaging beyond a simple chest x-ray to exclude occult pulmonary involvement should be performed according to clinical judgment. Extensive screening for visceral disease is not warranted in the absence of guiding symptoms or signs.

Prognosis has been broken down into two basic categories and is related as much to immunologic parameters as to tumor extent (Table 33.2). Immunologic control is a central feature of this highly immunologically sensitive tumor. In settings such as KS post-organ transplant, decreasing the dose of immunosuppressive agents can induce regression of KS. Similarly, in HIV-infected individuals, control of HIV infection has both reduced the incidence of new KS and resulted in regression of existing KS as CD4 cells climb. Although only limited information is available to date about the immunobiology of KSHV, further understanding of cytotoxic T-cell reactivity and epitopes they target may result in the development of vaccine or adoptive immunologic approaches to the disease.

Treatment

KS is a disease with a highly variable clinical course. There is no orderly progression and no certainty that progression will be inexorable. Some tumors do spontaneously remit or remain dormant for lengthy intervals suggesting that an aggressive approach to patients with minimal disease may be treated conservatively. However, some patients will develop rapidly progressive disease, with progressive pulmonary disease the one setting in which fatal complications have the greatest potential unless aggressively treated with cytotoxic chemotherapy. Deciding which patients require an aggressive tact versus those for whom observation may be appropriate depends on many features, but a simple guideline is whether the patient is symptomatic from something other than a cosmetic concern or if the patient has documented pulmonary parenchymal disease. Even among those with primarily cosmetic concerns, if large and disfiguring, the rapidity of response and excellent tolerance of systemic chemotherapy may justify its use.

All patients should have anti-HIV therapy reviewed and maximized. Response rates of KS to antiretroviral therapy have been reported to be as high as 85%, comparable to that of cytotoxic agents. Yet anti-HIV medications have no direct effect on KSHV, rather exerting their benefit through the secondary enhancement of immune function. The response of KS to anti-HIV medications may occur over prolonged intervals and be durable. One study demonstrated that 33 of 39 patients had control of KS exclusively with anti-HIV medications 24 months after initiating HAART. The interval between the time that antiretrovirals are begun and tumor response is generally measured in one to several months, but most patients will have demonstrated improvement by week eight and any patient with new lesions emerging after 12 weeks of HAART should move to other therapeutic options.

The possible approaches to KS are numerous, broadly categorized as those with local effect versus systemic therapies. Local therapies are generally reserved for patients with limited numbers of cutaneous or mucous membrane lesions. Lesions of small size may be amenable to local cryotherapy of intralesional injection of low dose vinblastine. Alternatively, topical 9-*cis* retinoic acid has been shown to be useful if patients can scrupulously apply the cream to avoid normal surrounding tissue, which can become quite inflamed. Radiation therapy can result in durable control, though expense and number of spot therapies may be prohibitive.

Those patients with KS-associated edema, extensive mucocutaneous disease, or symptomatic pulmonary or GI involvement should be considered for systemic therapy using cytotoxic chemotherapy. Responses to systemic chemotherapy have been variably reported in part due to the difficulty in applying standard response criteria. Due to the vascular nature of KS and leakage of red blood cells into tissue interstitium through the abnormal vasculature of KS, hemosiderin deposits may persist long after the proliferative component of a KS has regressed. Bidimensional measurements of the lesions of KS may therefore be quite misleading and criteria for response have been periodically modified. A recent scoring system using functional criteria has been developed by collaborative effort of the U.S.AIDS Malignancy Consortium, the NCI, and the Food and Drug Administration and is in the process of being prospectively assessed.

Combinations of bleomycin and vincristine or doxorubicin, bleomycin, and vincristine have been reported to result in tumor responses reported over a wide range (57–88%). Tolerability of these agents however is limited and alternatives have emerged that supplant these in clinical usefulness. Liposomal anthracyclines have been tested extensively and exploit the leaky vasculature of the KS lesions to result in local concentration of drug up to an order of magnitude greater than in nearby normal skin. The therapeutic ratio of these agents has been confirmed to be superior to that of traditional combination chemotherapy in several randomized phase III trials. Liposomal doxorubicin has also been shown to yield tumor response rates superior to standard chemotherapy. Liposomal anthracyclines are generally regarded as the reasonable first choice for systemic chemotherapy where cost and access are not prohibitive.

Another agent with exceptional activity in KS is the taxane tubuline stabilizer, paclitaxel, at low doses. A phase I trial involving 28 patients demonstrated a major response in 71% including individuals with heavily pre-treated, anthracycline treated KS. A phase II study observed a response rate of 59% with a longer duration of response than seen with other cytotoxic therapies for KS. This agent can be given at doses such as $100 \, mg/m^2$ every 2 weeks with excellent control of tumor over prolonged intervals (years).

Although a number of agents are active against KS, none is curative. Those patients who have an excellent response to chemotherapy will recur if therapy is interrupted and anti-HIV medications have not resulted in sufficient immune reconstitution. However, it is possible to reinstitute therapy quite successfully and it is a reasonable clinical practice to test the duration between chemotherapy cycles that can be tolerated to maintain a chemotherapy induced remission.

Alternatives to cytotoxic chemotherapy have long been sought and a number of agents have been through extensive testing. In particular, interferon alpha and beta have been demonstrated to be active in KS and may be useful even at low doses (1 million units/day) when combined with antiretroviral therapies. The basis for the effect may due to one or all of a number of different actions of interferon including immune modulation, antiviral, or antiangiogenesis effects. The toxicity of chronic interferon use can be quite prohibitive, however, and it appears to be active among those with relative preservation of immune function. Other agents with antiangiogenic effect have been tested and may be useful. These include thalidomide and the metalloproteinase inhibitor, col-3. These agents are being further developed and may be most appropriate for those with limited disease or in maintenance following chemotherapy.

FURTHER READING

Ballerini P, Gaidano G, Gong JZ, Tassi V, Saglio G, Knowles, DM, Dalla-Favera, R (1993) Multiple genetic lesions in acquired immunodeficiency syndrome-related non-Hodgkin's lymphoma. *Blood* 81:166–176.

Cesarman E, Chang Y, Moore PS, Said JW, Knowles DM (1995) Kaposi's sarcoma-associated herpesvirus-like DNA sequences in AIDS-related body-cavity-based lymphomas [see comments]. *N Engl J Med* 332:1186–1191.

Chang Y, Cesarman E, Pessin MS, Lee F, Culpepper J, Knowles DM, Moore PS. (1994) Identification of herpesvirus-like DNA sequences in AIDS-associated Kaposi's sarcoma [see comments]. *Science* 266:1865–1869.

Cingolani A, Gastaldi R, Fassone, L, Pierconti F, Giancola ML, Martini M, De Luca A, Ammassari A, Mazzone C, Pescarmona E, Gaidano G, Larocca LM, Antinori A (2000) Epstein-barr virus infection is predictive of CNS involvement in systemic AIDS-related non-Hodgkin's lymphomas. *J Clin Oncol* 18:3325–3330.

Gill P, Tulpule A, Espina B, Cabriales S, Bresnahan J, Ilaw M, Louie S, Gustafson N, Brown M, Orcutt C, Winograd B, Scadden D (1999) Paclitaxel is safe and effective in the treatment of advanced AIDS-related Kaposi's sarcoma. *J Clin Oncol* 17:1876–1883.

Gill PS, Levine AM, Meyer PR, Boswell WD, Burkes RL, Parker JW, Hofman FM, Dworsky RL, Lukes RJ (1985) Primary central nervous system lymphoma in homosexual men. Clinical, immunologic, and pathologic features. *Am J Med* 78:742–748.

Gill PS, Wernz J, Scadden DT, Cohen P, Mukwaya GM, von Roenn JH, Jacobs M, Kempin S, Silverberg I, Gonzales G, Rarick MU, Myers AM, Shepherd F, Sawka C, Pike MC, Ross ME (1996) Randomized phase III trial of liposomal daunorubicin versus doxorubicin, bleomycin, and vincristine in AIDS-related Kaposi's sarcoma. *J Clin Oncol* 14:2353–2364.

Grulich AE, Li Y, McDonald AM, Correll PK, Law MG, Kaldor JM (2001) Decreasing rates of Kaposi's sarcoma and non-Hodgkin's lymphoma in the era of potent combination antiretroviral therapy. *Aids* 15:629–633.

Hamilton-Dutoit SJ, Pallesen G, Franzmann MB, Karkov J, Black F, Skinhoj P, Pedersen C (1991) AIDS-related lymphoma. Histopathology, immunophenotype, and association with Epstein-Barr virus as demonstrated by in situ nucleic acid hybridization. *Am J Pathol* 138:149–163.

Kaplan LD, Straus DJ, Testa MA, Von Roenn J, Dezube BJ, Cooley TP, Herndier B, Northfelt DW, Huang J, Tulpule A, Levine, AM (1997) Low-dose compared with standard-dose m-BACOD chemotherapy for non-Hodgkin's lymphoma associated with human immunodeficiency virus infection. National Institute of Allergy and Infectious Diseases AIDS Clinical Trials Group. *N Engl J Med* 336:1641–1648.

Karcher DS, Alkan S (1997) Human herpesvirus-8-associated body cavity-based lymphoma in human immunodeficiency virus-infected patients: a unique B-cell neoplasm. *Hum Pathol* 28:801–808.

Kedes DH, Operskalski E, Busch M, Kohn R, Flood J, Ganem D (1996) The seroepidemiology of human herpesvirus 8 (Kaposi's sarcoma-associated herpesvirus): distribution of infection in KS risk groups and evidence for sexual transmission [see comments] [published erratum appears in *Nat Med* 1996 Sep. 2(9):1041]. *Nat Med* 2:918–924.

Krown SE, Testa MA, Huang J (1997) AIDS-related Kaposi's sarcoma: prospective validation of the AIDS Clinical Trials Group staging classification. AIDS Clinical Trials Group Oncology Committee. *J Clin Oncol* 15:3085–3092.

Levine AM, Seneviratne L, Espina BM, Wohl AR, Tulpule A, Nathwani BN, Gill PS (2000) Evolving characteristics of AIDS-related lymphoma. *Blood* 96:4084–4090.

Martin JN, Ganem DE, Osmond DH, Page-Shafer, KA, Macrae D, Kedes DH (1998) Sexual transmission and the natural history of human herpesvirus 8 infection. *N Engl J Med* 338:948–954.

Matthews GV, Bower M, Mandalia S, Powles T, Nelson MR, Gazzard BG (2000) Changes in acquired immunodeficiency syndrome-related lymphoma since the introduction of highly active antiretroviral therapy. *Blood* 96:2730–2734.

Northfelt DW, Dezube BJ, Thommes JA, Miller BJ, Fischl MA, Friedman-Kien A, Kaplan LD, Du Mond C, Mamelok RD, Henry DH (1998) Pegylated-liposomal doxorubicin versus doxorubicin, bleomycin, and vincristine in the treatment of AIDS-related Kaposi's sarcoma: results of a randomized phase III clinical trial. *J Clin Oncol* 16:2445–2451.

Pauk J, Huang ML, Brodie SJ, Wald A, Koelle DM, Schacker T, Celum C, Selke S, Corey L (2000) Mucosal shedding of human herpesvirus 8 in men. *N Engl J Med* 343:1369–1377.

Rabkin CS (2000). AIDS and cancer in the era of highly active antiretroviral therapy (HAART). *Eur J Cancer* 37:1316–1319.

Rabkin CS, Yang Q, Goedert JJ, Nguyen G, Mitsuya H, Sei S (1999). Chemokine and chemokine receptor gene variants and risk of non-Hodgkin's lymphoma in human immunodeficiency virus-1-infected individuals. *Blood* 93:1838–1842.

Ratner L, Lee J, Tang S, Redden D, Hamzeh F, Herndier B, Scadden D, Kaplan L, Ambinder R, Levine A, Harrington W, Grochow L, Flexner C, Tan B, Straus D (2001) Chemotherapy for human immunodeficiency virus-associated non-Hodgkin's lymphoma in combination with highly active antiretroviral therapy. *J Clin Oncol* 19:2171–2178.

Stewart S, Jablonowski H, Goebel FD, Arasteh K, Spittle M, Rios A, Aboulafia D, Galleshaw J, Dezube BJ (1998) Randomized comparative trial of pegylated liposomal doxorubicin versus bleomycin and vincristine in the treatment of AIDS-related Kaposi's sarcoma. International Pegylated Liposomal Doxorubicin Study Group. *J Clin Oncol* 16:683–691.

Straus DJ, Huang J, Testa MA, Levine AM, Kaplan LD (1998) Prognostic factors in the treatment of human immunodeficiency virus- associated non-Hodgkin's lymphoma: analysis of AIDS Clinical Trials Group protocol 142—low-dose versus standard-dose m-BACOD plus granulocyte-macrophage colony-stimulating factor. National Institute of Allergy and Infectious Diseases. *J Clin Oncol* 16:3601–3606.

Welles L, Saville MW, Lietzau J, Pluda JM, Wyvill KM, Feuerstein I, Figg WD, Lush R, Odom J, Wilson WH, Fajardo MT, Humphrey, RW, Feigal E, Tuck D, Steinberg SM, Broder S, and Yarchoan R (1998) Phase II trial with dose titration of paclitaxel for the therapy of human immunodeficiency virus-associated Kaposi's sarcoma. *J Clin Oncol* 16:1112–1121.

Yang TY, Chen SC, Leach MW, Manfra D, Homey B, Wiekowski M, Sullivan L, Jenh CH, Narula SK, Chensue SW, Lira SA (2000) Transgenic expression of the chemokine receptor encoded by human herpesvirus 8 induces an angioproliferative disease resembling Kaposi's sarcoma. *J Exp Med* 191:445–454.

CHAPTER 34

Oncological Emergencies

GLENN LIU and H. IAN ROBINS

University of Wisconsin, Comprehensive Cancer Center, Madison, Wisconsin

Cancer is so prevalent that almost everyone knows somebody who either currently has or has been previously diagnosed with a given malignancy. In fact, the lifetime risk that a man will develop invasive prostate cancer is 1 in 6. In women, the lifetime chance of developing breast cancer (in an average risk patient) is 1 in 8. Cancer statistics have also been showing increased incidence of colorectal cancer (42.3–60.8 per 100,000 people) as well as lung cancers (70 per 100,000 in the United States). With the steady increase in cancer diagnoses as well as treatment options, all physicians should be able to recognize and appropriately treat oncologic emergencies. Primary care physicians and emergency room doctors need be especially wary, as these situations can often precede the diagnosis of cancer.

Complications of cancer are the result of the underlying disease processes as well as secondary to therapeutic interventions. When a patient is undergoing treatment, whether surgery, chemotherapy, or radiotherapy, the physician has the responsibility to see that patient through any complications that may arise.

At times, supportive care may be the primary focus of intervention. In such case, a careful cost-benefit analysis should be addressed with the patient so that information is provided to allow for proper informed consent.

There are many methods to address certain commonly encountered oncological emergencies. The following represents a general approach to these issues.

SUPERIOR VENA CAVA SYNDROME

Superior vena cava syndrome (SVCS) is the clinical manifestation of blood flow obstruction to the superior vena cava (SVC). This was historically a more common

UICC Manual of Clinical Oncology, Eighth Edition. Edited by Raphael E. Pollock
ISBN 0-471-22289-5 Copyright © 2004 John Wiley & Sons, Inc.

TABLE 34.1. Malignant and Nonmalignant Causes of Superior Vena Cava Syndrome

Malignant (95%)
    Lung cancer (75%)
        Small cell cancer (50%)
        Squamous cell cancer (26%)
        Adenocarcinoma (14%)
        Large cell carcinoma (10%)
    Lymphoma (15%)
    Others (primary of metastatic) (10%)
Nonmalignant (5%)
    Granulomatous diseases
        Tuberculosis
        Syphilis
        Histoplasmosis
        Sarcoidosis
        Silicosis
    Goiter
    Aortic aneurysm
    Thrombosis
    Thymoma
    Teratoma
    Dermoid cyst
    Fibrosing mediastinitis

occurrence in the past, when syphilitic aortitis and tuberculous mediastinitis were more prevalent. Currently, over 95% of the cases of SVCS are due to malignancy, 75% of which are of lung origin. Of course, this means that not all cases of SVCS are malignant, thus establishing a diagnosis is of prime importance (Table 34.1).

This syndrome usually evolves insidiously, resulting in typical signs and symptoms. Most patients complain of shortness of breath, whereas many may experience a feeling of facial fullness or complain of chest pain or cough. Typically, examination will reveal neck venous distention, chest wall venous collateral distention, and often facial edema. Sometimes, facial plethora or cyanosis can also be seen (Table 34.2). Other associated symptoms can include hoarseness, syncope, and dizziness. Patients may also describe fullness that worsens with bending forward or lying down. At times, mental status changes can be seen, as well as pleural effusions.

It is extremely important to establish the diagnosis, as treatment can differ substantially. In the past, SVCS was considered a medical emergency in which immediate treatment was given, often even before a pathologic diagnosis was established. This led to difficulty in accurately diagnosing 50% of patients, which complicated follow-up treatment. We now recognize that the treatment of SVCS is medically urgent, as the process has generally been present for weeks. Thus, a thoughtful approach toward establishing a diagnosis and instituting appropriate

TABLE 34.2. Clinical Features of Superior Vena Cava Syndrome

Symptoms
  Dyspnea (63%)
  Facial swelling/fullness (50%)
  Cough (24%)
  Arm swelling (18%)
  Chest pain (15%)
  Dysphagia (9%)
Physical findings
  Neck vein distention (66%)
  Chest wall venous distention (54%)
  Facial edema (46%)
  Cyanosis (20%)
  Plethora (19%)
  Arm edema (14%)

therapy can be performed (unless the patient has significant respiratory compromise or central nervous system dysfunction). Again, not all SVCS is secondary to malignancy, thus a pathologic diagnosis is required.

Work-up of SCVS typically begins with a chest x-ray. More often than not, this will be abnormal, thus setting the stage for computed tomography (CT) and magnetic resonance imaging (MRI) scans, bronchoscopy, thoracoscopy, venograms, and possibly limited thoracotomy. Given the increased central venous pressure, the risk of bleeding during biopsy can be substantial. Therefore, the least invasive route to obtain a diagnosis is desirable. Often, sputum cytology, bronchoscopy with brushings, or limited biopsies can obtain the diagnosis around 60% of the time. Unfortunately, more invasive procedures sometimes are needed; thus, close observation for bleeding is warranted.

Treatment for SVCS can consist of chemotherapy, radiation therapy, thrombolytics or anticoagulation, expandable stents, balloon angioplasty, surgical bypass, steroids, and/or diuretics. In malignancy-associated SVCS, the choice of treatment depends on the tumor type. For example, lymphomas and small cell lung cancers can respond rapidly to chemotherapy alone, whereas other malignancies will likely require radiotherapy. One may elect to use combination chemoradiotherapy for small cell lung cancer or lymphoma, given the improved survival advantage seen in several studies as well as in improved local-regional control.

In general, with malignancy-associated SVCS, 75% of patients will show improvement in 3–4 days, with 90% having major improvements within 1 week. Patients that do not improve during that first week may have developed a central vein thrombus, thus requiring fibrinolytic or antithrombotic therapy. Given the increased central venous pressure and the fact that certain tumors are more friable, caution must be followed before anticoagulants are instituted. For this reason, prophylactic anticoagulation is not standard practice.

Occasionally, steroids can improve symptoms if the etiology of the SVCS is lymphoma. It can also decrease swelling while the patient is receiving radiation treatments for the SVCS. Benefits are usually minimal, however, if severe respiratory compromise is present, it would be a reasonable agent to use. Diuretics can provide symptomatic relief initially, but caution with regard to fluid status should be observed.

METASTASIS TO BRAIN AND SPINAL CORD

Brain metastasis occurs in 25–35% of patients with systemic cancer, most commonly in patients with cancers of the lung, breast, and in malignant melanoma. In general, brain metastases portend a poor prognosis with median survival ranges between 3 and 6 months with whole brain radiation alone. Now, with neurosurgical resection and stereotactic radiosurgery, survival has improved in selected patients. Generally, with current treatment strategies, median survival has increased to 6 months to 1 year from the onset of central nervous system (CNS) disease.

Common clinical signs and symptoms associated with brain metastases include headache, cranial nerve deficits, incoordination, muscle weakness, nausea, and mental status changes. Often, patients may present with a seizure, leading to the discovery of a metastatic lesion to the brain. On examination, one uncommonly sees papilledema reflecting increased intracranial pressure. This should be considered an emergent situation in which high-dose steroids (with or without mannitol or urea infusions) should be initiated immediately. Otherwise, a good neurological examination can help suggest whether symptomatic brain metastases are present, especially if focal findings are seen. These findings should then be confirmed with a CT scan of the head, or MRI scan (especially if cranial nerve findings suggest a brainstem lesion or exam suspicious for posterior fossa pathology).

Treatment typically begins with corticosteroids (e.g., dexamethasone 10 mg bolus intravenously (IV) or orally (PO), followed by 4 mg IV/PO every 6 hours), to decrease cerebral edema. This can result in improvements in symptoms within hours and prevent worsening symptoms once more definitive treatment is performed. Depending on the patient's functional status, number and location of metastatic lesion in CNS, and other end organ involvement, neurosurgical resection or stereotactic radiosurgery could be considered. Whether or not the patient is resectable, whole brain radiation should follow as the number of future neurological events has been shown to substantially decrease with radiotherapy.

Spinal cord metastasis with cord compression is a true oncological emergency in that delays in treatment can result in high morbidity with significant neurologic deficits. The natural history of disease is toward progressive pain, paralysis, sensory loss, and sphincter incontinence. Spinal cord compression is common. In general, 3–7.4% of patients with breast, prostate, or lung cancer will present to their physician with metastatic cord compression. In patients with advanced cancer, 5–10% of all patients will have evidence of cord compression at autopsy. Yet, despite its common occurrence, current treatment recommendations are largely empiric.

Clinically, patients typically present with back pain as the periosteum is invaded. In fact, 90% of patients with spinal metastases have localized pain. It is described as gradual in onset, and can be present for weeks to months before evidence of neurologic compromise. Other symptoms can include radicular pain or referred pain (e.g., sacroiliac pain in L1 compression). In some cases, patients present with weakness, sensory loss, or ascending numbness as pain may be masked by concurrent analgesic for other reasons. Late findings can include urinary retention and rectal sphincter dysfunction. Paraplegia is also an unfortunate late complication that may not resolve with appropriate therapy.

A MRI or CT scan easily confirms the diagnosis. Typically, the etiology is already known, but if the patient has no known diagnosis of cancer, appropriate work-up for a histologic diagnosis should be done. If tissue cannot be obtained in an appropriate time frame, and if neurologic compromise is already present, treatment should be initiated immediately as delays in therapy can substantially reduce the chance of full neurologic recovery and increase morbidity.

Treatment generally begins with high-dose corticosteroids. We prefer using dexamethasone 10 mg bolus, followed by 4 mg every 6 hours. Although some centers may use higher doses, there is no proven benefit to using higher doses of steroids, but side effects can increase substantially. Again, rapid improvements can be seen as symptoms secondary to surrounding edema can decrease within hours. This must be followed by more definitive treatment such as surgery or radiation as steroids alone are unlikely to stabilize the patient. Historically, laminectomy was the treatment of choice for malignant cord compression. With the advent in radiotherapy, improved local control rates were possible with less spinal instability as seen with laminectomy. With surgical improvements, vertebral body resection then became favored as spinal integrity was maintained. In general, radiation therapy is the treatment of choice as it has less treatment-associated morbidity. Indications for surgical intervention include evidence of bony compression (typically compression fracture >50%), spinal instability, or progression of symptoms despite radiotherapy.

One concern in a patient with malignant cord compression at a site that was previously irradiated is the development of radiation myelopathy if repeat radiotherapy is employed. It should be noted that if radiation myelopathy were to occur, it would typically present approximately 1 year after therapy. As most, such patients have a prognosis less than a year, and that progression of neurologic symptoms will inevitably occur without intervention, when considering the alternative (surgery or progressive cord compression), strong consideration for repeat radiation should be given.

Steroids can usually be tapered off over 2 weeks if symptoms are improving. Appropriate antifungal prophylaxis and antiulcer prophylaxis should always be provided as the high-dose steroids can cause thrush, gastritis, or a gastrointestinal bleed. Also, monitoring of blood glucose is important as the steroids can lead to a hyperglycemic response.

INFECTIONS

Antineoplastic therapy affects the cell-mediated and humoral immune systems, predisposing patients to infections. In addition, myelosuppression and mucositis from chemotherapy are both substantial risk factors toward developing a life-threatening infection. In immunocompromised hosts, infections can disseminate rapidly, leading to shock and death, so educating patients to be vigilant for fevers, or other signs of infection. In general, a single oral temperature of >38.3°C or temperature of ≥38.0°C for at least 1 hour should be considered a fever in a neutropenic patient. Although certain tumors (such as lymphomas, hepatic metastases, and tumor necrosis) can cause fevers, tumor fever needs to be a diagnosis of exclusion, and appropriate evaluation for an occult infection still needs to be performed.

Neutropenia is defined as an absolute neutrophil count of less than 1,000 per mm³. Once the neutrophil count falls below 500 per mm³, the chance for infection increases significantly. It is estimated that 50–60% of neutropenic patients will develop an established or an occult fever. Typical organisms include aerobic Gram-positive cocci (*streptococcus viridans*, coagulase-negative *staphylococcus*, or *S. aureus*) and aerobic Gram-negative bacilli (especially *Escherichia coli*, *Klebsiella pneumoniae*, or *Pseudomonas aeruginosa*).

Clinical signs or symptoms that may suggest infection can be subtle in a neutropenic host. This is likely secondary to the decreased inflammatory response that can be generated secondary to the lack of neutrophils. Therefore, special care in history taking and physical examination is performed to evaluate for a source of infection. In general, patients may only complain of fevers or rigors. The other typical clinical signs such as erythema, swelling, purulent drainage, and pain may be absent. Fortunately, relatively few anatomic sites are usually involved. Primary sites usually include the gastrointestinal tract (secondary to bacterial translocation from chemotherapy-damaged mucosa), skin (from vascular access devices), and possibly from periodontal, rectal, or respiratory infections (typically if more prolonged neutropenia). Therefore, special focus on examination should include the skin and venous access sites to look for erythema, tenderness, and discharge, the perianal region to look for a perirectal abscess or cellulitis, and the oropharynx to evaluate for leukoplakia, dental abscess, and stomatitis.

Initial work-up should include two sets of blood cultures (one from each lumen of the vascular access device if present plus a peripheral blood culture) prior to initiation of antibiotics, chest x-ray, and urine culture, as well as other clinically indicated studies or procedures. Routine cerebral spinal fluid (CSF) examination is not recommended, but should be performed if central nervous system infection is suspected. Unfortunately, with neutropenia, the typical pleocytosis during CSF infections may be absent. A complete blood count is also important as it quantifies the degree of neutropenia, and can allow the physician to estimate the time of neutropenia based on the patient's previous response and type of chemotherapy used. Measurement of other chemistries (liver function tests, creatinine, electrolytes, *etc.*) are important as it allows appropriate dosing of antibiotics and monitoring for potential drug toxicity.

Prompt administration of antibiotics is necessary, as current diagnostic tests cannot rapidly exclude an antimicrobial source of infection. Initial antibiotic therapy should be broad in spectrum and cover the common pathogens previously mentioned. Also, the initial selection should account for the local antibiotic resistance, patient drug allergies, and organ dysfunction that may limit the use of certain antibiotics. Drug interactions should also be considered as patients treated with potentially nephrotoxic chemotherapy (such as cisplatin) may receive added toxicity from the use of aminoglycosides. That being said, a standard regimen for empiric antibiotic selection follows.

We generally use regimens similar to the guidelines recommended by the Infectious Disease Society (*Clin. Infect. Dis.* 25:551–73, 1997). Typical combinations of empiric therapy can include an aminoglycoside plus an antipseudomonal β-lactam (such as pipercillin or ticarcillin). Monotherapy options can include carbapenems (like imipenum) or third-generation cephalosporins (like ceftazidime; not ceftriaxone secondary to inferior antipseudomonal efficacy). At our center, we typically use a fourth-generation cephalosporin (cefepime) at a dose of 2g IV every 8 hours when given as monotherapy (versus every 12 hours if used in combination with another antibiotic). Vancomycin is added only if the risk for a Gram-positive *Staphylococcus* infection is felt to be high (indwelling venous access device, severe mucositis, colonized with methacillin-resistant *S. aureus*) and is discontinued after 3–4 days if cultures are remain negative or susceptibility results are available (Figure 34.1).

Length of therapy depends mainly on the neutrophil count, response to therapy, and pathogen isolated. In general, if the patient remains afebrile and the neutrophil count exceeded 500/mm^3, we typically stop the antibiotic by day 7. If the patients becomes afebrile and the neutrophil count remains low, depending on the length of anticipated neutropenia, one can either continue the antibiotics until the neutropenia resolves or discontinue the antibiotics after 7 days with close observation. If a source for infection is identified (typically <50% of the time), longer antibiotic regimens (typically 10–14 days) are used. The initial broad-spectrum antibiotic started can then be adjusted to cover the isolated pathogen based on susceptibility data.

Fevers that persist after 3–4 days on initial broad-spectrum antibiotics implies either a nonbacterial infection, new infection, improper clearance of the initial infection (such as an abscess or infected vascular access device), inadequate antibiotic levels, drug fever, or tumor fever. A repeat search for the etiology of the fever should be done with focus on these possible causes. Changing antibiotics would not be unreasonable as well as adding amphotericin B (or fluconazole in certain situations) for a possible fungal infection.

Particular note should be made with regard to neutropenic patients who have abdominal pain or nausea. These patients can have typhilitis (necrotizing colitis of the cecum) and require anaerobic coverage and possibly a surgical consultation. Additionally, patients with prolonged neutropenia (such as those undergoing induction chemotherapy for leukemia or bone marrow transplantation) or on chronic steroids (such as brain cancer patients) can develop *Pneumocystis carinii*

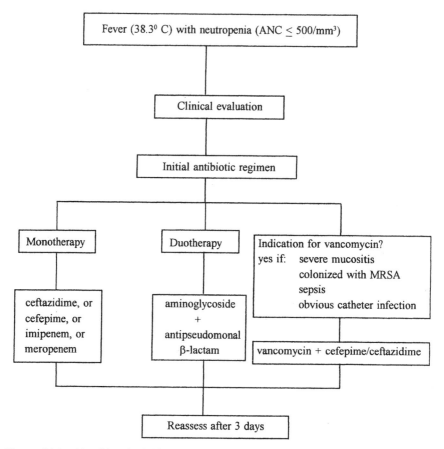

Figure 34.1 Algorithm for initial antibiotic regimen in neutropenic fever. ANC, absolute neutrophil count; MRSA, methacillin-resistant *S. aureus*.

infections if not on prophylactic therapy (e.g., trimethoprim/sulfamethoxazole or pentamidine inhaler).

Currently, the use of colony-stimulating factors has decreased the incidence and duration of neutropenia, and is currently being used prophylactically in many instances after an episode of neutropenic fever to prevent future occurrences. Although routine use is not recommended, colony-stimulating factors can be life saving in certain situations.

HYPERCALCEMIA

Hypercalcemia is the most common and potentially life-threatening metabolic emergency encountered in patients with cancer. It is seen in roughly 10–20% of all cancer patients. Most often, it is associated with breast, myeloma, lymphoma, lung, renal call, head and neck, and prostate cancer. Hypercalcemia can be secondary to destructive bony lesions as well as the release of parathyroid hormone-related peptide (PTHrP), prostaglandins, and various osteoclast-activating factors.

Typical symptoms include weakness, lethargy, and fatigue. Patients may also have nausea and vomiting, constipation, polyuria, anorexia, and dehydration. Occasionally, patients may present with confusion, seizures, or a coma. Examination may reveal mental status changes, dry mucus membranes, and muscle weakness. Deep tendon reflexes may be decreased or absent. An electrocardiogram may reveal a shortened QT segment or, less commonly, a first-degree AV block or intraventricular block. A serum calcium (corrected for hypoalbuminemia) or an ionized calcium level confirms the diagnosis.

Initial therapy with normal saline is the single most important step in treating hypercalcemia. This is because these patients are almost always dehydrated. Physiologically, 60% of plasma calcium is filtered by the glomerulus, 90% of that which is then reabsorbed in the proximal and thick ascending tubule coupled to sodium. Therefore, dehydration will lower the glomerular filtration rate (less calcium filtration) and cause increased calcium reabsorption (secondary to coupled Na^+/Ca^{++} transporters and an avid stimulus to retain sodium). This can lead to worsening hypercalcemia if fluid loss continues without adequate replacement. Thus, aggressive rehydration is always the first step. Immediate improvements in symptoms can be seen with a decrease in serum calcium within 12–24 hours.

Loop diuretics (furosemide) are often employed in the treatment of hypercalcemia as they enhance sodium excretion and, therefore, calciuresis. Again, the key is to correct the fluid deficit first. Once that is done, one can then add a loop diuretic, if necessary, with doses adjusted to maintain euvolemia. Loop diuretics can decrease serum calcium significantly in 1–2 days.

Bisphophonates are now evolving as the primary agents used in treating and preventing malignancy-associated hypercalcemia. They bind to bone minerals and help the bones resist breakdown by phosphatases from activated osteoclasts. Almost all patients with tumor-induced hypercalcemia with calcium >12 mg/dL should receive a bisphosphonate. Patients with calcium <12 mg/dL should also be treated with a bisphosphonate if symptomatic. We generally use pamidronate at a dose of 90 mg IV, as studies have shown that this dose can achieve normocalcemia in 90% of patients. Also, this dose appears necessary for humoral hypercalcemia (versus bone metastases induced).

Other treatment options for hypercalcemia include steroids (useful in hypercalcemia secondary to lymphoma or breast cancer) as well as calcitonin. Although calcitonin can decrease the serum calcium rapidly (within 2 to 4 hours), the peak effect is short lived as is usually seen within 2 days.

SYNDROME OF INAPPROPRIATE ANTIDIURETIC HORMONE SECRETION

Syndrome of inappropriate antidiuretic hormone secretion (SIADH) is usually seen in association with small-cell carcinoma of the lung. The tumor releases antidiuretic hormone, inappropriately resulting in hyponatremia and water retention, and an associated serum hypoosmolarity. Clinically, patients with SIADH have nausea, vomiting, and anorexia. They can be confused, lethargic, or weak and can also present with a seizure. In general, treatment involves correcting the underlying cause, in this case treating the small-cell lung cancer. Free water restriction can improve the sodium, although this is usually difficult to achieve in an uncontrolled setting. Drugs such as demeclocycline (300–600 mg twice a day) or lithium carbonate can improve symptoms by counteracting the effect of antidiuretic hormone by causing nephrogenic diabetes insipidus. These drugs can be especially useful in those who cannot follow or tolerate a fluid-restriction program, or in patients whose underlying malignancy if refractory to antineoplastic therapy.

HYPERURICEMIA AND TUMOR LYSIS SYNDROME

Hyperuricemia and tumor lysis syndrome (hyperuricemia, hyperkalemia, hyperphosphatemia, and hypocalcemia) can develop in patients with leukemia, lymphomas, and bulky small-cell carcinomas upon treatment with chemotherapy. This is due to the large breakdown of cells with therapy and the release of a large amount of purine precursors into circulation. The hyperuricemia can lead to urate crystal precipitatation in the kidney tubules leading to acute renal failure, and the electrolyte abnormalities can lead to cardiac irritability and even cardiac arrest. To prevent these complications, patients should be well hydrated and started on allopurinol before systemic treatment is begun. In addition, urine alkalization with sodium bicarbonate (to keep urine pH >7.0) can be considered to decrease urate crystal precipitation in the kidney tubules. Monitoring serum electrolytes and early treatment of electrolyte abnormalities are important during the first few days of therapy to prevent potential cardiac complications.

ADRENAL INSUFFICIENCY

Although metastatic involvement of the adrenals is not uncommon, particulary with breast and lung cancer, the development of adrenal insufficiency is rare. Clinical symptoms may include nausea, vomiting, apathy, abdominal pain, and hypotension. If suspected, steroid replacement should be started and appropriate work-up initiated. One situation that does occur commonly is the patient on chronic steroids with a suppressed adrenal gland secondary to negative feedback on the pituitary axis. These patients, when faced with a stressful event (such as infection or surgery), may develop symptoms of adrenal insufficiency because their adrenal gland cannot compensate for the added stressors to the body. In these cases, additional "stress-dose" steroids should be provided until the inciting event resolves.

Table 34.3. Common Presentations of Cancer-Related Thrombosis

Venous thromboembolism
    Deep venous thrombosis
    Migratory superficial thrombophlebitis
    Pulmonary embolism
    Catheter-related thrombosis
Arterial thrombosis
    Disseminated intravascular coagulation
    Marantic endocarditis

THROMBOSIS AND HYPERCOAGULABILITY

Laboratory evidence for coagulation abnormalities in cancer patients can be a common finding (up to 90% of cases). This can result in a hypercoagulable state as the various pathologic processes disturb the normal hemostatic balance. Typical processes can include thrombocytosis with increased vascular reactivity, increase in fibrin/fibrinogen degredation products, increase in tissue factor, and also hyperfibrinogenemia. Hypercoagulability may present as migratory thrombophlebitis, disseminated intravascular coagulation (DIC), marantic endocarditis, or a deep venous thrombosis (DVT) (Table 34.3). Classically, mucin-containg gastrointestinal malignancies and gliomas are associated with migratory thrombophlebitis, whereas DIC is associated with acute promyelocytic leukemia. It is reported that 10–15% of patients with cancer will develop a clinically significant thrombosis during the course of their disease. Interestingly enough, good percentages (up to 38%) of patients with an idiopathic DVT were later found to have an occult malignancy in some cohort studies, suggesting that a work-up for malignancy should be performed in patients with unexplained thrombosis. Occasionally, the risk of thrombosis is increased secondary to treatment (e.g., hormone therapy in breast cancer), but this can be difficult to sort out in many cases.

Initial therapy in general is parenteral heparin, followed by oral warfarin. The advent of low-molecular weight heparins (LMWH), with their improved safety profile and proven efficacy without need for frequent dose titration, have given physicians another alternative to intravenous heparin and has allowed treatment in an outpatient setting that was not previously possible. In fact, some data exists that suggests that LMWH may be more efficacious in malignancy-associated thrombosis and that extended therapy with LMWH instead of warfarin may be better and safer.

MALIGNANT EFFUSIONS

Malignant effusions can cause significant discomfort to the patient as well as increased morbidity. Potential anatomic sites (pericardium, pleural space, and peritoneum) should be evaluated if the patient complains of chest pain, shortness of breath, cough, shoulder pain, nausea, or abdominal distention as removing the fluid can improve symptoms immediately. Unfortunately, malignant effusions portend a poor prognosis but early treatment can improve survival and quality of life in many cases.

A malignant pericardial effusion develops in 5–15% of patients with cancer (typically leukemias, lymphomas, or breast cancer). This can be a true oncological emergency if tamponade physiology is achieved. Symptoms include dyspnea, chest pain, or cough, and examination can reveal distant heart sounds, a cardiac friction rub, and jugular venous distention. A pulsus paradoxus >10 mm Hg can be seen as well as systemic hypotention from decreased cardiac output. Diagnosis is suggested by a wide mediastinum on chest x-ray or low voltage (or electrical alternans) on the electrocardiogram. Echocardiography, CT, or MRI confirms the diagnosis. Treatment involves immediate pericardiocentesis with chemotherapy or radiation therapy directed toward the underlying etiology. Surgery with a pericardiectomy can also prevent fluid reaccumulation if necessary.

Malignant pleural effusions are common in advanced cancers. Symptoms are similar to pericardial effusions in that they can cause shortness of breath, pleuritic chest pain, cough, and orthopnea. All new effusions should be sampled to exclude more treatable etiologies like congestive heart failure and infections. Standard studies like a cell count and differential, lactate dehydrogenase, glucose, protein, pH, Gram stain and culture should be obtained. A sample for cytology should also be sent, but a negative cytology in no way excludes a malignant etiology. In general, an exudative effusion with negative cultures in a patient with known cancer is a malignant effusion until proven otherwise. This is because, if a malignant effusion remains untreated, continued growth of the tumor can cause encasement atelectasis and lead to a "trapped lung" that is unresponsive to chest tube placement or future thoracentesis. Removing the fluid and sending fluid for repeat cytology is an initial step. Once the diagnosis is made or suspected, treatment of the underlying disease can decrease fluid reaccumulation. Otherwise, repeat thoracentesis or pleurodesis can be performed for management of the recurrent malignant effusion. Occasionally, chest tubes can be left in place for drainage if pleurodesis fails or palliative measures are desired.

Malignant ascites are seen commonly in gynecological cancers, gastrointestinal cancers, and occasionally breast cancer. Many of these patients will have evidence for carcinomatosis by imaging or previous surgical staging. Symptoms are variable and patients can complain of anorexia, dyspnea with shallow breaths, nausea, abdominal pain and distension, and constipation. Again, these symptoms can greatly affect the quality of life and therefore need be addressed. Examination can show a fluid wave or evidence or peritoneal studding. The diagnosis is confirmed by CT (or MRI with carcinomatosis protocol) or ultrasound. Fluid sampling should be performed to exclude other causes such as cardiac, Budd-Chiari, or infection. As previously noted, if the effusion is exudative (even if the cytology is negative), malignancy is probably the cause. Treatment can be simple paracentesis to relieve symptoms. Medical management with diuretics and fluid restriction can at times control the ascites, and repeat paracentesis can always be performed as necessary. Unfortunately, frequent taps can result in peritonitis, protein depletion, and electrolyte disturbances. Occasionally, intraperitoneal chemotherapy has been used with fair response. More infrequently, peritovenous shunting has been performed for palliation of symptoms.

NAUSEA AND VOMITING

Patients consider chemotherapy- and radiotherapy-induced nausea and vomiting as among the most unpleasant of the acute side effects from their therapies. Patients sometimes develop anticipatory nausea and vomiting, which may require time-consuming interventions like hypnosis or behavior modification. Overall, these symptoms can be so profound that the decision to discontinue cancer treatment is requested.

The development of new, more effective antiemetics have allowed oncologists to administer more chemotherapy in an outpatient setting than was previously possible. These new agents have also decreased the frequency and severity of nausea, thus substantially improving patient comfort and quality of life. In general, tranquilizers (haloperidol), benzodiazepines (lorazepam), antihistamines (hydroxyzine), phenothiazines (prochlorperazine), antiserotonin agents (odansetron, granisetron, and dolasetron), corticosteroids (dexamethasone), and dopamine antagonists (metoclopramide) have all been used successfully in treating nausea. Rehydration of patients with nausea and vomiting is not only sound medically, but can help prevent post-therapy emetogenesis. When using highly emetogenic agents, the addition of steroids to an antiserotonin agent has been shown to have potentiating effects.

Occasionally, the symptoms of nausea and vomiting can be secondary to progressive cancer, with obstruction of a hollow viscous (bowel or ureteral obstruction, constipation), decreased bowel motility (from tense ascites or peritoneal carcinomatosis), metabolic disruption (hypercalcemia), or central nervous system disease (brain metastasis). In these cases, antiemetics can help control symptoms, but the inciting events should be corrected if possible.

USE OF TRANSFUSIONS AND CYTOKINES

Anemia

Anemia is often a result of antineoplastic therapy, but factors such as chronic disease, blood loss with iron deficiency, and marrow replacement by tumor can be important factors as well. In general, patients should receive blood transfusions if symptomatic or if their hematocrit <24% (hemoglobin <8 g/dL). Higher cut-off values should be allowed for patients with heart disease and/or pulmonary disease. The use of erythropoietin can decrease the need for blood transfusions in cancer patients if they develop chemotherapy-induced anemia. Unfortunately, the other causes of anemia in cancer patients respond less well. Given the cost of erythropoietin, judicious use is advised.

Thrombocytopenia

The pathophysiology of thrombocytopenia is similar to anemia. Occasionally, it may be then result of thrombosis, DIC, or splenic sequestration. In general, severe bleeding is uncommon if the patient's platelet count exceeds $20,000/mm^3$, but one can still see easy bruising or petechiae. The risk for severe bleeding (intracranial hemorrhage) does increase dramatically once the platelet falls under $10,000/mm^3$ so empiric transfusions are recommended when the platelet count falls below $20,000/mm^3$. Patients with uremia, brain tumor or metastases, or uncontrolled hypertension may require prophylactic transfusions at a higher cut-off threshold.

New platelet growth factors are being developed (e.g., IL-11), but more studies are needed to determine their efficacy.

Granulocytopenia

White-blood cell transfusions have had limited practical use in neutropenic patients. Thus, it is not considered standard practice. However, the use of granulocyte-colony stimulating factor (G-CSF) and granulocyte-macrophage colony stimulating factor (GM-CSF) have found a role in chemotherapy-induced neutropenia. They have been shown to decrease treatment-associated morbidity and helpful in preventing the number of episodes of neutropenic fevers and infections. Again, routine use of G-CSF or GM-CSF is not recommended, but in a high-risk patient with documented febrile neutropenia in the past, it should be considered for use.

CONCLUSION

Complications of cancer and its associated therapies can present in numerous ways to any physician in practice today. Given that these presentations can be the first sign of a malignancy, all physicians (not just oncologists) should be aware how to manage these problems. Prompt recognition and treatment cannot be overemphasized, as most of what we do is palliative in intent, and failure (or delay) in therapy can result in significant morbidity. The presentations of oncologic emergencies are usually a sign of progressive disease with a lack of effective treatment for the cancer patient, and can be emotionally the most stressful time during the patient's disease process. The physician's approach to patient care therefore needs to be thoughtful and compassionate, and therapy individualized to accommodate patient preference, comfort, and emotional well being.

FURTHER READING

Body JJ, Bartl R, Burckhardt P et al. (1998) Current use of bisphosphonates in oncology. *J Clin Oncol* 16:3809–3899.

Byrne TN (1992) Spinal cord compression from epidural metastases. *N Engl J Med* 327: 613–619.

Devita VT, Hellman S, Rosenberg S (eds) (1997) *Cancer—Principles and Practice of Oncology*, 5th edition, JB Lippencott, Philadelphia.

Gralla RJ, Osoba D, Kris MG et al. (1999) Recommendations for the use of antiemetics: Evidence-based clinical practice guidelines. *J Clin Oncol* 17:2971–2994.

Hughes WT, Armstrong D et al. (1997) Guidelines for the use of antimicrobial agents in neutropenic patients with unexplained fever. *Clin. Infect. Dis.* 25:551–573.

Lablaw DA, Laperriere NJ (1998) Emergency treatment of malignant extradural spinal cord compression: an evidence-based guideline. *J Clin Oncol* 16:1613–1624.

Prandoni P, Lensing A et al. (1992) Deep-venous thrombosis and the incidence of subsequent symptomatic cancer. *N Engl J Med* 327:1128–1132.

■■■■■ **CHAPTER 35**

Pain Management

BETTY R. FERRELL

City of Hope National Medical Center, Department of Nursing Research and Education, Duarte, California

This chapter reviews recent progress in the assessment and management of cancer pain with special considerations for chronic cancer pain management. Pain is viewed as a multidimensional problem requiring an interdisciplinary approach. Essential pharmacologic management is the cornerstone of pain relief. Fortunately, many recent advances in opioid pharmacology have improved our ability to greatly improve the relief of pain. Pain management is essential to quality of life and as a component of quality cancer care.

THE PROBLEM OF PAIN

Pain is a complex and distressing symptom impacting quality of life for the patient with cancer. Definitions of pain have emerged, from simple explanations of this symptom as a purely physiologic phenomenon to our current view of its multi-dimensional nature. The International Association for the Study of Pain (1986) provides a definition of pain as "an unpleasant sensory and emotional experience associated with actual or potential tissue damage, or described in terms of such damage." This definition acknowledges the multidimensional view of pain as an individual experience that includes physical and psychosocial perspectives.

The problem of cancer pain has been recognized as a major health care concern. Pain was identified by the World Health Organization (WHO) as an international priority in 1986 and continues as one of the WHO's chief priorities. The National Cancer Institute and other agencies in the United States have also designated the relief of cancer pain as a priority area for professional education and research. Other important advances in the United States have been the 1994 release of Chronic Cancer Pain guidelines developed by the Agency for Health Care Policy

UICC Manual of Clinical Oncology, Eighth Edition. Edited by Raphael E. Pollock
ISBN 0-471-22289-5 Copyright © 2004 John Wiley & Sons, Inc.

and Research (AHCPR) and pain guidelines published in 2001 by the National Comprehensive Cancer Network (NCCN). These cancer guidelines address the assessment and management of chronic cancer pain and recognize pain as an undertreated symptom impacting quality of life.

Many professional organizations throughout the world have begun assertive efforts to address the international problem of cancer pain. These efforts have resulted in clinical practice guidelines and a wealth of palliative care literature. The challenge for oncologists is to use this available knowledge to improve what has previously been a neglected area of cancer care. On a global scale, the WHO reports that of the 9 million new cancer cases each year, more than half are in developing countries and the majority of these patients have advanced disease at the time of diagnosis. Thus, improved pain management can result in benefit to a significant number of patients with cancer.

MECHANISMS OF PAIN

The physiology of pain is best explained by the perception and response of the individual to the noxious stimuli. There are several physiologic processes that result in the experience of pain. The first of these processes, transduction, begins when a noxious stimulus affects a peripheral sensory nerve ending that initiates the whole phenomenon of pain perception. Transmission, the next process, consists of the series of subsequent neural events that carry the electrical impulses throughout the nervous system, from peripheral to central. Modulation, the third process, is a neural activity that controls pain transmission neurons originating in the periphery and/or the central nervous system. The fourth process, perception, is the subjective correlate of pain that encompasses complex behavioral, psychological, and emotional factors that are little understood.

Pain in cancer is the result of multiple causes including direct tumor involvement, nerve compression or infiltration, or involvement of soft tissue. Pain also frequently results from treatments including chemotherapy, radiation therapy, and postsurgical syndromes such as postmastectomy pain. Pain resulting from stimulation of nerve receptors is nociceptive pain whereas pain resulting from damage to nerves is neuropathic pain. These classifications become important in selecting treatment options.

One of the most clinically important classifications of pain is the distinction between acute and chronic pain. Acute pain is defined as that of sudden onset and that generally has known cause and a limited duration. Acute pain, such as surgical or procedure related pain, is associated with activation of the autonomic nervous system. Patients in acute pain exhibit behaviors indicating their discomfort, and the pattern of this pain is predictable.

Chronic pain is characterized by adaptation of the autonomic nervous system that may result in the absence of outward behaviors in patients and/or the presence of other chronic illness behavior such as depression. Chronic pain is quite a distinct phenomenon from acute pain as the individual often can no longer recall its onset and knows there may be no end, other than eventual death. Chronic pain becomes far more subjective an experience, and is also associated with suffering. The longer lifespan of patients with cancer has also meant that many patients live for months and years with cancer pain.

CANCER PAIN AS A MULTIDIMENSIONAL PHENOMENON

Current conceptualizations of pain have moved from basic physiologic theories to a broad view of the pain experience through the perspective of quality of life (QOL). Pain interrupts physical well-being and is related to other physical symptoms such as fatigue or nausea. Pain is closely associated with psychological well-being and symptoms such as anxiety and depression. Patients often report that they are fearful of a future with pain and see it as a sign of progressive disease.

Pain is also a symptom that impacts the family as well as the patient experiencing the cancer. Social well-being is diminished as pain interferes with roles and relationships, sexuality, and appearance. Spiritual well-being includes religious beliefs and the dimension of suffering as well as the meaning of illness and pain to the patient.

BARRIERS TO PAIN RELIEF

At the time of diagnosis and continuing through active cancer treatment, 30–45% of cancer patients experience moderate to severe pain. The prevalence increases to approximately 75% in advanced cancer. Of patients with pain, 40–50% describe it as moderate to severe and 25–30% report very severe pain. Unfortunately, pain is not only a common problem of cancer but is also seriously undertreated. The AHCPR pain guidelines estimate that 50% of surgery patients receive inadequate pain management and that this undertreatment escalates to approximately 80% of chronic cancer-related pain. Table 35.1 summarizes the many barriers to adequate pain relief including problems of health care professionals, patients, and those related to the health care system.

The first category of barriers, problems related to health care professionals, recognized the importance of enhanced knowledge so that providers can improve the care provided to patients in pain. Previous studies have documented the deficiencies in the medical school curriculum and the need for improved formal and continuing education in palliative care. Beyond the barrier of knowledge, health care professionals also often have inappropriate fears of addiction and inadequate skills in pain assessment.

Frequently cited patient barriers to effective pain management include fears of respiratory depression, drug tolerance, and drug addiction, and inability to communicate pain. Treatment side effects, such as opioid-induced constipation and nausea, are also major reasons for patient noncompliance with analgesic regimens. In several studies, cancer patients have been found to consume only 50–60% of medications ordered even when the patient is experiencing unrelieved pain. Patient

TABLE 35.1. Barriers to Cancer Pain Management

Problems related to health care professionals
  Inadequate knowledge of pain management
  Poor assessment of pain
  Concern about regulation of controlled substances
  Fear of patient addiction
  Concern about side effects of analgesics
  Concern about patients becoming tolerant to analgesics

Problems related to patients
  Reluctance to report pain
    Concern about distracting physicians from treatment of underlying disease
    Fear that pain means disease is worse
    Concern about not being a "good" patient
  Reluctance to take pain medications
    Fear of addiction or of being thought of as an addict
    Worries about unmanageable side effects
    Concern about becoming tolerant to pain medications

Problems related to the health care system
  Low priority given to cancer pain treatment
  Inadequate reimbursement
    The most appropriate treatment may not be reimbursed or may be too costly for
      patients and families
    Restrictive regulation of controlled substances
    Problems of availability of treatment or access to it

From: Agency for Health Care Policy and Research (AHCPR). *Management of Cancer Pain. Clinical Practice Guideline* No. 9. AHCPR Publication No. 94-0592. Rockville, MD. U.S. Department of Health and Human Services, Public Health Services, March 1994.

noncompliance with pain medications is often due to fears of addiction, or respiratory depression, and a lack of understanding of principles of preventing pain through routine dosing of analgesics.

There are also many system barriers that inhibit adequate pain relief. The challenge to improve pain management occurs within a "just say no to drugs" social environment, often resulting in a lack of access to appropriate prescribing. The WHO has focused major efforts toward increased availability of opioids, which has been a major problem in many countries. Aggressive pain treatment is also limited by reimbursement and access of patients to specialized pain services or palliative care systems.

Despite the challenges, there is growing evidence that cancer pain can be successfully treated in the vast majority of patients. Efforts at implementation of the guidelines developed by the WHO and other associations has demonstrated that approximately 90% of cancer pain can be controlled through relatively simple means. Application of basic pain management principles can provide a foundation for optimum comfort throughout the course of cancer.

PRINCIPLES OF PAIN ASSESSMENT

Assessment of cancer pain is critical for all health care professionals because failure to assess pain leads to its undertreatment. The role of cancer pain assessment was emphasized in a 1993 study of 897 United States oncologists who, collectively in the previous 6 months, had managed more than 70,000 cancer patients. According to these physicians, poor pain assessment was the greatest barrier to effective cancer pain management in their own practices.

The initial evaluation of pain should include a detailed history, including an assessment of the pain intensity and character; physical examination, emphasizing the neurologic examination; psychosocial assessment; and appropriate diagnostic work-up to determine the cause of the pain.

One routine clinical approach to pain assessment and management was developed by the AHCPR cancer pain guideline panel and is summarized by the mnemonic "ABCDE":

A—*A*sk about pain regularly; *a*ssess pain systematically

B—*B*elieve the patient and family in their reports of pain and what relieves it

C—*C*hoose pain control options appropriate for the patient, family, and setting

D—*D*eliver interventions in a timely, logical, and coordinated fashion

E—*E*mpower patients and their families; *e*nable them to control their course to the greatest extent possible.

The pain assessment begins with evaluating pain intensity. Pain intensity is the assessment of the severity of pain experienced. A great deal of research has focused on use of various scales to measure pain intensity. Clinicians are encouraged to use pain scales, such as an ordinal scale in which patients are asked to rate their pain on a scale of 0 (no pain) to 10 (worst pain). Use of a pain rating scale assists in communicating pain and in evaluating changes in pain over time.

The assessment of the patient's pain and the efficacy of the treatment plan should be ongoing, and the pain reports should be documented. Pain should be assessed and documented at regular intervals after starting the treatment plan and with each new report of pain. Reassessment or evaluation of pain relief is equally important. At a suitable interval after each pharmacologic or nonpharmacologic intervention, the patient should again provide a pain rating to evaluate effectiveness of the interventions. In addition, patients should be taught to report changes in their pain or any new pain so that appropriate reassessment and changes in the treatment plan can be initiated.

Pain assessment is not a one-time occurrence but rather it is an ongoing process requiring constant attention to new pain. Changes in pain or the development of new pain should not be attributed to preexisting causes but should instead necessitate diagnostic evaluation. New pain may signal treatable problems such as infection or pathologic fracture. A change in pain often signals advancing disease, and because pain management relies on the treatment of the underlying disease, establishing a medical diagnosis is critical. One study conducted in a pain center revealed that a comprehensive pain assessment identified new causes of pain in 64% of 270 oncology patients with new pain complaints; most of the new diagnoses were neurologic. Thus, the need to reassess persistent pain to identify new causes cannot be overemphasized.

PAIN MANAGEMENT

The WHO, AHCPR, NCCN, and other organizations have emphasized that optimum pain management is based on a combined approach using nonsteroidal anti-inflammatory drugs (NSAIDs), opioids, and adjuvant medications. These pharmacologic approaches are used in combination with other treatments such as radiation therapy or invasive procedures. The three major classes—NSAIDs, opioids, and adjuvants—are described in the following sections.

Nonopioid Analgesics

The nonopioid analgesics include the NSAIDS, aspirin, and acetaminophen. They are useful for mild to moderate cancer pain and also are used in combination with opioids for moderate to severe pain. These drugs should not be used to replace the stronger opioid analgesics but are an important component of the pharmacologic regimen for optimum cancer pain relief.

Acetaminophen (paracetamol) has fewer side effects than other nonopioids and no effects on platelet function. The usual adult dose is limited to less than 4,000–6,000 mg per day, as doses exceeding that limit may cause severe hepatic toxicity. Aspirin is also an excellent analgesic and works by inhibiting prostaglandin synthesis. Adverse effects such as nausea or other gastrointestinal effects limit its use as does its inhibition of platelet aggregation. Many patients get excellent pain relief from acetaminophen or aspirin when used alone and others receive increased analgesia from opioids from these drugs.

Ibuprofen is an NSAID that is also used extensively in this category. The usual dose of 600–800 mg of ibuprofen given every 6–8 hours for a maximum daily dose of 2400 mg is suggested. There are many other NSAIDs widely used for cancer pain. The nonacetylated salicylates, including choline magnesium trisalicylate, are often used because of a minimal effect on platelet aggregation. The NSAIDs are often limited in use with cancer patients because of their gastrointestinal and renal effects. NSAIDs can cause renal insufficiency and are of special concern for the elderly or those with chronic renal or hepatic disease.

There are many NSAIDs to consider for those patients for whom the above agents are not effective. Prior experience with analgesics and a thorough history of gastrointestinal or hepatic-renal effects is important in selecting NSAIDs. Longer-acting NSAID analgesics can be important for patients to improve compliance, as it is well established that administering these drugs on a regular schedule for chronic pain helps to eliminate extreme episodes of pain when relief can be maintained in a steady state. Misoprostol has been used in conjunction with NSAIDs to minimize gastric ulcers, particularly for those who have been maintained on long-term administration of these analgesics. It is also important to assess the patient's overall drug regimen as many medications include NSAIDs and thus the combination of medications may exceed the dosage limits suggested for NSAIDs to avoid side effects. Patients should also be advised that use of NSAIDs, opioids, and adjuvants may often require several dosage titrations and several days of administration before benefits are seen. Another advance in the area of NSAID use has been the introduction of the COX-2 agents (e.g., Vioxx and Celebrex). These agents offer decreased incidence of gastrointestinal side effects as compared with other NSAIDs.

Opioid Analgesics

Opioid analgesics reduce pain primary through central mechanisms by binding to μ, δ, and κ receptors. The pure agonist opioids are preferred and morphine has been established as the gold standard for cancer pain analgesia. Other drugs from the pure agonist category recommended for cancer pain include hydromorphone, hydrocodone, oxycodone, methadone, and fentanyl. These drugs do have many adverse effects, the primary effects being nausea, constipation, and sedation. The selection and titration of an opioid requires a balance of pain relief with a minimum of side effects to truly enhance not only pain relief, but also quality of life.

There are many mixed agonist/antagonist opioids that are considered less appropriate for cancer pain management. Drugs such as pentazocine, butorphanol, and nalbuphine do not provide consistent analgesia like the agonists and also have a ceiling effect. These drugs often have side effects such as increased sedation, nausea, and confusion. The accepted standard of pain relief emerging over the past decade has been the use of a long-acting analgesic, morphine, along with short-acting opioids on an as-needed schedule for breakthrough pain. The WHO has established morphine as the standard of analgesia and many efforts are in place to increase the availability of morphine. Preparations that extend analgesia for 8, 12, or 24 hours have been acknowledged as providing a much improved relief of pain and quality of life by reducing interruptions in sleep and enhancing consistent relief. Patients on long-acting analgesics will need a short-acting analgesic available for those episodes of breakthrough pain that may occur between long-acting doses. The usual recommendation is for doses of approximately 10–15% of their 24-hour dose equivalent to be given on a every 2-hour schedule for breakthrough pain.

Hydromorphone is an alternative to morphine and is often used for those patients who cannot tolerate morphine. In some countries it is also available as a long-acting preparation. Hydromorphone is often used in subcutaneous infusions and is widely used in the oral route with several dosage forms available. Fentanyl is an analgesic that was used earlier in its history primarily in the surgical setting but has been extensively used in recent years for cancer pain because of its availability in the transdermal route. The transdermal fentanyl patch is applied for 48–72 hours duration. Fentanyl is a potent analgesic and is also used intravenously or epidurally.

Oxycodone is a very good analgesic used for moderate to severe pain. It is now available in a noncompounded form and also in a long-acting preparation. This drug is often an excellent choice for patients who are reluctant to take morphine and yet who require significant amounts of analgesia. Oxycodone is also available in several compounded formulations, usually combined with acetaminophen.

Many other strong analgesics are available. Methadone is a potent analgesic but its use is limited because of a long half-life that can cause accumulation and is of particular concern for the elderly or other patients for whom accumulation can create serious problems. Analgesics such as levorphanol are not used as frequently in recent years as the availability of better analgesics such as morphine and oxycodone has offered advantages, particularly as long-acting formulations in higher doses are available.

Meperidine is an opioid analgesic that is strongly discouraged for use in cancer pain management. Normeperidine, the active metabolite of meperidine, can accumulate as the drug is metabolized and is of particular concern with higher doses for any patient who will receive the drugs for more than a few days. Accumulation of normeperidine can result in central nervous system excitability, leading to seizures.

Table 35.2 includes dosing information for opioid analgesics. Knowledge of these key principles is important to provide the most aggressive pain relief possible.

Published tables vary in the suggested doses that are equianalgesic to morphine. Clinical response is the criterion that must be applied for each patient; titration to clinical responses is necessary. Because there is not complete cross-tolerance among these drugs, it is usually necessary to use a lower than equianalgesic dose when changing drugs and to retitrate to response.

Adjuvant Drugs

Adjuvant drugs are those medications used to enhance analgesic efficacy, treat concurrent symptoms, and provide independent analgesia for specific types of pain. The corticosteroids provide a range of effects including mood elevation, anti-inflammatory activity, antiemetic activity, and appetite stimulation. They may be beneficial in the management of cachexia and anorexia. They also reduce cerebral and spinal cord edema and are used in the emergency management of epidural spinal cord compression or severe, acute bone pain, such as in pathologic fracture.

Anticonvulsants are also used to manage neuropathic pain, especially lancinating or burning pain. Those drugs are used with caution in cancer patients undergoing marrow-suppressant therapies, such as chemotherapy and radiation. Antidepressants are useful in pharmacologic management of neuropathic pain. These drugs have innate analgesic properties and may potentiate the analgesic effects of opioids. The most widely reported experience has been with amitriptyline, but other agents such as imipramine or doxepin are also used. Neuroleptics, particularly metho-trimeprazine, have been used to treat chronic pain. Methotrimeprazine lacks opioid inhibiting effects on gut motility and may be useful for treating opioid-induced

TABLE 35.2. Dose Equivalents for Opioid Analgesics in Opioid-Naive Adults and Children ≥50 kg Body Weight[a]

	Equianalgesic Dose		Starting Dose	
Drug	Oral	Parenteral	Oral	Parenteral
Opioid Agonist[b,e]				
Morphine[c]	30 mg q 3-4 h (repeat around-the-clock dosing)	10 mg q 3-4 h	30 mg q 3-4 h	10 mg q 3-4h
Morphine, controlled release[c,d] (MS Contin, Oramorph)	90-120 mg q 12 h	N/A	90-120 mg q 12 h	N/A
Hydromorphone[c] (Dilaudid)	7.5 mg q 3-4 h	1.5 mg q 3-4 h	6 mg q 3-4 h	1.5 mg q 3-4 h
Levorphanol (Levo-Dromoran)	4 mg q 6-8 h	2 mg q 6-8 h	4 mg q 6-8 h	2 mg q 6-8 h
Meperidine (Demerol)[g]	300 mg q 2-3 h	75 mg q 3 h	N/R	N/R
Methadone (Dolophine, other)[h]	20 mg q 6-8 h	10 mg q 6-8 h	20 mg q 6-8 h	10 mg q 6-8 h
Combination Opioid/NSAID Preparations				
Codeine[f] (with aspirin or acetaminophen)	180-200 mg q 3-4 h	130 mg q 3-4 h	60 mg q 3-4 h	60 mg q 2 h
Hydrocodone (in Lorcet, Lortab, Vicodin, others)	30 mg q 3-4 h	N/A	10 mg q 3-4 h	N/A
Oxycodone (Roxicodone, also in Percocet, Percodan, Tylox, others)	20 mg q 3-4 h	N/A	10 mg q 3-4 h	N/A

[a] **Caution:** Recommended doses do not apply for adult patients with body weight less than 50 kg.

[b] **Caution:** Recommended doses do not apply to patients with renal or hepatic insufficiency or other conditions affecting drug metabolism and kinetics.

[c] **Caution:** For morphine, hydromorphone, and oxymorphone, rectal administration is an alternate route for patients unable to take oral medications. Equianalgesic doses may differ from oral and parenteral doses because of pharmacokinetic difference.

[d] Transdermal fentanyl (Duragesic) is an alternative option. Doses above 25 µg/h should not be used in opioid-naive patients.

[e] **Caution:** Doses of aspirin and acetaminophen in combination opioid/NSAID preparations must also be adjusted to the patients body weight. Aspirin is contraindicated in children in the presence of fever or other viral disease because of its association with Reye's syndrome.

[f] **Caution:** Codeine doses above 65 mg often are not appropriate because of diminishing incremental analgesia with increasing doses but continually increasing nausea, constipation, and other side effects.

[g] Demerol is not recommended for cancer pain but is included here for equivalence information.

[h] Methadone accumulates with repeated dosing, requiring decreases in dose size and frequency.

intractable constipation or other dose-limiting side effects. It also has antiemetic and anxiolytic effects.

Local anesthetics have also been used to treat neuropathic pain. Side effects for these may be greater than with other drugs used to treat neuropathic pain. Anxiety is a common symptom in patients with pain and hydroxyzine, a mild anxiolytic agent with sedating and analgesic properties, is useful in treating anxiety. This antihistamine also has antiemetic properties. Another common symptom in patients on opioids is sedation. This symptom can be treated by giving caffeine or caffeinated beverages, or psychostimulants may be useful in reducing opioid-induced sedation when opioid dose adjustment (i.e., reduced dose and increased dose frequency) is not effective. The bisphosphonates and radiopharmaceuticals are becoming more frequently used and offer improved analgesia for metastatic bone pain. Anticonvulsants (gabapentin, phenytoin, carbamazepine, sodium valproate, clonazepam) are useful for painful nerve syndromes often caused by cancer treatment.

Nonpharmacologic Strategies

Optimum pain relief is achieved through a combination of drug and nondrug techniques. Most patients will benefit from a combination of pharmacologic approaches used with physical or cognitive pain relief strategies such as heat, cold, distraction, or relaxation. Pain management also requires patient education to overcome patient fears of addiction or drug tolerance and to involve the patient and family with the goals of pain assessment and treatment. Recognition of the multidimensional nature of pain as depicted in Figure 35.1 also implies the need for an interdisciplinary approach to meet the complex physical and psychosocial needs of patients in pain.

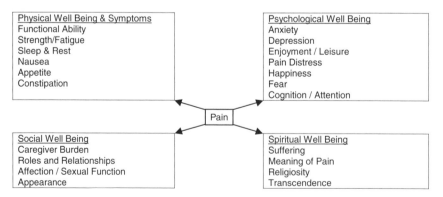

Figure 35.1 Pain impacts the dimensions of quality of life. (From Ferrell B R, Grant M. (2001) Copyright held by City of Hope National Medical Center.)

CONCLUSION

Cancer pain has been cited throughout the world as a seriously undertreated problem and one of enormous consequence for patients and their families. Advances in analgesia have provided the means to relieve the vast majority of pain using pharmacologic techniques and through recognition of the multidimensional nature of pain. Continued efforts are needed to eliminate barriers to adequate pain relief and to further close the gap between current practice and the potential for pain relief for all patients with cancer.

FURTHER READING

Agency for Health Care Policy and Research (AHCPR) (1994) *Management of Cancer Pain. Clinical Practice Guideline* No. 9. AHCPR Publication No. 94-0592. Rockville, MD. US Department of Health and Human Services. Public Health Service, March.

American Pain Society (APS) (1999) *Principles of Analgesic Use in the Treatment of Acute Pain and Chronic Cancer Pain*, 4th edition. American Pain Society, Skokie, IL.

Cherny NI, Portenoy RK (1994) The management of cancer pain. *CA Cancer J Clin* 44: 263–303.

Cleeland CS, Gonin R, Hatfield AK et al. (1994) Pain and its treatment in out-patients with metastatic cancer. *N Engl J Med* 330:592–596.

Doyle D, Hanks GWC, MacDonald N (eds.) (1998) *Oxford Textbook of Palliative Medicine*, 2nd edition. Oxford University Press, New York.

Ferrell BR (1995) The impact of pain on quality of life: A decade of research. *Nurs Clin NA* 30:609–624.

Ferrell BR, Ferrell BA, Ahn C, Tran K (1994) Pain management for elderly patients with cancer at home. *Cancer* 74:2139–2146.

Ferrell BR, Coyle N (2001) *Textbook of Palliative Nursing*. Oxford University Press, New York.

Ferrell BR, Rivera LM (1997) Cancer pain education for patients. *Semin Oncol Nurs* 13: 42–48.

International Association for the Study of Pain, Subcommittee on Taxonomy (1979) Part II. Pain terms: A current list with definitions and notes on usage. *Pain* 6:249–252 [updated 1982, 1986].

Levy MH (1996) Pharmacologic treatment of cancer pain. *N Engl J Med* 335:1124–1132.

McCaffery M, Pasero C (1999) *Pain: Clinical Manual*. Mosby, St. Louis.

Melzack R, Wall P (1982) *The Challenge of Pain*. Basic Books, New York.

National Comprehensive Cancer Network (NCCN), American Cancer Society (ACS) (2001) Cancer Pain Treatment Guidelines for Patients, Version 1, January [updated 2002, 2003].

Paice JA, Fine PG (2001) Pain at the end of life. In *Textbook of Palliative Nursing*. Ferrell BR, Coyle N (eds.) Oxford University Press, New York, pp 76–90.

Schug SA, Zech D, Door U (1990) Cancer pain management according to WHO analgesic guidelines. *J Pain Symp Manag* 5:27–32.

Twycross R. (1994). *Pain Relief in Advanced Cancer*. Churchill Livingstone, London.

Ventafridda V, Caraceni A, Gamba A (1990) Field-testing of the WHO Guidelines for Cancer Pain Relief: Summary report of demonstration projects. In *Advances in Pain Research and Therapy*, Vol 16. Foley KM, Bonica JJ, Ventafridda V (eds.) Proceedings of the Second International Congress on Pain. Raven Press, New York, pp 451–464.

Von Roenn JH, Cleeland CS, Gonin R, Hatfield AK, Pandya KJ (1993) Physician attitudes and practice in cancer pain management: A survey from the Eastern Cooperative Oncology Group. *Ann Intern Med* 119:121–126.

World Health Organization (1996) *Cancer Pain Relief*, 2nd edition. WHO, Geneva.

CHAPTER 36

Nutrition and Cancer

CHARLES A. STALEY and NICOLE M. DAIGNAULT
Emory University, Medical School–South Clinic, Atlanta, Georgia

WILEY W. SOUBA
University of Texas, M. D. Anderson Cancer Center, Houston, Texas

BRIAN I. LABOW
Massachusetts General Hospital, Division of Surgical Oncology, Boston, Massachusetts

Malnutrition is common in cancer patients and is an important cause of increased morbidity and mortality. The term *cancer cachexia* describes the clinical triad of weight loss, anorexia, and loss of lean body mass secondary to a growing malignancy. This condition is often accompanied by vitamin and trace mineral deficiencies, along with the most common form of nutritional depletion, protein calorie malnutrition. Cachexia is often exacerbated by chemotherapy, radiation therapy, and/or surgery, which can further compromise an already fragile nutritional status.

Recent developments have increased our understanding of the relationship between nutrition and metabolism in cancer patients. Severe malnutrition has been shown to have adverse effects on immune function and treatment tolerance of anticancer regimens, and is associated with increased postoperative complications in cancer patients who undergo surgery. In fact, weight loss itself is a predictor of therapeutic response and survival. Although limited weight loss in some cancer patients may be acceptable, many cancer patients develop significant malnutrition such that some form of nutritional support may be required. The rationale for such nutrition support is to prevent or reverse host tissue wasting, broaden the spectrum of therapeutic options, improve the clinical course, and ultimately prolong patient survival. Accordingly, oncologists should become familiar with the metabolic changes that develop in response to malignancy and with the indications for and delivery of nutritional support to the cancer patient.

UICC Manual of Clinical Oncology, Eighth Edition. Edited by Raphael E. Pollock
ISBN 0-471-22289-5 Copyright © 2004 John Wiley & Sons, Inc.

The purpose of this chapter is to examine the etiologies of and metabolic alterations that develop in cachectic patients and to establish a rationale for nutrition support in the malnourished cancer patient. In addition, the indications for the various means of nutrition support are examined. Portions of this review have been previously published (1–5).

CLINICAL MANIFESTATIONS OF CANCER CACHEXIA

Weight Loss

Most cancer patients develop weight loss at some point during the course of their disease and nearly half will have weight loss at the time of initial diagnosis. Published studies reported that patients who presented without weight loss had a significantly prolonged survival following therapy compared with similarly treated patients who had weight loss at presentation (Fig. 36.1) (6). These findings suggest that weight loss adversely affects survival following antineoplastic therapy and imply that appropriate nutritional therapy may be beneficial in certain patient groups. In addition, cancer patients with significant weight loss do not tolerate treatment regimens as well as an adequately nourished patient. Weight loss is dependent on the presence of the tumor, as curative surgical resection (or nonsurgical treatment) of the malignancy is almost invariably associated with a return to normal body weight. Although some weight loss following surgery may be expected because of postoperative ileus and increased metabolic demand, patients who do not regain their weight following surgical resection for cure should be investigated for metastatic or recurrent disease.

Anorexia and Other Factors Affecting Oral Intake

At some point during the course of their disease, most patients report a loss of appetite that includes alterations in taste, smell, and loss of appeal for most foods. Loss of appetite resulting in reduction in voluntary food intake is a central component of cancer cachexia, and, unfortunately oncologic therapies often initiate or worsen their anorexia. In some patients, this is reflected by an increase in resting energy expenditure without a compensatory increase in calorie intake. The combination of increased energy demand without increased food intake exacerbated weight loss and negative calorie and nitrogen balance. Early satiety, mechanical obstruction, and/or nausea are common in patients with malignances of the gastrointestinal tract, which often produce profound anorexia. However, digestive tract dysfunction cannot solely explain this phenomenon, as significant anorexia is also noted in patients with cancers that originate outside the abdominal cavity. In fact, careful studies using animal models of cachexia have clearly documented a decline in food intake in response to cancer. Proposed mechanisms for this "anorexia of malignancy" include local effects of the tumor, alterations in taste or palatability, hypothalamic dysfunction, modification of satiety mechanisms, and learned food aversion.

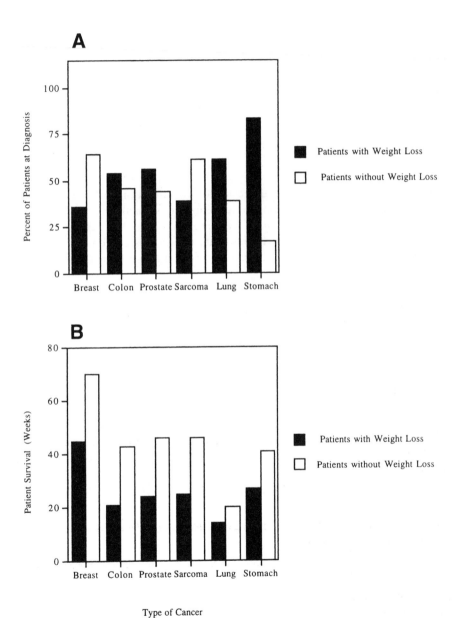

Figure 36.1   Prevalence of weight loss in cancer patients at the time of diagnosis (**A**) and its effect on survival following antineoplastic therapy (**B**), $p < 0.05$. (6)

Although tumors themselves may initiate or potentiate anorexia, many chemotherapeutic agents can also produce profound anorexia. Nausea, vomiting, mucositis, and/or gastrointestinal dysfunction often result from chemotherapy and radiation therapy. This "anorexia of therapy" may often contribute significantly to cachexia as well. Likewise, mechanical obstruction or dysphagia induced by gastrointestinal or oropharyngeal malignancies may inhibit oral intake. Another important consideration for the clinician is that during diagnostic evaluation, hospitalized cancer patients are often restricted from taking adequate nutrition. As a result, the patient may become iatrogenically malnourished prior to the initiation of oncologic treatment.

Weakness

With a loss of body cell mass and because of the effects of treatment regimens, cancer patients invariably develop a reduction in strength and a diminished functional capacity for physical work. Evidence for a central role of the tumor in the etiology of this weakness is derived from the clinical observation that successful management of the tumor almost always results in a return to preillness strength and work capacity.

CAUSES AND CONSEQUENCES OF CANCER CACHEXIA

An understanding of the metabolic mechanisms underlying cancer cachexia is imperative, as many cancer-related deaths are a consequence of malnutrition. Although the exact prevalence of cachexia is unknown, many studies have shown a high frequency of nutritional derangements in cancer patients. These studies have focused on findings such as weight loss or hypoproteinemia as indicators of cachexia. Consequently, the prevalence of cancer cachexia may be underestimated, as it is likely that subtle metabolic alterations precede these clinically apparent changes.

Many of the physiologic changes seen in cachectic patients resemble those of simple starvation, but it is clear that other derangements are also involved (Table 36.1). Instead of adapting to partial starvation by conserving lean body mass,

TABLE 36.1. Metabolic Differences Between the Response to Simple Starvation and to Advanced Malignant Disease

	Simple Staration	Advanced Malignant Disease
Basal metabolic rate	− or ↓	−, ↑, or ↓
Presence of mediators	−	+ + +
Hepatic ureagenesis	+	+ + +
Negative nitrogen balance	+	+ + +
Gluconeogenesis	+	+ + +
Muscle proteolysis	+	+ + +
Hepatic protein synthesis	+	+ + +

− indicates normal; + indicates slightly increased; + + + indicates a substantial increase.

the host continues to deplete its own muscle mass, probably to provide amino acids for tumor growth and to support hepatic gluconeogenesis and protein synthesis. Unfortunately, few studies have documented that aggressive feeding of cachectic cancer patients restores lean body mass. Furthermore, no consistent or clear association with duration of illness, stage of disease, or tumor histology has been demonstrated to correlate with the degree of cachexia. Although the demand for substrate may account in part for the loss of lean body mass, the actual energy and nitrogen demands of human tumors cannot account for the profound weight loss that is generally observed. For example, it is unusual for the total mass of the tumor to exceed 1% or 2% of total body weight, and yet patients with even much smaller tumors are often markedly cachectic. Many etiologies for cancer cachexia have been proposed, but no definitive explanation exists, and the etiology is likely to be multifactorial. Studies conducted over the last decade suggest that humoral factors such as cytokines may play a major role in mediating cachexia. Understanding the abnormalities in host intermediary metabolism and the effects of the mediators that produce them will hopefully allow the clinician to adopt a rational approach to therapy and will underlie efforts to develop better techniques to combat the devastating effect of malignancy.

ALTERATIONS OF INTERMEDIARY METABOLISM

Metabolic abnormalities affecting carbohydrate, protein and lipid utilization are characteristic of the tumor-bearing host. Although resting energy expenditure (REE) is variably affected by the presence of malignancy (7), even patients with no increase in metabolic rate can develop weight loss and negative nitrogen balance despite a normal food intake and in spite of a small tumor burden. In fact, some studies demonstrate that in some solid tumor-bearing patients, whole body protein turnover was increased 50%, despite no change in REE (8).

Glucose metabolism is often abnormal in cancer patients because of increased turnover. Furthermore, it has been shown that in patients with gastrointestinal malignancies, hepatic gluconeogenesis increases in proportion to tumor burden (9). Interestingly, patients with the largest tumors failed to suppress endogenous glucose production during glucose infusion, a response attributed to a reduction in insulin sensitivity. Other studies indicate that β-cell receptor sensitivity to glucose loading may also be diminished in the tumor-bearing host, in a manner similar to those with type II diabetes (10). These effects could contribute significantly to depletion of energy stores and tissue wasting.

Protein and amino acid metabolism is also altered in the tumor-bearing host. The changes observed are not simply the results of starvation. This has been demonstrated by studies comparing tumor-bearing patients, malnourished non-tumor-bearing patients, and healthy controls: protein turnover was found to be elevated only in the cancer group (11). In another study, patients with non-small-cell lung cancer were found to have increased whole body protein turnover, elevated 3-methylhistidine excretion, and increased muscle proteolysis (12). Tumor-bearing animal models also demonstrate increased whole body nitrogen turnover and increased liver protein fractional synthetic rate. In patients, studies measuring arterial and venous differences in amino acid content across a sarcoma-bearing limb, using the non-tumor-bearing limb as a control, have demonstrated that the tumor participates directly in augmenting protein metabolism (13). Compared with the non-tumor-bearing extremity, the tumor-bearing limb released lesser amounts of all amino acids, suggesting increased demand for amino acids to support neoplastic growth.

Lipid metabolism is also altered in the host with cancer. Kinetics studies using radiolabeled glycerol and fatty acids found cancer patients with weight loss had increased glycerol and fatty acid turnover when compared with weight stable patients (9). These cachectic patients were incapable of oxidizing endogenous fatty acids or intravenous lipids at normal rates and failed to suppress lipolysis during glucose infusion.

GLUTAMINE AND CANCER CACHEXIA

Glutamine metabolism in the tumor-bearing host has been extensively studied for three principle reasons: (1) glutamine is the principle fuel used by many cancers, (2) it is the most abundant amino acid in the body and its stores are quite labile, and (3) glutamine is a conditionally essential amino acid. Glutamine is a good substrate for oxidation by tumor cell mitochondria and glutamine extraction by tumors may be quite high. In fact, tumor-bearing rats demonstrate a progressive fall in plasma glutamine concentrations that correlate with tumor size (13). With time, blood glutamine levels may fall to less than 50% of normal, indicating an imbalance between rates of glutamine production and consumption. This reduction in circulating glutamine occurs despite increased muscle glutamine release, indicating either accelerated glutamine consumption by other tissues and/or tumor cells. Concomitantly, there are marked increases in tumor and hepatic glutamine uptake. Progressive tumor growth and glutamine depletion may accelerate muscle proteolysis, thereby exacerbating cachexia (14).

CYTOKINES: MEDIATORS OF CANCER CACHEXIA

An understanding of the mediators the produce the metabolic changes described above would help derive nutritional strategies that optimize the metabolic integrity of the host and allow antitumor therapies to be maximally effective. Cytokines, a class of paracrine/autocrine proteins that produce a wide array of physiologic responses, have been implicated by a number of recent studies, as important mediators of the host response to cancer. Cytokines can regulate both energy intake (i.e., appetite) and energy expenditure (i.e., metabolic rate) and thus play a pivotal role in determining the nutritional status of the tumor-bearing host.

Elevated concentrations of tissue and circulating cytokines have been demonstrated in patients with cancer (15) and enhanced hepatic cytokine gene expression has been demonstrated in tumor bearing animals. Administration of the cytokine tumor necrosis factor (TNF) to rodents and humans decreases food intake in a time- and dose-dependent manner (16,17). In patients receiving exogenous TNF, food intake was also diminished as predicted. However, nitrogen losses were not accelerated, indicating that the resultant negative nitrogen balance was due to starvation alone. These effects of TNF on appetite may account in part for the anorexia observed in cancer patients.

The cytokine interleukin-1 (IL-1) also suppresses food intake and its effect, like that of TNF, appears to be a direct effect on appetite via the central nervous system. Further evidence for IL-1 and TNF as mediators of energy balance in cancer comes from studies that demonstrated that treatment of tumor-bearing mice with antic-ytokine antibodies improved food intake and attenuated weight loss (18), and that mice implanted with tumors that secreted TNF showed marked reductions in weight loss, compared with animals with non-TNF secreting tumors (19).

In addition to their effects on appetite, cytokines also influence energy balance by stimulating basal metabolic rate (oxygen consumption). Studies indicate that patients receiving exogenous TNF may increase their metabolic rates by as much as 30% (20). Furthermore, cytokines have also been shown to influence the metabo- lism of carbohydrates, proteins, and lipids and thus may contribute to cancer cachexia via both energy consumption and derangement of host metabolism.

Effects on Glucose Metabolism

Studies evaluating the effects of cytokine administration on the circulating glucose concentration indicate that the plasma glucose level will rise or fall depending on the dose administered, the temporal nature of the measurement, and on the specific cytokine given.

In rats, sublethal doses of TNF that did not produce hemodynamic changes resulted in the development of hyperglycemia within 1 hour of administration (21). However, plasma glucose concentrations rose only 20% and were associated with an increase in circulating glucagon, adrenocorticotrophic hormone (ACTH), corti- costerone, and epinephrine all of which can cause hyperglycemia. When a lower dose of TNF was utilized, the plasma glucose did not change (22). Similar alterations in blood glucose levels were observed after IL-1 administration. Studies using relatively high IL-1 doses reported a 40% increase in plasma glucose concentration with 1 hour, with a return to basal levels by 2 hours (23). Interest- ingly, this transient increase in plasma glucose was paralleled by a severalfold increase in hindquarter glucose consumption. Other studies examining tissue glucose utilization *in vivo* in rats showed that following infusion of a nonlethal dose of TNF, glucose uptake was increased by 80–100% in liver, kidney, and spleen, 60% in skin, 30–40% in lung and ileum, and 150% increase in diaphragm muscle (24). No significant increase was observed in skeletal muscle, testis, or brain. These data indicate that TNF and IL-1 are capable of increasing whole body glucose utilization as well as plasma glucose concentration, and can certainly account in part for the alterations in carbohydrate metabolism seen in patients with cancer.

Effects on Protein/Amino Acid Metabolism

Marked changes in protein and amino acid metabolism are characteristic of cancer patients. A number of studies have evaluated the effects of cytokines on muscle protein metabolism and the results are conflicting. When recombinant TNF was infused in cancer patients, forearm amino acids efflux was accelerated, suggesting net skeletal muscle proteolysis, although the accelerated nitrogen release could also be accounted for by starvation effects (25). Similarly, infused radiolabeled leucine into rats receiving TNF and/or IL-1 led to an increase in muscle protein degradation in cytokine treated animals (26). However, when IL-1 activity was blocked with specific anti-IL-1 antibodies, the accelerated protein breakdown was not attenuated (27). Thus, although it is generally agreed that cytokine administration *in vivo* (at sufficient doses) stimulated net muscle proteolysis, it is unclear to what extent they act directly or via the effects of anorexia in cancer patients. In addition, *in vitro* studies (28) have failed to show a direct effect except in studies evaluating the effects of corticosterone on muscle protein breakdown. This glucocorticoid hormone, which accelerates protein degradation and diminishes protein synthesis, has a more potent effect in combination with TNF (29). However, TNF alone did not alter protein turnover.

Impact on Fat Metabolism

Altered fat metabolism is apparent clinically in cachectic patients from the observation that fat stores are diminished in association with weight loss. This may be due in part to the ability of TNF and IL-1 to mobilize fat stores. Bolus administration of TNF to rats increased serum triglyceride levels within 2 hours (20). The injection of IL-6 or TNF each reduced adipose tissue lipoprotein lipase (LPL) activity by more than 50% in tumor-bearing animals and both reduced heparin-releasable LPL activity *in vitro* in a dose dependent manner by 50–70% (30). Furthermore, TNF may also increase serum triglycerides via stimulation of hepatic lipid secretion in addition to its effects on adipocyte LPL activity (31).

NUTRITIONAL SUPPORT OF THE CANCER PATIENT

Rationale

Although it seems obvious that the provision of nutritional support to the malnourished patient with cancer is essential, evidence indicating that currently available nutritional formulas can maintain or reverse malnutrition is lacking. The rationale behind the provision of specialized nutrition support, whether enteral or parenteral, is the belief that such support will preferentially benefit the patient rather than stimulate tumor growth. Nutrition support would not be indicated if it could be clearly demonstrated that it did not favorably impact the response to antineoplastic therapies, lengthen disease-free survival, and/or improve quality of life. Interestingly, a consensus opinion regarding the role and efficacy of nutrition support in patients with cancer is lacking. Nonetheless, several well-designed clinical studies have allowed us to generate guidelines for the use of enteral and parenteral nutrition in patients with cancer. Most physicians and surgeons who care for patients continue to use nutrition support aggressively under specific circumstances.

Nutritional Assessment of the Cancer Patient

The nutritional assessment of the cancer patient encompasses the evaluation of many different parameters. A careful physical examination and complete medical history may help to ascertain potential nutrient deficiencies or illness-induced influence on requirements. A thorough diet history should include an assessment of food and supplement intake, food aversions or intolerances, appetite changes, and taste/smell alterations. Likewise, the assessment of gastrointestinal function can help determine the patient's ability to absorb and process nutrients. Energy deficits may be identified by changes in body weight, but loss of lean body mass may be masked by fluid retention if edema or ascites are present. Skinfold measurements may be useful to evaluate alterations in lean body mass or somatic fat stores, however, they have limited benefit in the clinical setting due to inconsistencies with measurements and influence of interstitial fluid accumulation. Nitrogen balance studies are also not routinely utilized in hospitalized patients due to difficulties in obtaining 24-hour urine collections an accurate records of other potential nitrogen losses such as stool, wound, respiratory and skin. Peripheral blood lymphocyte count and assessment of cellular immunity via skin delayed hypersensitivity to common antigens have been used as indicators of immunocompetence in the cancer patient. However, immunologic responses are not specific to nutritional deficiencies and are often observed in patients with advanced malignant disease who are adequately nourished. Serum albumin and transferrin levels are commonly measured serum proteins in nutritional assessment, but they have limited value in this setting. Instead, they are markers to reflect clinical outcome and morbidity risk due to alterations in their production and utilization induced by illness and catabolic stress. Other laboratory studies that may be useful include red blood cell indices to determine iron and micronutrient deficiencies, plasma glucose to assess insulin resistance, blood urea nitrogen and chemistry profile to determine renal and hydration status, and liver function tests.

The Role of Pharmacological Agents in the Treatment of Cancer Anorexia/Cachexia

The role of various pharmacological agents to alleviate cancer anorexia/cachexia have been investigated (75–84). The use of corticosteroids, cyproheptadine, and hydrazine has demonstrated only marginal success (78,79). The serotonin antagonist, cyproheptadine was shown to mildly enhance appetite in patients with advanced malignant disease, but had little impact on weight gain (75). Moertel was the first to demonstrate a temporary improvement with appetite in patients with advanced disease who were administered a low dose of dexamethasone, but failed to show a positive influence on weight gain (78). Others have indicated an improvement with quality-of-life indices and appetite with methylprednisolone (79,80,81).

There have been many documented reports demonstrating appetite stimulation and nonfluid weight gain in patients with cancer induced anorexia/cachexia treated with varying doses of megastrol acetate (MA) (75–78,82–85). Loprinzi et al. (85) established a dose response relationship with a dose range of 160–1,280 mg MA/day. MA intake of 800 mg/day was shown to induce the maximum benefit and above this dose no additional response was achieved. Due to the high expense of MA therapy and the positive results obtained with doses as low as 160 mg/day, the authors suggested an initial dose of 160 mg/day, which may be titrated accordingly to induce the desired response. No significant adverse effects or toxicity with the MA therapy were documented in the preceding studies, other than a slight trend toward thromboembolic events, a higher incidence of self-reported impotence in men, and mild edema in some patients. Additionally, the MA was noted to exhibit antiemetic properties. In comparison of the impact of a progestational agent, MA, versus a corticosteroid, dexamethasone, versus an anabolic corticosteroid, fluoxymesterone on cancer induced anorexia and cachexia, twice daily of fluoxymesterone (10 mg) was shown to have little influence on appetite or weight gain. Both 800 mg/day of MA and 0.75 mg dexamethasone four times per day were found to have similar positive effects on appetite stimulation and nonfluid weight gain, with only a nonsignificant trend in favor of the MA (78). This was consistent with the findings of a trial that compared 160 mg MA/day, 10 mg of prednisone, three times per day, and a placebo in cancer patients receiving pelvic radiation therapy. The authors concluded that in patients in whom a short-term benefit is desired, treatment with the corticosteroid might be more cost effective. However, the administration of MA is preferable in patients who may require a prolonged course of therapy (i.e., weeks to months) in order to avoid the toxicities associated with long-term corticosteroid use (78).

The Use of Enteral Nutrition in Cancer Patients

Numerous clinical trials have evaluated the use of aggressive enteral nutrition support as adjunctive therapy during the administration of antineoplastic regimens to cancer patients. Unfortunately, well-designed studies comprise a small fraction of these. Although these trials do not demonstrate any consistent benefit to the use of routine enteral nutrition, most authorities would agree that when and if nutrition support is required, the enteral route is preferred whenever the gastrointestinal tract is functional. This preference is based primarily on studies in which animals receiving exclusively parenteral nutrition developed intestinal changes including villous atrophy, alterations in gut flora, and bacterial translocation from the intestinal lumen to mesenteric lymph nodes (Table 36.2). Enteral feedings can be supplied via a number of routes including transnasal-gastric or duodenal catheters or via permanently placed gastrostomy or jejunostomy tubes. Feedings may be supplied as between meal supplements or may replace meals altogether if eating becomes impossible. Some of the better enteral feeding clinical trials in cancer patients (32–44) are listed (Tables 36.3–36.5).

TABLE 36.2. Proposed Benefits of Oral/Enteral Nutrition versus Parenteral Nutrition

1. Maintains gut mucosal mass
2. Maintains brush border enzyme activity
3. Supports gut immune function
4. Preserves gut mucosal barrier function
5. Maintains a balanced luminal microflora environment
6. Improves outcome after chemotherapy
   and radiation therapy

Peripheral Intravenous Feedings

Although less commonly used as a means of nutrition support, indications for peripheral intravenous feedings include: (1) supplement to partially tolerated enteral feedings, (2) as a method of nutrition support when the gastrointestinal tract must be kept relatively empty for short periods during diagnostic work-up, and (3) as preliminary feedings prior to central venous catheter insertion in patients requiring total parenteral nutrition (TPN). Peripheral veins must be used for infusion of glucose and amino acid solutions as well as fat emulsions. However, these solutions must be nearly isotonic to avoid peripheral vein sclerosis. Glucose solutions up to 10% by weight may be used and appear to increase the efficacy of amino acid utilization. Fat emulsions that provide an efficient fuel source can be administered simultaneously with glucose and amino acid infusions because they are isotonic. The major disadvantage of these peripheral administered mixtures is limited caloric delivery within tolerable fluid volumes.

Total Parenteral Nutrition in the Cancer Patient: General Recommendations

Although the initial enthusiasm for the use of (TPN) in cancer patients was considerable, it is now clear that TPN should only be provided to selected patients. Because of the failure of numerous clinical trials to yield a consensus with regard to the efficacy of TPN in cancer patients (35,45–69). (Tables 36.3–36.5), recently published articles have used meta-analysis to review these studies collectively and generate feeding guidelines. The general conclusion has been that parenteral nutrition appears to be of little benefit in most cancer patients. However, the most important factor to consider when making decisions regarding TPN is the response of the tumor to antineoplastic therapy. If there is limited or no response to chemotherapy, the potential complications of TPN therapy outweigh the benefits provided by the supplemental nutrition. However, there are certain patient populations that clearly benefit from the use of TPN and some guidelines for the use of TPN are listed (Table 36.6). These guidelines will likely undergo revision, as more effective antitumor regimens become clinically available.

TABLE 36.3. Results of Major Prospective Randomized Controlled Trials Evaluating Perioperative Nutrition

Author	Tumor Type	TPN Course	Number of Patients		Major Complications (%)		Perioperative Mortality (%)	
			TPN	Control	TPN	Control	TPN	Control
Parenteral Nutrition								
Holter and Fischer (45)	GI	3 d preop / 10 d postop	30	26	4 (13)	5 (19)	2 (7)	2 (8)
Heatley et al. (46)	Esophageal, gastric	7–10 d preop	38	36	2 (5) / 3 (8) / 9 (24)	3 (8) / 11 (31) / 16 (44)	6 (16)	8 (22)
Yamada et al. (47)	Gastric	18 d postop	18	16	1 (6)	5 (31)	0 (0)	1 (6)
Askanazi et al. (48)	Bladder	7 d postop	22	13	1 (5)	0 (0)	0 (0)	2 (15)
Muller et al. (49)	Esophageal	10 d preop	58	55	8 (14)	17 (31)	4 (7)	11 (20)
Bellantone et al. (50,51)	Oropharyngeal, esophageal, gastric, bladder	6 d postop	62	60	12	7	8 (13)	8 (13)
Buzby et al. (53)	GI Lung	7–15 d preop / 3 d postop	192	203	49 (26)	50 (25)	16 (8)	12 (6)
Sandstrom et al. (54)	GI, bladder	postop	150	150	227	163	12 (8)	10 (7)
von Meyenfeldt et al. (35)	Gastric, colorectal	10 d preop	51	50	5 (10)	8 (16)	not reported	not reported
Sciafani, et al. (55)	Pancreas	5–20 d postop	24	27	9 (38)	12 (44)	2 (8)	
Enteral Nutrition								
Shukla et al. (32)	GI, breast, oropharyngeal	10 d NG feeding preop	67	43	7 (10)	16 (37)	4 (6)	5 (12)
Smith et al. (33)	GI	10 d NCJ feeding postop	25	25	11 (44)	9 (36)	4 (17)	1 (4)
Foschi et al. (34)	Upper GI	12 d ND feeding postop	28	32	5 (18)	15 (47)	1 (4)	4 (13)
von Meyenfeldt et al. (35)	Gastric, colorectal	10 d preop	50	50	6 (12)	8 (16)	not reported	not reported

TABLE 36.4. Results of Prospective Randomized Controlled Trials in Patients Treated with Radiation Therapy

Author	Tumor Type	Number of Patients		Survival		Treatment Toxicity	
		NS	Control	NS	Control	Heme	GI
Parenteral Nutrition Trials							
Solassol et al. (5)	Ovarian	42	39	9 Month	8 Month (median)	Not reported	Better
Kinsella et al. (57)	Pelvic	17	15	47%	47%	Not reported	Not reported
Ghavimi et al. (58)	Childhood	14	14	27%	29%	Worse	Worse
Donaldson et al. (59)	Childhood	12	13	8%	8% (posttherapy)	Not reported	Worse
Enteral Nutrition Trials							
Douglass et al. (36)	GI	13	17	62%	76%	No difference	Not reported
Brown et al. (37)	Pelvic	30	17	Not reported	Not reported	Better	No difference
Boumous et al. (38)	Abdomen/pelvic	9	9	Not reported	Not reported	Better	Better
Daly et al. (39)	Head and neck	22	18	Not reported	Not reported	Not reported	Worse
Moloney et al. (40)	Various	42	42	36%	38%	Not reported	Not reported

TABLE 36.5. Results of Prospective Randomized Controlled Trials Evaluating Nutritional Therapy in Patients Receiving Chemotherapy

Parenteral Nutrition

Author	Tumor Type	Number of Patients		Survival		Tumor Response (%)		Treatment Toxicity		Infection Rate (%)	
		TPN	Control	TPN	Control	TPN	Control	Heme	GI	TPN	Control
Nixon et al. (60,61)	Colorectal	20	25	79	308 (Mean)	15	12	Worse	No difference	5	4
Samuels et al. (62)	Testicular	16	14	72%	77%(2.5 y)	63	79	Better	No difference	17	4
Shamberger et al. (63,64)	Sarcoma	14	18	13%	44% (4 y)	14	50	No difference	No difference	42	33
Valdivieso et al. (65,66)	Small-cell lung	30	35	11 mo	12 mo (median)	43	66	No difference	Worse	27	18
Clamon et al. (67)	Small-cell lung	57	62	51%	57% (1 y)	48	43	Better	Not reported	35	5
Issell et al. (68)	Squamous cell lung	13	13	Not reported	Not reported	31	8	Better	Better	Not reported	Not reported
Jordan et al. (69)	Adenocarcinoma lung	19	24	22 wk (median)	40 wk	12	30	Worse	No difference	32	8

Enteral Nutrition

Author	Tumor Type	Number of Patients		Survival		Tumor Response (%)		Treatment Toxicity	
		EN	Control	EN	Control	EN	Control	Heme	GI
Elkort et al. (41)	Breast	24	23	84%	87% (1 y)	No difference		No difference	No difference
Evans et al. (42)	Non-small cell	30	36	8 mo	6 mo (median)	28	15	Not reported	Not reported
Evans et al. (42)	Lung	30		7 mo		20		Not	
	Colorectal	21	33	9 mo	24 mo (median)	10	16	Not reported	No
Tandon et al. (43)	GI	31	39	94%	85%	35	21	Not reported	Better
Bounous et al. (44)	Metastatic	9	12	Not reported	Not reported	56	64	No difference	No difference

796

TABLE 36.6. Indications for the Use of TPN in the Cancer Patient

A. TPN for brief, in-hospital periods (7–10 days)

    1. TPN is not indicated:
        (a) In well-nourished or mildly malnourished patients undergoing chemotherapy, radiation therapy, or surgery.
        (b) In patients with rapidly progressive malignant disease who fail to respond to treatment and in those patients who have evidence of terminal disease and are not candidates for further antitumor therapy.
    2. TPN is indicated:
        (a) In severely malnourished patients who are responding to chemotherapy or in those in whom gastrointestinal or other toxicities preclude adequate enteral intake for 7–10 days or a longer period. Available evidence would suggest that patients who are candidates for TPN under these circumstances should, when feasible, receive TPN prior to or in conjunction with the institution of therapy.

B. Prolonged periods of in-hospital TPN or home TPN

    1. TPN is not indicated:
        (a) In patients with rapidly progressive tumor growth that is unresponsive to therapy.
    2. TPN is indicated:
        (a) In those patients for whom treatment associated toxicities preclude the use of enteral nutrition and represent the primary impediment to the restoration of performance status. Such patients will usually respond to antitumor therapy.
        (b) In selected malnourished cancer patients where the natural history of the disease can be expected to permit a period of normal or near normal performance status. Such patients should be receiving antitumor therapy with a reasonable anticipation of response, or the natural history of the untreated tumor is such that a reasonable quality of life can be expected (survival greater than 6–12 months).

Specific Indications for the Use of Total Parenteral Nutrition in the Cancer Patient

Acute Radiation and Chemotherapy Enteritis Cancer patients who receive abdominal/pelvic radiation or chemotherapy may develop severe and prolonged mucositis and enterocolitis that precludes the use of enteral feedings. Under these circumstances, TPN should be provided to malnourished patients until the enteritis resolves and enteral feeding can be resumed. Moreover, under circumstances where chemotherapy has been contraindicated secondary to severe malnutrition, TPN may improve nutritional status sufficiently to allow the chemotherapy to be initiated or resumed.

Patients undergoing radiation treatment may also develop malnutrition secondary to inadequate caloric intake or from an inability to eat. The potential side effects from radiotherapy are numerous and include nausea, vomiting, diarrhea, mucositis, xerostomia, dysphagia, and anorexia, which may all contribute to malnutrition. As stated previously, the enteral route is preferable for nutrition support whenever possible; however, in cases involving severe dysfunction of the gastrointestinal tract, TPN is indicated. TPN may allow the malnourished, high-risk patient to complete radiotherapy with less associated morbidity.

Nutrition Support in BMT Patients   Bone marrow transplantation (BMT) is a commonly used treatment for hematologic malignancies. The concomitant therapies associated with BMT, chemotherapy, and total body irradiation (TBI) and the potential complication of graft versus host disease (GVHD) may lead to increased catabolism and subsequent body protein losses. The potential toxic effects of the gut mucosa due to these treatment modalities may further compromise enteral nutritional intake, absorption, and metabolism. Protein-calorie malnutrition, which may result from increased losses and decreased intakes, may predispose these high-risk patients to infectious complications, whereas infection may further accelerate protein losses. Hence, parenteral nutrition (PN) support is often utilized in this setting. However, despite the fact that PN may help to diminish the rate of protein losses, most studies have failed to demonstrate a positive nitrogen balance as a result of the provision of adequate nutritional support. Likewise, the increased risk for infection associated with PN provokes further question as to its efficacy in this patient population.

Perioperative TPN in Cancer Patients   The use of preoperative TPN in cancer patients remains controversial and appears to depend highly on patient selection. One large prospective randomized clinical study strongly suggested that preoperative TPN should be limited to only the severely malnourished patient and only if the gastrointestinal tract could not be used for tube feedings (53,70). This study showed no difference in short-term or long-term survival and a higher rate of infectious complications including pneumonia, abscesses, and line sepsis in patients receiving TPN. Noninfectious complications (i.e., impaired wound healing) were significantly lower in those patients receiving TPN who were also severely malnourished (i.e., > 15% weight loss and serum albumin <2.8 mg%). A meta-analysis conducted to assess the efficacy of preoperative parenteral nutrition and when indicated, enteral nutrition support determined a small reduction in postoperative morbidity in response to nutritional intervention. The potential benefit of the nutrition support was found to be of such small magnitude that the cost-effectiveness of such interventions in this setting was questionable (86). Likewise, Bozzetti et al. (87) demonstrated the administration of preoperative and postoperative TPN to reduce the rate of complications and prevent morbidity in severely malnourished patients.

Postoperatively, TPN is often required in the well-nourished cancer patient who develops a complication that precludes enteral support, such as a postoperative ileus. In general, if the patient is unable to tolerate enteral feeding by the 7th postoperative day, TPN should be considered. Recent prospective studies have clarified both the indications for and contraindications to the use of TPN in the surgical patient with cancer (71). The authors concluded that the routine use of postoperative TPN was not indicated and may in fact have harmful side effects following pancreatic resection. It should be noted that many surgeons would elect to place a feeding jejunostomy in such patients.

Composition of TPN Formulations TPN solutions may be comprised of various combinations of amino acids, dextrose, and lipid in order to accommodate individual patient requirements. Dextrose content of TPN formulas should be limited to the maximum rate of glucose oxidation, 1–5 mg/kg/min. Amino acid concentration may vary according to patient needs, renal function, and liver function. Clinical practice of many nutrition support professionals is to limit lipid composition to <1 g/kg body weight due to the potential immunosuppressive effects of the long chain fatty acid oxidation.

TPN formulations may be highly concentrated in substrates and, when indicated, can provide a greater caloric and protein load in smaller volumes, as compared with peripheral regimens. These parenteral feedings are infused via a high flow central venous system to ensure tolerance and minimize the risk for venous sclerosis. According to the ASPEN (American Society for Parenteral and Enteral Nutrition) publication, "The Core Curriculum," the accepted recommendations regarding energy and protein requirements in the cancer patient are as follows:

Energy Requirements

- 20–25 kcal/kg: maintenance requirements for nonambulatory or sedentary patients
- 30–35 kcal/kg: for slightly hypermetabolic patients; requirements for anabolism/ weight gain
- 35 kcal/kg: for hypermetabolic, severely stressed patients or patients with intestinal malabsorption

Protein Requirements

- 0.8–1.0 g/kg: maintenance requirements
- 1.5–2.5 g/kg: for increased requirements due to hypermetabolism/stress, malnutrition/wasting, protein-losing enteropathy (88).

In addition, TPN formulas may be more concentrated in electrolytes than the respective peripheral regimens and may more appropriately satisfy specific patient needs. Electrolyte and micronutrient quantities of TPN administered to cancer patients may vary according to such factors as, nutritional status, gastrointestinal losses (i.e., emesis, diarrhea), and/or pharmacological interactions.

Potential Complications of TPN Advances in technology, monitoring, and catheter care have greatly reduced the incidence of complications associated with the use of TPN. The establishment of a nutrition support team (physician, dietitian, nurse, pharmacist) and the recognition of such a team as an important part of overall patient care has also been a key factor in reducing complications. Complications of TPN that occur in cancer patients can be divided into three types: (1) mechanical (i.e., pneumothorax, venous thrombosis, air embolization; (2) metabolic (i.e., hyperglycemia, azotemia, electrolyte aberrations, liver function test abnormalities; and (3) infectious (i.e., catheter related sepsis). Strict use of aseptic technique with placement and careful treatment of central venous catheters can help to minimize mechanical and infectious complications. Metabolic parameters including glucose, chemistry profiles, and liver function tests should be monitored routinely in patients receiving TPN.

Nutrition and Tumor Growth   With the introduction of specialized enteral and parenteral nutritional regimens into clinical medicine, aggressive nutritional support can now be provided to cancer patients who previously could not or would not eat. However, concerns regarding the stimulation of tumor growth persists. Although there are some animal studies that indicate that tumor growth may be enhanced with a high-protein diet and diminished by low-protein diets, studies in cancer patients are unclear. Until more data are available, nutrition support should continue to be used for those patients in whom its use is clearly warranted.

Improving the Efficacy of Current Feeding Regimens

Hormonal Therapy   The potential benefits of the administration of insulin, the primary anabolic hormone in the body, to the tumor-bearing host has been examined because of its role in stimulating amino acid uptake and protein synthesis in muscle. Studies indicate that treatment with insulin stimulates food intake and nitrogen retention without stimulating tumor growth. Likewise, the administration of insulin in combination with the glutamine antimetabolite acivicin to tumor-bearing rats receiving TPN preserved lean body mass (LBM) and retarded tumor growth. Whether these observations can be extrapolated to the clinical arena is unknown.

Recombinant human growth hormone (GH) has been shown to promote accrual of LBM, nitrogen retention, and improved wound healing in human and animal models. The administration of GH preoperatively in cancer patients was found to enhance net whole body protein balance, but demonstrated no significant improvement in skeletal kinetics. A subsequent trial investigated the efficacy of GH or GH in combination with insulin supplementation in patients receiving TPN. They found a significant increase in net whole body protein balance in response to the administration of GH with or without insulin. No additional benefit was derived by the combination of insulin and GH, however (89).

The potential for the anabolic agent GH to stimulate tumor proliferation raises some concern. Animal studies have demonstrated an increased aneuploid/diploid ratio in tumor cells, but no alterations in tumor weight or volume. Others have demonstrated a possible protective role in the reduction of metastatic lung deposits in animals affected with prostate tumors, as a result of GH treatment. Human data on long-term GH use in GH-deficient children with previously treated malignancies determined no association with tumor recurrence and GH therapy. Hence, a short-term course of GH therapy after curative resection or antineoplastic treatments for malignancies appears to be safe (89).

Glutamine There is a growing body of research focused on the modification of amino acid formulations to improve the efficacy and effectiveness of specialized nutrition support (90). Ziegler et al. (73,91) were the first to demonstrate a decreased morbidity in hospitalized BMT patients as a result of a specific nutritional modality. In a prospective, double-blinded, controlled trial, 45 patients receiving BMT for hematologic malignancies following a pretransplant regimen of high-dose chemotherapy with or without TBI, were studied. Patients were administered PN support with supplemental glutamine at a dose of 0.57 gm/kg/day or an isocaloric, isonitrogenous control, beginning the day after BMT. PN regimens were calculated to satisfy energy and protein requirements based upon a factor of 1.5 times basal energy expenditure and 1.5 gms protein/kg, for calories and protein, respectively. The glutamine-fortified PN regimens were administered without significant adverse effects for an average of 4 weeks, which confirmed earlier reports that established the clinical safety and dose response of L-glutamine (72,92). Patients who received glutamine-fortified PN formulas demonstrated a significant improvement in nitrogen balance, decreased incidence of infection and microbial colonization, and decreased length of stay (LOS), as compared with controls. Hence, the authors demonstrated an improved clinical outcome as a result of glutamine supplementation, in humans (91,118).

The results by Ziegler et al. are consistent with other human and animal studies, which show maintenance of skeletal muscle glutamine levels and protein synthesis in response to glutamine supplementation (118). Specifically, the heightened demand for the nonessential amino acid glutamine during times of catabolic stress and the lack of this nutrient in standard PN regimens due to its relative instability, has caused it to be studied extensively. The researchers attributed the decreased incidence of infection and colonization found in the glutamine supplemented group to the potential of glutamine to alter immune cell function, facilitate repair of the mucosal barrier and/or maintain tissue antioxidant status. Likewise, the attenuation of protein losses due to glutamine administration and the subsequent improvement in nutritional parameters was thought to play an additional role in reducing infection rates (91,118).

A follow-up study by Schloerb and Amare (93) failed to support the positive effects of PN supplemented glutamine. In a double-blinded, randomized trial, they studied 29 patients with hematologic malignancies and solid tumors who received either allogeneic or autologous BMT. Patient's received glutamine-enriched PN or an isocaloric, isonitrogenous control to provide estimated energy and protein requirements. Patients remained on PN for an average of 30 days without adverse effects. The results demonstrated a decreased length of stay (LOS) of approximately 5.8 days, but showed no significant difference in the incidence of infection or the number of positive blood cultures. The authors attributed their failure to confirm the clinical outcome findings of Ziegler et al. to a sicker study population, as evidenced by their higher mortality rate. A similar study evaluated the efficacy of enteral and parenteral glutamine supplementation in patients undergoing BMT versus isocaloric, isonitrogenous controls. They found no significant differences in hospital LOS, neutrophil recovery, sepsis, incidence of positive blood cultures, mocositis, or diarrhea. However, they noted a decreased requirement for PN and a trend toward improved long-term survival in glutamine-supplemented patients with hematologic malignancies (97). Others were unable to demonstrate a positive clinical outcome despite doses as high as 40 grams L-alanyl-L-glutamine in the experimental group (104,105).

Veno-occlusive disease (VOD) is believed to occur due to free radical damage to the endothelial cells of the sinusoids and small hepatic veins from by cytotoxic therapy given prior to BMT. As a result, levels of glutathione, the primary antioxidant of the cytosol, are depleted. Glutamine, the rate-limiting step in glutathione production and vitamin E, the major antioxidant of the cellular membrane, may help to counteract this problem. Case reports have documented success in treating VOD with the administration of 100 mm^3 of intravenous dipeptiven (20% solution of alanyl-L-glutamine dipeptide) and 200 mg oral vitamin E, or the oral intake of 20 g of glutamine powder and 400 mg vitamin E per day, respectively (94,95). Likewise, Brown et al. found that oral supplementation of 50 g glycyl-L-glutamine as compared with an isocaloric, isonitrogenous nonessential amino acid control resulted in a preservation of protein-C and albumin levels following BMT. Reduction in protein-C levels have been found to be predictive of VOD. Moreover, animal studies have demonstrated glutathione monoethylester supplementation prior to treatment with such agents as monocrotaline, BCNU, and cyclophosphamide to prevent against the potential lethal effects. The authors thus concluded that glutamine supplementation during BMT may have a protective role in the preservation of hepatic function (96,118).

The established role of glutamine as a primary fuel source for the enterocytes and an important nutritional parameter in the maintenance of intestinal growth and function has lead to a multitude of studies to investigate the ability of glutamine to counteract the gastrointestinal toxic effects of various treatment modalities. Anderson et al. (98) looked at patients administered 2 g/M (2) glutamine suspension or isonitrogenous placebo. Patients consumed the formulation twice daily, as a swish-and-swallow on the days of chemotherapy and for a minimum of 14 days afterwards. They found a significant decrease in the duration and severity of mucositis in the glutamine supplemented group. An additional study by Anderson et al. (99) evaluated the impact of a glutamine or isonitrogenous placebo swish-and-swallow regimen administered to patients receiving allogeneic or autologous BMT. This trial revealed improved incidence and duration of mucositis and a reduction in opiate use in patients undergoing autologous BMT. The failure to lessen mucositis in allogeneic recipients was attributed to the higher use of methotrexate in this group. Glutamine has been discovered to inhibit renal clearance of methotrexate and may, therefore, increase serum concentrations and subsequently worsen symptoms of mocositis. This group also found glutamine supplementation to improve 28-day survival, suggesting a possible protective role on the gastrointestinal tract. Others have confirmed previous reports of a reduction in the duration and severity of oral mucositis in response to administration of glutamine via the swish-and-swallow method or an oral mouth rinse without ingesting, in cancer patients receiving chemotherapy and primary or adjuvant irradiation (99,102,103,118).

Conversely, Okuno et al. (100) demonstrated no significant benefit of an oral swish-and-swallow regimen versus a placebo in alleviating mucositis induced by 5-fluorouracil treatment. All study patients were administered oral cryotherapy prior to the initiation of chemotherapy, which may have masked any positive results of glutamine. A prospective, randomized, double-blinded study, which examined oral glutamine supplementation versus a placebo in autologous or allogeneic BMT patients found no significant difference between the two groups with respect to nutritional status, PN days, LOS, mocositis, or diarrhea. The inconsistency of these results with those discovered in previous trials may be related to the dose received. The actual amount of glutamine consumed was found to be below the lower suggested and safe dose range of 0.285–0.57 g/kg/day due to the gastrointestinal intolerance caused by toxic BMT preparatory regimens (101,118).

There are many reports investigating the ability of glutamine administration to protect against radiation enteropathy and/or intestinal brush border damage induced by chemotherapy and radiation. Maintenance of the gastrointestinal tract in response to supplementation with oral glutamine during abdominal pelvic radiation therapy (XRT) has been demonstrated in animal models. Likewise, administration of 18 g of oral glutamine in chemotherapy patients led to a reduction in the severity and duration of diarrhea and a decreased requirement for PN. Others have found supplementation with parenteral glycyl-L-glutamine to significantly reduce gastric and duodenal mucosal ulcerations and mucositis in patients after chemotherapy. They noted an improved morphological appearance of the bowel mucosa as evidenced by increased villus height/depth ratio (106–111,118).

Additionally, oral glutamine has been shown to protect against the attenuation of gut permeability and falling lymphocytes induced by radiochemotherapy in esophageal cancer patients. This confirmed the findings of other trials in humans and animals, which implicated glutamine as a preferred fuel source for the enterocytes and lymphocytes (110). Thus, glutamine may play an important role in allowing patients with advanced disease to withstand more aggressive radiation and chemotherapy protocols. Others have failed to show an improvement with chemotherapy-induced diarrhea in response to oral glutamine supplementation (115). Further research is indicated to better assess the effect of glutamine on gut integrity and function in response to known gastrointestinal toxic regimens in oncology patients.

Glutamine is known to be essential for tumor growth. Markedly reduced levels observed in the cancer patient, are likely secondary to increased utilization by the tumor cells and cytokine-mediated alterations in host tissue glutamine metabolism. Experimental evidence indicates a relationship between glutamine administration and tumor proliferation (115). Much of the data used to support this belief, however, was derived from examination of *in vitro* systems (112). In many of these studies, tumor cells were incubated with air to facilitate an aerobic environment (112). It is known that the metabolic pathway for glutamine breakdown is oxygen dependent. It has been suggested that the reduced oxygen supply to the hypoxic or anoxic tumor tissue *in vivo*, limit the utilization of glutamine as an energy substrate (112). Klimberg et al. (113) investigated the impact of oral glutamine supplementation on muscle glutamine metabolism and tumor growth in animals. They found a significant increase in muscle glutamine content in animals fed the glutamine-enriched diet as compared with controls, but no effect on the rate of tumor growth. A study that employed the same tumor model examined the effect of PN-fortified glutamine versus an isocaloric, isonitrogenous control. Based on measured indices of tumor size, tumor DNA content, and tumor metabolism, they concluded that glutamine had no effect on tumor proliferation. However, an increased ratio of tumor cells to host infiltrating cells in the glutamine-treated group was noted (116). Additional studies have confirmed the absence of tumor stimulation as a result of oral or parenteral glutamine supplementation. Moreover, no progression of malignancy or inhibition of tumor response to cytotoxic therapy has been observed in clinical trials (115–118).

Immunostimulatory Agents There have been many studies to evaluate the role of nutritional modulation in the metabolic and immunological response to injury or physiological stress. Specifically, supplementation with arganine, omega-3-fatty acids, and RNA nucleotides have been investigated individually or in various combinations (119). Arganine, a nonessential amino acid, is termed "conditionally essential" due to the increased utilization and requirements during times of catabolic stress. It has been shown to improve wound healing and enhance immune function in human and animal models (130,132). It appears to have a dual role in its ability to influence metabolic activities directly at a cellular level and indirectly via hormonal interactions. Arganine stimulated the release of various hormones that play an integral part in T-cell proliferation, immune system activities, and post-injury metabolic functions, including growth hormone (GH), prolactin, and insulin. Likewise, it has been shown to directly increase T-cell proliferation, lymphokine-activated killer cell production, natural killer cell function, and macrophage tumor lysis (120). The omega-3 fatty acids (eicosapentaenoic acid/ "EPA" and docosahexaenoic acid/ "DHA") have also been shown to enhance immune function and reduce infectious complications post injury. They are believed to alter prostaglandin synthesis by inhibiting the production of the more immunosuppressive E2 (dienoic prostaglandin), while enhancing the production of the E3 (trienoic prostaglandin) form. This positive effect on immune function leads to an enhanced T-cell activity, natural killer cell function, and macrophage IL-1 (interleukin-1) production. Oral administration of EPA in patients with cancer cachexia resulted in a reduction in levels of the acute phase reactant, C-reactive protein (CRP). This was likely mediated by the EPA-induced IL-6 suppression (131). Finally, RNA nucleotides appear to play a role in protein synthesis and various T-cell mediated immunological activities. Animal studies have shown RNA supplementation to reduce infectious mortality and accelerate the return of immune function during protein repletion (121).

There is a considerable body of literature investigating the efficacy of immune-enhancing nutritional formulas (IEF) enriched with arganine, omega-3 fatty acids, and RNA nucleotides in surgical cancer patients. Studies have demonstrated decreased infectious complications (121–123,125) and hospital LOS (125) in response to the postoperative or perioperative administration of IEF versus an isocaloric, isonitrogenous control. Fortification with omega-3 fatty acids in the form of fish oil and medium-chain triglyceride–structured lipids was associated with a reduction in gastrointestinal complications and the incidence of infection (129). Supplementation with an IEF has demonstrated an augmentation of the immune depression induced by surgical trauma and a quicker recovery of immune function. Braga et al. (125) found an improvement with CRP, IL-6, prealbumin, and retinol binding protein levels in the supplemented group. Others have demonstrated the ability of the immune enhancing agents to modulate the acute phase response as evidenced by decreased TNF-α and IL-6 levels (120). Senkal et al. (119) identified a significant decrease in the occurrence of complications after postoperative day 5, but no significant difference in the early postoperative period. This is consistent with the findings of previous trials that exhibited a greater benefit of the IEF after postoperative day 7 (120,121,124,125). This suggests a minimum requirement for the IE agents in order to exert a clinical benefit (125). Moreover, the research indicates that the maximum benefit of the IEF is derived when it is administered during the preoperative and postoperative period, rather than the postoperative interval alone. This may in part explain the failure of Henslin et al. (133) to demonstrate a benefit of IEF when administered to patients following surgical resection for malignancies.

Several trials have compared the efficacy of the IE enteral formulas, isocaloric, isonitrogenous enteral feeding controls, and isocaloric, isonitrogenous PN. Provision of the IE feedings was shown to facilitate a quicker return of immunological function (124,126,127) and a reduction in postoperative infections and LOS (128). The initiation of early postoperative jejunal feedings was determined to be an acceptable nutrition modality in patients following major abdominal surgery. Likewise, the use of IEF is suggested to be more cost effective than standard enteral feedings or PN, despite the higher cost of the specialized enteral product (119,122,123,127). The route of feeding administration was also determined to influence clinical outcome. The greatest effect was derived from the IEF, whereas the PN demonstrated the least benefit (128). This may be the result of the protective effect of enteral nutrition in the preservation of gut barrier function and prevention of bacterial translocation, as described previously.

Antioxidants There is evidence that antineoplastic therapies induce the production of free radicals and depletion of tissue antioxidant stores (134,135). Plasma nutrient antioxidant levels of vitamin C, α-tocopherol, and β-carotene have been found to be reduced in BMT patients following the administration of high-dose cytotoxic therapies (135). Likewise, depleted plasma and hepatic levels of glutamine, an endogenous antioxidant known to act as a free radical scavenger, have been documented in human and animal models, receiving chemotherapy. Jonas et al. (135) demonstrated a significant decrease in plasma GSH-glutathione concentration and vitamin E levels in patients after high dose chemotherapy. They found no benefit of standard PN with micronutrients in the maintenance of antioxidant levels, as compared with the provision of micronutrients alone. Previous trials have documented the increased utilization of glutamine in response to the physiological stress induced by high-dose cytotoxic agents. Hence, glutamine may be the rate-limiting step for GSH-glutathione synthesis in this setting, as standard PN formulations are devoid of this amino acid. Moreover, the available data indicates that reactive oxygen species are generated in response to the peroxidation of the PUFA (polyunsaturated fatty acid) lipid emulsions in standard PN formulas (135,136). This may be counteracted, however, by adequate antioxidant supplementation. Specifically, the evidence suggests that the α-tocopherol requirements in PN patients may need to be adjusted according to the amount of intravenous PUFA's received daily. The provision of adequate doses of selenium to minimize susceptibility to oxidative stress is advised. Moreover, it appears that the levels of zinc, copper, and manganese contained in standard PN regimens are adequate to promote enhanced super oxide dismutase activity during exposure to oxidative stress (136). In a randomized, double-blind, placebo-controlled trial, glutathione administration was found to significantly reduce cisplatin-induced neurotoxicity without altering the clinical activity of the chemotherapeutic agent (137). Others have shown vitamin E, vitamin C, and N-acetylcysteine administration in cancer patients to reduce the cardiotoxic effects associated with chemotherapy or radiation treatment (135). The ability to counteract the harmful effects of free radical generation induced by anticancer therapies via nutritional antioxidant modulation is promising. More controlled trials are indicated to better evaluate the role and efficacy of antioxidant supplementation in this setting.

Nutrition Support for Cancer Patients and Health Care Reform

The impact of corporate medicine on nutrition support has recently been addressed (74). With the introduction of health care reform, nutrition support teams and the services they provide are now considered a cost center rather than a source of revenue. In the past, the costs required to pay the members of the nutrition support team have been offset by the reimbursements for the services provided, particularly the delivery of TPN. However, this is no longer the case. The challenge to nutrition support professionals is to coordinate efficient and early intervention and to document its efficacy and outcome. Some techniques to ensure that nutrition support is cost effective have been suggested in the literature (74). Others have demonstrated a cost savings and decreased metabolic and infectious complications as a result of patient management by a nutrition support team. It is imperative that the team be proactive and justify it added value to the institution in order to survive in this era of health care reform.

REFERENCES

1. Souba WW, Wilmore DW (1994) Diet and nutrition in the care of the patient with surgery, trauma, and sepsis. In *Modern Nutrition in Health and Disease*, 8th edition. Shils M, Young V (eds) Lea & Febiger, Philadelphia, pp. 1202–1240.

2. Souba WW (1993) Total parenteral nutrition. In *Current Practice of Surgery*. Copeland EM III, Levine BA, Howard RJ et al. (eds) Churchill Livingstone, New York.

3. Souba WW (1994) Cytokines: Key regulators of the nutritional/metabolic response to critical illness. *Curr Prob Surg* 31:577–652.

4. Hautamaki RD, Souba WW (1995) Principles and techniques of nutritional support in the cancer patient. In *Atlas of Surgical Oncology*. Karakousis CP, Copeland EM, Bland KI (eds) W. B. Saunders, Philadelphia PA, pp. 741–748.

5. Souba WW (1997) Nutrional support. In *Cancer Principles and Practice of Oncology*, 5th edition. Rosenberg S., Helman S, Devita V. (eds) Lippincott-Raven, Philadelphia, pp. 2841–2857.

6. DeWys WD, Begg D, Lavin PT et al. (1980) Prognostic effect of weight loss prior to chemotherapy in cancer patients. *Am J Med* 69:491–497.

7. Knox LS, Crosby LO, Feurer ID et al. (1983) Energy expenditure in malnourished cancer patients. *Ann Surg* 197:152–162.

8. Fearon KCH, Hansell DT, Preston T et al. (1988) Influence of whole body protein turnover rate on resting energy expenditure on patients with cancer. *Cancer Res* 48:2590–2595.

9. Shaw JHF, Wolfe RR (1986) Glucose and urea kinetics in patients with early and advanced gastrointestinal cancer: The response to glucose infusion, parenteral feeding, and surgical resection. *Surgery* 101:181–191.

10. Lundholm K, Edstrom S, Karlberg I et al. (1982) Glucose turnover, gluconeogenesis from glycerol, and estimation of net glucose cycling in cancer patients. *Cancer* 50:1142–1150.

11. Jeevanandam M, Lowry SF, Horowitz GD et al. (1984) Cancer cachexia and protein metabolism. *Lancet* 1:1423–1426.

12. Heber D, Chlebowski RT, Ishibashi DE et al. (1982) Abnormalities in glucose and protein metabolism in noncachectic lung cancer patients. *Cancer Res* 42:4815–4819.

13. Norton JA, Burt ME, Brennan MF (1980) In vivo utilization of substrate by human sarcoma bearing limbs. *Cancer* 45:29–34.

14. Souba WW (1993) Glutamine and cancer. *Ann Surg* 218:715–728.

15. Balkwill F, Osborne R, Burke F et al. (1987) Evidence for tumor necrosis factor/cachectin production in cancer. *Lancet* 2:1229.

16. Michie HR, Sherman ML, Spriggs DR et al. (1989) Chronic TNF infusion causes anorexia but not accelerated nitrogen loss. *Ann Surg* 209:19–24.

17. Darling G, Fraker DL, Jensen C et al. (1990) Cachectic effects of recombinant human tumor necrosis factor in rats. *Cancer Res* 50:4008–4013.

18. Sherry BA, Gelin J, Fong Y et al. (1989) Anticachectin/tumor necrosis factor-α antibodies attenuate development of cachexia in tumor models. *FASEB J* 3:1956–1962.

19. Oliff A, Defeo-Jones D, Boyer M et al. (1987) Tumors secreting human TNF/cachectin induce cachexia in mice. *Cell* 50:555–563.

20. Starnes HF, Warren RS, Jeevanandem M et al. (1988) Tumor necrosis factor and the acute metabolic response to injury in man. *J Clin Invest* 82:1321–1325.

21. Darling G, Goldstein DS, Stull R et al. (1989) Tumor necrosis factor: immune endocrine interaction. *Surgery* 106:1155–1160.

22. Arbos J, Lpoz-Soriano FJ, Carbo N et al. (1992) Effects of tumor necrosis factor-α (cachectin) on glucose metabolism in the rat. *Mol Cell Biochem* 112:53–59.

23. Fischer E, Marano M, Barber AE et al. (1991) Comparison between effects of interleukin-1α administration and sublethal endotoxemia in primates. *Am J Physiol* 261:R442–R452.

24. Meszaros K, Lang CH, Bagby GJ (1987) Tumor necrosis factor increases in vivo glucose utilization of macrophage-rich tissues. *Biochem Biophys Res Commun* 149:1–6.

25. Warren RS, Starnes HF, Gabrilove JL et al. (1987) The acute metabolic effects of tumor necrosis factor administration in humans. *Arch Surg* 122:1396–1400.

26. Flores EA, Bistrian BR, Pomposelli JJ et al. (1989) Infusion of tumor necrosis factor/cachectin promotes muscle catabolism in the rat. *J Clin Invest* 83:1614.

27. Fong Y, Moldawer LL, Marano M et al. (1989) Cachectin/TNF or IL-14α induces cachexia with redistribution of body proteins. *Am J Physiol* 256:R659–R665.

28. Moldawer LL, Svanninger G, Gelin J et al. (1987) Interleukin-1 and tumor necrosis factor do not regulate protein balance is skeletal muscle. *Am J Physiol* 253:C766–C773.

29. Hall-Angeras M, Angeras U, Zamir O et al. (1990) Interaction between corticosterone and tumor necrosis factor stimulated protein breakdown in rat skeletal muscle, similar to sepsis. *Surgery* 108:460–466.

30. Greenberg AS, Nordan RP, McIntosh J et al. (1992) Interleukin 6 reduces lipoprotein lipase activity in adipose tissue of mice in vivo and in 3T3-L1 adipocytes: A possible role for interleukin 6 in cancer cachexia. *Cancer Res* 52:4113–4116.

31. Memon RA, Feingold KR, Moser AH et al. (1992) Differential effects of interleukin-1 and tumor necrosis factor on ketogenesis. *Am J Physiol* 263:E301–E309.

32. Shukla HS, Rao RR, Banu N et al. (1984) Enteral hyperalimentation in malnourished surgical patients. *Indian J Med Res* 80:339–346.

33. Smith RC, Hartemink RJ, Holinshead JW et al. (1985) Fine bore jejunostomy feeding following major abdominal surgery: A controlled randomized clinical trial. *Br J Surg* 72:458–461.

34. Foschi, D. Cavagna G., Callioni, F et al. (1986) Hyperalimentation of jaundiced patients on percutaneous transhepatic biliary drainage. *Br J Surg* 73:716.

35. von Meyenfeldt MF, Meyerink WJ, Soeters PB et al. (1991) Perioperative nutritional support results in a reduction of major postoperative complications especially in high risk patients [Abstract]. *Gastroenterology* 100:A553.

36. Douglass HO, Milliron S, Nava H et al. (1978) Elemental diet as an adjuvant for patients with locally advanced gastrointestinal cancer receiving radiation therapy: A prospectively randomized study. *JPEN* 2:682–686.

37. Brown MS, Buchanan RB, Karran SJ (1980) Clinical observations on the effects of elemental diet supplementation during irradiation. *Clin Radiol* 31:19–20.

38. Bounous G, LeBel E, Shuster J et al. (1975) Dietary protection during radiation therapy. *Strahlentherapie* 149:476–483.

39. Daly JM, Hearne B, Dunaj J et al. (1984) Nutritional rehabilitation in patients with advanced head and neck cancer receiving radiation therapy. *Am J Surg* 148:514–520.

40. Moloney M, Moriarty M, Daly L (1983) Controlled studies of nutritional intake in patients with malignant disease undergoing treatment. *Hum Nutr Appl Nutr* 37A:30–35.

41. Elkort RJ, Baker FL, Vitale JJ et al. (1981) Long-term nutritional support as an adjunct to chemotherapy for breast cancer. *JPEN* 5:385–390.

42. Evans WK, Nixon DW, Dlay JM et al. (1987) A randomized study of oral nutritional support versus ad lib nutritional intake during chemotherapy for advanced colorectal and non-small cell lung cancer. *J Clin Oncol* 5:113–124.

43. Tandon SP, Gupta SC, Sinha SN et al. (1984) Nutritional support as an adjunct therapy of advanced cancer patients. *Indian J Med Res* 80:180–188.

44. Bounous G, Gentile JM, Hugon J. (1971) Elemental diet in the management of the intestinal lesion produced by 5-fluorouracil in man. *Can J Surg* 14:312–324.

45. Holter AR, Fischer JE (1977) The effects of perioperative hyper-alimentation complications in patients with carcinoma and weight loss. *J Surg Res* 23:31–34.

46. Heatley RV, Williams RH, Lewis MH (1979) Pre-operative intravenous feeding: A controlled trial. *Postgrad Med J* 55:541–545.

47. Yamada N, Koyama H, Hioki K et al. (1983) Effect of postoperative total parenteral nutrition (TPN) as an adjunct to gastrectomy for advanced gastric carcinoma. *Br J Surg* 70:267–274.

48. Askanazi J, Hensle TW, Starker PM et al. (1986) Effect of immediate postoperative nutritional support on length of hospitalization. *Ann Surg* 203:236–239.

49. Müller JM, Keller HW, Brenner U et al. (1986) Indications and effects of preoperative parenteral nutrition. *World J Surg* 10:53–63.

50. Bellantone R, Doglietto GB, Bossola M et al. (1988) Preoperative parenteral nutrition in the high risk surgical patient. *JPEN* 12:195–197.

51. Bellantone R, Doglietto, G, Bossola M et al. (1988) Preoperative parenteral nutrition of malnourished surgical patients. *Acta Chir Scand* 154:249–251.

52. Woolfson AM, Smith JA (1989) Elective nutritional support after major surgery: A prospective randomized trial. *Clin Nutr* 8:15–21.

53. The Veterans Affairs Total Parenteral Nutrition Cooperative Study Group (1991) Perioperative total parenteral nutrition in surgical patients. *N Engl J Med* 325:525–532.

54. Sandstrom R, Drott C, Hyltander A et al. (1993) The effect of post-operative intravenous feeding (TPN) on outcome following major surgery evaluated in a randomized study. *Ann Surg* 217:185–195.

55. Sclafani LM, Shike M, Quesada E et al. (1991) A randomized prospective trial of TPN following major pancreatic resection or radioactive implant for pancreatic cancer. Presented at the Society of Surgical Oncology, March, Orlando, FL.

56. Solassol C, Joyeux J, Dubois JB (1979) Total parenteral nutrition (TPN) with complete nutritive mixtures: An artificial gut in cancer patients. *Nutr Cancer* 1:13–18.

57. Kinsella TJ, Malcolm AW, Bothe A et al. (1981) Prospective study of nutritional support during pelvic irradiation. *Int J Radiat Oncol Biol Phys* 7:543–548.

58. Ghavimi F, Shils ME, Scott BF et al. (1982) Comparison of morbidity in children requiring abdominal radiation and chemotherapy, with and without total parenteral nutrition. *J Pediatr* 101:530–537.

59. Donaldson SS, Wesley MN, Ghavimi F et al. (1982) A prospective randomized clinical trial of total parenteral nutrition in children with cancer. *Med Pediatr Oncol* 10:129–139.

60. Nixon DW, Moffitt S, Lawson DH et al. (1981) Total parenteral nutrition as an adjunct to chemotherapy of metastatic colorectal cancer. *Cancer Treat Rep* 65(Suppl 5):121–128.

61. Nixon DW, Heymsfield SB, Lawson DH et al. (1981) Effect of total parenteral nutrition on survival in advanced colon cancer. *Cancer Detect Prev* 4:421–427.

62. Samuels ML, Selig DE, Ogden S et al. (1981) IV hyperalimentation and chemotherapy for stage II testicular cancer: a randomized study. *Cancer Treat Rep* 65:615–627.

63. Shamberger RC, Brennan MF, Goodgame JT et al. (1984) A prospective, randomized study of adjuvant parenteral nutrition in the treatment of sarcoma: results of metabolic and survival studies. *Surgery* 96:1–12.

64. Shamberger RC, Pizzo PA, Goodgame JT et al. (1983) The effect of total parenteral nutrition on chemotherapy-induced myelosuppression. *Am J Med* 74:40–48.

65. Valdivieso M, Frankmann C, Murphy WK et al. (1987) Long-term effects of intravenous hyperalimentation administered during intensive chemotherapy for small cell broncho-genic carcinoma. *Cancer* 59:362–369.

66. Valdivieso M, Bodey GP, Benjamin RS et al. (1981) Role of intravenous hyperalimenta-tion as an adjunct to intensive chemotherapy for small cell bronchogenic carcinoma. *Cancer Treat Rep* 65(Suppl 5):145–150.

67. Clamon GH, Feld R, Evans WK et al. (1985) Effect of adjuvant central IV hyper-alimentation on the survival and response to treatment of patients with small lung cancer: A randomized trial. *Cancer Treat Rep* 69:167–177.

68. Issell BF, Valdivieso MD, Zaren HA et al. (1978) Protection against chemotherapy toxicity by IV hyperalimentation. *Cancer Treat Rep* 62:1139–1143.

69. Jordan WM, Valdivieso M, Frankman C et al. (1981) Treatment of advanced adeno-carcinoma of the lung with ftorafur, doxorubicin, cyclophosphamide, and cisplatin (FACP) and intensive IV hyperalimentation. *Cancer Treat Rep* 65:197–205.

70. Fan ST, Lo CM, Lai ECS et al. (1994) Perioperative nutritional support in patients undergoing hepatectomy for hepatocellular carcinoma. *N Engl J Med* 331:1547–1552.

71. Brennan MF, Pisters PWT, Posner M et al. (1994) A prospective randomized trial of total parenteral nutrition after major pancreatic resection for malignancy. *Ann Surg* 220:436–444.

72. van der Hulst RRWJ, van Kreel BK, von Meyenfeldt MF et al. (1993) Glutamine and the preservation of gut integrity. *Lancet* 341:1363–1365.

73. Ziegler TR, Young LS, Benfell K et al. (1992) Glutamine-supplemented parenteral nutrition improves nitrogen retention and reduces hospital mortality versus standard parenteral nutrition following bone marrow transplantation: a randomized, double-blind trial. *Ann Intern Med* 116:821–828.

74. Nelson, J (1995) The impact of health care reform on nutrition support—the practitio-ner's perspective. *Nutr Clin Prac* 4:1–7.

75. De Conno F, Martini C, Zecca E et al. (1998) Megastrol acetate for anorexia in patients with far-advanced cancer: a double-blind controlled clinical trial. *Eur J Cancer* 34:1705–1709.

76. Westman G, Bergman B, Albertsson M et al. (1999) Megastrol acetate in advanced, progressive, hormone-insensitive cancer. Effects on the quality of life: a placebo-controlled, randomized, multicentre trial. *Eur J Cancer* 35:586–595.

77. Erkurt E, Erkisis M, Tunali C (2000) Supportive treatment in weight-losing cancer patients due to the additive adverse effects of radiation treatment and/or chemotherapy. *J Exp Clin Cancer Res* 19:431–439.

78. Loprinzi CL, Kugler JW, Sloan JA et al. (1999) Randomized comparison of megastrol acetate versus dexamethasone versus fluoxymesterone for the treatment of cancer anorexia/cachexia. *J Clin Oncol* 17:3299–3306.

79. Kardinal CG, Loprinzi CL, Schaid DJ et al. (1990) A controlled trial of cyproheptadine in cancer patients with anorexia and/or cachexia. *Cancer* 65:2657–2662.

80. Della Cuna GR, Pellegrini A, Piaazzi M (1989) Effect of methylprednisolone sodium succinate on quality of life in preterminal cancer patients: a placebo-controlled, multi-center study. *Eur J Clin Oncol* 25:1817–1821.

81. Popiela T, Lucchi R, Giongo F (1990) Methylprednisolone as palliative therapy for female terminal cancer patients. *Eur J Clin Res* 25:1823–1829.

82. Tchekmedyian NS, Tait N, Moody M et al. (1987) High-dose megastrol acetate; a possible treatment for cachexia. *JAMA* 257:1195–1198.

83. Bruera E, Macmillan K, Kuehn N et al. (1990) Controlled trial of megastrol acetate on appetite, caloric intake, nutritional status, and other symptoms in patients with advanced cancer. *Cancer* 66:1279–1282.

84. Loprinzi CL, Ellison NM, Schaid DJ et al. (1990) Controlled trial of megastrol acetate for the treatment of cancer anorexia and cachexia. *J Natl Cancer Inst* 82:1127–1132.

85. Loprinzi CL, Michalak JC, Schaid DJ et al. (1993) Phase III evaluation of four doses of megastrol acetate as therapy for patients with cancer anorexia and/or cachexia. *J Clin Oncol* 11:762–767.

86. von Meyenfeldt MF (1999) Nutritional support during treatment of biliopancreatic malignancy. *Ann Oncol* 10:S273–S277.

87. Bozzetti F, Gavazzi C, Miceli R et al. (2000) Perioperative total parenteral nutrition in malnourished, gastointestinal patients: a randomized, clinical trial. *JPEN J Parenter Enteral nutr* 24:7–14.

88. Bloch AS. Cancer. In *Nutrition Support Dietetics Core Curriculum*, 2nd ed. Gottschlich MM, Matarese LE, Shronts EP, eds. Silver Spring, MD: The American Society for Parenteral and Enteral Nutrition; 1993; 213–227.

89. Berman RS, Harrison LE, Pearlstone DB et al. (1999) Growth hormone, alone and in combination with insulin, increases whole body and skeletal muscle protein kinetics in cancer patients after surgery. *Ann Surgery* 229:1–10.

90. Iqbal N, Salzman D, Lazenby AJ et al. (2000) Diagnosis of gastrointestinal graft versus-host disease. *Am J Gastoenterol* 95:3034–3038.

91. Ziegler TR, Young LS, Benfell K et al. (1992) Clinical and metabolic efficacy of glutamine-supplemented parenteral nutrition after bone marrow transplantation: a randomized, double-blind, controlled study. *Ann Intern med* 116:821–828.

92. Ziegler TR, Benfell K, Smith RJ et al. (1990) Safety and metabolic effects of l-glutamine administration in humans. *JPEN J Parenter Enteral nutr* 14(Suppl): 137S–46S.

93. Schloerb PR, and Amare M (1993) Total parenteral nutrition with glutamine in bone marrow transplantation and other clinical applications (a randomized, double-blind study). *JPEN J Parenter Enteral nutr* 17:407–413.

94. Goringe AP, Brown S, Callaghan UO et al. (1998) Glutamine and vitamin E in the treatment of hepatic veno-occlusive disease following high-dose chemotherapy. *Bone Marrow Transplant* 21:829–832.

95. Nattakom TV, Charlton A, Wilmore DW (1995) Use of vitamin E and glutamine in the successful treatment of severe veno-occlusive disease following bone marrow transplantation. *Nutr Clin Prac* 10:16–18.

96. Brown SA, Goringe A, Fegan C et al. (1998) Parenteral glutamine protects hepatic function during bone marrow transplantation. *Bone Marrow Transplant* 22:281–284.

97. Schloerb PR, Skikne BS (1998) Oral and parenteral glutamine in bone marrow transplantation: a randomized, double-blind study. *JPEN J Parenter Enteral Nutr* 23:117–122.

98. Anderson PM, Schroeder G, Skubitz KM (1998) Oral glutamine reduces the duration and severity of stomatitis after cytotoxic cancer chemotherapy. *Cancer* 83:1433–1439.

99. Anderson PM, Ramsay NKC, Shu XO (1998) Effect of low-dose oral glutamine on painful stomatitis during bone marrow transplantation. *Bone Marrow Transplant* 22:339–344.

100. Okuno SH, Woodhouse CO, Loprinzi CL et al. (1999) Phase III controlled evaluation of glutamine for decreasing stomatitis in patients receiving fluorouracil (5-FU)-based chemotherapy. *Am J Clin Oncol* 22:258–261.

101. Coghlin Dickson TM, Wong RM, Negrin RS et al. (2000) Effect of oral glutamine supplementation during bone marrow transplantation. *JPEN J Parenter Enteral Nutr* 24:61–66.

102. Cockerham MB, Weinberger BB, Lerchie SB (2000) Oral glutamine for the prevention of oral mucositis associated with high-dose paclitaxel and melphalan for autologous bone marrow transplantation. *Ann Pharmacother* 34:300–303.

103. Huang E, Leung SW, Wang C et al. (2000) Oral glutamine to alleviate radiation-induced oral mucositis: a pilot randomized trial. *Int J Radiat Oncol Biol Phys* 46:535–539.

104. Van Zaanen HCT, Van der Lelie H, Timmer JG et al. (1994) Parenteral glutamine dipeptide supplementation does not ameliorate chemotherapy-induced toxicity. *Cancer* 74:2879–2884.

105. Jebb SA, Maughan TS, Mohideen N et al. (1994) 5-fluorouracil-induced mucositis: no effect of oral glutamine supplementation. *Br J Cancer* 70:732–735.

106. Jensen JC, Schaefer R, Nwokedi W et al. (1994) Prevention of chronic radiation enteropathy by dietary glutamine. *Ann Surg Oncol* 1:157–163.

107. Muscaritoli M, Micozzi A, Conversano L et al. (1997) Oral glutamine in the prevention of chemotherapy-induced gastrointestinal toxicity. *Eur J Cancer* 33:319–320.

108. Decker-Baumann C, Buhl K, Frohmuller S et al. (1999) Reduction of chemotherapy-induced side-effects by parenteral glutamine supplementation in patients with metastatic colorectal cancer. *Eur J Cancer* 35:202–207.

109. Yoshida S, Matsui M, Shirouzu Y et al. (1998) Effects of glutamine supplements and radiochemotherapy on systemic immune and gut barrier function in patients with advanced esophageal cancer. *Ann Surg* 227:485–491.

110. Ziegler TR, Daignault NM (2000) Glutamine regulation of human immune cell function. *Nutrition* 16:458–461.

111. Blijlevens NMA, Donnelly PP, De Pauw BE (2000) Mucosal barrier injury: biology, pathology, clinical counterparts and consequences of intensive treatment for haematological malignancy: an overview. *Bone Marrow Transplant* 25:1269–1278.

112. Kallinowski F, Runkel S, Fortmeyer HP et al. (1987) L-glutamine: a major substrate for tumor cells in vivo? *J Cancer Res Clin Oncol* 113:209–215.

113. Klimberg VS, Souba WW, Salloum RM et al. (1990) Glutamine-enriched diets support muscle glutamine metabolism without stimulating tumor growth. *J Surg Res* 48:319–323.

114. Austgen TR, Dudrick PS, Sitren H et al. (1992) The effects of glutamine-enriched total parenteral nutrition on tumor growth and host tissues. *Ann Surg* 215:107–113.

115. Bozzetti F, Biganzoli L, Guavas C et al. (1997) Glutamine supplementation in cancer patients receiving chemotherapy: a double-blind randomized study. *Nutrition* 13:748–751.

116. Bartlett DL, Charland S, Torosian MH. (1995) Effect of glutamine on tumor and host growth. *Ann Surg Oncol* 2:71–76.

117. Souba WW (1993) Glutamine and cancer. *Ann Surg* 218:715–728.

118. Ziegler TR (2001) Glutamine supplementation in cancer patients receiving bone marrow transplantation and high dose chemotherapy. *J Nutr* 131:2578S–2584S.

119. Senkal M, Mumme A, Eickhoff U et al. (1997) Early postoperative enteral immunonutrition: clinical outcome and cost-comparison analysis in surgical patients. *Crit Care Med* 25:1489–1496.

120. Senkal M, Kemen M, Homann H et al. (1995) Modulation of postoperative immune response by enteral nutrition with a diet enriched with arganine, RNA, and Omega-3 fatty acids in patients with upper gastrointestinal cancer. *Eur J Surg* 161:115–122.

121. Daly JM, Weintraub FN, Shou J et al. (1995) Enteral nutrition during multimodality therapy in upper gastrointestinal cancer patients. *Ann Surg* 221:327–338.

122. Senkal M, Zumtobel V, Bauer K et al. (1999) Outcome and cost-effectiveness of perioperative enteral immunonutrition in patients undergoing elective upper gastointestinal tract surgery. *Arch Surg* 134:1309–1316.

123. Snyderman CH, Kachman K, Molseed L et al. (1999) Reduced postoperative infections with an immune-enhancing nutritional supplement. *Laryngoscope* 109:915–921.

124. Kemen M, Senkal M, Homann H et al. (1995) Early postoperative enteral nutrition with arganine-ω-3 fatty acids and ribonucleic acid-supplemented diet versus placebo in cancer patients: an immunologic evaluation of Impact. *Crit Care Med* 23: 652–659.

125. Braga M, Gianotti L, Radaelli G et al. (1999) Perioperative immunonutrition in patients undergoing cancer surgery. *Arch Surg* 134:428–433.

126. Braga M, Vignali A, Gianotti L et al. (1996) Immune and nutritional effects of early enteral nutrition after major abdominal operations. *Eur J Surg* 162:105–112.

127. Gianotti L, Braga M, Vignali A et al. (1997) Effect of route of delivery and formulation of postoperative nutritional support in patients undergoing major operations for malignant neoplasms. *Arch Surg* 132:1222–1230.

128. Braga M, Gianotti L, Vignali A et al. (1998) Artificial nutrition after major abdominal surgery: impact of route of administration and composition of the diet. *Crit Care Med* 26:24–30.

129. Kenier AS, Swails WS, Driscoll DF et al. (1996) Early enteral feeding in postsurgical cancer patients; fish oil structured lipid-based polymeric formula versus a standard polymeric formula. *Ann Surg* 223:316–333.

130. Barbul A, Lazarou SA, Efron DT et al. (1990) Arginine enhances wound healing and lymphocyte immune responses in humans. *Surgery* 108:331–337.

131. Wigmore SJ, Fearon KCH, Maingay JP et al. (1997) Down-regulation of the acute-phase response in patients with pancreatic cancer cachexia receiving oral eicosapentaenoic acid is mediated via suppression of interleukin-6. *Clin Sci.* 92:215–221.

132. Kirk SJ, Hurson M, Regan MC et al. (1993) Arginine stimulates wound healing and immune function in elderly human beings. *Surgery* 114:155–160.

133. Heslin MJ, Latkany L, Leung D et al. (1997) A prospective, randomized trial of early enteral feeding after resection of upper gastrointestinal malignancy. *Ann Surg* 226: 567–579.

134. Weijl NI, Cleton FJ, Osanto S (1997) Free radicals and antioxidants in chemotherapy-induced toxicity. *Cancer Treat Rev* 23:209–240.

135. Jonas CR, Puckett AB, Jones DP et al. (2000) Plasma antioxidant status after high-dose chemotherapy: a randomized trial of parenteral nutrition in bone marrow transplantation patients. *Am J Clin Nutr* 72:181–189.

136. Pironi L, Ruggeri E, Zolezzi C et al. (1998) Lipid peroxidation and antioxidant status in adults receiving lipid-based home parenteral nutrition. *Am J Clin Nutr* 68:888–893.

137. Cascinu S, Cordella L, Del Ferro E et al. (1995) Neuroprotective effect of reduced glutathione on cisplatin-based chemotherapy in advanced gastric cancer: a randomized double-blind placebo-controlled trial. *J Clin Oncol* 13:26–32.

CHAPTER 37

Rehabilitation of the Cancer Patient

THERESA A. GILLIS

Oncology Rehabilitation Services, Helen F. Graham Cancer Center,
Christiana Care Health System, Newark, Delaware

Rehabilitation may be defined as the process of restoring or maximizing the quality of life of an individual through attention to their physical, psychological, social, and vocational functions and the societal roles they experience. To achieve the goal of preventing or limiting functional loss in cancer patients, aggressive symptom management, psychosocial interventions, application of physical interventions and adaptive equipment, wise utilization of resources, and patient and caregiver education are essential. Use of objective, standardized, and validated measures of function will advance understanding of rehabilitation's impact on the abilities of cancer patients, their quality of life, and the burden of care associated with diminished independence and satisfaction in these domains.

THE ROLE OF CANCER REHABILITATION

The rehabilitation philosophy fundamentally values independence and self-determination, and through these goals hopes to maximize quality of life. Rehabilitation interventions may be indicated at different points across the continuum of cancer treatment. Commonly, rehabilitation will be considered when a structural loss has occurred, as in resection of a tumor that involves an organ or functional unit such as a limb. Rehabilitation is also often employed when an **obvious** functional impairment is encountered, such as a gait pattern abnormality (e.g., limp or foot drop), speech production or articulation deficit, hemiparesis, or other gross limitation is apparent. These are traditional triggers for rehabilitation interventions that are easily identified, and the interventions themselves may not be markedly distinct from those used for patients with similar deficits from nononcologic origins.

UICC Manual of Clinical Oncology, Eighth Edition. Edited by Raphael E. Pollock
ISBN 0-471-22289-5 Copyright © 2004 John Wiley & Sons, Inc.

Less commonly, rehabilitation will be considered for patients with a generalized decline in the speed, ease, or acuity of their functional abilities, in the absence of an overt organ, or structural compromise. Patients with fatigue related to radiation treatment, overall loss of endurance related to immobility and the deconditioning syndrome, or distal muscle weakness and sensory loss related to chemotherapy may not have referral to rehabilitative interventions despite the often-severe functional limitations that result. Functional decline may be viewed by the physician and patient as a necessary component of the disease or treatment. If the decline is identified as a problem, neither the physician nor the patient may know how to intervene effectively in these situations.

In the landmark study by Lehman and colleagues, over 800 hospitalized cancer patients were assessed to detect problems amenable to rehabilitation interventions. More than 30% had problems with activities of daily living (ADLs) or general weakness. Ambulation was a problem for nearly a quarter of the sample. The majority of patients were not prescribed rehabilitation interventions due to several identified issues including: (1) failure of the healthcare team to identify that such problems were present in their patients; (2) a lack of physician and team awareness regarding the availability of helpful rehabilitation interventions; and (3) insufficient knowledge within the team as to how to access such interventions. These barriers are gradually being brought down through the concerted educational efforts of rehabilitation professionals, the growing consumer advocacy of patients who expect and demand attention to quality of life concerns, and the increasing number of enlightened cancer treatment centers.

In the cancer setting, rehabilitation takes on an additional, unique importance due to the use of functional characterizations as criteria for receiving chemotherapy or other cancer treatments. Performance status measures often include specific functional criteria such as independent gait or self-care skills. In some situations, patients slip below a target performance status rating and become ineligible for standard or investigational treatment protocols. In some of these cases, rehabilitation may in fact facilitate achievement of cure or remission by enabling patient access to another line of treatment though restoration of abilities. Thus, the rehabilitation goal expands beyond that of amelioration of, or adaptation to, a functional deficit, to incorporate life-prolongation and cancer cure as a potential outcome of the rehabilitation plan.

Another distinctive characteristic of rehabilitation in the oncology setting is the need for rehabilitative interventions in the face of advancing and incurable cancer. Palliative rehabilitation is not unique to cancer; rehabilitation care is employed for those with amyotrophic lateral sclerosis, Duchenne's muscular dystrophy, and other mortal illnesses. In many of these diagnoses, however, the patterns of decline are fairly uniform and demise occurs within rather predictable timelines. In contrast, many cancer patients face waxing and waning functional levels, with multifactorial etiologies for losses. Additionally, some of the etiologies of decline are transient or amenable to medications or other interventions.

As an example, consider a patient with myeloma who experiences a slow, progressive decline in mobility and cognition. The mobility changes may be the result of painful bone disease and impending fractures, coupled with proximal weakness caused by prolonged use of corticosteroid therapy. Cognitive decline may originate from analgesic or benzodiazepine side effects, depression, or a metabolic delirium from hypercalcemia. Some of these impairment etiologies are readily remediable, others are not, and some may require sequential interventions that will take some time to bring the patient back to a state of equilibrium.

The oncology rehabilitation team does not withhold attempts to mobilize the patient, facilitate communication, and maximize nutritional intake while the underlying problems are addressed. The rehabilitation team also strives to prevent the complications of immobility that would often accompany the symptom burden in a patient such as the one described above.

The oncology and rehabilitation team may struggle at times to know what are realistic functional goals for a patient, and particularly so when systemic or/or multiorgan symptomatology is present. Generally, it is beneficial to aim for higher achievements from these patients, for otherwise they can fall to the level of too-limited expectations. Sequential assessments over time will best facilitate the determination that goals are not realistic, that cancer may be progressing, or other factors are inhibiting the recovery of function.

When the etiologies of functional decline are irreversible, the rehabilitation team continues its goals of prevention of complications and facilitation of self-determination and expression of needs, but also revises the goals of physical or cognitive independence. Goal revision in the face of advancing disease usually occurs in discussion with patients and their families, and is usually, but not always addressed when the oncology treatment shifts to a purely palliative intent. These discussions may be painful for the patient, family, and rehabilitation specialist. However, the reiteration of the team's goal to facilitate independence of spirit and body, despite the expanding cancer, in a respectful and supportive manner is usually comforting and reassuring to the patient and her or his family/caregiver network.

The greatest challenges in oncology rehabilitation, therefore, are (1) the identification of remediable etiologies for impairment, and oncology-specific complications of therapy and disease; (2) determining the appropriate functional goals for a specific patient; (3) recognizing when goals must be revised, which may occur when cancer control is lost; and (4) understanding and accepting palliative goals when that transition has occurred for a patient.

REHABILITATION METHOD

Interventions may be brief or sustained, comprehensive or limited in scope. Inpatient or outpatient venues may be utilized. Treatment may require frequent hands-on therapy by one or more rehabilitation professionals from a variety of disciplines, or a one-time instruction leading to self-directed restorative or preventive activities by the patient. Patients cared for in a multidisciplinary, comprehensive manner are often managed in a team structure, involving physiatrists (rehabilitation physician specialists), therapists, nurses, and other specialists

TABLE 37.1. The Multidisciplinary Oncologic Rehabilitation Team

Physician: physiatrist, oncologist, primary care physician
Physical therapist
Occupational therapist
Speech pathology specialist
Chaplain
Psychologist
Oncology nurse
Social worker
Nutritionist

As needed:
    Respiratory therapist
    Orthotist: specialist in fabrication/design/fitting of devices that support the
        function of a weak or otherwise compromised structure
    Prosthetist: specialist in fabrication/design/fitting of devices that replace an
        absent structure
    Dentist
    Wound ostomy care nurse

(Table 37.1). Other disciplines may be involved as dictated by patient-specific needs. A particular patient's team may shift in composition over time as some functional problems remit and others emerge. For example, a breast cancer patient may have need of intensive physical therapy for a brief period after mastectomy, with psychological support due to stress and grief reactions to her new diagnosis, and nursing and physician support for treatment of postmastectomy pain. If her disease progresses to a more advanced stage involving a brain metastasis to her frontal lobe, speech pathology and neuropsychology input and assistance may be helpful to address cognitive changes. A chaplain may facilitate spiritual self-appraisal and mortality fears; a social worker can identify alternate financial support if she is unable to return to her job. Physical therapy may not be required at that later point, but occupational therapy may, in order to enhance her safety during showering, or reduce fatigue during activities of daily living.

Rehabilitation disciplines should be involved in the early stages or inception of the cancer treatment plan. Preventive techniques may be employed in situations where functional decline is expected or a high risk of disability is present. Examples of such interventions include exercise programs during the bone marrow transplantation process, shoulder flexibility exercises begun following axillary dissection, or strengthening exercises initiated when corticosteroid medications are prescribed.

Once impairment occurs, therapies may seek to reverse it or to prevent disability through compensatory techniques. Impairments in the setting of rapidly advancing, aggressive disease may be addressed in a palliative sense, where reversal or avoidance of disability are not goals. In these cases, psychosocial support, enhanced coping abilities for the patient and family, and avoidance of preventable impairments and unpleasant symptoms such as decubitus ulcers or untreated pain may be the goals.

IMPAIRMENT, DISABILITY, AND HANDICAP

The World Health Organization has provided a model to describe the impact of disease or injury to an individual. *Impairment* is the loss or abnormality of psychological, physiological, or anatomic structure or function. *Disability* is any restriction or lack, resulting from impairment, in one's ability to perform in the manner or within the range considered normal for a human. *Handicap* is the disadvantage for an individual, resulting from their impairment or disability, which then limits or prevents the fulfillment of a normal or usual role for that individual. A clinical example to clarify these concepts can be described as follows.

A woman with melanoma of the proximal lower extremity undergoes resection and lymph node resection followed by local radiation. Although she recovers well without evidence of disease, due to her scar and soft tissue changes she has *impairment* in flexibility at her ipsilateral hip joint. The *disability* she experiences as a result is that she is unable to flex the hip to 90 degrees or adduct it to neutral, causing an inability to sit in a standard chair in a normal posture. The presence or absence of a *handicap* then depends entirely upon her unique situation. If this patient is employed in manufacturing, and stands throughout the day at an assembly line station, she may experience no employment-related handicap. However, if she is a professional dancer, her range of motion restriction at the hip creates complete handicap *in that role*. This same patient may also have a handicap with regard to social roles, if she plays bridge in a league as an avocational, enjoyable activity. An inability to sit comfortably for any duration might impede this patient's participation in her social role. Rehabilitation professionals categorize and interpret functional changes within this framework and thus develop interventions appropriate to the patient's concerns and values as well as the physical findings.

It must also be recognized that cancer patients most often experience disability and handicap not through a single, severe impairment, but rather an accumulation of several less-profound impairments. A leukemia patient may experience a sensory peripheral neuropathy as a result of treatment, which makes ambulation more tedious and uncomfortable. This same patient may have cognitive changes, such as diminished concentration, as a result of alpha interferon therapy. The combination of the distracting discomfort and the impaired ability to focus attention may create severe handicap in a patient who might otherwise do well.

Thus, the rehabilitation assessment includes not only the patient's physical and cognitive impairments, but also the social, vocational, and avocational environment around that individual. The physical environment and resources available to a patient are also essential to understanding potential barriers to independence as well as avenues for assistance. The interpersonal support of family, friends, or others may also be critical to achieve a patient's optimal level of function. An understanding of a patient's financial circumstances and an awareness of charitable and governmental resources will also allow the clinician to direct interventions in the manner most advantageous to patients within the constraints of their situation.

CHALLENGES IN CANCER REHABILITATION

There are obvious similarities between the rehabilitation philosophy, goals and techniques utilized for cancer and noncancer patients with disability. The fundamental difference in the treatment of cancer patients is the concern, anxiety, or uncertainty regarding prognosis faced by the rehabilitation professionals and the patients themselves. For example, patients who survive a cerebrovascular accident face significant mortality risks over the ensuing months and years. However, generally the patient, family, and treatment team do not question the fullest application of rehabilitation interventions, and do not ruminate over the very real risk of a sudden cardiac death or severe cardiovascular event and whether resources should be directed toward the rehabilitation of a stroke patient. However, many cancer patients face discrimination from health care systems that limit access to rehabilitation resources, and rehabilitation professionals reluctant to accept cancer patients, based on misguided beliefs about imminent death or inexorable functional decline associated with cancer. In a world of limited health care resources, this bias leads to the denial of services for many patients.

The diagnosis of cancer encompasses a broad range of diseases, with different impairments and survival statistics. Even among patients with a specific tumor pathology, the individual patterns of relapse, complications, and recovery lead to difficulty anticipating a given patient's disease course. Determining whether a patient will be able to overcome an impairment or benefit significantly from sustained rehabilitation interventions can be challenging. When a patient fails to make meaningful progress toward a functional goal, the team must review whether adverse symptoms (e.g., pain, nausea), cognitive or psychological changes, or recurrent or progressive disease are present. Remediable problems are addressed, but if success is not met, the rehabilitation goals should be altered. Limited physician skills in symptom assessment and management, and uncertainty regarding prognosis, add to the reluctance of oncologists and rehabilitationists to utilize rehabilitation interventions. It is most reasonable to pursue trials of rehabilitation, with a limited, predetermined number of sessions or duration of therapy followed by a reassessment, whenever it is unclear whether a patient with impairment will benefit from therapy.

SPECIFIC PROBLEMS

General Fitness and Immobility

The immobility syndrome has been well characterized, with some of the relevant work contributed as a result of space exploration research. Immobility and reduced weight-bearing situations have definite and severe consequences to the human body. Unfortunately, these sequelae are sometimes viewed as inevitable in the course of care for cancer patients. Recent research utilizing exercise interventions during chemotherapy and radiation therapy regimens, as well as studies of patients immediately after stem cell and marrow transplantation, have shown encouraging results. Functional capacity as measured by maximal oxygen uptake has been shown to improve, and unintended benefits of enhanced nausea control and reduced psychological distress have also been suggested. Patients also have generally high levels of acceptance and tolerance for exercise and functional expectations. It is possible that a greater emphasis on preventive exercise regimens will develop as an outcome of these studies.

Other common, and thus commonly overlooked or unidentified, sequelae of cancer treatment can include neuromuscular complications. Peripheral neuropathies associated with chemotherapies can result in sensory and motor deficits. The functional consequences may include reduction in ambulation and thus endurance and/or independence, inability to perform fine-motor skills such as dressing or eating independently, or an increased risk of skin injury and infection. Access to physical and occupational therapy interventions and patient education are important to prevent functional decline. Autonomic neuropathies can manifest as diminished peristalsis, urinary incontinence or retention, and orthostatic hypotension. Symptoms may be treated with medications or mechanical interventions such as suppositories, urinary collection devices, and compression garments, respectively.

Steroid-induced myopathies are encountered in patients receiving glucocorticoids, typically for hematological cancers or for control of edema around central nervous system tumors. The presentation is that of proximal extremity weakness, with patients noting inability to climb stairs or arise from a bed or chair. Steroid receptor density within muscular cytoplasm increases in muscles with disuse and this may explain why inactive patients appear to be more vulnerable to pronounced steroid-related weakness. Patient education emphasizing the importance of maintenance of activity, and a program of strengthening exercise for the affected muscles, should be provided at the time steroid therapy is initiated.

Fatigue

Cancer-related fatigue is certainly a widespread complaint among cancer patients. It has been considered by some authors to be a unique phenomenon, separate from fatigue complaints related to depression, or experienced in otherwise healthy patients. It may, conversely, possess a pathophysiologic process equivalent to or closely resembling that of other chronic, immune-related diseases such as rheumatoid arthritis.

Contributors to fatigue such as anemia and hypothyroidism are rather easily corrected but are infrequently present. Depression or mood disorders are not strongly associated with the fatigue complaint in several studies, but should be assessed. Asthenia and overt neuromuscular pathology are not usually present. Inefficiencies of function, described by Donovan as "energy leaks" are not well recognized but may be contributing factors. Mild foot drop, impaired balance or vision, upper limb incoordination, or pain are but a few possible examples of impairments that make ordinarily simple tasks more energy consuming and fatiguing, both mentally and physically. Correction or compensation for such leaks is helpful. Exploration of sleep and activity patterns and determination of the presence and intensity of pain may lead to specific means of lessening the fatigue severity. Limiting naps or rest breaks to periods shorter than an hour has been recommended. Use of aerobic exercise, or even frequent low-intensity activities such as gardening, walking, and household tasks have been proposed as helpful. Cognitive impairments including diminished executive functions, attention, and order/hierarchy constructions may be subtle, and have been described as a sequelae of interferon therapies. These impairments can manifest as a fatigue complaint as well. Stimulants, ranging from caffeine to amphetamines, have been employed by some practitioners to counteract fatigue. Nutrition and hydration are likely to play significant roles in fatigue even in noncachectic patients, but there is little specific scientifically-based information for guidance in this area.

Neck, Shoulder, and Upper Extremity Dysfunction

Impairments of the neck and shoulder region are frequently encountered in cancer patients. Imbalance of the multiaxial shoulder joint can arise through sequelae of surgery or radiation, as well as direct tumor involvement. Bone and soft tissue (muscle, connective tissue, lymphatic) tumors, whether primary or metastatic, are more readily recognized etiologies for shoulder pain. Scarring, weakness or paralysis of muscle, contracture of the shoulder capsule, or scarring and fibrosis of the chest wall or neck soft tissues may all result from treatment of tumors in the forequarter and are more subtle etiologies.

Trapezius denervation is typically associated with many head and neck cancer surgeries, due to the frequent loss or partial, devascularization injury of the spinal accessory nerve (SAN) during cervical node dissections. Neuropraxia causing temporary or incomplete SAN injury can also occur even with attempts to spare the nerve. Both the trapezius and sternocleidomastoid muscles are innervated by the SAN, but the trapezius has a particularly critical role in active shoulder flexion, abduction, or weight carrying. The trapezius anchors the scapula to the posterior thorax, and during abduction elevates the scapula while it rotates the scapular acromion in a cephalad direction. At rest, when the arm is hanging at the side, the scapula has unopposed pull by gravity and is thus laterally deviated on the chest wall. When the arm is attempting to rise in flexion or abduction, the rotator cuff muscles become compressed by the acromioclavicular ligament against the humeral head. The impingement is lessened in a supine position as the scapula is better anchored by the compressive weight of the body against the bed. The traction of unopposed gravity upon the arm can lead to brachial plexus irritation and subsequent dysesthesias throughout the affected arm. Unweighting the arm can reduce pain, as can limiting attempts to flex, abduct, and carry loads with that limb (Table 37.2).

TABLE 37.2.   Management of Shoulder Dysfunction Secondary to Spinal Accessory Nerve Loss

Avoid attempts to raise arm above shoulder height
Do not attempt to single-arm carry more than 5 kg on affected side
Only rarely attempt to carry more than 5 kg using both arms
Use upward pressure of humerus at shoulder with:
   Arm rests and table tops
   Placement of hand on chair seat with elbow extended
   Rest hand in pocket, waistband, or belt loop when walking
Strengthen remaining scapular stabilizers: serratus anterior, levator scapulae, rhomboids
Strengthen cervical and mid-upper thoracic paraspinal muscles
Stretch pectoralis minor
Use of shoulder orthoses in selected cases

Restrictive scarring in the chest soft tissues may follow mastectomy or thoracotomy. Classically, a scapula may be "trapped" in an elevated, laterally deviated position by a thoracotomy scar, or can be tethered by a contracted pectoralis muscle following breast surgery. In either case, rotator cuff impingement can occur as the humerus abducts against the scapular acromion that fails to move in a normal upward rotation. Consistent stretching and mobilization of the soft tissues can usually relieve the problem if imposed before scar maturation. Ideally, preventive stretching would be prescribed following such surgical approaches.

Neck motion can be drastically reduced following surgical resection or irradiation of tumors in the head and neck region, due to nerve loss or soft tissue contracture. Sternocleidomastoid paralysis will result from SAN loss. Paraspinal muscle strength and skin sensation can be reduced by resection of posterior cervical tumors through direct tissue loss or by resection of cervical root posterior branches. Fibrosis itself can restrict the motion of the head, particularly in extension, side-bending, and rotation. In all these cases, preventive stretching programs are essential. When posterior muscular support is lost, a cervical orthosis must be used to prevent a fixed, severe, cervical flexion deformity caused by unopposed pull of the anterior cervical muscles.

Tumors of the spine, humerus, clavicle, scapulae, ribs, and sternum may all adversely affect upper-extremity function. Metastatic plexus lesions generally cause both pain and weakness, whereas radiation plexopathy tends to cause weakness and discomfort. Upper limb orthoses may be used to immobilize or support painful limbs. Sling devices and waist-affixed shelf-like supports are commercially available and can enable patients with severe bone and soft tissue disease in the forequarter to remain ambulatory with less pain. Slings should always be removed when the patient reclines or is supine.

Distal arm weakness and pain may also arise through peripheral neuropathy. Edema related to neuropathy or lymphedema may cause sensory changes as well, with complaints of stretching, pulling, or electrical sensations. Static orthoses can hold the wrist and hand in positions of comfort or positions of function. Dynamic orthoses can assist with grip or with finger and wrist extension. Dynamic orthoses may be well tolerated for limited periods but are usually not sustained due to their bulk. Massage and edema control may allow the patient better function, and strengthening and desensitizing exercises may be worthwhile. Adaptive equipment such as built-up utensils, brushes, rocker knives, and innumerable other gadgets can help patients manage reduced grip strength or dexterity. Shoulder, elbow, and hand range of motion should be preserved whenever possible, but if pain is extreme and the goals of care are palliative, and life expectancy is brief, pain relief will supplant mobility as the goal.

Nodal Dissection and Irradiation

Inguinal, pelvic, axillary, and cervical nodal basin injury can create significant impairment through several means. These basins are all in close proximity to important neural structures, raising the risk of denervation injury as a direct consequence of treatment, or secondary neural compromise through soft-tissue scarring. Joint motion can also be severely compromised due to soft-tissue changes. Lymphedema risks increase with manipulation of the nodal basins and lymphatic vessels. Edema pressure can create entrapment neuropathy-like pain, muscular fatigue, and imbalance due to the excessive limb weight, and obviously dangerous sequelae from increased risk of infections. Stretching programs to inhibit restrictive scarring and lymphedema management should become standard components of aftercare for patients undergoing nodal manipulation.

Lymphedema Management

Preventive education is included in the concept of lymphedema management. Although there is no way to definitively prevent lymphedema, reasonable steps to reduce risks of infection and further injury to an affected lymph drainage zone should be encouraged in at-risk patients. Prohibition of exercise and heavy use of an unaffected but at-risk limb may not be reasonable as the etiologic associations between lymphedema and lifestyle factors (vocational and avocational) have not been studied in any serious manner.

Lymphedema treatment includes lymphatic massage of the affected drainage basin and stimulation of unaffected contra- or ipsilateral basins that might assist in relieving lymphatic congestion. Compressive bandaging follows massage sessions, and exercises are generally performed while the limb is bandaged in order to promote lymphatic flow from the limb back into the arteriovenous circulation. After lymphedema has been reduced or controlled, compressive garments are generally used to help maintain these gains. Numerous resources are available for further reading on this topic. Pneumatic compression pumps can be used with multichamber, gradient sleeve, or stocking devices. Use of these devices has declined out of concern that they fail to address the problem of an already-overwhelmed proximal lymph basin, which they press lymph and intravascular volume toward.

Disorders of Communication, Speech, and Swallowing

Rehabilitation interventions are commonly utilized following treatment for head and neck cancers that disrupt the anatomical structures participating in functions of speech, phonation, mastication, and/or swallowing. Much has been written in numerous texts regarding the management of laryngectomized patients. Options for speech following laryngectomy include tracheoesophageal puncture prostheses, which utilize a one-way valve to direct air into the esophagus for phonation; esophageal speech, which involves swallowed air and vibration of the oropharyngeal soft tissues; or artificial larynx use such as an intraorally or externally applied electrolarynx.

Patients with other tumor pathologies are less commonly assessed for these impairments, but many interventions are available. Patients with primary or metastatic tumors of the brain, including leptomeningeal disease, can commonly develop communication abnormalities, ranging from aphasia to dysarthria. Delirium and dementia have been mistakenly diagnosed in the presence of severe hearing loss. Dysphonia and hoarseness can occur whenever the recurrent laryngeal nerve in the neck is compressed by cervical adenopathy. Speech and language pathologists are helpful in both the diagnosis and the management of these problems.

Dysphagia is an extremely common problem among cancer patients. Oral candidiasis and esophagitis can create pain but also mechanical failure of the coordinated swallow. Patients with generalized debility may develop dysphagia that is secondary to pharyngeal weakness rather than incoordination. The use of a deeply flexed cervical spine ("chin tuck"), double-swallows, or hard swallows is often helpful in minimizing aspiration and propelling the oral bolus through the pharynx more efficiently. Rotation of the head toward the weaker side or tilting the head toward the stronger side can help those with asymmetric or unilateral weakness by directing food to the stronger side of the pharynx. Patients may not report an abnormal sensation or complaint, and therefore a high degree of suspicion should be maintained for those "at risk" due to the above factors. Even bedside evaluations of swallowing safety can miss some aspirating patients, so therefore, those at highest risk, and certainly those with exams suggesting possible aspiration, should be evaluated by videofluoroscopy swallowing studies.

Spinal Cord and Brain Disorders

Patients with injury to the central nervous system due to cancer have impairments and rehabilitation needs similar to those with spinal and brain injury problems of traumatic etiology. However, patterns of recovery and the social implications of the cancer diagnosis do differ from other etiologies. When a patient develops weakness, sensory changes or other complaints originating from a tumor compressing normal brain or spinal tissues, and the tumor is removed before frank ischemia and necrosis have developed, the neurological deficits may resolve completely within hours or days. Other patients have a more incomplete recovery, but this variability in outcome and abbreviated timeline differ from most traumatic injuries of the same structures.

For those with incomplete recovery, the rehabilitation team may face conflicting goals. Brain or epidural spinal cord metastases are harbingers of progressive disease and are thus particularly associated with limited life expectancy. Thus, it may be difficult to balance the efforts required of both patient and treatment team to regain higher levels of independence against the patient's limited lifespan and the limited resources available. The functional goals set by the patient simply may not be achievable within their remaining lifespan. The unique context of the patient's desires, their ability to comprehend and cope with the uncertainty and the certainty of death, and their sense of quality of life can help guide the rehabilitation team to a treatment plan comfortable to all parties.

Pelvic and Lower-Extremity Impairments

Tumors of the pelvis and lower extremities often affect ambulation abilities due to pain and or weakness. Pelvic tumors including bulky retroperitoneal nodal disease may cause pain with activation or stretch of the iliopsoas muscle, making upright stance and advancing the leg during gait or stair-climbing painful or impossible. Femoral nerve injury or quadriceps group tumors cause instability of the knee during gait and increase the risk of falls, so a knee extension orthosis or brace is warranted. Sciatic nerve injury or peripheral neuropathy will often result in weakness or loss of ankle dorsiflexion and toe extension, with stumbling caused by catching the toes on the floor or obstacles. Ankle instability may also be present. An ankle-foot orthosis (AFO) can be fabricated to hold the ankle in a position of comfort and mechanical advantage to avoid toe drag. This brace not only increases safety but also can reduce the energy cost of ambulation and thus reduce fatigue. AFOs are sometimes useful for the allodynia associated with neuropathy, as the brace provides pressure and sensory feedback. Hip girdle weakness can be detected by a characteristic waddling gait. Peripheral neuropathy may cause disorders of balance due to the lack of proprioceptive feedback. Adaptive equipment such a raised toilet seats, tub benches or chairs, and other devices enhance safety and thus independence. In both proximal and distal weakness, a gait assist device such as a cane or walker may reduce the effort of walking and enhance safety. Wheeled walkers allow a more rapid pace and consistent weight bearing through the arms, reducing pain and effort in the affected lower extremity. Gait assist devices, adaptive equipment, orthoses, and exercise programs may enable patients to compensate safely for a host of lower-extremity impairments.

Bowel and Bladder Concerns

Bowel and urinary function are almost universally affected during the course of cancer. Incontinence of urine is multifactorial, involving sensory feedback, autonomic nervous system pathways, cognitive awareness, and also muscle strength and coordination for the effort of using a commode or bedpan. Not only is incontinence unpleasant, but skin breakdown is enhanced in the presence of urine due to excessive moisture and chemical burn of the skin. Amenable factors include treatment of infection, access, and assistance to use a commode. Urinary collection devices are sometimes required, unfortunately.

Urinary retention is, by contrast, often silent. Some patients may have a sense of incomplete emptying as the only clue to its presence. Prostatic hypertrophy, urinary infection, bowel impaction, detrusor muscle weakness, detrusor-urinary sphincter incoordination (dyssynergia), or excessive sphincter tone due to medications are usual etiologies. Dyssynergia arises with injury to the neural pathways in the spinal cord, such as with spinal cord compression or irradiation injury. Urine may be under high pressure within the bladder due to detrusor contraction against a tightly closed urinary sphincter, with the result of urine backflow toward the kidneys and increased risk of infection and renal compromise. Reversible causes of retention should be ruled out. Indwelling or intermittent urinary catheterization may be necessary.

Constipation and diarrhea are battled by many patients throughout the course of their disease. Opioid- and chemotherapy-induced constipation can be treated with promotility agents, stool softeners, enhanced water intake, use of caffeine, prunes, or other dietary stimulants. Diarrhea accompanies many chemotherapies and radiation treatments and fluid intake and electrolyte management are essential.

Skin

Skin is particularly vulnerable in immobile patients and those with insensate areas, or in areas exposed to excessive moisture. Reduced muscle bulk and subcutaneous fat over bony prominences, such as around the spine and sacrum, can particularly predispose a patient toward skin breakdown. Inadequate protein intake will slow healing of wounds.

Pressure relief through frequent turns and avoidance of friction, reduced weight bearing on bony prominences through cushioning and weight distribution, enhanced nutrition, and localized wound care efforts are essential. Keeping the wound clean, with adequate but not excessive moisture, removal of eschar, and edema management are components of skin management. Patients must be taught to protect insensate skin, avoid burns and trauma, and inspect the skin daily to identify new injuries.

Functional Assessment and Quality of Life

A variety of tools and instruments have been developed to measure function in humans. Other instruments have been created to assess health status, whereas still others attend to quality of life. Interest in the impact of cancer and cancer treatment on these domains is increasing worldwide. Patients, clinicians, researchers, and payers struggle to measure the value of oncology therapy beyond reduction cure or control of disease, and to understand the outcomes of successful treatment from the patients perspective.

Confusion regarding the terminology has led to misuse of instruments and, at times, faulty conclusions. Quality of life tools generally include some assessment of function, but the opposite is not always the case. Conclusions have sometimes erroneously equated quality of life and performance or health status when those associations have not been studied. There has been limited coordination of efforts across the disciplines of psychology, public health, rehabilitation, and oncology, and thus a host of instruments have been devised. When attempting to include the domains of function, quality of life, and health status in oncology outcomes research, the number and variety of instruments available can be overwhelming.

Several tools are clinician assessments of global function, such as the Karnofsky and Zubrod instruments. The rater may ask questions of the patient regarding their daily function, or may observe their physical status and infer a level of function. A possible limitation of these tools is their subjective nature, and the ability of a patient to "put on their best face" for an encounter with the physician treating their cancer. Functional outcome assessments may sometimes define function in an anatomical or physiological sense, rather than a behavioral manner. Strength, range of motion, extent of edema, and similar parameters do not necessarily correlate with functional performance of daily activities and other functions relevant to the individual. Functional outcome studies must improve their investigation of the disablement (or lack thereof) of patients in returning to their own usual roles.

Quality of life instruments are often devised with functional abilities and role performance as only one aspect of life satisfaction. Understanding the time frame of reference is crucial for interpreting studies using such measures. For example, an instrument may inquire about various domains within the past week, or within the past month. Symptom burdens and functional capacities may change rapidly over brief periods during treatment. Patient perceptions of their own abilities are susceptible to mood and the perceptions of other's opinions. Coupling subjective ratings with objective functional performance may enhance understanding and accuracy when studying specific outcomes of treatment.

CONCLUSION

Rehabilitation interventions promote independence, enhanced patient awareness, understanding, and participation in management of impairments, and they minimize disability and handicap among cancer patients. Preventive programs can be devised to address anticipated impairments. Therapies should be provided to restore functional capacity in those undergoing treatments associated with fatigue and immobility. The multifactorial causes of impairment and variability in disease course necessitate frequent, ongoing assessments for rehabilitation-amenable deficits, and may create unique challenges for the rehabilitation team. Increased recognition of oncology-related impairments and utilization of rehabilitation interventions will lead to improved patient function, and, as future research may show, enhanced survival and quality of life.

FURTHER READING

Cheville A (2001) Rehabilitation of patients with advanced cancer. *Cancer* 92(4 Suppl): 1039–48.

Cheville AL (2001) Pain management in cancer rehabilitation. *Arch Phys Med Rehabil* 82(3 Suppl 1):S84–7.

Cheville AL, McGarvey CL, Petrek JA, Russo SA, Taylor ME, Thiadens SR (2003) Lymphedema management. *Seminars Rad Oncol* 13(3):290–301.

Courneya KS, Friedenreich CM, Quinney HA, Fields AL, Jones LW, Fairey AS (2003) A randomized trial of exercise and quality of life in colorectal cancer survivors. *Europ J Cancer Care* 12(4):347–57.

Dimeo FC (2001) Effects of exercise on cancer-related fatigue. *Cancer* 92(6 Suppl):1689–93.

Dimeo F, Fetscher S, Lange W, Mertelsmann R, Keul J (1997) Effects of aerobic exercise on the physical performance and incidence of treatment-related complications after high-dose chemotherapy. *Blood* 90(9):3390–4.

Dimeo F, Schwartz S, Fietz T, Wanjura T, Boning D, Thiel E (2003) Effects of endurance training on the physical performance of patients with hematological malignancies during chemotherapy. *Support Care Cancer* 11(10):623–8.

Dimeo FC, Stieglitz RD, Novelli-Fischer U, Fetscher S, Keul J (1999) Effects of physical activity on the fatigue and psychologic status of cancer patients during chemotherapy. *Cancer* 85(10):2273–7.

Gillis TA (2003) Rehabilitation medicine interventions. In *Cancer Pain*. Bruera E, Portenoy RK (eds) Cambridge University Press, New York.

Gillis TA, Donovan ES (2001) Rehabilitation following bone marrow transplantation. *Cancer* 92 (4 Suppl):998–1007.

Gillis TA, Yadav RA (2002) Rehabilitation of the patient with soft tissue sarcoma. In *American Cancer Society Atlas of Clinical Oncology Soft Tissue Sarcoma*. BC Decker, Hamilton, Ontario.

Gillis TA, Yadav R, Guo Y (2002) Rehabilitation of patients with neurologic tumors and cancer-related central nervous system disabilities. In *Cancer in the Nervous System*, 2nd edition, Levin VA (ed) Oxford University Press, New York.

Huang ME, Cifu DX, Keyser-Marcus L (2000) Functional outcomes in patients with brain tumor after inpatient rehabilitation: comparison with traumatic brain injury. *Am J Phys Med Rehabil* 79(4):327–35.

Janjan NA, Payne R, Gillis T, Podoloff D, Libshitz HI, Lenzi R, Theriault R, Martin C, Yasko A (1998) Presenting symptoms in patients referred to a multidisciplinary clinic for bone metastases. *J Pain Symp Manage* 16(3):171–8.

Lehmann JG, DeLisa JA, Warren CG, deLateur BJ, Bryant PL, Nicholson CG (1978) Cancer rehabilitation: assessment of need, development, and evaluation of a model of care. *Arch Phys Med Rehabil* 59(9):410–9.

Marciniak CM, Sliwa JA, Heinemann AW, Semik PE (2001) Functional outcomes of persons with brain tumors after inpatient rehabilitation. *Arch Phys Med Rehabil* 82(4):457–63.

Tunkel RS, Lachmann EA (2002) Rehabilitative medicine. In *Palliative Care and Supportive Oncology*, 2nd edition. Berger AM, Portenoy RK, Weissman DE (eds) Lippincott Williams and Willkins, Philadelphia.

WHO (1980) *International Classification of Impairments, Disabilities and Handicaps*. WHO, Geneva.

Winningham ML, Barton-Burke M (eds) (2000) *Fatigue in Cancer: A Multidimensional Approach*. Jones and Bartlett, Sudbury, Massachusetts.

CHAPTER 38

Supportive Care and Quality of Life Assessment

VITTORIO VENTAFRIDDA, ELENA SCAFFIDI, ALBERTO SBANOTTO, and ARON GOLDHIRSCH

World Health Organization Collaborating Center for Cancer Control and Palliative Care, European Institute of Oncology, Milan, Italy

The majority of cancer treatments are prescribed focusing on the illness rather than on the patient and his or her subjective perceptions, such as quality of life (QOL). When QOL evaluations are considered as an integral part of cancer care and health professionals take care of its assessment and evaluation, the outcomes in terms of satisfaction for the cure are immediately perceived, from both the patient/family and the care team. The endpoints, which are easier to measure, such as survival, disease-free survival time, response duration, treatment-associated toxicity, and tumor response, are increasingly complemented by some QOL measures. Several studies have shown that successful treatment might lead to prolongation of life, yet there is a need to define success of therapy as prolongation of life with preserved quality. Cancer is the most of the time a chronic disease; that's why it is very important to make the patient aware of this dimension, giving him or her, at the same time, new and efficient tools to bear the personal effort required to face, manage, and control the disease over time. In addition, the benefits from cancer treatments are often difficult to define due to subjective side effects, which influence QOL. Information about toxicities of treatment and details on disease-related symptoms is generally assessed using the physician's perspective, whereas recently introduced QOL measures have the advantage of incorporating the patient's perspective as well. This aspect is particularly important in phase II and III studies, which often involve patients with advanced disease, and in which clinical decisions should take into account patients' preferences. Even though QOL research instruments are available, QOL evaluation is often lacking in many studies. It is therefore

UICC Manual of Clinical Oncology, Eighth Edition. Edited by Raphael E. Pollock
ISBN 0-471-22289-5 Copyright © 2004 John Wiley & Sons, Inc.

preferred that a proper QOL indicator be prominently included in the decision-making process for tailoring treatments in cancer medicine.

Despite increasing interest, no consensus has been reached concerning the definition of QOL. Many definitions exist, for example, the World Health Organization (WHO) Quality of Life Group defines it as "an individual's perception of his position in life in the context of the culture and value systems in which he lives and in relation to his goals, expectations, standards and concerns."

All authors agree that QOL is a subjective phenomenon. We can refer to a conceptual definition and to an operational one. With the former, we consider it an amalgam of satisfactory functioning in essentially four domains:

- Social
- Psychological and spiritual
- Occupational
- Physical

It is closely related to well being, human values, and to the WHO concept of health as a global, multidimensional view of health status. Different authors have suggested evaluating the single components of QOL, but it still remains difficult to achieve an overview of these different parts.

The operational definition of QOL refers to a patient's evaluation of his or her health compared with what he or she thinks could be possible or ideal. It has been pointed out that in clinical studies QOL is not related to happiness, satisfaction, or living standards, but rather considers the impact of treatment, positive or negative, on some dimensions of life. Different approaches to define QOL have been recognized; some of them refer to psychological aspects; some to a patient's preference; and some are related to basic concepts of life or to reintegration to normal living, or to the gap between the hopes and the expectations of patients.

One relevant aspect of QOL of cancer patients is related to communication problems. A complete knowledge of the illness, stage, and planned treatment are important factors that allow a patient to decide about his or her future. This is extremely important in advanced and terminal phases of disease, when treatment is often of little benefit and QOL becomes the major issue. A patient-centered communication model should be used where patient's ideas can be explored and concerns about health and health care can be addressed. Sharing decisions and support to improve the patient's ability to take choices complete this approach. Doctors, nurses, and other professionals have a range of individual skills that can be used to achieve these tasks, and specific programs should be implemented to improve their ability to communicate.

Regular assessment of patient's satisfaction with care will allow care providers and hospital management to identify the most relevant issues to be focused on for improvement and progress in different domains of care (clinical, doctor-patient relationship, communication, psychological aspects of cancer, nursing, etc.).

MEASURING QOL

Two types of instruments may be used to measure QOL, which can be either disease specific or generic. Disease-specific instruments refer to measures used for one disease or for a narrow range of illnesses, whereas generic ones are used for a wide range of domains. The instruments may be either designed specifically to cover one item, may be more general, or specifically designed for measuring QOL in cancer patients. Usually, generic measures are less reliable for assessing the specific effects of a treatment, although they might allow the detection of its unexpected consequences. Generic measures may allow easier comparisons between studies. It is important to clearly identify which dimension of QOL is under scrutiny in a specific study and for which subgroup of individuals it is used. Most QOL instruments rely upon visual analogue scales, asking the patient to mark on a 10-cm line, according to the intensity of the symptom, or upon Likert scales, where values are related to discrete ranges of intensity. In general, patients understand Likert scales more easily. Several instruments have been used for the measurement of QOL in cancer patients (Table 38.1).

An interesting approach has been undertaken by the European Organization for Research and Treatment of Cancer (EORTC), by a modular assessment strategy. The EORTC-QLQ-C30 is a generic questionnaire that can be completed by specific modules (e.g., lung, breast) to obtain more specific measures. Another example of

TABLE 38.1. Some QoL Instruments

Instrument	Administration	Items	Notes
EORTC-QLQ-C30 (3)	Self-report	30 Likert questions	Can be supplemented with site-specific questions. Cross-validated for different languages
Functional Assessment of Cancer Therapy (FACT) (4)	Self-report	29 Likert questions	Can be supplemented with site-specific questions. Cross-validated and available in different languages.
Functional Living Index Cancer (FLIC) (5)	Self-report	22 Likert/Analog scale	Especially suitable for physical and psychological factors. Indicated for outpatients. Site-specific questions not available.
Quality of Life— Cancer (6)	Self-report	30 Likert/Analog scale	Especially used in cancer nursing research. Some site-specific versions available.

this modular strategy is the Functional Assessment of Cancer-Therapy QOL questionnaire (FACT). The International Breast Cancer Study Group (IBCSG) developed a visual-analogue questionnaire that can be easily used by patients with breast cancer to evaluate different chemotherapy and endocrine treatment regimens, giving the possibility to make comparisons of women's QOL perception in each treatment option. These questionnaires are suitable for study purposes, but are also adaptable to general patient care. A QOL questionnaire should allow the investigation of at least four domains: physical, psychological, social, and the so-called "performance status." Physical functions, in particular, including pain and other symptoms, mood, and social support should be evaluated from the time of diagnosis to terminal illness. Owing to the subjective nature of QOL, its evaluation should be obtained through a self-administered questionnaire. In a palliative care setting, where communication might be scanty or impossible, the rating of relevant aspects of QOL by individuals close to the patient on his or her behalf might be useful and relevant.

PSYCHO-ONCOLOGY: GENERAL ASPECTS

Psycho-oncology is a subspecialty in oncology encompassing issues of psychological care in cancer medicine. Its recent increasing relevance is due to several changes of medical science, life style, and communication. Earlier diagnosis and progress in scientific knowledge have lead to improved efficacy of treatments. New treatments often influence patient's QOL: improvement in disease control might be associated with relevant costs in terms of physical and psychological side effects and might be associated with significant social and economical distress. Thus, survival of cancer patients has been prolonged and cancer survivors have considerably increased, issues of rehabilitation and other patients' needs have increasingly emerged. The need to control side effects of treatment is underlined. Psychological disorders may result from a cancer diagnosis or its treatment. They are generally ranging in the spectrum of adjustment disorders, but psychiatric complications have been reported in cancer populations as well. The psychological impact of the decision-making process and the compliance to treatments is immense. The need for psychosocial care and rehabilitation has therefore been recognized. In addition, the role of behavioral factors in cancer risks, early detection, compliance with treatment, and survival were acknowledged. Psychologists actively involved in cancer medicine are often solicited to provide expert opinion when information campaigns or psychosocial projects are planned or conducted. Examples for such programs are antismoking interventions or cancer-screening campaigns. The function of the psychologist in the oncology team is to counsel the patient on some practical aspects of the disease and care, provide psychological support for patients and their families in order to ease adjustment, and help cope with cancer and its related problems. The psycho-oncologist has an important role in training of care providers on psychological aspects of cancer (related to patients, family, and staff), on enhancement of communication skills.

Psycho-oncologists may have a substantial role in training volunteers and helping the patient to find psychosocial help after hospital discharge. Assessment and evaluation of psychological dimensions in patients with cancer, such as anxiety and depression, sexuality after treatments, overall quality of life, and satisfaction with care, are typically included among the duties of a psycho-oncologist.

PALLIATIVE CARE: GENERAL ASPECTS

According to the WHO, in the next years there will be a great increase in new cases and cancer deaths, which will be much more concentrated in the developing countries. In fact, the data show that in 1985 in all countries (including both developed and developing countries) there were 5 million deaths and 9 million new cases and by 2015 the projection would be about 9 million deaths and 15 million new cases (with the bigger percentage in developing countries). Cancer is still a major worldwide problem. In 1996, there were an estimated 17.9 million persons with cancer surviving up to 5 years after diagnosis. Each year about 6 million deaths are due to this illness, and the percentage of cure remains still low, especially in developing countries. For this reason, the domain of palliative care is paramount. Palliative care can be defined as the active total care of patients whose disease is not responsive to a specific curative treatment. The targeted control of symptoms, especially pain, and of psychological, social, and spiritual problems is extremely important. The proper support for all these domains of human suffering and distress should, however, be applied at any stage of disease and should not be denied even at the early phases of cancer, in conjunction with anticancer treatment. On the other hand, specific antineoplastic therapies play a major role in palliative care, when control of symptoms outweighs the disadvantages of side effects of treatments. More than 50% of cancer patients live in developing countries, where less than 10% of resources committed to cancer therapies are available. Most resources are devoted to curative (and usually expensive) treatments, with little attention given to training health personnel. For this reason a better allocation of resources is needed, especially in those countries where financial constraints are significant (Fig. 38.1).

Different palliative care programs have been developed, according to local resources and problems:

- *Home care.* Palliative care experts consider the home as the best place to take care of advanced cancer patients. Whenever possible, a patient's autonomy and self-esteem, independent of an institution, should be sought and the presence of a primary health care team may greatly facilitate this approach. However, existing funding does not always allow the equitable distribution of resources in many countries. Home care usually increases the costs for families, both financially and emotionally. The dedicated caring for a relative at home should not be taken for granted, and expansion of home nursing services and provision for financial support are needed in many countries.

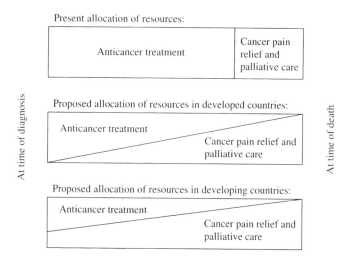

Figure 38.1   Proposed allocation of cancer resources. With permission, WHO, Technical Report Series 804, 1990 (8).

- *Inpatient care.* Hospice and palliative care units represent this program. These settings are devoted to controlling pain and other manifestations of physical and social distress, and offer respite care for patients and families.
- *Consultation service.* Small teams, usually composed of nurses, a social worker, and a consulting physician, can provide specific consultation for different wards and hospitals. These programs also offer proper educational opportunities for involved health workers.
- *Day-hospice.* Day-care programs may provide a proper framework to alleviate the burden of home care for relatives in offering therapy adjustments, physiotherapy, and social opportunity. Patients living alone may also benefit from these programs.
- *Hospice.* A structure for terminally ill patients represents an alternative care setting, either at the hospital or at home. The first palliative care programs began in United Kingdom in the 1970s and were developed thanks to the creation of the first hospices. Their impact on patient care was immense due of their educational contribution in improving attitude toward death and dying. These hospices have inspired many health professionals who have then spread these models in various parts of the Anglo-Saxon world. In the United States, together with the majority of the European countries, hospices are becoming a real alternative by hosting patients and their family members in an appropriate setting, where professional expertise is focused on patient's well-being during his or her last period of life.
- *Bereavement support.* Trained health personnel, usually social workers and volunteers, may help relatives to cope with bereavement. Psychological support should be available both for the dying than for his or her family members, especially when they are young and unable to express autonomously feelings, emotions and concerns.

- *End of life care.* This is a cardinal aspect of palliative care, though typically neglected due to scanty scientific knowledge and to cultural attitude. A major aspect, which requires specific attention, is communication, not only between patients and members of their family, but obviously also between patient/ family and the multiprofessional care team. For the high level of denial linked with death-related issues, communication among health professionals on these specific aspects is strongly recommended.

- *Family counseling in palliative care.* Continuity of care is an essential element of palliative care, although often neglected. Palliative care heavily relies on prevention of distress related to symptoms. For this reason, family members should be trained regarding specific aspects of care, such as administration of analgesics, prevention of decubitus ulcers, injection techniques, and dealing with proper diet. Clear guidelines for drug administration and for emergencies should be explained and clearly written instructions should be left at patient's home. Ignorance concerning even small problems may be a cause of failure of an otherwise efficient program of care.

Palliative care is directed to maintain or improve QOL of patients. We have already discussed its essence and assessment. In the palliative care setting, it is crucial that methods to appraise QOL be simple and not increase the workload of care providers, who should concentrate on patient support rather than on administering questionnaires. The subjective assets of most measures of QOL is therefore appropriate and does not represent a limitation. Physical symptoms and performance, psychological state, and social interactions are the aspects usually evaluated. Some aspects, often omitted, include sexuality, spiritual features, the meaning of the illness, and its impact on patient's family. A better knowledge of QOL in advanced and terminal phases could also help to convince policy makers to develop more balanced interventions in cancer care, with a different allocation of resources.

Education of Health Professionals

Several reports show that health professionals lack education in palliative care (e.g., cancer pain management). Education is a priority to guarantee successful implementation of a palliative care program. Several data indicate that enhanced knowledge in palliative care can be transferred and integrated in existing health care systems. Education should include the following domains:

1. *Attitudes, values, and beliefs.* Philosophy of palliative care, attitude toward illness and death, and multidisciplinary teamwork are some of the topics related to this aspect.
2. *Knowledge (basic).* Refers to the core of topics to be included, such as psychological needs, pathophysiology of symptoms, or spiritual distress.
3. *Skills.* Relates to the application of learned knowledge, through communication, discussions, role-playing, and practice.

The educational program should be part of courses leading to basic professional qualification, academic education, and should be included in postgraduate programs.

Such effort should be made by joint public and private agencies, including health care associations. Also, the public should be made aware of these topics, especially those concerning the meaning of illness and relief of suffering. It is also important to ensure the availability of drugs needed for proper palliative care; this is especially the case for opioids, such as morphine. These drugs should be widely available, together with the education on their use and easy prescription.

MANAGEMENT OF SYMPTOMS: THE CULTURE OF PAYING ATTENTION TO PAIN AND OTHER SYMPTOMS

The most relevant aspect of a symptom is the patient's own perception of it. Such features can be best evaluated by using either analogical or categorial (Likert) scales. A care provider should select the most proper instrument, according to the symptom(s), taking into account specific characteristics of the patient (e.g., age), his or her life, culture and care environment, and features and disease (e.g., advanced stage).

Pain is one of the most important medical aspects of QOL. The evaluation of pain, similarly to the evaluation of all other symptoms, should be meticulously documented in the medical records (when available) or communicated to the person in charge for the patient's care, to allow assessment of treatment effects and to be able to tune therapies according to patient's needs. If at all possible, specific cultural and educational programs should be developed to alert health professionals on the relevance of specific problems/symptoms (particularly pain), to guide and update the concepts of their management. Specifically, each member of a team of care providers should be conscious about his or her role in allowing a proper assessment of (using a uniform set of instruments), communication, management of symptoms, verification of a beneficial outcome of treatment, and the burden of side effects. Frequent and regular assessments may guarantee a proper therapeutic coverage allowing each member of the care providers to responsibly intervene to lessen suffering. Health structures should promote and economically sustain continual medical education (CME) programs on this subject as an activity of high priority. This should lead to training of health professionals and increase their awareness on these issues. Specific information for the general public should be also endorsed through the media or, if necessary, by brochures, booklets, or other means focused on escalating awareness on the main issues related to cancer symptoms' management (e.g., opioids for control of pain).

General Strategy

Cancer patients suffer from a variety of physical symptoms. Important examples are pain, dyspnea, constipation, nausea, hiccups, and several others. As in other areas of cancer medicine, the emphasis is on prevention of symptoms and their early diagnosis. Many symptoms, such as constipation due to opioids, pressure sores, and stomatitis, can be prevented if the care program includes prophylactic treatment and regular longitudinal assessment. Attention to detail is essential. Discussion with relatives is important. It also allows evaluation of the level of cooperation and of participation of the family in the procedures of care. Communication with family members makes it possible to depict the main side effects of treatments, and to educate to a proper strategy for their prevention. These features of care are particularly important when the patient is at home. Some principles for controlling symptoms should be underlined:

- Global evaluation
- Thorough explanation of care programs to patient and family, followed by a check and assessment of the degree of understanding and compliance
- Individualized therapies
- Attention to detail
- Regular assessment of effects

According to the WHO, the regular administration of drugs is particularly important (e.g., for pain management or for constipation), as is the availability of specific drugs for rescue medication or for emergencies (e.g., sedatives for agitation or analgesia for breakthrough pain). The medication program should include the minimal number of drugs necessary to achieve a satisfactory treatment effect, to ensure compliance, and lessen opportunities for unexpected drug interactions. "Standard doses" and long-term prescription of supportive medications are unrealistic. The individualized titration of drugs is, in fact, particularly important (e.g., for pain management). The program for drug administration should take into account the physical and behavioral characteristics of the patient. It is often necessary to accept that some symptoms are not fully controlled (e.g., fatigue), despite proper attempts to their treatment. Continuity of care should remain a first priority, guaranteeing the beneficial effect of several subjective aspects of care and reassuring the patient against a common devastating sensation of being abandoned. It is important to stress that at some stage of the disease, technical skills are of marginal usefulness, whereas psychosocial and spiritual aspects are paramount. Making the last hours of life more peaceful, and sustaining the family in their bereavement, are the major goals of this phase of the disease.

COMMON SYMPTOMS AND THEIR TREATMENT

In this section, we deal with some of the other common symptoms affecting advanced and terminal cancer patients. Pain, which is one of the most frequent and important, has been discussed previously.

Dyspnea

Dyspnea is defined as an unpleasant awareness of difficulty in breathing. The subjective essence of this symptom is stressed in the definition, which is important, especially when dealing with patients who present with breathlessness. Dyspnea may affect about 50% of terminal cancer patients, and up to 70% of the patients with lung cancer. Its incidence increases during the last weeks of life. Dyspnea may be related to cancer and its treatment or, often, preexisting conditions of restrictive or obstructive pulmonary disease. Treatment choice requires establishing the cause of this symptom and whether it is reversible or not. Specific means such as radiotherapy, antibiotics, or pleural drainage should be considered. Irreversible causes of dyspnea, frequently observed in advanced or terminal phases, should be treated with proper support (e.g., correct positioning in the bed and/or the use of oxygen) and respiratory sedatives introduced, aimed at improving perception of breathlessness. Morphine is the main respiratory sedative in use. It has respiratory and analgesic properties, and is thus particularly useful in patients with concomitant pain (e.g., pathologic fracture of ribs), and it may be administered in different routes. Starting doses are usually 20–40 mg daily by mouth. In circumstances of acute dyspnea, intravenous or subcutaneous routes are more efficacious. Usually, if the patient is already on morphine for pain, it might be sufficient to increase the dose by 30–50 mg. In cases of acute attacks of dyspnea, the use of nebulized morphine may be tested; usually 20 mg of morphine sulfate in 10 mL of saline solution is administered by a common nebulizer in air or oxygen. The rate of absorption of the drug is negligible. Oxygen by nasal prongs or mask is usually not helpful in most cancer patients, and a trial of therapy is the best way to determine benefit. Patients with respiratory panic attacks benefit from regular oral morphine as well as from additional means, including regular lorazepam or diazepam (although an unpredictable interaction with morphine is possible).

Constipation

Constipation is a very common problem in advanced cancer patients, with a prevalence of approximately 40% in patients referred to hospices. Up to 90% of those receiving opioids complain of this symptom. Constipation may be due to various causes and a preventive approach represents the best way of dealing with this symptom. The clinical history and examination are helpful for identifying concurrent causes for the symptom like reduced intestinal motility, bowel obstruction, presence of hard and impacted feces, and chronic use of laxatives. Patients treated with opioids almost always complain about constipation and an intensive prevention of this symptom and its treatment should rely upon the following:

- Dietary measures: it is often not practical to prescribe a high-fiber diet. Fluid intake should be increased to a reasonable maximum.
- Whenever possible, activity and mobilization should be encouraged.
- Nursing measures, such as raising the toilet seat, privacy, warm bathroom, or the use of a commode, might be important.
- Regular use of laxatives (especially when treated with opioids).

- If needed, measures such as glycerin suppositories, enemas, or manual evacuation might be needed. Different laxative regimens are available, and it is usually advisable to start with a stool softener such as docusate in association with a bowel stimulant such as senna or bisacodyl.

Delirium

Delirium may be defined as an acute, organic global impairment of mental function. It differs from chronic, progressive loss of memory and intellectual functions, which are typical for dementia. The onset of delirium may be acute, within a few hours, but may develop during several days. Its course may fluctuate and it is often worse at night. Hallucinations may be present and disorientation and agitation are common. Its prevalence ranges from 20 to 70% of patients with advanced cancer, and more than 90% during the last days of life. Advanced age, hospitalization, and advanced disease are all risk factors for developing delirium, which generally is a multifactorial disorder. It is important to evaluate competing features when dealing with an apparently delirious patient. Sometimes a deaf or anxious patient might be interpreted as drowsy and confused. Common problems, which might lead to consciousness disorders in advanced cancer patients (hypercalcemia, severe anemia, sepsis, meningitis, and brain metastases), must be ruled out prior to discussing specific therapies. In most cases, an empirical approach is required:

- If possible, stop or reduce as many drugs as possible, especially sedatives and analgesics. Withdrawal syndromes such as those following abrupt withdrawal of steroids should be dealt with.
- Reassure patient and family by explaining, for example, the pathophysiology of the disorder. Choose for the patient, if necessary, a quiet environment. Reorientating techniques may be useful (e.g., familiar objects, calendar, clock, some physical activity, if applicable).
- Adjust metabolic imbalance and treat specific causes (e.g., correct hypercalcemia, give steroids and anticonvulsants for brain metastases).
- Treat agitation with haloperidol, by oral or parenteral route. If sedation is required, add midazolam or diazepam by continuous intravenous infusion. Midazolam may be conveniently administered subcutaneously.

Inform the family about the severity of the clinical status and its impending course. In patients with advanced cancer, acute confusional state is often a landmark of imminent death.

Nausea and Vomiting

These symptoms may be present in up to 60% of patients with advanced cancer. Nausea and vomiting are frequent side effects of most chemotherapy regimens. In the recent years, management of nausea and vomiting during treatments has substantially improved, even though they should not be neglected, especially during the administration of sustained and high-dose chemotherapy. Nausea and especially vomiting are closely linked with anxiety and fear. Psychological approaches might be helpful and may involve a psycho-oncologist or other care provider (nurse, social worker, volunteer, physician). This may include verbalization of the patient's physical distress helping to overall concerns. These symptoms may be more frequently observed in patients starting on opioid treatment: tolerance to this side effect usually develops within 2 weeks. Nausea is an expression of the stimulation of the autonomic nervous system, whereas vomiting is a complex reflex involving different muscles and neurological functions. The vomiting center, located in the brainstem, receives afferents from the chemoreceptor trigger zone. This region is very sensitive to different stimuli such as cytotoxic agents, various metabolic products (e.g., in case of hepatic or renal failure or acidosis), radiation therapy, and various drugs (e.g., digitalis). Several other stimuli reach the vomiting center from the upper gastrointestinal tract via sympathetic and vagal routes (e.g., effects of chemotherapy, gastrointestinal metastasis), whereas others arrive from cerebral and vestibular areas. A clinical assessment is important in order to identify a potential cause of these symptoms, and a proper diagnostic work-up might be complex. With this regard, some specific issues might help in defining a presumed cause for nausea and vomiting:

- Determine the pattern of nausea and vomiting (e.g., relationship with food ingestion)
- Check for neurological symptoms evocative for intracranial hypertension
- Review the drug schedule
- Make an accurate clinical examination, including rectal examination, when applicable
- Laboratory tests might be useful (e.g., creatinine, calcium, albumin, some drug level, when appropriate)
- In case of gastrointestinal obstruction, evaluate role of palliative surgery. If not amenable to surgery, treat conservatively (see below)

Besides medication, actions include frequent small meals and dietary advice, and providing the patient, if applicable, a calm and reassuring environment. Reversible causes of nausea and vomiting should be treated whenever possible (e.g., hypercalcemia, gastritis, intracranial hypertension, etc.).

The pharmacological treatment of nausea and vomiting is most likely to succeed especially if given with a preventive intent, usually by mouth. If the patient is already experiencing nausea and vomiting, suppositories or parenteral medication are obviously preferable. Continuous intravenous and subcutaneous administration are commonly used. In terminally ill patients, the following points about management may be useful:

- Metclopramide, 10–20 mg every 6–8 hours, is a typical starting therapy.

- If no relief is reached or if the patient suffers brain metastases, the addition of dexamethasone, 16–36 mg/day might be useful.
- In case of liver failure, uremia, or opioid-induced vomiting, haloperidol at a dose of 1–4 mg/day may improve the symptoms.

In patients with nausea and vomiting unable to take oral medications, starting a subcutaneous or intravenous continuous infusion with metclopramide, 30–60 mg, plus haloperidol, 2 mg, in 24 hours might provide relief. These infusions might be administered via a simple syringe-driver or by applying a hypodermoclysis (which is even cheaper). Patients equipped with a permanently implanted intravenous line, might clearly benefit from the use of this device.

Gastrointestinal Obstruction

Gastrointestinal obstruction may affect about 3–5% of hospice patients, but it is particularly common in advanced ovarian cancer and in colorectal cancer, ranging from 25 to 40% and 10 to 15%, respectively. Tumor is the main cause of obstruction in about 60% of patients, but nonmalignant causes and second tumors are also frequent in 25% and 10% of the patients, respectively. It is mandatory to distinguish between operable and inoperable bowel obstruction. This might often be a very arduous task, particularly in patients who have had previous surgery. If the patient is inoperable, the site of obstruction will dictate management.

- Higher sites of obstruction (duodenum) may require a gastrostomy or nasogastric tube to obtain relief of vomiting.
- Lower sites of obstruction generally do not require mechanical decompression, and can be satisfactorily managed with pharmacological agents (see below), which find indication also for a higher level obstruction too. Nasogastric tube and intravenous fluids are recommended in the management of terminally ill patients only in the context of relief of the symptoms of dehydration. Such treatment is generally uncomfortable for the patient, interferes with social functions, and creates a barrier between the patient and the surrounding environment.

The principles of pharmacological treatment of inoperable obstructions rely upon the following combined approaches:

- Controlling pain, both colicky and continuous
- Reducing intraluminal fluids, to alleviate nausea and vomiting with antisecretive drugs
- Reducing nausea and vomiting with antiemetics.

Pain control is properly obtainable with opioids, mainly morphine. Nausea and vomiting may be relieved with haloperidol, 2–6 mg/day and antisecretory drugs such as hyoscine *N*-butylbromide, 60–240 mg/day or the synthetic somatostatin analogue octreotide, 0.3–1 mg/day, which is substantially more expensive. This last drug also increases the reabsorption of intraluminal fluids. These different drugs may be mixed in the same solution and administered as a continuing subcutaneous/intravenous infusion, by syringe-driver, or hypodermoclysis. Steroids may be added. Metclopramide and other prokinetic agents might be useful when intestinal continuity is maintained. In the case of complete bowel obstruction, they may increase colicky pain and, thus, are not indicated.

The Terminal Phase

The main goals of care during the last days and hours of life may be summarized as follows:

- Keep the dying person as comfortable as possible, maintaining his or her dignity.
- Prepare the patient's family for the coming event and support them.
- Intervene to relieve symptoms and respect the process of dying, not trying to shorten or prolong it (as a main focus of intervention).

Explain to relatives that antemortem symptoms, such as changes in breathing, are not perceived by the patient, and thus do not require specific therapeutic intervention. Restlessness or agitation should be either prevented or treated (usually with parenteral haloperidol). Regular and frequent checks for unnecessary medications should be done to avoid their use. Drugs might be easier to administer by subcutaneous or intravenous routes. Opioids, sedatives, and antiemetics are typically the drugs in use during the last hours. Enteral and parenteral feeding should be stopped and parenteral fluids should be avoided: hydration can increase cough, pulmonary congestion, peripheral edema, vomiting, and urinary distress. These aspects have to be clearly explained to the family. The death rattle may be reduced by adding, upon its onset, SC/IV hyoscine, 60–120 mg/day, and by correct positioning of the patient. If agitation or restlessness is present, continuing SC haloperidol (4–10 mg/day) or midazolam (10–30 mg/day) might be useful.

Ethical Aspects

Oncologists (as any other care provider in medicine) should seek an acceptable balance between the advantages and the disadvantages of treatment, especially during the advanced and terminal phases of the illness. The ethical principle of offering care while minimizing harm reflects an accepted approach. Three other principles apply:

- Respect for life
- Respect for patient autonomy
- Fairness in the use of limited resources

When facing situations of uncertainty, the patient's preferences are the most important consideration. When the general condition of the patient deteriorates, freedom from pain and from other subjective symptoms are the pillars of "death with dignity." If, for example, shortening of life results from the use of proper doses of analgesics, this should not be considered as intentionally terminating life by overdose. Life-prolonging treatments also present ethical problems. Preservation of life at any cost is not always the wished for and suitable choice, especially if the burden of side effects and personal costs appears unacceptable for the patient. Moreover, life-supporting therapies often reduce patient's freedom in communication and in other elementary needs of a human being. In many countries, health professionals have come to accept this notion, and the ethic of allowing cancer patients to die peacefully has become current practice. This approach involves withholding or discontinuing aggressive interventions, such as respiratory support, systemic antitumor medications, or parenteral nutrition. The patient's will is to be considered first and respected. Three other ethical and philosophical principles are relevant:

- The principle of proportion
- The principle of equivalence
- The relativity principle

In brief, they help us to accept the limits of medicine and the resources of a patient. The patient's perception of our efforts as a prolongation of dying, rather than an enhancement of living, justifies discontinuing life-prolonging techniques. Moreover, stopping a treatment is ethically not different from never starting it. The principle of relativity affirms that life is not an absolute good and that even death should be accepted as a "normal" event. Medicine should respect personal values and life-prolonging therapies should give way to other kinds of care.

However, even when controlling pain, confusion, respiratory distress, and the other symptoms according to the guidelines, our work is only half-way through. We should recall that at that specific moment, in every patient, there might be a perception that death is approaching. Nonmedical support might be proper and necessary according to the wishes of the patient. Dying patients (probably most of the patients who suffer regression appearing with the disease and hospital stay) have a strong desire of physical expression of caring: touching, hugging, kissing. They might also still be involved in the control of decision of care and would like to be involved in the discussion of practical issues, such as finances and family future. One of their worries is personal appearance: they know their aspect is changing and should be helped to keep clean, dry, and good smelling. They usually appreciate the presence of caring individuals to avoid isolation and increase communication. Aspects related to the desire of the sincerity (e.g., truth about their conditions), spirituality, and religion should be taken into account.

An essential aspect of care is related to touching, which enhances communication and promotes comfort and could be instrumental: washing, mobilizing, gentle massage, and so on are all typically appreciated.

A frequently raised ethical dilemma concerns euthanasia. Palliative care is a strong and modern answer to this problem: reducing physical and psychosocial suffering is surely a practicable alternative to euthanasia. Efforts then should be made to implement national palliative care programs. In our opinion, euthanasia might also be considered a failure of palliative care, being requested most of the time because the dying patient (and his or her family) is not benefiting from proper physical and psychological support. The debate about euthanasia should be continued with the understanding that proper palliative care might significantly change its terms.

FURTHER READING

Aaronson NK, Ahmedzai S, Bergman B et al. (1993) The European Organization for the Research and Treatment of Cancer: A quality of life instrument for use in international clinical trials in oncology. *J Natl Cancer Inst* 85:365–376.

Batel-Copel LM, Kornblith AB, Batel PC, Holland JC (1997) Do oncologists have an increasing interest in the quality of life of their patients? A literature review of the last 15 years. *Eur J Cancer* 33:29–32.

Berger AM, Portenoy RK, Weissman DE (1998) *Principles and Practice of Supportive Oncology.* Lippincott-Raven, Philadelphia.

Cella DF, Tulsky DS, Gray G et al. (1993) The Functional Assessment of Cancer Therapy (FACT) Scale: Development and validation of the general version. *J Clin Oncol* 11:570–579.

Holland J (ed) (1998) *Psycho-Oncology.* Oxford University Press.

Meuser T, Pietruck C, Radbruch L, Stute P, Lehmann KA, Grond S (2001) Symptoms during cancer pain treatment following WHO guidelines: a longitudinal follow-up study of symptom prevalence, severity and etiology. *Pain* 93:247–257.

Padilla GV, Presant C, Grant MM, Metter G, Lipsett J, Heide F (1983) Quality of life index for patients with cancer. *Res Nurs Health* 3:117–126.

Schipper H, Clinch J, McMurray A et al. (1984) Measuring the quality of life of cancer patients: The Functional Living-Index Cancer: development and validation. *J Clin Oncol* 2:472–483.

Vainio A, Auvinen A (1996) Prevalence of symptoms among patients with advanced cancer: An international collaborative study. *J Pain Symptom Manage* 12:3–10.

Ventafridda V, Tamburini M, Caraceni A, De Conno F, Naldi F (1987) A validation study of the WHO method for cancer pain relief. *Cancer* 59:850–856.

Weiss SC, Emanuel LL, Fairclough DL, Emanuel EJ (2001) Understanding the experience of pain in terminally ill patients. *Lancet* 357:1311–1315.

WHO QOL Group (1993) Study protocol for the World Health Organization project to develop a quality of life assessment instrument. *Qual Life Res* 2:143–159.

World Health Organization (1990) *Cancer Pain Relief and Palliative Care.* Technical Report Series, No. 804, WHO, Geneva. p. 16.

World Health Organization (1997) Annual Report 1996. WHO, Geneva.

Waller A, Caroline NL (1996) *Handbook of Palliative Care in Cancer.* Butterworth-Heinemann, Boston.

Zech DFL, Grond S, Lynch J et al. (1995) Validation of WHO guidelines for cancer pain relief: a 10 year prospective study. *Pain* 68:65–76.

CHAPTER 39

Cancer in the Elderly

RICCARDO A. AUDISIO

Whiston Hospital, Prescot, Merseyside, United Kingdom

LAZZARO REPETTO

Oncology Unit, Istituto Nazionale di Riposo e Cura per Anziani, Rome, Italy

VITTORINA ZAGONEL

Department of Oncology and Oncology Unit, Fatebenefratelli Hospital, Rome, Italy

There is a steady increase in the number of elderly subjects suffering from cancer; this is an emerging problem for industrialized countries (1).

There are three reasons for this progressive increase:

1. Median age is rising, and the number of cardiovascular conditions is decreasing for the elderly
2. The risk of cancer increases proportionally with age
3. Anticancer treatments are more effective, thus rendering cancer a "chronic" disease

The elderly subject with a malignant condition requires a holistic approach; we should reject the attitude of dealing with only the malignant condition (2). A modern approach to the oncogeriatric subject is aimed to improve his or her global well being by means of the integration of active and supportive treatments (Fig. 39.1) (3). The nursing team also plays a major role. Peculiar aspects should be considered, too, such as a different natural history and cancer behavior, which affect our decision-making process (4).

Oncologists are looking for adequate and more specific answers for these patients, whom we know little about, apart from the fact that they are dramatically increasing in number (5).

UICC Manual of Clinical Oncology, Eighth Edition. Edited by Raphael E. Pollock
ISBN 0-471-22289-5 Copyright © 2004 John Wiley & Sons, Inc.

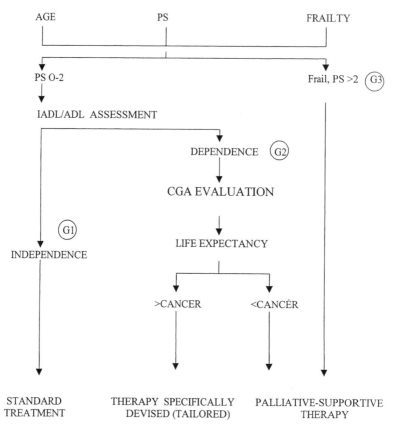

Figure 39.1   Algorithm for the management of cancer in patients 70 years of age or older.

EPIDEMIOLOGY

Median life expectancy within all industrialized countries has dramatically increased in recent years. Average life expectancy was 40 years at the end of the 19th century; presently, life expectancy has doubled (81 years expected survival for females in Italy, and 76 years for males). Life expectancy averages 24 years for a 60-year-old subject, and 6 years for the 80-year-old one (5).

In 1990, those 65 and older composed 15% of the whole population; they presently account for the 21%, and they are expected to represent 40% of the population by the year 2035 (6).

The risk of developing cancer increases proportionally with age. According to the EUCAN (Cancer Incidence, Mortality and Prevalence in the European Union) 90 data, approximately 58% of cancers, and 69% of cancer deaths, affect subjects aged 65 years or more. When all tumors are taken into account, the ratio between cancer incidence in those older than 65 versus those 55–64 years, is 2.9 for males and 2.2 for females (the risk of developing cancer among persons older than 65 is 2.9-fold for males and 2.2 for females, in comparison with persons 55–64 years old) (6).

According to the SEER (Surveillance, Epidemiology, and End Results) data the prevalence of cancer is 207.4 cases per 100,000 in those younger than 65 years old, and 2,163.9 per 100,000 in those older than 65 year old. Mortality is 68.8 and 1,076.2 per 100,000 subjects, respectively. This means that cancer prevalence and mortality are 10 and 15 times higher in the >65-year-old subjects, respectively (5).

The International Agency for Research on Cancer (IARC) data show how the most prevalent cancers for the European elderly subjects are the same as the younger patients, though a change in their order of prevalence is noticeable: prostate, lung, and colorectal cancers most frequently affect the male population, followed by bladder and gastric tumors, kidney, head and neck, pancreas, liver, and so on (6). Females are most frequently affected by breast cancer, colorectal, lung, and gastric tumors. The ITACARE data (7) demonstrate a progressive increase for the age group 75–84 years old, in keeping with the European data; a slight reduction in prevalence is recorded for both genders after 84 years of age. The incidence data collected by the 11 cancer registries in Italy, for the period 1976–1992, show that the prevalence is six times higher in the elderly (8).

Using data from Italy's National Health System, records from 7 million inhabitants were analyzed: 44,000 subjects >65 years old had a diagnosis of malignancy over the last 5 years, and 13,300 within the last year (7). It was also shown that the elderly have a worse 1- and 5-year survival for all cancer types, the difference being more obvious at 1 year. The delay in diagnosis may play a relevant role in the older patients, when the stage at diagnosis is the most robust prognostic factor for all cancer types (7).

Elderly males show a similar 5-year survival, after an initial disadvantage (in the 1-year survival), possibly related to a higher mortality for those patients presenting with more advanced disease. The minimal variability of mortality rates for lung cancers is balanced by the extremely unfavorable prognosis, no matter the patient's age, and the more favorable biological behavior in the elderly (9). The SEER data support the European data, showing a significant inverse relation between stage and age, with less aggressive histotypes being detected in the elderly (10).

The picture is even worse for female patients, particularly with gynecological cancers. The relative risk of death averages between 1.94 and 2.01 at 1 year, and 1.43–1.76 at 5 years, when compared with the younger group. Again, late diagnosis plays a pivotal role; this highlights the lack of screening programs for the elderly, in addition to restrictions to surgical treatment. When breast cancer is taken into account, female patients show a 1.7 increase in the relative risk, although the 5-year prognosis is similar to the younger age group (RR = 1.09) (8).

Both genders show a worse prognosis for urinary tract cancers, particularly bladder cancers, and non-Hodgkin's lymphomas (NHL).

The good news is that a progressive increase in survival has been shown: when the 1978–1981, 1982–1985, 1986–1989 periods were analyzed, an increased survival was shown for males (from 22% to 30%) as well as females (from 34% to 42%), a possible consequence of a improved diagnosis and treatment over recent years (8).

ASSESSING HEALTH STATUS IN THE ELDERLY

Comprehensive Geriatric Assessment

Functional status, depression, cognitive impairment, nutritional status, and insufficient social support have all been demonstrated to affect the survival of elderly cancer patients, with relative risks of death often increased two to four times (11). The most effective evaluation of the clinical importance of functional limitations and disability is provided by the Comprehensive Geriatric Assessment (CGA). Broad agreement exists on the areas that should be tested in a CGA (Table 39.1), though the format of CGA is not standardized (12). CGA is based on a series of validated scales such as Katz's Activities of Daily Living (ADL) (13) and Lawton's Instrumental Activities of Daily Living (IADL) (14), which assess functional status; the geriatric depression scale (GDS) (15), which assesses mental status; the folstein Mini Mental Status (MMS) for cognitive status (16), and nutritional assessment. CGA is routinely employed in geriatric clinics and nursing homes, and is now being increasingly used by oncologists. In patients treated for neoplasia, the ability to the cancer center, to reach the responsible physician or nurse by phone in case of complications, and to take the prescribed drugs at home is very important and correlates with adherence to treatment plan. In 1996, a CGA scale was developed and validated by Monfardini et al. (17) for the first time in an oncology setting. From 1995 to 1996, the Italian Group of Geriatric Oncology (GIOGer) has prospectively assessed the efficacy of this instrument in a large multi-institutional series of elderly cancer patients and elderly noncancer subjects (18). Six hundred and fifty-five subjects aged 65 or older were prospectively evaluated: 363 neoplastic

TABLE 39.1. Areas of Assessment and Related Instruments for the Comprehensive Geriatric Assessment

Domain	Instrument
Demographic	Age, sex
Health	Number of co-morbid conditions (Satariano's index)
	Co-morbidity indices: Charlson's, CIRS-G
Function	Performance status,
	Activities of daily living (ADL): eating, dressing, continence, grooming, transferring, going to the bathroom
	Instrumental activities of daily living (IADL): use of transportation, shopping, management of money and medications, ability to provide own meals, to perform laundry, house management, and use of telephone
Cognition	Folstein Mini Mental Status (MMS)
Emotions	Geriatric Depression Scale (GDS)
Nutrition	Serum albumin, triceps skinfold, transferrin
Social and economic	Living conditions, effective caregiver, income, marital adjustment, access to transportation

CIRS-G, Cumulative Illness Rating Scale–Geriatric.

patients and 292 noncancer patients as controls. Of the 269 cancer patients with a good performance status (PS) (i.e., lower than 2), 37.7% had IADL and 9.3% ADL limitations, 13% presented with two or more co-morbid conditions, and approximately 30% of patients had limitations in their mental or emotional status (18). CGA, as proposed by GIOGer, adequately collects homogeneous information on functional and emotional status and disability, thus allowing the recognition of persons at higher risk for treatment-related complications in a group of patients not discriminated by PS (18). Controversy remains about whether cancer is an independent determinant of the functional status among older patients, and very little is known about the interrelation between cancer and other co-morbid conditions. The evaluation of physical function provides critical information in the decision-making process because it may help estimating tolerance to treatments. In general, a low IADL index (i.e., high degree of physical impairment) identifies a patient with high risk of developing complications from antineoplastic treatment (19–21).

Another experience underway at the Lee Moffit Cancer Center in Tampa, Florida, showed that elderly patients with breast and colon cancer who had CGA showed a better prognosis expressed in terms of progression-free survival than non-CGA patients. Likewise, CGA contributed to the preservation of functional status in elderly cancer patients (20).

Assessment for Co-morbidity

A reliable assessment of co-morbidity is also essential in elderly cancer patients to establish the benefits and risks of specific antineoplastic agents and to grossly estimate survival. The prognostic impact of associated diseases may be different according to their severity (e.g., diabetes). A few validated scales exist for assessing co-morbidity in older cancer patients (20). The Cumulative Illness Rating Scale–Geriatric (CIRS-G) (22), was compared with the Charlson co-morbidity scale (23) in 203 patients who received a CGA in a Lee Moffit Cancer Center evaluation program (SAOP) (20). This study demonstrated that co-morbidity and functional status are poorly correlated in older cancer patients. Whether co-morbidity was defined in a restrictive way (Charlson), or a comprehensive way (CIRS-G), it displayed no correlation with ADL, IADL, and ECOG PS. In the GIOGer study, three or more co-morbid conditions, as measured by the Satariano's index (24), were present in 43.7% of noncancer patients and 31.8% of cancer patients (18). Several groups have shown that the survival of patients with tumors such as breast, colon, prostate, and head and neck cancers is significantly modified by co-morbidity (11). Satariano showed a significant correlation between the number of selected co-morbid conditions and the risk of death due to noncancer-related conditions, whereas the risk of cancer-related death was the same regardless of co-morbidity (24). Yancik et al. (25) evaluated co-morbidity and age in 1,610 patients, 55 years and older, with colon carcinoma as predictors of early mortality and concluded that co-morbidity affects survival. In this study, 28% of patients had died within 2 years of diagnosis and about 30% of patients died from noncancer-related causes. More than 50% of the total deaths occurred in stage IV (25). For these reasons, co-morbidity should be distinguished from functional status and needs to be measured separately in elderly cancer patients (26).

Correlation Between PS and CGA

The ECOG or Karnofsky scales of PS have been shown to be effective predictors of outcome in several oncologic studies. However, their application to patients over 70 years of age has limited utility and may underrepresent the degree of functional impairment (18,27). The GIOGer study suggests that among elderly cancer patients many aspects of physical limitations are not totally recognized by PS, in particular those aspects collected through IADL, and that may affect adherence to diagnostic and therapeutic protocols. Similar results are reported by Exterman (20): ECOG PS, ADL, and IADL, are moderately correlated with a slight advantage for IADL. Though a correlation exists among co-morbidity, PS, ADL and IADL, this correlation is not strong enough to be reflected in a single parameter. Therefore, each of these areas should be independently explored. The evaluation of the global health of elderly patients affected by cancer may assist oncologists in making the most appropriate therapeutic decision for each patient, and may became of the utmost importance in clinical practice (Fig. 39.1).

Which Patients Benefit from CGA?

Figure 39.1 summarizes the clinical application of CGA in oncological patients. The frail elderly, as defined by Winograd et al. (28) presents conditions that prevent independent living and are associated with reduced life expectancy. The average life expectancy of the frail person, even in the absence of cancer, is limited but not negligible, being longer than 2 years. Though frail persons may die with cancer rather than of cancer, they are likely to experience severe cancer-related symptoms causing deterioration of quality of life (29). Therefore, even the condition of frailty may not prevent effective cancer treatment. Indeed, the clinical management of frail patients has to be evaluated on an individual basis considering all the information obtained with CGA. To optimize the definition of the frail elderly is one of the major goals of both oncological and geriatric research.

The systematic introduction of CGA into both clinical research and practice in oncology settings can contribute to a common language and may help the management of older cancer patients in at least three important areas: assessment of life expectancy of the patient, identification of frail persons, and prediction of antineoplastic treatment tolerance. Further investigations might help to achieve a wider consensus on the CGA with the aim of optimizing and standardizing the appraisal of co-morbidity and disability in elderly cancer patients.

From a practical point of view, CGA allows us to distinguished three groups of patients:

Group 1: healthy elderly: PS 0–2, age ≥75 years, IADL and ADL independent with no severe co-morbidity. These patients are candidates for standard cancer treatments, with the only exception of bone marrow transplantation.

TABLE 39.2. Criteria of Fraility*

Age more than 85 years
Dependence in one or more ADLs
Presence of three or more co-morbid conditions
Presence of one or more geriatric syndromes (dementia, delirium, depression, incontinence,
  falls, osteoporosis, neglect and abuse, failure to thrive)
Psychological problems

*According to Winograd (28).
ADLs, Activities of daily living.

They might require more intensive supportive therapies, in order to minimize treatment-related toxicities (e.g., growth factors administered as a prophylactic intent, rather than with therapeutic finality) (all conditions present).

Group 2: not eligible for categories 1 and 3.

Group 3: frail subjects: IADL and/or ADL dependent; two or more co-morbidities; one or more geriatric syndrome (at least one condition). They are candidates to receive supportive-palliative treatments, including anticancer treatment, with the aim of improving or maintaining quality of life (Table 39.2) (30,31).

BIOLOGICAL FEATURES OF CANCER IN THE ELDERLY

Just as aging in the general population alters the demographics of cancer, aging in the individual patient alters the biology of cancer. These biological changes affect the risk of cancer, tumor activity, and the response to treatment (32). There is no general rule, and age plays a different role according to each specific cancer type (32). For several tumors, most notably breast, prostate, and lung cancer, there is good evidence that the tumors may be different. A difference in the growth pattern and doubling time, hormonal receptor status, DNA ploidy, angiogenesis, percentage of cells in S-phase, p53 expression, and extracellular matrix proteins expression, has been noticed and confirmed (33). Senescent tissues in general may also provide a microenvironment less capable of supporting rapid tumor growth. Thus, histologically identical tumors in older patients are likely to be different than those in younger patients. In fact, Age has different implications in different tumor sites. The astute oncologist soon learns that the age of the cancer patient at diagnosis may have everything or very little (or somewhere in between) to do with the biology of the cancer.

TARGETING TREATMENT

The decision-making process on how best to treat the elderly cancer patient is quite complex; it requires a careful evaluation of the different variables that might affect the final result (Table 39.3).

TABLE 39.3. Decision Making in Elderly Cancer Treatment

First step	Patient	Age
		PS, ADL/IADL
		CGA
Second step	Cancer	Biologic characteristic
		Stage
		Symptoms
		Therapeutic options
Third step	Target	Life expectancy
		Quality of life
Fourth step	Final decision	Treatment (standard, tailored)
		Palliative supportive therapies

PS, performance status; ADL, activities of daily living; IADL, instrumental activities of daily living; CGA, Comprehensive Geriatric Assessment.

We should ask ourselves: Will the patient die of cancer, or with cancer? Will he or she tolerate cancer treatment? To what extent will the treatment impact on his or her quality of life? Life expectancy for most of these patients is frequently longer than cancer-related survival; thus, the options of any cancer treatment should be considered with the aim of improving the quality of life and life expectancy. Unfortunately, real life is quite different: a redundancy of data is to prove the minimal accrual of elderly subjects into cancer trials, both in Europe (34,35) and in North America (36). This results in a dramatic lack of knowledge concerning the feasibility of treatment protocols for elderly patients.

A recent report from the meeting of the American Society of Clinical Oncology (ASCO) (GALGB study) investigated the impact of patient age on entering clinical trials. Patients and physicians were asked the reasons for entering (or not entering) into clinical investigations. Fifty percent of adult women surveyed were asked to take part to the trial, whereas only 35% of the elderly ones were invited ($p = 0.06$). Interestingly, they were not entered because of the physician's choice, on the assumption that the elderly subjects were not sufficiently reliable; co-morbidities and patient's refusal were never the issue (36).

The Southwest Oncology Group retrospectively analyzed 16,396 subjects entered between 1993 and 1996 in 164 trials according to sex, race, and age under or over 65 years (37). These rates were compared with the corresponding rates in the general population of patients with cancer. The overall proportion of women <65 years was similar to the estimated proportion in the U.S. population of patients with cancer. In contrast, patients 65 years age or older were significantly underrepresented. The underrepresentation was particularly notable in trials of treatment for breast cancer (9% vs. 49%, $p < 0.001$). The authors suggested the adoption of policy measures to promote the accrual of elderly subjects into clinical trials (37).

A global and harmonized approach to the elderly with cancer requires the geriatrician, family doctor, oncologist, and health workers to work together, integrating care according to the specific clinical problem, as related to cancer progression (Fig. 39.2) (37).

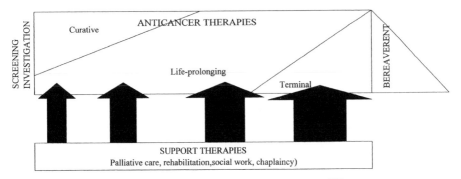

Figure 39.2 Model of cancer management (37).

All specialists involved (surgeon, medical oncologist, and radiotherapist) are invited to plan the most appropriate treatment. The patient, together with his or her family, should be involved in the decision-making process. The patients socio economic situation, and the presence or lack of effective caregiver should also be taken into account (37).

SUPPORTIVE TREATMENT

There is evidence that the elderly with cancer have a shorter survival, receive inadequate treatment, and manifest a greater incidence and severity of toxic effect from chemotherapy. Thus, we might ask ourselves if they are being offered the most appropriate supportive treatment.

Aging is associated with a progressive decline in the functional reserve of multiple organ systems, which may lead to enhanced susceptibility to stress such as that caused by cancer chemotherapy. Myelodepression is the most common and most commonly fatal complication of antineoplastic drug therapy, and may represent a serious hindrance to the management of cancer in older individuals (31,38). Supportive care should differ between adults and elderly receiving the same treatment. Nutritional status plays a pivotal role. The reasons for the frequent malnourishment in these subjects is not clear, although we suspect they can be partially due to the malignancy, to the patient himself, and to the cancer treatment. The caloric intake should be distributed in at least five or six meals per day, and 2 liters of water are required to avoid weight loss.

Anemia is the second most important factor affecting treatment and prognosis of cancer patients (39). Anemia may also be associated in older patients with a number of other complications that may precipitate functional dependence, including fatigue. It often has a multifactorial etiology, as recent studies show that fatigue is the symptom most frequently affecting quality of life, after pain. Hemoglobin levels progressively decrease during chemotherapy's courses. Suboptimal hemoglobin levels may affect the outcomes of treatment for some tumor types (40), and tissue hypoxia, secondary to anemia, may select a radioresistant cellular cancer phenotype (40,41). The management of chemotherapy-related anemia with erythropoietin improves energy levels and quality of life when hemoglobin is maintained at 12 g/dL. In the elderly, the most frequent type of anemia is a consequence of folate and–or vitamin B_{12} deficiencies, and is macrocytic and myelodisplasia related. Thus, erythropoietin should be supported by folic acid and vitamin B_{12} administration, rather than iron administration (31).

Hematopoietic growth factors, such as granulocyte colony-stimulating factor (G-CSF) are recommended in a prophylactic setting during standard chemotherapy such as CHOP or CMF (31,38,42–44). Different reports in NHL patients suggest that the prophylactic use of G-CSF in older patients may turn out to be of actual clinical value by inducing a significant reduction in the number of chemotherapy courses delayed due to neutropenia. In addition, patients receiving the first chemotherapy course without G-CSF displayed not only a longer and more marked neutropenia following chemotherapy, as expected, but also a reduced neutrophylic response when G-CSF was administered in subsequent courses (31). Whatever the underlying biologic mechanisms, this study suggests that in patients 70 years old or more, G-CSF should be given from the very beginning of chemotherapy, instead of being reserved for hematological toxicity. This treatment also may prevent costly complications, such as neutropenic infections and functional dependence, and, thus, both medical and economic considerations suggest the use of growth factors in older individuals treated with standard chemotherapy, in a prophylactic setting (38,45).

The recent availability of the broad-spectrum cytoprotective agent amifostine has provided the dreamed of opportunity to use a single drug that appears theoretically able to protect normal tissues from most of the toxicities elicited by different classes of anticancer agents (46). ASCO warmly recommends amifostine in preventing platinum-induced nephrotoxcicity and mucosytis in head and neck cancer patients treated with radiation therapy (47). Amifostine can also successfully accelerate the hemopoietic recovery as a consequence of a prolonged survival, and overall increase in hemopoietic progenitor cells, which also takes place in the aged subjects (31). When the >70 year old subjects are compared with the younger age group, the adminstration of amifostine in combination with chemotherapy was associated with an acceptable toxicity profile in patients over 70 years of age (48). Owing to the capacity of amifostine to provide multiorgan protection, this drug appears promising in the prevention of chemotherapy side effects in older patients. Prospective controlled clinical trials of amifostine plus chemotherapy in the elderly are lacking and should be rapidly designed to evaluate the actual impact of the cytoprotection strategy in such patients' subsetting. A large number of compounds are available to minimise chemo- and radioinduced toxicity; this will require specifically tailored prospective studies in the elderly (31).

SPECIFIC CANCER TREATMENT

Breast Cancer

Surgical treatment should not differ significantly with respect to patient's age, provided no major contraindication for a general anesthesia is evident (49). A large number of clinical investigations has conclusively shown how "optimal surgery," namely the radical removal of breast cancer in free margins, achieves control and cure in up to 80% cases (50). Breast-preserving surgery should be considered, as the interest in conservative management is constantly increasing.

Patients with no evidence of lymph node involvement on clinical assessment might take advantage of radiotherapy to the axilla, and their survival can be improved up to 84% (51). It must also be said that surgical oncologists, as well as most general surgeons, have recently been familiarized with the axillary dissection, so that level I and II clearance should be considered as a first option, in order to avoid the side effects of radiotherapy. Patients with no clinical evidence of axillary lymph node involvement and tumors <2 cm might avoid axillary dissection, and even the use of radiotherapy might be reserved to selected patients. The recently introduced sentinel lymph node technique is another option to avoid undue axillary dissection and reduce surgery-related morbidity.

Hormonal treatment is presently accepted as the first-line therapy for estrogen receptor–positive patients, both as an adjuvant and for stage IV conditions. The same indications as for adult postmenopausal patients should be considered. It might be appropriate to associate cardioaspirin with tamoxifen to avoid the vascular side effects in patients older than 70 years. Ongoing randomized trials comparing aromatase inhibitors, pure antiestrogens, and tamoxifen as an adjuvant might provide evidence that the former treatment is more appropriate in the older age subgroup due to a similar efficacy and lower toxicity.

Chemotherapy is suggested for estrogen receptor–negative and metastatic (or locally advanced) disease. CMF is so far the most popular cocktail, although this choice should be reassessed on the basis of the most recent results. Both CMF efficacy and tolerability were reduced in patients older than 65 years, according to the International Breast Cancer Study Group Trial VII (52), where the elderly have shown 17% grade III toxicity hematological and mucosal toxicities and all severe toxicities were significantly worse in the >65 years group compared with 7% in the younger group. The amount of drug effectively delivered was also reduced in the elderly, where 5-year survival is 63% for the CMF plus tamoxifen group versus 61% for tamoxifen only. No significant advantage was detected when adding chemotherapy to hormonal treatment in the elderly. Gelman and Taylor (53) proposed a methotrexate and 5-fluorouracil dose adjustment, aimed to better tolerate this multidrug treatment. Several different associations appear to be more reliable, effective, and handy. A recent ICCG (International Collaborative Cancer Group) study has shown the relapse rate was reduced by 27% when epiribicine was added to tamoxifen in postmenopausal node-positive women (54). Toxicity was significantly increased in the group receiving the treatment, although no long-term cardiac toxicity was detected.

Ibrahim et al. (55) examined 1,011 breast cancer patients treated with anthra-cyclines: the comparison between the two age groups (50–63 vs. ≥64 years) identified a higher response rate for the younger age group; similar toxicity, as well as overall and disease-free survivals were recorded. Taxanes have also been given on a 3-week schedule in association with G-CSF (56): weekly schedules have shown promising results in the elderly with regard to tolerability and efficacy.

In conclusion, chemotherapy is feasible and advisable in the advanced elderly breast cancer patient, even if a reduced efficacy was shown.

Colorectal Cancer

Recent investigations show that, after the age of 85, colorectal cancer accounts for 30% of all cancers (57). Although radical surgery remains the most effective treatment for colorectal malignancies, fewer elderly patients actually receive major surgery than their younger counterparts (58). This can be related to outdated reports on poorer outcomes and higher operative risk. Recent advances in anesthetics and surgery have led to the view that surgery can and should be considered as a first option. Surgical management of the elderly under elective conditions has been shown to expose the patient to a similar risk as for the younger patients; it was also shown to be cost effective (59). Given the present life expectancy of the 70–75-year-old patient, adjuvant chemotherapy should be considered for Dukes' C stages. The disease-specific survival of elderly patients who have had no postoperative chemotherapy was not significantly different from that of younger subjects similarly treated (60). A recent meta-analysis of 1,365 subjects with advanced disease, who were entered into 13 randomized studies (5-FU based protocols vs. supportive treatment), has pointed out a 35% decrease in the risk of death, with a 3.7-month increase in median survival, for those who had chemotherapy (61). 5-FU is still the most popular treatment, both as an adjuvant and for advanced disease. The elderly patient shows a reduced tolerance to 5-FU (62,63); a dose reduction is sometimes advisable, particularly when creatinine clearance is reduced. Mucositis (small bowel and oral cavity) should be carefully looked for; most frequently, it can be avoided by means of prophylactic medications. Sargent et al. (64) conducted a meta-analysis of 3,351 subjects entered into 5-FU plus folic acid/levamisole adjuvant treatment protocols (Dukes' stages B2 and C); an increased 5-year survival was noticed for the >70-year-old subjects who received adjuvant treatment in comparison with controls (71% vs. 64%). The incidence of toxicity except for neutropenia was not increased in patients older than 70 in comparison with younger patients (64).

Continuous 5-FU infusion is advisable (after de Gramont), because it is better tolerated than bolus. Where no disability is detected (IADL), and no serious comorbidity is present, the new and recently introduced cocktails for the treatment of metastatic disease (5-FU plus irinotecan or oxaliplatin) can be utilized as an adjuvant as well as for advanced disease. There is not conclusive data as yet regarding tolerability and efficacy with respect to any of these combinations.

Lung Cancer

More than 50% of all lung cancer cases are diagnosed in patients aged 65 years or above, and more than 30% occur in those older than 70 (10). However, conventional surgical risk increases over age 65. As a result, surgical procedures for lung cancer are far less frequent in elderly patients. Many clinicians avoid surgery, or minimize surgical procedures on the basis of chronological age. Recent advances in preoperative risk assessment, as well as surgical and anesthetic techniques, have resulted in a significant decrease in operative mortality and morbidity for the elderly population. The treatment of lung cancer in elderly patients should no longer be based upon previous bias. Every effort should be made to assess risk and optimize treatment for this large and expanding portion of the population. A joint surgical and anesthesiological assessment is advisable where the disease is likely to be localized (49). A surgical approach can be considered, regardless of the chronological age of the patient, when alveolar ventilation is able to provide carbon dioxide elimination and oxygen exchange is well maintained at rest and in exercise situations (65). Selection of surgical candidates by these new concepts may explain the recent decline in expected operative mortality following lung resection in patients older than 70 years, falling from a range of 5–20% in the period from 1970 to 1980, to as low as 3–6% in more recent reports (66–68). Video-assisted thoracic surgery (VATS) had a notable impact on the elderly population; however, the technique is not yet well established and there are some documented differences between studies (68). Therefore, these results must be confirmed in studies with larger samples of elderly patients with lung cancer, because they represent the subset group of patients most likely to benefit from this approach. Pneumonectomy represents a feasible surgical option for elderly patients, though careful selection is mandatory.

Limited resections appear to be promising for elderly lung cancer patients because of the higher prevalence of stage I disease and the potential reduction in postoperative complications. At least for the first postoperative years, limited resections do not carry an increased risk of recurrence or death, thus potentially benefiting elderly patients with lower life expectancy than the younger population. Although there is not enough data to suggest the use of limited resections in every patient with early lung cancer, these procedures are reasonable alternatives for the elderly with high operative risk, cardiopulmonary impairment, and other co-morbid diseases.

Radiotherapy has an important role for locally advanced, inoperable disease. Both palliative and curative radiotherapy has shown good compliance among subjects aged >80 years, who could successfully complete their treatment in 80% cases (69–71).

Chemotherapy is indicated in symptomatic patients with advanced disease. Platinum-based combinations are generally avoided in older than subjects 70 years old (72,73). Rosvold et al. (74) has recently shown a reduced efficacy for platinum and taxol in the elderly. They recorded 32% objective responses versus 50% in the younger group, whereas toxicity and survival were similar. Vinorelbine and gemcitabine are frequently employed in single-agent treatment. Two retrospective investigations of gemcitabine have shown similar efficacy, tolerability, and survival as for the younger patients; an even better response rate was noticed for stage IV elderly patients (37% vs. 13%) (74–76).

Vinorelbine treatment can achieve 12–39% objective responses, with a median survival of 21–40 months (73). Gridelli lead a comparative study (ELVIS), showing how vinorelbine can improve quality of life (as measured with the EORTC C30 and LC13 questionnaire). Also, treated patients had a better survival than best supportive care (28 vs. 21 weeks, $p = 0.04$) (77). A recent meta-analysis showed a similar survival advantage to what could be achieved in adult subjects receiving platinum-based schedules (78). A randomized clinical study for stages IIIB–IV non–small-cell lung cancer NSCLC, comparing vinorelbine versus gemcitabine versus vinorelbine plus gemcitabine, developed after the ELVIS study, have now been completed. The preliminary results of MILES (Multicenter Italian Lung Cancer in the Elderly Study) study showed no survival advantage of the combination arm in comparison with single agent (79). Thus, single-agent treatments represent the standard regimen, further investigations are needed to establish if selected group of patients may benefit from combination treatment and the single agent of choice. The weekly administration of taxanes as a single agent has shown a good tolerability and efficacy for the >65-year-old patients (80). More clinical data is required to draw final conclusion.

Prostate Cancer

For organ-confined prostate cancers, treatment options include observation, radical prostatectomy, external beam or interstitial radiation, and cryoablation. The appropriate therapeutic decision is based on analysis of multiple factors, namely grade, stage, and CGA.

Radical prostatectomy produces acceptable results in T3 patients with well/moderately differentiated tumors, whereas patients with T3G3 (poorly differentiated) cancers have early progression and need adjuvant treatment (81). Radical prostatectomy with androgen ablation therapy is a viable option for patients with stage III disease, in view of the excellent local control and low mortality.

Complication rates of external beam radiation therapy, interstitial radiotherapy, and radical prostatectomy have decreased during the last decades (82). Cryosurgery has widely been practiced in the aging subjects. Patient-reported complications compared favorably to those for radical prostatectomy and external beam irradiation; patient satisfaction can be up to 96% (83). The introduction of prostate-specific antigen (PSA) has revolutionized the epidemiology, diagnosis, treatment, and follow-up of prostate cancer. Early stages are increasingly been detected, whereas rectal examination and/or transanal ultrasound, associated with PSA 1- or 2-year monitoring has been recommended (84). Rietbergen et al. (85) studied 20,632 volunteers aged 55–76 years, and 2,262 subjects alternatively receiving PSA or rectal examination and/or ultrasound had a prostatic biopsy. A total of 474 prostate cancers were detected, of which 78% had localized disease. Another recent study analyzed all causes of death for subjects suffering from prostate cancer, revealing how cancer-related mortality decreases with the age of the patient; besides, the neoplasm does not modify age-related life expectancy for early stages (86).

Recently, the American Urological Association reviewed 12,501 publications from 1955 to 1992 to shed light on radiotherapy- and surgery-related complications. Median age at diagnosis was shown to be significantly increased, whereas prevalence of morbidities decreased (87). Postoperative radiotherapy for patients with positive margins and/or high PSA postoperative levels improved disease control (73). The therapeutic plan for localized disease is based on Gleason score (G), where 15-year survival for subjects with G <5 not receiving further treatment averages 7%. To the opposite, mortality progressively increases with G (G5: 6–11%, G6: 18–30%, G7: 42–70%, G8–G10: 60–87%). Further treatment is thus advisable for these subsettings (88). Newschaffer et al. (89) analyzed all causes of death in two cohorts of elderly subjects, affected or not affected by prostate malignancy. It was shown how an aggressive treatment policy increased non-cancer-related death to 51%; conversely, a "watchful waiting" decreases it by 34%. Thus, there is extensive evidence showing how the treatment plan should be based on the tumor extension, delivering aggressive treatment to those subjects with advanced disease. A recent meta-analysis evaluated 27 randomized studies comparing androgenic suppression plus and minus antiandrogens (90). A total of 8,275 patients were entered into this investigation, and no 5-year survival advantage was shown in favor of this combination. Chemotherapy has shown some advantage in pain control, quality of life, and time to progression in two randomized trials comparing methotrexate versus steroids (91,92). The combination of vinblastine and estramustine was shown to achieve better biochemical response rates (PSA), and time to progression, when compared with estramustine alone. A nonsignificant advantage in survival was also noticed (93). Thus, objective response and symptom palliation can be obtained, while chemotherapy regimens for metastatic disease should be considered. Several ongoing studies will assess the effectiveness of chemotherapy for localized disease with an high recurrence risk (G >8, positive margins, extracapsular invasion, or positive pelvic lymph-nodes). The role of radiotherapy should not be dismissed for pain control and bone metastasis.

Hematologic Malignancies

Specifically designed studies for the elderly have been developed over the last few years, on the basis of the increased chemosensitivity and potential curability of some hematologic malignancies, besides the high prevalence of these conditions in the last decades of life. Unfortunately, the therapeutic results are still dismal (94).

Age represents one of the most important adverse prognostic factors in acute myeloid leukemia (AML). As opposed to the consistent progress achieved over the last two decades in the treatment of AML in younger adults, the prognosis of AML arising in individuals older than 60 years remains poor, and the current therapeutic results for patients accrued into clinical trials of intensive chemotherapy are largely unsatisfactory (complete remission rates rarely superior to 50–60%; median relapse-free survival usually less than 12 months). Because only 30–40% of elderly patients are actually entered into intensive chemotherapy trials, the overall failure of current treatment strategies appears even more disappointing when considered in the context of the whole population of older individuals with AML (95). The poor clinical outcome of AML in the elderly appears primarily due to intrinsic differences in the biology of leukemia itself, but also to host factors (i.e., the reduced tolerance to intensive chemotherapy) and co-morbid conditions linked to the chronological age of patients. AMLs arising in older subjects display significant biological overlaps with secondary AMLs (drug- or myelodysplasia-related), as indicated by a high frequency of multilineage clonal involvement, immature phenotype of leukemic cells, presence of unfavorable cytogenetic abnormalities, high levels of expression, and elevated functional activity of multidrug resistance genes. Despite the considerable efforts to improve clinical results by adopting a variety of different therapeutic approaches, new drugs, and hemopoietic growth factors, the optimal treatment of AML in the elderly remains highly controversial as to both induction and postremission strategies. The emerging role of biologically based prognostic factors may now help to select among the heterogeneous population of elderly AML patients those who may actually benefit from aggressive chemotherapy, probably including stem cell transplantation procedures, from those who should be offered attenuated/palliative treatments or enrolled in trials testing completely new biologic and immunologic strategies. Hopefully, the information most recently gained on the biology of the disease together with newer therapeutic developments will be of help to offer a "risk-adapted" strategy aimed at improving disease-free survival and/or quality of life for elderly AML patients with different risk profiles (95).

Non-Hodgkin's lymphoma (NHL) is the most common and most extensively studied of the age-related hematologic malignancies (96). If NHL prevalence rates remained relatively stable in patients younger than 45 years, they increased at least 100% for each 10-year age cohorts between 45 and 75 during the last 40 years, and increased by nearly 400% in patients older than 75 years. Different studies in the last years showed that older patients with aggressive NHL derive benefit from treatment comparable to that derived by younger patients, and that older patients should be treated similarly to younger patients, with the intent to cure (97–99). In fact, once complete remission was reached, the disease-free survival did not differ significantly between adult and older patients, emphasizing the importance of achieving complete remission. An increasing number of treatment regimens have been proposed and clinically assessed in older patients, in particular for a diffuse large cell lymphoma, a potentially curable disease, also, in the elderly. The standard treatment remains CHOP or CHOP-like regimens, whatever the age of the patient, provided that the subject does not present with an ADL-IADL dependence, or severe co-morbidity. In this situation, the collective evidence consistently points to the conclusion that otherwise-healthy, elderly patients can obtain the same benefits from standard chemotherapy as can younger patients.

New chemotherapy regimens, tailored for the elderly with ADL or IADL dependence or co-morbidity are required (99,100). The randomized trials in the elderly have reaffirmed the value of CHOP and emphasize the need for adequate dosing, maintaining schedules, and anthracyclines (99). The prophylactic use of G-CSF reduces the incidence, severity, and duration of chemotherapy-induced neutropenia, thereby helping maintain adequate dose intensity. The cost-effectiveness of using G-CSF as prophylaxis against neutropenia is also been demonstrated (42–45).

Early evidence that older and younger patients with NHL have comparable response to chemotherapy came about somewhat unexpectedly. Conversely, the results obtained for high-grade NHL have significantly been related to the dose intensity (24,36). Prognosis is not different for the elderly, when affected by the similar histotypes and International Prognostic Index (IPI), and similarly treated (36). Supportive treatments should be optimized, to enable these patients completing the treatment plan. quite a few age-oriented schedules have been published, as well as dose-adjusted standard treatments (CHOP, CHOP-like) (36,83,84). The former ones have been shown to be less effective than the latter (85), thus reinforcing the idea that an adequate dose intensity is required to achieve a lasting result. CHOP remains the best and key treatment, even for the aged patient (36,84–86). All means of treatment (prophylactic growth factors, cardioprotective drugs, or less toxic anthracyclines) should be undertaken when treating lymphomas, in order to improve the patient's compliance with standard treatments (23). CGA has been proven useful in orienting treatment plans in the older lymphoma patients (87). Intensified schedules for standard chemotherapy schemes are presently under investigation for patients aged 65–75 years. It has also been noticed that an adequate number of $CD34^+$ hematopoietic cells can be collected between 60 and 70 years (23,83). Prospective investigations are ongoing to better understand the feasibility of the reinfusion of $CD34^+$ cells in order to allow CHOP high dosages (86).

Follicular NHL deserves a special comment, because it is a common idea that only the symptomatic patient requires treatment (86). There is now a redundancy of effective immunological treatments, which have proven to be capable of slowing down the progression of disease at its early stages. Nevertheless, the patients' symptoms should not be underestimated, because they might be related to the disease progression (i.e., anemia, pneumonia, etc), requiring targeted intervention. An evaluation of the presently available biological treatments for hematological tumors is likely to obtain adequate response rates to the treatment of these malignancies when affecting the elderly subject.

CONCLUSION

The time bomb of the elderly patients soon representing the largest proportion of cancer subjects is no news. Increased attention to this problem has been seen over the last few years, together with the holistic aspects that it implies. Nevertheless, these efforts have not sufficiently improved the management of the elderly patient with cancer. Large funds are needed to provide them the most appropriate specific and supportive treatments, with the two-fold target: optimizing quality of life and increasing life expectancy. Forthcoming gene and biological therapies will be appropriate for this subgroup of cancer patients; there are expectations for them to largely replace conventional chemotherapy, which is only marginally beneficial to them. An integrated and targeted multidisciplinary treatment plan is nevertheless required for now, in keeping with the disease's complexity. Each different stage of the disease in each patient requires the harmonization of diversified experiences, with respect to cancer progression, patient health conditions, and quality of life.

REFERENCES

1. Silverberg E, Lubera JA (1988) Cancer statistics. *CA Cancer J Clin* 38:5–22.
2. Exterman M (1999) Assessment of the older cancer patient. *Proc Am Soc Clin Oncol*, p. 353.
3. Ahmedzai SH, Walsh D (2000) Palliative medicine and modern cancer care. *Semin Oncol* 27:1.
4. Cohen HJ (1999) Management of cancer in the older person: introduction. *Proc Am Soc Clin Oncol*, p. 339.
5. Lag R, Eisner MP, Kosary CL et al. (eds). *SEER Cancer Statistics Review* 1973–1997.
6. Cancer in the European Union 1995. Lyons, France, IARC, 1999.
7. Vercelli M, Quaglia A, Parodi S, Crosignani P (1999) Cancer prevalence in the elderly. ITAPREVAL Working Group. *Tumori* 85:391.
8. Vercelli M, Quaglia A, Casella C, Parodi S, Capocaccia R, Martinez Garcia C (1998) Relative surival in elderly cancer patients in Europe. EUROCARE Work Group. *Eur J Cancer* 34:2264.
9. Vercelli M, Quaglia A, Casella C, Mangone L (1997) The ITACARE Working Group. Cancer patient survival in the elderly in Italy. *Tumori* 83:490.
10. Havlik RJ, Yancik R, Long S et al. (1994) The National Cancer Institute on Aging and the National Cancer Institute SEER. Collaborative study on comorbidity and early diagnosis of cancer in the elderly. *Cancer* 74:2101.
11. Extermann M (1999) Assessment of the older cancer patient. In: Perry MC, ed. American Society of Clinical Oncology 1999 Educational Book, 35th Annual Meeting. Alexandria, American Society of Clinical Oncology Publications, pp. 353–360.
12. National Institutes of Health Consensus Development Conference Statement (1988) Geriatric assessment methods for clinical decision-marking. *J Am Geratr Soc* 36: 342–347.
13. Katz S, Akpom CA (1976) A measure of primary sociological function. *Int J Health Serv* 6:493–507.
14. Lawton MP, Brody EM (1969) Assessment of older people: self-mantaining and instrumental activities of daily living. *Gerontologist* 9:179–186.
15. Brink TL, Yesavage JA, Lum O, Hevesuma PH, Adey M, Rose TL (1982) Screening test for geriatric depression. *Clin Gerontol* 1:37–44.
16. Folstein MF, Folstein Se, McHugh PR (1975) Mini Mental State. A practical method for grading the cognitive state of patients for the clinicians. *J Psychiat Res* 12:189–198.
17. Monfardini S, Ferrucci L, Fratino L, Del Lungo I, Serraino D, Zagonel V (1966) Validation of a multidimensional evaluation scale for use in elderly cancer patients. *Cancer* 77: 395–401.
18. Repetto L, Fratino L, Audisio RA et al. (2002) The comprehensive geriatric assessment adds information to ECOG Performance Status in elderly cancer patients: a GIOGer Study. *J Clin Oncol* 20:494–2002.

19. Fratino L, Serraino D, Zagonel V (1998) The impact of cancer on the physical function of the elderly and their utilisation of health care. *Cancer* 83:589–590.

20. Exterman M, Overcash J, Lyman GH, Parr J, Balducci L (1998) Comorbidity and functional status are independent in older cancer patients. *J Clin Oncol* 16: 1582–1587.

21. Extermann M, Chen H, Cantom AB et al. (2000) Predictors of toxicity from chemotherapy in older patients: a prospective pilot study. *Proc Am Soc Clin Oncol* 617:2430.

22. Miller MD, Paradis CF, Houck PR et al. (1992) Rating chronic medical illness burden in geropsychiatric practice and research: application of the Comulative Illness Rating Scale. *Psychiatry Res* 41:237–248.

23. Charlson ME, Pompei P, Ales K et al. (1987) A new method of classifying prognostic comorbidity in longitudinal studies: development and validation. *J Chronic Dis* 40: 373–383.

24. Satariano WA, Ragland DR (1994) The effect of comorbidity on 3-year survival of women with primary breast cancer. *Ann Intern Med* 120:104–110.

25. Yancik R, Wesely MN, Ries L et al. (1998) Comorbidity and age as predictors of risk for early mortality of male and female colon carcinoma patients. A population-based study. *Cancer* 82:2123–2134.

26. Monfardini S, Repetto L, Fratino L et al. (2000) Less age-associated comorbidity and better performance status in cancer versus non-cancer elderly patients. *Proc Am Soc Clin Oncol* 618, 2433.

27. Fratino L, Zagonel V, Serraino D et al. (2000) Does the measurement of physical limitations add information to performance status among elderly cancer patients? *Proc Am Soc Clin Oncol* 603:2375.

28. Winograd CH, Gerety MB, Chung M et al. (1991) Screening for fraility: criteria and predictors of outcomes. *J Am Geriat Soc* 39:778–784.

29. Balducci L, Extermann M (2000) Management of the frail person with advanced cancer. *Crit Rev Oncol Hematol* 33:143–148.

30. Zagonel V (2001) Importance of a comprehensive geriatric assessment in older cancer patients. European Cancer Conference, 11, Lisbon, 21–25 October.

31. Zagonel V, Pinto A, Monfardini S (1988) Strategies to prevent chemotherapy related toxicity in the older person. In *Comprehensive Geriatric Oncology*, Balducci L, Lyman GH, Ershler WB (eds). Harwood Academic Publishers, Amsterdam, p. 481.

32. Trimble EL (2000) Cancer biology and aging. *Proc Am Soc Clin Oncol* 96.

33. Ershler WB (2000) Do old people get old tumors? *Proc Am Soc Clin Oncol* 87.

34. Monfardini S (1996) What do we know on variables influencing clinical decision-marking in elderly cancer patients? *Eur J Cancer* 32A:12.

35. Hutchins LF et al. (1999) Underrepresentation of patients 65 years of age or older in cancer treatment trials. *N Engl J Med* 341:2061.

36. Kemeny M, Muss HB, Kornblith AB, Peterson B, Wheeler J, Cohen HJ (2000) Barriers to participation of older women with breast cancer in clinical trials. *Proc Am Soc Clin Oncol* 19:2371.

37. Ahmedzai SH, Declan W (2000) Palliative medicine and modern cancer care. *Semin Oncol* 27:1–6.

38. Balducci L, Yates J (2000) General guidelines for the management of older patients with cancer. *Oncology (Huntingt)* 14:221–227.

39. Pecotelli S (2000) Suboptimal hemoglobin levels: do they impact patients and their therapy? *Semin Oncol* 27(2 Suppl 4):1–3.

40. Pederson D, Sogaard H, Overgaard J et al. (1995) Prognostic value of pretreatment factors in patients with locally advanced carcinoma of the uterine cervix treated by radiotherapy alone. *Acta Oncol* 34:787.

41. Kim CY, Tsai MH, Osmanian C et al. (1997) Selection of human cervical epithelial cells that possess reduced apoptotic potential to low-oxygen conditions. *Cancer Res* 57:4200.

42. Balducci L (2001) Patients aged ≥70 are at high risk for neutropenic infection and should receive hemopoietic growth factors when treated with moderately toxic chemoterapy. *J Clin Oncol* 19:1583–1584.

43. Monfardini S, Sacco C, Babare R et al. (1994) VP16, mitoxantrone and prednimustine (VMP) with or without G-CSF in patients with non-Hodgkin's lymphoma (NHL) older than 70 years (yrs). *Proc Am Soc Clin Oncol* 13:1277.

44. Zinzani PL, Storti S, Zaccaria A et al. (1999) Elderly aggressive histology non-Hodgkin's lymphoma: first line VNCOP-B regimen experience on 350 patients. *Blood* 94:33.

45. Zagonel V, Babare R, Merola MC et al. (1994) Cost-benefit of granulocyte colony-stimulating factor administration in older patients with non-Hodgkin's lymphoma treated with combination chemiotherapy. *Ann Oncol* 5:127.

46. Capizzi RL (1999) Recent developments and emerging options: the role of Amifostine as a broad-spectrum cytoprotective agent. *Semin Oncol* 26(2 Suppl 7):1–2.

47. Hensley ML, Schuchter LM, Lindsley C, Meropol NJ, Cohen GI, Broder G, Gradishar WI, Green DM, Langdon RJ, Mitchell RB, Negrin R, Szatrowski TP, Thigpen JT, Von Hoff D, Wasserman TH, Winer EP, Pfiste DG (1999) American Society of Clinical Oncology clinical practice guidelines for the use of chemotherapy and radiotherapy protectants. *J Clin Oncol* 17:3333.

48. Spath-Schwalbe E, Lange C, Genvresse I, Schweigert M, Harder H, Possinge K (2000) The cytoprotective agent amifostine is well tolerated by patients ≥70 years. *Proc Am Soc Clin Oncol* 19:2428.

49. Audisio RA, Zbar AP (2002) updates in surgical oncology for elderly patients. *Crit Rev Oncol Hemat* 43:209–217.

50. Martelli G, De Palo G (1999) Breast cancer in elderly women (> or = 70 years): which treatment? *Tumori* 85:421–424.

51. Wazer DE, Erban JK, Robert NJ et al. (1994) Breast conservation in elderly women for clinically negative axillary lymph nodes without axillary dissection. *Cancer* 74:878–883.

52. Crivellari D, Bonetti M, Castiglione Geertsch M et al. (2000) Burdens and benefit of adjuvant cyclophosphamide, methotrexate, and fluorouracil and tamoxifen for elderly patients with breast cancer: The International Breast Cancer Study Group Trial VII. *J Clin Oncol* 18:1412.

53. Gelman RS, Taylor SG (1984) Cyclophosphamide, methotrexate and 5-fluorouracil chemotherapy in women more than 65 years old with advanced breast cancer: the

elimination of age trands in toxicity by using doses based on creatinine clearance. *J Clin Oncol* 2:1406.

54. Wils JA, Bliss JM, Marty M et al. (1999) Epirubicin plus tamoxifen versus tamoxifen alone in node positive postmenopausal patients with breast cancer: A randomized trial of the international collaborative cancer group. *J Clin Oncol* 17:1988.

55. Ibrahim NK, Frye DK, Budzar AU et al. (1996) Doxorubicin-based chemotherapy in elderly patients with metastatic breast cancer. Tolerance and outcome. *Arch Intern Med* 156:882.

56. Constenla M, Lorenzo I, Carrete N et al. (2000) Docetaxel (TXT) monotherapy and G-CSF for advanced breast cancer (ABC) in elderly patients (EP). *Proc Am Soc Clin Oncol* 19:425.

57. Grobovsky L, Kaplon M, Krozser-Hamati A, Karnard AB (2000) Feature of cancer in frail elderly patients (Pts) ($\geq$85 years of age). *Proc Am Soc Clin Oncol* 19:2469.

58. Arveux I, Boutron MC, El Mrini T et al. (1997) Colon cancer in the elderly: evidence for major improvements in health care and survival. *Br J Cancer* 76:963–967.

59. Audisio RA, Cazzaniga M, Robertson C et al. (1997) Elective surgery for colorectal cancer in the aged: a clinical economical evaluation. *Br J Cancer* 76:382.

60. Puig-La Calle J Jr, Quayle J, Thaler HT et al. (2000) Favorable short-term and long-term outcome after elective radical rectal cancer resection in patients 75 years of age or older. *Dis Colon Rectum* 43:1704–1709.

61. Colorectal Meta-analysis Collaboration. Palliative chemotherapy for advanced or metastatic colorectal cancer. *Cochrane Database Syst Rev* 2000;(2):CD001545.

62. Stein BN, Petrelli NJ, Douglass HO et al. (1995) Age and sex are independent predictors of 5-fluorouracil toxicity. *Cancer* 75:11.

63. Zalcherg J, Kerr D, Seymour L, Palmer M (1998) Haematological and non-haemato-logical toxicity after 5-fluorouracil and leucovorin in patients with advanced colorectal cancer is significantly associated with gender, increasing age and cycle number. Tomudex International Study Group. *Eur J Cancer* 34:1871.

64. Sargent D, Goldberg R, Jacobson SD, MacDonald J, Labianca R, Haller D, Shepard L, Seitz KF, Francini G (2001) A pooled analysis of adjuvant chemotherapy for colon cancer in elderly patients. *N Engl J Med* 345:1091–1097.

65. Johnson BD, Badr MS, Demsey JA (1994) Impact of the aging pulmonary system on the response to exercise. *Clin Chest Med* 15:229–246.

66. Yellin A, Benfield JR (1985) Surgery for bronchogenic carcinoma in the elderly. *Am Rev Respir Dis* 131:97.

67. Jack CIA, Lye M, Lesley P, Wilson G, Donnelly RJ, Hind CRK (1997) Surgery for lung cancer: age alone in not a contraindication. *Int J Clin Pract* 51:423–426.

68. Poulin EC, Labbè R (1997) Fully thoracoscopic pulmonary lobectomy and specimen extraction through rib segment resection. *Surg Endosc* 11:354–358.

69. Olmi P, Ausili-Cefaro G (1997) Radiotherapy in the elderly: a multicentric prospective study on 2060 patients referred to 37 italian radiation therapy centers. Rays 22:53.

70. Zagonel V, Pinto A, Serraino D et al. (1994) Lung cancer in the elderly. *Cancer Treat Rev* 20:315.

71. Lichtman SM, Gupta V, Wasil T, Rush S (2000) Clinical evaluation of radiation therapy in cancer patients 80 years of age and older. *Proc Am Soc Clin Oncol* 19:2494.

72. Gridelli C, Perrone F, Monfardini S (1997) Lung cancer in the elderly. *Eur J Cancer* 33:2313.

73. Gridelli C (2000) Chemotherapy of advanced non small cell lung cancer in the elderly: an update. *Crit Rev Oncol Hematol* 35:219.

74. Rosvold E, Langer CJ, McAleer C et al. (1999) Advancing age does not exacerbate toxicity or compromise autcome in non small cell lung cancer (NSCLC) patients (pts) receiving paclitaxel carpoplatin (P-C). *Proc Am Soc Clin Oncol* 18:478a.

75. Sheperd FA, Abratt RP, Andreson H et al. (1997) Gemcitabine in the treatment of elderly patients with advanced non small cell lung cancer. *Semin Oncol* 24:s7.50.

76. Martin C, Ardizzoni A, Rosso R (1997) Gemcitabine: safety profile and efficacy in non small cell lung cancer unaffected by age. *Aging* 9:297.

77. The Elderly Lung Cancer Vinorelbine Italian Study Group (1999) Effect of vinorelbine on quality of life and survival of elderly patients with advanced non small cell lung cancer. *J Natl Cancer Inst* 91:66.

78. Non Small Cell Lung Cancer Collaborative Group (1995) Chemotherapy in non small cell lung cancer: a meta-analysis using update on individual patients from 52 randomized clinical trials. *Br Med J* 311:899.

79. Gridelli C, Perrone F, Cigolari S et al. (2001) The MILES (Multicenter Italian Lung Cancer in the Elderly Study) Phase 3 trial: Gemcitabine + Vinorelbine vs Vinorelbine and vs Gemcitabine in elderly advanced NSCLC patients. *Proc Am Soc Clin Oncol* 20:1230.

80. MsKay CE, Hainswoth JD, Burris HA et al. (2000) Weeky docetaxel in the tratment of elderly patients with advanced nonsmall cell lung cancer (NSCLC). A minnie pearl cancer research network phase II trial. *Proc Am Soc Clin Oncol* 19:1964.

81. Diab SG, Freeman S, Faragher D, Dibella N (2000) Favorable outcome of elderly patients with early stage breast and prostate carcinomas. Analysis of the surveillance epidemiology and end results (SEER) registry. *Proc Am Soc Clin Oncol* 19:2427.

82. van den Ouden D, Hop WC, Schroder FH (1998) Progression in and survival of patients with locally advanced prostate cancer (T_3) treated with radical prostatectomy as monotherapy. *J Urol* 160:1392–1397.

83. Thompson IM, Middleton RG, Optenberg SA et al. (1999) Have complication rates decreased after treatment for localized prostate cancer? *J Urol* 162:107–112.

84. Badalament RA, Bahn DK, Kim H et al. (1999) Patient-reported complications after cryoablation therapy for prostate cancer. *Urology* 54:295–300.

85. Rietbergen JB, Hoedemaeker RF, Kruger AE et al. (1999) The changing pattern of prostate cancer at the time of diagnosis: characteristics of screen detected prostate cancer in a population based screening study. *J Urol* 161:1192–1198.

86. Thompson IM, Middleton RG, Optenberg SA et al. (1999) Have complication rates decreased after treatment for localized prostate cancer? *J Urol* 162:107.

87. Vicini FA, Ziaja EL, Kestin LL et al. (1999) Treatment outcome with adjuvant and salvage irradiation after radical prostatectomy for prostate cancer. *Urology* 54:111.

88. Albertsen PC, Hanley JA, Gleason DF et al. (1998) Competing risk analysis of men aged 55 to 74 years at diagnosis mamaged conservatively for clinically localized prostate cancer. *JAMA* 280:975.

89. Newshaffer CJ, Otani K, McDonald MK, Penberthy LT (2000) Causes of death in elderly prostate cancer patients and in a comparison nonprostate cancer cohort. *J Natl Cancer Inst* 92:613.

90. Prostate Cancer Trialists' Collaborative Group (2000) Maximun androgen brockade in advanced prostate cancer: an overview of the randomised trials. *Lancet* 335:1491.

91. Osoba D, Tannock IF, Ernst DS, Neville AJ (1999) Health-related quality of life in men with metastatic prostate cancer treated with prednisolone alone or mitoxantrone and prednisone. *J Clin Oncol* 17:1654.

92. Kantoff PW, Helabi S, Conawau M et al. (1999) Hydrocortisone with or without mitoxantrone in men with hormonerefractory prostate cancer: result of the Cancer and Leukemia Group B 9182 study. *J Clin Oncol* 17:2506.

93. Hudes G, Einhorn L, Ross E et al. (1999) Vinblastine versus vinblastine plus oral estramustine phosphonate for patients with hormone-refractory prostate cancer: A Hoossier Oncology Group and Fox Chase Network phase III trial. *J Clin Oncol* 17:3160.

94. Zagonel V, Monfardini S et al. (2001) Management of hematologic malignancies in the elderly: 15 year experience at the Aviano Cancer Center. *Crit Rev Oncol Hematol* 39:289–305.

95. Pinto A, Zagonel V, Ferrara F (2001) Acute myeloid leukemia in the elderly: biology and therapeutic strategies. *Crit Rev Oncol Hematol* 39:275–287.

96. Coiffier B (1998) Non-Hodgkin's lymphoma in the elderly: therapeutics strategies and result in clinical trials. *Ann Oncol* 9(Suppl 3):019.

97. Tirelli U, Zagonel V, Errante D et al. (1998) Treatment of lymphoma in the elderly: an update. *Hematol Oncol* 16:1.

98. Gaynor ER, Dahlberg S, Fisher RI (1994) Factors affecting reduced survival of the elderly with intermediate and high grade lymphoma: an analysis of SWOG-8516 (INT 0067)—the National High Priority Lymphoma Study: a randomized comparison of CHOP vs m-BACOD vs ProMACE-CytaBOM vs MACOP-B. *Proc Am Soc Clin Oncol* 13:1250.

99. Tirelli U, Errante D, Van Glabbeke M et al. (1998) CHOP is the standard regimen in patients of 70 years of age of more with intermediate and high grade non-Hodgin's lymphoma: results of a randomized study of the EORTC Lymphoma Cooperative Study Group. *J Clin Oncol* 16:27.

100. Lichtman SM (2000) Aggressive lymphoma in the elderly. *Crit Rev Oncol Hematol* 33:119–128.

UICC Manual of Clinical Oncology, Eighth Edition. Edited by Raphael E. Pollock
ISBN 0-471-22289-5 Copyright © 2004 John Wiley & Sons, Inc.